Applied Pathophysiology

FOR THE ADVANCED PRACTICE NURSE

Lucie Dlugasch, PhD, MSN, APRN

Associate Clinical Professor
Adult Gerontology Program Leader
Nicole Wertheim College of Nursing
 and Health Sciences
Florida International University

Lachel Story, PhD, RN

Associate Dean, Research and Graduate Education
Director, School of Leadership and Advanced Nursing Practice
Associate Professor
College of Nursing and Health Professions
The University of Southern Mississippi

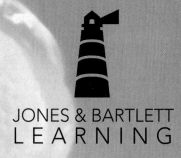

JONES & BARTLETT
LEARNING

World Headquarters
Jones & Bartlett Learning
5 Wall Street
Burlington, MA 01803
978-443-5000
info@jblearning.com
www.jblearning.com

Jones & Bartlett Learning books and products are available through most bookstores and online booksellers. To contact Jones & Bartlett Learning directly, call 800-832-0034, fax 978-443-8000, or visit our website, www.jblearning.com.

Substantial discounts on bulk quantities of Jones & Bartlett Learning publications are available to corporations, professional associations, and other qualified organizations. For details and specific discount information, contact the special sales department at Jones & Bartlett Learning via the above contact information or send an email to specialsales@jblearning.com.

18292-7

Production Credits
VP, Product Management: Amanda Martin
Director of Product Management: Matthew Kane
Product Manager: Tina Chen
Product Assistant: Melina Leon-Haley
Project Specialist: Alex Schab
Digital Project Specialist: Angela Dooley
Senior Marketing Manager: Jennifer Scherzay
Production Services Manager: Colleen Lamy
Product Fulfillment Manager: Wendy Kilborn

Composition: S4Carlisle Publishing Services
Cover Design: Kristin E. Parker
Text Design: Kristin E. Parker
Senior Media Development Editor: Troy Liston
Rights Specialist: John Rusk
Cover Image (Title Page, Part Opener, Chapter Opener): © Yurchanka Siarhei
Printing and Binding: LSC Communications
Cover Printing: LSC Communications

Library of Congress Cataloging-in-Publication Data
Names: Dlugasch, Lucie, author | Story, Lachel, author. | Based on (Work):
   Story, Lachel. Pathophysiology.
Title: Applied pathophysiology for the advanced practice nurse / Lucie
   Dlugasch & Lachel Story.
Description: Burlington, Massachusetts : Jones & Bartlett Learning, [2020] |
   Includes bibliographical references.
Identifiers: LCCN 2019014108 | ISBN 9781284150452
Subjects: | MESH: Pathology | Physiology | Advanced Practice Nursing | Nurses
   Instruction
Classification: LCC RB113 | NLM QZ 140 | DDC 616.07--dc23
LC record available at https://lccn.loc.gov/2019014108

6048

Printed in the United States of America
24 23 22 21 20   10 9 8 7 6 5 4 3 2

Contents

Preface

Pathophysiology is a critical foundational course for all nurses. Advanced pathophysiology is a core course that must be included in all graduate nursing curriculums preparing nurses in direct care roles. These roles are varied and include nurse practitioners, nurse anesthetists, nurse midwives, clinical nurse specialists, and nurse educators. This text includes content across the life span and content to meet the needs of advanced practice population areas including pediatrics, psychiatric mental health, and gerontology and incorporates information from an acute and primary care focus.

Many pathophysiology books are geared toward undergraduate nursing students and often lack the requisite content and focus to prepare advanced practice nurses. Educators teaching this course often have to create supplementary materials to ensure their students are better prepared for their advanced practice roles. Some of these books are also unwieldly and contain too much information, and educators must often edit texts' content to make it manageable and understandable. Without a dedicated pathophysiology text available for advanced practice nursing, students are often overwhelmed, and educators are frustrated when teaching this course. This text was developed with these issues in mind and takes a comprehensive yet concise approach to presenting the content.

The text was also developed with the awareness that graduate students have a foundation in pathophysiology yet have different experiences. Students enter advanced pathophysiology with varying numbers of years since they took basic sciences and nursing courses. Therefore, this text serves as a bridge between their basic education and clinical experience and the advanced knowledge necessary for their new advanced roles. Concepts in pathophysiology can be difficult to understand and remember. In this text, concept descriptions are repeated several times within a chapter and between different chapters. As an example, there is an extensive discussion pertaining to osmosis in the cellular function chapter. The concept of osmosis is then briefly described again when discussing the process in the vascular and renal systems. This repetition serves as a prompt for students to remember and see concepts in different contexts, disorders, and practice situations.

Advanced pathophysiology is usually one of the courses students must take in the beginning of their academic programs. This text was written in a format so that students can start to transition into their new roles and think like an advanced practice nurse. Advanced practice nurses must have the ability to understand and compare and contrast presenting signs and symptoms and then discern between one diagnosis and another. Choices must then be made pertaining to necessary diagnostic tests, and treatment plans need to be developed. The text contains information and examples in a way that helps students to begin mastering these competencies. In each chapter, there are several Application to Practice activities. Within these application activities are case studies that I have developed from real-life scenarios accumulated from 35 years as a practicing nurse (24 of those as an advanced practice registered nurse) and educator. These cases represent common encounters an advanced practice nurse may face in practice. Some of the cases were developed by other faculty who are also expert practicing clinicians and educators. The content in the cases is concise, mimicking typical clinical encounters. These shorter cases allow students to practice what they just read and help them gain understanding and confidence. Several of the application activities have multiple cases that have common features, yet the diagnosis or clinical manifestations may be different. These activities allow the students to develop knowledge necessary to differentiate between clinical presentations, pathogenesis, diagnosis, and treatment.

The chapters are written in a format providing students with information pertaining to the most common scenario and likely underlying disorder. Chapters are organized with overarching concepts and disorders organized by underlying pathophysiologic processes. Disorders that have a common presentation are discussed in a common section as patients come in with concerns and clinical manifestations, not diagnoses. The grouping of common presentations with varying diagnoses is another technique to help students think like an advanced practice nurse and develop critical thinking skills. As an example, when a patient is complaining of a sore throat the various possible diagnoses can include viral pharyngitis, streptococcal pharyngitis, and infectious mononucleosis. Infectious mononucleosis in other texts is often discussed in hematology chapters, and in this text, it is discussed with other common pharyngitis causes. Providing information in this format sets the stage for future courses and clinical encounters where students need to establish a diagnosis based on a patient's presentation. Tables are also provided to help students understand differentiation between disorders.

Diagnostic links are another tool found throughout each chapter. These diagnostic links provide the student with a background for commonly used diagnostic tests in practice. The links are strategically placed in the chapter where content pertaining to the diagnostic test was just discussed to maximize understanding. As examples, a reticulocyte count is discussed with a description of hematopoiesis or clotting studies are discussed with hemostasis.

The strength of this text is that the content is written in a format linking together multiple concepts from an applied pathophysiologic perspective; a style that is often lacking in other pathophysiology texts. This text is written to answer the how, when, and why to how things can go wrong, along with guidelines for diagnosis and treatment. With this practical approach to discussing the complex topic of pathophysiology, the student will gain confidence and be prepared to make sound decisions.

Sources

APRN Consensus Work Group & National Council of State Boards of Nursing APRN Advisory Committee. (2008). The *Consensus Model for APRN Regulation: Licensure, Accreditation, Certification, Education*. Retrieved Dec. 9, 2019 from https://www.ncsbn.org/Consensus_Model_for_APRN _Regulation_July_2008.pdf

AACN. (2011). *The essentials of master's education in nursing*. Retrieved from http://www.aacn.nche.edu/education -(2011). *The essentials of master education in nursing*. American Association of Colleges of Nursing.

American Association of Colleges of Nursing and National Organization of Nurse Practitioner Faculties. (2016). *Criteria for evaluation of nurse practitioner programs: A report of the National Task Force on quality nurse practitioner education*.

Acknowledgments

I would like to thank my husband, Philip, for supporting me during all my career endeavors such as writing this book. You are not only my husband but are also my best friend and are one of the most passionate fellow nurse practitioners I know. Thank you for reviewing many sections in my book. The personal sacrifices you have made for me are immeasurable and have been noticed, and for this I am so grateful. To my daughters, Nicole and Lauren, I thank you for your words and gestures of encouragement and pushing me along the way when I was tired and doubted myself. To Analise, my daughter in heaven who now lives as an eternal part of my soul, I was able to find inspiration in my memories of how passionately you lived your life. I was also fueled by the drive and dedication you displayed in all your pursuits. To my friends and colleagues, thank you for listening and instilling confidence in my abilities. To my mom and stepdad, thanks for picking up the pieces, bringing me food, helping me with the house and just always being there for me; I am lucky to be the recipient of your tireless generosity. I love you both so much. To all my students, I am happiest when I am with you in the classroom. Our discussions, even the contentious ones, energize me and remind me how in health care, information is always evolving and learning is lifelong. Although we may become weary, we must never rest, as we are charged and entrusted with caring for the most important thing in life and that is the health of others.

A big thank you to Lachel Story, my coauthor, who enabled me to embark on this journey, provided much encouragement, and guided me along the way. I am also thankful to the team at Jones & Bartlett Learning: Anna Maria Forger, Tina Chen, and Alex Schab, and many behind-the-scenes people who were supportive and flexible with me throughout this process.

Lucie Dlugasch

First, I would like to thank my husband, Tom, and children, Clayton and Mason, for their never-ending love and encouragement. I would also like to express my deepest gratitude to my mom, Carolyn, and dad, Tommy, because I would not be who I am today without them. I would also like to acknowledge all my students past, present, and future for constantly teaching me more than I could ever teach them and for all their feedback—I heard it and I hope this is more what you had in mind. Finally, I would like to convey my appreciation to my colleagues for their gracious mentoring and support.

Lachel Story

Contributors

Philip Dlugasch, MSN, APRN, ACNP-BC
Intensive Care Unit APRN
Jackson Memorial Hospital
Adjunct Nursing Instructor
University of Miami School of Nursing
Lt. Colonel, Retired
Chief Nurse
United States Air Force

Derrick C. Glymph, CNAP, CRNA, APRN, COL., USAR
Nicole Wertheim College of Nursing and Health Sciences
Florida International University
Miami, Florida

Deana Goldin, PhD, DNP, MSN, APRN, FNP-BC
Assistant Clinical Professor and Family Nurse Practitioner Program Leader
Nicole Wertheim College of Nursing and Health Sciences
Florida International University
Miami, Florida

Dana Sherman, DNP, MSN, APRN, ANP-BC, FNP-BC
Assistant Clinical Professor
Nicole Wertheim College of Nursing and Health Sciences
Florida International University
Miami, Florida

Reviewers

Nicole R. Clark, DNP, FNP-BC
Oakland University
Rochester, Michigan

Angie M. Fetsko, BSN, RN-BC
Greater Waco Advanced Health Care Academy
Waco, Texas

Julian L. Gallegos, PhD, RN, FNP-BC, CNL
Touro University
Vallejo, California

Mary Knowlton, DNP, RN, CNE
Western Carolina University
Cullowhee, North Carolina

Leanna R. Miller, DNP, CCRN-CMC, PCCN-CSC, CEN, CNRN, CMSRN, NP
Western Kentucky University
Bowling Green, Kentucky

Katie Morales, PhD, RN, CNE
Berry College
Mount Berry, Georgia

Tonya Sawyer-McGee, DNP, MBA, MSN, RN, ACNP
Abilene Christian University
Abilene, Texas

Crystal Slaughter, DNP, APRN, CNS
Saint Francis Medical Center College of Nursing
Peoria, Illinois

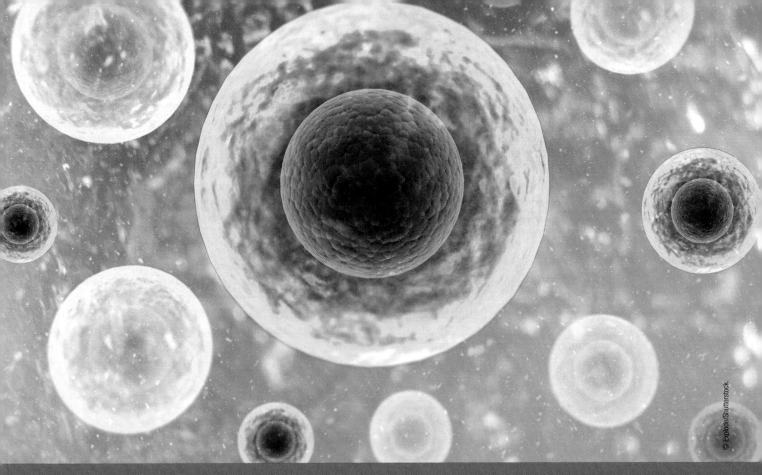

CHAPTER 1
Cellular Function

LEARNING OBJECTIVES

- Analyze the purpose and function of cellular structures.
- Analyze how various substances cross the cell membrane.
- Explain cellular energy sources and production.
- Discuss the process of protein synthesis.
- Summarize how cells are organized.

- Analyze mechanisms of cellular proliferation, differentiation, and adaptation as they relate to disease development.
- Describe the correlation between genetics, epigenetics, and environment in disease development.
- Evaluate patterns of inheritance and compare how various disorders are inherited.
- Differentiate genetic and congenital disorders.

Pathophysiology inquiry begins with exploring the basic building blocks of living organisms. Cells give organisms their immense diversity. Organisms can be made up of a single cell, such as with bacteria or viruses, or billions of cells, such as with humans. In humans, these building blocks work together to form tissues, organs, and organ systems. Alterations and maladaptation in these basic units of life are also the foundation for the development of disease.

The impact of disease is evident from the cellular level up to the system level. Knowledge of cellular-level mechanisms, genetics, genomics, and epigenetics have led to scientific breakthrough in the understanding of disease and treatment strategies. Therefore, understanding basic cellular function and dysfunction are core and essential to understanding pathophysiology.

Basic Cell Function and Structure

Cells are complex miniorganisms resulting from millions of years of evolution. Individual cells are part of a network of other cells that are grouped together to serve a function and purpose. These groupings of cells are organized into tissues. Groups of tissues then form organs, and groups of organs are organized into systems. Survival of an organism is dependent on these groupings and not just on individual cells. Cells, therefore, must coexist and communicate with each other to proliferate and survive. When this communal environment does not exist, then adaptation or disease occurs. Cells can arise only from a preexisting cell, and through the process of differentiation, cells become specialized to perform certain functions. Cells will vary greatly in size and shape in order to perform certain functions. Despite having varying functions and features, cells have several commonalities such as a nucleus, cytoplasm, and organelles. Cells also have the remarkable ability to exchange materials with their immediate surroundings, obtain energy from organic nutrients, synthesize complex molecules, and replicate themselves.

Cellular Components

The basic components of cells include the cytoplasm, organelles (including the nucleus),

and cell membrane. The cytoplasm, or protoplasm, is a colorless, viscous liquid containing water, nutrients, ions, dissolved gases, and waste products; this liquid is where the cellular work takes place. The cytoplasm supports all the internal cellular structures called *organelles* (FIGURE 1-1), which are little organs that perform the work that maintains the cell's life (TABLE 1-1). The cytoplasm also surrounds the nucleus. The nucleus is usually the largest and most prominent cellular compartment and is the control center of the cell. The nucleus contains all the genetic information (deoxyribonucleic acid, or DNA) and is surrounded by a double membrane. The nucleus regulates cell growth, metabolism, and reproduction. The cell membrane, also called the *plasma membrane*, is the semipermeable boundary containing the cell and its components (FIGURE 1-2). A lipid bilayer, or fatty double covering, makes up the membrane. The interior surface of the bilayer is uncharged and primarily made up of lipids. The exterior surface of the bilayer is charged and is less fatty than the interior surface. This fatty cover protects the cell from the aqueous environment in which it exists, while allowing it to be permeable to some molecules but not others.

Exchanging Material

Cellular permeability is the ability of the cell to allow passage of some substances through the membrane, while not permitting others to enter or exit (Figure 1-2). To accomplish this process, cells have gates that may be opened or closed by proteins, chemical signals, or electrical charges. Being selectively permeable allows the cell to maintain a state of internal balance, or homeostasis. Some substances have free passage in and out of the cells, including enzymes, glucose, and electrolytes. Enzymes are proteins that facilitate chemical reactions in cells, while glucose is a sugar molecule that provides energy. Electrolytes are chemicals that are charged conductors when they are dissolved in water. Passage across the cell membrane is accomplished through several mechanisms, including diffusion, osmosis, active transport, endocytosis, and exocytosis. Failure of these exchange mechanisms can lead to the development of disease.

Diffusion is the movement of solutes—that is, particles dissolved in a solvent—from an area of higher concentration to an area of

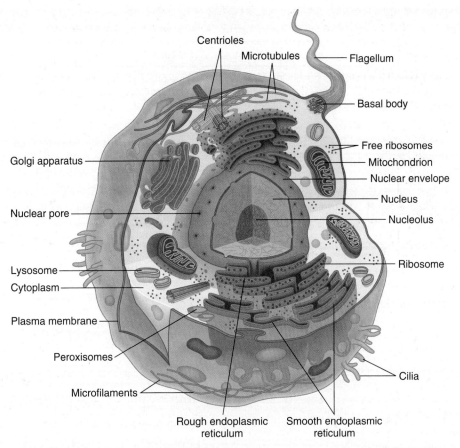

Centrioles

Microtubules

Flagellum

Basal body

Free ribosomes

Mitochondrion

Nuclear envelope

Nucleus

Nucleolus

Golgi apparatus

Nuclear pore

Ribosome

Lysosome

Cytoplasm

Plasma membrane

Peroxisomes

Cilia

Microfilaments

Rough endoplasmic
reticulum

Smooth endoplasmic
reticulum

FIGURE 1-1 The cytoplasm contains several organelles.

TABLE 1-1	Overview of Cell Organelles	
Organelle	**Structure**	**Function**
Nucleus	Round or oval body. Surrounded by nuclear envelope. Largest organelle. Has membrane with pores to allow communication with the cytoplasm.	Contains the genetic information (DNA and histones). Histones (proteins) bind DNA into tight, threadlike packages called *chromosomes*. Necessary for control of cell structure, function, and replication. Genes are sections of DNA that contain hereditary information.
Nucleolus	Round or oval body in the nucleus.	Produces ribosomal ribonucleic acid (RNA) subunits (rRNA) and transcribes, processes, and assembles these subunits which are then sent out to the cell to form into ribosomes.
Endoplasmic reticulum (ER)	Network of membranous tubules in the cytoplasm of the cell. Continuous with nuclear and cell membrane. Smooth endoplasmic reticulum (SER) contains no ribosomes. Rough endoplasmic reticulum (RER) is studded with ribosomes.	SER is involved in the production of phospholipids and has many different functions depending on the cells. RER is the site of the synthesis of lysosomal enzymes and proteins for intracellular and extracellular use.
Ribosomes	Small particles found in the cytoplasm. Made of rRNA and ribosomal proteins.	Aid in protein production on the RER and polysomes (messenger RNA and ribosomes). The ribosome along with transfer RNA (tRNA) interpret messenger RNA (mRNA), which carries the genetic material from the DNA.
Golgi complex	Series of flattened sacs usually located near the nucleus.	Sorts, chemically modifies, and packages proteins produced on the RER.

(continues)

TABLE 1-1   Overview of Cell Organelles (*continued*)

Organelle	Structure	Function
Secretory vesicles	Membrane-bound vesicles containing proteins produced by the RER and repackaged by the Golgi complex. Contain protein hormones or enzymes.	Store protein hormones or enzymes in the cytoplasm awaiting a signal for release to the outside of the cell.
Food vacuole	Membrane-bound vesicle containing material engulfed by the cell.	Stores ingested material and combines with lysosomes. Site of digestion and degradation of engulfed materials (i.e., autophagy).
Lysosome	Round, membrane-bound structure containing digestive enzymes (i.e., hydrolases).	Combines with food vacuoles and digests materials engulfed by cells. Lysosome membrane separates digestive enzymes from cytoplasm.
Peroxisomes	Small structures containing enzymes.	Break down various potentially toxic intracellular molecules and involved in nerve cell myelin sheath development.
Mitochondria	Round, oval, or elongated structures with a double membrane. The inner membrane is shaped into folds.	Contains enzymes to convert food into energy. Complete the breakdown of glucose, producing nicotine adenine dinucleotide and adenosine triphosphate (ATP), which is the cell's fuel source.
Cytoskeleton	Network of microtubules and microfilaments in the cell.	Gives the cell internal support, helps transport molecules and some organelles inside the cell, and binds to enzymes of metabolic pathways.
Cilia	Small projections of the cell membrane containing microtubules; found on a limited number of cells.	Propel materials along the surface of certain cells.
Flagella	Large projections of the cell membrane containing microtubules. In humans, found only on sperm cells.	Provide motile force for sperm cells.
Centrioles	Small cylindrical bodies composed of microtubules arranged in nine sets of triplets. Found in animal cells, not plants.	Help organize spindle apparatus necessary for cell division.

Modified from Story, L. (2017). Pathophysiology: A Practical Approach (3rd ed.). Burlington, MA: Jones & Bartlett Learning.

Learning Points

Solution

A solution is made of a solvent and solutes. Solvents dissolve solutes. In the human body, the solvent is usually water, and the solutes are particles such as sodium, potassium, glucose, urea, and oxygen.

lower concentration (**FIGURE 1-3**). Simple diffusion will occur until the concentration gradient, which is the difference in concentrations of substances on either side of the membrane, is equal on each side. How fast diffusion will occur depends on the size and polarity of particles and on lipid solubility. Particles that are smaller, such as water, and particles that are lipid soluble, such as steroids, will diffuse faster. The outer charged cell membrane (mainly Ca^{++}) repels polar particles; therefore, diffusion is slower with ions and polarized molecules, such as Na^+ and K^+, and faster for nonpolarized particles like oxygen. Diffusion is a passive process and cell energy is not expended. **Facilitated diffusion** is also the movement of substances from an area of higher concentration to an area of lower concentration, but as opposed to simple diffusion, it occurs with the assistance of a carrier molecule (**FIGURE 1-4**). Energy is not required for this process, and the number of molecules that can be transported in this way is directly equivalent to the concentration of

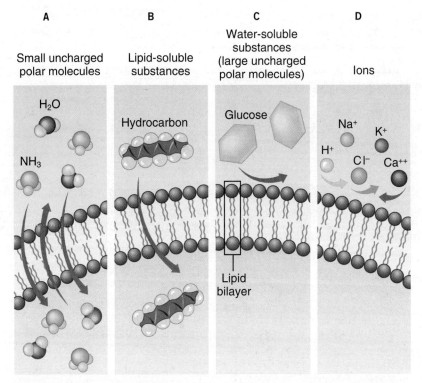

A Small uncharged polar molecules

B Lipid-soluble substances

C Water-soluble substances (large uncharged polar molecules)

D Ions

H_2O

NH_3

Hydrocarbon

Glucose

Na^+ K^+ H^+ Cl^- Ca^{++}

Lipid bilayer

FIGURE 1-2 A selectively permeable membrane maintains homeostasis by allowing some molecules to pass through, while others may not. **(A, B, D)** Simple diffusion. **(C)** Facilitated diffusion.

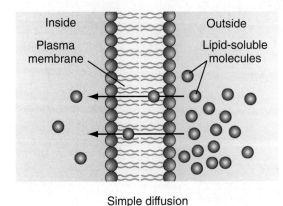

Inside

Plasma membrane

Outside

Lipid-soluble molecules

Simple diffusion

FIGURE 1-3 Lipid-soluble substances pass through the membrane directly via simple diffusion from high to low concentration and without a transport protein or ATP.

the carrier molecule. Insulin transports glucose into the cells using this method.

Water is an important solvent—a substance that dissolves solutes (i.e., dissolved particles)—and intracellular amounts must be balanced to maintain cellular health. Water amount across various body compartments is mediated by the process of **osmosis** (**FIGURE 1-5**). Osmosis is the movement of water or any other solvent across the cellular membrane from an area of low solute concentration or high water to an area of high solute concentration or low water. The membrane is permeable to the solvent (e.g., water) but not to the solute (e.g., Na^+, Cl^-). The movement of the solvent (water) usually continues until concentrations of the solute equalize on both sides of the membrane. The solute concentration is the determinant of the ability to attract water, which is termed *osmotic pressure*. The higher the solute concentration, the higher the osmotic pressure, and more water is drawn into the cell. Osmotic pressure can be used to describe the concentration of a solution. A solution consists of solvent, such as water, and solute, such as Na^+, Cl^-. Cellular balance of water is critical to cell health because the cell will swell and burst (lysis) if too much water enters the cell membrane. If too much water moves out of the cell, the cell will shrink (crenation). Like simple and facilitated diffusion, osmosis is passive. Osmolality and osmolarity are units of measure of osmotic activity/pressure, and both measures reflect water and electrolyte balance. Osmotic pressure decreases with

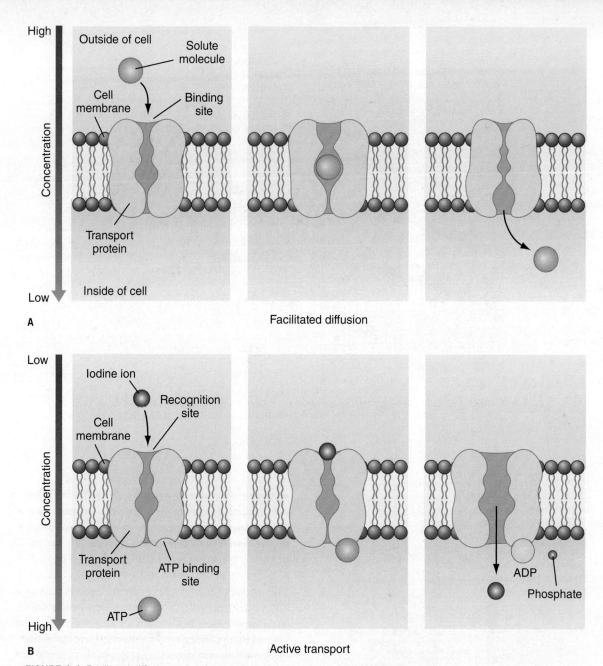

FIGURE 1-4 Facilitated diffusion and active transport use a transport protein. **(A)** Water-soluble molecules can also diffuse through membranes with the assistance of proteins but without ATP in facilitated diffusion. **(B)** Other proteins use energy from ATP to move against concentration gradients in a process called *active transport*.

too much water (e.g., excess hydration, inappropriate antidiuretic hormone—too much causes a person to retain water) and increases with less water or more solutes (e.g., dehydration, hypernatremia).

In addition to osmotic pressure, hydrostatic pressure, and colloid osmotic pressures (i.e., oncotic pressure) are also factors that affect filtration (movement out) and reabsorption (movement in). Hydrostatic pressure is created by water pushing against the cellular membrane, forcing the water out, which is the opposite of osmotic pressure, which, when higher, draws water in. Osmotic and hydrostatic pressure help regulate fluid balance in the body; an example can be found in the functioning of the kidneys. Oncotic pressure is created by plasma proteins—particularly albumin—and is similar to osmotic pressure as higher pressure draws water in.

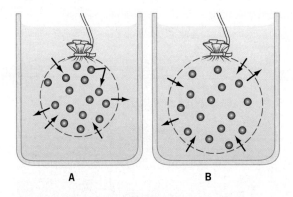

● Sucrose molecules

FIGURE 1-5 (A) When a bag of sugar water is immersed in a solution of pure water, **(B)** water will diffuse into the bag toward the lower concentrations of water, causing the bag to swell.

Like osmotic pressure, oncotic pressure is in opposition to hydrostatic pressure. Patients with low albumin levels (e.g., liver failure) therefore, have a low oncotic pressure and have an inability to draw water into the cell, so the water stays in the interstitial space, resulting in edema.

Diagnostic Link

Osmolality and Osmolarity and Osmolar Gap

Osmolality and osmolarity are units of measure of osmotic activity/pressure. The results reflect body water and electrolyte balance (sodium in particular) and, therefore, can be used as a reflection of hydration status. Clinically, the terms are used interchangeably, but there are differences. Osmolality is expressed as milliosmoles of solute/1 kilogram of solvent. The numerator is a reflection of solutes (intracellular and extracellular), mainly sodium and other ions (e.g., bicarbonate, chloride), glucose, and urea. The denominator is the solvent, which is water in urine or water in plasma (serum). The osmolality can be measured with an osmometer or calculated. Normal serum range is 270–300 mosm/kg (mmol/kg). Sodium, glucose, and blood urea nitrogen are used in the calculation. *Osmolality* is the preferred term when referring to fluids inside the body. Osmolarity is expressed as milliosmoles of solute/1 liter of solution. The denominator is a solution, which is different than the osmolality denominator. The osmolarity is a calculation. Normal serum range is 282–295 mosm/kg (mmol/kg). Osmolarity is best used to describe fluids outside the body. The osmolal gap is a difference between the measured osmolality and the calculated osmolality. Normal gap is about 6 mosmol/L. A high (> 10 mosmol/L) osmolal gap usually occurs with the ingestion of ethanol or toxic alcohols such as methanol (e.g., in windshield wiper fluid) or ethylene glycol (e.g., in anti-freeze products).

Active transport is the movement of a substance from an area of lower concentration to an area of higher concentration, against a concentration gradient (Figure 1-4). This movement involves a carrier molecule, like facilitated diffusion, but energy, usually in the form of adenosine triphosphate (ATP), is required because of the effort necessary to go against the gradient. The sodium-potassium (Na^+-K^+) pump is an example of active transport (see chapter 4).

Learning Points

Diffusion

To illustrate diffusion, consider an elevator filled beyond capacity with people. When the door opens, the people near the door naturally fall out—moving from an area of high concentration to an area with less concentration with no effort, or energy. In the body, gases are exchanged in the lungs by diffusion. Unoxygenated blood enters the pulmonary capillaries (low concentration of oxygen; high concentration of carbon dioxide), where it picks up oxygen from the inhaled air of the alveoli (high concentration of oxygen; low concentration of carbon dioxide), while dropping off carbon dioxide to the alveoli to be exhaled.

Reproduced from Story, L. (2017). *Pathophysiology: A Practical Approach* (3rd ed.). Burlington, MA: Jones & Bartlett Learning.

Learning Points

Osmosis

To understand osmosis, envision a plastic bag filled with sugar water (solute) and with holes punched in it that allow only water to pass through them. If this bag is submerged in distilled water (contains no impurities), the bag will begin to swell because the water is attracted to the sugar. The water shifts to the areas with higher concentrations of sugar (i.e., high solute) in an attempt to dilute the sugar concentrations (Figure 1-5). So, the high sugar area with low water has a high osmotic pressure attracting water. Osmotic pressure is determined by the solute concentration, not the water amount. In our bodies, osmosis allows the cells to remain hydrated.

Modified from Story, L. (2017). *Pathophysiology: A Practical Approach* (3rd ed.). Burlington, MA: Jones & Bartlett Learning.

Endocytosis is the process of bringing a substance into the cell that is too large to go by other mechanisms (**FIGURE 1-6**). The cell membrane surrounds the particles, engulfing them.

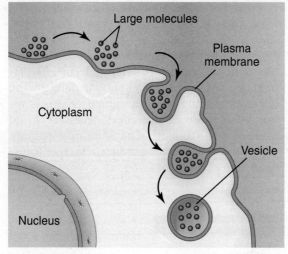

A Endocytosis

B Phagocytosis

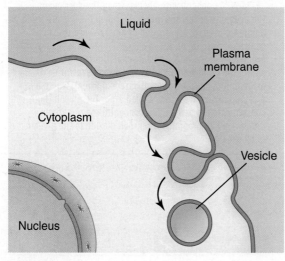

C Pinocytosis

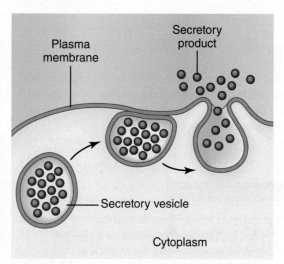

D Exocytosis

FIGURE 1-6 (A–C) Cells can engulf large particles, cell fragments, liquids, and even entire cells. **(D)** Cells can also get rid of large particles.

Phagocytosis, or cell eating, occurs when this process involves solid particles. Pinocytosis, or cell drinking, takes place when this process involves a liquid. Components of the immune system use endocytosis, particularly phagocytosis, to consume and destroy bacteria and other foreign material. **Exocytosis** is the release of materials (typically large particles) from the cell onto the cell membrane, usually with the assistance of a vesicle (a membrane-bound sac) (Figure 1-6). The materials that are deposited onto the cell membrane will either function to replace the part of the membrane that was used during endocytosis or is released. Often glands secrete hormones using exocytosis.

Learning Points

Active Transport

To understand active transport, consider the overfilled elevator again. If the door opens and someone from outside the elevator attempts to get in, it will require a great deal of effort (energy) to enter the full elevator. The sodium-potassium pump is an example of active transport in the body. Energy is required to move sodium out of the cell where the concentrations are high and move potassium into the cell where the concentrations are high.

Reproduced from Story, L. (2017). *Pathophysiology: A Practical Approach* (3rd ed.). Burlington, MA: Jones & Bartlett Learning.

Energy Production

Energy is needed to fuel cellular activity. Cells can obtain energy from two main sources—the breakdown of glucose (a type of carbohydrate) and the breakdown of triglycerides (a type of fat). Food enters the gastrointestinal tract, where it is broken down into sugars, amino acids, and fatty acids. These substances then are either converted to larger molecules (e.g., glucose to glycogen, amino acids to proteins, and fatty acids to triglycerides and fats), stored until needed, or metabolized to make ATP. When used to make ATP, all three sources of energy (amino acids, sugars, fatty acids) must first be converted. Sugars, through the process of glycolysis (splitting), becomes pyruvate in the cytoplasm. If oxygen is present (i.e., through an aerobic process), pyruvate then becomes acetyl coenzyme A (acetyl CoA). Acetyl CoA is also derived from amino acids and fatty acids. The acetyl CoA then enters the Krebs cycle (i.e., citric acid cycle or tricarboxylic cycle), which is a high-electron-producing process that occurs in the mitochondria. During the Krebs cycle, these molecules go through a complex series of reactions that result in the production of large amounts of ATP. If there is no oxygen present (i.e., anaerobic process), the process of glycolysis will result in a less efficient pathway to create ATP, and the pyruvate becomes lactic acid rather than acetyl CoA. Lactic dehydrogenase (LDH) is the enzyme that catalyzes the conversion of pyruvate to lactic acid. Lactate is produced from lactic acid and can be used as a measure of disease severity. The inefficient anaerobic pathway provides energy to cells with no mitochondria (e.g., red blood cells) or is used during times when oxygen delivery is inadequate, such as during exercise or with tissue hypoxia from disease.

Diagnostic Link

Lactate Levels

Lactate forms predominantly from muscle cells and is cleared by the liver. Lactate levels can rise and can eventually lead to lactic acidosis. Lactate levels are used as a measure of disease severity and outcome or as a measure of response to therapy. Elevated levels occur when there is an increased production or decreased excretion. Common causes of increased production of lactate include hypoxia from inadequate oxygen uptake from lungs (e.g., respiratory failure), decreased perfusion of oxygen to tissues (e.g., shock), or a combination of both. Lactate levels can also rise even when uptake and perfusion are adequate but demand for oxygen is increased (e.g., exercise). Liver and renal dysfunction can result in decreased metabolism and excretion. Lactate levels are measured in serum or cerebrospinal fluid.

Chromosomes, DNA, and Genes

When the cells are replicating, information is being produced and transmitted. That information is packaged in **chromosomes**, which are in the nucleus of the cell (FIGURE 1-7). A chromosome consists of deoxyribonucleic acid (**DNA**) and histone and nonhistone proteins. Chromosomes have a well-defined structure. The centromere is an area where the chromosomes are attached. The centromere gives a chromosome its shape, and because of the shape, genes can be more easily located. DNA consists of a **nucleotide** where genetic codes are stored. The nucleotide is a double helix strand (it looks like a twisted rope ladder) made of a sugar molecule and phosphate (forms the ladder sides) attached to a nitrogen containing base (forms the ladder steps). If you were to stretch out DNA, it would be up to six feet long. However, DNA is tightly coiled and wound around proteins (like a spool), and it all fits into every cell nucleus. The DNA that is combined and wrapped around the histone proteins is called **chromatin**. About 99% of DNA is in the nucleus (i.e., nuclear DNA), while less than 1% of DNA is in the mitochondria.

The nitrogen bases (steps) of the nucleotide are either purine (adenine and guanine) or pyrimidine (thymine and cytosine). These four nitrogen bases act as letters in an alphabet. These letters come together to form words and sentences (i.e., a person). The bases are in pairs and packaged into the 46 chromosomes of each cell. Adenine pairs only with thymine, and guanine pairs only with cytosine for DNA replication; however, RNA bases are different for transcription (a step to protein building) (FIGURE 1-8 and FIGURE 1-9). Each of these pairings (e.g., adenine/thymine) is called a **base pair**. There are 3 billion nucleotide base pair sequences available inside the 46 chromosomes (i.e., 23 pairs) located in each cell nucleus. On the DNA are small parts or sections on the double helix known as **genes** (like tags hanging from the rope ladder). Genes are made of DNA, and multiple genes are on DNA; hence, multiple genes are on a chromosome. Genes are the physical and functional units passed on to offspring and, therefore, form the basis of inheritance. This transmitted gene information forms the **genotype** or blueprint (**karyotype**) of a person. The complete set of DNA and genes (i.e., genetic instructions) is called a **genome**.

Gene function and expression is influenced by many factors, such as the environment. The

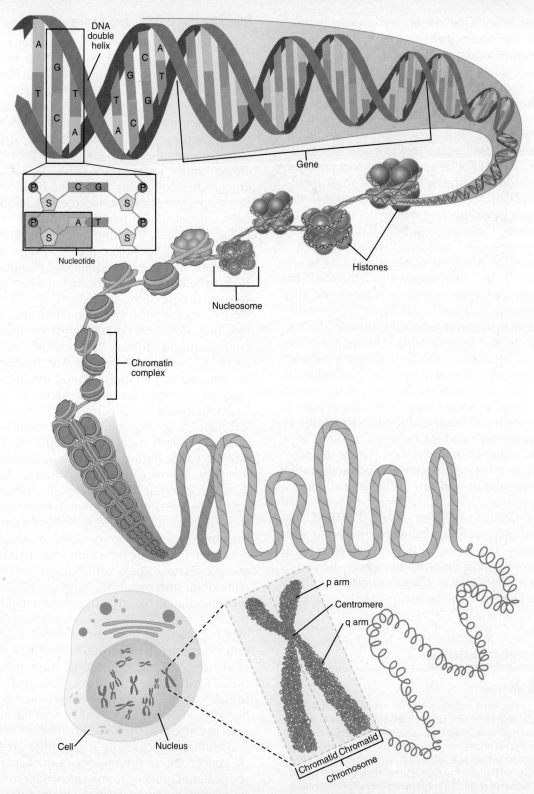

FIGURE 1-7 Diagram of a cell demonstrating that genetic material in the form of DNA is organized into chromosomes. Each chromosome contains thousands of genes in tightly coiled strands of DNA.

detectable outward expression of the genotype is termed **phenotype**. About 20,000–25,000 genes have been identified in nuclear DNA and about 37 genes in mitochondrial DNA.

Approximately 1% of nuclear DNA genes serve as instructions (code) to make the body's basic building blocks and proteins, and the remaining 99% of DNA are noncoding proteins. It is

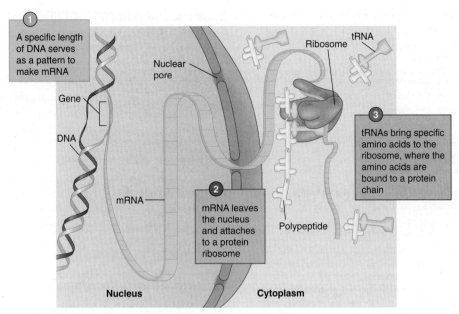

FIGURE 1-8 Termination of protein synthesis.

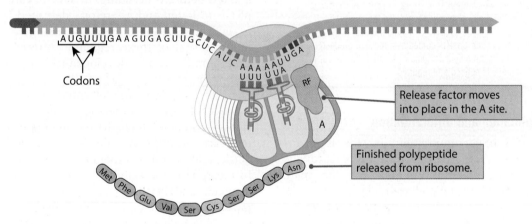

FIGURE 1-9 Protein synthesis.

not clear what all these noncoding proteins do, but they are thought to control gene activity such as enhancing or repressing transcription. In other words, only about 1% of DNA has genes that make up a person.

Learning Points

Chromatin Versus Chromosome Versus Chromatid

Chromatin is used to refer to the DNA coiled up in histone proteins. Chromatin is also loose inside the nucleus waiting for transcription (protein formation). The term chromatin is also used to refer to the structure inside a chromosome. The coiled-up chromatin loops that are structured are what make up a **chromosome**. When the chromosome replicates, it creates an identical version of itself, and the pairs attach to each other through a centromere. Each of those separate individual copies is called a **chromatid** (they are also known as sister chromatids), and the two copies together are called a *chromosome*.

Learning Points

Genetic Engineering

Genetic engineering (i.e., genetic modification or manipulation) is the process of genetic or genome alteration with the intent of creating a new genotype and phenotype. The alteration may involve changing a base pair and adding or deleting whole genes. DNA can be taken from one organism and combined with another organism, which is termed *recombinant DNA*. Genetic engineering has been used in many areas including developing resilient crop varieties that have a high nutritional value or to allow sheep to produce a protein in their milk that patients with cystic fibrosis can consume. Genetically engineered organisms are called *transgenic organisms* or more commonly, *genetically modified organisms* (GMO). The use of GMO for food sources is an area of significant bioethical discussion. While the intent of genetically modifying food is to produce a better food product; the potential long-term clinical consequences are an area of concern. Pharmacologic agents are produced through recombinant DNA approaches and a common example is insulin. A piece of human insulin gene is inserted into a loop (plasmid) of bacteria DNA, this combined piece is returned to the bacteria (now a recombinant bacterium), and insulin is produced.

Some examples of insulin produced in this manner include insulin glargine and regular insulin. Genetic engineering is a broad term associated with several other concepts such as gene cloning, which is making identical copies of DNA. Polymerase chain reaction (PCR) is a technique to make many copies of a specific DNA segment. PCR is used in laboratory diagnostic tests to identify pathogens or forensic DNA analysis.

Replication and Differentiation

A cell's basic requirement for life is ensuring that it can reproduce. Many cells divide numerous times throughout the life span, whereas others die and are replaced with new cells. Proliferation is the regulated process by which cells divide and reproduce. The process of growth and division is regulated by protein growth factors known as cytokines and genetic material. Cells do not decide to divide on their own but rather wait for a stimulus from growth factors that comes from neighboring cells. Genes such as proto-oncogenes within the cell direct production of growth factor receptor sites on the cell membrane. Tumor suppressor genes and some growth factors inhibit cell division and differentiation. Replication control and balance is important to prevent abnormal proliferation, termed *neoplasms*, which can become cancer. While most mature cells can replicate and divide, some are incapable of division and replication, and these cells are found in nerves, muscles, and eye lenses. Cells have a finite number of times in which they can divide, and then they die.

The most common form of cell division, in which the cell divides into two separate cells, is mitosis (FIGURE 1-10). Mitosis is the way somatic (nongamete) cells divide. Meiosis, the second type of cell division, is the way sperm and ova cells (gametes) divide.

The cell cycle is divided into two key stages: interphase and mitosis (FIGURE 1-11). Interphase is the phase prior to mitosis and is the time when the cell grows and prepares for division by producing many substances such as RNA and DNA. Interphase is a crucial phase in the cell cycle and can last anywhere from 18 to 23 hours. Some cells divide quickly, but others divide slowly and can remain in the beginning of interphase from days to years. During interphase, various checkpoints serve as a cell quality control mechanism. Progression through the cell cycle does not occur until the genome is checked and found ready to move into mitosis. As an example, at one of these checkpoints, a tumor suppressor protein (known as p53) ensures that damaged DNA is fixed before proceeding. In several cancers, p53 is mutated and, therefore, damaged DNA is replicated. A focus in tumor biology is the identification of these regulatory proteins so that therapies can be developed to stop abnormal proliferation.

After interphase, the cell enters mitosis. This process, which lasts about 1 hour, occurs in four steps—prophase, metaphase, anaphase, and telophase. In prophase, the chromosomes condense, and the nuclear membrane disintegrates. In metaphase, the spindle fibers attach to centromeres, and the chromosomes align. The chromosomes separate and move to opposite poles in anaphase. Finally, the chromosomes arrive at each pole, and new membranes are formed in telophase. The result in mitosis is the division of one cell, which results in two genetically identical (homologous) and equal diploid daughter cells. Cytokinesis is cytoplasm division.

Meiosis is a form of cell division that occurs only in mature sperm and ova (Figure 1-10). Meiosis also has two key stages—interphase and meiosis (prophase, metaphase, anaphase, telophase). The processes of ova development (oogenesis) and sperm development (spermatogenesis), while similar, have some key differences. Sperm are continually produced, while the ova are not. All the ova in the ovaries remain in a state of prophase for as long as 45 years. Meiosis completion in egg cells occurs during fertilization. As a woman gets older, the ova released are also older. There is a greater risk for abnormal meiosis in these older ova resulting in chromosomal abnormalities and congenital diseases.

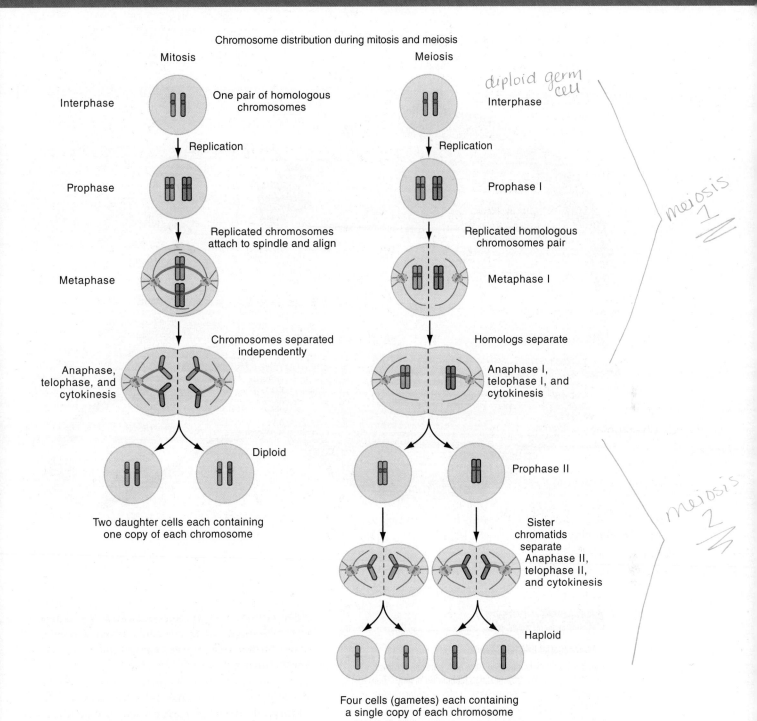

Chromosome distribution during mitosis and meiosis

Mitosis

Interphase — One pair of homologous chromosomes

Replication

Prophase

Replication

Replicated chromosomes attach to spindle and align

Metaphase

Chromosomes separated independently

Anaphase, telophase, and cytokinesis

Diploid

Two daughter cells each containing one copy of each chromosome

Meiosis

Interphase — diploid germ cell

Replication

Prophase I

Replicated homologous chromosomes pair

Metaphase I

Homologs separate

Anaphase I, telophase I, and cytokinesis

Prophase II

Sister chromatids separate
Anaphase II, telophase II, and cytokinesis

Haploid

Four cells (gametes) each containing a single copy of each chromosome

meiosis 1

meiosis 2

FIGURE 1-10 Mitosis and meiosis.

After meiosis, an ovum produces 1 daughter cell, sperm produces 4 daughter cells, and each contains 23 chromosomes, which are called *haploid cells*. The haploid cells are not yet paired with other chromosomes. When the sperm and ova join, a single-cell zygote is formed and becomes diploid during sexual reproduction. The zygote is a mixture of traits with 23 chromosomes transmitted from the mother and 23 from the father. The result is a total of 23 chromosomes pairs (46 total chromosomes). Of the 23 pairs, one pair are sex chromosomes. A homologous XX chromosome will be present if female, and a nonhomologous XY chromosome will be present if male. The other 22 pairs of autosome (somatic) cells are homologous. In summary, each body cell has 23 pairs of chromosomes (46 total), and in each cell are 22 autosome pairs (total 44) and 1 sex chromosome pair (total 2).

CELL CYCLE

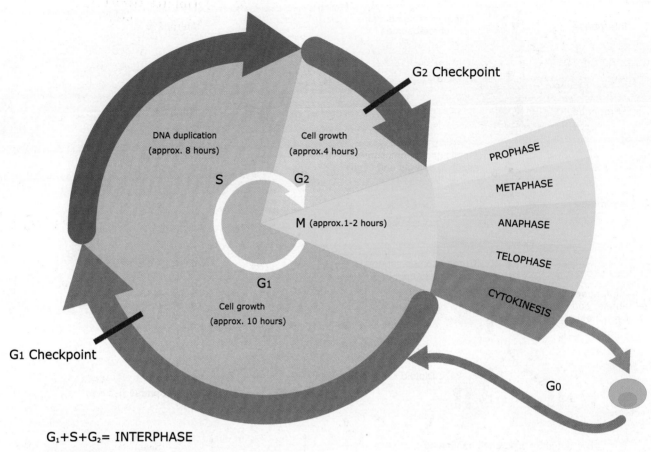

$G_1 + S + G_2 =$ INTERPHASE

$M =$ Mitosis

FIGURE 1-11 Cell cycle.

© ellepigrafica/Shutterstock.

Differentiation (cell maturation) is a process by which cells become specialized in terms of cell type, function, structure, and cell cycle. After fertilization, the zygote starts to divide by mitosis into a blastocyst. Inside this blastocyst is an inner cell mass (embryonic stem cells). Embryonic stem cells go on to become the embryo. The primitive, undifferentiated embryonic stem cells are called **pluripotent**, as they develop into any kind of cells and ultimately will develop into the over 200 specialized cells (e.g., cardiac cells, nerve cells) of the adult human. During this early development after fertilization, the embryo is the most susceptible to damage from environmental influences. While embryonic stem cells were used to essentially build a human, the adult stem cells are important in the maintenance and repair of tissue such as skin regeneration or hematopoiesis. Adult stem cells are called *multipotent* because they can only make cells from their same germ layer. Therefore, **multipotent** adult stem cells from blood (a mesoderm tissue) can only make other blood cells and not liver cells, which is endodermal tissue. Some adult stem cells are called **unipotent** as they can only make a single cell type such as precursors to egg or sperm cells. All stem cells, whether embryonic or adult stem cells, can self-produce into more undifferentiated stem cells and can differentiate. Clinically, embryonic cells have been used for therapeutic uses such as retinal disease, spinal cord injury, and diabetes mellitus type 1 because they can make any cells. Cord and placental blood stem cells have been used to treat leukemias. A mature cell that was differentiated can be genetically manipulated to reverts to a pluripotent embryonic type stem cell. These cells are termed *induced pluripotent stem (iPS) cells*. The iPS cells have been used in Huntington disease and are being evaluated for use in other diseases.

Learning Points

Germ Layers

During ovum development, cells branch out into two groups—a peripheral and inner group. The peripheral group forms tissue that maintains the embryo (e.g., placenta), while the inner group divides into three levels (ectoderm, mesoderm, endoderm), called *germ layers*. Each of these layers form different organs and tissues. The ectoderm is the outer, the middle is the mesoderm, and the inner is the endoderm. For example, the brain and spinal cord arise from the ectoderm, while the endoderm forms the digestive system epithelial lining.

Learning Points

Stem Cell Sources

Embryonic stem cells are derived from embryos in vitro and not from a pregnant woman. These pluripotent cells are taken from the blastocyst at about 4–5 days after fertilization. Cord blood cells are not from embryos but, rather, from cord and placental blood after birth. These cells are adult multipotent hematopoietic stem cells.

Cellular Organization

Types of Tissue

Individual cells do not function in isolation. Each cell is part of a complex community that performs specific functions. Tissues are a group of cells with a common structure and function. There are four major types of tissue—epithelial, connective, muscle, and neural. Groups of tissue form organs such as the liver and kidneys, which have a specific function. A system is a grouping of organs that work together to perform similar and complementary functions, such as the cardiovascular or endocrine system. In order for tissues and organs to form, the cells must recognize, adhere, and migrate toward each other and retain their distinct identity from other cells.

Epithelial Tissue

Epithelial tissue lines the outside and all interior areas of the body. Epithelial tissue structure varies depending on the location and function. A single layer of cells is termed *simple epithelium*, and multiple layers are referred to as *stratified epithelium*. The epithelial cells can also have different shapes, and there are three types— squamous, cuboidal, and columnar. Epithelial cells have a protective function, such as the stratified squamous epithelia of the skin and other orifices that open to the outside, such as the mouth, esophagus, and vagina. The outer layer of the skin has a fibrous protein called *keratin*, and through keratinization, these cells shed and are replenished rapidly. Irritants, chemicals, pressure, and other factors can lead to the overproduction of keratin (hyperkeratosis), which is manifested in conditions such as calluses, warts, and eczema. Other functions of the epithelia include absorption, secretion, and excretion.

Connective Tissue

Connective tissue is made up of a large extracellular matrix and fibroblast cells that produce several types of fibers. These fibers are in various parts of the body and serve different functions. Connective tissue most commonly functions to support, attach, and store. The three types of fiber are collagen, elastic, and reticular.

Muscle Tissue

Muscle tissue is made of fibers, termed *myocytes*, that consists of the contractile proteins actin and myosin. These proteins bind to each other causing a shortening and lengthening action. At a neuromuscular junction, the neurotransmitter acetylcholine stimulates the muscle fiber.

The fiber stimulation leads to an action potential, which causes depolarization and the release of calcium. The calcium binds to troponin, and this binding uncovers the actin-binding sites and allows for myosin strands (myosin heads) to pull the actin, leading to contraction. Binding requires energy in the form of ATP. Relaxation occurs when there is no longer a signal or no ATP, calcium is pumped back in, and tropomyosin covers the actin-binding sites.

Muscle fibers are either smooth, cardiac, or skeletal and can be under voluntary (e.g., skeletal movement) or involuntary control (e.g., heart contraction or blood vessels diameter). In general, muscle cells are incapable of replication.

[handwritten margin note: transitional found epithelium in lining of bladder, kidneys, ureters]

Neural Tissue

Neural tissue is composed of neural (nerve) cells called *neurons* (FIGURE 1-12) whose chief function is to process and transmit information. Neurons have specialized characteristics in comparison to other cells. Neurons have a cell body (i.e., soma), an axon that conduct impulses away from the cell body, and dendrites, which tend to conduct impulses toward the cell body. In addition to neurons, the second type of neural cells are neuroglial (glial) cells. These cells are more numerous than neurons and function in a supporting role. Neuroglial cells consist of astrocytes, oligodendrocytes, Schwann cells, microglia, and ependymal cells. Astrocytes form the framework of the brain and spinal cord and form the blood–brain barrier. Ependymal cells form the epithelial lining of the central nervous system and produce cerebrospinal fluid. The oligodendrocytes are responsible for the development of myelin in the central nervous system. Myelin covers and protects nerves and speeds transmission of impulses. Schwann cells produce myelin, but in the peripheral nervous system. Microglia have phagocytic activities. Nerve cells, like muscle cells, are incapable of division and replication.

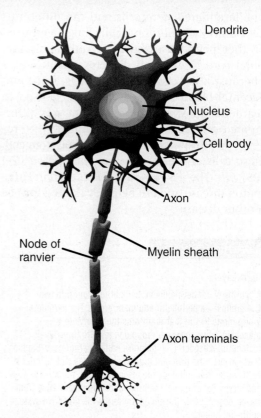

FIGURE 1-12 A motor neuron structure.
© Ducu59us/Shutterstock.

BOX 1-1 Application to Practice

Understanding the cellular organization is important in understanding diseases and therapies. Read the following scenarios and identify the tissue level discussed.

Scenario 1: A 40-year-old woman has a cervical cytology report with the following findings: Atypical squamous cells of undetermined significance. Choose the tissue level the findings refer to:

a. Epithelial
b. Connective
c. Muscle
d. Neural

Scenario 2: A 55-year-old woman would like to get hyaluronic injection fillers for her "laugh lines." Choose the tissue level the injections are administered in:

a. Epithelial
b. Connective
c. Muscle
d. Neural

Scenario 3: A 40-year-old man is diagnosed with a glioblastoma. Choose the tissue level the disease is affecting:

a. Epithelial
b. Connective
c. Muscle
d. Neural

Scenario 4: A 72-year-old woman has a cystoscopy/biopsy report with the following findings: transitional cell carcinoma of the bladder. Choose the tissue level the disease is affecting:

a. Epithelial
b. Connective
c. Muscle
d. Neural

Cellular Adaptation and Damage

Cellular Adaptation

Cells are constantly exposed to a variety of environmental factors that can cause damage. Cells attempt to prevent their own death from environmental changes through adaptation. They may modify their size, numbers, or types in an attempt to manage these changes and maintain homeostasis. Adaptation may involve one or a combination of these modifications. These modifications may be normal or abnormal depending on whether they were mediated through standard pathways. They may also be permanent or reversible. Nevertheless, adaptation ceases once the stimulus is removed. Specific types of adaptive changes include atrophy, hypertrophy, hyperplasia, metaplasia, and dysplasia (FIGURE 1-13).

Atrophy occurs because of decreased work demands on the cell. The body attempts to work as efficiently as possible to conserve energy and resources. When cellular work demands decrease, the cells decrease in size and number. These atrophied cells utilize less oxygen, and their organelles decrease in size and number. Causes of atrophy include disuse, denervation, endocrine hypofunction, inadequate nutrition, and ischemia. An example of disuse atrophy can be seen when a muscle shrinks in an extremity that has been in an immobilizing cast for an extended period. Denervation atrophy is closely associated with disuse; it can be seen when a muscle shrinks in a paralyzed extremity. Atrophy because of a loss of endocrine function (e.g., reduced estrogen) can be seen when the reproductive organs (e.g., ovaries) of postmenopausal women shrink. When these organs are not supplied with adequate nutrition and blood flow, cells shrink due to a lack of substances necessary for their survival—much like when water and fertilizer are withheld from a plant.

The opposite of atrophy is hypertrophy. Hypertrophy occurs when cells increase in size (not number), leading to an increase in the affected organ size. Hypertrophy occurs in an

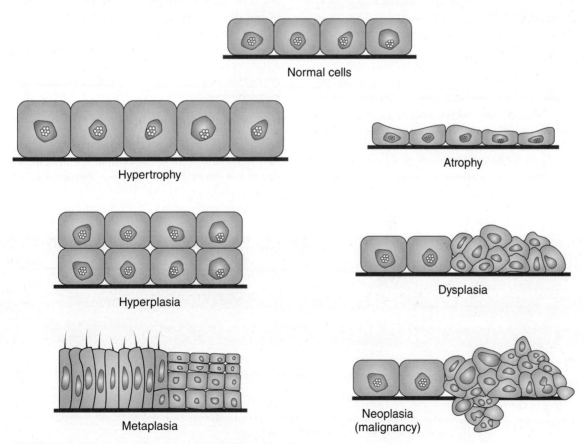

Normal cells

Hypertrophy

Atrophy

Hyperplasia

Dysplasia

Metaplasia

Neoplasia (malignancy)

FIGURE 1-13 Cellular adaptation: abnormal cellular growth patterns.

attempt to meet increased work demand. This size increase may result from either normal or abnormal changes. Such changes are commonly seen in cardiac and skeletal muscle. For example, consider what happens when a body builder diligently performs biceps curls with weights—the biceps gets larger. This type of hypertrophy is a normal change. An abnormal hypertrophic change can be seen with hypertension. Just as the biceps muscle grows larger from increased work, the cardiac muscle will thicken and enlarge when an increased workload is placed on it because of hypertension. The biceps muscle increases in strength and function when its workload is increased; however, over time the heart loses the flexibility to fill with blood and pump the blood when the cardiac muscle increases in size. This abnormal hypertrophic change can lead to complications such as cardiomyopathy and heart failure (see chapter 4).

Hyperplasia refers to an increase in the number of cells (not size of cell) leading to an increase in the affected organ/tissue size. This increase occurs only in cells that can perform mitotic division, such as epithelial cells. The hyperplasia process can be the result of normal or abnormal stimuli. Examples of normal or beneficial hyperplasia include menstruation, liver regeneration, wound healing, and skin callouses. Hyperplasia can also be pathologic, and under these circumstances is usually the result of abnormal hormonal stimulation. Some examples include endometrial (inner uterine lining) hyperplasia, which can be the result of oversecretion of estrogen leading to an imbalance with progesterone. The endometrial hyperplastic cells can become malignant. While hyperplasia is different from hypertrophy, these processes often occur together because they have similar triggers.

The process in which one adult cell is replaced by another cell type that is less mature is called *metaplasia*. This change is usually initiated by chronic irritation and inflammation, such that a more virulent cell line emerges. The cell types do not cross over the overarching cell type. For instance, epithelial cells may be converted into another type of epithelial cell, but they will not be replaced with nerve cells. Metaplastic changes can occur in the airway when the protective columnar cells that usually secrete mucus and have cilia change to stratified squamous epithelium, which does not have the same protective function. In the airway, this metaplasia usually occurs due to chronic smoking or vitamin A deficiency. Metaplasia, just like hyperplasia, does not necessarily lead to cancerous changes; however, if the stimulus is not removed, cancerous changes will likely occur.

The final cellular adaption is dysplasia, which is also called *atypical hyperplasia*. In dysplasia, cells mutate into cells of a different size, shape, and appearance. Although dysplasia is abnormal, it is potentially reversible by removing the trigger. Dysplastic changes are often implicated as precancerous cells. Areas in the reproductive tract such as the cervix or respiratory tract are common sites for this type of adaptation because of their increased exposure to carcinogens (e.g., human papillomavirus and cigarette smoke).

Cellular Injury and Death

Death is a normal part of the human existence, and it is no different at the cellular level. Cellular death can occur due to injury or a programmed

BOX 1-2 Application to Practice

Review and interpret the following endometrial biopsy reports that were done for two women with postmenopausal bleeding.

Report 1: Atrophic endometrium

Report 2: Atypical adenomatous hyperplasia

Review and interpret the following esophagus biopsy reports that were done for two people with history of persistent gastroesophageal reflux disease despite therapy.

Report 1: Low-grade dysplasia

Report 2: Intestinal metaplasia

cell death, termed *apoptosis*. Cellular injury can occur in many ways and is usually reversible up to a point. Whether the injury is reversible or irreversible usually depends on the severity of the injury and intrinsic factors (e.g., blood supply, nutritional status). The vulnerability and tolerance of the cell in adverse conditions can influence survival. Brain and cardiac cells can only last a few minutes without oxygen, while connective tissue can last longer. Cell injury can occur for multiple reasons and can include 1) physical agents such as mechanical forces and extreme temperature; 2) chemical injury such as pollution, lead, and drugs; 3) radiation; 4) biologic agents such as viruses, bacteria, and parasites; 5) nutritional imbalances; 6) hypoxia; 7) genetics; and 8) free radicals. In general, ATP is depleted when cells are injured and a whole cascade of events leads to cell membrane dysfunction. Free radicals (unstable atoms in the body) also cause membrane and cellular destruction. The membrane dysfunction causes imbalances in intracellular calcium, further damaging the membrane. Normal substances such as water, carbohydrates, lipids, and proteins are no longer in a homeostatic state. Metabolic internal substances or external toxins (e.g., infectious organisms, lead) accumulate. As a result of this cellular dysfunction, the cells either produce abnormal substances or phagocytic cells engulf the abnormal substance and store them throughout the body or in certain organs. A clinical example of the consequence of the storage problem is proliferation of macrophages that can cause enlargement of the spleen.

Hypoxia is a common cause of cellular injury and is often the result of ischemia, which refers to inadequate blood flow to tissue or an organ. This lack of blood flow essentially strangles the tissue or organ by limiting the supply of necessary nutrients and oxygen. Ischemia can leave cells damaged to the extent that they cannot survive, a condition called *infarction*. Myocardial infarction and cerebrovascular accidents (cerebral infarction) are life-threatening diseases as a result of ischemia. Another type of cellular death that can occur from ischemia is called *necrosis* (FIGURE 1-14). Infarction is tissue death from lack of blood supply, and necrosis is tissue death from injury, disease, or lack of blood supply. (See chapter 4 and chapter 11.)

Necrosis can take one of several pathways (FIGURE 1-15, FIGURE 1-16, and FIGURE 1-17). Liquefaction necrosis occurs when caustic enzymes dissolve and liquefy necrotic cells. The most common site of this type of necrosis is the brain, which contains a plentiful supply of these enzymes. Caseous necrosis (Figure 1-15) occurs when the necrotic cells disintegrate, but the cellular debris remains in the area for months or years. This type of necrosis has a cottage cheese–like appearance, and it is most commonly noted with pulmonary tuberculosis. Fat necrosis occurs when lipase enzymes break down intracellular triglycerides into free fatty acids. These fatty acids then combine with magnesium, sodium, and calcium, forming soaps. These soaps give fat necrosis an opaque, chalky appearance. Fat necrosis can occur with injury to breast from trauma or radiation or with acute pancreatitis. Coagulative necrosis usually results from an interruption in blood flow. In such a case, the pH drops (acidosis), denaturing the cell's enzymes. This type of necrosis most often occurs in the kidneys, heart, and adrenal glands.

Gangrene is a form of coagulative necrosis that represents a combination of impaired blood flow and a bacterial invasion. Gangrene usually occurs in the legs because of arteriosclerosis (hardening of the arteries) or in the gastrointestinal tract. Gangrene can take any of three forms—dry, wet, and gas. Dry gangrene (Figure 1-16) occurs when bacterial presence is minimal, and the skin has a dry, dark brown, or black appearance. Wet gangrene (Figure 1-17) occurs with liquefaction necrosis. In this condition, extensive damage from bacteria and white blood cells produces a liquid wound. Wet gangrene can occur in extremities and internal organs. Gas gangrene develops because of the presence of *Clostridium*, an anaerobic bacterium. This type of gangrene is the most serious and has the greatest potential to be fatal. The bacterium releases toxins that destroy surrounding cells, so the infection spreads rapidly. The gas released from this process bubbles from the tissue, often underneath the skin.

Another important mechanism of cellular injury is reactive oxygen species (ROS), which are types of free radicals. Free radicals are injurious, unstable agents that can cause cell death. A single unbalanced atom initiates this pathway, which can rapidly produce a wide range of damage. Such an atom has an unpaired electron, making it unstable (electrons are stable in pairs). In an attempt to stabilize itself, the atom borrows an electron from a nearby atom, usually rendering it unstable. This newly unstable atom will then borrow an electron

Necrosis versus Apoptosis

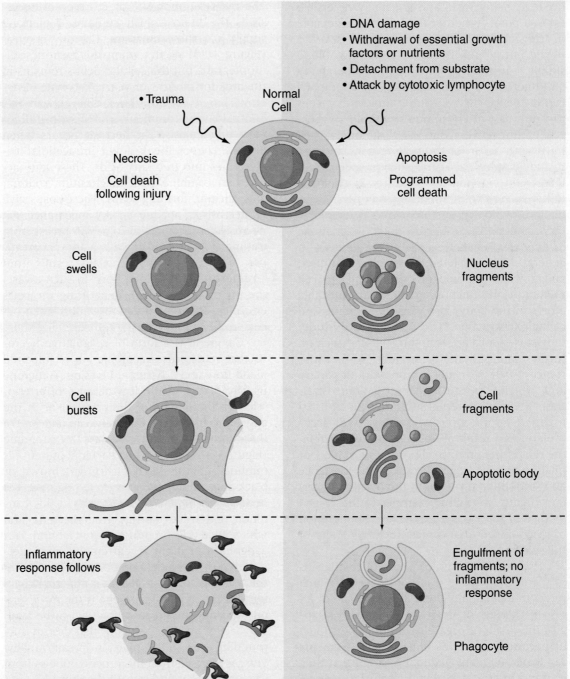

- Trauma

Normal
Cell

- DNA damage
- Withdrawal of essential growth factors or nutrients
- Detachment from substrate
- Attack by cytotoxic lymphocyte

Necrosis

Cell death
following injury

Apoptosis

Programmed
cell death

Cell
swells

Nucleus
fragments

Cell
bursts

Cell
fragments

Apoptotic body

Inflammatory
response follows

Engulfment of
fragments; no
inflammatory
response

Phagocyte

FIGURE 1-14 Cellular damage can result in necrosis, which has a different appearance than apoptosis, as organelles swell and the plasma membrane ruptures.

from its neighbor, creating a domino effect that continues until the atom giving the electron is stable without it. The free radicals that are most concerning are those derived from oxygen and, therefore, called *ROS*. These ROS are formed through oxidation, which is a process of losing electrons, and oxygen is one of the key oxidizers. The body can generally handle a certain number of ROS; however, excesses from stress, pollution, smoking, and poor diet can lead to disease. Protective antioxidant systems (e.g., vitamins C and E, transferrin, and

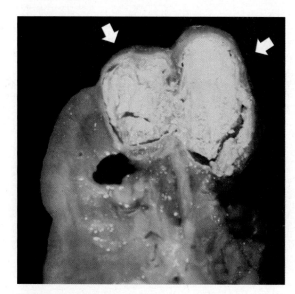

FIGURE 1-15 Caseous necrosis.

Reproduced from Gibson, M. S., Pucket, M. L., & Shelly, M. E. (2004). Renal tuberculosis. *Radiographics, 24*(1), 251–256.

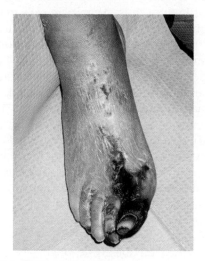

FIGURE 1-16 Dry gangrene.

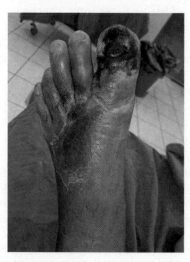

FIGURE 1-17 Wet gangrene.

© Krit_manavid/Shutterstock.

enzymes) are unable to overcome the deleterious effects of ROS leading to oxidative stress. ROS are a cause or contributor to many deleterious effects in the inflammatory and vascular systems. ROS are a major influence in the development and correlation of hypertension, diabetes, and heart disease. ROS have also been linked to cancer, aging, and a variety of other conditions.

Learning Points

Antioxidants

Antioxidant is a general term for molecules that can protect against oxidation, which is how free radicals/ROS can develop. Oxidative processes, however, can be normal, such as when glucose oxidizes to carbon dioxide and oxygen to water. Additionally, not all free radicals generated are dangerous such as when phagocytes release free radicals to fight off infections. Regardless, many free radicals/ROS are deleterious and associated with disease. Many types of antioxidants are marketed as preventing and/or fighting disease and preventing aging. Antioxidants are in food, or in supplements whether in pill form or topical agents. There are over 100 antioxidants, and examples of common ones include vitamin A, C, E, and beta carotene. While antioxidants are beneficial, they can cause disease in excess. An example is the excess use of vitamin E has been associated with an increased prostate cancer risk.

In addition to injury, cell death occurs due to apoptosis. Apoptosis is a programmed cell death and is the process by which unwanted cells (damaged or stressed) are eliminated (Figure 1-14). Programmed cell death is genetically controlled and occurs at a specific point in development. Apoptosis occurs because of morphologic (structure or form) cell changes. Apoptosis as a mechanism of cell death is not limited to certain times in development, but may also result from environmental triggers (e.g., ultraviolet rays, chemotherapy). Apoptosis is important in tissue development, immune defense, and cancer prevention. However, apoptosis can result in inappropriate destruction of cells if it is unregulated. Inappropriate apoptosis (too much or not enough) can lead to degenerative neurologic diseases such as Alzheimer disease, ischemia, and autoimmune disorders. Several therapeutic agents (e.g., anticancer) are geared toward altering apoptotic pathways. While apoptosis and necrosis both result in cellular death, they cause different cellular morphologic changes. In apoptosis, the cells condense or shrink; in necrosis, the cells swell and burst (Figure 1-14). Necrosis and apoptosis can occur at the same time together or independently.

Neoplasms

During cellular division, DNA is being copied and transmitted to the cell being reproduced. From the time of embryonic development forward, cellular division is a constantly occurring process, and while errors occur, they are usually corrected. Cellular repair mechanisms, however, can fail and lead to a DNA nucleotide sequence mutation (variation). Many different types of mutations can occur. Mutations can occur in multiple nucleotides (copy number variants) or in a single nucleotide (single nucleotide variants). Sometimes mutations have no health effects, but, at times, mutations can lead to the development of disease or predispose a person to the development of disease. Chromosomal numbers and structure can be altered and lead to disease such as in Down syndrome, when there is an extra copy (trisomy) or as in cri du chat syndrome where there is a chromosomal deletion. Pieces of one chromosome can translocate to another chromosome such as in leukemia.

Mutations alone are usually insufficient to cause disease. Epigenetic and environmental factors contribute to mutational alterations. Epigenetics involves determining gene expression (how the genes are read) as opposed to genetics, which involves the actual DNA sequence. Epigenetics changes, in other simple terms, can determine whether a gene is "on or off." Many chemical compounds attach or are on (i.e., epi) the genome, and therefore these compounds are termed *epigenomic* or *epigenetic*. Environmental factors include infections, smoking, and eating patterns, can cause genetic mutations or these factors can alter the epigenome

Gene mutations or variations can be hereditary or acquired. If mutations occur in the germline cells (ovum and sperm), the mutation will be inherited from either parent or both, and the mutation will occur in every body cell of the offspring. Acquired mutations occur in somatic cells and do not affect all the cells in the body. Somatic mutations are not inherited. As the understanding of the human genome increases, evidence emerges that most diseases, whether inherited or acquired, have a genetic component.

Cancer is one of the 10 leading causes of death and is discussed in the next section as an example of how a combination of genetic, epigenetic, and many other factors culminate into disease. Congenital disorders, or birth defects, and patterns of inheritance with select inherited disorders all originate from genetic insult and are also discussed. More in-depth information on cancer and congenital disorders will be discussed in respective system chapters, such as leukemia in chapter 3 and congenital urologic disorders in chapter 8.

Benign and Malignant Neoplasms

When the process of cellular proliferation or differentiation goes wrong, neoplasms (abnormal cells) can develop. A neoplasm, or tumor, is a cellular growth that is no longer responding to normal regulator processes, usually because of a mutation. The loss of differentiation that occurs with cells is referred to as *anaplasia*. Anaplasia occurs in varying degrees. The less the cell resembles the original cell, the more anaplastic the cell is. Anaplastic cells may begin functioning as completely different cells, often producing hormones or hormonelike substances.

The two major types of neoplasms are benign and malignant (**TABLE 1-2**; FIGURE 1-18). Malignant neoplasms are called *cancer*. Tumors can occur anywhere in the body and are generally named based on the organ, tissue, or cell origin. Benign tumor prefixes provide information pertaining to the location (*lipo-* refers to fat, *osteo-* to bone, and *chondro-* to cartilage). Therefore, a benign tumor from fat tissue would be a lipoma, and a benign bone tumor would be an osteoma. Malignant tumors are categorized into three groups based on the tissue origin—carcinoma (epithelial), sarcoma (connective), and leukemia/lymphoma (hematopoietic). Other descriptors can be added to these three cancer categories. Carcinomas and sarcomas can be further identified by the origin, such as osteosarcoma (bone), adenocarcinoma (glands), or the epithelial layer such as squamous cell carcinoma.

Benign tumors usually consist of differentiated (less anaplastic) cells that are reproducing more rapidly than normal cells. Because of their differentiation, benign tumors (e.g., lipoma, leiomyoma) are more like normal cells and cause fewer problems. Benign cells are usually encapsulated and are unable to metastasize. The tumor, however, can compress surrounding tissue as it grows. Benign tumors can cause problems due to that compression. Regardless of its size, the tumor can cause devastating problems if it arises in a sensitive area, such as the brain or spinal cord.

TABLE 1-2	Characteristics of Benign and Malignant Tumors	
	Benign tumors	**Malignant tumors**
Cells	Similar to normal cells Differentiated Mitosis normal	Varied in size and shape Many undifferentiated Mitosis increased and atypical
Growth	Relatively slow Expanding mass Frequently encapsulated	Rapid growth Cells not adhesive, infiltrate tissue No capsule
Spread	Remains localized	Invades nearby tissue or metastasizes to distant sites through blood and lymph vessels
Systemic effects	Rare	Common
Life threatening	Only in certain locations (e.g., brain)	Yes, by tissue destruction and spread

Reproduced from Story, L. (2017). *Pathophysiology: A Practical Approach* (3rd ed.). Burlington, MA: Jones & Bartlett Learning.

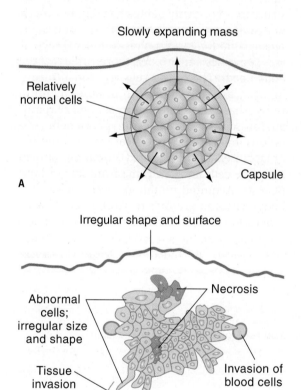

FIGURE 1-18 Characteristics of **(A)** benign and **(B)** malignant tumors.

TABLE 1-3	Common Sites of Metastasis
Cancer type	**Main sites of metastasis***
Bladder	Bone, liver, lung
Breast	Bone, brain, liver, lung
Colorectal	Liver, lung, peritoneum
Kidney	Adrenal gland, bone, brain, liver, lung
Lung	Adrenal gland, bone, brain, liver, other lung
Melanoma	Bone, brain, liver, lung, skin/muscle
Ovary	Liver, lung, peritoneum
Pancreas	Liver, lung, peritoneum
Prostate	Adrenal gland, bone, liver, lung
Stomach	Liver, lung, peritoneum
Thyroid	Bone, liver, lung
Uterus	Bone, liver, lung, peritoneum, vagina

*In alphabetical order.

Reproduced from National Cancer Institute. (2017). Metastatic cancer. Retrieved from http://www.cancer.gov /about-cancer/what-is-cancer/metastatic-fact-sheet

Benign tumors are discussed in various chapters based on their location (e.g., leiomyoma in chapter 7).

Malignant Neoplasms

Malignant tumors usually are undifferentiated (more anaplastic), nonfunctioning cells that are reproducing rapidly. Malignant tumors often penetrate surrounding tissue and spread to secondary sites (**TABLE 1-3**). Some malignant tumors become solid (e.g., sarcoma, carcinoma), while other malignancies are not solid tumors (e.g., leukemia). Cancer's key features include rapid, uncontrolled proliferation and a loss of differentiation (**FIGURE 1-19**). Thus, cancer cells differ from normal cells in size, shape, number, differentiation, purpose, and function.

Cancer is the second leading cause of death in the United States and in many countries following cardiovascular disease (CDC, 2016). Cancer can affect many organs and tissues throughout the body. Over 100 diseases are classified as cancers. Some cancers (e.g., pancreatic cancer) are aggressive and/or difficult to manage and significantly shorten life span, while others (e.g., basal cell carcinoma) are not as aggressive and easier to cure. Cancer

incidence increases with age, and with a continuing rise in the number of people living longer, many people will develop the disease.

Cancer development, invasion, and metastasis (spread) are caused by genetic, epigenetic, and microenvironmental factors. Cancer development, therefore, is not one single event but, rather, results due to a series of events. Carcinogenesis, the process by which cancer develops, has some common features and can be described as occurring in three phases—initiation, promotion, and progression (FIGURE 1-20).

Initiation involves the exposure of a normal cell to an environmental substance or event (e.g., chemicals, viruses, or radiation) that causes DNA damage or mutation. While a mutation is a change in DNA structure, DNA can also be damaged without the structure necessarily being changed. In cancer, one single cell has many **genetic** alterations. This cell no longer responds to normal regulatory processes and proliferates regardless of the body needs. The cancer cells are clonal (meaning they are cells derived from other identical cells), share the same genotype, and perpetuate this same abnormal genotype. Genetic mutations that can lead to cancer can be inherited or acquired. The inherited mutations are in germline cells and can come from one or both parents. Acquired mutations occur in somatic body cells and are due to DNA errors during replication or repair. These mutations can also be due to carcinogen exposure (e.g., chemicals, viruses, or radiation). Acquired cancer mutations are often sporadic and nonfamilial

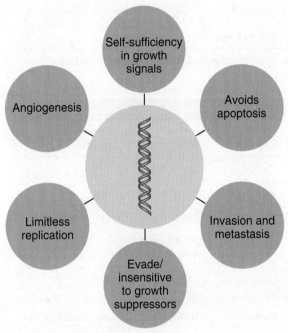

FIGURE 1-19 The hallmarks of cancer.

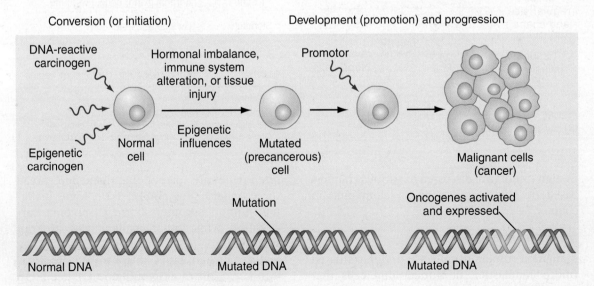

FIGURE 1-20 Carcinogenesis: the stages leading to cancer.

and are more common than inherited (i.e., familial) mutations which account for approximately 5–15% of cancers. Somatic mutations occur regularly in the body. Enzymes detect the damage or mutations and repair the cell or cause apoptosis. If the event is overlooked, the mutation can become permanent, irreversible, and passed onto that cell's future cellular generations. The germline or somatic mutated cells are vulnerable, and further insults may lead to cancer development. Many errors and faulty repair systems occur as the body ages, which is probably one of the reasons for a higher rate of cancer with aging. With cancer, many types of DNA mutations, including frameshift, missense, and nonsense, as well as chromosomal changes such as rearrangements and deletions are possible.

Learning Points

Mutagens and Carcinogens

Mutations are errors in a cell's DNA and can lead to abnormal protein production. Chemical (e.g., poison) or physical (e.g., ultraviolet light) mutagens can cause these DNA structural changes (i.e., mutations). Carcinogens are cancer-causing substances, and some are mutagens. Some carcinogens, however, are not mutagenic, and they damage DNA without affecting the DNA structure.

Mutations can occur on many genes, but mutations in several specific classes of genes are likely to lead to cancer. These genes are normally involved in the proliferation and differentiation process; in other words, they are involved in the cell-cycle regulatory process (i.e., interphase–telophase). These regulatory genes can be divided into two broad categories—proto-oncogenes and tumor suppressor genes.

Proto-oncogenes are involved in normal cellular growth and division. When mutation occurs, they are called *oncogenes* and can cause cancer. The oncogenes (i.e., mutated proto-oncogenes) act like accelerators, and the cell is said to gain function. Oncogene mutations are on somatic cells as opposed to germline cells, so they are not inherited. Over 100 oncogenes exist, and only some oncogenes are associated with cancer. Examples of proto-oncogenic proteins that are mutated and become oncogenic as well as the associated cancer include RAS—pancreatic cancer, c-sis—glioblastoma, c-Myc—oral cancer, and BCR-ABL—chronic granulocytic leukemia. The cancer-causing oncogenes affect several different areas of the cell

cycle. As an example, the RAS proto-oncogene in its inactive form is bound to guanosine diphosphate (GDP) during normal cell growth and when activated, becomes guanosine triphosphate (GTP). The activated RAS triggers transcription factors that facilitates progression through the cell cycle. RAS then reverts from GTP to GDP. A mutation in RAS prevents GTP from reverting to its inactive state GDP, thereby keeping transcription turned on and causing proliferation.

Tumor suppressor genes have an opposite role of proto-oncogenes and are involved in suppressing cellular growth and division and act as the brakes on the cell cycle. Some tumor suppressor genes regulate the cell cycle and cell apoptosis while others are involved in maintenance and repair of DNA. Mutations in tumor suppressor genes cause a lost or diminished braking ability. Tumor suppressor gene mutations, therefore, lead to a loss of function. Tumor suppressor gene mutations can be on germline (inheritable) or somatic cells. Several tumor suppressor gene mutations are associated with cancer development, such as the retinoblastoma gene and the *TP53* gene associated with colon, breast, and lung cancer. The *TP53* gene normally produces the protein p53, which regulates whether mutated genes can be repaired or apoptosis should occur. The *TP53* gene, therefore, is called the *guardian of the genome*. *TP53* gene mutation allows mutated genes to survive and multiply. Breast carcinoma 1 and 2 (*BRCA1* and *BRCA2*) are two other well-known tumor suppressor genes that when mutated are associated with breast, ovarian, and other cancers.

Genes become mutated (initiation), but this mutation is not usually sufficient for carcinogenesis. The second phase of carcinogenesis, **promotion**, involves the mutated cells' exposure to factors (e.g., hormones, nitrates, or nicotine) that promote growth. This phase may occur just after initiation or years later, and it can be reversible if the promoting factors are removed. Several therapeutic agents are geared at removing promoting factors.

Epigenetic abnormalities can lead to cancer development. During transcription and translation (Figures 1-8 and 1-9), many things can go wrong. With epigenetics abnormalities, DNA sequence is intact, but gene expression, which can be described as the turning on and off of genes, is altered. Epigenetic expression normally changes throughout life to activate or inactivate different genes depending on body needs. During pregnancy, for example, various processes need to change to accommodate a developing fetus, so some genes are turned on and others are turned off. Genes are passed down to children, but epigenetic factors can also be hereditary. In the last few decades, research and knowledge in the field of epigenetics has increased dramatically. The same factors that can mutate genes (DNA sequence), such as smoking and diet, can lead to abnormalities in epigenetic mechanisms. Epigenetic changes can be reversible, and how to cause this reversal is an exciting area in the development of cancer therapies.

Epigenetic mechanisms can be grouped into three categories—DNA methylation, histone modification, and microribonucleic acids. Gene expression regulation is modulated by the cell so that protein expression occurs in an efficient manner and at appropriate times. **DNA methylation** (FIGURE 1-21) involves the addition of a methyl group to DNA cytosine. DNA methylation causes a gene to become inactive or silent, leading to inhibition of transcription. This process is essential for normal development. Methylation is different depending on the type of cell (e.g., skin versus muscle). Demethylation

is the removal of the methyl group. Some cancer cells have been found to have changes in the normal methylation/demethylation process on genes.

Histones are proteins that basically are the spools that DNA wraps itself around. These packaged repeating spools of protein and DNA are called *nucleosomes*. There are four different types of histones. Histones can change how tightly or loosely the DNA is coiled and bound around them. The process of histone uncoiling is called *acetylation* (Figure 1-21) and involves the enzyme histone acetyltransferase. The uncoiling is necessary to allow access for transcription for the expression of genes (turn on). Deacetylation is the process of binding that involves the enzyme histone deacetylase (HDAC). Deacetylation leads to less transcription (turning off). In cancer cells, some histones (e.g., H3 and H4) have modifications that affect the process of transcription. Therapeutic agents used in cancer therapy, such as HDAC inhibitors, block deacetylation and through complex processes keep normal genes active, arrest cancer cell growth, and increase apoptosis. Examples of some HDAC inhibitor agents include panobinostat, which is used in multiple myeloma and vorinostat for T-cell lymphoma. HDAC inhibitors are also used in neurologic disorders.

MicroRNA are noncoding proteins whose function is decreasing mRNA translation or stability. MicroRNA, in essence, function as regulators. There are many types of microRNA; some types have an oncogenic effect, leading to cancer. Tumor suppressive types of microRNA are not as abundant in cancer cells. An area of microRNA research is focused on determining if microRNAs can be clinically used as tumor markers to aid in diagnosis and prognosis of cancer. Development of therapeutic applications of microRNA is also under investigation.

Cancer cells live in a microenvironment (like a neighborhood) that also includes noncancer cells (like neighbors) and other components in the extracellular matrix (like sidewalks, parks, etc.). The neighboring noncancer cells and other surroundings influence cancer cell proliferation, survival, metastasis, and treatment response. The microenvironment includes all kinds of cell types (e.g., macrophages, endothelial cells). Some cells in the microenvironment, such as myofibroblasts, form an environment facilitating cancer cell growth and survival. Other cells in the microenvironment may promote angiogenesis

Methylation of DNA and histones causes nucleosomes to pack tightly together. Transcription factors cannot bind the DNA, and genes are not expressed.

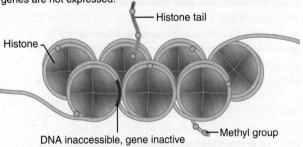

Histone tail

Histone

DNA inaccessible, gene inactive

Methyl group

Histone acetylation results in loose packing of nucleosomes. Transcription factors can bind the DNA and genes are expressed.

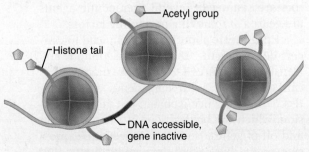

Acetyl group

Histone tail

DNA accessible, gene inactive

FIGURE 1-21 DNA methylation and histone acetylation.

OpenStax, Biology. OpenStax CNX. 23 Mar 2016. Retrieved from https://cnx.org/contents /GFy_h8cu@10.8:ES2pStNH@5/Eukaryotic-Epigenetic-Gene-Regulation (growth of new blood vessels) or metastasis. Further understanding of the microenvironment will lead to continued improvements in diagnosis and treatment strategies.

Learning Points

Precision Medicine

Precision medicine is an approach to treatment and prevention strategies that take into account the similarities and differences among individuals. The traditional approach to care is a standardized treatment for all. In contrast, the individual's genes, environment, and lifestyle are considered when determining treatment strategies with precision medicine. Targeted molecular drugs or therapy, also called *precision drugs*, are available for several diseases such as cystic fibrosis. In cancer, several types of targeted drug therapies are available, such as monoclonal antibodies (immunotherapy) and hormones. In comparison to traditional chemotherapy, these drugs are designed to attack only the cancer cells with less effect on normal cells.

The third phase of carcinogenesis is progression, which is when the tumor invades, metastasizes, and becomes drug resistant. This final phase is permanent or irreversible. Most cancer deaths are due to **metastasis**, but not all tumors can metastasize. The tumor's ability to metastasize (**FIGURE 1-22** and **FIGURE 1-23**) depends on its ability to access and survive in the circulatory or the lymphatic system. Most commonly, the tumor metastasizes to tissue or organs near the primary site, but some tumor cells may travel to distant sites (Table 1-3). The tumor at the site of metastasis has the same cells as the primary site, so the cancer continues to be named by the primary site. As an example, if cancer cells are found in the lungs and they came from the primary breast cancer, then the diagnosis is breast cancer with metastasis to lung or metastatic breast cancer. A second primary cancer can develop but is rare.

The mechanism of metastasis is a multistep process, and similar genetic, epigenetic, and microenvironment abnormalities induce and contribute to metastasis just like in proliferation and differentiation. Regardless of the type of tumor, several factors are essential for the tumor's progression and survival in the new environment. The tumor must have an adequate blood supply, and sometimes it will divert the blood supply from surrounding tissue and grow new blood vessels (**angiogenesis**) to meet those needs. The tumor will grow only as large as the blood supply will support. Location is critical because it determines the cytology of the tumor as well as the tumor's ability

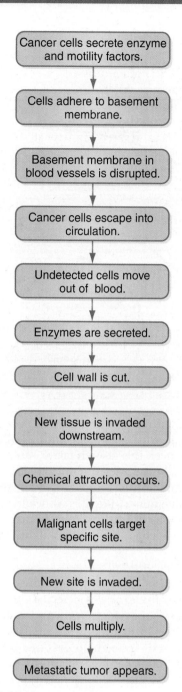

FIGURE 1-22 How cancer metastasizes.

to survive and metastasize. Host factors including age, gender, health status, and immune function will also affect the tumor. Alterations in some of these host factors can create a prime environment for the tumor to grow and prosper. Metastatic cells can also remain in an inactive state and potentially reactivate or never reactivate. Therapies are limited in the treatment of metastasis since the process is not fully understood. One example of a drug targeting metastasis is the monoclonal antibody trastuzumab (Herceptin). This drug targets human

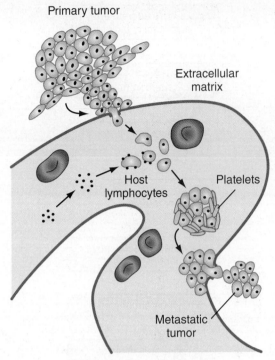

Primary tumor

Extracellular matrix

Host lymphocytes

Platelets

Metastatic tumor

FIGURE 1-23 Pathogenesis of metastasis.

epidermal growth factor receptor-2 (HER-2). In breast cancer, this growth factor receptor malfunctions and causes multiple copies of genes (gene amplification) leading to overexpression and proliferation. HER-2 is associated with an aggressive breast cancer. Trastuzumab binds to HER-2, thereby inhibiting proliferation.

Clinical Manifestations

In most cases, a patient's prognosis improves the earlier the cancer is detected and treated. Healthcare providers, patients, and family members detect many cases of cancer first through the recognition of manifestations. Heeding these warning signs is vital to initiating treatment early. Unfortunately, people often ignore or do not recognize the warning signs for a variety of reasons (e.g., denial and symptom ambiguity).

As the cancer progresses, the patient may present with manifestations of advancing disease, including anemia, cachexia, fatigue, infection, leukopenia, thrombocytopenia, and pain. Anemia can be a result of the blood-borne cancers (e.g., leukemias), chronic bleeding, malnutrition, chemotherapy, or radiation. Cachexia, a generalized wasting syndrome in which the person appears emaciated, often occurs due to malnutrition. Fatigue, or feeling of weakness, is a result of the parasitic nature of a tumor, anemia, malnutrition, stress, anxiety, and

chemotherapy. Factors that can increase the risk for infection include bone marrow depression, chemotherapy, and stress. Leukopenia (low leukocyte levels) and thrombocytopenia (low platelet levels) are common side effects of chemotherapy and radiation due to bone marrow depression. Pain is often associated with cancer due to tissue pressure, obstructions, tissue invasion, visceral stretching, tissue destruction, and inflammation. Cancers have many different clinical manifestations depending on the type, and these manifestations will be discussed in the appropriate chapter (e.g., lung cancer in chapter 4).

Diagnosis and Treatment

Diagnosis of cancer is complex and is specific to the type of cancer suspected. This section provides a basic overview of cancer diagnostic procedures; more specifics are presented in other chapters as specific cancers are discussed. A set of diagnostic procedures usually follows a thorough history and physical examination. These diagnostic procedures may vary depending on the type of cancer suspected. The intention of these diagnostic tests is to identify cancer cells, establish the cytology, and determine the primary site and any secondary sites; however, all these goals are not always accomplished. The healthcare provider will gather as much information as possible to paint the clearest and most complete picture possible of the patient to develop an appropriate treatment plan.

Screening tests and procedures are used for early detection of cancer prior to the development of any symptoms (**TABLE 1-4**). Some of the criteria for determining whether a screening test is recommended are age, gender, behavioral risk behaviors (e.g., tobacco), family history, and ethnicity/race. Screening test recommendations vary based on the organization. As an example, the American Cancer Society recommends offering annual screening mammograms from the age of 40 while the United States Preventive Services Task Force recommends screening mammograms every 2 years starting at the age of 40. If the screening tests are abnormal, further confirmatory tests (e.g., biopsy) may be needed for diagnosis. In addition to screening tests, various other types of diagnostic tests are used in cancer diagnosis such as X-rays, radioactive isotope scanning, computed tomography scans, endoscopies, ultrasonography, magnetic resonance imaging, positron emission tomography scanning, biopsies, and blood tests. Some of the blood tests

TABLE 1-4 Selected Cancer Screening Guidelines Based on Age, Gender, and Risks (Asymptomatic)*

Screening	Routine	Risks—most listed; family or personal history often dictates earlier screening in asymptomatic individuals
Breast		
Mammogram Clinical and self-breast exam	Yearly age 40 and older *or* 50–74 every 2 years can stop at 75 and over unless expect to live longer than 10 years No clear benefit but women should get to know their breasts and notify provider of change	Yearly—Age 30 if: *BRCA1* or *BRCA2* gene mutation (self or 1st-degree relative) Radiation therapy to chest ages 10–30 Lifetime risk ≥ 20% based on family history
Breast and ovarian		
BRCA1 and *BRCA2* genetic screen and testing	No	If at risk based on a screening questionnaire then do BRCA1 and BRCA2 blood test
Cervix		
Cytology (Pap) and human papillomavirus (HPV)	Cytology only every 3 years ages 21–65 Cytology if with HPV co-testing can increase to every 5 years between the ages of 30–65; HPV co-testing not recommended ages 21–29	Continue after 65 under certain circumstances (e.g., history of precancer or cancer within 20 years)
Endometrium		
Endometrial biopsy or pelvic ultrasound	No	Consider at 35 if history of oligomenorrhea (times of no menses or long intervals between menses) or 1st-degree relative with uterine, colon, or ovarian cancer Potential benefits vs. harm inconclusive
Prostate		
Prostate-specific antigen Digital rectal exam	Consider at age 50 and older Potential benefits vs. harm inconclusive	Consider at 45 if African American, or father/brother with prostate cancer before 65
Lung		
Low-dose computed tomography (CT)	No	Age 55–74 with 30-pack year smoking history (current smoker or quit smoking in past 15 years)
Colorectal		
Colonoscopy (gold standard); if unable, other tests (e.g., sigmoidoscopy, fecal test) may be done	Age 50–75 or 45–75 every 10 years	Consider younger than 45 if family history of colorectal or personal history of colorectal cancer or polyps, inflammatory bowel disease, or abdominal/pelvic radiation

*Guidelines may vary based on recommending organization. These were based on American Cancer Society and United States Preventive Services Task Force recommendations accessed in 2018.

Modified from Story, L. (2017). *Pathophysiology: A Practical Approach* (3rd ed.). Burlington, MA: Jones & Bartlett Learning.

may include tumor markers—substances secreted by the cancer cells—for specific cancers (**TABLE 1-5**). These tumor markers not only aid in cancer detection but also assist in tracking disease progression and treatment response.

Malignant cancer cells are classified based on the degree of differentiation (grading) and extent of disease (staging). The grading system determines the degree of differentiation on a scale of 1 to 4, in order of clinical severity. For

TABLE 1-5 | **Common Tumor Cell Markers**

Marker	Malignant condition	Nonmalignant condition
Alpha fetoprotein	Liver cancer Ovarian germ cell cancer Testicular germ cell cancer	Ataxia telangiectasia Cirrhosis Hepatitis Pregnancy
Anaplastic lymphoma kinase	Lung cancer Large-cell lymphoma	Unknown
BCR-ABL	Chronic myeloid leukemia Acute lymphocytic leukemia	Unknown
β_2-microglobulin	Multiple myeloma Chronic lymphocytic leukemia Some lymphomas	Kidney disease
Carcinoembryonic antigen	Bladder cancer Breast cancer Cervical cancer Colorectal cancer Kidney cancer Liver cancer Lung cancer Lymphoma Melanoma Ovarian cancer Pancreatic cancer Stomach cancer Thyroid cancer	Inflammatory bowel disease Liver disease Pancreatitis Chronic obstructive pulmonary disease Rheumatoid arthritis Tobacco use
CA 15-3	Breast cancer Lung cancer Ovarian cancer Prostate cancer	Benign breast disease Endometriosis Hepatitis Lactation Benign ovarian disease Pelvic inflammatory disease Pregnancy
CA 19-9	Bile duct cancer Colorectal cancer Pancreatic cancer Stomach cancer	Thyroid disease Rheumatoid arthritis Cholecystitis Inflammatory bowel disease Cirrhosis Pancreatitis
CA 27-29	Breast cancer Colon cancer Kidney cancer Liver cancer Lung cancer Ovarian cancer Pancreatic cancer Stomach cancer Uterine cancer	Benign breast disease Endometriosis Kidney disease Liver disease Ovarian cysts Pregnancy (first trimester)

Marker	Malignant condition	Nonmalignant condition
CA 125	Colorectal cancer Gastric cancer Ovarian cancer Pancreatic cancer	Endometriosis Liver disease Menstruation Pancreatitis Pelvic inflammatory disease Peritonitis Pregnancy
Human chorionic gonadotropin	Choriocarcinoma Embryonic cell carcinoma Liver cancer Lung cancer Pancreatic cancer Stomach cancer Testicular cancer	Marijuana use Pregnancy
Lactate dehydrogenase	Almost all cancers Ewing sarcoma Leukemia Non-Hodgkin lymphoma Testicular cancer	Anemia Heart failure Hypothyroidism Liver disease Lung disease
Neuron-specific enolase	Kidney cancer Melanoma Neuroblastoma Pancreatic cancer Small-cell lung cancer Testicular cancer Thyroid cancer Wilms tumor	Unknown
Prostatic acid phosphatase	Prostate cancer	Benign prostate conditions
Prostate-specific antigen	Prostate cancer Multiple myeloma Lung cancer	Benign prostatic hyperplasia Prostatitis

instance, grade 1 cancers are well differentiated, meaning they are less likely to cause serious problems because they are more like the original tissue. By comparison, grade 4 cancers are undifferentiated, meaning they are highly likely to cause serious problems because they do not share any characteristics of the original tissue. The TNM staging system evaluates the tumor size, nodal involvement, and metastatic progress (FIGURE 1-24).

Cancer treatment usually consists of a combination of chemotherapy, radiation, surgery, targeted therapy, hormone therapy, immunotherapy, hyperthermia, stem cell transplants, photodynamic therapy, and laser treatment. Additionally, other strategies may include watchful waiting and alternative therapies, including herbs, diet, and acupuncture. The goal of treatment may be either curative (eradicate the disease), palliative (treat symptoms to increase comfort), or prophylactic (prevent the disease).

When surgery is undertaken, attempts are made to remove the tumor and surrounding tissue. Chemotherapy involves the administration of a wide range of medications that destroy replicating tumor cells. Radiation includes the use of ionizing radiation to cause cancer cellular mutation and interrupt the tumor's blood supply. Radiation may be administered by external sources or through internally implanted sources. Targeted therapy is a treatment that uses drugs to identify and attack cancer cells while sparing normal cells; this drug therapy differs from traditional

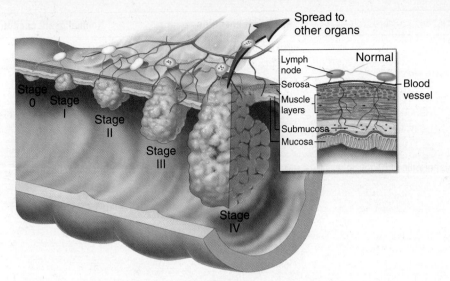

FIGURE 1-24 TNM staging system. The example shown is staging of colorectal cancer.
© 2005 Terese Winslow, U.S. Govt. has certain rights.

chemotherapy but is often used in combination. Hormone therapy involves administering specific hormones that inhibit the growth of certain cancers. Immunotherapy involves administering specific immune agents (e.g., interferons and interleukins) to alter the host's biologic response to the cancer. Hyperthermia precisely delivers heat to a small area of cells or part of the body to destroy tumor cells. This technique can also increase the effectiveness of radiation, immunotherapy, and chemotherapy. Stem cell transplants may include peripheral blood, bone marrow, or umbilical cord blood. These transplants are used to restore stem cells in bone marrow destroyed by disease or treatment. In photodynamic therapy, specific drugs are combined with light to kill cancer cells; these drugs work only when certain types of light activate them. Lasers may be used to shrink or destroy a tumor through application of heat, perform precise cuts in surgery, or activate a chemical.

Learning Points

Gene Therapy

Gene therapy is aimed at treating the basic cause of a disease by using DNA to treat a person's disease-causing DNA. Gene therapy is still limited to a few diseases but is an area under investigation for several disorders. One effective gene therapy is for melanoma called *talimogene laherparepvec* (T-VEC). The medication is a herpes simplex 1 virus that has been modified and is unable to cause the usual cold sores. Instead the virus causes the immune system to target the cancer cells in the tumor and elsewhere in the body.

Prognosis

A cure for cancer is usually defined as a 5-year survival without recurrence after diagnosis and treatment. Prognosis refers to the patient's likelihood for surviving the cancer. Prognosis is heavily dependent on the cancer's ability to metastasize. The more the cancer spreads to other sites by way of the circulation or lymph system, the worse the patient's prognosis. Early diagnosis and treatment usually improve the prognosis by treating the cancer before metastasis has occurred. Fewer treatment options are available once metastasis has occurred. Remission refers to a period when the cancer has responded to treatment and is under control. Remission may occur with some cancers, and generally the patient does not exhibit any manifestations of cancer during that time.

Many cancers are preventable, so health-promoting education (e.g., smoking cessation, proper nutrition, and weight management) is vital to decrease the incidence and prevalence of all cancers. Although the likelihood of these cancers can be diminished with these strategies, it is noteworthy that cancer can develop in people with no risk factors. This unpredictable development contributes to the mystery and challenges surrounding cancer.

Genetic and Congenital Disorders

Genetic and congenital defects are important to understand because of the encompassing nature of these disorders. These diseases affect

TABLE 1-6	Genetic Disorders and Inheritance	
Single-gene disorders	**Multifactorial disorders**	**Chromosomal disorders**
Autosomal dominant	Anencephaly	Cri du chat syndrome
Adult polycystic kidney disease	Cleft lip and palate	Down syndrome
Familial hypercholesterolemia	Clubfoot	Monosomy X (Turner syndrome)
Huntington disease	Congenital heart disease	Polysomy X (Klinefelter syndrome)
Marfan syndrome	Myelomeningocele	Trisomy 18 (Edwards syndrome)
	Schizophrenia	
Autosomal recessive	Alcoholism	
Albinism	Breast cancer	
Color blindness		
Cystic fibrosis		
Phenylketonuria		
Sickle cell anemia		
Tay-Sachs disease		
X-linked recessive		
Duchenne muscular dystrophy		
Hemophilia A		

Reproduced from Story, L. (2017). *Pathophysiology: A Practical Approach* (3rd ed.). Burlington, MA: Jones & Bartlett Learning.

people in all age groups and can involve almost any system. These disorders can result in serious disability or death. Genetic disorders are caused by changes in DNA sequence (mutations) with cancer just discussed as an example of one of many diseases with a genetic basis. Genetic disorders may or may not be present at birth. Congenital defects, often referred to as *birth defects*, usually develop during the prenatal phase of life, are apparent at birth or shortly thereafter, and are often due to genetic or chromosomal abnormalities. Genetic and congenital defects can be hereditary (e.g., cystic fibrosis) or acquired (e.g., Down syndrome). Genetic disorders can be separated into three categories (**TABLE 1-6**)—single-gene (monogenic) disorders, chromosome disorders, and multifactorial inheritance disorders. Multifactorial inheritance disorders are the most common types of genetic disorders. Some disorders also fall into two categories such as fragile X syndrome, which is a single-gene disorder with chromosomal duplication abnormalities. Patterns of inheritance and select genetic disorders (hereditary and acquired) from each category are discussed in this chapter, while many others are discussed throughout the respective chapters (e.g., cystic fibrosis in chapter 5).

Patterns of Inheritance

During reproduction, each parent contributes one set of chromosomes to the fertilized egg. Some characteristics, or traits, and diseases be can determined by one single gene (monogenic) such as cystic fibrosis or a widow's peak on hair. Some traits are determined by multiple genes (polygenic) such as height and skin color (**FIGURE 1-25**). Genes are located on a specific area of the chromosome called a *locus*. That locus has a function (e.g., hair color, skin color, height, protein expression). The locus function and location are the same on each chromosome transmitted from each parent. At the locus, however, the base pairs (nucleotide) vary, and this base pair variation is the allele. Traits are a pair of alleles. When looking at the gene locus for hair color, the mother's allele on this locus may be brown hair and the father's may be blond hair. Therefore, the gene locus function is hair color, but different versions of the hair color gene are possible, such as shades of brown (allele). A person who has identical alleles of each chromosome is homozygous for that gene; if the alleles are different, then the person is said to be heterozygous for that gene.

For unknown reasons, one allele on a chromosome may be more influential than the other in determining a specific trait. The more powerful, or dominant, allele is more likely to be expressed in the offspring than the less influential, or recessive, allele. The dominant allele is symbolized by a capital letter and the recessive by a lowercase letter. Offspring will express the dominant allele in both homozygous (e.g., AA) and heterozygous (e.g., Aa) allele pairs. In contrast, offspring will express the recessive allele only in homozygous pairs (aa). Alleles can be codominant, which means

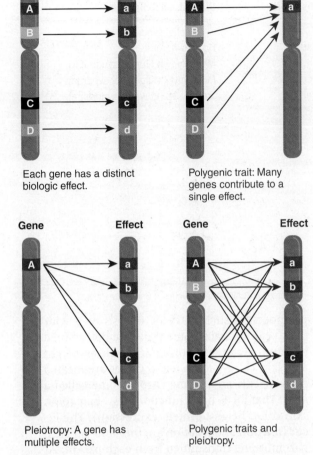

Each gene has a distinct biologic effect.

Polygenic trait: Many genes contribute to a single effect.

Pleiotropy: A gene has multiple effects.

Polygenic traits and pleiotropy.

FIGURE 1-25 Single single gene/multiple genes

a heterozygote has two dominant alleles (e.g., AB) like in a blood type or sickle cell disease. Single-gene (monogenic) trait inheritance follow principles of dominance and recessiveness. Single-gene patterns are sometimes called *Mendelian inheritance patterns* after Gregor Mendel. Polygenic traits are more complex and do not follow usual single-gene inheritance patterns. These polygenic genes and traits are often a product of genetic and environmental factors (see Table 1-6). An example of a polygenic trait is blood pressure. The blood pressure trait is affected by environmental factors, such as diet and exercise.

If a person has a diseased allele but does not express the disease (phenotype normal), then the person is called a *carrier*. Carriers can transmit diseases to offspring.

The sex chromosomes (X and Y) can pass on genes when they are linked, or attached, to one of the sex chromosomes. For example, a male will transmit one copy of each X-linked gene to his daughter but none to his son, whereas a female will transmit a copy of her X-linked gene to each offspring, male or female. X-linked disorders follow the inheritance pattern of dominance and recessive.

Single-Gene Disorders

An estimated 4,000 diseases are caused by single-gene alterations. Most single-gene disorders are hereditary and transmitted more commonly on autosomes in comparison to the X chromosome. Inheritance patterns for these single-gene disorders, like single-gene traits (Mendelian traits), follow the traditional dominant versus recessive allele transmission. The four types of modes of inheritance are autosomal dominant, autosomal recessive, X-linked dominant, and X-linked recessive. On the Y chromosome there is very little genetic material and few genes that cause disease. Diseases of the Y chromosome primarily affect male fertility. Autosomal dominant disorders and, less commonly, autosomal recessive disorders can have a genotype but features (phenotype) of the disorder may never develop. This lack of development is termed **incomplete penetrance**. **Variable expressivity** refers to having a genetic disorder, but the clinical manifestations vary widely among affected individuals. Incomplete penetrance and variations in expression are thought to occur due to epigenetics, environmental factors, or differences in the mutation.

Learning Points

Hereditary Versus Acquired Mutations

Hereditary mutations are usually on single genes (particularly autosomes), and this mutated gene is in all body cells of the mother and/or father. The mother and/or father, depending on the gene mutation (e.g., dominant or recessive), may be a carrier or have the disease. During reproduction, this mutation may be passed on to all cells of the child. Hereditary mutations may have also existed in other biologic family members. Hereditary mutations are also called *germline mutations* as they are passed on through the germline cells (from precursors, ovum, or spermatozoa cells).

Acquired mutations were not in a mother's and/or father's body cells, so they are not passed on. These mutations occur on somatic cells (nongametes) and occur spontaneously or due to an insult (e.g., radiation, infection), and they are called *de novo mutations*. These mutations can occur during embryonic development or after birth. No family history of the mutation is present. Chromosomal abnormalities are often not hereditary and often are a result of a failure of separation during meiosis (i.e., nondisjunction). If this happens during gametogenesis then during fertililzation the zygote will have a chromosomal abnormality.

Autosomal Dominant Disorders

Autosomal dominant disorders are single-gene mutations that are passed from an affected parent to an offspring regardless of sex. When a child has an autosomal dominant disorder, one of the parents must have the trait. Male and female are equally capable of transmission to offspring. Autosomal dominant disorders occur with both homozygous (e.g., AA) and heterozygous (e.g., Aa) allele pairs. Depending on the disease, a homozygous-affected fetus may not survive. If the infant does survive, he or she will likely have a more severe expression of the disorder, compared to children with the heterozygous pair, because the homozygous pair provides a double dose of the gene.

Autosomal dominant disorders typically involve abnormalities with structural proteins. Recurrence risks can be evaluated with a diagram (Punnett square) to predict gene combinations of recessive and dominant traits in offspring (FIGURE 1-26). The recurrence risks for an autosomal disorder being transmitted when one parent is heterozygous and the other is normal is 50% for each child, and the risk remains 50% for each subsequent birth. If both parents are affected (not as common of a union), the risk remains 50% even though one allele of the four possibilities will be homozygous dominant (AA). A homozygous-dominant (AA) infant is unlikely to survive. Even with two affected parents, each birth is an independent event; therefore, the recurrence risk continues to be 50%.

If both parents do not have the trait or any family history but a child is born with an autosomal dominant disorder, then a new mutation occurred in one of the parent's genes during reproduction. In these circumstances, all the other cells in the parents are normal, so next time there is a pregnancy, the risk is the same as the general population. Examples of autosomal dominant disorders include Marfan syndrome and neurofibromatosis.

How to Use a Punnett Square for Autosomal Dominance

1. In autosomal dominance, the capital letter (A) is the representation of the mutated gene. Since the disease is rare, the most likely scenario is a pairing of a normal parent (does not have disease trait so homozygous (a) is the normal) and an affected heterozygous parent (most homozygous dominant people do not survive or are severely affected and not likely to reproduce).
2. By reviewing the square, you can see that there is a 50% chance of an offspring being affected (disease) and a 50% chance of being unaffected in this typical mating scenario.

Marfan Syndrome

Marfan syndrome is one of the more common inherited degenerative generalized disorders of the connective tissue with an incidence of 1 in 5,000 persons (FIGURE 1-27). Most cases of Marfan syndrome are inherited in an autosomal dominant pattern, but 25% are a result of new mutations (no family history). The condition results from a single-gene mutation (*FBN1*) on chromosome 15, and in less than 10% of cases, no mutations on the *FBN1* are present, but, rather, other genetic abnormalities (e.g., allele deletion) occur. The *FBN1* gene provides instructions for making a protein called *fibrillin-1*. Fibrillin-1 binds to other fibrillin-1 proteins and other molecules to form threadlike filaments called *microfibrils*. Microfibrils provide strength and flexibility to connective tissue as well as store and release growth factors to control growth and tissue repair. The mutation causes excess growth factors to be released, and elasticity in many tissues is decreased; together, these two processes lead to overgrowth and instability of tissues.

Clinical Manifestations

The manifestations of Marfan syndrome vary widely in their severity, timing of onset, and rate of progression. The defects in Marfan syndrome produce a variety of classic ocular, musculoskeletal, and cardiovascular disorders. The lungs, skin, and central nervous system,

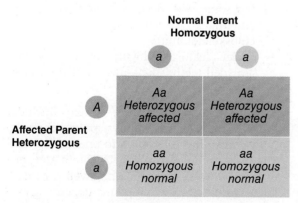

FIGURE 1-26 Punnett square for autosomal dominant disorder. Typical mating scenario.

BOX 1-3 Application to Practice

Case 1: Mary and John want to have a second child. They have a 10-year-old with Down syndrome, and they have questions about the risks of having a second child with Down syndrome.

Explain the risks for the development of Down syndrome and the recurrence risk in a second pregnancy.

Case 2: A 5-year-old boy was just diagnosed with red–green color blindness. His parents are concerned and want clarification regarding how their son got this disorder as they have a daughter who does not have the disorder. Answer the following questions his parents have about the new diagnosis.

1. How is red–green color blindness inherited?
2. Why doesn't our daughter have the disorder?

Case 3: Draw a Punnett square for cystic fibrosis (both parents are carriers) and Marfan syndrome (one parent is affected and one is unaffected) and discuss the gender distribution, risks of being a carrier, or affected. Discuss risks for subsequent births.

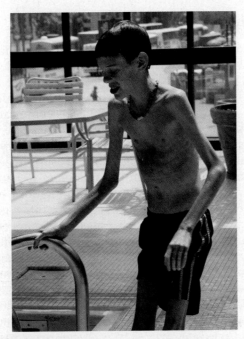

FIGURE 1-27 Marfan syndrome.
Courtesy of Rick Guidotti/Positive Exposure/National Marfan Foundation.

however, can also be affected. The classic manifestations include the following:

Cardiovascular
- Aortic defects (coarctation, aneurysm, dissection, aortic regurgitation) (most life threatening because it can lead to aortic rupture and internal bleeding)
- Mitral valvular defects (e.g., redundancy of leaflets, stretching of the chordae tendineae, mitral valve regurgitation)

Ocular
- Ectopia lentis (lens displacement) which is an ocular hallmark
- Increased tendency for cataracts, glaucoma, and retinal detachment

Musculoskeletal
- Great height (tall and slender)
- Long extremities (e.g., arm span-to-height ratio is increased)
- Arachnodactyly (long, spiderlike fingers)
- Sternum defects (e.g., funnel chest [pectus excavatum] or pigeon breast [pectus carinatum]
- Spine deformities (e.g., scoliosis or kyphosis)
- Pes planus (flat feet)
- Acetabulum protrudes (seen on imaging such as computed tomography, magnetic resonance imaging)
- Hypotonia and increased joint flexibility but some with decreased mobility (elbow and fingers), which can predispose to musculoskeletal injury
- Facial features (highly arched palate, crowded teeth, small lower jaw, thin, narrow face)

Manifestations in other systems include lung disorders such as emphysematous changes with bullae that predispose to pneumothorax. The skin can develop striae. The brain and spinal cord dura can enlarge and swell (i.e., dural ectasia), causing symptoms depending on location (e.g., low back pain, perineal pain, headaches).

Diagnosis and Treatment

A thorough history and physical examination are vital in diagnosing Marfan syndrome. In most cases, the family history is positive for the disease or the symptoms. A physical examination would reveal the presence of the hallmark lens displacement and other symptoms of the disease. Diagnostic procedures may include a skin biopsy that would be positive for fibrillin, X-rays that would confirm the skeletal abnormalities, an echocardiogram that would reveal the cardiac abnormalities, and a DNA analysis for the gene. Marfan manifestations may mimic other disorders. To improve diagnostic accuracy, defined criteria (e.g., Ghent nosology) are established and take into consideration family history. With the Ghent nosology, numerous manifestations are possible, and each manifestation is assigned points (e.g., dural ectasia +2). The criteria and easy to use calculators can be found at www.marfan.org/dx/home.

Clinical care usually involves a comprehensive multidisciplinary team. Typical treatment focuses on relieving symptoms and may include the following measures:

- Surgical repair of aneurysms and valvular defects
- Surgical correction of ocular deformities
- Steroid and sex hormone therapy to aid in closure of long bones, thereby, limiting height
- Beta-adrenergic blocking agent or angiotensin receptor blockers (which decrease blood pressure and heart rate) to limit complications from cardiac deformities
- Bracing and physical therapy for mild scoliosis and surgical correction for severe cases

Other strategies include avoiding contact sports, supportive care for the patient and family, and frequent checkups. Relatives at risk should be tested.

Neurofibromatosis

Neurofibromatosis is a condition involving neurogenic (nervous system) tumors that arise from Schwann cells and other similar cells. Schwann cells are a type of neuroglial cells that keep peripheral nerve fibers alive through functions such as forming and maintaining the myelin sheath in motor and sensory axons. Although most cases of neurofibromatosis are inherited, 30–50% occur

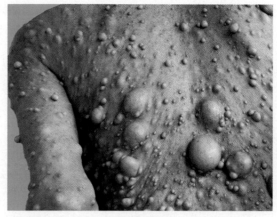

FIGURE 1-28 Neurofibromatosis type 1.
© Chiewr/iStock/Getty Images.

spontaneously. There are three main types—type 1 and type 2 neurofibromatosis and schwannomatosis.

Type 1 neurofibromatosis (von Recklinghausen disease) (**FIGURE 1-28**) is the most common of the 3 types and occurs in 1 in 3,000–4,000 people. Type 1 neurofibromatosis results from mutations in the *NFI* gene on chromosome 17. This gene provides instructions for making a protein called *neurofibromin* present in many tissues such as the brain, kidney, and spleen. Neurofibromin acts to suppress tumor development. The defect caused by the mutations results in lesions that may include and typically appear in this order with aging—café au lait spots (brown pigmented birthmarks), freckling, iris elevated with tan nodules (Lisch nodules), and neurofibromas. Manifestations are different from person to person with some developing tumors compressing nerves leading to pain and loss of function, while others may only have café au lait spots.

Type 2 neurofibromatosis results from mutations in the *NF2* gene on chromosome 22. This gene provides the instructions for making a protein called *merlin* that acts to suppress tumor development. The defect caused by the mutations results in bilateral acoustic (eighth cranial nerve) tumors, called *vestibular schwannomas* or *acoustic neuromas*, that cause hearing impairment (loss and tinnitus) and balance issues. Intracranial and spinal meningiomas can also develop, and manifestations will vary depending on the location and size. The clinical manifestations usually appear around the age of 20, and if diagnosed in children, they have a more severe presentation. Type 2 neurofibromatosis occurs in 1 in 33,000 people.

Schwannomatosis causes multiple benign tumors along the nerve sheaths with no skin or vestibular involvement. The genetic mutation is of the *SMARCB1* or *LZTR1* tumor suppressor gene located on chromosome 22. The manifestations are multiple tumors with nerve symptoms, such as tingling and weakness, that will vary depending on the tumor location. Chronic pain is common and may or may not be tumor related. The incidence is like type 2 and occurs in about 1–40,000 afflicted individuals. The signs appear in adulthood (25–30 years old) with an average age of diagnosis around 40 years.

People with neurofibromatosis can be affected in many ways. For example, this genetic disorder is associated with an increased incidence of learning disabilities and seizure disorders. Vision, skeletal, and cardiac issues including optic gliomas and cataracts, scoliosis, and hypertension may also be present, particularly with type 1. Cognitive impairments, seen in type 1 and schwannomatosis, are not associated with type 2. Some individuals with type 1 neurofibromatosis, but not type 2, develop cancerous tumors such as neurofibrosarcoma, and neurofibromatosis increases risk of developing other cancers (e.g., brain and leukemia). The appearance of the lesions varies between individuals, and the lesions can be disfiguring in some cases. There is no cure for neurofibromatosis, but regular tumor surveillance (e.g., annual brain magnetic resonance imaging) is important. Surgeries may be necessary to remove the lesions for palliative or safety reasons. Pain management is important. Targeted tumor therapy with drugs such as monoclonal antibodies are another area of investigation. Screening at-risk family members is recommended.

Autosomal Recessive Disorders

Autosomal recessive disorders are single-gene mutations passed from an affected parent to an offspring regardless of sex, but they occur only in homozygous (aa) allele pairs. Those persons with heterozygous (Aa) pairs are only carriers and exhibit no symptoms (phenotypically normal). The usual scenario for transmission will be two carrier (heterozygous) parents, and a recessive defective gene from each will be passed down in order to result in the disease. By looking at the Punnett square (**FIGURE 1-29**), we see that 25% of offspring will get the disease and 50% will become carriers. If one parent is a carrier and one is not a carrier or unaffected then no disease will be produced,

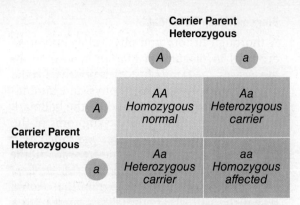

FIGURE 1-29 Punnett square for autosomal recessive disorder. Typical mating scenario.

but 50% will be carriers. If both parents have the disease, then all offspring will have the disease. As opposed to dominant disorders, recessive traits usually continue from generation to generation as they are hidden in normal carriers. Consanguinity, which refers to relation by blood, is often implicated in recessive disorders as both may share the recessive allele passed down from ancestors. The age of onset for these disorders is usually early in life, and they occur most commonly as deficiencies in enzymes and inborn errors in metabolism. Examples of autosomal recessive disorders include cystic fibrosis, phenylketonuria (PKU), and Tay-Sachs disease.

How to Use a Punnett Square for Autosomal Recessiveness

1. In autosomal recessive disorders, the lowercase letter (a) represents the recessive gene mutation. For an offspring to get the disease, both parents have to be carriers (the most common mating scenario).
2. By reviewing the square, we see that with two carriers, there is a 25% chance of an offspring being affected (disease); a 50% chance an offspring will be a carrier, and a 25% chance an offspring will be unaffected. Another mating scenario is if one parent is a carrier and one is unaffected, then the disease will not be inherited but 50% will be carriers.

Phenylketonuria

PKU is a deficiency of phenylalanine hydroxylase, the enzyme necessary for the conversion of phenylalanine to tyrosine, due to a mutation in the *PAH* gene on chromosome 12. Phenylalanine is a building block of proteins that is obtained in the diet (proteins and aspartame), and it plays a role in melanin production. A deficiency of phenylalanine hydroxylase leads to toxic levels of phenylalanine in the blood, causing central nervous system damage. The occurrence of PKU varies worldwide, but it is found in 1 in 10,000–15,000 newborns.

Clinical Manifestations

If untreated, PKU leads to severe intellectual disability. Symptoms develop slowly and can go undetected. Because untreated cases almost always lead to intellectual disability, all newborns in the United States are screened for PKU shortly after birth by testing for high serum phenylalanine levels. If untreated, children can develop the following clinical manifestations:

- Failure to meet milestones
- Microcephaly
- Progressive neurologic decline
- Seizures
- Hyperactivity
- Electrocardiograph abnormalities
- Learning disability
- Mousy or musty-smelling urine, skin, hair, and sweat
- Lighter skin and hair than unaffected family members
- Eczema
- Behavioral problems (e.g., hyperactivity disorders)
- Psychiatric disorders

Diagnosis and Treatment

In addition to diagnosis after birth, prenatal screening through chorionic villus sampling and amniocentesis can be done for at-risk women. Treatment for PKU involves consumption of a diet low in phenylalanine. Newborns may be breastfed, but the quantity of breastmilk taken in has to be monitored. Special infant formulas are available for supplementation. Dietary restrictions include avoiding proteins and aspartame as well as minimizing starches. Oral medications are available to lower phenylalanine (e.g., sapropterin [Kuvan]). Additionally, gene and enzyme therapy have demonstrated promise in treating PKU.

Tay-Sachs Disease

Tay-Sachs disease is a progressive disorder that results from a mutation in the *HEXA* gene on chromosome 15. This gene provides the instructions for making part of a lysosomal enzyme called *beta-hexosaminidase A*. The enzyme is necessary to metabolize certain lipids called *gangliosides*. With *HEXA* gene mutation, lipids accumulate in the lysosomes of nerve cells and gradually destroy and demyelinate nerve cells. This destruction of nerve cells leads to a progressive mental and motor deterioration, often causing death by 5 years of age.

Tay-Sachs disease is rare in the general population and almost exclusively affects individuals of Ashkenazi Jewish descent, of whom about 1 in every 27 is a carrier. The mutation is also more common in certain French Canadian communities in Quebec, the Old Order Amish community in Pennsylvania, and the Cajun population in Louisiana.

Clinical Manifestations

Tay-Sachs disease is divided into three forms based on symptom onset—infantile (most common), juvenile, and adult (extremely rare). Clinical manifestations of Tay-Sachs disease usually appear between 3 and 10 months and include the following:

- Exaggerated Moro reflex (startle reflex) at birth
- Apathy to loud sounds by age 3–6 months
- Inability to sit up, lift head, or grasp objects
- Difficulty turning over
- Progressive vision loss
- Deafness and blindness
- Seizure activity
- Paralysis
- Spasticity
- Pneumonia

Diagnosis and Treatment

This genetic disorder is diagnosed by a thorough history and physical examination as well as evaluating for deficient serum and amniotic beta-hexosaminidase A levels. Because of the devastating nature of Tay-Sachs disease, genetic counseling is important for persons of Jewish ancestry and individuals with a positive family history. No cure for the disease exists; most treatments are supportive. Those supportive approaches include seizure control, parenteral nutrition, pulmonary hygiene including suctioning and postural drainage, skin care, laxatives, and psychological counseling.

Sex-Linked Disorders—Recessive or Dominant

Genes located on the sex chromosomes cause a variety of genetic disorders. Most sex-linked disorders are X linked as the Y chromosome carries little genetic material.

X-linked disorders may be either recessive or dominant, with recessive disorders being more common. In general, with X-linked disorders, males are more affected than females. Males tend to have a more severe presentation than females. In terms of inheritance, the patterns are somewhat different than autosomal disorders, and there are also differences between dominant and recessive X-linked disorders.

There are differences in the inheritance patterns between X-linked disorders (dominant vs. recessive) between males and females. In X-linked recessive disorders, a female becomes a carrier when inheriting only one copy of a defective allele from its carrier or from an affected mother or an affected father. For a female to get the disease, she needs to get two recessive alleles (one from her mother and one from her father). In dominant X-linked disorders, the female needs only one mutated X copy to get the disease. The other normal X effects are dominated by this dominant mutated allele. This mutated dominant allele can come from the mother or father.

All males who get the disease with X-linked recessive disorders do so because they only have one X chromosome and do not have a normal other X allele to counteract. Males, therefore, cannot be carriers. Fathers only give a Y chromosome to their sons, so they never transmit the disease to their sons. The disease is transmitted from their mother. X-linked dominant disorders are rare except for fragile X syndrome. This disorder has a more complicated inheritance pattern and males can be carriers. Fragile X inheritance will be discussed in the next section. Examples of X-linked recessive diseases include Duchenne muscular dystrophy and hemophilia.

Fragile X Syndrome

Fragile X syndrome (**FIGURE 1-30**) is an X-linked dominant disorder associated with a single trinucleotide gene sequence (*FMR1*) on the X chromosome. The *FMR1* gene provides the instructions for making a protein called *familial mental retardation protein* (FMRP) that regulates production of other proteins and plays a role in synapse development. Synapses are critical in relaying nerve impulses. Normally, this trinucleotide sequence is repeated about 5–40 times, but in people with fragile X syndrome, it is repeated more than 200 times. The increased repetitions lead to turning off or silencing of the *FMR1* gene and FMRP production stops.

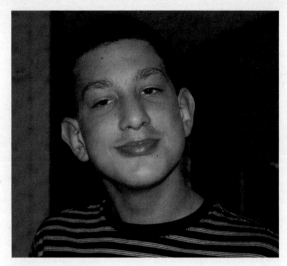

FIGURE 1-30 Fragile X syndrome.
© Courtesy of Nikki Deal.

The more repeats of this gene sequence, the more severe the disease.

Fragile X syndrome is considered the second most common cause of intellectual disability following Down syndrome. Fragile X syndrome is more common and usually more severe in males (it occurs in 1 in 4,000 males and 1 in 8,000 females). There are a few differences in fragile X syndrome inheritance pattern and X-linked recessive disorders. Males who are not carriers of X-linked recessive disorders can be carriers of fragile X and be phenotypically normal. Males can become carriers because there is incomplete penetrance. The *FMR1* gene goes through stages as it is passed down in families. The gene can start off as normal, then premutate, and then fully mutate. Other X-linked disorders do not have a premutation stage. Sometimes, alleles have 45–54 sequence repeats and are termed *gray area* alleles. These alleles are a bit unstable and may result in a premutation. A premutation is defined as 55–200 sequence repeats, and a person with such a premutation is said to be a carrier. A full mutation and disease occur with over 200 trinucleotide sequence repeats. Females with premutations are at risk of passing on the abnormal genes; the more sequence repeats, the higher the risk and the more likely the premutation will be a full mutation. Some females with premutation have health issues such as menstrual irregularities, infertility, and premature ovarian failure. Males with premutations will pass this carrier gene to all their daughters but not the full mutation. Some males with the premutations may develop tremors and ataxia with aging.

Clinical Manifestations

Clinical manifestations of fragile X syndrome, particularly language and developmental delays, are usually seen by age 2. The average age of diagnosis for males is 36 months, and for females it is 42 months. The manifestations include the following:

- Intellectual, behavioral, and learning disabilities
- Prominent jaw and forehead
- Long, narrow face with long or large ears
- Connective tissue abnormalities (e.g., flexible fingers, flat feet)
- Large testes
- Hyperactivity, inattentiveness, and anxiety
- Seizures
- Speech and language delays
- Tendency to avoid eye contact
- Autism spectrum disorders

Diagnosis and Treatment

Diagnosis of fragile X syndrome involves the identification of clinical manifestations and a positive genetic test. No cure for this condition exists, so treatment focuses on controlling individual symptoms. Genetic counseling is appropriate for persons with a positive family history. Behavioral and psychological support may be indicated for both parents and the affected child. Other supportive interventions include physical, speech, and occupational therapy. The earlier the interventions, the better the outcomes.

Chromosomal Disorders—Number or Structural

Chromosomal disorders are a major category of genetic disorders that result most often from alteration in chromosomal number or structure. These alterations can occur on autosomes or X chromosomes. These disorders often occur in utero because of some environmental influences (e.g., maternal age, drugs, infections). The most vulnerable time for the fetus is at 15–60 days' gestation. This period immediately follows fertilization and implantation, when much of the cellular differentiation is occurring. More than 60 disorders fall in this category, many of which result in first-trimester spontaneous abortions.

Chromosomal aberrations include those with an abnormal number of pairs or copies of chromosomes. **Polyploidy** is the term used when there is more than the normal (euploid)

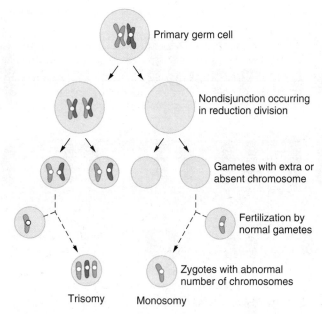

FIGURE 1-31 Chromosome nondisjunction abnormality.

23 pairs in a cell. Types of polyploidy include triploidy, which occurs when there are 3 copies of each pair, or tetraploidy, where there are 4 copies of each pair (4 × 23 = 92 pairs of chromosomes). These conditions are not compatible with life, so fetuses or newborns die. **Aneuploidy** is another term that has to do with chromosomal numbers. Aneuploidy occurs due to nondisjunction (**FIGURE 1-31**), which is an abnormal separation during cell division leading to too many or too few chromosomes.

An aneuploidy, such as monosomy, occurs when there is only one copy of a chromosome inside a pair, so there are 45 chromosomes. Autosomal monosomy is not compatible with life; therefore, the fetus will not survive. Those individuals with X-linked monosomy (e.g., Turner syndrome), however, can survive. If there is no X chromosome at all, then there is no zygote survival (males cannot survive with Y only). With aneuploidy, an extra copy within a pair, such as trisomy where there are 47 chromosomes, may be present (**FIGURE 1-32**).

Autosomal trisomies, as opposed to autosomal monosomy, can survive; trisomy 21 (Down syndrome) and trisomy 13 (Patau syndrome) are examples. X-linked trisomies include disorders such as Klinefelter syndrome (e.g., XXY), but there can be 3 or 4 copies of X (e.g., 45, XXXY). Females can also have too many X chromosomes (e.g., XXX) and have reproductive disorders and other manifestations.

With aneuploidy, all or part of a chromosome may be lost. **Chromosomal mosaicism**

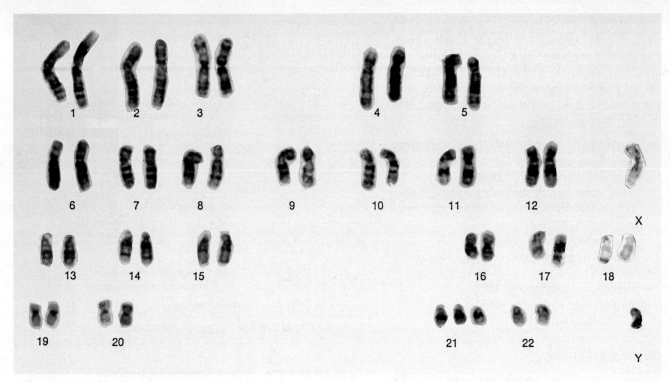

FIGURE 1-32 Karyotype with trisomy 21.

© Jens Goepfert/Shutterstock.

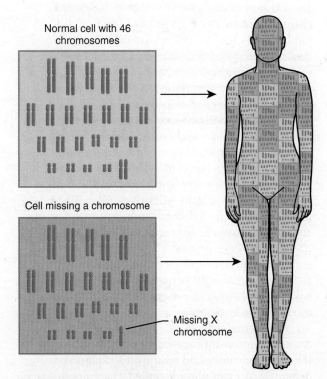

FIGURE 1-33 Chromosomal mosaicism.

Help Me Understand Genetics Mutations and Health, Genetic Home Reference, April 2 2019, U.S. National Library of Medicine.

is when the aneuploidy only occurs in some of the body cells of the offspring, but others are normal (**FIGURE 1-33**). Mosaicism can occur in many disorders such as Turner, Klinefelter, and Down syndromes. Individuals with mosaicism are affected by the abnormal chromosomes.

Since polyploidy and aneuploidy have to do with numbers, it can be easy to confuse them. One way to remember is polyploidy has to do with pairs and aneuploidy has to do with individual chromosomes inside the pair. With aneuploidy, there are always 23 pairs, but the number of individual chromosomes goes up or down. Individuals with polyploidy and aneuploidy with fewer chromosomes (except for X-linked monosomies) usually do not survive.

Autosomal Aneuploidy

Trisomy 21

Trisomy 21, or Down syndrome, is a spontaneous chromosomal mutation that results in three copies of chromosome 21 (Figure 1-32 and **FIGURE 1-34**). These extra copies are thought to disrupt the course of normal development. Trisomy 21 occurs in about 1 in 800 births. The risk of this mutation increases with greater parental age and environmental teratogen exposure. Up to 95% of Down syndrome cases are due to nondisjunction of the maternal egg, and most of the remaining cases are due to paternal sperm cell nondisjunction (Figure 1-31). Less commonly (about 4% of cases), the cause of the mutation is due to translocation (**FIGURE 1-35**), which is the exchange of genetic material

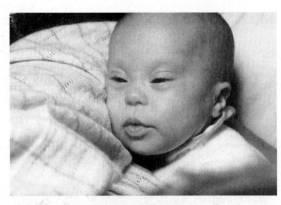

FIGURE 1-34 Down syndrome.

Courtesy of Sarah Coulter-Danner.

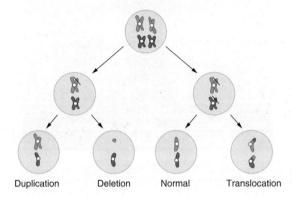

Duplication   Deletion   Normal   Translocation

FIGURE 1-35 Chromosome breaks.

between different chromosomes. In the case of Down syndrome caused by translocation, chromosome 21 fuses and exchanges material with chromosome 14. While most Down syndrome cases are not hereditary, some translocations can be passed on to offspring. Those individuals with a stable translocation can be unaffected yet they can pass down the stable abnormal translocation to an offspring. In an offspring, the once stable translocation can become unstable and cause Down syndrome.

Clinical Manifestations

Clinical manifestations can vary widely and are apparent at birth and often in utero. These manifestations typically include the following characteristics:

- Hypotonia
- Distinctive facial features (e.g., low nasal bridge, epicanthic folds, protruding tongue, low-set ears, and small, open mouth)
- Congenital heart defects
- Single crease on the palm (simian crease)
- White spots on the iris

- Varying intellectual disability that typically worsens with age
- Developmental delay
- Behavioral issues (e.g., inattention, obsessive/compulsive behavior, stubbornness, and tantrums)
- Strabismus and cataracts
- Poorly developed genitalia and delayed puberty

Early death can occur due to cardiac and pulmonary complications (e.g., hypertension and pneumonia). Persons with trisomy 21 have increased susceptibility to leukemia and infections. These individuals are also at increased risk for developing gastrointestinal (e.g., intestinal obstruction, gastroesophageal reflux disease, and celiac disease) and thyroid issues (e.g., hypothyroidism). Approximately half of all persons with trisomy 21 will develop Alzheimer disease, usually starting around the age of 50.

Diagnosis and Treatment

Clinical manifestations can be detected using four-dimensional ultrasounds. Other prenatal testing includes amniocentesis and serum hormone levels. No cure for trisomy 21 exists. Treatment strategies focus on symptom and complication management.

X-Linked Aneuploidy
Turner Syndrome

Monosomy X, or Turner syndrome, is the result of a deletion of part or all of an X chromosome. This abnormality is due to nondisjunction and usually occurs spontaneously (not inherited) during the formation of reproductive cells (eggs and sperm) in the parents. When transmitted, all cells of the child are affected. At times, however, only some of the cells are affected during early fetal division, and other cells have a full two copies of the XX. This event is known as mosaic Turner syndrome. While most cases of Turner syndrome are not inherited, partial X deletions can be inherited. It is not completely understood which genes on the X chromosome are associated with the features of Turner syndrome. This condition occurs in about 1 of every 2,500 live births but is much more common among pregnancies that do not continue to term.

Clinical Manifestations

Turner syndrome affects only females as males cannot live without an X chromosome. Affected females develop gonadal streaks instead of ovaries; therefore, they will not menstruate. A small percentage, however, will retain normal ovarian function. Intelligence is usually normal. Clinical presentation can vary and includes the following:

- Short stature
- Lymphedema (swelling) of the hands and feet
- Broad chest with widely spaced nipples
- Low-set ears
- Small lower jaw
- Drooping eyelids
- Increased weight
- Small fingernails
- Webbing of the neck
- Coarctation of the aorta
- Horseshoe kidney
- Ear infections
- Reduced bone mass

Complications of monosomy X include vision (e.g., cataracts), skeletal (e.g., osteoporosis, pathologic fractures, and scoliosis), hearing, metabolic (e.g., diabetes and thyroid), cardiac (e.g., hypertension and valvular defects), and renal (e.g., kidney failure) issues.

Diagnosis and Treatment

Diagnosis is usually accomplished through a history, physical examination, serum hormone levels, and genetic testing (either before or after birth). Turner syndrome is treated by administering female sex hormones to promote development of secondary sex characteristics and skeletal growth. Growth hormones may also be administered to improve skeletal growth. Identification of this condition is often delayed until late childhood or early adolescence if the clinical presentation is subtle, but chromosomal analysis can confirm the diagnosis. Early treatment allows for early hormone replacement to minimize problems and detect complications.

Klinefelter Syndrome

Polysomy X, or Klinefelter syndrome, is a relatively common abnormality that results from one or more extra X chromosomes and at least one Y. The karyotype would be XXY (trisomy) sex chromosome. Klinefelter syndrome is not inherited and occurs due to spontaneous mutation in reproductive cells due to nondisjunction. If this mutation is passed on, then all of the offspring's cells will be affected. Because of the presence of a Y chromosome, persons with this syndrome are male (**FIGURE 1-36**). Klinefelter

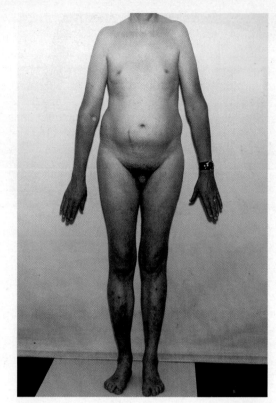

FIGURE 1-36 Klinefelter syndrome.
Courtesy of www.dermnet.com

syndrome affects 1 in 500 to 1,000 newborn males. The syndrome usually becomes apparent at puberty when testicles fail to mature, rendering affected boys infertile. The extra copies of the X chromosome interfere with male sexual development. Health issues worsen with each additional X chromosome (e.g. 48, XXXY or 49, XXXXY).

Clinical Manifestations

Clinical manifestations of Klinefelter syndrome include the following:

- Small penis, prostate gland, and testicles
- Sparse facial and body hair
- Sexual dysfunction (e.g., impotence, decreased libido)
- Gynecomastia (femalelike breasts)
- Long legs with a short, obese trunk
- Tall stature
- Behavioral problems
- Learning disabilities
- Delayed speech and language development
- Increased incidence of pulmonary disease and varicose veins

Other problems that can develop include osteoporosis and breast cancer.

Diagnosis and Treatment

Diagnostic procedures consist of a history, physical examination, hormone levels, and chromosomal testing. Treatment includes male hormone replacement to promote secondary sex characteristics. A mastectomy may be performed in cases of gynecomastia and breast cancer. Psychological counseling and support may be beneficial to the patient and the parents.

Chromosomal Structural Disorders

Chromosomal structural disorders can occur during cellular division and can result in disease. These breaks occur spontaneously or due to environmental factors (e.g., radiation, infections), inherited traits or a combination. The types of breakage are deletions, duplications, translocations (Figure 1-34), inversions, substitution, and fragile sites.

Deletions result in missing a part of genetic material (e.g., multiple myeloma chromosome 13). Duplications result in extra genetic material. With translocations, part of one chromosome exchanges place with another. In chronic myeloid leukemia, a translocation on chromosome 22 and 9 called the *Philadelphia chromosome* (discovered in Philadelphia) is present. With inversions, the chromosome breaks off and reattaches in a different manner (e.g., cancer).

Multifactorial Disorders

Single-gene and chromosomal abnormalities can be devastating but are far less prevalent than multifactorial disorders. Most multifactorial disorders are the result of an interaction between multiple genes (polygenic) and environmental factors. These disorders can be inherited or acquired (e.g., cancers). If inherited, these disorders do not follow a clear-cut pattern of inheritance. Risks of transmission and/or development of the disease are often based on epidemiologic data. These disorders may be present at birth (congenital), as with cleft lip or palate, or they may be expressed later in life, as with hypertension or diabetes. Environmental factors that play roles in these disorders may include any of a number of teratogens (birth defect–causing agents) such as infections, chemicals, or radiation.

Researchers are discovering that most diseases have a multifactorial component. Some diseases have a higher incidence or prevalence and seem to occur more often in some families, certain ethnicities, or geographic regions. With multifactorial disorders, the influences are multiple and may include diet, age, exercise, smoking, and many other lifestyle choices that impact health. Various principles and some common congenital and adult disorders are discussed in the upcoming sections.

When evaluating for multifactorial inherited diseases, ascertaining a history of blood relatives is important. Higher risk for inheriting a disease that is multifactorial include things such as the relationship to the relative. The closer the relationship (e.g., mother, daughter, or siblings), the higher the chance for inheriting the disorder. A high number of members in a family who have the disease can increase the inheritance risk.

Learning Points

Single Nucleotide Polymorphisms and Diseases

The completion of the Human Genome Project (2003) and the International HapMap Project (2005) provided the human genome sequence and map of genetic variation. There is only 0.1% genome sequence variation among people, or, in other words, 99.9% of the genome sequence is identical for all people. The variances in the human genome could account for disease and even more benign differences such as eye and hair color. The site where the variation occurs in a single DNA base pair is known as single nucleotide polymorphism (SNPs or snips). About once for every 1,000 base pairs a SNPs occurs. These human variance points are like genetic markers. The two major completed projects paved the way for the Genome Wide Association Studies (GWAS), which involves a comparison of large groups (e.g., thousands) of people with disease and without disease who are matched for various criteria such as age and sex. The groups' genomes are analyzed to evaluate SNPs. GWAS have found SNPs associated with disease, increased risk of disease, and SNPs that may influence a response to a drug. Most SNPs have no effect on health.

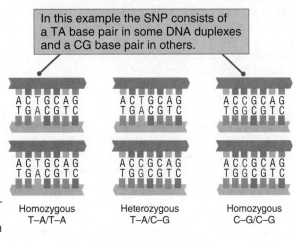

In this example the SNP consists of a TA base pair in some DNA duplexes and a CG base pair in others.

A C T G C A G
T G A C G T C

A C T G C A G
T G A C G T C

Homozygous
T–A/T–A

A C T G C A G
T G A C G T C

A C C G C A G
T G G C G T C

Heterozygous
T–A/C–G

A C C G C A G
T G G C G T C

A C C G C A G
T G G C G T C

Homozygous
C–G/C–G

CHAPTER SUMMARY

Cells are the basic units of life, and they face many challenges in their struggle to survive. These challenges include hypoxia, nutritional changes, infection, inflammation, and chemicals. Cells adapt to the challenges in an attempt to prevent or limit damage as well as death. This adaptation may be reversible or permanent.

Neoplasms arise from abnormal cellular proliferation or differentiation. They can be either benign or malignant. Benign neoplasms are more differentiated; therefore, they are more like the parent cells. Benign tumors are less likely to cause problems in the host or metastasize except in terms of location. Malignant tumors are less differentiated; therefore, they are less like the parent cells. Malignant tumors are more likely to cause problems in the host and metastasize.

Genetic and congenital disorders can develop from factors that disrupt normal fetal development or interact with defective genes. These factors, or teratogens, can include radiation, infections, or chemicals. Genetic and congenital disorders may be present at birth or may not appear until later in life. Many diseases have a genetic basis in their development. New discoveries and information are evolving rapidly regarding the understanding of complex gene–gene interactions, epigenetics, and environmental factors. Exploring these basic cellular and genetic concepts and issues lays the foundation for understanding where disease begins.

REFERENCES AND RESOURCES

AAOS. (2004). *Paramedic: Anatomy and physiology.* Sudbury, MA: Jones and Bartlett Publishers.

Baig, S., Seevasant, I., Mohamad, J., Mukheem, A., Huri, H. Z., & Kamarul, T. (2016). Potential of apoptotic pathway-targeted cancer therapeutic research: Where do we stand? *Cell Death and Disease, 7*(1), e2058. doi:10.1038/cddis.2015.275

Berry, T., & Workman, L. (2011). *Genetics and genomics in nursing and health care.* Philadelphia, PA: F. A. Davis.

Centers for Disease Control and Prevention (CDC). (2016). Leading cause of death. Retrieved from https://www.cdc.gov/nchs/fastats/leading-causes-of-death.htm

Chiras, D. (2015). *Human biology* (8th ed.). Burlington, MA: Jones & Bartlett Learning.

Crowley, L. (2017). *An introduction to human disease: Pathology and pathophysiology correlations* (10th ed.). Burlington, MA: Jones & Bartlett Learning.

Eckschlager, T., Plch, J., Stiborova, M., & Hrabeta, J. (2017). Histone deacetylase inhibitors as anticancer drugs. *International Journal of Molecular Sciences, 18*(7), 1414. doi.org/10.3390/ijms18071414

Elling, B., Elling, K., & Rothenberg, M. (2004). *Anatomy and physiology.* Sudbury, MA: Jones and Bartlett Publishers.

Hartl, D. L. (2020). *Essential genetics and genomics* (7th ed.). Burlington, MA: Jones & Bartlett Learning.

Jacob, M., Varghese, J., & Weil, P. (2018). Cancer: An overview. In V. W. Rodwell, D. A. Bender, K. M. Botham, P. J. Kennelly, & P. Weil (Eds.), *Harper's illustrated biochemistry* (31st ed.). New York, NY: McGraw-Hill.

Lewin, B., Cassimeris, L., Lingappa, V., & Plopper, G. (Eds.). (2007). *Cells.* Sudbury, MA: Jones and Bartlett Publishers.

Mosby's dictionary of medicine, nursing, and health professionals (9th ed.). (2012). St. Louis, MO: Mosby.

Murphy, S. L., Xu, J., Kochanek, K. D., Curtin, S. C., Arias, E., for the Division of Vital Statistics, CDC. (2017). *National vital statistics reports: Deaths, final data for 2015, 66*(6), 1-75.

National Human Genome Research Institute. (n.d.). Frequently asked questions about genetic disorders. Updated November 10, 2015. Retrieved from https://www.genome.gov/19016930/faq-about-genetic-disorders/

National Institutes of Health: National Center for Complementary and Integrative Health. (2013). Antioxidants: In depth. Retrieved from https://nccih.nih.gov/health/antioxidants/introduction.htm

National Institutes of Health: U.S. National Library of Medicine. (2019). What Is DNA? Retrieved from https://www.ghr.nlm.nih.gov

Porth, C. (2014). *Essentials of pathophysiology* (9th ed.). Philadelphia, PA: Lippincott Williams & Wilkins.

Professional guide to pathophysiology (3rd ed.). (2010). Philadelphia, PA: Lippincott Williams & Wilkins.

Schropfer, E., Rauthe, S., & Meyer, T. (2008). Diagnosis and misdiagnosis of necrotizing soft tissue infections: Three case reports. *Cases Journal, 1,* 252.

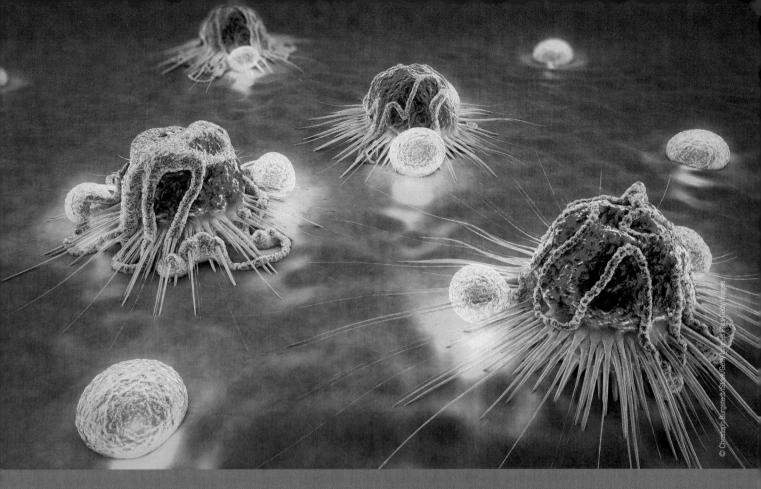

CHAPTER 2
Immunity

LEARNING OBJECTIVES

- Explain the role of the body's normal defenses in preventing disease.
- Describe the similarities and differences between innate and adaptive immunity.
- Discuss the various types of vaccines and their use in different clinical scenarios.
- Compare and contrast the pathogenesis of hypersensitivity by mechanism and antigen.

- Apply understanding of altered immune responses when describing and discussing common disorders such as systemic lupus erythematosus and human immunodeficiency virus (HIV)/acquired immune deficiency syndrome (AIDS).
- Identify factors that enhance and impair the body's defenses.
- Develop diagnostic and treatment considerations for various immune disorders.

The body is under constant assault by life-threatening microbes and environmental toxins. Although the vast majority of microbes and toxins are harmless, occasionally they are not. The immune system is responsible for protecting the body against an array of microorganisms (e.g., bacteria, viruses, fungi, protozoans, and prions) as well as removing damaged cells and destroying cancer cells. The immune system provides this protection through two major actions—defending and attacking. A functioning immune system is essential for survival. Optimal immunity requires intact nonspecific defenses (e.g., skin, mucous membranes, phagocytes, complement systems), a functional lymphatic system, an efficient innate immune response, an operational inflammatory response, and an appropriate and adaptive acquired immunity. Innate immunity provides immediate protection and is nonspecific, meaning it provides protection against all invaders. Adaptive or acquired immunity can take 7–10 days to provide protection, but it is specific to the antigen. Antigens are any substances that the body recognizes as foreign and can include microorganisms, environmental substances, drugs, and transplanted tissues. Fundamental to a properly functioning immune system is the ability to recognize and respond to a foreign agent or antigen. Some immune cells circulate constantly, always on alert for an invasion, whereas others remain passively in tissue and organs, waiting to be activated (**TABLE 2-1**). Additionally, some of the body's structures serve as barriers to antigens, preventing invasion, and some components are designed to manage the degree of the immune response, as an overzealous response can also be deleterious.

TABLE 2-1	Major Components of the Immune System
Antigen	A foreign agent that triggers the production of antibodies by the immune system.
Antibody (immunoglobulin)	A protein used by the immune system to identify and neutralize foreign agents, such as viruses and bacteria.
Autoantibody	An antibody made by the immune system that attacks an individual's own proteins.
Thymus	A gland located in the anterior superior mediastinum; develops T lymphocytes and thymosins.
Lymphatic tissue	Connective tissue containing many lymphocytes; transports immune cells, antigen-presenting cells, fatty acids, and fats; filters body fluids.
Bone marrow	Soft, fatty tissue found inside of bones; contains stem cells and leukocytes.
Cells	
Neutrophils	Infection-fighting agents; usually the first to arrive on the scene of an infection; attracted by various chemicals released by infected tissue; escape from the capillary wall; migrate to the site of infection; and phagocytize microorganisms.
Basophils	White blood cells that bind immunoglobulin E (IgE) and release histamine in specific inflammatory responses (e.g., anaphylaxis).
Eosinophils	White blood cells involved in allergic reactions.
Monocytes	White blood cells that replenish macrophages and dendritic cells in normal states and respond to inflammation by migrating to infected tissue to become macrophages and dendritic cells; their conversion elicits an immune response.
Macrophages	White blood cells within tissues, produced by differentiation of monocytes; phagocytize and stimulate lymphocytes and other immune cells to respond to pathogens.
Mast cells	Connective tissue cells that contain histamine, heparin, hyaluronic acid, slow-reacting substance of anaphylaxis, and serotonin.
B cells (B lymphocytes)	Cells that mature in the bone marrow, where they differentiate into memory cells or immunoglobulin-secreting (antibody) cells, eliminate bacteria, neutralize bacterial toxins, prevent viral reinfection, and produce immediate inflammatory response.
Memory B cells	B cells that stimulate a quick response with subsequent exposures to an antigen; recall of the antigen as foreign leads to rapid antibody production.
Plasma cells	White blood cells that develop from B cells and produce large volumes of specific antibodies.

TABLE 2-1	Major Components of the Immune System
T cells (T lymphocytes)	Produced in the bone marrow and mature in the thymus, hence *T* cell; include two major types that work to destroy antigens—regulator cells and effector cells.
Killer T cells	T cells that destroy cells infected with viruses by releasing lymphokines that degrade cell walls; also called *cytotoxic cells* and *effector cells*.
Helper T cells	Regulator cells that activate, or call up, B cells to produce antibodies.
Natural killer lymphocytes	Cells that destroy cancer cells, foreign cells, and virus-infected cells.

Innate Immunity

Barriers

The first innate or nonspecific approach relies on physical and chemical barriers that indiscriminately protect against all invaders. The most prominent barriers used in this approach are the skin and mucous membranes. The skin is a thick, impermeable layer of epidermal cells overlying a rich vascular layer known as the *dermis*. Newly produced skin cells push the dead ones outward while also removing bacteria. The dead cells produce a protective, waterproof layer because of the keratin contained in those dead cells. Although the skin protects the human body from microbe invasions, some passageways (respiratory, gastrointestinal, and genitourinary tracts) allow direct access to the body's interior. These passageways are lined with a protective mucous membrane that is not as thick as skin but does provide a moderate layer of protection. The epithelial cells are constantly turning over and are thereby preventing microorganisms from residing on the surfaces of these passageways. The passageways have an ability to mechanically wash off their surfaces from microorganisms. Vomiting, as an example, can be an attempt to remove a noxious substance such as a toxin or microorganism from the gastrointestinal tract.

The physical barriers also include chemical barriers to prevent invasion. The skin, for example, produces a slightly acidic substance that inhibits bacterial growth. Hydrochloric acid in the stomach destroys many ingested bacteria. Tears and saliva contain lysozyme, an enzyme that dissolves bacterial cell walls. The epithelial layers also secrete several proteins known as *cathelicidins* and *defensins* that serve as antimicrobials and can stimulate the adaptive immune system.

Even microorganisms participate in innate immunity to benefit humans. The human microbiome consists of bacteria and some fungi (collectively referred to as *normal flora*) which reside on the skin, gastrointestinal, and genitourinary tracts. Normal flora do not usually cause disease unless there is an imbalance or immunocompromise. Microorganisms can contribute to immune defenses by secreting chemicals, blocking pathogenic attachment, and secreting protein molecules. Therefore, the human microbiome is involved in health and disease states. When reviewing results of samples sent for microbial evaluation, consider whether the microbe is part of the normal flora; it can lead to disease even if it is part of normal flora. Review the culture report to determine what is pathogenic and what promotes pathogenicity.

Diagnostic Link

Sample Collection for Infection

Specimen quality to evaluate for infection is critical as improper collection can lead to difficulties in interpretating whether the results are due to contamination, normal residing organisms, or infection. There are three ways to obtain specimens to evaluate for infection: 1) direct sampling, 2) indirect sampling, and 3) microbiota sampling. Direct sampling involves collecting a specimen from sterile tissue such as from the lung or cerebrospinal fluid and is usually done surgically or with a needle aspiration. Direct sampling specimens are the most accurate in diagnosing infection as they usually only contain the pathogen. The technique, however, is invasive and is the riskiest to obtain. The second technique is indirect sampling, which is a local sampling that is normally sterile such as from the lungs (sputum) or the bladder (urine). With indirect sampling the specimen has to go through normal flora to be obtained, so normal flora and contamination may be present and must be considered with interpretation. The third technique is microbiota sampling such as from the throat or vagina, which has normal flora (usually several different) mixed in with pathogens. Since there are usually several normal bacteria, the specimen may require handling with special media. This media is necessary do determine which organisms are nonresident (e.g., beta-hemolytic streptococci in the throat) and which are normal nonpathogenic organisms.

The Human Microbiome

Microbes are all around us. There are 10 times more bacteria in the body than human cells, and 1,000 more genes in the microbiome than in the human genome (NIH Human Microbiome Project, 2016). Usually, microbes have been studied as a specie and in an artificial laboratory environment. The science of metagenomics, however, has transformed the ability to study microbes and understand genomes collected from microbial communities in their natural environment as opposed to in a culture dish. This knowledge has contributed to understanding the critical role of microbes in disease and health leading to exciting information about diagnosis, prevention, and treatment. Key points about the human microbiome include:

- The composition of the microbiome starts prenatally and changes over the years with growth, development, and aging.
- The microbiome each person has is influenced by many other factors, such as genetics, environment, and physiology.
- Alterations in the microbiota have been linked to many diseases of the gastrointestinal system and metabolic functioning as well as neuropsychiatric disorders. Most diseases demonstrate some evidence of microbiota changes, although the meaning of these changes is still unclear.
- Several areas of research continue to explore the causal link, ratio of microbiota (between flora and host) in terms of disease and health, and the implications of a lack of diversity in flora.

The physical and chemical barriers are not completely impenetrable. Tiny breaks in the skin or in the lining of the respiratory, gastrointestinal, or genitourinary tract may permit an antigen invasion. When the barriers are penetrated, blood-borne innate defenses are in place to respond to those antigens through the activation of the inflammatory response.

Inflammatory Response

When cells and body tissues are injured, regardless of the cause (e.g., microorganisms, chemical irritants, immune/genetic defects, hypoxia), a series of reactions referred to as the *inflammatory response* is triggered. As part of the innate immune response, the inflammatory reaction is nondiscriminatory. The same sequence of response occurs no matter the type of injury or prior exposure as there is no memory involved. The acute phase of the inflammatory response starts immediately after the injury and continues until the threat is eliminated (usually hours to days), or a chronic inflammatory response takes over until healing and repair are complete (usually weeks or months). Acute or chronic inflammation leads to local or systemic effects—a common vascular response and the release of a series of cellular and plasma mediators that create and regulate the inflammatory response.

Vascular Response and Cellular Mediators

The acute inflammatory response consists mainly of a vascular response that creates the cardinal signs of erythema, edema, heat, and pain at the site of injury (**FIGURE 2-1**). These clinical manifestations are the result of the release of preformed mediators and the synthesis of new biochemical mediators from mast cell degranulation (**TABLE 2-2**). Mast cells are white blood cells (granulocytes) that are abundantly found in areas exposed to the environment such as the skin, gastrointestinal tract, and respiratory tract and are central to the inflammatory process. The mast cells release several preformed mediators such as histamine, which stimulates vasodilation causing erythema, edema, and heat. Mast cells also cause synthesis of other mediators such as prostaglandins, which stimulate pain receptors in the area. Prostaglandin and another mediator, leukotriene, causes vasodilation and increased vascular permeability. Platelet-activating factor acts similarly to leukotrienes and also activates platelets. While the preformed mediators are released immediately, the newly synthesized mediators start 15 minutes to hours after activation. Several other mediators that continue to contribute to the inflammatory process are released and/or synthesized.

Immediately after an injury, arterioles in the area of injury briefly go into spasm and constrict to limit bleeding and the extent of the injury. The brief vasoconstriction is immediately followed by vasodilation. The vasodilation increases blood flow to the injured area in an attempt to dilute toxins and provide the area with essential immune cells (predominantly neutrophils), nutrients, and oxygen. The vasodilation, however, also increases capillary permeability, leading to edema. As permeability increases, leukocytes line the vessel wall in preparation for migration into the surrounding tissue. While the leukocytes are lining the vessel walls and accumulating (i.e., margination), endothelial cells in the vessel walls react to biochemical mediators that cause these vessels to retract. This retraction gives the leukocytes enough room to migrate (i.e., transmigration) into the interstitial space and begin the cleanup process of phagocytosis, or the engulfing and digestion of foreign substances and cellular debris.

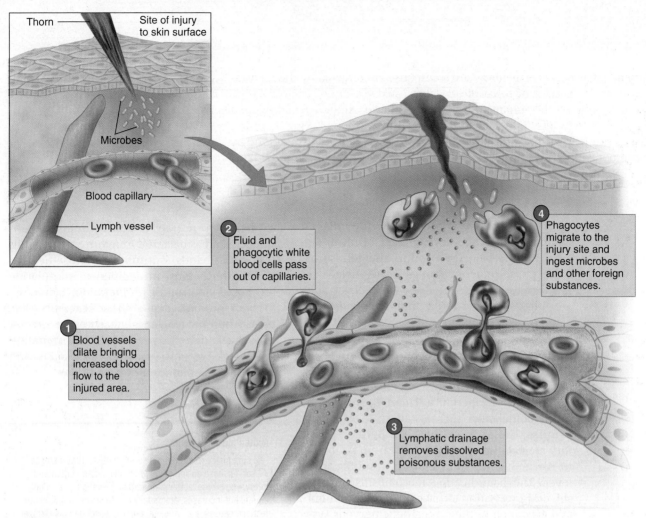

FIGURE 2-1 Inflammatory response.

TABLE 2-2	Mediators From Mast Cell Degranulation

Mediator/category*	Key effect**
Histamine/preformed	H$_1$ receptors—increased vascular permeability, vasodilation, bronchial and smooth muscle contraction H$_2$ receptors—increased vascular permeability, increased gastric secretion
Proteoglycans (heparin and chondroitin sulfate)/preformed	Heparin—anticoagulant, promotes new blood vessel growth (angiogenesis) Chondrotin sulfate—affects kinin pathway. Bradykinin is key component produced and causes vasodilation and works with prostaglandin
Tryptase/preformed	Inactivates fibrinogen and inhibits fibrinogenesis (leads to bleeding); recruits eisonophils; increases interleukin 8 response (i.e., neutrophil chemotactic factor)—attraction of neutrophils, stimulate phagocytosis, promotes angiogenesis
Cytokines and chemokines (e.g., interleukins, tumor necrosis factor-alpha, tumor growth factor-beta)/both	Involved in multiple processes such as B cell proliferation, antibody development, white blood cell recruitment
Leukotrienes/newly synthesized	Bronchoconstriction, increased vascular permeability, and pain in conjunction with prostaglandins
Platelet activating factor/newly synthesized	Attract white blood cells (eosinophils, neutrophils, monocytes, macrophages); bronchoconstriction, increased vascular permeability
Prostaglandins/newly synthesized	Pain, bronchoconstriction, increased vascular permeability, inhibit platelet aggregation, attract neutrophils, and activate eosinophils

*Categories can overlap. ** Key effects—partial list

BOX 2-1 Application to Practice

Various pharmacotherapeutics are used in the treatment of the clinical manifestations of the inflammatory response. Review the following scenario. Describe which mediators and/or components of the inflammatory response are targeted by the medications listed.

Scenario: A 20-year-old woman has asthma. She is taking albuterol by inhaler as needed; fluticasone by inhaler every day; and montelukast orally every day. She states that she notes that her asthma is worse when she exercises so she is prescribed cromolyn inhaled.

The systemic response to the acute inflammation includes the development of fever, elevated white blood cell count, and release of acute phase proteins. Pyrogens are molecules that cause the systemic response of fever and are either endogenous (e.g., interleukin, prostaglandin E_2) or exogenous (e.g., pathogens). Endogenous pyrogens cause fever in response to a pathogen or even in the absence of a pathogen. Pyrogens travel to the hypothalamus, the portion of the brain primarily responsible for controlling body temperature. There, they turn up the hypothalamic "thermostat" in a regulated manner. The body, through its thermoregulatory mechanisms, attempts to heat up the body to reach this new temperature, resulting in a fever. The body-heating mechanisms include shivering, cessation of sweating, vasodilation, and activation of the sympathetic nervous system to increase heat production. Fever is distinguished from other forms of hyperthermia (e.g., heat stroke) because the body temperature increase is regulated and thermoregulatory mechanisms of heating and cooling are functioning. Hyperthermia from heat stroke involves a dysfunctional unregulated increase in temperature along with an inability of the body to cool itself. Fever creates an unpleasant environment for bacterial growth. Mild fevers cause the spleen and liver to remove iron from the blood, which is required by many bacteria to reproduce. Fever increases metabolism, which facilitates healing and accelerates phagocytosis. In addition to the benefits of fever, there can also be deleterious effects such as the denaturation of vital proteins, especially enzymes, needed for biochemical reactions.

During the acute inflammatory process, the complement system and interleukin along with other mediators stimulates the bone marrow to produce more leukocytes, particularly neutrophils. The neutrophils phagocytize, release antimicrobials, and release their nucleus content to form traps to destroy injurious substances such as bacteria. Immature neutrophils (known as bands) outnumber mature neutrophils. Interleukins, in addition to stimulating fever and neutrophil proliferation, cause the liver to produce acute phase reactants. The most common reactants measured in the serum to evaluate the presence of inflammation are C-reactive protein (CRP), fibrinogen, and erythrocyte sedimentation rate (ESR).

Diagnostic Link

Acute Phase Reactants

Acute phase reactants are serum proteins that increase or decrease during acute or chronic inflammation and injury. The ESR reflects inflammation. Elevations, especially significant increases, are usually due to infection, but noninfectious causes (e.g., anemia, renal disease) can also trigger elevations. CRP's normal levels are not known, and formulas can be used to obtain an approximation for men or women based on age. Infections, particularly bacterial, tend to cause moderate to high increases. CRP rises and falls more rapidly than ESR. Fibrinogen, which is a major component of a clot, is elevated during inflammatory states. Acute-phase reactants that decrease are albumin, transferrin, and transthyretin.

Interferons

Interferons are small proteins released from cells infected by viruses (FIGURE 2-2). These molecules diffuse from the site of invasion through the interstitial tissue and bind to receptors on the plasma membranes of uninfected cells. The binding of interferons to uninfected cells triggers the synthesis of enzymes that inhibit viral replication. Consequently, viruses cannot replicate and spread when they enter the previously uninfected cells. Interferons do not protect cells already infected by a virus but rather stop the spread of the virus to new cells. In essence, interferon production is the dying cell's attempt to protect other cells.

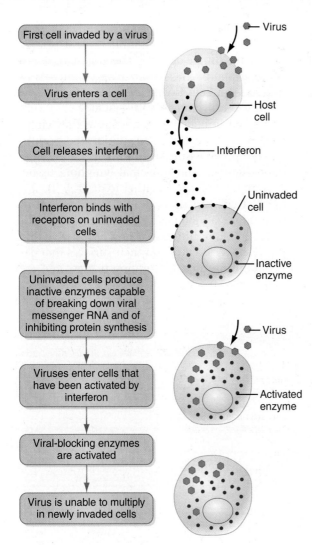

First cell invaded by a virus

↓

Virus enters a cell

↓

Cell releases interferon

↓

Interferon binds with receptors on uninvaded cells

↓

Uninvaded cells produce inactive enzymes capable of breaking down viral messenger RNA and of inhibiting protein synthesis

↓

Viruses enter cells that have been activated by interferon

↓

Viral-blocking enzymes are activated

↓

Virus is unable to multiply in newly invaded cells

Virus — Host cell — Interferon

Uninvaded cell — Inactive enzyme

Virus — Activated enzyme

FIGURE 2-2 How interferon works.

Plasma Protein Mediators

In addition to the cellular mediators, proteins that are part of the inflammatory response are continuously circulating within the plasma. The proteins are part of three systems—complement, clotting, and kinins. The complement system is a process that involves approximately 20 blood plasma proteins and enhances the action of antibodies. Complement proteins circulate in the blood in an inactive state. When foreign substances invade the body, these proteins become activated, and several pathways are taken to enhance pathogen destruction and participate in the inflammatory response. Only a few activities in this complex process are described here.

Five complement system proteins join together to form a large molecule, or membrane attack complex. The membrane attack complex becomes embedded in the plasma membrane of bacteria, creating an opening into which water flows. The influx of water causes the bacterial cells to swell, burst, and die. Other complement proteins stimulate vasodilation in an infected area as a part of the inflammatory response. Some complement proteins increase the permeability of vessels, allowing white blood cells and plasma to pass quickly through them to the infected area. Other complement proteins serve as chemical attractants, drawing macrophages, monocytes, and neutrophils to the infected area where they phagocytize foreign cells. Still other complement proteins bind to microbes, forming a rough coat on the invader that promotes phagocytosis.

The clotting system is activated during infection and injury. Like the complement system, various pathways are taken. The pathways ultimately participate in the inflammatory response by attracting (chemotaxis) neutrophils to the site of injury and causing increased vascular permeability. Part of the clotting system includes the transformation of fibrinogen into fibrin. This fibrin is used to wall off the injured area so that foreign substances are contained. A meshwork of new cells form to provide support for the healing process. Blood clotting begins if blood vessels have been damaged. Kinin system activation primarily leads to the development of bradykinin. Similar to histamine and prostaglandins released from mast cell degranulation, bradykinin causes pain, increased vascular permeability through vasodilation, neutrophil recruitment, and smooth muscle contraction (i.e., bronchoconstriction).

Chronic Phase of the Inflammatory Response

The outcome of the acute inflammatory phase may be resolution or progression to chronic inflammation. The chronic phase can last weeks to months. This phase usually occurs because the acute response was not effective in eliminating or repairing the injury or infection. Under certain circumstances, microorganisms are resistant to phagocytosis or even live within macrophages such as with *Mycobacterium tuberculosis* (tuberculosis) or *Treponema pallidum* (syphilis), and, thereby, there is a minimal acute inflammatory response. Other organisms such as *Corynebacterium diphtheriae*, *Clostridium tetani*, and *Clostridium botulinum* release toxins that remain after their death. The process of chronic inflammation, in contrast to acute inflammation, mainly consists of infiltration with monocyte macrophages and lymphocytes. The neutrophil and monocyte macrophages continue the cleanup. Granulomas, which consist

Complement System

Clotting System

Kinins

of macrophages and lymphocytes, develop in an attempt to separate and contain the infection. Some infectious granulomatous diseases include tuberculosis, syphilis, leprosy, and brucellosis. Syphilis, leprosy, and brucellosis can also survive within macrophages and avoid clearance. Granuloma formation is not to be confused with granulation tissue development which is a step in tissue repair. Granulation tissue is a mixture of new vasculature and fibroblasts, which produces connective tissue fibers and collagen.

Adaptive Immunity

Adaptive or acquired defenses are the body's own individual immune system. These defenses recognize and attack antigens that make it through the innate defenses. Adaptive defense mechanisms are often stimulated and primed during the innate defense. There are two major adaptive approaches—cellular and humoral immunity. Key cells involved in these approaches are the T cells and B cells (**FIGURE 2-3**). T cells and B cells mingle with antigens as they circulate throughout the body's fluids and peripheral lymphoid tissue, such as the tonsils, lymph nodes, spleen, and intestinal lymphoid tissue. This interaction serves either to destroy the antigen (T-cell function or cellular immunity) or to produce antibodies against the antigen (B-cell function or humoral immunity). T cells and B cells have receptors on their surfaces that develop during their maturation process and are prepared to recognize antigens.

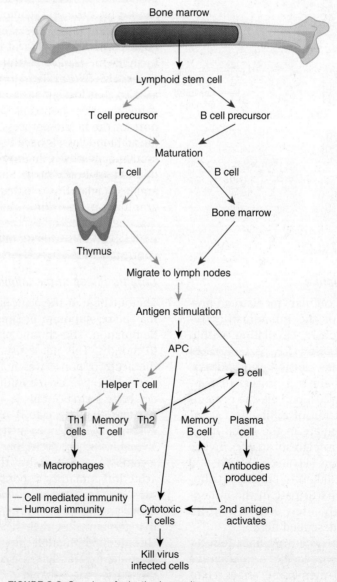

FIGURE 2-3 Overview of adaptive immunity.

Modified from Gould, B. (2014). Pathophysiology for the health professions (5th ed.). Philadelphia, PA: Elsevier. Copyright Elsevier 2015.

Cellular Immunity

Cellular immunity is a defense approach that is mediated by T cells. T cells are produced in the bone marrow, but then they enter the bloodstream and travel to the thymus for maturation, hence the name "T" cells. Two major types of T cells work to destroy antigens: 1) regulator cells, including helper T cells and suppressor T cells; and 2) effector cells, or killer T cells (i.e., cytotoxic cells) (Figure 2-3). Helper cells can further be subdivided into T-helper (Th) 1 and Th 2. The Th 2 cells activate, or call up, B cells to produce antibodies while the Th 1 cells are involved in the inflammatory process and the activation of macrophages. Helper cells secrete a protein termed *CD4+*, which is a major target of the human immunodeficiency virus (HIV).

The second type of regulator cells, suppressor T cells, turn antibody production off. Effector killer cells, or cytotoxic cells, destroy cells infected with viruses by releasing lymphokines that degrade cell walls. Cytotoxic cells are marked by the CD8+ protein on their surface. T cells work to protect the body against viruses, fungi, parasites, intracellular bacteria, and cancer cells. T cells are responsible for hypersensitivity reactions and transplant rejection.

Antigens must be processed and presented to the cell receptor for proper recognition by the T cells. This recognition system is important for the body to distinguish self from nonself. For some antigens, presentation can be accomplished by any cell, but for other antigens to be recognized by T cells, specialized antigen-presenting cells (APCs) are required. The dendritic cells from the bone marrow are important APCs. They are located all over the skin, respiratory system, and gastrointestinal system. Macrophages and B lymphocytes are two other key APCs. The antigen that is in the APC further binds to the major histocompatibility complex (MHC). The MHC encompasses a group of genes involved in immune function. The MHC genes include various cell markers, proteins, and antigens bound to a protein that then presents the antigen to the T cells. In humans, the MHC is called the *human leukocyte antigen* (HLA) system as the genes are expressed on the surface of the white blood cell. The human MHC and human HLA are synonymous. MHC genes are located on chromosome 6, and two different antigens will be on the cell surfaces—class I and II (i.e., regions). Class I cells include HLA-A, HLA-B, and HLA-C and are located on cells throughout. Class II cells are HLA-D, which are mainly in the immune system (B lymphocytes and monocytes), and are expressed on dendritic cells, macrophages, and B cells (all APCs). Class II cells present to the CD4+ helper T cells while class I cells present to the CD8+ suppressor and cytotoxic T cells. The adaptive system is often dependent on APCs. The MHC/HLA system is critical to understanding organ transplantation and the predisposition to diseases (e.g., rheumatoid arthritis, type 1 diabetes mellitus). Antigen recognition and antigen binding triggers a response by other immune cells. Class III region consist of components of the complement system and class IV has other immune genes such as tumor necrosis factors.

Humoral Immunity

B cells mature in the bone marrow where they differentiate into either memory cells or plasma cells, which produce immunoglobulins (Ig; antibodies) (**TABLE 2-3**). These cells eliminate extracellular bacteria, neutralize bacterial toxins, prevent viral reinfection, and produce an immediate inflammatory response. Each B cell has receptor sites for a specific antigen; when it encounters this antigen, the B cell becomes activated and multiplies into either plasma cells or memory cells. The antibody-producing cells produce millions of antibody molecules during their 24-hour life span. B cells can begin this antibody production within 72 hours after initial antigen exposure. Subsequent exposures

TABLE 2-3	Immunoglobulins and Their Functions
IgG	Second response after IgM. Main defense against bacteria and can cross the placenta to protect the fetus against infections, giving it passive immunity. Eventually replaces IgM.
IgM	First Ig formed in response to antigen. Fights blood infections and triggers additional production of IgG. Present in lymphocyte cells and the first antibody made by a developing fetus.
IgA	Found in membranes of the respiratory and gastrointestinal tract, tears, saliva, mucus, and colostrum. Important in local immunity.
IgE	Protects the body through its presence in mucous membranes and skin and is attached to mast cells and basophils. Responds to parasites and triggers allergic reactions.
IgD	Present in blood serum in small amounts and on B-cell surfaces. Receptor for antigens and helps anchor cell membranes.

Modified from Gould, B. (2014). *Pathophysiology for the health professions* (5th ed.). Philadelphia, PA: Elsevier. Copyright Elsevier 2015.

TABLE 2-4	Types of Acquired Immunity		
Type	Mechanism	Memory	Example
Natural active	Pathogens enter the body and cause illness; antibodies form.	Yes	Person has rubella once.
Artificial active	Vaccine (live or attenuated organisms) is injected into the body. No illness results, but antibodies form.	Yes	Person receives measles vaccine.
Natural passive	Antibodies are passed directly from mother to child to provide temporary protection.	No	Passage through placenta during pregnancy; consumption of breastmilk; lasts about 1 year.
Artificial passive	Antibodies are injected into the body (antiserum) to provide temporary protection or to minimize the severity of an infection.	No	Gamma globulin injection to treat immunologic disease, such as idiopathic thrombocytopenia purpura; human immunoglobulin to treat hepatitis A and B.

Acquired (handwritten, left of Natural active row)
Acquired (handwritten, left of Natural passive row)

Modified from Gould, B. (2014). *Pathophysiology for the health professions* (5th ed.). Philadelphia, PA: Elsevier. Copyright Elsevier 2015.

to the antigen then trigger a quick response because memory cells recall the antigen as foreign and antibody production occurs rapidly. This reaction is referred to as acquired immunity (**TABLE 2-4**).

Learning Points

Microorganisms

Viruses: Viruses only survive and multiply by invading host cells, and, therefore, are similar to obligate bacteria. Viruses reside in neurons until they are reactivated. There are debates concerning whether viruses are living creatures or simply molecules. Examples of viruses include herpes simplex 1 (e.g., oral sores).

Bacteria: Bacteria invade the extracellular (EC) or intracellular (IC) environments. EC bacteria cannot survive in the harsh intracellular conditions, and some penetrate tissue while others live on epithelial surfaces secreting toxins. Examples of EC bacteria include *Pseudomonas aeruginosa* (e.g., causes pneumonia, septicemia), *Staphylococcus aureus* (e.g., causes skin infections), *Streptococcus pyogenes* (e.g., causes pharyngitis), and *Haemophilus influenzae* (e.g., causes pneumonia).

IC bacteria can be facultative or obligate. IC bacteria that are facultative invade host cells and have mechanisms to shield themselves from destructive IC lysozymal enzymes and humoral antibodies. Examples of IC facultative bacteria include *Neisseria gonorrhoeae* (e.g., causes sexually transmitted diseases), *Legionella* (e.g., causes pneumonia), and *Mycobacterium* (e.g., causes tuberculosis). IC bacteria that are obligate cannot live on their own and are dependent on the host cell for survival. Examples of IC obligate bacteria include *Chlamydia trachomatis* (e.g., causes sexually transmitted diseases).

Fungi: Fungi cause disease in the form of yeast in humans. An example is *Candida albicans* (e.g., causes oral thrush, vaginal candidiasis).

Protozoa: When they invade human body, they develop a parasitic relationship living off a host. Examples are *Plasmodium* (e.g., causes malaria), *Giardia lamblia* (e.g., causes giardiasis), *Cryptosporidium* (e.g., causes waterborne diseases and diarrhea), *Toxoplasma gondii* (e.g., causes toxoplasmosis).

Diagnostic Link

Evaluating Microorganisms

Laboratory diagnosis of microorganisms is usually accomplished through microscopic direct visualization, culture, antigen–antibody binding, or antigen or antibody detection. Organisms require microscopy in order to be visualized (except for some parasites) and some organisms require staining for identification. Bacteria usually require staining, and the two key types are the gram stain and acid-fast techniques. A culture is another common method of microorganism identification. A culture involves growing the microorganism, usually bacteria, in vitro (i.e., outside the organism). There are various media and techniques used to identify the organism; some of these can be accomplished within a relatively short period (e.g., 2 hours). Antigens bind with antibodies in a specific manner, and antigens and antibodies can be detected because of this binding. When reading a microorganism report, identify what was evaluated and how the evaluation was conducted—determine whether the evaluation was of the antibodies to an antigen (e.g., IgG, IgM for hepatitis), whether the organism was grown (e.g., as a culture for *Streptococcus*), and whether the organism was stained (e.g., acid-fast bacillus for *Myobacterium tuberculosis*).

Diagnostic Link

IgG and IgM

IgM and IgG are often measured to evaluate the immune response to a pathogen or vaccine. IgM is the first to respond and, therefore, rises after exposure. An elevated IgM is generally a marker of acute infection and will decrease with time. IgG, on the other hand, is found throughout the body and responds later than IgM. Elevated IgG is a marker of long-term immunity and will be positive for life after exposure. A way to remember which indicates which is that with IgM, the immune system is creating memory (*M*), and with IgG, the infection is gone (*G*).

Active acquired immunity refers to immunity gained by actively engaging with the antigen—that is, through invasion or vaccination. In active immunity, the body makes antibodies, and protection is usually long term. Examples of active immunity include getting a varicella infection (chickenpox), and not getting the disease again or when a person receives the varicella vaccine and never gets varicella.

Passive acquired immunity refers to immunity gained by receiving antibodies made outside the body by another person, animal, or recombinant DNA. In passive immunity, the person is not actively producing antibodies and protection is short lived. Examples of passive immunity include mother-to-fetus transfer through the placenta and breastfeeding transference of antibodies. Exposure to rabies infection is often treated with a combination of immunoglobulin (passive) and a killed form of the virus (active).

The adaptive defenses change naturally with aging. These changes make older adults and the elderly more susceptible to developing infections and having worse outcomes. Diseases such as diabetes or heart failure, which are more prevalent with aging, further contribute to immune dysfunction because they directly impair aspects of the immune system or deplete the body's reserves. The deterioration of the immune system as a result of aging is termed *immune senescence*. These changes include a reduced production of T cells and B cells and altered functioning of mature lymphocytes. Hematopoietic stem cells that differentiate into lymphocytes are fewer. B cells and T cells proliferate less and apoptosis rates are higher. The thymus gland involutes affecting T-cell maturation. Beneficial cytokine production decreases. B cells have a decreased capacity to produce immunoglobulins. More immune complexes and autoantibodies are present.

Other age-related adaptive immune system differences are evident in newborns who are also more susceptible to infections while their immune systems mature. Normal term newborns have maternal antibodies, specifically IgG. Around 3 months, the maternal IgG drops, and the infant continues producing its own IgG. However, levels are remain low until about 6 months when newborn production becomes adequate. During this 3–6 months the infant is said to have a benign, physiologic hypogammaglobulinemia. T cells are not transferred from mother to newborn; however,

the newborn produces T cells. Newborn T-cell function is limited; therefore, newborns are susceptible to infections.

Vaccines

While getting an infection is the best way to get lifelong immunity against a pathogen, the outcome of an infection may be too risky, causing significant morbidity and even death. Vaccines were developed to stimulate the immune system to provide protection against infection and avoid the consequences of getting an infection. Vaccination response is influenced by 1) antigen characteristic and dose, 2) administration route (e.g., inhaled, oral), and 3) adjuvants added to enhance and modulate response (e.g., aluminum-based material, oil-in-water emulsions). Vaccines fall into two categories— 1) live, attenuated and 2) inactivated. **Live, attenuated** vaccines are created from weakened wild viruses or bacteria that can replicate without causing diseases. Live, attenuated vaccines create an almost identical immune response as active infection. Some examples of live viral vaccines include paramyxovirus (mumps), rubella (German measles), varicella-zoster (chickenpox), and live bacterial vaccines include *Salmonella* serotype typhi (typhoid) and bacillus Calmette-Guérin (tuberculosis). Live vaccines tend to give longer immune protection; however, oral versions of live vaccines may not give as long-term protection as parenteral versions. Some people do not respond to one dose of a live vaccine, so multiple doses need to be given (e.g., measles, mumps, rubella). Live, attenuated vaccines can cause infections and are contraindicated in those who are immunocompromised. Live vaccines are fragile and must be protected from heat and light and stored properly.

Inactivated vaccines are made from whole or fractions of viruses or bacterial antigen or the toxin produced by the bacteria. The response stimulated is mainly humoral with little or no stimulation of cellular immunity. The organisms with inactivated vaccines do not replicate, and multiple doses and boosters are usually necessary. Whole virus vaccine examples include polio, rabies, and hepatitis A. Whole inactivated bacterial vaccines (e.g., cholera, plague, typhoid) are not available in the United States.

Fractional vaccines are either toxoid or subunit. There are three types of subunits— protein based, polysaccharide, and conjugate based. Toxoids, like one of the subunits, are protein-based vaccines (e.g., diphtheria and tetanus), and these are made by modifying the toxins produced by some bacteria; the modification does not cause disease. Subunit fractional vaccines are made from the antigenic part of a pathogen (purified antigen) as opposed to the whole pathogen that has been killed. Subunits can be protein based by using a protein component to present the antigen (e.g., acellular pertussis, hepatitis B). Other subunits are only made from the polysaccharide wall that surrounds some bacteria (e.g., pneumococcus, meningococcal bacteria). The third type of fractional subunit vaccine are those made by conjugating a piece of the polysaccharide wall with a protein carrier (e.g., *Haemophilus influenzae* type b, meningococcal vaccine, or pneumococcal vaccine). The pure, polysaccharide (i.e., carbohydrate) -only based vaccines tend to be less effective than live vaccines or inactivated vaccines with a protein base. Additionally, the polysaccharide vaccines are often not very immunogenic. Children younger than 2 years do not respond consistently to these types of vaccines due to their immature immune systems, and these vaccines are, therefore, not effective or recommended in the young. An example is the pneumococcal polysaccharide vaccine 23, which is recommended after the age of 2. The antibody produced with polysaccharides is mainly IgM, which does not confer long-term protection. Inactivated vaccines do not cause disease from infection even in immunocompromised people.

Recombinant vaccines are those developed through genetic engineering technology and can include the use of the pathogen's DNA, genetic medication of a pathogen, and a viral vector which is a virus that has been modified to insert genetic material into cells. Examples of recombinant vaccines include hepatitis B, human papillomavirus, and some influenza. Vaccine development and technology is rapidly changing, and the most up-to-date information and recommendations can be accessed at www.cdc.gov/vaccines.

Altered Immune Response

A malfunction at any point in any of the numerous and highly complex immune responses can create a pathologic state. Malfunctions may include exaggeration (hypersensitivity), failure of self-recognition (autoimmunity), or diminution (immunodeficiency).

Hypersensitivity

Hypersensitivity is an inflated or inappropriate response to an antigen. The result is inflammation and destruction of healthy tissue. Hypersensitivity reactions may be immediate, occurring within minutes to hours of reexposure to the antigen, or delayed, occurring several hours after reexposure. Hypersensitivity reactions can be categorized by the disease mechanism, of which there are four types—type I (IgE mediated), type II (tissue specific), type III (immune complex–mediated), and type IV (cell mediated) (**TABLE 2-5**). Hypersensitivity reactions can also be categorized by the type of antigen the immune system is responding to, such as self-antigens (autoimmunity), antigens from another person (alloimmunity), or environmental antigens (allergy). When a hypersensitivity reaction occurs, more than one mechanism can contribute. Hypersensitivity reactions can cause a localized or widespread response.

Hypersensitivity by Mechanism
Type I Hypersensitivity

With type I hypersensitivity (**FIGURE 2-4**), allergens activate T cells (usually helper cells), which bind to mast cells. These T cells stimulate B cells to produce IgE antibodies specific to the antigen, which are commonly environmental. A reaction to an environmental antigen is termed *allergy*. The difference between a normal immune response and a type I hypersensitivity response is that the antibody produced is IgE instead of IgA, IgG, or IgM. The IgE coats the mast cells and basophils, making them sensitive to the allergen. At the next exposure to the same antigen, the antigen binds with the surface IgE. The binding of the antigen with the IgE causes mast cell degranulation and mediator (e.g., histamines, cytokines, and prostaglandins) release. The degranulation and mediator release further activates the inflammatory process, attracting neutrophils and eosinophils and triggering the complement system. Histamine is the mediator causing many symptoms. The effects of type I reactions include immediate inflammation and pruritus. Repeated exposure to relatively large doses of the allergens is usually necessary to cause this response. The reaction can be localized as occurs in asthma, allergic rhinitis, and food allergies. See chapter 5.

Widespread, immediate systemic reactions resulting from sudden release of mast cell and

TABLE 2-5 Overview of the Hypersensitivity Reactions

Hypersensitivity type	Origin of hypersensitivity	Antibody involved	Cells involved	Mediators involved	Evidence of hypersensitivity	Examples
Type I IgE mediated	B lymphocytes	IgE	Mast cells, basophils	Histamine, serotonin, leukotrienes, prostaglandins	Immediate (30 minutes or less); or delayed (e.g., hours)	Allergic rhinitis; systemic anaphylaxis; asthma
Type II cytotoxic	B lymphocytes	IgG, IgM	RBCs, WBCs	Complement	5–8 hours	Transfusion reactions; hemolytic disease of newborns
Type III immune complex	B lymphocytes	IgG	Host tissue cells	Complement	2–8 hours	Serum sickness; Arthus phenomenon; SLE; rheumatic fever; rheumatoid arthritis
Type IV cellular	T lymphocytes	None	Host tissue cells	Cytokines	1–3 days	Contact dermatitis; infection; Crohn disease

RBCs, red blood cells. WBCs, white blood cells. SLE, systemic lupus erythematosus.

Reproduced from Story, L. (2017). *Pathophysiology: A Practical Approach* (3rd ed.). Burlington, MA: Jones & Bartlett Learning.

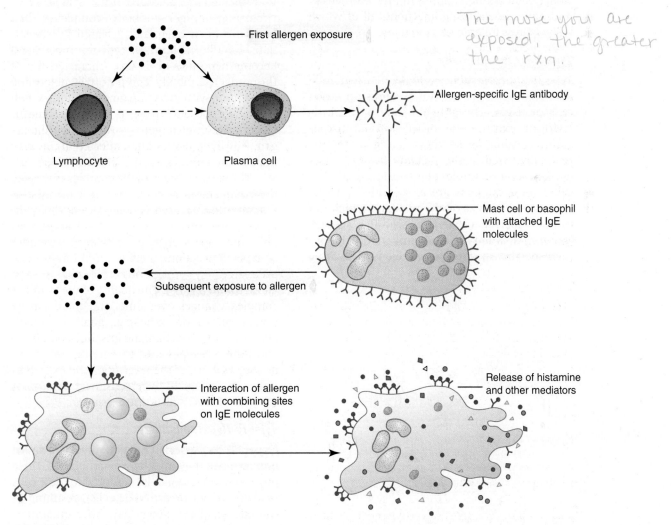

The more you are exposed, the greater the rxn.

FIGURE 2-4 Pathogenesis of an allergy.

basophil mediator release is termed *anaphylaxis*. Anaphylaxis is usually the result of an IgE event, but IgG and immune complex/complement reactions may also occur. These three types of reactions are termed *immunologic anaphylaxis*. Mast cells and basophils may be activated without IgE, IgG, or immune complexes and the reaction is termed *nonimmunologic anaphylaxis* (formerly *anaphylactoid*). Examples of nonimmunologic reactions are red man syndrome, caused by vancomycin administration or erythema; pruritus; and edema with exposure to cold (cold urticaria). Clinically, the underlying immune event in anaphylaxis is often difficult to determine. While most environmental allergies are type I IgE mediated, some are type II and type III, such as when gluten from wheat causes gastrointestinal symptoms (e.g., celiac disease) with a penicillin allergy. Poison ivy, although an environmental allergen, causes a type IV hypersensitivity (see Table 2-5). Treatment of type I reactions may include epinephrine, antihistamines, corticosteroids, and desensitizing injections, all of which will suppress inflammatory activity.

Type II Hypersensitivity

Type II hypersensitivity (FIGURE 2-5) generally involves the destruction of antigens on target cells or tissue. The antigens may be intrinsic (self) or extrinsic (absorbed through exposure). The human leukocyte antigens (MHC/HLA) discussed in the *Adaptive Immunity* section are some examples of intrinsic antigens on cells. Some antigens are also located on certain tissues, such as on the prostate, which has prostate-specific antigen. In type II reactions, IgG or IgM antibodies bind with an individual's own specific cell or tissue antigens, activating

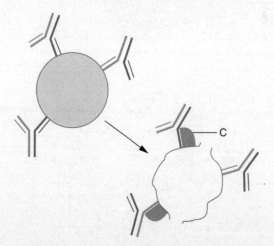

FIGURE 2-5 Type II hypersensitivity reaction with lysis of red blood cells. Antibody reacts with cell surface antigens, resulting in complement fixation (c) and cell lysis.

the complement system. The end result is destruction or a malfunctioning cell. Recognition of these cells by macrophages triggers antibody production. Type II hypersensitivity mechanisms include complement activation, leading to cell lysis, phagocytosis, and neutrophil or cytotoxic (natural killer) cells destroying the targets. Another type II mechanism involves an antibody binding with a cell surface receptor and blocking the action of this receptor. Examples of type II reactions include blood transfusion reactions and erythroblastosis fetalis. Treatment for these two reactions focuses on prevention and includes ensuring blood compatibility prior to transfusions, administering medication to suppress immune activity (e.g., corticosteroids and cyclosporine), and preventing maternal antibody development (e.g., $Rh_o[D]$ with immune globulin [RhoGAM]).

Type III Hypersensitivity

In **type III hypersensitivity** (FIGURE 2-6), circulating antigen-antibody complexes that have not been adequately cleared by the innate blood-borne immune cells accumulate and become deposited in tissues. Characteristics of the antigen-antibody complex will determine where and with what tissue the complex will bind. As opposed to type II reactions, type III reactions are not targeted toward a specific organ. However, tissues often affected in this way include the kidneys, joints, skin, and blood vessels. The accumulation of the complexes triggers the complement system, causing local inflammation and increased vascular permeability; in turn, more complexes accumulate as neutrophils and macrophages are activated. Examples of type III reactions include autoimmune disorders (e.g., systemic lupus erythematosus and glomerulonephritis). The quality of the immune complex changes over time, and there can be several types at one time (e.g., small, intermediate, or large). The changing immune complexes and different types lead to varying symptomatology and causes the remissions and exacerbations seen in type III hypersensitivity. Treatment for type III reactions is disease specific.

Type IV Hypersensitivity

Type IV hypersensitivity involves a delayed processing of the antigen by macrophages. Once processed, the antigen is presented to the T cells (usually helper or cytotoxic cells), resulting in the release of cytokines that cause inflammation and antigen destruction. As opposed to the other types of hypersensitivity, type IV is not

Blood vessel wall

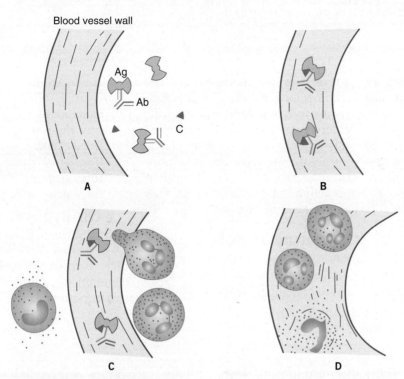

FIGURE 2-6 Type III allergic hypersensitivity reaction. **A.** Antigen (Ag) and antibody (Ab) form complexes in the presence of excesss antigen **B.** The complexes are deposited in the vessel wall and fix complement (c). **C.** Activated components of complement cause release of vasoactive materials from mast cells and chemotaxis of polymorphonuclear leukocytes. **D.** The end result is acute inflammation and destruction of the vessel wall.

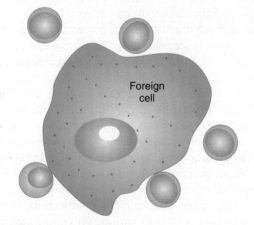

FIGURE 2-7 Sensitized T lymphocytes attach foreign cells."

antibody mediated (**FIGURE 2-7**). These reactions can cause severe tissue injury and fibrosis. Examples of type IV reactions include tuberculin skin testing, transplant reactions, and contact dermatitis from poison ivy. Treatment for type IV reactions is disease specific.

Hypersensitivity by Antigen
Alloimmunity

The immune system's protective nature presents challenges for patients who require tissue and organ transplants and blood transfusions. Ensuring the best possible tissue match is critical for transplant success. Four types of tissue transplants are possible—allogeneic, syngeneic, autologous, and xenogenic. Allogeneic transplants are those in which the tissue used is from the same species and is of similar tissue type, but it is not identical. Most transplants use allogeneic tissue. Syngeneic transplants use tissue from the identical twin of the host. With autologous transplants, the host and the donor are the same person. An example of this type of transplant is someone storing up his or her own blood prior to a scheduled surgery. Xenogenic transplants use tissue from another species. An example of this type of transplant is the use of pig heart valves to replace diseased valves in a human. Donors may be live or a cadaver, but no matter the source used, making a close tissue match is fundamental to preventing rejection.

In organ transplantation, the immune system of the host targets the major histocompatibility complex on donor cell surfaces (see the *Cellular Immunity* section). The T cells are activated, cytotoxic cells begin destruction, and T cells facilitate B cell antibody production.

Rejection reactions are classified based on their timing. Hyperacute tissue rejections occur

BOX 2-2 Application to Practice

Case 1: A 20-year-old woman comes in concerned that she has genital herpes as she has been having unprotected sex. She does not have any lesions but wants to be tested. An antibody test is done and the results revealed the following:

HSV 1 IgG type-specific antibody: < 0.90 (negative)
HSV 2 IgG type specific antibody: > 1.10 (positive)

How would you explain these results to her? Can you tell if this is a recent or past infection? Can you tell how long ago she was infected?

Case 2: A patient arrives in the emergency department with possible anaphylaxis. An epinephrine intramuscular injection is administered. Describe the therapeutic actions of epinephrine as they apply to immune alterations in anaphylaxis.

Activity 1: There are many kinds of fungal infections. Describe the location and most common organism for the following diagnoses:

Vulvovaginitis
Balanitis
Balanoposthitis
Onychomycosis
Tinea capitis
Tinea cruris
Tinea corporis
Tinea pedis

Activity 2: What are the differences between gram-negative and gram-positive bacteria? Which are more pathogenic? List examples of common organisms that are negative or positive.

---

immediately to 3 days after the transplant. Such reactions occur due to a complement response in which the recipient has antibodies against the donor tissue. This complement response triggers a systemic inflammatory reaction. The response is so quick that often the new tissue has not had a chance to establish vascularization; as a result, the tissue becomes permanently necrotic.

Acute tissue rejections are the most common and treatable type of rejection. These reactions usually occur between 4 days and 3 months following the transplant. Acute reactions are cell mediated with mainly Th 1 cells producing interleukin 2 and interferon gamma, causing macrophage stimulation and resulting in transplant cell destruction (lyses) or necrosis. The patient exhibits manifestations of the inflammatory process including fever, redness, swelling, and tenderness at the graft site. Additionally, the patient may experience impaired functioning of the transplanted organ.

Chronic tissue rejection occurs from about 4 months to years after the transplant. This reaction is most likely due to an antibody-mediated immune response. Antibodies and complement molecules become deposited in the transplanted tissue vessel walls, resulting in decreased blood flow and ischemia.

Most rejection reactions are classified as host-versus-graft rejection; in other words, the host is fighting the graft. The graft fights the host in another type of reaction, known as *graft-versus-host rejection*. This potentially life-threatening type of reaction occurs with bone marrow or stem cell transplants. The immunocompetent graft cells recognize the host cells as foreign due to the host having antigens that are not on the graft and organize a cell-mediated (primarily T-cell) attack. The host is usually immunocompromised and unable to fight the graft cells' actions.

Identifying the rejection reaction quickly is crucial to reversing it. Assessment including manifestations of a healthy and unhealthy transplant organ is paramount. For example, decreased urine output may indicate a failing kidney transplant. Diagnostic procedures include laboratory tests to identify immune and inflammatory activity (e.g., white blood count and erythrocyte sedimentary rate) and specific tests to determine functioning of the transplanted organ (e.g., renal panel and urinalysis).

Treatment for transplant rejection usually begins with prevention. Prevention starts with ensuring a tissue match and initiating immunosuppressive therapy (e.g., corticosteroids and cyclosporine). The transplant patient will likely require immunosuppressive therapy for life. Once a rejection is suspected, immunosuppression therapy is intensified to reverse it.

Autoimmunity

More than 80 diseases are classified as autoimmune disorders. Some common disorders are systemic lupus erythematosus, inflammatory bowel disease (i.e., Crohn disease and ulcerative colitis), type 1 diabetes mellitus, and rheumatoid arthritis. In autoimmune diseases, the body's normal defenses become self-destructive—that is, they fail to identify self-antigens within the host from nonself foreign antigens. Under normal circumstances, the immune system has the capacity to tolerate self-antigens and regulate them to avoid a maladaptive immune response. These mechanisms are central and peripheral tolerance. Central tolerance occurs in primary lymphoid tissue (e.g., thymus for T cells and bone marrow for B cells) when lymphocytes are maturing. With central tolerance, B or T cells that are autoreactive (bind to self) are destroyed or suppressed. In the secondary lymphoid tissue (e.g., lymph nodes, spleen) where B and T cells migrate, peripheral tolerance and self-antigens are simply not recognized. With a healthy immune system, self-recognition and tolerance are important mechanisms in shaping the adaptive immune system and maintainence as apoptotic cells and tissue debris needs to be removed. In addition to tolerance, self-antigens are often sequestered, and the immune system has regulatory mechanisms (e.g., B and T cells, cytokines) that limit the degree of immune reactivity.

Autoimmune disease can occur when things go wrong with tolerance, sequestration, and regulatory mechanisms. Reasons for tolerance failure and a misdirected response are unclear. However, an exogenous trigger and endogenous abnormalities (e.g., viral, genetic, medicinal, hormonal, environmental) with multiple mechanisms likely contribute to autoimmune disease development. The exogenous trigger may cause autoimmunity when the antigen (e.g., pathogen) looks like an antigen already present (a process called *molecular mimicry*). The immune system attacks the foreign antigen as well as the self-antigen because they look so similar. Some antigens such as viruses or bacteria act as superantigens and have the ability to bind to T cells that are nonspecific and mount an immune response. Some antigens modify the immune response (e.g., adjuvant effect) by increasing the immunogenicity (provoking immune response).

Several endogenous abnormalities can contribute to autoimmunity and can include abnormal antigen presentation. The immune system may have problems clearing cellular debris such as apoptotic cells. Other endogenous abnormalities include B cells and T cells responding inappropriately to signals or defects in autoantibody production. Imbalances in cytokines, such as tumor necrosis factor and interleukin, can derail the immune system.

Autoimmune disorders affect women more often than men, pointing to a possible hormonal influence in autoimmune development. Many autoimmune diseases can have family tendencies, pointing to genetic influences. Inheriting a gene can lead to susceptibility for acquiring a disease. The susceptibility, coupled with other factors such as an infection or other environmental stimuli, can lead to autoimmune disorders. Some gene polymorphisms lead to several autoimmune disorders, while other gene mutations are only associated with one condition. Autoimmune disorders are more prevalent with aging as self-recognition regulatory systems become less effective.

In autoimmune disorder, there are two key ways the immune system attacks itself: by autoantibody or T-cell mechanisms. Some autoantibodies can mark an antigen for phagocytosis. This marking, called *opsonization*, occurs in diseases such as autoimmune thrombocytopenic purpura or hemolytic anemia. Autoantibodies can block receptors. As an example, autoantibodies can block insulin receptors, which leads to insulin-resistant diabetes mellitus. In Graves disease, an autoimmune hyperthyroid disorder, the autoantibodies-thyrotropin receptor antibodies (TRAb) which are also known as thyroid-stimulating immunoglobulins bind to thyrotropin receptors, leading to excess thyroid hormone production (thyroxine/T4 and triiodothyronine/T3).

Characteristics of autoimmune diseases can affect any tissue or organ in the body, such as the thyroid in Hashimoto thyroiditis, as well as multiple systems, such as rheumatoid arthritis. At times, having one autoimmune disorder can predispose or lead to the development of another. Some autoimmune disorders have the presence of multiple autoantibodies that do not cause pathology. An example is in myasthenia gravis, where rheumatoid factor or antithyroid antibodies are present yet cause no pathology. Autoimmune disorders are characterized by frequent progressive periods of exacerbations (worsening of symptoms) and remissions (easing of symptoms). Physical and emotional stressors frequently trigger exacerbations. Exacerbations are common, particularly in autoimmune disorders such as systemic lupus erythematosus and rheumatoid arthritis.

Because of the somewhat mysterious nature of autoimmune disorders, diagnostic procedures often begin by eliminating all other causes. In general, diagnostic tests such as laboratory autoimmune antibody tests can be difficult to interpret. There are laboratory tests that are specific to the suspected autoimmune disorder (e.g., rheumatoid factor for rheumatoid arthritis), but these tests, as seen in the myasthenia gravis example, are not always specific. Treatment for autoimmune disorders is disease specific. Systemic lupus erythematosus is one of the most common autoimmune disorders and will be discussed in the next section while other autoimmune disorders will be discussed in the appropriate system chapter (e.g., autoimmune thyroiditis in chapter 10).

Systemic Lupus Erythematosus

Systemic lupus erythematosus (SLE) is a chronic, inflammatory, autoimmune disorder that can affect any connective tissue. SLE occurs more often in women than in men. In adults, the female-to-male ratio can range from 7:1 to 15:1. SLE is more common in Asians, Blacks, and Hispanic Americans in comparison to Whites. The incidence has increased dramatically due to improved diagnostic testing. Disease onset in 65% of cases is between the ages of 16 and 55. The disease is different in terms of ethnicity, gender, and age of onset. Men, for example, have a lower incidence but worse outcome. Manifestations are also different in men, who have a higher incidence of renal disease and hypertension, in comparison to women, who have a higher incidence of Raynaud phenomenon.

Other examples of variances include worse renal outcomes for Black and Hispanic Americans and worse symptomatology in children.

Genetic alterations, such as the presence of susceptibility genes and absence of protective genes, predispose to the development of SLE, and SLE development is more likely when coupled with epigenetic influences. The higher incidence in women is attributed to X chromosome issues and to the effects of estrogen, progesterone, and prolactin on the immune system. Most of the hormonal effects can lead to heightened immune response and autoantibody production.

In SLE, B cells are thought to be activated and autoantibodies will bind with autoantigens (e.g., antinuclear antibodies) and form immune complexes. These immune complexes fight against the body's own tissues, such as nucleic acids, red blood cells, platelets, and lymphocytes. Hyperactive helper T cells and subdued suppressor T cells are thought to create a prime environment for B cells to overproduce.

Clinical Manifestations

Usually the symptoms a person has at the beginning of the disease or within the first few years remain throughout the course of their disease. SLE is an unpredictable disorder but most often affects the heart, joints, skin, lungs, blood vessels, liver, kidneys, hematologic function, and nervous system (**TABLE 2-6**).

TABLE 2-6	Common Manifestations of Systemic Lupus Erythematosus
Systemic	**Fatigue**, **fever**, weight change (usually loss)
Musculoskeletal	Myalgia, **polyarthritis** (migratory, symmetrical) with swollen and painful joints, without damage; **arthralgia**
Skin	**Butterfly rash** with erythema on cheeks and over nose, or rash on body; photosensitivity— exacerbation with sun exposure; usually painless ulcerations in oral mucosa; hair loss
Kidneys	**Glomerulonephritis** with antigen–antibody deposits in glomerulus, causing inflammation with marked proteinuria and progressive renal damage, nephrotic syndrome
Lungs	Pleurisy—inflammation of the pleural membranes, causing chest pain
Heart	Carditis—inflammation of any layer of the heart, commonly pericarditis
Blood vessels	Raynaud phenomenon—periodic vasospasms in fingers and toes, accompanied by pain and vasculitis throughout (e.g., skin lesions, hepatic, coronary)
Central nervous system	Psychoses, depression, mood changes, seizures
Hematologic	Anemia of chronic disease, leukopenia, thrombocytopenia, lymphadenopathy, splenomegaly, thrombus (venous or arterial)

In bold: greater than 35% incidence at onset.

Diagnosis and Treatment

[handwritten: order ANA test if (+) do reflex helps to determine etiology]

Because patients with SLE can have a wide variety of symptoms and different combinations of organ involvement, diagnosis can be challenging. Clinical criteria have been developed to improve diagnostic accuracy. These criteria continue to evolve in attempts to get a universal consensus. Some patients suspected of having SLE may never develop enough of the criteria to qualify for a definite diagnosis; other patients accumulate enough criteria to merit SLE diagnosis only after months or years. When a person has four or more of the criteria, the diagnosis of SLE is strongly suggested. When evaluating a patient, these criteria can be used in patients presenting with common SLE symptoms (Table 2-6) although some are vague (e.g., fatigue, fever) and can be present in many other disorders.

Clinical Criteria for SLE Diagnosis

[handwritten mark: ✳]

Skin: Acute/subacute cutaneous—Malar rash ("butterfly" rash over the cheeks of the face), photosensitivity; Chronic cutaneous lesions—(e.g., discoid lupus—rough, scaly, raised, red circular)

Oral ulcers—look like aphthous ulcer (i.e. cold sore) but can also be in nose

Alopecia—usually patchy

Synovitis—joint inflammation causes pain, swelling usually symmetrical, two or more joints and can migrate

Serositis (inflammation of the serous membranes that line the lungs [pleura], heart [pericardium], and inner abdomen [peritoneum])

Hemolytic anemia

Leukopenia ($< 4,000/mm^3$)

Lymphocytopenia ($< 1,000/mm^3$)

Thrombocytopenia ($100,000/mm^3$)

Neurologic disorder (e.g., brain irritation manifested as seizures or psychosis)

Renal: RBC casts, Proteinuria (>0.5 g/24 hours), Positive biopsy (nephritis), even if no other criteria is present

RBC casts

Protein/creatinine (> 0.5)

Positive biopsy, even if no other criteria is present

In children and older adults, some clinical manifestations will vary. The diagnosis is usually made after the age of 5 years but is often present after the age of 10. While children can have the same clinical manifestations as adults, they most often present with fever, malaise, weight loss, small-joint arthritis, and renal disease. Additionally, their symptoms are usually more severe. Older adults usually have a milder presentation with higher incidence of sicca (e.g., dry eyes, dry mouth), serositis, and lung and musculoskeletal manifestations.

In addition to the common presentation and criteria, other tests can be helpful in evaluating patients for SLE. Routine laboratory tests would include a complete blood count and differential to evaluate for anemia and white blood cell and platelet abnormalities. A chemistry profile can evaluate renal function. A urinalysis may reveal casts and proteinuria. Immunologic tests for autoantibodies—of which at least one needs to be positive for diagnosis—will include testing for antinuclear antibodies, which is usually positive in most people with SLE; antibodies that are specific to SLE including anti–double-stranded DNA; and anti-Smith antibodies, which are very specific. Antiphospholipid antibodies are not unique to SLE, but it is one of the criteria. Low C3 and C4 complement levels (proteins that promote immune and inflammatory response) or a complete complement test (CH50), which checks all complements 1–9, can be done. A positive direct Coombs (measure of antibody bound to RBCs) test also can count as one criterion. Other appropriate testing procedures, such as liver function tests and echocardiography are selected for the patient on an individual basis. Tissue biopsies may also be necessary (e.g., of the skin and kidneys).

[handwritten margin: Diagnostic testing]

Treatment of SLE is directed at symptom management. General strategies include stress reduction, exercise, and sleep. Medications include nonsteroidal anti-inflammatory drugs (NSAIDs) to reduce pain and inflammation in joints, muscles, and other tissues. Corticosteroids may also be used to treat SLE. Corticosteroids are more potent than NSAIDs in reducing inflammation and restoring function when the disease is active and particularly when internal organs are affected. Corticosteroids, however, have multiple side effects (e.g., weight gain, risk for infection, hyperglycemia, and high blood pressure) that must be considered. Biologic disease-modifying antirheumatic drugs reduce pain and tissue damage as a result of inflammation. These drugs are more potent than NSAIDs and corticosteroids, but they carry significantly more risks, such as the risk for infection or organ damage. As the disease progresses, use of these agents may be necessary to prevent severe complications of SLE. Antimalarial drugs can treat fatigue, joint pain, rashes, and pleural inflammation by suppressing the immune system. Immunosuppressants may be used for patients with kidney and nervous system involvement. Additionally, plasmapheresis can remove antibodies and other immune substances from the blood to suppress immunity.

Immunodeficiency

A diminished or absent immune response increases susceptibility to infections. Immunodeficiencies may be primary (reflecting a defect with the immune system) or secondary (reflecting an underlying disease or factor that is suppressing the immune system). Primary deficits involve basic developmental failures, many of which result from genetic or congenital abnormalities (e.g., hypogammaglobulinemia). Secondary or acquired immunodeficiency refers to a loss of immune function because of a specific cause; such causes may include infection, splenectomy, malnutrition, hepatic disease, drug therapy, or stress. The problem may be either acute or chronic. The most common forms of immunodeficiency are caused by viral infections or are iatrogenic reactions to therapeutic drugs (e.g., corticosteroids and chemotherapy). The human immunodeficiency virus (HIV) and acquired immunodeficiency syndrome (AIDS) are reviewed in this chapter, while other secondary immune disorders such as leukemia, multiple myeloma, and viral hepatitis will be discussed in other chapters as appropriate.

Primary Immunodeficiency

Over 350 disorders are classified as primary immunodeficiency diseases (PID). Many deleterious genetic mutations are associated with these disorders. Some disorders are hereditary. These chronic disorders are rare. Innate defects such as dysfunctional, inadequate, or absent phagocytic capacity (e.g., asplenia, severe congenital neutropenia) can be present. Receptors on cells and the ability of cells to trigger important cellular processes can become defective, and the complement system can also be deficient (e.g., C3 deficiency). In the adaptive system, antibodies can be deficient (e.g., IgG and IgA disorders), or there can be B cell defects (e.g., IgA deficiency, hyper-IgM syndrome) or T cell defects (e.g., DiGeorge syndrome, Wiskott-Aldrich syndrome). Combined B cell and T cell defects may also be present, and often many classifications overlap. It is beyond the scope of this text to discuss each defect/disorder but a general overview is provided.

Clinical Manifestations

Manifestations of PID can occur early in the newborn or in infancy as potential life-threatening infections. Children and adults with PID have a susceptibility to infections. Everyone gets an infection at some point in time. Normal frequency of infections in children usually include two or fewer respiratory infections (e.g., otitis media, bronchitis) in a year. PID presentation in adults is not as common, but normal frequency for adults is usually three or fewer infections (e.g., sinusitis, pneumonia) requiring antibiotics within a year. In PID, infections tend to be recurrent and/or chronic.

Regardless of frequency, a summary for suspicion for PID includes infections that are:

- Severe—requires hospitalization or intravenous antibiotics
- Persistent—will not completely clear up or clears very slowly
- Unusual—caused by an uncommon organism
- Recurrent—keeps coming back
- Familial—others in the family with a similar susceptibility to infection (www.primaryimmune.org)

Diagnosis and Treatment

Newborn screening is recommended (and in some states mandated) for severe T-cell immunodeficiency. Diagnosis is based on clinical suspicion. A referral to an immunologist is warranted. Diagnosis and management is best handled by immunologists working with PID patients. Some laboratory tests are specific to the infection (e.g., site and organism). A complete blood count with differential will give information on lymphocytes and neutrophils. Flow cytometry can give detailed information pertaining to B cells and T cells. Testing may include antibody deficiencies by checking IgG, IgM, and IgA as well as complement testing (e.g., CH50). Vaccines may be given to evaluate if the person has developed antibodies (a normal, expected response). Carbohydrate and protein-based vaccine responses will be evaluated as a person may respond to one but not another. Genetic testing is often completed to identify the cause.

Prevention of infection is crucial in patients with PID and may include prophylactic antibiotic administration. Vaccine administration is not contraindicated for all patients with PID, but updates and guidelines need to be reviewed carefully. Treatment may include immunoglobulin replacement therapy, stem cell therapy, and gene therapy. Patients should get regular healthcare maintenance, such as dental care and primary care visits. Frequent illness can be burdensome, and mental health issues can be dealt with through counseling and support groups.

Secondary Immunodeficiency: HIV and AIDS

AIDS is a deadly, sexually transmitted disease caused by the HIV, a retrovirus. HIV attacks and weakens the immune system. There are two primary strains of the virus—HIV-1 is the most prevalent strain in the United States, and HIV-2 is the most prevalent strain in Africa.

According to the Centers for Disease and Control and Prevention (CDC), in 2016, approximately 36.7 million people worldwide and 1.2 million people in the United States were living with HIV, but 1 in 8 (13%) of these people did not know they were infected. HIV is the seventh leading cause of death in individuals 25 to 44 years of age in the United States, down from the number one cause of mortality in this age group in 1995. Most individuals infected are men, particularly gay, bisexual, or having sex with men. In 2014, men having sex with men accounted for 70% of all new cases of HIV infections. Diagnoses of new cases among women have declined 40% since 2005. Heterosexual contact is the most common (87%) mode of transmission for women. Cases involving female-to-female transmission (women having sex with women) are rare. In 2014, Blacks made up only 12% of the United States population but accounted for 44% of all new cases (particularly Black men) of HIV infections; however, Black women are also disproportionately affected. Of all women diagnosed with HIV in 2015 (CDC, 2017), 59% were Black, 17% White, and 19% Hispanic/Latina. The incidence of HIV in children is low, and 122 cases were diagnosed in 2016. For children under 13, most cases are transmitted from their mother. In terms of regional presence of HIV in the United States, the South accounted for most new HIV and AIDS diagnoses (54%/53%), persons living with HIV/AIDS diagnoses (44%), and AIDS deaths (47%) (CDC, 2017).

HIV is transmitted through direct contact with infected blood or body fluids (e.g., breastmilk, rectal and vaginal secretions, preejaculate/semen). HIV is contracted when these body fluids come in contact with mucous membranes located in the rectum, vagina, penis, or mouth. Contact usually occurs during sexual intercourse with receptive anal sex being the highest incidence followed by insertive anal sex and then penile–vaginal sex. The risk of contracting HIV

from penile–vaginal sex is higher for women in comparison to men. Oral sex is a rare mode of transmission with fellatio conferring the highest risk, but the presence of blood and open areas in areas of contact would increase risks.

Ranking after sexual intercourse, injection drug use involving needle or syringe sharing, and other equipment sharing is the next highest mode of transmission in the United States. The risk of acquiring HIV from an accidental needlestick is minimal (1 in 300 or 0.3%), but the risk of transmission from sharing needles is significantly greater (1 in 150). From 1985–2013, 58 confirmed cases of occupational transmission to a healthcare worker and 150 possible exposures were reported. Of the 58 confirmed cases, 57 occurred before 1999, and only one new case occurred after 1999 (Joyce, Kuhar, & Brooks, 2015). However, underreporting is possible because such reporting is voluntary. There is a 13–40% chance of an infected mother transmitting infection to her child. The risk of transmission decreases to 1% with the administration of antiretroviral therapy early in the pregnancy. The antiretroviral drug most commonly used to prevent maternal transmission is Retrovir (zidovudine), which has a high safety index. HIV status can even be checked during labor and delivery, so antiretroviral therapy can be given during labor or within hours of delivery to reduce the incidence of transmission. Cesarean delivery can further decrease the risk of HIV transmission to the fetus, but vaginal delivery can occur under certain circumstances (e.g., on treatment with low viral load). Breastfeeding is also another method of mother-to-child transmission.

Other less common methods of transmission include the transfusion of blood or blood products or organ/tissue transplant. This risk is negligible due to extensive prescreening. Any contact of an open wound or bleeding from any source (e.g., gums) with another open area or mucous membrane, although rare, can lead to transmission. This mode of transmission is often dependent on such factors as amount of blood and entrance into the bloodstream. HIV is not transmitted by saliva alone, but if there is blood in the saliva, it may occur.

As a retrovirus, HIV requires a host to survive. The life cycle of HIV is important to understand as most pharmacologic agents are targeted toward a part of the cycle (FIGURE 2-8 and FIGURE 2-9). Once it gains access to the body, the virus targets macrophages, dendritic

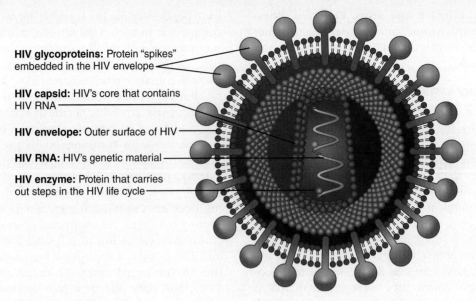

HIV glycoproteins: Protein "spikes" embedded in the HIV envelope

HIV capsid: HIV's core that contains HIV RNA

HIV envelope: Outer surface of HIV

HIV RNA: HIV's genetic material

HIV enzyme: Protein that carries out steps in the HIV life cycle

FIGURE 2-8 HIV cell.

Reproduced from U.S. Department of Health and Human Services. The HIV Life Cycle. (2018). Retrieved from https://aidsinfo.nih.gov/understanding-hiv-aids/fact-sheets/19/73/the-hiv-life-cycle-

cells, and **CD4+ helper T cells.** The HIV outer surface has a **glycoprotein 120 (GP-120)** that binds to the CD4+ on dendritic cells (an antigen-presenting cell located on skin and mucosal tissue). Macrophages are also a target, and the virus GP120 needs to bind with a coreceptor known as **chemokine receptor (CCR5)** in addition to the CD4+ cells. To attach to the T cells, the virus GP120 must attach to another receptor called **CXCR4** and the CD4+. Once attached and bound, the second part of the life cycle is known as **fusion,** which is the joining of the virus protein (glycoprotein 41), and the CD4+ membrane, which then allows entry. Once inside the CD4+ cells, it uses an enzyme, **reverse transcriptase,** to convert the viral RNA to DNA. The viral DNA then becomes integrated into the CD4+ cell's own DNA with the help of another viral enzyme known as **integrase.** The infected CD4+ cell reproduces new viral RNA, viral capsid, and other HIV building blocks (protein chains). The HIV RNA and building blocks go to the surface of the cell to assemble into immature and noninfectious HIV. Once out of the cell, another enzyme, protease, breaks up the protein into smaller chains, which then form mature, infectious HIV. Meanwhile, the virus replicates and infects susceptible cells, releasing millions of viral copies into the bloodstream. Unfortunately, there is no HIV immune response. Each viral copy then attaches to a new CD4+ cell to start the process over again.

Clinical Manifestations

Once infected, an individual may not experience any symptoms, or they may be subtle and missed. Up to about 60% of individuals will develop flulike symptoms (e.g., fever, malaise, headache, sore throat, myalgia/arthralgia, nausea, diarrhea, rash, and lymphadenopathy). If the symptoms are prolonged or there are mucocutaneous lesions (e.g., shallow, demarcated ulcers with a white base and red area in the mouth, anus, penis or esophagus), then the suspicion even becomes higher for HIV. The stage with these clinical manifestations is referred to as the **acute retroviral syndrome.** This syndrome usually occurs within 4 weeks after infection. At this time, there will be a high viral load (e.g., > 1 million copies), decreased CD4+, and a high transmission potential (**FIGURE 2-10**). During this acute period, viral load fluctuates and then reaches a set point. After this brief early infection episode, the individual may remain asymptomatic for months to years, and the virus continues replicating but not as fast as during the acute phase. This stage is known as the **clinical latency or chronic HIV infection stage.** Depending on other health factors and behaviors, individuals can be in this stage for up to 10 years until they move into the late stage of infection and develop **AIDS.** The virus is methodically infecting and destroying CD4+ cells. As more and more CD4+ cells are destroyed, the individual

The HIV Life Cycle

HIV medicines in seven drug classes stop (🛑) HIV at different stages in the HIV life cycle.

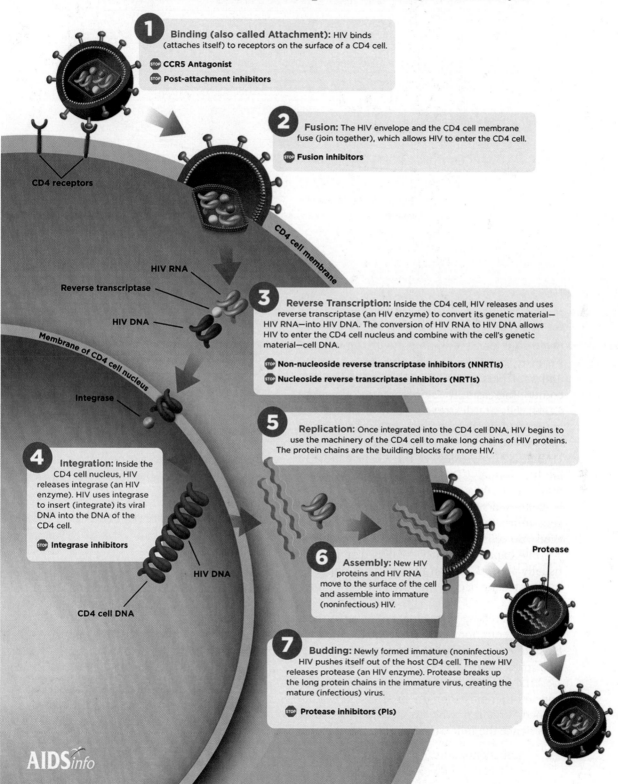

1 Binding (also called Attachment): HIV binds (attaches itself) to receptors on the surface of a CD4 cell.

🛑 **CCR5 Antagonist**
🛑 **Post-attachment inhibitors**

2 Fusion: The HIV envelope and the CD4 cell membrane fuse (join together), which allows HIV to enter the CD4 cell.

🛑 **Fusion inhibitors**

3 Reverse Transcription: Inside the CD4 cell, HIV releases and uses reverse transcriptase (an HIV enzyme) to convert its genetic material—HIV RNA—into HIV DNA. The conversion of HIV RNA to HIV DNA allows HIV to enter the CD4 cell nucleus and combine with the cell's genetic material—cell DNA.

🛑 **Non-nucleoside reverse transcriptase inhibitors (NNRTIs)**
🛑 **Nucleoside reverse transcriptase inhibitors (NRTIs)**

4 Integration: Inside the CD4 cell nucleus, HIV releases integrase (an HIV enzyme). HIV uses integrase to insert (integrate) its viral DNA into the DNA of the CD4 cell.

🛑 **Integrase inhibitors**

5 Replication: Once integrated into the CD4 cell DNA, HIV begins to use the machinery of the CD4 cell to make long chains of HIV proteins. The protein chains are the building blocks for more HIV.

6 Assembly: New HIV proteins and HIV RNA move to the surface of the cell and assemble into immature (noninfectious) HIV.

7 Budding: Newly formed immature (noninfectious) HIV pushes itself out of the host CD4 cell. The new HIV releases protease (an HIV enzyme). Protease breaks up the long protein chains in the immature virus, creating the mature (infectious) virus.

🛑 **Protease inhibitors (PIs)**

CD4 receptors

CD4 cell membrane

HIV RNA
Reverse transcriptase
HIV DNA

Membrane of CD4 cell nucleus

Integrase

HIV DNA

CD4 cell DNA

Protease

AIDS*info*

FIGURE 2-9 The HIV life cycle.

Reproduced from U.S. Department of Health and Human Services. The HIV Life Cycle. (2018). Retrieved from https://aidsinfo.nih.gov/understanding-hiv-aids/fact-sheets/19/73/the-hiv-life-cycle-

Blood test for HIV antibody for diagnosis, also test for viral load.

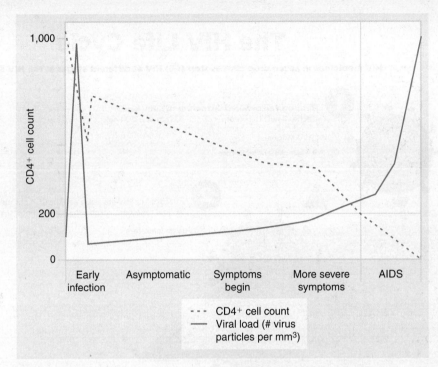

FIGURE 2-10 CD4+ cell count and viral load following HIV infection.

begins to have symptoms (e.g., lymphade-nopathy, diarrhea, weight loss, fever, cough, and shortness of breath). The individual becomes increasingly symptomatic as more CD4+ cells are destroyed. AIDS is defined as a CD4 count of less than 200 cells/mm³ or the development of an opportunistic infection (**TABLE 2-7**) regardless of the CD4+ count. In adults, normal CD4+ counts range between 500 and 1,500 cells/mm³. In children, AIDS is diagnosed when the CD4+ is less than 500 cells/mm³ (in 1- to 5-year-olds) and less than 750 cells/mm³ (in those < 1 year old).

Life expectancy once AIDS is diagnosed is usually about 3 years unless a severe opportunistic infection occurs, and then life expectancy can decrease to 1 year. This disease trajectory can be altered by managing HIV with antiretroviral medications and developing a healthy lifestyle (e.g., exercise, healthy nutrition, safe sex, stress reduction).

HIV infection in infants and children may appear differently than the progression just described. Children who are HIV positive may experience the following manifestations:

- Lymphadenopathy with hepatosplenomegaly early in the course
- Difficulty gaining weight
- Difficulty growing normally
- Problems walking
- Delayed mental development

TABLE 2-7	Opportunistic Infections

Bacterial pneumonia, recurrent (≥ 2 episodes in 12 months)
Candidiasis of the respiratory tract and esophagus
Invasive cervical cancer
Fungal infections
Parasitic and protozoan infections (> 1-month duration)
Cytomegalovirus disease
Encephalopathy
Herpes simplex: chronic ulcers (> 1-month duration)
Histoplasmosis
Kaposi sarcoma
Lymphoma
Mycobacterium avium complex
Mycobacterium tuberculosis
Pneumocystis jirovecii (formerly *carinii*) pneumonia
Progressive multifocal leukoencephalopathy
Salmonella septicemia
Toxoplasmosis of the brain
Wasting syndrome due to HIV (involuntary weight loss > 10% of baseline body weight) associated with either chronic diarrhea (≥ 2 loose stools per day ≥ 1 month) or chronic weakness and documented fever ≥ 1 month)

- Severe forms of common childhood illnesses such as ear infections (otitis media), pneumonia, and tonsillitis

Opportunistic infections that are more prevalent in children include pneumocystis

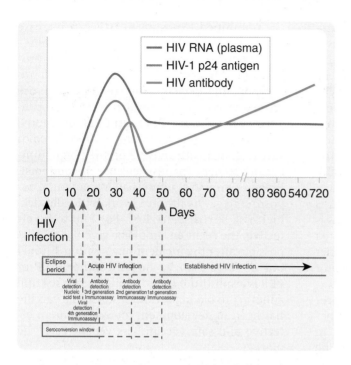

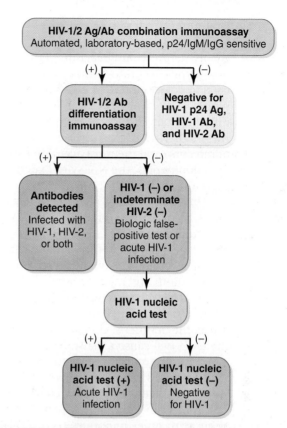

FIGURE 2-11 Antibody-only testing, combination antigen and antibody testing, and viral detection.

Centers for Disease Control and Prevention and Association of Public Health Laboratories. Laboratory Testing for the Diagnosis of HIV Infection: Updated Recommendations. Available at http://dx.doi.org/10.15620/cdc.23447. Published June 27, 2014.

pneumonia, wasting syndrome, oral candidiasis, encephalopathy, cytomegalovirus infections, and frequent bacterial infections.

Diagnosis and Treatment

Diagnosis is established through a set of laboratory tests as early as 2 weeks after exposure to the virus. There are three categories of testing—antibody-only testing, combination antigen and antibody testing, and viral detection (**FIGURE 2-11**). Antibody tests detect antibodies IgM and IgG against HIV-1 and HIV-2, usually within 3 weeks, but the time from HIV exposure to the test detecting the antibodies (i.e., the window period) can be up to 12 weeks (third-generation immunoassay).

Antibody-only tests can be completed on saliva or blood. Antibody testing can be done at home or in a laboratory, and results can be obtained in less than 20 minutes for some tests. Most home tests evaluate antibodies. The HIV-1 Western blot and enzyme-linked immunoassay (ELISA) are first-generation immunoassay antibody tests for IgG only and are no longer recommended to establish diagnosis.

The next category (termed *fourth generation*) are combination antigen and antibody tests. The antibodies tested are for HIV-1 and HIV-2 and include IgG and IgM. The p24 protein makes up the capsid or viral core HIV, and antigen testing detects this HIV protein (see Figure 2-8 and Figure 2-9). The p24 antigen testing is for HIV-1 detection. This test can become positive within 6 weeks after infection. The fourth-generation combination test is recommended by the CDC (2014) as the initial screening test. If the test is negative, then no further testing is necessary. If the test is positive, then an HIV-1/HIV-2 antibody differentiation immunoassay (not Western blot or ELISA) should be done to confirm and detect whether there is an infection due HIV 1, HIV 2, or both. If the test is negative (for HIV-1 and/or HIV-2) or there is an indeterminate (HIV-1), then a viral RNA should be done. Viral detection is the third category of HIV test. Viral detection tests include the p24 antigen and HIV genetic material. Of the genetic testing, HIV RNA is the most commonly used and other tests include HIV DNA and nucleic acid sequence based amplification. Viral detection occurs before antibodies are detected. Viral RNA testing is accomplished through a qualitative (nonnumeric) test referred to as *nucleic acid testing* (NAT) that checks for HIV-1. NAT uses a polymerase chain reaction (PCR) technology. Other laboratory methods can also be used to detect viral RNA other than PCR techniques. The viral RNA NAT test can be positive between 7 and 28 days after infection. Although viral RNA is the earliest indication of infection and the most accurate early in the infection period, the NATs are expensive and, therefore, not first line.

Once HIV/AIDS is confirmed, viral RNA is measured quantitatively, also with NAT; this is known as a *viral load measurement*. The plasma viral load, or number of viral particles per milliliter of blood, is mainly used to monitor disease status and management.

Viral detection testing is the most appropriate test for infants and young children because the mother's circulating antibodies in the child will cause a "false" positive test. The aim of antiretroviral therapy is to reduce the viral load to a point that the body's immune system can keep the virus in check. Viral load can also be an indicator of treatment success, along with other indicators (e.g., CD4+ count and presence of opportunistic infections).

Although there is no cure for AIDS, antiretroviral therapy is used to control the reproduction of the virus and slow the progression of the disease. Highly active antiretroviral therapy (HAART)—the recommended approach—includes three or more antiretroviral medications from different classes. The approved classes include nucleoside/nucleotide reverse transcriptase inhibitors, nonnucleoside reverse transcriptase inhibitors, protease inhibitors, integrase strand transfer inhibitors, fusion inhibitors, CCR5 antagonists, and postattachment inhibitors (see Figure 2-8). Pharmacokinetic enhancers may also be used to increase the effectiveness of the medication regimen. HAART has been very effective in suppressing HIV replication, but resistance can occur if the patient does not strictly adhere to the prescribed regimen. Genetic tests that can determine whether the patient's particular HIV strain is resistant to a particular drug are available, and this information can be used to ensure that the best possible combination of drugs is prescribed. Other treatment strategies include medications to treat specific opportunistic infections as they arise, management of the numerous drug side effects (e.g., high cholesterol and blood glucose), and prevention of reexposure.

Continued exposure to HIV can increase the viral load and introduce another strain—both factors can accelerate the disease's progression. Medications can also be taken to prevent the development of HIV and are termed *preexposure prophylaxis* (PrEP) and *postexposure prophylaxis* (PEP). PrEP can be offered to individuals who have a higher risk of exposure (e.g., sex with an HIV+ partner, high number of partners, inconsistent use of condoms). PEP is offered in situations after a potential exposure (e.g., healthcare worker needlestick, high-risk sexual behavior). For PEP to be effective, the regimen should be given as soon as possible after the incident (e.g., within 1 hour) but no later than 72 hours. Neither PrEP or PEP is a substitute for engaging in safe sex and adhering to blood precautions. An HIV vaccine has been in development for years, but an effective and safe vaccine has yet to reach the market.

Preventing HIV transmission is a worldwide public health priority. Prevention includes the following strategies:

- Avoiding contact with bodily fluids
- Avoiding activities that increase risk of exposure to those bodily secretions (e.g., drug use and multiple sexual partners)
- Education
- Using condoms with every sexual experience
- PrEP and PEP
- Male circumcision (reduces the risk of female-to-male transmission of HIV and other sexually transmitted infections)

Learning Points

Antibiotic Stewardship

Antibiotic resistance is a major public health threat. Some bacteria are resistant to more than one antibiotic in multiple classes. When resistance occurs, more toxic antibiotics often have to be used. In the United States, an estimated 2 million people a year are diagnosed with a serious infection that is not responsive to usual antibiotic treatment. Healthcare providers too often prescribe antibiotics unnecessarily, such as for the common cold or inappropriately, such as choosing the wrong antibiotic. Antibiotic stewardship involves using antibiotics appropriately and safely. Efforts have been under way to target healthcare providers, patients, policy makers, and administrators to improve antibiotic prescribing. Antibiotic stewardship examples include using rapid diagnostic testing techniques to determine if an infection is viral, rendering antibiotics unnecessary. Other efforts to promote antibiotic stewardship include a recommendation to switch patients from intravenous to oral antibiotics as soon as possible.

BOX 2-3 Application to Practice

Case 1: Mr. Jones, a 45-year-old man, is concerned that he has HIV as he had unprotected receptive anal sex with a man. Answer the following questions:

1. Which HIV test would be conducted first?
2. If he contracted HIV, how many days after exposure would be needed before the test would be positive?
3. Would you consider offering him PEP or PrEP, and, if so, why and when?

Case 2: Mary, a 20-year-old woman, comes to the clinic complaining of unintentional weight loss and fatigue. She also states her knees and wrists are achy at times and she feels stiff in the morning for a few minutes. She feels like they are a bit swollen. She also noticed a rash around her cheeks. She had the symptoms for about 1 month. She has no past medical or surgical history. She takes no medications. Her physical exam is normal except for a malar rash and mildly edematous joints with pain upon range of motion. The tentative diagnosis is SLE.

1. A complete blood count, complete chemistry profile, and what other laboratory tests can be done to evaluate for SLE?
2. What laboratory findings would correlate with SLE?
3. Which clinical manifestations does Mary have that support the diagnosis of SLE?

Developing a Strong Immune System

The key to preventing infectious diseases is building a strong immune system. Many people assume that the best way to stay healthy is to avoid exposure. However, the immune system requires early exposure to antigens to operate optimally because it is a memory system. Exposure to microbes is limited today because of small family units, good sanitation, and widespread antibiotic use. Research suggests that avoiding oversanitizing our environment can increase exposure to microbes earlier and help develop a stronger immune system.

Myth Busters

Despite efforts to educate the public, many misconceptions persist regarding HIV/AIDS.

Myth 1: I can get HIV by being around people who are HIV positive.

Facts: Evidence has consistently demonstrated that HIV cannot be spread through touch, tears, or saliva. In addition, HIV is not stable outside the body. The virus cannot be transmitted through toilet seats, water fountains, eating utensils, exercise equipment, hugging, or kissing.

Myth 2: I can get HIV from mosquitoes.

Facts: Although HIV spreads through blood, several studies have shown that mosquitoes cannot transmit HIV even in areas with high numbers of mosquitoes and HIV cases. Mosquitoes do not inject the blood they consume into the next person they bite, and the virus lives only a short time in the insect.

Myth 3: If I'm receiving treatment, I cannot spread HIV.

Facts: Effective treatment can decrease the viral load in the blood, even to the point that the virus cannot be detected by a blood test. However, the virus can hide in other areas of the body, waiting for an opportunity to increase its replication again. The risk of transmission is lower when the viral load is lower, but transmission is still possible.

Myth 4: My partner and I are both HIV positive, so there is no reason to practice safer sex.

Facts: Continued exposure to HIV can increase the viral load and introduce another strain—both factors that can accelerate the disease's progression. Practicing safer sex (e.g., wearing condoms and using other barriers) can limit exposure to HIV and other sexually transmitted infections.

Myth 5: You cannot get HIV from oral sex.

Facts: It is true that the risk of transmission through oral sex is lower than with other types of sex, but HIV can be transmitted by having oral sex with either a man or woman who is HIV positive.

BOX 2-4 Application to Practice

Let us put the things you have learned about the body's defenses into practice. Which of the following individuals would be at highest risk for impaired immune function?

- A 23-year-old female who weighs 5% more than her ideal body weight
- A 78-year-old male with poorly controlled diabetes mellitus
- An 89-year-old male with controlled hypertension
- A 45-year-old female who was recently widowed

When considering this type of question, you start by counting things that might impair the immune system. The patient with the most risk factors is at the greatest risk. Eliminate any information that does not increase risk. For instance, being male or female does not impair immune function, so eliminate that factor from your consideration.

Let us look at each of the example patients. The 23-year-old is not in an increased age range and is fairly close to her ideal body weight; she has no risk factors. The 78-year-old is assigned one risk factor for his increased age and another for his chronic disease. Go ahead and give him another risk factor because his diabetes is uncontrolled—now he has three risk factors. The 89-year-old has one risk factor for his increased age and another for having a chronic disease, but his hypertension is controlled. He has two risk factors. Finally, the 45-year-old has only one risk factor, the stress of being recently widowed. After examining all of these patients, the 78-year-old male is at the most risk for impaired immune function owing to his three risk factors.

At-risk individuals and states, medications, or habits that specifically put individuals at risk for an impaired immune system include the following:

- Being very young or very old
- Poor nutrition
- Impaired skin integrity
- Circulatory issues
- Alterations in normal flora due to antibiotic therapy
- Chronic diseases, especially diabetes mellitus
- Corticosteroid therapy
- Chemotherapy
- Smoking
- Alcohol consumption
- Immunodeficiency states

The following strategies can be employed to build a healthy immune system:

- Increasing fluid intake
- Eating a well-balanced diet
- Increasing antioxidants and protein intake
- Getting adequate sleep
- Avoiding caffeine and refined sugar
- Spending time outdoors
- Reducing stress

Modified from Story, L. (2017). *Pathophysiology: A practical approach* (3rd ed.). Burlington, MA: Jones & Bartlett Learning.

CHAPTER SUMMARY

Humans are in a constant state of warfare with often unseen enemies. The body takes a multilevel approach to prevent attacks and eliminate invaders. Problems can occur at any of these levels that can lead to overreactions, underreactions, and inappropriate reactions. These altered reactions can produce disease states that negatively affect the body. Multiple conditions can impair the body's ability to battle, but when armed with the appropriate weapons, the body becomes a fighting machine that can withstand many a fierce invader.

REFERENCES AND RESOURCES

Ahmed, Z., Kawamura, T., Shimada, S., & Piguet, V. (2014). The role of human dendritic cells in HIV-1 infection. *Journal of Investigative Dermatology, 135*, 1225–1233; advance online publication, doi:10.1038/jid.2014.490

Centers for Disease Prevention and Control (CDC). (2014). HIV Surveillance Report. Retrieved from https://www.cdc.gov/hiv/pdf/library/reports/surveillance/cdc-hiv-surveillance-report-2017-vol-29.pdf

Centers for Disease Prevention and Control (CDC). (2017). HIV/AIDS. Retrieved from Centers for Disease Control and Prevention and Association of Public Health Laboratories. (2014, June). Laboratory testing for the diagnosis of HIV infection: Updated recommendations. http://dx.doi.org/10.15620/cdc.23447

Chiras, D. (2015). *Human biology* (8th ed.). Burlington, MA: Jones & Bartlett Learning.

Elling, B., Elling, K., & Rothenberg, M. (2004). *Anatomy and physiology*. Sudbury, MA: Jones and Bartlett Publishers.

Gladman, D. D. (2018). Overview of the clinical manifestations of systemic lupus erythematosus in adults. In D. S. Pisetsky (Ed.), *Uptodate*. Retrieved from https://www.uptodate.com/contents/overview-of-the-clinical-manifestaions-of-systemic-lupus-erythematosus-in-adults

Gould, B. (2015). *Pathophysiology for the health professions* (5th ed.). Philadelphia, PA: Elsevier.

Immune Deficiency Foundation. (2019). Retrieved from www.primaryimune.org

Joyce, M. P., Kuhar, D., & Brooks, J. T. (2015). Notes from the field: Occupationally acquired HIV infection among health care workers- United States, 1985-2013,

Lu, W., Mehraj, V., Vyboh, K., Cao, W., Li, T., & Routy, J.-P. (2015). CD4:CD8 ratio as a frontier marker for clinical outcome, immune dysfunction and viral reservoir size in virologically suppressed HIV-positive patients. *Journal of the International AIDS Society, 18*(1), 20052. http://doi.org/10.7448/IAS.18.1.20052

McQuenn, C. (2017). *Comprehensive Toxicology* (3rd ed.). St. Louis, MO: Elsevier.

Montecino-Rodriguez, E., Berent-Maoz, B., & Dorshkind, K. (2013). Causes, consequences, and reversal of immune system aging. *The Journal of Clinical Investigation, 123*(3), 958–965. http://doi.org/10.1172/JCI64096

National Institutes of Health, Human Microbiome Project (2019). Retrieved from https://www.hmpdacc.org/overview/

National Research Council (U.S.) Committee on Metagenomics: Challenges and Functional Applications. (2007). *The new science of metagenomics: Revealing the secrets of our microbial planet: Why metagenomics?* Washington, DC: National Academies Press. Retrieved from: https://www.ncbi.nlm.nih.gov/books/NBK54011/

Pommerville, J. C. (2013). *Alcamo's fundamentals of microbiology* (10th ed.). Burlington, MA: Jones & Bartlett Learning.

Porth, C. (2010). *Essentials of pathophysiology* (3rd ed.). Philadelphia, PA: Lippincott Williams & Wilkins.

Principles of laboratory diagnosis of infectious diseases. In K. J. Ryan (Ed.), *Sherris medical microbiology* (7th ed.). New York, NY: McGraw-Hill. Retrieved from http://accessmedicine.mhmedical.com.ezproxy.fiu.edu/content.aspx?bookid=2268&sectionid=176081782

Professional guide to pathophysiology (3rd ed.). (2010). Philadelphia, PA: Lippincott Williams & Wilkins.

Pulendran, B., & Ahmed, R. (2011). Immunological mechanisms of vaccination. *Nature Immunology, 12*(6), 509–517.

Rogers, G. B. (2014). The human microbiome: Opportunities and challenges for clinical care. *Internal Medicine Journal, 45*(9), 889–898.

Surana, N. K., Kasper, D. L. (2018). The human microbiome. In J. Jameson, A. S. Fauci, D. L. Kasper, S. L. Hauser, D. L. Longo, & J. Loscalzo (Eds.), *Harrison's principles of internal medicine* (20th ed.). New York, NY: McGraw-Hill. Retrieved from http://accessmedicine.mhmedical.com.ezproxy.fiu.edu/content.aspx?bookid=2129&sectionid=192534978

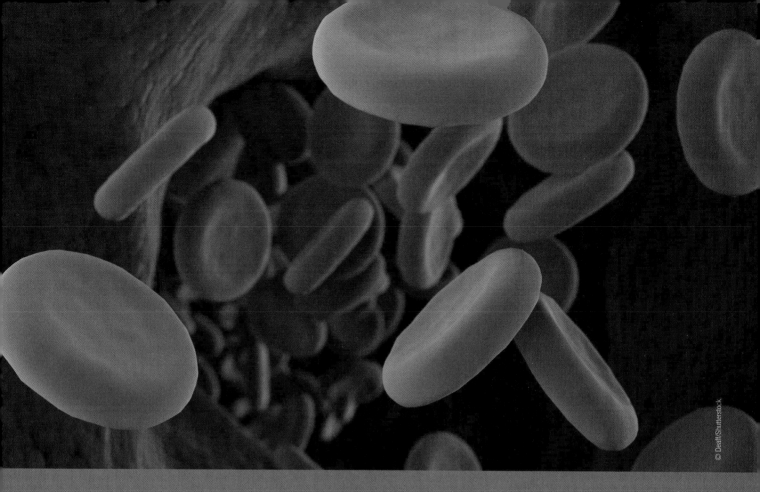

CHAPTER 3
Hematopoietic Function

LEARNING OBJECTIVES

- Explain the process of normal hematopoietic function.
- Describe the structure and role of the lymphoid system.
- Compare and contrast the pathogenesis of blood cell alterations and disorders.
- Apply knowledge of hematopoietic and lymphoid system alterations, including various common

disorders such as leukemia, lymphoma, anemia, and coagulopathy.
- Explain the clinical consequences of common blood cell disorders.
- Develop diagnostic and treatment plans for various blood cell disorders.

Blood is the life fluid of the human body, and it is essential for health and homeostasis. The approximately 5 liters of blood continuously circulating in the human body provides nutrients and oxygen to tissues while aiding in the excretion of waste products. Blood consists of plasma, blood cells, and platelets. Disease occurs when there are too few, too many, or dysfunctional blood components. These conditions can result from many causes that may be congenital, genetic (whether acquired or inherited), and environmental factors, but they can also be iatrogenic. Blood disorders often present with manifestations in multiple systems; therefore, an understanding of normal blood function, formation, and hemostasis are requisite to understanding how abnormalities develop.

Hematopoietic System

Blood is both a viscous fluid and a connective tissue. Blood accomplishes its functions through its various components—the plasma (liquid protein), leukocytes (white blood cells), erythrocytes (red blood cells), and thrombocytes (platelets) (**FIGURE 3-1**) (**TABLE 3-1**). Plasma is a transport medium that carries the

blood cells as well as antibodies, nutrients, electrolytes, hormones, lipids, and waste products. The most abundant of the plasma proteins is albumin, which creates colloid oncotic (osmotic) pressure as one mechanism to maintain fluid balance in blood vessels.

Leukocytes are key players in the inflammatory response and infectious process. Leukocytes consist of neutrophils, eosinophils, basophils, and mast cells. These cells are called *granulocytes* because of the granules in their cytoplasm. Because of their multiple nuclear lobes, they are also called *polymorphonuclear leukocytes*. The two other leukocytes are monocytes and lymphocytes whose nuclei are not multilobular and, therefore, are called *mononuclear cells* or *agranulocytes* (absence of cytoplasm granules). Granulocytes and monocytes are also phagocytes. Monocytes are precursors and differentiate into tissue macrophages, which are phagocytes. In adults, neutrophils are the most abundant type of leukocyte followed by lymphocytes. Infants during the first year of life, however, have an abundance of monocytes and eosinophils. Lymphocyte function diminishes with aging.

Erythrocytes are disk-shaped cells that carry oxygen to tissues and transport carbon

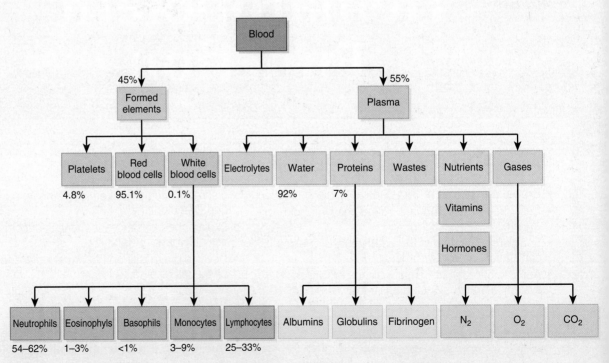

FIGURE 3-1 Blood composition.

TABLE 3-1   Summary of Blood Cells

Name	Light micrograph	Description	Concentration (number of cells/mm³)	Life span	Function
Red blood cells (RBCs)		Biconcave disk; no nucleus	4–6 million	120 days	Transport oxygen and carbon dioxide
White blood cells (WBCs)					
Neutrophil Granulocyte, polymorphonuclear		Approximately twice the size of RBCs; multilobed nucleus; clear-staining cytoplasm	3,000–7,000	6 hours to a few days	Phagocytizes bacteria
Eosinophil Granulocyte, polymorphonuclear		Approximately same size as neutrophil; large pink-staining granules; bilobed nucleus	100–400	8–12 days	Phagocytizes antigen-antibody complex; attacks parasites
Basophil Granulocyte, polymorphonuclear		Slightly smaller than neutrophil; contains large, purple cytoplasmic granules; bilobed nucleus	20–50	A few hours to a few days	Releases histamine during inflammation
Monocyte Agranulocyte, mononuclear		Larger than neutrophil; cytoplasm is grayish blue; no cytoplasmic granules; U- or kidney-shaped nucleus	100–700	Lasts many months	Phagocytizes bacteria, dead cells, and cellular debris
Lymphocyte Agranulocyte, mononuclear		Slightly smaller than neutrophil; large, relatively round nucleus that fills the cell	1,500–3,000	Naïve 1–3 months; Exposed Can persist for many years	Involved in immune protection, either attacking cells directly or producing antibodies
Platelets		Fragments of megakaryocytes; appear as small, dark-staining granules	250,000	5–10 days	Play several key roles in blood clotting

Modified from Story, L. (2017). *Pathophysiology: A Practical Approach* (3rd ed.). Burlington, MA: Jones & Bartlett Learning.

dioxide out of the tissues for its subsequent removal from the body. Erythrocytes contain proteins such as hemoglobin, which binds to oxygen, giving blood its red color. The brighter the shade of red, the more the blood is saturated with oxygen. Hematocrit refers to how much of the blood volume comprises erythrocytes.

Thrombocytes, along with clotting factors, control coagulation. Carried passively in the blood, thrombocytes are coated with a sticky material that causes them to adhere to irregular surfaces. Clotting is a quick chain reaction stimulated by the release of thromboplastin from damaged cells lining the blood vessels in the area of an injury. In conjunction with the initiation of the clotting cascade, platelets containing contractile proteins pull the edges of the wound together. Blood clots do not persist indefinitely; if they did so, they would clog up the entire circulatory system. Plasmin is an enzyme that dissolves clots once healing has occurred.

Hematopoiesis

Hematopoiesis is the process of blood formation, and it occurs primarily in the bone marrow (**FIGURE 3-2**). Hematopoiesis requires an adequate supply of hematopoietic stem cells. These primitive cells are considered multipotent cells as they can differentiate into all blood cell types. The hematopoietic stem cells differentiate into myeloid and lymphoid progenitor cell lines. Differentiation leads to varying

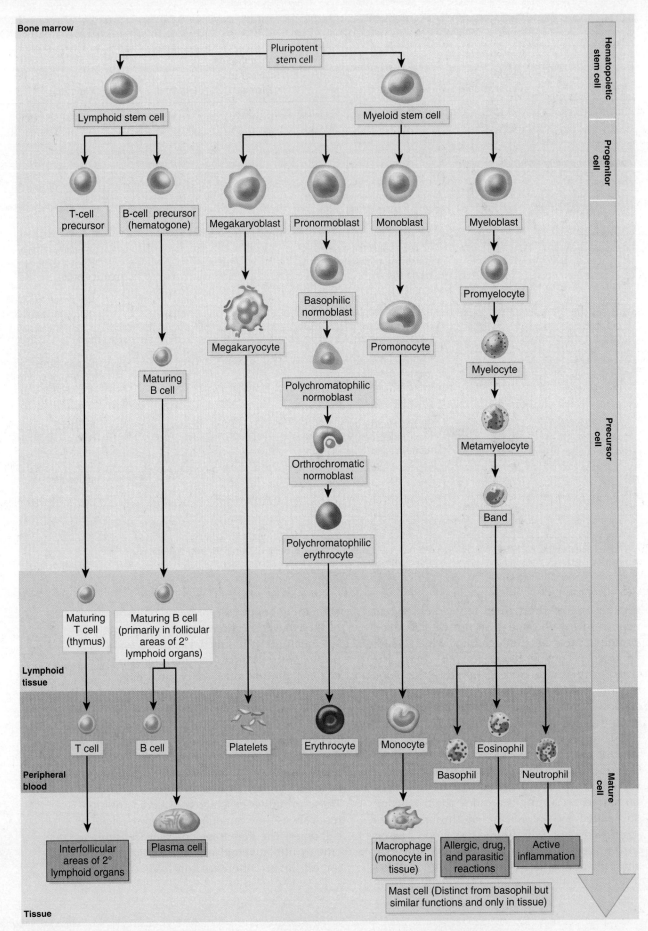

FIGURE 3-2 Hematopoiesis.

precursors for each of the different blood cells. Maturation of the various blood cells occurs in different areas such as the thymus (T lymphocytes), the bone marrow (B lymphocytes), peripheral blood (granulocytes, monocytes, erythrocytes), or tissue (plasma).

Hematopoietic stimulus for red blood cell production may include hypoxemia and blood loss, while the stimulus for white blood cell production may be infection and inflammation. In response to reduced oxygen supply, the kidneys (liver in the fetus) produce the growth factor **erythropoietin** (EPO). EPO is a physiologic regulator of red blood cell production. Erythropoietin is essential for erythropoiesis as it amplifies signals in the cells for continued development and differentiation of the progenitor and precursor cells. Recombinant erythropoiesis-stimulating agents, epoetin and darbepoetin, are synthetic versions of EPO. Synthetic EPO is used in some anemias such as those caused by chronic renal failure or chemotherapy. Erythrocytes come from the progenitor myeloid stem line. These myeloid cells develop into a pool of erythroblast precursors (e.g., proerythroblast).

While the red blood cell is developing, **vitamin B$_{12}$** and **folic acid** are necessary in addition to EPO. Vitamin B$_{12}$ and folic acid are necessary for cellular DNA synthesis. Deficiencies can lead to several abnormalities, such as the inability of the cell to undergo nuclear division, premature apoptosis, and phagocytosis of precursor cells. Folic acid and vitamin B$_{12}$ come from dietary sources. Folate is the natural form in food, and folic acid is the supplement added to foods. Both terms are often used interchangeably. Inadequate intake of folic acid (e.g., inadequate diet), impaired absorption (e.g., celiac disease, alcoholism), and impaired folic acid action (e.g., caused by phenytoin) lead to deficiency. Vitamin B$_{12}$ absorption is reliant on a protein called *intrinsic factor*. This protein secreted by gastric parietal cells binds to the vitamin B$_{12}$ and is then absorbed in the small intestine. Small amounts of folic acid are stored in the body, but vitamin B$_{12}$ can be stored in the liver for long periods until needed. Both these vitamins are water soluble and excesses are excreted in the urine.

While the erythrocytes are developing, iron is needed for the heme portion of hemoglobin. Iron is either in a ferric (3+ oxidation) state or ferrous (2+ oxidation) state. Iron is obtained from dietary sources with heme iron (Fe^{2+} in heme) found mostly in animal products, while nonheme (Fe^{3+} nonheme) is mainly in plant foods and dairy products. Heme iron (ferrous) is more readily absorbed, but the nonheme (ferric) with Fe^{3+} must be reduced to ferrous 2+ for absorption. Nonheme and heme are absorbed through different mechanisms (**FIGURE 3-3**).

Once the iron is absorbed, it is in a free form and is labile (Fe^{3+} form). This labile iron cannot remain in this state because damaging reactive oxygen species can develop. The labile iron (Fe^{3+} form), the form that moves around, needs to be bound and used, transported, or stored. In the duodenum, several things occur with this labile iron. The iron can bind with apoferritin in the duodenum and become ferritin. The iron can be carried across the duodenal membrane to the blood by ferroportin. The ferritin binds to transferrin, which is the protein in blood that transports iron around the circulation. Some iron remains in the cell mitochondria for use to develop enzymes or heme. Most of the iron is taken to the bone marrow to make more hemoglobin during erythropoiesis, and about 75% of iron is in hemoglobin. Some iron is also taken to the liver where it binds to transferrin receptors and gets stored as ferritin. Iron is also in the spleen where old red blood cells (RBCs) are broken down by macrophages releasing iron to be reused.

Hepcidin is a protein in the liver that tightly regulates dietary iron uptake and transport in several places such as the duodenum, liver, or spleen (**FIGURE 3-4**). The liver and spleen membranes also have ferroportin, which transports iron (Fe^{2+}) across the cell membrane back into the blood where again it binds with transferrin (Fe^{3+}) to be taken where needed. Iron is often going from a stable, usable ferrous (Fe^{2+}) to labile, mobile ferric (Fe^{3+}) state and then vice-versa. Hepcidin acts as a ferroportin inhibitor. When iron levels are high, hepcidin increases and binds to ferroportin, inhibiting the transport action across the cell membrane so less iron is absorbed. Low levels of iron leads to less hepcidin production and more can be absorbed. Many clinical disorders, such as chronic hepatitis C infection, alcoholism, chronic kidney disease, infections, and inflammation can alter hepcidin levels and lead to iron absorption problems (too much or too little). The only other mechanism for iron elimination is

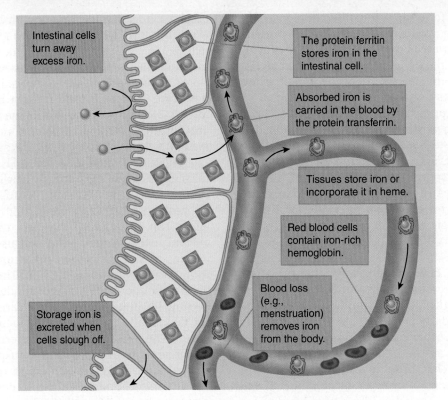

FIGURE 3-3 Iron absorption in the gastrointestinal tract.

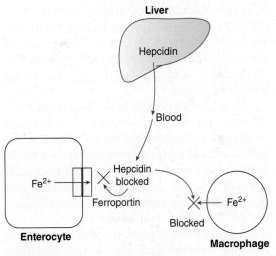

FIGURE 3-4 Role of the liver hormone hepcidin in iron absorption. Hepcidin will block iron absorption when iron stores are sufficient.

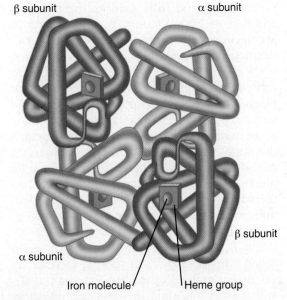

FIGURE 3-5 Porphyrin ring.

through normal processes such as menstruation, small amounts from desquamation in intestines, or disorders (e.g., hemorrhage).

Hemoglobin is the protein that carries oxygen and is made while the RBCs are developing. Hemoglobin has four separate subunits, and each subunit consists of a heme (iron and porphyrin ring) and a one-globin chain (alpha, beta, or delta) (FIGURE 3-5). Hemoglobin A comprises about 97–98% of the type of hemoglobin in a normal adult and consists of two subunits that are alpha chains and two that are beta chains. The remaining 2–3% is composed of hemoglobin A_2 and consists of two alpha and two delta chains. For oxygen to be transported and released, the iron in hemoglobin needs to be in the ferrous (Fe^{2+}) state. Some diseases (e.g., hereditary methemoglobinemia or toxic ingestions of nitrites) and drugs (e.g., benzocaine) cause the normal oxygen-carrying ferrous state to become a noncarrying oxygen ferric state. The abnormal hemoglobin is called *methemoglobin*.

During erythrocyte development, the cell gets smaller and loses its nucleus once most

Diagnostic Link

Reticulocyte Count

A reticulocyte count can be useful to evaluate bone marrow function or to distinguish between different types of anemia. The values are expressed as a percentage of RBCs or an absolute number and are a reflection of recent bone marrow activity. A corrected reticulocyte count is often calculated and takes hematocrit value into account and is more accurate with anemia. The results should be evaluated in context of other diagnostic tests such as the hemoglobin, hematocrit, or the complete blood count. If there is an anemia due to blood loss or RBC destruction (e.g., hemolytic disease), the reticulocyte count will be high as the bone marrow tries to compensate. Low reticulocyte counts occur if the bone marrow is dysfunctional, as in bone marrow suppression, indicating a production problem. A low reticulocyte count may occur when the bone marrow is able to produce but does not have the proper requisites to make red blood cells such as iron, folic acid, vitamin B_{12}, or erythropoietin. These deficiencies might occur with iron deficiency anemia, alcoholism, celiac disease or Crohn disease, or kidney disease, respectively. Reticulocyte counts are not diagnostic of any particular disease but rather are indicators of the status of RBC production.

of the hemoglobin is synthesized. At this stage, the cell is called a *reticulocyte*. The time from the first precursor, proerythroblast, to development into a reticulocyte in the circulation is about 5 days. Once in the circulation, the reticulocytes complete their differentiation into mature erythrocytes whose life span is approximately 4 months.

Hemostasis

Hemostasis is the process by which bleeding from an injury is stopped. The coagulation process needs to be limited to the area of injury so that blood flows in an unimpeded manner to unaffected areas. Hemostasis requires factors that promote coagulation as well as factors that inhibit coagulation. Normal hemostasis requires endothelial lining integrity and platelets. Hemostasis can be divided into two processes—primary and secondary (**FIGURE 3-6**).

When a vessel is injured, the goal is to decrease blood loss. The blood vessel quickly vasoconstricts reflexively under the influence of **endothelin** secreted by endothelial cells. Under normal circumstances, platelets are blocked from adhering to the cell membrane by **nitric oxide** and **prostacyclin**, which are also secreted by the endothelial cells. During injury, nitric oxide and prostacyclin decreases, allowing platelet adhesion. The endothelial lining secretes **von Willebrand factor (vWF)**, which, in response to injury, binds to the basement membrane. The platelet binds to the vWF via the Ib receptor, one of the two glycoprotein receptors on the platelet. The vWF is the glue

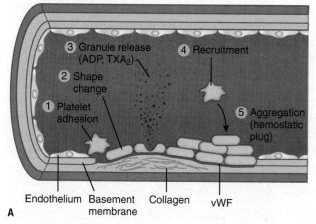

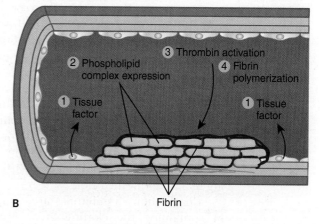

FIGURE 3-6 Primary and secondary hemostasis.

or link between the platelets and the area of injury. The bound platelets then become active and change their shape. The platelets release various substances, which include vWF, **serotonin** (a vasoconstrictor), and **adenosine diphosphate** to activate platelets which all lead to aggregation (clustering). The platelets also release **fibrinogen** and **calcium**, which are both necessary for secondary hemostasis. The activated platelets release **thromboxane A^2**, a potent vasoconstrictor, that acts in opposition to prostacyclin. Thromboxane A^2 promotes further platelet activation and aggregation. The second glycoprotein receptor on the platelet, IIb/IIIa, binds with fibrinogen circulating in the blood, leading to further aggregation and resulting in what is termed a *platelet plug*.

This platelet plug is relatively weak and is strengthened by **fibrin**, an insoluble protein. The form of fibrin that is circulating through blood is fibrinogen, which is soluble. Fibrinogen becomes fibrin through activation of the coagulation cascade with the enzyme **thrombin** as a key mediator. This process represents secondary hemostasis. The coagulation factors involved in the cascade are in an inactive form. In this cascade, one factor activates another factor, which then activates the next factor, hence the term *coagulation cascade*. Two important cofactors, fibrinogen and calcium, are necessary for the coagulation cascade. The aggregated platelets (i.e., platelet plug) have a phospholipid surface where secondary hemostasis reactions occur. Inactive precursor coagulation factors such as prothrombin become active thrombin. Calcium released by activated platelets is necessary for some of the coagulation factors (II, VII, IX, and X) to be activated. Vitamin K produced by the liver produces the inactive (precursors) for these same factors (II, VII, IX, and X).

The coagulation cascade can be divided into the intrinsic and extrinsic pathway that both lead to a common pathway (**FIGURE 3-7**). The injured blood vessel triggers the extrinsic pathway tissue factor, which activates factor VII and, in turn, activates factor X. Activation of X leads to thrombin activation. Thrombin then activates intrinsic pathways going back up (XI, VIII, V, and VII), all contributing to fibrinogen becoming fibrin. The fibrin strands attach to the platelet plug (factor XIII) resulting in a fibrin meshed clot.

Coagulation inhibitors are important in containing the clotting area. Protein C and S along with antithrombin III inactivate

Diagnostic Link

Assessing Clotting or Hemostasis

The partial thromboplastin time (PTT) and activated clotting time are used to evaluate the intrinsic to common pathway (XII to I). The PTT is commonly used for managing heparin infusion dose. The prothrombin time (PT) is used to evaluate the extrinsic pathway except for tissue factor (III), so from VII, X, V to II to I. The PT is used to monitor warfarin dose. Thrombin time is used to measure how much time it takes for a clot to form and evaluates fibrinogen activity. While PT, PTT, and activated clotting time are quantitative studies, thromboelastography is used to qualitatively evaluate coagulopathic bleeding. Thromboelastography measures the physical properties of the clot in whole blood and shows the interaction of platelets with the coagulation cascade (e.g., aggregation, clot strengthening, fibrin linking, and fibrinolysis). The clinician can use results of thromboelastography to pinpoint the cause of the hemorrhaging and determine which transfusion agents are warranted (e.g., cryoprecipitate, platelets, or fresh frozen plasma).

coagulation factors. The fibrin clot needs to be dissolved through the fibrinolytic system, which is activated during the coagulation process. Thrombin that activated the coagulation process also triggers the fibrinolytic system by stimulating inactive plasminogen to become active plasmin. Plasminogen is also activated by tissue plasminogen activator (t-PA) and urokinase. Plasminogen activators can be produced and used as therapeutic fibrinolytic agents (e.g., recombinant t-PA [alteplase]; streptokinase) that are used for myocardial infarction (t-PA, streptokinase) or ischemic stroke (t-PA).

Lymphoid System

All the lymphoid organs connect the hematologic and immune systems. The components include the thymus, which is the site of T cell maturation, and the bone marrow, which is the site of hematopoiesis. From the bone marrow, the cells are released into the circulation. Other lymphoid organs include the spleen and lymph nodes. The spleen acts as a blood filter clearing out old or abnormal RBCs and any foreign material from the bloodstream.

Lymph nodes, which are masses of lymphocytes and fibers, are interspersed throughout the body along lymphatic channels. As lymph flows through these channels, foreign substances and microorganisms are destroyed, and the immune system is activated. The tonsils and adenoids are composed of lymphoid

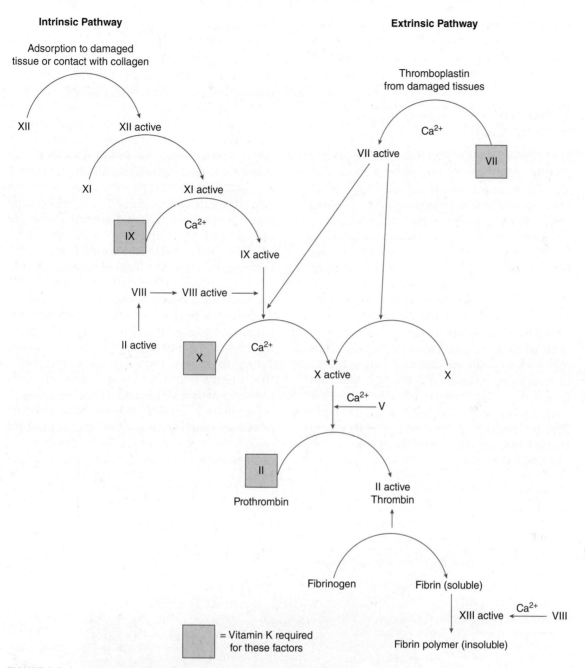

Intrinsic Pathway

Adsorption to damaged
tissue or contact with collagen

XII → XII active

XI → XI active

IX   Ca²⁺
IX active

VIII → VIII active →

II active

X   Ca²⁺

Extrinsic Pathway

Thromboplastin
from damaged tissues

Ca²⁺

VII active   VII

X active   X

Ca²⁺
← V

II
Prothrombin

II active
Thrombin

Fibrinogen   Fibrin (soluble)

XIII active   Ca²⁺ ← VIII

= Vitamin K required
for these factors

Fibrin polymer (insoluble)

FIGURE 3-7 Cascade of events leading to the activation of insoluble fibrin, which provides the structural foundation for a blood clot.

BOX 3-1 Application to Practice

Activity: Identify the part of the coagulation cascade in which the following medications have an effect and describe the effect: low molecular-weight heparin, unfractionated heparin, warfarin, direct thrombin inhibitors, and vitamin K.

tissue that form part of the immune system by trapping microorganisms that enter the nose or mouth. Lymphoid tissue such as Peyer patches is also found in the intestines.

Diseases of the White Blood Cells

Leukocytes are a diverse group of cells that trigger the inflammatory process and combat infections. Normal white blood cell (WBC) levels range from 5,000 to 10,000 cells/mL^3 of blood. Leukocytosis describes states characterized by increased WBC levels, and leukocytopenia refers to decreased WBC levels. Leukocytosis can indicate an active infectious process, whereas leukocytopenia can indicate an immune deficiency state (e.g., bone marrow suppression). The blood, by way of the circulatory system, transports leukocytes to the site of an infection. When the leukocytes arrive at the scene, they leak through the capillary wall to the site of trauma or invasion (FIGURE 3-8). Most leukocyte disorders originate from deficiencies of one or more of the varying leukocytes. Disorders are a result of increased production, increased destruction, alteration in function, or a combination.

Neutrophils

Usually the first responders to arrive on the scene of an infection or inflammation, neutrophils are attracted by various chemicals released by infected tissue (FIGURE 3-9). The increased number of neutrophils is known as *neutrophilia*. The term *granulocytosis* is often used to describe neutrophilia as neutrophils are the most abundant of granulocytes. The infection triggering neutrophil release is usually bacterial, but some viruses or fungi can also stimulate neutrophils. These cells escape from the capillary wall and migrate to the site of infection. Once they get to the site, neutrophils phagocytize microorganisms, preventing the infection from spreading. As the neutrophils are fully used, the infected cells die and become part of the yellowish wound drainage, or pus. When the demand for neutrophils is higher than the supply, the bone marrow starts releasing immature leukocytes. When there are increased immature cells, the balance is disrupted, and clinically, it is termed a *leukemoid reaction*. If the infection or inflammation subsides and the bone marrow produces more granulocytes, the neutrophil counts go back up. Physiologic transient increases can occur with stress or exercise

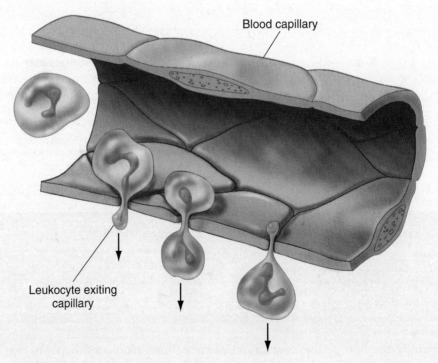

Blood capillary

Leukocyte exiting capillary

FIGURE 3-8 Leukocyte movement.

1. Foreign invaders signal nearby neutrophils to squeeze through endothelial cells that line the blood vessel and enter the infected tissue.

2. Through a cell-eating process known as phagocytosis, the neutrophil ingests the bacteria and releases toxic products that kill the bacteria.

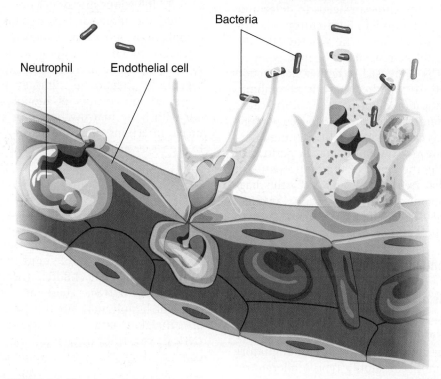

Bacteria

Neutrophil   Endothelial cell

FIGURE 3-9 The role of neutrophils.

or during the third trimester of pregnancy and labor.

Neutropenia is the opposite of neutrophilia and refers to a decrease in circulating neutrophils to fewer than 1,500 cells/mL (the normal range is 2,000–7,500 cells/mL). When fewer of these first responders are available, the body is poorly equipped to fight infections. The degree to which the body can fight infections, especially bacterial infections, is related to the severity of the neutropenia. In other words, the lower the neutrophil count, the lower the body's ability to fight infections. Causes of neutropenia may include infection and inflammation that are severe and/or prolonged. With severe and prolonged conditions, the usage of neutrophil increases and the bone marrow cannot keep up with the demand. The bone marrow may also be suppressed due to therapies (e.g., radiation, immunosuppressants, chemotherapy) or diseases such as aplastic anemia and leukemia, which will all cause neutropenia. Periodic or cyclic congenital conditions are usually associated with defects in production. Neutropenia can be due to inadequate amounts of vitamins and other nutrients such as vitamin B_{12} and folate, which are necessary for hematopoiesis. At times, demand may be normal and production intact, but the cells are being destroyed in the circulation or sequestered. Hemodialysis, autoimmune disorders, and splenic disorders such as Felty syndrome lead to increased destruction.

Clinical Manifestations

Clinical manifestations of neutropenia initially include signs and symptoms of bacterial and fungal infections (e.g., malaise, chills, and fever). The respiratory tract is the most common site of infection. Mouth ulcerations are also often associated with neutropenia, as are ulcerations of the skin, vagina, and gastrointestinal tract. Other manifestations of neutropenia will be dependent on the cause. Clinical manifestations of neutrophilia are also dependent on the cause (e.g., fever with infections).

Diagnosis and Treatment

Diagnostic procedures center primarily on serum neutrophil levels and determining the cause of the neutropenia or neutrophilia. For neutrophilia, the clinician needs to determine why the demand is high. For neutropenia, the clinician needs to determine whether the demand is higher than what can be met, whether production is decreased, whether destruction is increased, or whether there is a combination. Identification and treatment of the cause are important, particularly with neutropenia as low levels can lead to life-threatening infections. A bone marrow biopsy may be performed to determine the cause of the neutropenia or neutrophilia. Treatment is guided by the diagnosis. Antibiotic therapy is used to treat infections as they develop. Hematopoietic growth factors such as granulocyte colony-stimulating factor may be used to stimulate maturation and differentiation of neutrophils.

Eosinophils and Basophils

The number of eosinophils and basophils in circulation is low in comparison to neutrophils. Eosinophils are involved in the inflammatory response, most commonly type 1 allergic responses and asthma. These cells help control and augment the inflammatory response. Eosinophils can be high with parasitic infections as they have toxins that can destroy parasites. Eosinophilia can also occur with malignancies or drugs. Basophils are involved in the inflammatory response and release histamine and other mediators. Basophilia can occur during immediate hypersensitivity reactions such as food allergies or hives. Since eosinophil and basophil counts are already low, the significance of eosinopenia or basopenia is usually clinically insignificant.

Lymphocytes and Monocytes

Lymphocytes are one of the key cells involved in the immune response. Increased lymphocytes (lymphocytosis) is more likely to occur with viral infections such as hepatitis, herpes, or cytomegalovirus but may also occur with some bacterial infections such as pertussis. Since lymphocytes are derived from the lymphoid stem cells, lymphocytosis can occur with lymphocytic leukemia and lymphoma. Decreased lymphocytes (lymphocytopenia) occurs in immunodeficiency syndromes such as AIDS or due to destruction such as what occurs from radiation or chemotherapy. Lymphocyte

disorders that are nonhematologic are covered in various respective chapters. Infectious mononucleosis which is commonly caused by the Epstein-Barr virus (EBV), causes a lymphocytosis. In infectious mononucleosis, the pharynx is often the target and pharyngitis the initial complaint. Monocyte alterations (monocytosis) often accompany neutrophil alterations. Since monocyte counts are normally low, monocytopenia in isolation is clinically insignificant. Repeated low counts of monocytes can occur with bone marrow failure or some leukemias. Infectious mononucleosis is discussed in the *Upper Airway* section of chapter 5.

Lymphomas

Lymphomas are cancers that develop from malignant lymphocytes in the lymphoid tissues. They are the most common blood cancers, and lymphoma is the seventh most common cancer in adults and the fifth most common cancer in children (American Cancer Society, 2018). There are several subtypes of lymphoma, but the two main types are Hodgkin and non-Hodgkin lymphoma (NHL). Non-Hodgkin lymphoma is far more common than Hodgkin lymphoma (HL). Risk factors for both types of lymphoma include infection with the human immunodeficiency virus (HIV) or EBV. Additional risk factors for non-Hodgkin lymphoma include 1) the presence of an inherited immune or autoimmune condition, 2) infection with *Helicobacter pylori* or human T-cell leukemia/lymphoma virus type 1 (HTLV-1), and 3) exposure to pesticides.

Hodgkin Lymphoma

Hodgkin lymphoma can start in any lymph node of the lymphatic system, but most often arises in the lymph nodes of the upper body (e.g., neck, chest, and upper arms). The affected lymph nodes swell and compress surrounding tissue. Systemically, the cancer cells spread from one lymph node to the next through the lymphatic vessels. In rare cases, the disease spreads into the blood vessels and other structures, in a process that continues until late in the disease.

The two main types of HL are classical Hodgkin lymphoma (four subtypes), which accounts for 95% of HL, and nodular lymphocyte predominant Hodgkin lymphoma, which accounts for the remaining 5%. The types of lymphoma differ in the way the cancer cells appear under a microscope. Identification of which type the patient is experiencing is important because they

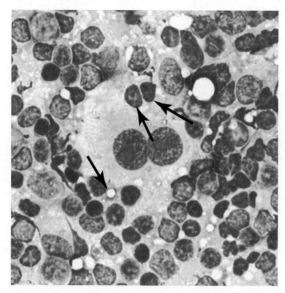

FIGURE 3-10 Reed-Sternberg cells associated with Hodgkin lymphoma.

© David A. Litman/Shutterstock.

grow and spread in different ways, and they are often treated differently.

The cancer cells of classic HL are unique; they are called *Reed-Sternberg cells* or *Hodgkin cells* (FIGURE 3-10). These cells are an abnormal type of B lymphocyte that is much larger than normal lymphocytes and do not look or function like normal B cells. The Reed-Sternberg cells, while low in numbers, can attract other cells; the cells become mixed together and the other cells become part of the neoplasm. The Reed-Sternberg cells are thought to arise from germinal centers and then proliferate into the lymphoid tissue. The germinal center is the location in lymph nodes or the spleen where mature B lymphocytes proliferate and differentiate into memory B cells or plasma cells. The germinal center is also the site where hypermutation of B cells' immunoglobulin genes occurs, so they can recognize and bind to antigens. During hypermutation (i.e., normal gene rearrangements), the cells are at risk for mutations that become oncogenic. Errors in immunoglobulin gene arrangement result in defective lymphocytes. In HL, T lymphocytes also appear to have defects, contributing to a total lymphocyte decrease.

The incidence of classic HL is on the decline. Classic HL occurs primarily in adults 20–40 years of age, with equal prevalence across genders. A second peak occurrence is seen in men older than 55 years of age. Due to improvements in the treatment of classic HL, mortality has decreased by nearly 50% over the past 25 years. Over the same period, incidence has

remained relatively steady. Prognosis is further improved when the disease is localized and is treated early, with many cases considered cured.

Nodular lymphocyte predominant Hodgkin lymphoma, in contrast to classic HL, has a different type of Reed-Sternberg cell called *lymphohistiocytic cells*. These cells retain normal B cells' features and function, and the pathogenesis is unclear. The Epstein-Barr virus is implicated in classic HL but not nodular lymphocyte predominant HL. This type of HL tends to be more localized and grows slowly. Males are affected more than females. As in classic HL, there is peak incidence in children and then again in adults (around 30–40 years). The survival rate is high (> 80%).

Clinical Manifestations

In up to 80% of patients, HL presents with a painless, enlarged lymph node in the neck and/or supraclavicular area. The other areas of lymphadenopathy include the axilla or inguinal nodes. The second most common initial presentation is the finding of a mediastinal mass on a chest X-ray. The mass may cause symptoms of retrosternal chest pain, cough, and difficulty breathing. Mediastinal nodes, which are not accessible on physical exam, are often seen on imaging studies. Although not as common, lymphadenopathy can occur in areas not accessible on physical exam (e.g., retroperitoneal area, mesentery) and in palpable areas (e.g., popliteal and epitrochlear areas). Persistent fever (> 100.4°F), night sweats, and unexplained weight loss (> 10% over 6 months) are called *B symptoms*. B symptoms can occur over weeks to months and are a sign of more advanced HL disease. Fatigue, malaise, and splenomegaly may occur. Pruritus, when associated with cancer, is termed *paraneoplastic pruritus* and occurs before or during the development of the cancer. In 10–30% of patients with HL, pruritus develops at some point during their disease course.

Clinical manifestations of the less common, nodular lymphocytic-predominant HL, vary from the classic. Most patients at presentation are in the early stages. Lymphadenopathy tends to be chronic. A mediastinal mass or B symptoms are not as common on initial presentation.

Diagnosis and Treatment

Diagnostic procedures primarily center on biopsy of the affected lymph node. Biopsy samples reveal the presence of Reed-Sternberg

Fever
Wt loss
Night sweats

cells for classic HL or lymphohistiocytic cells for nonclassic HL. Other diagnostic procedures consist of a physical examination, complete blood count, and chest X-rays.

A staging system is used to grade the severity and progression of the disease (FIGURE 3-11):

- **Stage I:** The lymphoma cells are in one lymph node group (such as in the neck or the underarm), or if the lymphoma cells are not in the lymph nodes, they are in only one part of a tissue or an organ (such as the lung).
- **Stage II:** The lymphoma cells are in at least two lymph node groups on the same side of (either above or below) the diaphragm, or the lymphoma cells are in one part of a tissue or an organ and the lymph nodes near that organ (on the same side of the diaphragm). Lymphoma cells may be in other lymph node groups on the same side of the diaphragm.
- **Stage III:** The lymphoma cells are in lymph nodes above and below the diaphragm. Lymphoma cells may be found in one part of a tissue or an organ (such as the liver, lung, or bone) near these lymph node groups. The cells may also be found in the spleen.
- **Stage IV:** Lymphoma cells are found in several parts of one or more organs or tissues, or the lymphoma cells are in an organ (such as the liver, lung, or bone) and in distant lymph nodes.
- **Recurrent:** The disease returns after treatment.

Staging is determined through the use of a computed tomography scan, magnetic resonance imaging, positron emission tomography scan, and bone marrow biopsy. Other staging procedures may include biopsies of other lymph nodes, the liver, or other tissue. After diagnosis, cancer treatment includes a combination of chemotherapy and radiation. Other treatments include bone marrow or stem cell transplant. With treatment, cure is likely in 75% of cases.

Non-Hodgkin Lymphoma

Non-Hodgkin lymphoma (NHL) consists of a diverse group of malignancies. NHL can start at any age and in any lymph node but is more common in middle-aged to older adults. NHL accounts for 90% of lymphomas, while HL accounts for the remaining 10%. Non-Hodgkin lymphoma is more common in Whites compared to other ethnic groups. NHL malignancies are derived from mature B cells or T cells or their precursors and less commonly from natural killer cells. Each category of NHL has many subtypes. Approximately 5% of all childhood cancers are NHL, and three subtypes account for almost all pediatric cases of

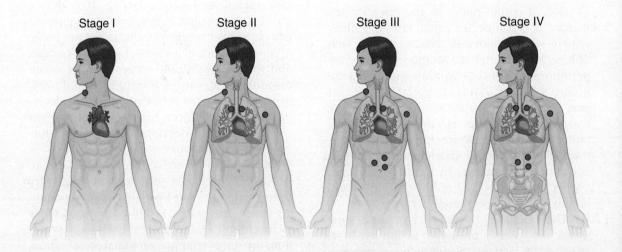

Stage I   Stage II   Stage III   Stage IV

● Site of lymphoma

FIGURE 3-11 Stages of Hodgkin lymphoma.

NHL (**TABLE 3-2**). Childhood NHL tends to be aggressive and fast growing. As with HL, B cells at the germinal center and T cell receptors must undergo normal gene rearrangements to be effective in the immune system. Errors can lead to defective lymphocytes. Three viruses associated with some NHL subtypes include Epstein-Barr virus, HTLV-1, and human herpesvirus 8. These oncogenic viruses integrate their genome into target cells. The genetic alterations that occur are mainly chromosomal translocations. With NHL, no Reed-Sternberg cells are present. Risk factors associated with non-Hodgkin lymphoma development include 1) the presence of an inherited immune or autoimmune condition, 2) infection exposure such as *Helicobacter pylori*, 3) toxins such as hair dyes or agricultural pesticides, 4) obesity, and 5) inflammatory gastrointestinal diseases such as Crohn disease or celiac disease.

Clinical Manifestations

NHL can be divided into aggressive (fast-growing) and indolent (slow-growing) types. Aggressive types (e.g., diffuse, large B-cell lymphoma, Burkitt lymphoma) will usually present acutely, with rapid mass growth, and B symptoms. Death can result within a few weeks without treatment. Indolent types (e.g., follicular lymphoma) may present with slowly developing lymphadenopathy, hepatomegaly, or splenomegaly. Patients may present with gastrointestinal tract lymphoma with symptoms such as anorexia, nausea, vomiting, and weight loss. Patients may have central nervous system lymphoma and present with headache, seizures, and lethargy. Other symptoms vary greatly across patients and some symptoms, such as pruritus, fatigue, and malaise, are similar to HL. In comparison to HL, NHL involves multiple nodes scattered throughout the body, and metastasis occurs in an unorganized manner. Metastasis is often present at diagnosis.

Diagnosis and Treatment

Diagnostic tests and staging are similar to HL. Other diagnostic tests may include tumor markers, immunoglobulin studies, lumbar puncture, and serology tests for HIV and hepatitis. Treatment is dependent on the subtype and can include chemotherapy, radiation therapy, immunotherapy, or a combination of these. The prognosis for patients with this disease varies with each subtype, but it is worse than HL. While treatments are improving, survivors are at risk for long-term complications of therapy such as secondary malignancies, cardiovascular disorders, or endocrine disorders.

TABLE 3-2	Non-Hodgkin Lymphoma in Children and Adolescents		
Type	**Epidemiology U.S.**	**Common clinical presentation**	**Special notes**
Burkitt lymphoma Origin: B lymphocytes Most linked to EBV	40% More common in males Age 5–10 years; peak 4–6 years	Abdominal mass, pain, nausea, vomiting, and change in bowel patterns Rapid growing head and neck lymphadenopathy	One of the most aggressive fast-growing cancers Cases in Africa account for almost all NHL. Over 50% of childhood cancers develop in the jaw or other facial bones
Lymphoblastic lymphoma Origin: precursor B or precursor T lymphocytes (T more common)	25–30% Males 2× more likely Median diagnosis 12	T cell: thymus—retrosternal or anterior tracheal mass with difficulty breathing, chest pain; susceptibility to infections B cell: painless lymphadenopathy in the neck Both: B symptoms	Aggressive, fast growing > 25% bone marrow lymphoblast categorized as acute lymphocytic leukemia
Large-cell lymphoma Origin: Mature T cells Anaplastic or mature B cell for diffuse large B cell	Older children and teens Anaplastic: 10% (median age 12) Diffuse large B cell: 15%	Mass anywhere in the body Diffuse large B cell: mediastinal mass or neck/abdomen lymph nodes Anaplastic: painless lymphadenopathy, fever, malaise	Not as aggressive as other lymphomas with rare metastasis to brain

Multiple Myeloma

Multiple myeloma (MM) is a cancer of the plasma cells that most often affects older adults. Because the plasma cells originate from B cells, MM is classified as a type of NHL. According to the American Cancer Society (2018), multiple myeloma is the third most common type of blood cancer. Over the past 20 years, incidence and mortality rates have remained relatively stable. The median age at diagnosis is 66, and rates are low before the age of 50 (10%). MM is more common in men than women. Additionally, Blacks have about twice the incidence and mortality rates of Whites.

In most cases, prior to the develop of MM and for unclear reasons, normal plasma cells begin to respond abnormally to antigens. The abnormal plasma cells make monoclonal (one type of) antibodies, and at this stage, the disorder is called *monoclonal gammopathy of undetermined significance*. These abnormal plasma cells are vulnerable, and if exposed to further insults such as genetic mutations, the condition can progress to MM. Other less common precursor plasma cell abnormalities such as smoldering myeloma or solitary plasmacytomas can also lead to MM, but monoclonal gammopathy of undetermined significance is the most common. The abnormal plasma cells overproduce abnormal immunoglobulins that are intact or in fragments. The type of abnormal immunoglobulin that is usually produced is IgG and at times IgA. The most common chromosomal abnormalities in MM, as in many other hematologic cancers, are translocations. Deletions (e.g., of chromosome 17) and chromosomal number alterations (e.g., trisomy-47 chromosomes) can also cause MM. In MM, proto-oncogenes (e.g., *RAS*) are activated and tumor suppressor genes such as p53 are inactivated. The genetic alterations seem to occur during B-cell development in the bone marrow. After leaving the bone marrow, the abnormal B cells become activated by an antigen and differentiate into abnormal plasma cells with stimulation from T helper cells in germinal centers. The abnormal plasma cells then migrate back to the bone marrow, which normally contains 5% of plasma cells but after migration are > 10% in the bone marrow. The result of this bone marrow infiltration is bone destruction. In the bone marrow, the malignant plasma cells bind to bone marrow stromal cells, which regulate hematopoiesis.

Under normal circumstances, bone-building cells called *osteoblasts* regulate bone resorption by bone-chiseling osteoclasts. Osteoblasts regulate resorption by secreting the protein RANKL, which binds to RANK on the osteoclast, leading to osteoclastic activity. Osteoblasts can also secrete osteoprotegerin, which inhibits binding and, therefore, decreases osteoclastic activity. Various cytokines are produced, which affect osteoblastic and osteoclastic activity, and there is an abnormal response by the plasma cells in MM. Interleukin 3, as an example, leads to decrease osteoblast production. Interleukin 6 and tumor factor MIP1 α stimulates osteoclastic activity. The malignant plasma cells of MM secrete substances that decrease osteoprotegerin production and increase RANKL; therefore, osteoclastic activity increases. Ultimately, the balance is tipped toward increased bone resorption causing bone thinning, fractures, and bone pain. The bone breakdown causes calcium to be released, resulting in hypercalcemia.

The plasma cell interactions with the stromal bone marrow cells provide an excellent environment for proliferation, survival, and migration of the malignant plasma cells. The abnormal immunoglobulin produced by the plasma cells are called *paraproteins* or *M proteins*, with the *M* standing for *monoclonal antibody*. While albumin is usually the most common protein in blood, the M protein predominates due to the proliferation of malignant plasma cells. Immunoglobulins are glycoproteins that consist of two heavy chains that are different in each of the five classes (e.g., IgA or IgD) and two light chains. In MM, plasma cells produce not only abnormal immunoglobulins but also free light chains. The free light chains are small and pass through the kidneys. In the kidneys, amyloid deposits are formed, and these are detected in the urine as Bence Jones proteins. The free light chains can also build up in the liver, spleen, and heart. Increased infections occur due to suppression of normal B cells by the malignant cells.

Clinical Manifestations

The onset of multiple myeloma is usually insidious, and malignancy is often well advanced upon diagnosis. Clinical manifestations of multiple myeloma can be remembered with use of the acronym CRAB (hypercalcemia [using the *C*], renal failure, anemia, bone lesions). Hypercalcemia causes neuromuscular dysfunction. Anemia, due to decreased erythropoiesis and renal failure, causes manifestations such as fatigue, pallor, dyspnea, and decreased activity tolerance. Bone lesions cause bone pain, and on imaging studies such as X-rays, lytic or punched-out lesions can be seen. The bones involved in MM are usually the vertebrae, ribs, pelvis/femur, clavicle, and scapula. Infections of the lungs (e.g., pneumonia) and urinary tract (e.g., pyelonephritis) are more common due to leukopenia.

Diagnosis and Treatment

The diagnosis of multiple myeloma is often made incidentally during routine blood tests or imaging studies that are done while evaluating other conditions. The criteria for multiple myeloma includes monoclonal antibodies in bone marrow, urine, or blood as well as one or more of the CRAB features. Patients with suspected multiple myeloma should all have a serum protein electrophoresis which is used to analyze monoclonal proteins. The serum protein electrophoresis can detect the presence of M-protein and allows for measurement of the size of the M protein. The higher the amount of M protein, the higher the disease burden. Several other tests can be performed such as serum immunofixation to further determine whether the type of monoclonal protein is heavy or light chain. Bence Jones proteins may be present in urine or serum and are characteristic of MM. X-rays can be done but are not sensitive in detecting lesions. Imaging is important in the evaluation of MM and should consist of whole body, computed tomography, positron emission tomography or magnetic resonance imaging to evaluate bone destruction.

Multiple myeloma is not considered curable, but chemotherapy improves the remission rate. Additional treatments may include corticosteroids, angiogenesis inhibitors, targeted therapies, stem cell transplant, biologic therapy, radiation therapy, and supportive care. The median survival time is 3 years. Analgesics are used to treat bone pain. Blood dyscrasias, hypercalcemia, and renal impairment are treated as needed.

Myelodysplastic Syndrome

Myelodysplastic syndrome (MDS) is characterized as a group of hematopoietic stem cell neoplasms that result in abnormal cell growth, differentiation, and maturation. The cells affected can include red blood cells, platelets, and mature granulocytes. Nearly one in three people with MDS will develop acute myeloid leukemia (AML). MDS was once considered a preleukemia and a disorder of low malignant potential, but with increasing evidence, it is now considered a hematologic malignancy. The incidence of MDS increases greatly with age especially after 40 years, and the median age at diagnosis is 72 years. The overall incidence and prevalence is not clear as there have been inconsistent classifications and underreporting of cases; however, MDS is considered a common hematologic malignancy. Most cases of MDS are thought to occur from years of acquired accumulated somatic mutations that occur with aging. Over 50 recurrently mutated genes have been identified, and people with MDS have at least one and often more than one mutation. Other less common causes include mutation caused by environmental exposure (e.g., radiation, chemotherapy) or inherited mutations predisposing a person to myeloid disorders such as leukemia. The somatic mutations occur in the multipotent myeloid progenitor cell. These mutations cause change in precursor and mature cell morphology (e.g., shape, structure), abnormal differentiation, and, ultimately, various cytopenias (e.g., anemia, leukopenia, thrombocytopenia). The mutated cells' microenvironment and host immune response will significantly influence the clinical manifestations of the disease. There are six main types of MDS recognized by the World Health Organization classification of 2016, each with varying diagnostic criteria and prognosis.

Clinical Manifestations

Patients can be asymptomatic. Clinical manifestations are related to the type of cytopenia. Anemia manifestations, depending on the severity, may cause pallor, weakness, fatigue, and shortness of breath. Thrombocytopenia may cause bleeding disorders. Those individuals with neutropenia will have a higher chance of infections and manifest symptoms such as fever. Generalized arthralgia and bone pain can be an initial complaint. Weight loss and anorexia may be present.

Diagnosis and Treatment

A complete history and physical examination are necessary. Diagnosis is based on the presence of one or more cytopenias that is otherwise unexplained. A complete blood count will often reveal anemia, which is present in 85% of patients, and neutropenia in approximately 50% of patients. Thrombocytopenia is evident in 25–50% of cases. Bone marrow biopsy will be conducted and a high blast cell percentage (>5- ≤ 19%) will be present. Genetic testing will reveal various mutational abnormalities. In order

BOX 3-2 Application to Practice

Match the case/descriptors with the most likely disorder.

	Case/descriptor	Disorder
A	Usually presents as painless, enlarged lymph node in neck	Hodgkin lymphoma A
C	Bence Jones proteins	Non-Hodgkin lymphoma B
A	Reed-Sternberg cells	Multiple myeloma C
C	Hypercalcemia, bone pain	Myelodysplastic syndrome D
D	One third of cases progress to acute myelogenous leukemia	
D	Most will present with anemia and neutropenia	
B	Lymphohistiocytic cells	
B	Burkitt lymphoma is a type	
C	Black men more commonly affected than White men	
C	Metastasis often present at diagnosis	

to diagnose MDS, the clinical manifestations and diagnostic findings cannot be explained by another disorder such as human immunodeficiency virus (HIV), autoimmune disorders (e.g., systemic lupus erythematosus, immune thrombocytopenic purpura), or leukemia. Estimating prognosis is important to determine the likely course of the disease and inform treatment. Prognosis-estimating systems (e.g., World Health Organization prognostic scoring system) can be used to determine disease outlook. Risks and benefits of treatment need to be considered relative to the disease prognosis. Treatments may include observation only and supportive care such as antibiotics for infections or transfusions (e.g., platelet, red blood cell). Treatments can also include hematopoiesis growth factors such as erythropoiesis-stimulating agents, chemotherapy, and stem cell transplant.

Leukemias

Leukemia is a cancer of the leukocytes. With this disease, the bone marrow stem cells make abnormal leukocytes, or leukemia cells, that then travel through the vascular system affecting different organs. The proliferation and differentiation issues occur in mature or primitive leukocytes. Unlike normal blood cells, leukemia cells do not die when they should, so they sometimes begin crowding normal leukocytes, erythrocytes, and thrombocytes. This crowding makes it difficult for normal blood cells to function properly. The exact cause of leukemia is unknown.

According to the American Cancer Society (2018), leukemia is the ninth most common cancer in adults. Leukemia, specifically acute lymphoblastic leukemia, is the most common cancer among children; although, it affects 10 times as many adults as children. Incidence rates remained relatively consistent from 1999 to 2018, but the mortality rates decreased. Men are more likely to develop leukemia than are women. Other risk factors include exposure to chemical, viral, and radiation mutagens; smoking; use of chemotherapies; certain disease conditions (e.g., Down syndrome); and immunodeficiency disorders.

Leukemias are grouped on the basis of their cell line (myeloid or lymphoid) and as either acute (mostly primitive cells) or chronic (mostly mature cells). Acute leukemias tend to have a more rapid onset and progression. Chronic leukemias, in contrast, are more insidious in onset and less aggressive. The four most common types of leukemia include:

- Acute lymphoblastic leukemia (ALL)
- Acute myeloid leukemia (AML)
- Chronic lymphoid leukemia (CLL)
- Chronic myeloid leukemia (CML)

Acute Leukemias

The acute leukemias are characterized by abnormalities in immature (precursor) leukocytes. These immature cells are termed *blast* cells and are categorized based on their progenitor stem cell line origin—myeloblasts are from the myeloid line while lymphoblasts are from the lymphoid line (B progenitor cells or T progenitor cells). Of the acute leukemias, the incidence of AML is approximately 80% for adults and 20% in children. In children, the highest incidence occurs before the age of 1 and declines thereafter but increases with age again. The median age of diagnosis is 65–70. The overall incidence of AML in comparison to other cancers is rare. ALL is more common in children. ALL accounts for 75% of all leukemias and 29% of all types of cancers in children (CDC, 2014). The median age for diagnosis is 13, but the risk is highest in children less than 5 years of age. ALL peaks again after age 50 and accounts for approximately 20% of the acute leukemia incidences in adults. Slightly more males are affected with AML and ALL, and non-Hispanic Whites have the highest incidence.

The general pathogenesis of the acute leukemias involves genetic and epigenetic changes in precursor cells that lead to abnormal proliferation, differentiation, maturation, and resistance to apoptosis (cell death). A small pool of cells amongst the leukemic cells have stem cell–like properties and can self-renew and maintain the leukemic state. The leukemic cells can crowd out the bone marrow, or normal hematopoiesis can be inhibited leading to a reduction in erythrocytes, thrombocytes, and other leukocytes.

The acute leukemias are genetically and phenotypically heterogenous. There are numerous subtypes of ALL and AML. Chromosomal alterations can include deletions (e.g., chromosome 5, 7, 9), inversions (e.g., 16), and translocations (swapping of DNA—the most common alteration). Some examples of translocations in adults with ALL include the translocation at 4 and 11 or a translocation of chromosome 9 and 22, which is known as the *Philadelphia chromosome*. Other examples of genetic alterations include defects in tumor protein p53 or Wilms tumor 1 gene (tumor suppressor genes) allowing for proliferation. Most mutations are not inherited but rather acquired or are new (*de novo*). Identification of the subtype is important as it defines severity, influences prognosis, and guides treatment.

Several risk factors are associated with the development and/or are causes of acute leukemia. Environmental factors include radiation exposure, chemotherapy, tobacco, or toxins such as benzene. The presence of other blood disorders such as myelodysplastic syndrome can lead to AML. Familial genetic or congenital abnormalities such as Down syndrome (trisomy 21), neurofibromatosis, or Fanconi anemia can increase risk. Other disorders that increase risks include HIV infection or thyroid disease. Obesity may be a risk factor. Despite the various risk factors, often exposure to an antecedent is not present and no etiologic factor is found.

Clinical Manifestations

Acute leukemia clinical manifestations can be a result of the cytopenias. Anemia will cause pallor, fatigue, weakness, dyspnea, and dizziness. These symptoms are often out of proportion to the anemia. Thrombocytopenia may cause bruising, petechiae, and increased bleeding, such as from the nose and gums. Infections can be minor or recurrent, and fever may be present. Infections are related to the degree of neutropenia. Various other symptoms may include unintentional weight loss and anorexia. Bone and joint pains are more common in ALL, particularly in children. Physical findings, which are more common in ALL, include lymphadenopathy, hepatomegaly, and splenomegaly. Extramedullary sites of accumulated leukemic cells may lead to a variety of systemic manifestations such as leukemia cutis or cutaneous lesions. Although not as common, other systems such as the central nervous system can be affected. If the central nervous system is involved, the patient may complain of headache, seizures, and vision and balance problems. Other organ involvement can include the gonads and eyes. Since ALL and lymphoma originate from B cell or T cell disease, the two types of lymphoid cancers have many overlapping features (see *Lymphomas* section).

Diagnosis and Treatment

Diagnostic procedures include a history, physical examination, peripheral blood smears, complete blood count, and bone marrow biopsy. Laboratory findings will include anemia and thrombocytopenia. Leukemic blast cells (e.g., myeloblasts or lymphoblasts) will be present. Bone marrow biopsy and aspirate will reveal blast cells ($\geq$ 20% for leukemia), chromosomal abnormalities, and abnormal morphology. Histiochemical staining of blood or bone marrow will be used to identify the type of leukemia.

The goal of treatment is complete remission. Maintenance therapy may be necessary. Chemotherapy is the mainstay of treatment for leukemia, and several courses may be necessary to eradicate the cancer. Chemotherapy is more effective for the acute types of leukemia than for the chronic types. Bone marrow transplants may be attempted if chemotherapy is unsuccessful. Other treatments may include targeted therapy, radiation, biologic therapy, surgery, and donor lymphocyte infusion.

Chronic Leukemias

The chronic leukemias are characterized by abnormal proliferation of more mature cells. The cells have a similar appearance to normal cells but function abnormally. These leukemic cells are present in blood and bone marrow. CLL is the most common leukemia in adults. As with ALL, considerable overlap exists between CLL and lymphomas. Distinctions are made primarily by whether proliferation is in the blood (CLL) or is nodal (lymphoma). The median age of diagnosis is 70 years old, and CLL is rarely diagnosed in people under 40 years old. CML is more common in adults and almost all cases are in people over 50 years old. In both CLL and CML, risk is slightly higher in men and Whites have a higher incidence than other ethnicities.

The general pathogenesis of CLL involves proliferation of mostly mature malignant B cells. T cell involvement is rare. Hematopoiesis may be affected but is not as severe as in ALL. How the B cells transform is not well understood; however, CLL development is considered to be an interplay between genetics, epigenetics, and the microenvironment. Genetic factors are more likely than environmental risks such as pesticide exposure in the cause or risk for CLL.

CML is characterized by proliferation of mostly mature and maturing granulocytes that are fairly well differentiated. The several forms of CML depend on the lineage (e.g., neutrophils, eosinophils). CML is classified as myeloproliferative along with polycythemia vera, essential thrombocytosis, and primary myelofibrosis. In CML, the Philadelphia chromosome is present in 95% of patients, while in other leukemias, the chromosome is present but at a much lower rate (e.g., ALL 5–30%). The abnormal chromosome is created during a translocation of a segment on chromosome 9, known as the Abelson (ABL) proto-oncogene, with a region on chromosome 22, known as the breakpoint cluster region (BCR). This translocation results in a *BCR-ABL* fusion gene on chromosome 22—the Philadelphia chromosome. The gene causes abnormal production of myeloid cells, which then leads to the start of CML.

Clinical Manifestations

Most patients with CLL are asymptomatic at time of presentation. The most common abnormal physical finding is local or general lymphadenopathy with the upper part of the body (such as the cervical or axillary areas) frequently affected. Hepatomegaly and/or splenomegaly may be present. Other symptoms that are not as common at initial presentation include B symptoms which includes fever, night sweats, and unexplained weight loss. Neurologic or gastrointestinal involvement are not common. Manifestations at presentation will depend on the patient's current disease stage.

CML has three clinical phases—chronic, accelerated, and blast crisis phase. At diagnosis, most CML cases are in the chronic phase and are asymptomatic or have very few manifestations. While there are a few criteria for each phase, the phases are generally determined by the blasts in peripheral blood and bone marrow. The chronic phase consists of < 10% blasts, accelerated consists of 10–19% blasts, and blast crisis phase has > 20% blasts. As a person progresses through the phases, manifestations become more prevalent and may include fatigue, malaise, weight loss, diaphoresis, abdominal pain and fullness, hepatomegaly, and splenomegaly. Blast crisis in CML is similar to AML. Progression from one phase to the next may be slow in the beginning (e.g., 1–2 years) but progresses faster with aging.

Diagnosis and Treatment

Diagnosis of chronic leukemia is often made when a routine blood count comes back abnormal. CLL blood counts will reveal lymphocytosis; granulocytosis and monocytosis will be present with CML. Anemia or thrombocytopenia or thrombocytosis are usually mild. A peripheral blood smear and immunophenotyping will be done. Bone marrow aspirate and biopsy or nodal biopsy may be conducted. In CLL, immunoglobulins are not produced because plasma B cells do not differentiate; therefore, hypogammaglobulinemia (e.g., decreased IgG, IgA, or IgM) may occur.

BOX 3-3 Application to Practice

Review the case. Which type of leukemia (acute lymphocytic vs. acute myelogenous or chronic lymphocytic vs. chronic myelogenous) is most likely? Discuss the data supporting your decision.

Case

- A 13-year-old female presents with the recent onset of fatigue, fever 100°F, and epistaxis over the past week.

- She has no past medical history except for mononucleosis last year. She is generally very healthy.
- Physical exam findings unremarkable except for:
  - Pale conjunctiva
  - Multiple petechiae on lower legs
  - Abdomen soft with hepatosplenomegaly
  - Labs:

CBC	Result	Normal range
WBC	12.0 x10^3/mL	4.8–10.8 x10^3/mL
Hgb	8.0 g/dL	12.0–15.6 g/dL
Hct	25%	35–46%
RBC	5.0 x 10^6/mL	4.5–5.9 x10^6/mL
MCV	90 x µL/red cell	80–96.1 x µL/red cell
MCH	32 pg/red cell	27.5–33.2 pg/red cell
MCHC	31 g/L	33.4–35.5 g/L
Platelets	45,000/mL	150–400,000/mL
Blasts	85%	0%

CBC = complete blood count; WBC = white blood cells; Hgb = hemoglobin; Hct = hematocrit; RBC = red blood cells; MCV = mean corpuscular volume; MCH = mean corpuscular hemoglobin; MCHC = mean corpuscular hemoglobin concentration

Treatment may vary from observation to aggressive management with various therapeutic agents such as monoclonal antibodies, chemotherapy, radiation, and stem cell transplantation. Targeted therapy, such as tyrosine kinase inhibitors, which block BCR-ABL, are standard treatment for chronic-phase CML. Survival and prognosis is variable and dependent on the type of CLL or the phase of diagnosis for CML. Patients in the advanced CML phase are less responsive to treatment.

Diseases of the Red Blood Cells

Erythrocytes are the most prevalent blood cell in the human body—millions can be found in a single drop of blood (the normal range is 4.2–5.9 million cells/mL). These cells function primarily to transport oxygen to the tissue and the waste products for excretion. Most diseases of the red blood cells (RBCs) are related to the quantity or quality of the erythrocytes. Too few RBCs cause anemia and too many cause polycythemia vera.

Anemia

Anemia is a common acquired or inherited disorder of the erythrocytes that impairs the oxygen-carrying capacity of the blood. This condition can result from 1) a decreased production of RBCs such as from lack of requisites such as iron or bone marrow dysfunction and 2) increased loss of RBCs such as would occur with destruction or blood loss. Anemias can be classified in different ways. One classification is by the cause of the anemia (e.g., increased destruction, blood loss, inadequate production); however, these categories can overlap (**TABLE 3-3**). Another common classification

TABLE 3-3	Anemias by Etiology

Inadequate production	Examples
Lack of requisites—bone marrow functioning	• Iron: dietary lacking, chronic blood loss, decreased absorption, decreased release • B$_{12}$: dietary lacking, absorption • Folic acid: dietary lacking, absorption
Bone marrow dysfunction	• Anemia of chronic disease/inflammation • Reduced precursors: not maturing (e.g., aplastic anemia) • Bone marrow suppression: drugs, chemotherapy, irradiation
Excessive loss	
Blood loss	External or internal
Defects shortening survival	Hemolytic anemia (e.g., sickle cell disease, thalassemia)

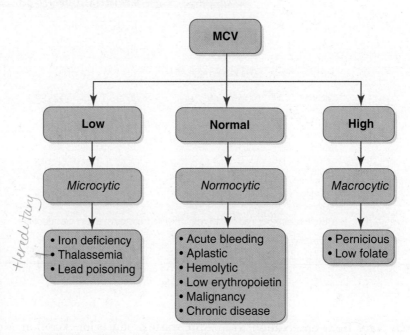

FIGURE 3-12 Mean corpuscular volume changes with anemia.

is by the morphology or hemoglobin content of the RBCs (e.g., microcytic-hypochromic) (**FIGURE 3-12**) (**TABLE 3-4**). In clinical practice, morphology is the more common classification used. Some anemias respond quickly to treatment and cause no sequelae; whereas others can cause lifelong problems. The clinical manifestations of anemia reflect the decreased oxygen-carrying capacity. Regardless of the cause of anemia, manifestations include weakness, fatigue, pallor, syncope, dyspnea, and tachycardia. The degree of symptomatology correlates with the severity of the anemia, with mild anemia causing fewer problems. Severe anemia can cause more pronounced symptoms, and compensatory mechanisms can become overwhelmed, resulting in an anemia that is life threatening. Compensatory mechanisms will involve the hematologic, cardiovascular, and respiratory systems by way of increased erythropoiesis, vasodilation to increase blood flow, and increased respiratory rate, respectively.

Anemia is diagnosed in adults (> 18 years of age) when hematocrit is less than 41% in males and less than 37% in females; that is, hemoglobin concentration falls to less than 13.5 g/dL in males and less than 12 g/dL in females. Hematocrit is the percentage of RBCs in whole blood and the hemoglobin is the concentration of hemoglobin in whole blood (Table 3-4). The RBC count is the number of red blood

TABLE 3-4	Common Labs in Anemia	
Test	**Purpose**	**Interpretation**
Hemoglobin (Hgb)	Amount of hemoglobin in blood	Low: anemia High: polycythemia
Hematocrit (Hct)	Percent of intact RBCs in whole blood	Low: anemia High: polycythemia
Mean corpuscular volume (MCV)	Average volume of patient RBCs	Low: microcytic High: macrocytic Normal: normocytic
Mean corpuscular hemoglobin concentration (MCHC)	Average concentration of hemoglobin per RBC (size of RBC taken into account)	Low: hypochromic High: hyperchromic Normal: normochromic
Mean corpuscular hemoglobin (MCH)	Amount of Hgb per RBC	Alterations same reasons as MCV
Red cell distribution width	Variations in sizes of the RBCs (i.e., anisocytosis)	Low: uniformity in size High: large variation in RBC size or shape (i.e., poikilocytosis)
Reticulocyte count	Immature erythrocytes	Low: problems with production of RBCs High: increased need for RBCs
Plasma iron	Requisite for Hgb synthesis (heme component)	Low: increased need, lack of intake, poor absorption High: increased absorption, excess intake
Total iron-binding capacity (TIBC)	Amount of iron capable of binding to transferrin (indirect measure of transferrin availability)	Low: excess iron High: deficiency in iron
Transferrin	Transports iron around circulation (TIBC can be used as indirect measure)	Low: excess iron High: deficiency in iron
Transferrin saturation	Amount of transferrin saturated with iron	Low: deficiency in iron High: excess iron
Ferritin	Stored iron	Low: deficiency in iron High: excess iron; acute phase reactant so may be high independent from iron stores
B_{12}	Requisite for RBC production	Low: B_{12} deficiency High: liver disease; myeloproliferative disorders
Folate	Requisite for RBC production	Low: folate deficiency

cells in the volume of whole blood. Normal values vary by age under the age of 18. Treatment depends on the specific type of anemia experienced.

Decreased Production of RBCs

When the bone marrow is functioning properly, a decrease in RBCs will result in precursor increase and an acceleration of erythropoiesis to make more reticulocytes. The factors necessary for stimulation of RBC production are erythropoietin and nutrients such as iron, vitamin B_{12}, and folic acid. Deficiencies in any of these will result in a decreased production leading to anemia. Bone marrow dysfunction in the form of suppression or inadequate precursors from disease or treatment will result in decreased RBC production. Iron deficiency anemia and megaloblastic anemia are disorders of decreased RBC production.

Iron Deficiency Anemia—Microcytic

According to the World Health Organization (2016), iron deficiency anemia is the most widespread anemia in the world. This type of anemia is most commonly seen in women of childbearing age, children younger than 2 years of age, and the elderly. Iron deficiency anemia occurs when the supply of iron necessary to produce hemoglobin is inadequate to meet the demand of hemoglobin production. It may be caused by decreased iron consumption, decreased iron absorption, or increased loss because of bleeding (e.g., menstruation, gastrointestinal cancer). Decreased iron intake is a common cause of deficiency, particularly in developing countries.

Iron is ingested through animal and plant sources. Although the average American ingests more than 10 mg of iron each day, which is within the recommended daily allowance, only about 10% of the ingested iron is actually absorbed. Infants, children, and adolescents need a higher intake of iron to meet the demands of rapid growth and increased muscle mass. In children, inadequate iron intake is usually the cause of anemia. Blood loss, whether overt or occult, is a more likely cause in U.S. adults as iron intake is usually adequate. Menstrual blood loss can cause approximately 1 mg of iron to be lost per day. Blood loss can occur acutely (e.g., as a result of trauma) or chronically (e.g., from gastrointestinal bleeding). Blood loss may not be overt, and evaluation for gastrointestinal malignancy is warranted with adults over 50 years old, nonmenstruating women, or those at risk for colorectal cancer. Problems of iron absorption are not as common as deficiencies due to decreased intake or blood loss. Absorption of iron occurs in the upper gastrointestinal tract (maximum in duodenum). Various disorders such as celiac disease, atrophic gastritis, *Helicobacter pylori* infection, and bariatric surgery affect the mucosal cells responsible for absorption through different mechanisms. When an iron deficiency exists, hemoglobin synthesis diminishes. Erythrocytes will become pale (hypochromic) because the cells have less hemoglobin and small (microcytic) because the cell is trying to accommodate to the decreased hemoglobin (**FIGURE 3-13**).

Clinical Manifestations

In addition to the previously mentioned anemia signs and symptoms (e.g., fatigue), the following clinical manifestations may be associated with iron deficiency anemia: cyanosis of sclera, brittle nails, spoon-shaped nails (koilonychia), decreased appetite especially in children, headache, irritability, stomatitis, unusual food cravings (pica), and delayed healing. Neurocognitive impairments can occur in the elderly, often manifested as confusion and memory loss. Children may develop irreversible neurologic damage without adequate iron, and manifestations could include slower visual and auditory processing, decreased attention span, learning difficulties, and motor impairment.

Diagnosis and Treatment

Diagnosis of iron deficiency anemia is made by conducting a history and physical as well as evaluating laboratory findings. Diagnostic procedures for iron deficiency anemia include a complete blood count, serum ferritin, serum iron, and transferrin saturation (see Table 3-4). Serum ferritin and iron levels will be low. Transferrin will be high as the body is trying to compensate for the low iron levels by increasing transport. TIBC is high so that more iron can be delivered. Despite an attempt to increase binding and transportation of iron, there is not enough iron to actually bind to transferrin so the transferrin saturation is low. Additional tests such as fecal occult blood test, colonoscopy, and endoscopy may be performed to determine the cause (see Figure 3-12). The American Academy of Pediatrics recommends

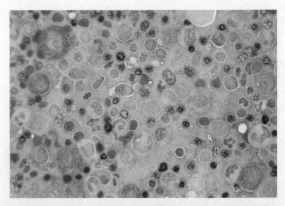

FIGURE 3-13 Iron deficiency anemia.
Courtesy of Dr. Gordon D. McLaren/CDC.

BOX 3-4 Application to Practice

Case 1: Mr. Hernandez is a 59-year-old Hispanic man who presents for an annual physical exam. He has no complaints or concerns at the visit.

Past medical history: hypertension.

Medications: lisinopril 10 mg orally every day.

Allergies: penicillin (causes hives).

Social history: truck driver, divorced. Quit smoking 5 years ago after smoking one pack per day for 20 years, drinks three to four beers a week.

Vital signs: temperature 98.6°F; pulse 74 beats per minute; respirations 18 breaths per minute; blood pressure 124/76 mm/Hg; body mass index 31.

Health maintenance: refuses the influenza shot; has never had a colonoscopy.

Family history: he is adopted.

His physical exam is unremarkable. Mr. Hernandez's complete metabolic profile was within normal limits and his complete blood count with differential revealed the following results:

CBC	Result	Normal range
WBC	9.0×10^3/mL	$4.8–10.8 \times 10^3$/mL
Hgb	10.6 g/dL	14–18.0 g/dL
Hct	32%	42–52%
RBC	3.20×10^6/mL	$4.7–6.1 \times 10^6$/mL
MCV	78 x μL/red cell	80–96.1 x μL/red cell
MCH	32 pg/red cell	27.5–33.2 pg/red cell
MCHC	31 g/L	33.4–35.5 g/L
Platelets	278/mL	150–400,000/mL

CBC = complete blood count; WBC = white blood cells; Hgb =hemoglobin; Hct = hematocrit; RBC = red blood cells; MCV = mean corpuscular volume; MCH = mean corpuscular hemoglobin; MCHC = mean corpuscular hemoglobin concentration

Answer the following questions based on this scenario:

Describe the type of anemia present (e.g., microcytic, macrocytic, normocytic) and list the results that support your decision.

Describe additional diagnostic tests to be ordered and explain why they will be ordered.

Describe the top two most likely diagnoses and explain why you made these choices.

Case 2: A 22-year-old man comes in because he was shaving and felt a lump on his neck. He states the lump is not painful and he noticed it about 2 weeks ago. He states he's been more tired than usual for the past month and attributes this to his hectic schedule with work and school. He has not noticed any other changes in his health and denies other symptoms such as fever, weight loss, and difficulty swallowing. The remainder of his history is as follows:

- Past medical and surgical history: tonsillectomy and adenoidectomy; mononucleosis
- Medications: none
- Allergies: none
- Social history: smokes pot two to three times a week and uses no other drugs; drinks four to five beers on weekends; denies tobacco use; business major in college; not in a relationship for past 6 months.

A complete physical exam was done and is unremarkable except for the presence of a cervical lymph node that is 2 centimeters, rubbery, and fixed.

Hodgkin lymphoma is suspected.

Answer the following questions based on this scenario:

- What other clinical manifestations are consistent with Hodgkin lymphoma?
- What are other possible diagnoses to explain these manifestations?
- What diagnostic tests (e.g., CBC) will be done, and what are the expected findings if the diagnosis is Hodgkin lymphoma?

routine screening for anemia in children at 1 year of age, but other organizations such as the U.S. Preventive Services Task Force do not recommend screening due to a lack of evidence of the benefits.

Treatment includes the identification and resolution of the underlying cause of the iron deficiency anemia. Other strategies to increase iron levels include increasing consumption of iron-rich foods (e.g., liver; red meat; fish; beans; raisins; and green, leafy vegetables) or administering oral or intravenous iron replacement. Additionally, foods or supplements high in vitamin C should be increased because vitamin C increases the absorption of iron. Infants below the age of 1 may get adequate intake from breast milk but need supplementation with the introduction of food. Cow's milk is not a good source of iron and should be avoided. Iron-rich formula is recommended.

Megaloblastic Anemia—Macrocytic

Vitamin B_{12} (cobalamin) and folic acid are necessary for the normal development of RBCs and other bone marrow cells such as thrombocytes and leukocytes. The impaired DNA synthesis, due to vitamin B_{12} and folic acid deficiency, is characterized by delayed nuclear development but normal cytoplasm development (i.e., nuclear-cytoplasmic aysynchrony). The aysynchrony causes large developing cells called megaloblasts and large mature cells that are macrocytic (FIGURE 3-14). Cell color is unaffected, and, therefore, the anemia is normochromic. Vitamin B_{12} and folic acid deficiencies also cause premature precursor cell death

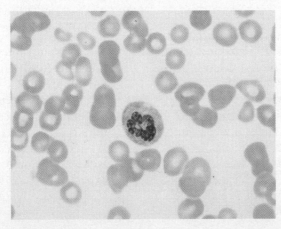

FIGURE 3-14 Pernicious anemia.
© LindseyRN/Shutterstock.

through phagocytosis or apoptosis. While there are commonalities in causes of these two deficiencies, the mechanisms are different and are discussed separately.

Folic Acid

Folic acid as a water-soluble B vitamin is eliminated in urine, and a small quantity (0.5 to 20 mg) is stored in the body. Therefore, folic acid must be regularly replenished through dietary intake. Folic acid is the supplement added to foods, and folate is the natural form in food. Both terms are often used interchangeably. Deficiencies can occur within a short period, such as weeks, depending on the degree of insufficiency or if demand is high. Inadequate dietary intake, while not as common in countries that fortify foods with folic acid such as the United States, occurs usually due to poor overall food intake or lack of a varied diet. Poor intake is common in chronic alcohol use, anorexia nervosa, or malnutrition from illness. Deficiencies can also be due to states of increased needs such as during pregnancy, lactation, or hemodialysis. Absorption of folic acid occurs in the small intestines—duodenum and jejunum. Dysfunctional intestinal surfaces or removal of intestinal surfaces can cause malabsorption. Patients who have undergone gastric bypass or other intestinal surgery or have an inflammatory gastrointestinal disorder such as Crohn disease, ulcerative colitis, or celiac disease are at higher risk for deficiency. Commonly used medications that interfere with folate metabolism include methotrexate for rheumatoid arthritis and several cancers, or antibiotics such as trimethoprim or antiseizure drugs such as carbamazepine. Genetic disorders that affect folate are rare.

Vitamin B_{12}

Vitamin B_{12} absorption requires intrinsic factor, which is a glycoprotein produced by gastric parietal cells. The binding of vitamin B_{12} and intrinsic factor is facilitated by pancreatic enzymes in the duodenum. The bound vitamin B_{12}-intrinsic factor complex is then absorbed by the ileum and carried through the bloodstream. As opposed to folic acid, vitamin B_{12} stores (about 5 mg) are more abundant, and deficiencies can take longer to develop (e.g., 1 year or longer). Inadequate dietary intake can lead to deficiencies. Good dietary sources of vitamin B_{12} are in meats and dairy products;

therefore, patients who restrict intake of these products (e.g., vegans) may become deficient. However, foods can be fortified with vitamin B_{12} as different forms (e.g., cyanocobalamin, methylcobalamin). Deficiencies due to dietary intake are less common and absorption issues are more likely.

The most common cause of deficiency is known as pernicious anemia. At one time, this anemia was fatal, and the term *pernicious*, which means harmful or destructive, was used to describe this anemia. With pernicious anemia, autoantibodies target gastric parietal cells. The autoantibodies impair production and cause destruction of intrinsic factor and other gastric secretions, causing gastric mucosal atrophy. The immune response is thought to involve CD4+ T cells. Autoimmune diseases such as chronic (metaplastic) atrophic gastritis, Hashimoto thyroiditis, Graves disease, and diabetes mellitus type 1 are comorbid illnesses associated with pernicious anemia. Prior *Helicobacter pylori* infection is thought to elicit the autoimmune response as the bacteria produces antibodies that react with enzymes on parietal cells.

In addition to autoantibodies, vitamin B_{12} absorption can be affected by other disorders through a different mechanism. Gastric surgery such as bariatric surgery or gastric cancer surgery causes a reduced secretion of intrinsic factor and decreased absorption. Surgery or diseases affecting the small intestine (e.g., Crohn disease, celiac disease) reduces absorption. Pancreatic diseases such as pancreatic insufficiency or chronic pancreatitis affect absorption by not providing the necessary enzymes for vitamin B_{12} to dissociate from food proteins. Several medications reduce absorption. Long-term use of medications such as antacids (H_2 receptor blockers and proton pump inhibitors) reduce gastric acid, thereby, affecting vitamin B_{12} ability to bind to intrinsic factor. Calcium is another element that is needed for normal vitamin B_{12}-intrinsic factor complex to be absorbed. Metformin reduces vitamin B_{12} absorption by altering calcium action, predisposing users to B_{12} deficiency. In patients with preexisting B_{12} deficiency, the use of nitrous oxide (i.e., laughing gas), whether as an anesthetic or recreationally (e.g., whippets), may inactivate B_{12} and precipitate an acute onset of anemia and neurologic or psychiatric symptoms. Genetic disorders as a cause of deficiency are rare.

Food cobalamin malabsorption is a term used to describe a disorder where vitamin B_{12} deficiency occurs as a result of an inability to absorb dietary vitamin B_{12} despite adequate intake. The disorder is common in older adults and often does not result in anemia. Predisposing risk factors for malabsorption are similar to those that cause megaloblastic anemia such as atrophic gastritis, antacid use, and chronic alcohol use.

Clinical Manifestations (Vitamin B_{12} and Folic Acid)

Manifestations of vitamin and folic acid deficiency can be similar to other anemias (e.g., fatigue, shortness of breath, glossitis). With vitamin B_{12} and folic acid deficiencies, as with other anemias, the worse the severity, the worse the symptoms. Vitamin B_{12} deficiency manifestations take longer to develop in comparison to folic acid deficiency. Vitamin B_{12} deficiency is associated with the development of neuropsychiatric symptoms that are generally not present in folic acid deficiency. These symptoms can become irreversible. The neurologic manifestations can include symmetrical paresthesias more often in the lower extremities with decreased vibratory sense. Proprioception (awareness of body position) and gait can be altered. Several other neuropsychiatric manifestations can include memory and mood alterations such as irritability, depression, or personality changes. Although the exact mechanism is not clear, the neurologic problems occur because of a breakdown in myelin. The neurologic effects may be seen before anemia is diagnosed.

Diagnosis and Treatment

Diagnostic tests for megaloblastic anemia include a complete blood count and peripheral blood smear. The results will reveal macrocytic RBCs (high MCV) with a low reticulocyte count. Other tests include serum vitamin B_{12} and folate levels. Homocysteine (an amino acid) levels are elevated in both deficiencies. Vitamin B_{12} is a cofactor with methylmalonic acid (MMA), resulting in the production of coenzyme A that is necessary for cellular function. If there is insufficient vitamin B_{12}, then the MMA levels will rise as the MMA is not being used. MMA is normal with folic acid deficiency. Testing for antibodies to intrinsic factor (i.e., anti-IF) can be used to detect pernicious anemia. Antibody testing for parietal cells (i.e., anti-parietal cell antibodies) can be conducted, but the tests are not as specific for pernicious anemia or gastritis. The Schilling test, which measures vitamin B_{12} absorption, was commonly used but has been replaced by the other antibody tests. Other diagnostic tests may be necessary to identify underlying causes such as Crohn disease or ulcerative colitis. Treatment consists of replacement with oral or parenteral vitamin B_{12} or folate. Vitamin B_{12} is also available in sublingual and nasal preparations. If the B_{12} deficiency is due to absorption problems, parenteral replacement is recommended. Periconceptional folic acid supplementation is recommended for women planning to become pregnant to prevent neural tube defects.

Anemia of Chronic Disease/Inflammation—Normocytic

Anemia of chronic disease (ACD), also known as anemia of chronic inflammation, is the second most common anemia, after iron deficiency anemia. The anemia is caused by many different chronic diseases or inflammation (e.g., cancer, chronic kidney disease, congestive heart failure, and infections). ACD has similar features regardless of whether it is caused by disease or inflammation. These features include a decreased RBC production by the bone marrow and shortening of RBC survival. Several mechanisms underlie ACD. The chronic inflammation results in cytokine release (e.g., interleukin 1, interleukin 6, tumor necrosis factor). These inflammatory cytokines may lead to RBC precursor apoptosis, decreased erythropoietin receptor on progenitor cells, and decreased erythropoietin secretion by the kidney cells. Iron storage and transport become dysfunctional. The cytokines, particularly interleukin 6, cause increased release of hepcidin by the liver. Hepcidin under normal circumstances regulates iron uptake by inhibiting ferroportin (transports iron across the cell membrane). With increased levels of hepcidin in ACD, less iron is absorbed and iron becomes trapped in macrophages. Transferrin and ferritin dysfunction may also contribute to iron trapping. The anemia produced by ACD is often mild to moderate. RBCs are produced and develop to maturity so the RBCs are normocytic and normochromic. In approximately 25% of patients, ACD can be microcytic and hypochromic. Clinical manifestations of ACD contribute a little to the symptomatology of whatever underlying disease is causing the anemia. In other words, the underlying disease, which might be chronic kidney disease or cancer, is probably causing most of the patient's manifestations.

Diagnosis and Treatment

Diagnosis is usually made by completing a history and physical, which will reveal chronic disease or chronic inflammation. Anemia is usually mild to moderate with ACD. The reticulocyte count is usually low reflecting a decrease in bone marrow production. Inflammatory markers and acute phase reactants such as erythrocyte sedimentation rate may be elevated, reflecting inflammatory process. Other studies such as iron, total iron-binding capacity, and transferrin are low as iron is not absorbed or is sequestered. Transferrin saturation is normal. Iron levels are low with iron deficiency anemia and ACD; however, the transferrin saturation is low and the total iron-binding capacity is high with iron deficiency anemia. Ferritin is normal, but it is also an acute phase reactant, so ferritin levels may be high. Treatment includes resolving the underlying disorder and the anemia if it becomes severe.

Aplastic Anemia—Normocytic

Aplastic anemia is a rare but serious type of anemia that is a result of the bone marrow failing to produce multipotent hematopoietic stem cell precursors. This leads to a lack of erythrocytes, leukocytes, and platelets, which is referred to as *pancytopenia*. The cells that are present, while low in numbers, are mature, normocytic, and normochromic. A lack of these blood cells leads to a series of complications that could include infections, bleeding, hypoxia, fatty replacement of marrow, and death. Aplastic anemia may be temporary or permanent. Causes of aplastic anemia include the following:

- Idiopathic conditions
- Autoimmune conditions (e.g., systemic lupus erythematosus and rheumatoid arthritis)
- Medications and treatments (e.g., chemotherapy and radiation)
- Viruses
- Toxins (e.g., pesticides, arsenic, and benzene)
- Genetic abnormalities (e.g., myelodysplastic syndrome)
- Infectious diseases (e.g., EBV, cytomegalovirus, parvovirus, and HIV)
- Pregnancy (the anemia often resolves after delivery)
- Cancer

Clinical Manifestations

Clinical manifestations include signs and symptoms of general anemia (e.g., weakness, pallor, and dyspnea), leukocytopenia (e.g., recurrent infections), and thrombocytopenia (e.g., bleeding). As blood cell levels decline, clinical manifestations worsen.

Diagnosis and Treatment

Diagnostic tests for aplastic anemia include a complete blood count and bone marrow biopsy. Prompt treatment of the underlying causes and any complications as they arise is crucial for positive outcomes. Treatment of underlying causes may include discontinuation of medications or treatments. Treatment of complications may include the following measures:

- Oxygen therapy
- Infection control measures (e.g., hand washing, avoiding groups, and avoiding fresh flowers)
- Infection treatment (e.g., antibiotics)
- Bleeding precautions (e.g., electric razors, soft-bristle toothbrushes, and injury prevention)
- Hematopoietic stimulants (e.g., erythropoietin and colony-stimulating factors)
- Immunosuppressant therapy (e.g., cyclosporine and methylprednisolone)
- Anti-infectives (e.g., antibiotics and antiviral medications)
- Blood and platelet transfusions
- Bone marrow transplants

Excessive Loss of RBCs

Erythropoiesis may remain relatively intact, and anemia can be due to loss of RBCs as a result of acute blood loss (see the *Iron Deficiency Anemia—Microcytic* section for information on chronic anemia). RBC loss may be due to various disorders that cause RBC destruction in the intravascular space (e.g., disseminated intravascular coagulation, transfusion reaction, hemoglobinuria) or extravascular space (e.g., autoimmune hemolytic anemia) or there can be defects shortening the life span (e.g., megaloblastic, thalassemia major). Acute blood loss due to trauma will cause a normocytic, normochromic anemia as the bone marrow increases normal production to replace the RBCs and compensate for the loss. Destruction of RBCs occurs with hemolytic anemias. Due to the accelerated destruction, the bone marrow may not be able to keep up with the demand.

Causes of hemolytic anemia may be idiopathic, autoimmune, genetic, infectious (e.g., malaria), blood transfusion reactions, and blood incompatibility in the neonate. There are several types of hereditary hemolytic anemias.

These hereditary disorders can be categorized into those that cause enzyme deficiencies (e.g., glucose-6-phosphate dehydrogenase), plasma membrane mutations/defects (e.g., hemoglobinuria), and hemoglobin abnormalities (e.g., sickle cell disease and anemia, as well as thalassemia). Specifics in regard to pathogenesis, clinical manifestations, diagnosis, and treatment vary based on type. Two of the more common hemolytic anemias, sickle cell disease and thalassemia, are discussed.

Sickle Cell Disease

Abnormality in the genes coding for the globin portion of hemoglobin characterize the group of hereditary disorders known as sickle cell disease (SCD). In the United States, SCD is considered one of the most common inherited blood disorders. SCD is much more common in Blacks (1 out of every 500 births). Sickle cell disease is also seen in people from South America and Central America (1 in 1,000–1,400), the Caribbean, the Middle East, and the Mediterranean. Hemoglobin A comprises about 97–98% of the type of hemoglobin in a normal adult. The globin portion of hemoglobin consists of two α-globin chains and two β-globin chains, and, therefore, hemoglobin A is designated as $\alpha_2\beta_2$. (See Figure 3-4). The remaining type of hemoglobin in an adult is hemoglobin A_2, which has alpha and delta chains, and hemoglobin F, which has alpha and gamma chains. The hemoglobin F is the main type in fetal blood. In SCD, a mutation occurs in the *HBB* gene, which provides instructions for making the β-globin chain. While the mutation of *HBB* can cause different abnormal hemoglobin, one of the clinically significant types is hemoglobin S (HbS). The HbS changes the shape of the red blood cell into a sickle (**FIGURE 3-15**). The HbS is designated as $\alpha_2\beta S_2$, reflecting that the two β-globin chains have an *S* mutation. The allele for the sickle cell gene is codominant—so if a person inherits one abnormal gene (HbS) and one normal gene (HbA), then the hemoglobin will be HbAS and the person has sickle cell trait and is a heterozygous carrier. Persons with sickle cell trait do not usually have symptoms of SCD because fewer than half of their erythrocytes are sickled. However, conditions of increased oxygen demand (e.g., high-intensity exercise, high altitude) or dehydration can precipitate sickling, which then causes hemolysis and vascular occlusions due to the clumping of the sickled cells. Awareness of being a carrier is also important for preconception counseling.

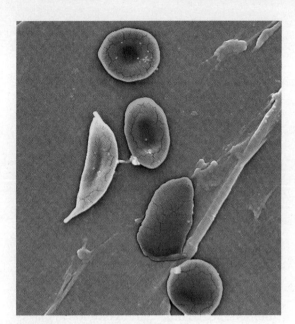

FIGURE 3-15 Sickle cell anemia.

Courtesy of Janice Haney Carr/Sickle Cell Foundation of Georgia: Jackie George, Beverly Sinclair/CDC.

The mode of SCD transmission follows an autosomal recessive pattern (see chapter 1).

A child from two heterozygous parents would have a 25% of no disease, 25% chance of SCD, and 50% chance of having the trait. As opposed to the trait, those with SCD will inherit two abnormal hemoglobin genes that replace the two β-globin chains. In SCD, at least one needs to be HbS, and there are various other types of SCD, which include:

- Hemoglobin Sβ0 thalassemia—absent β-globin production; common
- Hemoglobin Sβ+ thalassemia—reduced (but not absent) β-globin production; common
- Hemoglobin SC, α_2 CS_2—common
- Hemoglobin SD—not common
- Hemoglobin SE—not common
- Hemoglobin SS, α_2 βS_2 sickle cell anemia; most common and most severe disease

Regardless of the type of hemoglobin S (e.g., SD, SE, SC), the shape of erythrocytes are distorted, especially when the body's supply of oxygen is low. The erythrocytes have an abnormal crescent or sickle shape (sickling) (Figure 3-15). These fragile, sickle-shaped cells deliver less oxygen to the body's tissues. These cells also can clog easily in small blood vessels and break into pieces that disrupt blood flow (vasoocclusive crisis). These sickled RBCs have a short survival time. Hemolysis occurs as does anemia due to decreased RBCs. SCD clinical manifestations, clinical course, and treatment vary depending on the type. The most common type with the most severe manifestations, sickle cell anemia, will be discussed next.

Sickle Cell Anemia—Normocytic

Those persons who inherit the hemoglobin S gene from both parents, creating a homozygous allele pair, have sickle cell anemia. Sickle cell anemia is the most common of the sickle cell disease types, and the disease is more severe because almost all of the individual's erythrocytes are abnormal. Sickle cell anemia and SCD are sometimes used interchangeably, but SCD is best used as an umbrella term for patients with at least one sickle hemoglobin S. With sickle cell anemia, the RBCs are normocytic and normochromic as erythropoiesis is not affected.

Clinical Manifestations

Clinical manifestations (**FIGURE 3-16**) usually do not appear in newborns because fetal hemoglobin (i.e., hemoglobin F) protects the red blood cells from sickling. The fetal hemoglobin is replaced by adult hemoglobin, however, when a child reaches 4 to 5 months of age. Swelling and pain in the hands and feet (dactylitis), often in conjunction with a fever, is usually the first symptom of sickle cell anemia in the infant. The swelling results from the sickled cells occluding the blood vessels and blocking blood flow in and out of the hands and feet. Manifestations due to hemolysis include fatigue, irritability, pallor, and jaundice. Most patients, in addition to the signs of hemolytic anemia, will experience acute painful episodes, or crises, that can last for hours to days. Pain is caused by obstruction of small blood vessels as the sickled cells clog up the vessels, leading to ischemia and necrosis. The pain during these vasoocclusive crises is usually described as sharp, intense, and stabbing. The common location of pain is the lower back, chest, abdomen, and long bones. The number and severity of these crises vary among patients, but episodes can be triggered by dehydration, stress, high altitudes, fever, menses, and extreme temperatures. Underlying acute complications, some of which have severe morbidity and mortality, must be considered when a patient is having an episode of acute pain. In between the intermittent acute pain episodes that can be erratic at times is underlying chronic pain that most experience. The chronic pain has more of a neuropathic component with hyperalgesia, sensitization to pain, and opiod hyperalgesia. Neuropathic

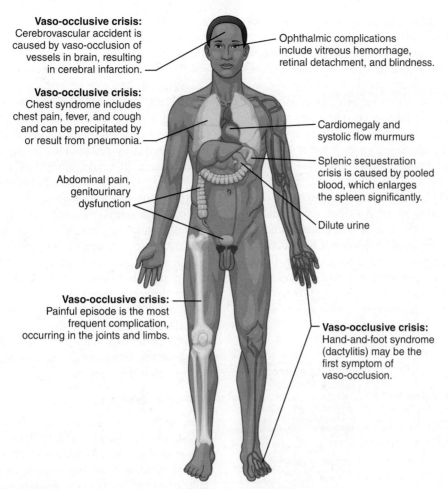

Vaso-occlusive crisis:
Cerebrovascular accident is caused by vaso-occlusion of vessels in brain, resulting in cerebral infarction.

Vaso-occlusive crisis:
Chest syndrome includes chest pain, fever, and cough and can be precipitated by or result from pneumonia.

Abdominal pain, genitourinary dysfunction

Vaso-occlusive crisis:
Painful episode is the most frequent complication, occurring in the joints and limbs.

Ophthalmic complications include vitreous hemorrhage, retinal detachment, and blindness.

Cardiomegaly and systolic flow murmurs

Splenic sequestration crisis is caused by pooled blood, which enlarges the spleen significantly.

Dilute urine

Vaso-occlusive crisis:
Hand-and-foot syndrome (dactylitis) may be the first symptom of vaso-occlusion.

FIGURE 3-16 Pathophysiology of sickle cell disease.

pain develops more as the patient gets older. Sensitization means a person has a heightened sensitivity to pain and has more pain with less provocation. Opioid hyperalgesia refers to a phenomenon where a patient becomes more sensitive to certain painful stimuli with opioid administration. Chronic complications can develop in many systems (Figure 3-16). Because of improved disease understanding and management, most patients with sickle cell anemia now live into their 50s.

Diagnosis and Treatment

Carriers of the defective sickle cell gene can be identified by hemoglobin electrophoresis, a simple blood test that measures and identifies types of abnormal hemoglobin. Additionally, the sickle cell test can determine whether the hemoglobin is normal or sickled. A complete blood count and bilirubin test are useful in determining diagnosis and progression.

There is no single best treatment for all people with SCD. Stem cell transplants are the

option for a cure. Medications such as hydroxyurea and l-glutamine are available to reduce the frequency of crises. Avoidance of sickling triggers is also helpful. Other strategies include the following measures:

- Oxygen therapy
- Hydration
- Pain management (e.g., nonopioids and opioids, relaxation techniques, distraction)
- Infection control measures
- Vaccinations
- Blood transfusions
- Bone marrow transplants
- Genetic counseling for those persons with sickle cell trait

Thalassemia—Microcytic

Thalassemia is another hereditary type of hemolytic anemia, which results in abnormal hemoglobin. The abnormal hemoglobin is a result of an abnormal quantity of one of the two protein chains, resulting in α-thalassemia or β-thalassemia. Thalassemia occurs most frequently in persons of Mediterranean descent. Other ethnic groups affected by thalassemia include those of Asian, and Indian descent and Blacks.

β-Thalassemia, as in SCD, is caused by a mutation in the *HBB* gene. The most common mode of inheritance is an autosomal recessive pattern, and some cases present in an autosomal dominant pattern. The *HBB* mutation can cause a complete absence of β-globin (β^0) synthesis. The *HBB* mutation can also cause a reduced amount of β-globin (β^+) synthesis (FIGURE 3-17). There can be some normal hemoglobin A or none. β-Thalassemia is categorized by the severity of symptoms. Major thalassemia (Cooley anemia) is a more severe type of anemia with increased symptomaticity while minor/intermediate types cause a less severe

anemia and disease. Thalassemia minor is also called thalassemia trait. The severity is determined by whether the mutation is heterozygous (e.g., β^+/β^0) or homozygous (e.g., β^0/β^0).

With an absence or reduction in β-globin chains in β-thalassemia, alpha chains accumulate and become excessive. The α-globin is unstable and precipitates, causing destruction of erythroblasts by phagocytes in the bone marrow. Mature RBC with abnormal α-globin are destroyed in the spleen. The anemia produced is microcytic and hypochromic.

α-Thalassemia is not as common as β-thalassemia. α-Thalassemia occurs due to mutations in the HBA1 and HBA2 genes of which there are two copies each. These genes direct α-globin chain synthesis. There are many different types of α-thalassemia, such as hydrops fetalis (loss of all α-globin genes) and HbH disease (loss of three of four α-globin genes). Inheritance patterns are complex because of the different number of gene combinations that may occur.

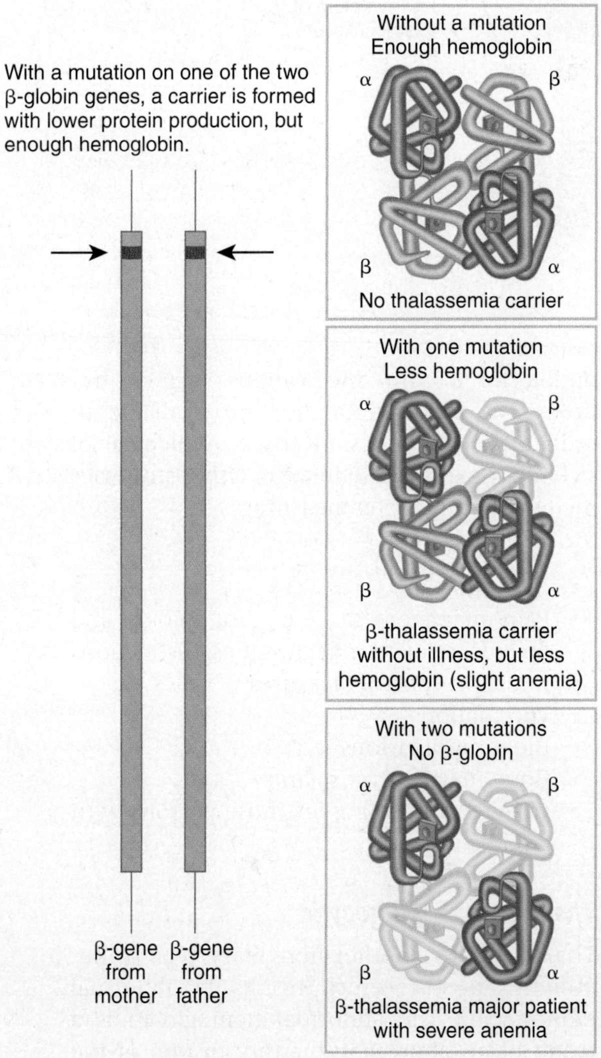

Clinical Manifestations

Patients with α- or β-thalassemia minor or the traits may be asymptomatic or have milder anemia symptoms (e.g., pallor, weakness, fatigue). The symptoms may not appear until later in childhood. Patients with β-thalassemia major or some variants of α-thalassemia (e.g., HbH) have more severe anemia manifestations and complications. In these severe anemias, symptoms appear at a younger age (e.g., less than 2 years old). Infants with hydrops fetalis, which is also known as α-thalassemia major, are usually stillborn or die shortly after birth due to heart failure and severe anemia. In β-thalassemia major, the manifestations and complications include delayed growth and development. Children will have skeletal deformities such as dental malocclusion and prominent facial bones. Iron overload (hemosiderosis and hemochromatosis) occurs due to too much absorption as the body tries to compensate for ineffective erythropoiesis and is also a result of treatment from blood transfusions. Iron overload causes hepatomegaly and liver disorders. Splenomegaly occurs because of the increased RBC destruction. With treatment, some of the manifestations may not be evident. Heart failure can lead to early death.

Diagnosis and Treatment

A positive family history and physical findings supported by laboratory studies are used

With a mutation on one of the two β-globin genes, a carrier is formed with lower protein production, but enough hemoglobin.

β-gene from mother   β-gene from father

Without a mutation
Enough hemoglobin
No thalassemia carrier

With one mutation
Less hemoglobin
β-thalassemia carrier without illness, but less hemoglobin (slight anemia)

With two mutations
No β-globin
β-thalassemia major patient with severe anemia

FIGURE 3-17 *HBB* mutation.

to diagnose thalassemia. Erythrocytes will appear microcytic and hypochromic. They vary in size and morphology (e.g., target cells, teardrop cells). Iron deficiency presents with a microcytic-hypochromic anemia like thalassemia (particularly minor); therefore, recognition of differences are important. RBC levels are high in thalassemia but may be low in iron deficiency anemia. Iron levels in thalassemia major or intermedia tend to be high, but the levels may be normal in thalassemia minor. In iron deficiency, the iron levels will be low. Hemoglobin electrophoresis will be conducted, and hemoblobin abnormalities will be present with thalassemia. Treatment may not be necessary in mild cases of thalassemia. Severe cases, however, can cause early death due to heart failure, usually between the ages of 20 and 30. The heart failure occurs due to myocardial iron deposition. If treatment is warranted, it includes blood transfusion, chelation therapy, bone marrow transplants, and splenectomy.

Polycythemia

Polycythemia is the term used to describe above-normal increases in RBCs and hemoglobin. Two types include primary polycythemia, also known as polycythemia vera (PV) and secondary polycythemia. Any disease or circumstance that leads to decreased oxygen levels triggers a compensatory increased erythropoietin release from the kidneys, leading to RBC production. People living in high altitudes have a physiologic polycythemia. In relative polycythemia, there is not a true increase in RBC and hemoglobin but, rather, the appearance due to a reduction in plasma (e.g., dehydration, obesity). Chronic heart and lung conditions such as chronic obstructive lung disease, pulmonary fibrosis, and congenital heart disease are associated with decreased oxygen levels and may result in polycythemia.

PV is a primary disorder in which the bone marrow produces too many blood cells. This primary polycythemia is referred to as "true" PV. This rare condition is considered a neoplastic disease because of the uncontrolled proliferation of cells. PV falls into the category of myeloproliferative neoplasms along with chronic myeloid leukemia, essential thrombocythemia, and primary myelofibrosis.

PV occurs due to a mutation in the *JAK2* gene which is present in all patients with PV, but the mutation is also present in other myeloproliferative disorders. The role of the *JAK2* gene is controlling cellular growth from hematopoietic stem cells. The mutated clone cells develop without the usual necessary erythropoietin. In addition to increased RBCs, thrombocytes and leukocytes are increased to a lesser degree. The exact cause of this mutation, which occurs most frequently in men, is unknown. Most cases of PV are acquired and inheritance is rare. The most common age for diagnosis is around 60 years old, and the disorder is rare in children or young adults. As blood cell numbers increase, so does the blood volume and viscosity. Blood vessels become distended and blood flow is sluggish.

Clinical Manifestations

The following manifestations may be present at or prior to diagnosis. The manifestations (in relative order of frequency) are visual disturbances (e.g., ophthalmic migraine, transient blindness), hypertension, and splenomegaly. Pruritus after contact with water is present in about one-third of patients and can be present up to 3 years prior to diagnosis. The cause of pruritus is not clear. Theories include histamine release along with other cytokines or cool water contact causing vasoconstriction with prostaglandin and platelet aggregation. Some patients' pruritus is relieved with aspirin. Vasomotor and microvascular thrombotic changes can lead to symptoms such as burning pain in the hands or feet with erythema, pallor, or cyanosis (erythromelalgia), and paresthesias. Serious complications such as arterial and venous thrombosis (e.g., myocardial infarction, stroke) or hemorrhaging or transformation to other neoplasms (e.g., acute myeloblastic leukemia) are not common. Gouty arthritis is also associated with PV due to the high turnover of RBCs causing increased uric acid production. Gastrointestinal disease (e.g., peptic ulcer disease, erosions) are attributed to changes in blood flow and inflammatory response (e.g., histamine release).

Diagnosis and Treatment

Diagnosis is often made incidentally when a complete blood count, as part of routine exam or done for other reasons, reveals an increased hemoglobin. PV should be suspected under those circumstances unless the polycythemia can be attributed to a disorder of chronic hypoxemia or other secondary disorders. Erythromyalgia and aquagenic pruritus are characteristic and indicative of PV. Low serum erythropoietin and peripheral blood mutation of *JAK2* are considered diagnostic of

PV. With other causes of increased RBCs and hemoglobin, erythropoietin levels are usually normal or high. Bone marrow aspiration and biopsy may be conducted depending on findings and for further confirmation. Treatment is not curative, and goals are to relieve symptoms and improve survival through prevention of complications. Strategies are centered on risk stratification based on age and history of clotting. Treatment may include phlebotomy and low-dose aspirin, which should be administered cautiously with bleeding. Chemotherapy/cytoreductive agents, specifically hydroxyurea, is first line of treatment. Gout, hypertension, and other associated disorders are managed per usual guidelines, taking into consideration PV treatment potential interactions.

Iron Overload

Iron overload can be a result of increased intake or absorption. Multiple packed cell transfusion as therapy in disorders such as thalassemia, SCD, or myelodysplastic syndromes can cause iron overload. While not as common, administration of iron or iron-containing products, either in excess or therapeutically, can lead to overload. Diseases that increase absorption can include inherited anemias such as thalassemia and SCD; therefore, the disorder and the treatment can lead to iron overload. Liver disease such as chronic hepatitis causes inflammation and increased ferritin along with other acute phase reactants and the release of iron stored in the liver, causing iron increases. Hereditary hemochromatosis is a genetic disorder caused by several mutations on genes (e.g., *HFE*, *HAMP*) that regulate iron absorption, transport, and storage. Hereditary hemochromatosis has four types, with types 1 and 4 occurring in adult men around the age of 40–60 and type 2 occurring in childhood. Type 1 in women usually occurs after menopause as women compensate with increased iron loss with menstruation, pregnancy, or lactation. Type 3 occurs somewhere in between these ages. Of the types of hemochromatosis, type 1 is the most common, and types 2, 3, and 4 are rare.

Excess iron saturates transferrin until capacities are exceeded. The iron starts binding to other proteins such as albumin. The nontransferrin-bound iron excesses are absorbed by cells that have mechanisms to take in the iron in this form. The liver, heart, endocrine organs (e.g., pancreas), and joints can all take in this extra iron. The iron then gets chemically transformed in affected organs and become a reactive oxygen species causing tissue damage, inflammation, and fibrosis.

Clinical Manifestations

Iron overload manifestations are often nonspecific and develop slowly. At times, manifestations become evident once there is organ damage such as heart failure or hepatic fibrosis. The multiple manifestations are usually related to the damage caused by the excess iron and dependent on which organs are affected. Patients can present with symptoms of diabetes, hypothyroidism, osteoporosis, and integumentary conditions such as hyperpigmentation. Type 2 hemochromatosis (juvenile-onset disorder) may manifest due to alterations in sex hormones, leading to symptoms such as delayed sexual maturation or amenorrhea after a period of normal menstruation.

Diagnosis and Treatment

The complete blood count may be normal or reveal different anemias depending on the underlying cause of the iron overload. Iron levels, ferritin, and transferrin saturation are high. The total iron-binding capacity (indirect measure of transferrin) will be low reflecting the inability to bind. Hepatic enzymes may be altered with liver involvement. Magnetic resonance imaging of the heart or liver may reveal iron deposition. A liver biopsy may also be done. Phlebotomy can aid in diagnosis and treatment, as every 500 milliliters removed is equivalent to approximately 200–250 milligrams of iron. Patients with iron overload might have 5,000 milligrams stored. If phlebotomy (usually a few times a week) leads to a decrease in ferritin level, then this decrease is consistent with a diagnosis of iron overload. Chelation therapy is another treatment option. The goal of treatment is prevention of organ damage caused by iron overload.

Diseases of the Platelets

Platelets are vital components of the coagulation process. Normal platelet levels range from 150,000 to 350,000 cells/mL^3. Diseases of the platelets include issues in quantity and quality of platelets. Thrombocytosis refers to increased platelet levels, and thrombocytopenia describes decreased platelet levels. Thrombocytosis increases the risk of thrombus formation, while thrombocytopenia increases the risk of bleeding and infection. Qualitative issues refer to alterations in how the platelet functions. In these circumstances, platelet count is normal but bleeding time is prolonged. Congenital disorders that alter platelet function are rare (e.g., Bernard-Soulier syndrome, Scott syndrome). More commonly, platelet function alterations are due to drug effects (e.g., aspirin), system diseases (e.g., those of the liver or kidney), or other hematologic disorders (e.g., leukemia).

Thrombocytopenia

Thrombocytopenia refers to low platelet levels. The lower the number of platelets, the higher the risk for life-threatening bleeding. Levels below 15,000 cells/mL^3 can result in spontaneous bleeding with no trauma. The bleeding can result in mucous membrane manifestations such as petechiae (< 3 mm pinpoint capillary hemorrhage), purpura ($\geq$ 3 mm, < 1 cm), and ecchymoses (large area > 1 cm). Bleeding from other systems such as the gastrointestinal tract (e.g., hematochezia) or respiratory tract (e.g., hemoptysis) can also occur. Thrombocytopenia occurs due to a decreased production or increased destruction of platelets or a combination of both. Bone marrow disorders will lead to a decreased production and occurs with nutritional deficiencies in iron, B$_{12}$, or folate. Alcohol use, whether acute or chronic, may cause impaired hematopoiesis. Many drugs such as quinidine, acetaminophen, and methyldopa can lead to an immune drug-dependent antibody binding that causes platelet destruction. A medication history, therefore, is important when evaluating for causes of thrombocytopenia. During pregnancy, up to 10% of women can develop a transient benign reduction in platelets (usually to 100,000–150,000/µL), but more severe syndromes such as preeclampsia or hemolysis, elevated liver function tests, low platelets syndrome may be present with lower values. Fluid resuscitation or massive blood transfusion (e.g., > 10 units of packed cells) can cause a dilutional thrombocytopenia. Platelets may be decreased due to blood loss. The most common cause of thrombocytopenia that is isolated (no other disorders) is primary immune thrombocytopenia. Disorders can also stimulate autoimmune antiplatelet antibodies leading to secondary immune thrombocytopenia.

Learning Points

Heparin-Induced Thrombocytopenia (HIT)

Administration of heparin can lead to life-threatening thrombocytopenia and thrombosis. The reaction is more common with unfractionated (4%) versus low molecular weight (0.1%) heparin. Antibody IgG, with no IgM response, attacks platelet factor IV with resultant platelet activation and thrombin activation. Increased platelets lead to thrombosis with opposing increase in platelet consumption and subsequent decrease in platelets. Heparin can cause a mild, inconsequential decrease in platelets to 100,000/µL, but HIT usually causes a 50% decrease. HIT onset can be as early as 4 days and up to 10 days after administration of heparin. The treatment is withdrawal and switching to a nonheparin anticoagulant with precaution due to the continued risk of bleeding.

Immune Thrombocytopenic Purpura

Immune thrombocytopenic purpura (ITP) is a hypocoagulopathy state resulting from the immune system destroying its own platelets (autoimmunity). The disorder can be primary and not associated with an underlying disorder or secondary occurring due to another condition. The condition causing the ITP is usually written in parenthesis in secondary ITP (such as hepatitis C associated). Secondary ITP causes include autoimmune diseases (e.g., systemic lupus erythematosus), immunizations from a live vaccine, infections (e.g., HIV, hepatitis C, *Helicobacter pylori*), and cancer.

ITP development is autoantibody mediated. The key mechanism is circulating IgG produced by B cells reacting with the surface glycoprotein IIb/IIIa. The platelets are then destroyed in the spleen with some destroyed in the liver and bone marrow. Other mechanisms, such as autoreactive cytotoxic T cells, impair production.

Primary ITP (i.e., idiopathic thrombocytopenia purpura) is the most common cause of isolated thrombocytopenia and occurs due to increased platelet destruction and decreased production. Primary ITP can be either acute or chronic (> 12 months). Acute ITP is more common in children, and the peak age of presentation is 2–4 years old. This form of the disease typically has a sudden onset and is self-limiting, often lasting less than a week and usually resolving within 6 months. Chronic ITP is more common in adults aged 20–50 years and in women, has a slower onset, and spontaneous resolution is rare. After age 65 years, there is a higher incidence in men. Severe bleeding does not usually occur in adults and in children occurs in < 10% of cases. Prognosis is usually good for both acute and chronic ITP.

Clinical Manifestations

Adults and children with ITP are often asymptomatic. Manifestations, when present, include abnormal bleeding (e.g., petechiae, epistaxis, and hematuria). Purpura lesions are usually in distal dependent areas and are nonpalpable and nonblanchable.

Diagnosis and Management

Thrombocytopenia is often an incidental finding during laboratory evaluation, whether done routinely or for evaluation of other reasons. Diagnostic procedures will be directed toward identifying possible causes of the decreased platelets. The history, physical, and complete blood count may provide apparent reasons (e.g., anemia). Isolated thrombocytopenia is usually a diagnosis after other possibilities for the thrombocytopenia have been excluded. Examples of diagnostic tests may include hepatitis profile, HIV testing, bone marrow biopsy, and humoral studies.

The overall goal of treatment is to increase the platelet count to a level to prevent severe bleeding, and if present, manage the severe bleeding. Thrombocytopenia treatment may not always be necessary. Therapies are often individualized. Treatment strategies may include glucocorticoid steroids and immunoglobulins to prevent further platelet destruction. Rituximab can reduce B cells in autoimmune disorders or thrombopoietin receptor agonists can stimulate platelet production. Splenectomy, plasmapheresis, and plateletpheresis can be considered.

Thrombotic Thrombocytopenic Purpura

Thrombotic thrombocytopenic purpura (TTP) is a coagulation disorder resulting from a deficiency of an enzyme, a disintegrin and metalloproteinase with thrombospondin domain 13 enzyme (ADAMTS13), which is necessary for cleaving von Willebrand factor (vWF). The result is platelets aggregating around the large vWF molecules and increased clotting, which decreases available platelets. Fewer platelets can lead to bleeding; therefore, TTP is characterized by microthrombi in the microvasculature, thrombocytopenia, and bleeding. The clots are composed of vWF and platelets. Causes include hereditary mutations of *ADAMTS13* gene, and the mode of transmission is autosomal recessive. Hereditary TTP is rare, and a worldwide registry has 150 families.

Hereditary TTP is more common in infants and children. Acquired disorders are the most common causes of TTP and are due to autoantibodies IgG inhibiting the ADAMTS13 enzyme. Acquired TTP may occur with conditions such as bone marrow transplants, cancer, pregnancy, infections, or medications.

Clinical Manifestations

TTP manifestations can be acute or insidious. Multiple systems can be involved. Neurologic manifestations can include memory changes, headache, confusion, and changes in consciousness. The individual may present with renal insufficiency, renal failure, or fever. Cardiovascular manifestations can include chest pain, congestive heart failure, and myocardial infarction. Gastrointestinal symptoms include pain, nausea, vomiting, and diarrhea. The pancreas, adrenal glands, and spleen may also be affected while the lungs are usually spared.

Diagnosis and Treatment

Diagnostic procedures for TTP include a history, physical examination, complete blood counts, peripheral blood smears, lactate dehydrogenase (LDH) levels, and bilirubin. LDH levels are high, reflecting tissue injury along with high indirect bilirubin. Reticulocytes are also high. Fragments of RBCs, called *schistocytes*, may be present on RBC smears. In addition to thrombocytopenia, a microangiopathic (small vessel disease) hemolytic anemia is present. Coagulation tests are usually normal. Plasmapheresis is the treatment for TTP. Additionally, a splenectomy and glucocorticoid steroids may be necessary.

Thrombocythemia

Thrombocythemia (i.e., thrombocytosis) refers to an increase in platelet count. Secondary thrombocytosis can occur due to pooling of platelets in the circulation after splenectomy or as a reactive response to infections and inflammations. Secondary thrombocytosis is usually self-limiting with no sequelae. Primary thrombocytosis (i.e., essential thrombocythemia) is a myeloproliferative neoplasm. Polycythemia vera, primary myelofibrosis, and chronic myeloid leukemia are malignancies associated with thrombocytosis.

Diseases of Coagulation or Hemostasis

Coagulation factor disorders, like platelet diseases, can increase bleeding. Impairments in one factor, such as in hemophilia, are usually inherited. Disorders of multiple coagulation factors are usually due to alterations in synthesis (e.g., liver disease) or inappropriate activation of coagulation (e.g., disseminated intravascular coagulation). Thrombophilia are disorders that lead to hypercoagulability. Several inherited and possible genetic mutations are associated with increased risk for thrombosis.

Hemophilia

Hemophilia A, or classic hemophilia, involves a deficiency or abnormality of clotting factor VIII. Hemophilia B involves abnormality of clotting factor IX. Hemophilia A is more common, with an incidence of 1 in 5,000 males worldwide, and hemophilia B occurs in 1 in 20,000 males worldwide. Both are X-linked recessive bleeding disorders. Factor VIII and IX are part of the intrinsic pathway that lead to factor X activation. The severity of the disorder varies depending on the amount of factor present in the blood, but those with hemophilia A usually have a more severe disease than hemophilia B.

Clinical Manifestations

Severe forms of hemophilia become apparent by 1 month, and milder forms are usually diagnosed by 1 year of age. Bleeding is the main symptom of the disease and sometimes occurs when an infant is circumcised. Additional bleeding problems may be seen when the infant starts crawling and walking. Mild cases may go unnoticed until later in life, when they are detected during surgery or trauma. Internal bleeding may happen anywhere, and bleeding into joints, or hemarthrosis, is common. Other manifestations include petechiae, bruising, gastrointestinal bleeding, and hematuria.

Diagnosis and Treatment

Diagnosis of hemophilia includes examination of bleeding studies. Platelets, bleeding time, and prothrombin time are usually normal, but partial prothromboplastin time, activated partial prothromboplastin time (aPTT), and coagulation time are prolonged. However, aPTT may be normal, in mild cases. Serum levels of factor VIII and IX are low. Genetic testing is done to identify the gene mutation (i.e., F8 for hemophilia A and F9 for hemophilia B).

Treatment strategies include replacing clotting factors through transfusions that are plasma derived or recombinant such as Advate (antihemophilic factor, a recombinant DNA product) for hemophilia A. To prevent a bleeding crisis, patients can be taught to give factor VIII or IX concentrates at home prophylactically or at the first signs of bleeding. People with severe forms of the disease may need regular preventive treatment. Mild hemophilia may be treated with desmopressin (DDAVP), which helps the body release factor VIII that is stored within the lining of blood vessels. Additionally, bleeding precautions should be employed (e.g., electric razors, soft-bristle toothbrushes, and injury prevention).

Von Willebrand Disease

Von Willebrand disease is the most common hereditary bleeding disorder. It results from a deficit of von Willebrand factor, which ordinarily causes platelets to aggregate and adhere to the vessel wall in times of injury. Mild cases are often undiagnosed, but incidence is estimated at 1 in 100 to 10,000. Several forms of von Willebrand disease are distinguished:

- **Type 1 von Willebrand disease** is the most common (70–80%) and mildest form. It follows an autosomal dominant inheritance pattern. The level of von Willebrand factor in the blood is reduced. Because this form is often very mild, most cases go undiagnosed. Type 1 does not usually cause spontaneous bleeding, but significant bleeding can occur with trauma or surgery.
- **Type 2 von Willebrand disease** occurs in 15–20% of cases. It can be either autosomal dominant or recessive, and four subtypes exist. In type 2, the building blocks (multimers) that make up the von Willebrand factor are smaller than usual or break down easily. Bleeding with this type are usually moderate to severe.
- **Type 3 von Willebrand disease** follows an autosomal recessive inheritance pattern. Severe bleeding problems are seen with this type due to the lack of measurable von Willebrand factor and factor VIII. Type 3 is the rarest form.
- **Acquired type von Willebrand disease** occurs in persons with Wilms tumor, congenital heart disease, systemic lupus erythematosus, and hypothyroidism.

Clinical manifestations of von Willebrand disease include abnormal bleeding. Diagnosis requires bleeding studies (e.g., bleeding time, prothrombin time, and partial prothromboplastin time) and factor VIII levels. Treatment, if needed, includes infusions of cryoprecipitate or administration of desmopressin; desmopressin increases the release of von Willebrand factor and factor VIII. Clotting factor concentrates of vWF and factor VIII can be administered. Additionally, measures are used to control bleeding and prevent injury, such as using pressure dressings.

Disseminated Intravascular Coagulation

Disseminated intravascular coagulation (DIC) is a life-threatening disorder that occurs as a complication of other diseases and conditions, such as serious acute infections. The incidence is estimated at 1% of tertiary hospital admissions. Normally, during injury, clotting factors (Figure 3-7) become activated and travel to the injury site to help stop bleeding, and then through fibrinolysis, the clot is dissolved. However, in persons with DIC, coagulation and fibrinolysis become abnormally active. In fact, they may become active as an inappropriate immune reaction. Consequently, small blood clots form within the blood vessels, and some of these clots can occlude blood supply to tissue and organs. Over time, the clotting factors become used up. When this happens, the person is at risk for serious bleeding from even a minor injury.

Learning Points

DIC bleeding pattern

In DIC, hypercoagulation uses up all the available clotting factors. Once available clotting factors are utilized, the patient begins excessively bleeding. In other words, the individual clots, clots, clots, and then bleeds, bleeds, bleeds!

Reproduced from Story, L. (2017). *Pathophysiology: A Practical Approach* (3rd ed.). Burlington, MA: Jones & Bartlett Learning.

It is not clear why certain disorders lead to DIC. In DIC, various disorders may expose the blood to procoagulant stimuli through different mechanisms. Bacteria, as an example, may activate coagulation; while with sepsis from meningococci, particles of tissue factor are found in the blood. Trauma from burns and head injury causes damage and possible release of procoagulants. Other conditions associated with DIC include:

- Blood transfusion reaction
- Cancer (e.g., leukemia, aplastic anemia, and metastatic carcinoma)
- Pregnancy complications (e.g., retained placenta after delivery, abruptio placentae, and eclampsia)
- Recent surgery or anesthesia
- Sepsis
- Severe liver disease
- Cardiac arrest
- Poisonous snake bites

Clinical Manifestations

Clinical manifestations of DIC can be multisystem. Tissue and organ ischemia occur from microvascular and macrovascular thrombosis. DIC affects the cardiovascular, pulmonary, renal, hepatic, and central nervous systems. Manifestations of multisystem organ damage can include altered mentation, seizure, angina, tachycardia, hypotension, and oliguria. Cyanosis is usually symmetrical and can occur in fingers, toes, and breasts. Underlying organ damage may not be evident immediately, and often bleeding is the first sign that something is wrong. The patient may start bleeding from intravenous sites or other invasive areas. Petechiae, epistaxis, hematuria, and other signs of bleeding may occur.

Diagnosis and Treatment

Diagnostic procedures for DIC consist of complete blood counts. Platelet counts decrease rapidly. Coagulation studies such as thrombin time, prothrombin time, and partial prothromboplastin time will reveal prolonged clotting times. Many other disorders can alter these tests, and they are not specific to DIC. Fibrin degradation products are the most specific and includes a D-dimer test, which is a protein fragment produced from clot breakdown. DIC causes high D-dimer levels. Fibrinogen function can be measured; levels would be low, reflecting the consumption of clotting products that occurs in DIC. Anticoagulation factors such as antithrombin III, protein C, and protein S are also consumed and would be decreased. Management of DIC is complicated but starts with the identification and treatment of the underlying cause. The treatment of the DIC disorder itself is a delicate balance between preventing clots and treating bleeding (FIGURE 3-18).

Thrombophilia

Thrombophilia refers to a state of increased coagulation. Thrombophilia is due to an abnormality in the coagulation system that leads to the tendency to form venous thromboembolisms. Antiphospholipid syndrome is an acquired type of thrombophilia. This syndrome is caused by a primary autoimmune disorder or may occur with other autoimmune disorders such as systemic lupus erythematosus. Women are more commonly affected, and diagnosis is usually between the ages of 30 and 40 years. Arterial and venous clots are a complication, and women often have miscarriages or are predisposed to preeclampsia. Inherited causes of thrombophilia are commonly due to factor V Leiden and prothrombin mutations. Other less

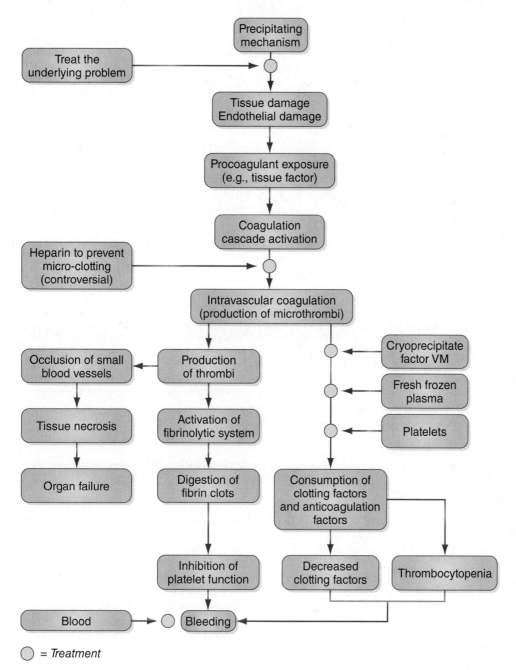

FIGURE 3-18 Understanding DIC and its treatment.

common causes are elevated factor VIII, hyperhomocysteinemia, and deficiencies in antithrombin, protein C, and protein S.

Whether the disorder is inherited or acquired, most individuals who have the disorder develop a clot in the presence of another inciting or prothrombotic state like immobilization or cancer. While there is a higher tendency for a person with the disorder to develop a clot, this tendency alone is insufficient to cause a clot. Those individuals with inherited thrombophilia will develop venous thromboembolism at a younger age, may have a strong

family history of clots, or develop a clot in an unusual site like the portal, hepatic, or mesenteric veins. Some individuals also have a history of recurrent spontaneous clots. However, a first episode may not happen until a person is older and has a case of a venous thromboembolism.

Treatment is dependent on the degree of risk for thrombosis and may include aspirin, dipyridamole, warfarin, heparin, or supplemental concentrates of the deficient factor (e.g., protein C, antithrombin III). Further discussion of venous and arterial thrombosis is covered in chapter 4.

BOX 3-5 Application to Practice

Case: Parents recently received confirmation that their 2-month-old son has sickle cell anemia. They are somewhat anxious. Answer the following questions:

1. The parents brought in a hemoglobin electrophoresis report and want you to explain the results. Which of the following indicates sickle cell anemia?

   a. HgAS
   b. HgAC
   c. HgSS
   d. HgSD

2. They are confused because they are both Hispanic and they thought this was a disease that only occurred in Black children. Explain the ethnic/racial distribution of this disease. Explain the inheritance pattern.

3. The parents want to know symptoms of the disease. Explain the signs and symptoms that may be seen in an infant with sickle cell anemia.

4. Discuss healthcare education you will provide the parents regarding how to care for their child.

CHAPTER SUMMARY

Blood serves many purposes in the body. If this life fluid does not function properly, the body cannot maintain health and homeostasis; therefore, problems with any types of blood cells can lead to widespread and life-threatening problems. Hematologic problems can result from a variety of origins but usually lead to abnormal cell numbers or function. Timely identification and treatment of these disorders is vital for positive health outcomes.

REFERENCES AND RESOURCES

American Cancer Society. (2018). Cancer facts and statistics 2018. Retrieved from https://www.cancer.org/content /dam/cancer-org/research/cancer-facts-and-statistics /annual-cancer-facts-and-figures/2018/cancer-facts-and -figures-2018.pdf

Centers for Disease Control and Prevention (CDC). (2014). Epstein-Barr virus and infectious mononucleosis. Retrieved from http://www.cdc.gov/epstein-barr/

Chiras, D. (2015). *Human biology* (8th ed.). Burlington, MA: Jones & Bartlett Learning.

Copstead, L., & Banasik, J. (2014). *Pathophysiology* (5th ed.). St. Louis, MO: Elsevier.

Dean, L. (2006, April 26). Mutations and blood clots: How point mutations in clotting factor genes conspire to increase the risk of thrombosis. In L. Dean & J. McEntryre (Eds.), *Coffee break: Tutorials for NCBI tools.* Retrieved from http://www.ncbi.nlm.nih.gov/books/NBK2318

DeBruin, M., Dorresteijn, L., van't Veer, M., van der Pal, H., Kappelle, A., Alman, B., & van Leeuwen, F. (2009). Increased risk of stroke and transient ischemic attack in 5-year survivors of Hodgkin lymphoma. *Journal of National Cancer Institute, 101*(13), 928–937.

Elling, B., Elling, K., & Rothenberg, M. (2004). *Anatomy and physiology.* Sudbury, MA: Jones and Bartlett Publishers.

Girelli, D., Nemeth, E., & Swinkels, D. W. (2016). Hepcidin in the diagnosis of iron disorders. *Blood, 127*(23), 2809–2813. http://doi.org/10.1182/blood-2015-12-639112

Kaushansky, K., Lichtman, M. A., Prchal, J. T., Levi, M. M., Press, O. W., Burns, L. J., & Caligiuri, M. (Eds.). *Williams hematology* (9th ed.). New York, NY: McGraw-Hill. Retrieved from http://accessmedicine.mhmedical.com.ezproxy.fiu .edu/content.aspx?bookid=1581&sectionid=94301148

Porth, C. (2014). *Essentials of pathophysiology* (9th ed.). Philadelphia, PA: Lippincott Williams & Wilkins.

Professional guide to pathophysiology (3rd ed.). (2010). Philadelphia, PA: Lippincott Williams & Wilkins.

Schick, P. K. (2006). Anemia. Retrieved from https://www .ashacademy.org/Product/index/98006810

U.S. Cancer Statistics Working Group. (2018). U.S. cancer statistics data visualizations tool, based on November 2017 submission data (1999–2015): U.S. Department of Health and Human Services, Centers for Disease Control and Prevention and National Cancer Institute. Retrieved from www.cdc.gov/cancer/dataviz

World Health Organization. (2016). Micronutrient deficiencies. Retrieved from https://www.who.int/nutrition /topics/vad/en/

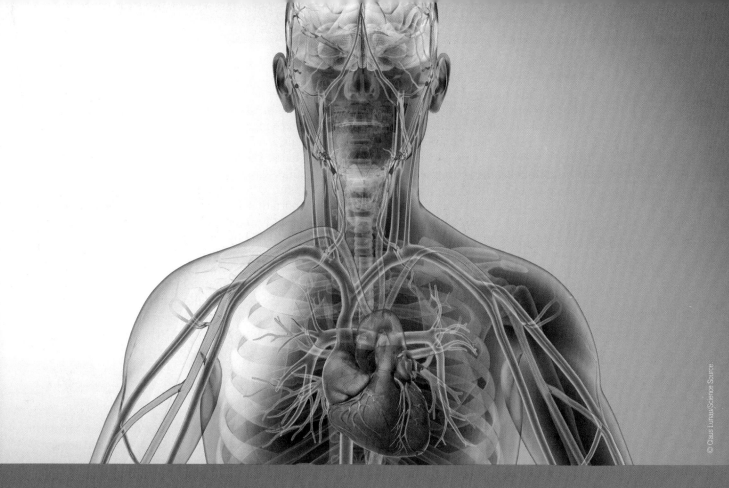

© Claus Lunau/Science Source.

CHAPTER 4
Cardiovascular Function

he cardiovascular system is composed of the heart, blood vessels, lymphatic system, and blood. This chapter focuses on normal and abnormal states of the heart and blood vessels. The components of the cardiovascular system work together to maintain life. Additionally, these components play a crucial role in the functioning of other systems. This pivotal role begins early in life when the fetus is about 4 weeks old and lasts until the end of life. Disorders of the cardiovascular system are common and complex, as they often affect other systems. Cardiovascular disorders will likely be encountered in any clinical setting and often occur in association with other disorders.

Anatomy and Physiology

The cardiovascular system is similar to the plumbing in a house. Both have a pump (the heart), a network of pipes (the blood vessels), and fluid (blood). The cardiovascular system delivers vital oxygen and nutrients to cells, removes waste products, and transports hormones. Circulation is divided into two branches—pulmonary and systemic (**FIGURE 4-1**). In the pulmonary circulation, the waste product—carbon dioxide—is exchanged for oxygen in the lungs through diffusion (**FIGURE 4-2**). In the systemic circulation, blood carries oxygen and nutrients to all cells and waste products to the kidneys, liver, and skin for excretion. To accomplish these transportation functions, the cardiovascular system requires a properly functioning heart to propel the blood by rhythmic contractions. The blood circulates through three types of vessels—arteries, capillaries, and veins. The lymphatic system assists in maintaining homeostasis by returning excess fluid from the body's tissues to the circulatory system as well as by playing a vital role in the immune system. The following sections review the basic anatomy and physiology of the cardiovascular system. (See chapter 2 for a discussion of immunity.)

Heart

Roughly the size of a closed fist, the heart is a muscular organ that pumps blood throughout the body. Men's hearts are usually slightly

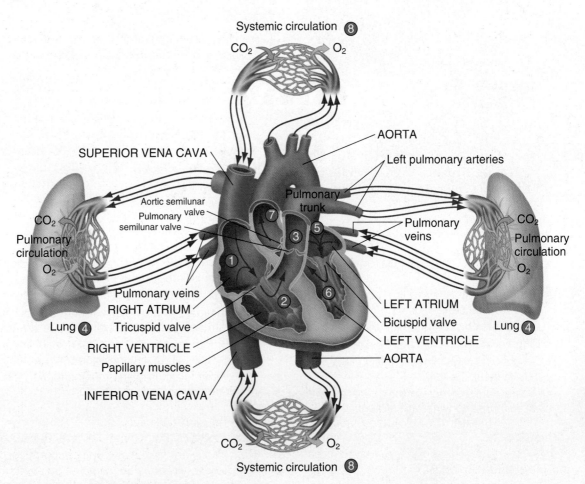

FIGURE 4-1 The cardiovascular system.

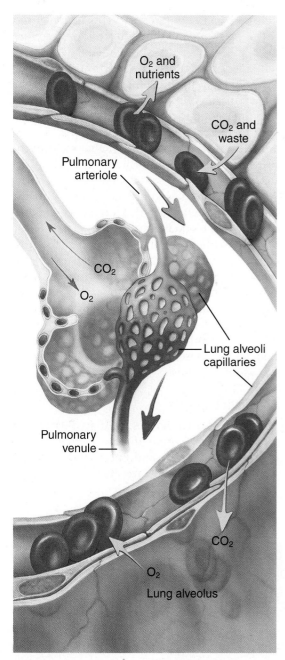

FIGURE 4-2 Pulmonary gas exchange.

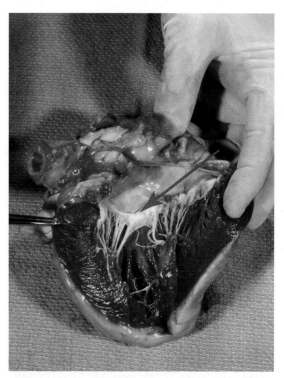

FIGURE 4-3 Heart valves.
© Phil Degginger/Alamy Stock Photo.

larger at 0.45% of body weight while women's are 0.40% of body weight. The heart is the workhorse of the cardiovascular system, pumping blood through the body's 50,000 miles of blood vessels and beating approximately 100,000 times per day. If you received a dollar for every heartbeat, you would be a millionaire in just 10 days. The heart can quickly adjust its rate to meet the ever-changing needs of the body.

The heart is in the thoracic cavity between the lungs and behind the sternum. The pericardial sac, or pericardium, encloses the heart to provide protection and support. Between the two layers of the pericardium (inner visceral and outer parietal) there is pericardial fluid. The amount of fluid contained in the pericardial space is approximately 50 mL. This fluid protects the heart against trauma from surrounding structures, invasions of foreign organisms, and friction from the constant movement. The pericardium provides support in terms of anchoring the heart and prevents overdistention. The pericardium contains receptors that can reflexively cause a change in blood pressure and heart rate.

The outer layer of the heart wall is the epicardium. The myocardium, the middle layer of the heart, is the muscle portion of the organ. The walls of the ventricles, especially the left ventricle, are thicker than the atrium because of the distance and pressures against which those chambers must pump blood. The atria are receiving chambers that pump blood to their respective ventricles. The ventricles pump blood to the low-pressure lungs and the high-pressure systemic circulation (15 mmHg and 92 mmHg, respectively).

The endocardium is the inner epithelial layer of the heart that makes up the cardiac valves; these valves function to ensure one-way flow of blood through the heart (FIGURE 4-3).

Cardiac Cycle

Understanding the blood flow through the heart is essential to understanding structural alterations and appreciating how they result in decreased cardiac output and/or altered tissue perfusion (FIGURE 4-4). As illustrated in blue in Figure 4-4, blood low in oxygen and rich in carbon dioxide enters the right side of the heart from the systemic circulation through the superior vena cava and the inferior vena cava. These veins empty blood directly into the right atrium. From the right atrium, blood flows quickly during ventricular diastole (i.e., atrial systole) through the tricuspid valve to the right ventricle. At the end of diastole, the atria contracts (i.e., *atrial kick*) to push the last amount of blood to the right ventricle. At this time, right ventricular pressure increases, and the tricuspid valve closes. The right ventricle pressure is higher than pulmonary artery pressure, causing the pulmonic valve to open, and ventricular contraction (i.e., systole) causes blood flow to the pulmonary arteries. The pulmonary arteries then carry the blood to the lungs for oxygenation. Pressure and volume in the right ventricle drop, and ventricular relaxation causes closure of the pulmonic valve.

The newly oxygenated blood returns from the lungs to the heart through the pulmonary veins. From the pulmonary veins, blood enters the left atrium, and the same cycle as described on the right occurs simultaneously through left-sided structures. The left atrium blood flows quickly through the mitral valve to the left ventricle, and the atrial kick forces the remaining blood through. Left ventricular pressure increases, causing mitral closure. The left ventricle pressure becomes higher than aortic pressure, opening the aortic valve, and ventricular contraction causes blood flow to the aorta. At this point, the blood is transported to the body. The coronary arteries receive oxygenated blood when blood is going from the atria to the ventricles (diastole) and not when the ventricles are contracting, supplying the rest of the body. The reason for the supply time being reversed for the coronaries is that when the ventricles are contracting there is high pressure in the chambers and most of the coronary vessels are closed. Both atria fill and contract simultaneously; likewise, both ventricles fill and contract simultaneously.

Conduction System

Left to their own devices, cardiac muscle cells would contract individually, which would create a disorderly and ineffective contraction. The muscle cells are able to contract in

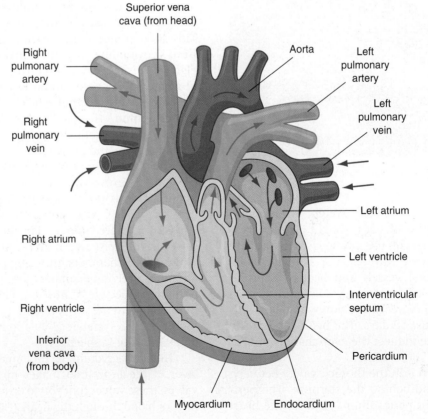

FIGURE 4-4 Blood flow through the heart.

an organized manner, however, due to the internal electrical stimulus initiated by a pacemaker. These electrical impulses are called *action potentials*. Basically, the heart's pacemaker acts like a generator creating an impulse for every heartbeat. Conductivity is the ability of cells to transmit electrical impulses. The ability of the cells to respond to electrical impulses is referred to as *excitability*. Cardiac cells are able to generate an impulse to contract even with no external nerve stimulus, a process called *automaticity*. When impulses travel through the cardiac cells, the result is a shortening of muscle fibers, which then causes contraction and pumping out of blood (i.e., systole). Between impulses, the fibers rest and go back to their usual length, which is when filling (i.e., diastole) occurs. See chapter 1 for further discussion of cellular function.

All cardiac muscle cells can initiate impulses, but normally the conduction pathway originates in the sinoatrial (SA) node located high in the right atrium (**FIGURE 4-5**). The SA node generates impulses faster than other areas (e.g., atrioventricular [AV] node, His bundle, Purkinje fibers) with pacemaker and automaticity capacity. Therefore, the SA node takes the lead and is the pacemaker of the heart, and other areas follow. Impulses originating in the SA node travel through the right

and left atria, resulting in atrial contraction. The SA node automatically generates impulses ranging from 60 to 100 beats per minute (sinus rhythm). The impulse then travels to the AV node, which is located in the right atrium adjacent to the septum. Although it does not usually initiate impulses unless the SA node begins failing, the intrinsic rate of impulses in the AV node is 40–60 beats per minute. The impulses are delayed, or move slowly, through the AV node so that the atria contracts right before the ventricle to allow for complete ventricular filling.

Next, the impulses move in rapid succession through the bundle of His; right and left bundle branches, which divide into the left anterior and posterior bundles; and Purkinje network of fibers. The flow of this impulse stimulates ventricular contraction. If the impulses fail to fire from the SA or AV node, the ventricles will attempt to pace themselves. The ventricles can generate impulses at 20–40 beats per minute, which may not result in adequate cardiac output because the ventricles may beat before they have a chance to fill with blood. These optional pacemakers in the heart function as a fail-safe mechanism to sustain life.

The conduction of the cardiac impulse produces an electric current that can be read by electrodes attached to the skin at various

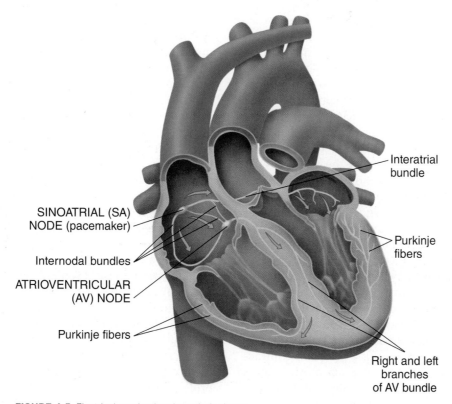

SINOATRIAL (SA)
NODE (pacemaker)

Internodal bundles

ATRIOVENTRICULAR
(AV) NODE

Purkinje fibers

Interatrial
bundle

Purkinje
fibers

Right and left
branches
of AV bundle

FIGURE 4-5 Electrical conduction through the heart.

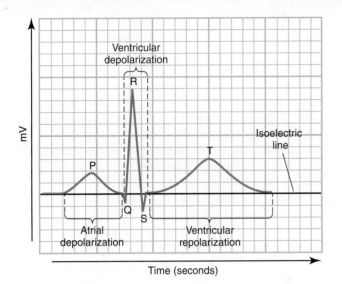

FIGURE 4-6 Characteristic features of a normal electrocardiogram.

P = atrial depolarization, which triggers atrial contraction.
QRS = depolarization of AV node and conduction of electrical impulse
through ventricles. Ventricular contraction begins at R.
T = repolarization of ventricles.
P to R interval = time required for impulses to travel from SA node to ventricles.
ST segment = complete ventricular depolarization.
Q to T interval = complete electrical systole.

points of the body, producing an electrocardiogram (EKG) (**FIGURE 4-6**). Organized depolarization (an increase in electrical charge through the exchange of ions across the cell membrane) of the cardiac cells generates cardiac muscle contraction. On the EKG reading, atrial contraction is represented by depolarization in the P wave, and ventricular contraction is represented by depolarization in the large QRS complex. The more intense the contraction, the higher the wave or complex. Because the force required for the atria to pump blood into the ventricles is minimal compared to the force required for the ventricles to pump blood to the entire body, the P wave is smaller than the QRS complex. The T wave represents repolarization, or recovery, of the ventricles. In repolarization, the ions line up on both sides of the cell membrane in preparation for depolarization. Repolarization of the atria does not appear on an EKG because it is hidden by the other, more prominent waveforms. Abnormal variations in the EKG, known as *arrhythmias* or *dysrhythmias*, may indicate acute problems, such as infarction or electrolyte imbalances.

Cardiac muscle cells require sodium (Na^+), potassium (K^+), calcium (Ca^+), and chloride (Cl^-) ions to initiate and conduct electrical signals as well as the resulting muscular contraction (see **FIGURE 4-7**). Pharmacologic agents have an effect on different phases of the action potential. To initiate the depolarization that creates contraction, the sodium–potassium pump shifts these ions to generate a charge. Ca^+ balance is required for muscle contractility, especially in a muscle that contracts many times each minute. Additionally, the neurologic system controls cardiac function, and it requires Na^+ balance to function properly.

The brain (specifically the medulla) monitors and controls cardiac function through the autonomic nervous system, endocrine system, and cardiac tissue. These functions include the rate of contraction (chronotropic effect), rate of electrical conduction (dromotropic effect), and strength of contraction (inotropic effect). Receptors in the brain, heart, blood vessels, and kidneys continuously monitor body functions to maintain homeostasis. Chemoreceptors detect chemical changes in the blood, and baroreceptors, located in the carotid arteries, detect pressure in the heart and arteries. If homeostasis is interrupted, receptors begin to fire, and neurotransmitters or hormones that activate either the sympathetic nervous system (SNS) or the parasympathetic nervous system (PNS) are released. Stimulating the SNS releases norepinephrine from nerve endings on the heart and other catecholamines (e.g., epinephrine), which circulate through the bloodstream and bind with receptors on the heart. The beta (β) and alpha (α) receptors are the most abundant and have more of an effect. The beta-1 receptors are located on the conduction system and myocardium and beta-2 are on the myocardium and smooth muscles (e.g., bronchial smooth muscle). When stimulated, heart rate and contractility increase (beta-1, beta-2) and the blood vessels will vasodilate (beta-2). The beta-2 effects on the vascular tone is small as beta 1 is the predominant receptor on the heart. Beta-2 stimulation also leads to bronchodilation. An opposing receptor is beta-3, and stimulation of this receptor leads to reduced contractility. The alpha receptors cause vasoconstriction (alpha-1) or centrally mediated vasodilation (alpha-2) to keep blood pressure in balance. Several medications to lower heart rate and blood pressure act through these receptor mechanisms. Some examples include beta-adrenergic blocking agents, which block beta-1 and beta-2 receptors (first generation nonselective beta blockers), thereby decreasing heart rate and contractility. Second generation beta blockers are cardioselective, blocking mainly beta 1 receptors (e.g., atenolol, bisoprolol). Another class of beta blockers (e.g.,

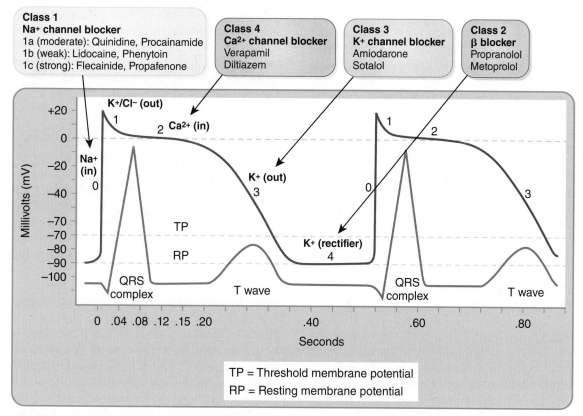

FIGURE 4-7 Cardiac action potential of myocardial cells.

carvedilol) which are nonselective are also alpha-1 receptor blockers thereby dilating blood vessels. Nonselective beta blockers, because they block the beta-2 receptors, can cause bronchoconstriction. Parasympathetic nervous system stimulation, specifically the vagal nerve, causes release of acetylcholine, which decreases heart rate and reduces contractile strength. Vagal nerve stimulation, which may occur with emotional distress from any situation like blood drawing, will cause a drop in heart rate and blood pressure referred to as a *vagal* or *vasovagal* reaction.

Blood Vessels

The heart's blood is supplied by the coronary arteries (see **FIGURE 4-8**). Two main arteries arise from the root of the aorta and divide into the right (RCA) and left (LCA) coronary arteries. These vessels branch out several times throughout the heart and the percent of flow and pattern of their branching varies among individuals. The LCA divides into the anterior descending artery, which supplies the front of the heart, the left and right ventricles, and the interventricular septum. The second LCA division is the circumflex, which supplies the

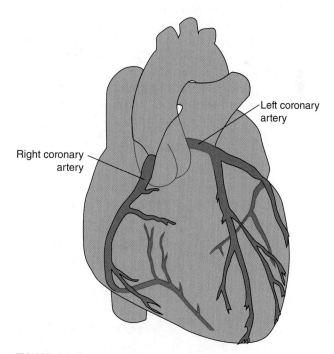

FIGURE 4-8 Coronary arteries.

left atrium and lateral left ventricle wall. The RCA supplies the right atrium and right ventricle and posterior part of the heart including the back of the interventricular septum. The coronary arteries have multiple connections within and between each other called *anastomoses*. The flow through the anastomosis provides critical collateral circulation when it is not sufficient from the RCA or LCA for various reasons such as occlusions. New collateral vessels can even be formed when there are problems with flow. Understanding coronary artery supply is necessary to be able to interpret 12-lead EKG (there are 12 tracings each reflecting various areas of the myocardium) and understand consequences of a coronary artery occlusion. As an example, an occlusion in the left anterior descending artery can result in left ventricular damage., This damage will be reflected in the V_3, V_4 tracings on the 12-lead EKG as these leads represent the myocardium that is supplied by the left anterior descending artery (left ventricle).

The systemic blood vessels are the intricate highway system along which the blood travels. Arteries carry blood away from the heart, while veins carry blood back to the heart. Left ventricular contractions project blood through the arteries, while valves in the veins assist in moving the blood back to the heart against gravity. The veins that have valves are those in the arms and legs. Once arteries leave the heart, they begin branching into smaller vessels called *arterioles* (FIGURE 4-9). These vessels continue branching into even smaller, thin-walled vessels called *capillaries*. Their thin walls allow oxygen and nutrients to shift out of the capillaries into the cells. Additionally, carbon dioxide and waste products shift from the cells into the capillaries. This exchange occurs through diffusion. Once blood is utilized at the cellular

level, the blood moves through the capillaries and transitions into larger vessels known as *venules*. The venules continue to merge into larger vessels until they become veins, much as small streams unite to form a river. (See chapter 1 for a discussion of cellular function.)

Generally, arteries carry blood rich in oxygen and nutrients, while veins carry blood saturated with carbon dioxide and metabolic waste. One exception to this pattern occurs in the pulmonary arteries and veins. The pulmonary arteries carry oxygen-depleted blood away from the right side of the heart to the lungs for gas exchange (Figure 4-2). Following gas exchange in the lungs, the oxygen-saturated blood returns to the left side of the heart through the pulmonary veins.

The walls of the blood vessels consist of three layers (FIGURE 4-10). The composition of the three layers varies among the different type of blood vessels. In general, the tunica intima is the smooth, thin, inner layer of the blood vessels known as the endothelium. The tunica media, the middle layer, is composed of smooth muscle that is responsible for the vessel's ability to change diameter. The outer layer, the tunica adventitia, consists of elastic and fibrous connective tissues that provide the necessary elasticity to accommodate the rush of blood with each cardiac contraction. Arteries also have a layer of elastic fiber in the tunica media and adventitia (externa) of some arteries that allow them to accommodate for high pressures. The small venules, capillaries, and arterioles do not have this elastic tissue, making them susceptible to damage when pressure increases. Large veins and arteries also have blood vessels called *vasa vasorum* and nerve endings on the adventitia that are not present on other vessels. The smooth muscle layer of arteries and arterioles is also much thicker than veins. Capillaries only have an endothelial layer.

Blood Pressure and Cardiac Output

The heart, conduction system, and blood vessels and their functions are all interconnected and influenced by many variables (FIGURE 4-11). The pressure within the walls of blood vessels created by blood flowing through is what is known as blood pressure. The pressure in the artery when the left ventricle contracts is systole, and the pressure in the arteries at rest is diastole. This pressure is described as a fraction with the systolic measurement as the numerator and the diastolic measurement as the denominator. According to the American Heart

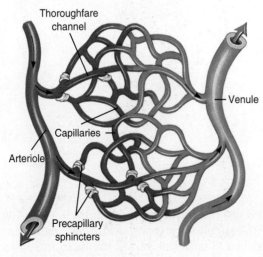

FIGURE 4-9 The circulatory system.

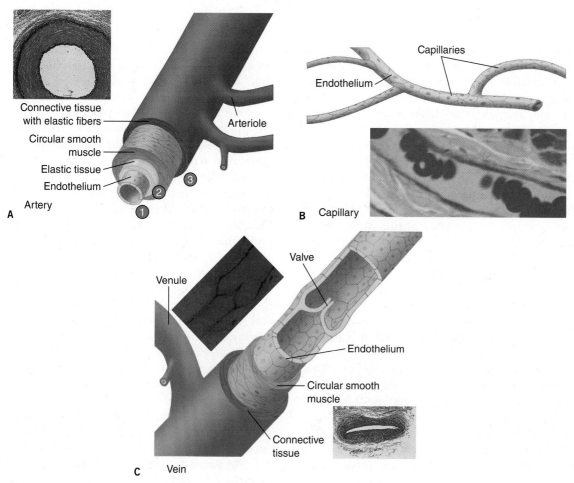

FIGURE 4-10 The walls of the blood vessels are composed of three layers of tissue: the endothelium, elastic tissue, and the connective tissue. **A** Artery; **B** capillary; **C** vein.

Artery photo: © Cabisco/Visuals Unlimited, Inc.; Capillary photo: © Ed Reschke/Photolibrary/Getty Images; Vein photos: © Cabisco/Visuals Unlimited, Inc. and © Dr. John D. Cunningham/Visuals Unlimited, Inc.

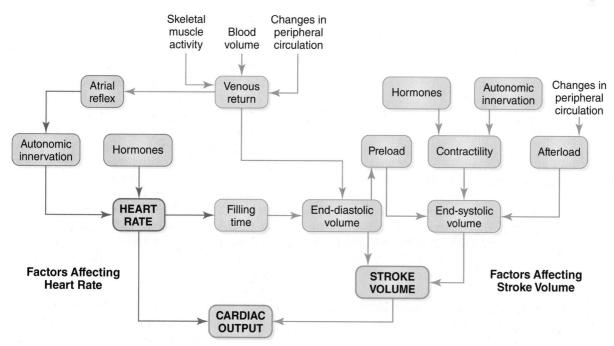

FIGURE 4-11 Factors affecting cardiac output.

Association (2017), a normal blood pressure reading should be less than 120/80 mmHg to maintain health and limit chronic disease risk. The average pressure in the arteries in one systole–diastole cycle is the mean arterial pressure and is considered an overall average pressure in the arteries. The mean arterial pressure as opposed to blood pressure can be used as a determinant of adequate perfusion. **Pulse pressure** is the difference between the systolic and diastolic pressures and represents the force the heart generates each time it contracts. The pulse pressure gives an indication of the stroke volume and the elasticity of the arterial wall. Various control mechanisms are in place to keep blood pressure at a range that is adequate for tissue perfusion.

Cardiac output and systemic vascular resistance significantly affect blood pressure ($BP = CO \times SVR$, where BP is blood pressure, CO is cardiac output, and SVR is systemic vascular resistance). Cardiac output refers to the amount of blood the heart pumps in one minute. This amount is determined by stroke volume and heart rate ($CO = SV \times HR$, where SV is stroke volume, and HR is heart rate) (Figure 4-11). Stroke volume is the amount of blood ejected from the heart with each contraction. Not all the blood in the heart is ejected. The amount pumped out with each cycle relative to how much blood volume there is at the end of diastole is called the *ejection fraction* (EF), and it is expressed as a percentage. The ejection fraction is a commonly used measurement to determine how well the ventricle is functioning. Various imaging techniques such as an echocardiogram or computed tomography (CT) can measure the EF. The stroke volume is influenced by the preload, afterload, and contractility. The pressure created in the left ventricle by the volume of blood at the end of diastole (left ventricular end diastolic pressure) is what constitutes the preload. Concepts in reference to pressure and volume are generally centered around the left side of the heart; however, the right side of the heart also responds similarly to the left. The preload pressure causes the cardiac muscle fibers to lengthen and the tension relationship to change. The fibers change and shorten to provide the best contraction. The preload will vary depending on how much blood volume blood is going into the left ventricle and how much volume stays in the ventricle after it contracts (systole). A key determinant of preload is volume, and measurements can be used as a gauge for ventricular volume.

Afterload is the pressure (resistance) the ventricle must overcome to eject blood (aortic pressure for the left ventricle and pulmonary pressure for the right ventricle). The left ventricle afterload is not only impacted by the aortic pressure and aortic valve functioning but also the systemic vascular resistance (SVR). The afterload is inversely related to contractility and preload because the afterload creates opposition to muscle fiber shortening. Afterload is often equated with SVR. The resistance that is created is dependent on whether the arterioles are constricted (increasing SVR) or dilated (decreasing SVR). The diameter changes are under the influence of the sympathetic nervous system. Neurotransmitter binding with alpha-1 receptors leads to vasoconstriction and binding with beta-2 receptors leads to vasodilation.

The third variable affecting stroke volume and, in turn, cardiac output and ultimately blood pressure, is the contractility of the heart. The end-diastolic volume (left preload) causes the ventricle muscle to stretch and contract. Norepinephrine is a dominant catecholamine that increases contractility along with epinephrine and dopamine. Acetylcholine, another neurotransmitter, depresses contractility. Hormonal influences from the thyroid will increase contractility.

The Frank-Starling law explains the myocardial length–tension relationship and preload. The law states that the more the myocardial stretch, the greater the contraction. The myocardial stretch is created by the end-diastolic volume and the muscle fibers. The muscle fibers reach a certain length at a certain speed, and these factors will determine the force of contraction. The principle is similar to when you stretch a rubber band. The more you stretch a rubber band the more forceful the snap when released. There is, however, a limit to this law, and beyond a certain point the muscle fibers will lose contractile ability. Overstretching over time will eventually cause the rubber band to lose elasticity; when stretched and released, it will barely snap. The same is true with heart muscle fibers—if they are already dilated from heart disease (i.e., unable to stretch), the heart will not contract effectively.

Laplace's law can explain factors influencing afterload, which is a pressure that is opposite to preload. In Laplace's law, wall stress (i.e., tension) is due to pressure in the ventricle and the radius (i.e., diameter), which is inversely related to wall thickness. In other words, the wall stress is influenced by pressure, diameter, and wall thickness. Wall stress affects metabolic demands, and the higher the wall stress the greater the metabolic demand. As an example, the ventricle has to increase its contractile force to overcome the increased pressure within the chamber. If the diameter of the blood vessel or heart chamber has an increased radius, then the heart has to increase its contractile force to supply the larger diameter. When the ventricle wall thickness increases, the opposite happens, and like a bodybuilder's big muscle, the heart does not have to contract as hard. To summarize, increasing radius or pressure increases wall stress, and increasing wall thickness decreases wall stress. Cardiac disorders can disrupt this balance, leading to increased wall stress with resulting increased metabolic demands and decreased perfusion.

Other factors can influence blood pressure by directly or indirectly regulating systemic vascular resistance, contractility, or blood volume. Baroreceptors located throughout the body (e.g., carotid, aorta) and changes in blood pressure due to position or volume changes will trigger vessel diameter and heart rate changes and contractility. The baroreceptors sense drops in blood pressure, causing the heart rate to increase, vessels to constrict, and the contractility to increase to maintain perfusion. The reverse happens with an increased blood pressure. Aging causes changes to these receptors that make them less effective and leads to a slower response. When an elderly person changes position from sitting to standing, the receptors do not respond as quickly (i.e., blood pressure does not rise) and hypotensive signs such as dizziness or blurred vision occur. This response is termed *postural hypotension*.

Aside from the adrenal gland hormones (epinephrine and norepinephrine), other hormones involved in blood pressure regulation include antidiuretic hormone (ADH), aldosterone, and angiotensin II. ADH, also known as vasopressin, increases water reabsorption in the kidney, which increases blood volume. Additionally, ADH is a vasoconstrictor, which increases SVR.

The renin–angiotensin–aldosterone system (RAAS) in the kidneys is a vital control and compensatory mechanism that becomes activated when renal blood flow is decreased, as is often the case in hypotensive states (**FIGURE 4-12**). When renal blood flow decreases, renin is released from the kidneys, activating angiotensin I, which is then converted to angiotensin II (a vasoconstrictor) through the actions of angiotensin-converting enzyme in the lungs.

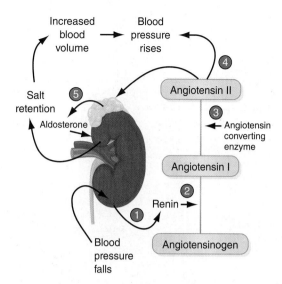

FIGURE 4-12 Role of kidneys in blood pressure.

Aldosterone secretion is also stimulated. Aldosterone (from the adrenal cortex) increases the reabsorption of Na^+ and Cl^- in the kidneys; Na^+ attracts water, which, like ADH, increases blood volume. In hypotensive states, this mechanism raises blood pressure and maintains the blood supply to vital organs. In chronic disease states such as hypertension, this mechanism is inappropriately activated because of reduced blood flow (vasoconstriction) to the kidneys, further contributing to the hypertension. In contrast to ADH and aldosterone, natriuretic hormones (e.g., atrial natriuretic peptide) cause loss of Na^+, Cl^-, and water.

The endothelial lining of blood vessels releases various vasoactive chemicals. The chemicals either cause vasoconstriction (e.g., thromboxane, prostaglandin) or vasodilation such as nitrous oxide or endothelium-derived relaxing factor. Angiotensin II is in the vascular tissues and blocks vasodilators (e.g., nitrous oxide).

Lymphatic System

The lymphatic system is an extensive network of vessels and glands that returns excess fluid (about 3 liters per day) in body tissue to the circulatory system and works with the immune system. Interstitial fluid surrounds cells and provides a medium through which nutrients, gases, and wastes can diffuse between the capillaries and the cells. Capillaries are continuously replenishing this fluid. Normally, the fluid outflow from the capillaries exceeds the fluid returned. Lymph capillaries absorb the excess fluid (**FIGURE 4-13**). This fluid, or lymph, drains from these capillaries into larger vessels and ducts (right lymphatic duct and thoracic duct)

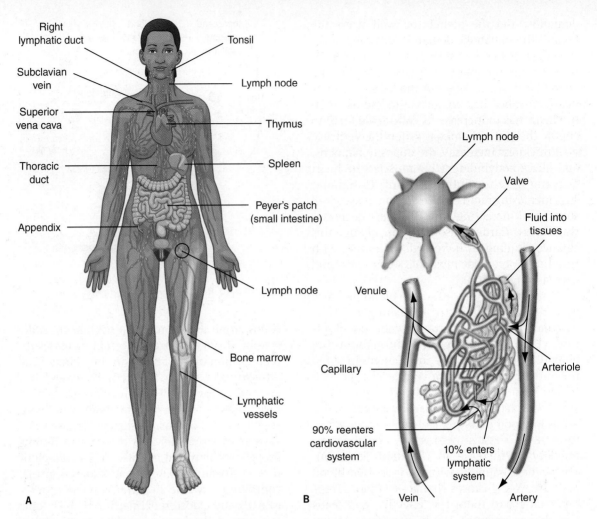

FIGURE 4-13 The lymphatic system. **(A)** The lymphatic system consists of vessels that transport lymph—that is, excess tissue fluid—back to the circulatory system. **(B)** Lymph is picked up by lymphatic capillaries that drain into larger vessels. Like the veins, the lymphatic vessels contain valves that prohibit backflow. Lymph nodes are interspersed along the vessels and serve to filter the lymph.

that empty into large subclavian veins at the base of the neck. The movement of lymph occurs in much the same way that blood travels through the veins, with the assistance of valves and body movement. (See chapter 2 for a discussion of immunity.)

The lymphatic system also includes several organs and tissue—lymph nodes, the spleen, the thymus, the bone marrow, and tonsils. These organs primarily function in the immune response. Lymph fluid contains antigen-presenting cells and lymphocytes that go from node to node waiting to respond to antigens. Located in clusters throughout the body, lymph nodes are a network of fibers and irregular channels that slow down the lymph flow. As the lymph passes through the nodes, the fibers filter out bacteria, viruses, and cellular debris. Numerous macrophages line the channels to phagocytize microorganisms and other material.

Normally, the rate at which lymph is produced equals the rate at which it is removed. In some body states, the amount of lymph produced exceeds the capacity of the system. For example, burns can cause extensive damage to capillaries, causing them to leak fluid into the tissues. This flooding results in excessive fluid in the tissue, or edema. Fluid can also leak into the tissues as a result of lymphatic vessels becoming occluded, often because of infection.

Understanding Conditions That Affect the Cardiovascular System

When considering alterations in the cardiovascular system, organizing them based on basic structures such as the pump (heart) and the vasculature can increase understanding.

Disorders of either of these basic structures can lead to impaired cardiac output or tissue perfusion and often a combination of both. Alterations in pump function can occur due to disorders in the valves, conduction system, and the various layers of the heart wall. The vasculature system can be categorized by disorders of the veins and arteries (including the coronary arteries). Since the vasculature is located throughout the body, most diseases will involve the vasculature. Many diseases of the heart and vasculature are life threatening, so quickly determining the source of the problem will lead to appropriate intervention. Prevention and maintenance of cardiovascular health are crucial to maintain quality of life and reduce the burden of so many diseases associated with cardiovascular dysfunction.

Impaired Cardiac Output: Heart Disease

Pericarditis

Pericarditis refers to an inflammation of the pericardium—the sac that surrounds, protects, and supports the heart. This inflammation is most commonly triggered by viral infections (usually after a respiratory infection), but it may result from bacterial, fungal, or parasitic infections. Some common viruses implicated are coxsackievirus and other echoviruses, herpes simplex, cytomegalovirus, and human immunodeficiency virus. Other causes are noninfectious and can be related to myocardial infarction, thoracic

trauma including those that are iatrogenic (e.g., surgery, postcardiac interventions, radiation) or noniatrogenic (e.g., accident). Malignancy can cause pericarditis, whether from primary tumors or, more commonly, secondary tumors, particularly from the breast, lung, or lymphoma. Other causes of pericarditis include autoimmune conditions, particularly systemic lupus erythematosus, rheumatoid arthritis, scleroderma, and, rarely, metabolic disorders (e.g., uremia or myxedema) and various pharmacologic agents (e.g., procainamide or phenytoin).

During the inflammatory process, fluid shifts from the capillaries to the space between the pericardial sac and the heart. The fluid type may be a clue to the underlying cause. The fluid may be serous, as with heart failure; purulent, such as with infections; serosanguinous, as occurs with neoplasms or uremia; or hemorrhagic, as seen with aneurysms or trauma. As the pericardial tissue becomes inflamed, the swollen pericardial tissue rubs against the swollen cardiac tissue, creating friction.

Fluid can accumulate slowly or quickly in the pericardial cavity, creating a pericardial effusion. Usually conditions that cause a rapid effusion can progress to life-threatening cardiac tamponade. Slower, larger effusions or even those loculated and not affecting the whole pericardium can also lead to tamponade (**FIGURE 4-14**). In cardiac tamponade, the fluid accumulates in the pericardial cavity to the point that it compresses the heart. This compression prevents the heart from stretching and filling during diastole, initially affecting

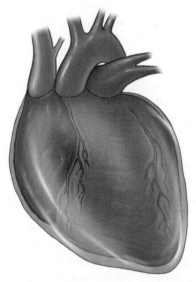
Normal heart

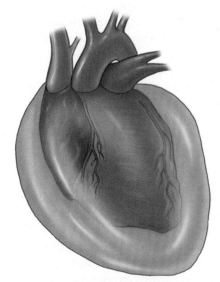
Cardiac tamponade

FIGURE 4-14 Cardiac tamponade.

the right side of the heart due to its lower pressure. The decreased right-side stretching and filling causes blood to back up into the venous circulation, causing right-sided heart failure and a reduction in left ventricle filling. The result is a decreased cardiac output. Arterial pressures then fall (because of the decreased cardiac output), venous pressures rise (because of the accumulation of blood within the systemic circulation), and the pulse pressure narrows (because of the arterial and venous pressure changes). Additionally, the heart sounds are muffled upon auscultation because the excess fluid drowns out the sound. Heart failure, cardiogenic shock, and death can result from cardiac tamponade.

Pericardial inflammation that becomes chronic can lead to constrictive pericarditis. In constrictive pericarditis, the pericardium becomes thick and fibrous from the chronic inflammation and causes the visceral and parietal layers to adhere. The constriction results in a situation similar to tamponade with reduced cardiac filling, decreasing cardiac output, and systemic congestion. Tamponade due to constrictive pericarditis develops slowly as opposed to other causes of tamponade that develop quickly.

Clinical Manifestations

Clinical manifestations of pericarditis include the following symptoms: dyspnea and chest pain. The pain is usually in the anterior chest and is described as sharp and sudden. The pain increases with deep inspiration or lying flat (when the pericardium is closest to the chest wall) and decreases when the patient sits up and leans forward. Flulike symptoms including fever, chills, malaise, and myalgia may be present depending on the cause. Physical examination findings include a pericardial friction rub, which is a grating sound heard usually between the lower left sternal border and cardiac apex when the breath is held. The rub may be intermittent. If there is an effusion, the heart sounds may be muffled. Sudden acute tamponades present as shock with a low blood pressure, jugular vein distention, and muffled heart sounds—referred to as *Beck's triad*. Tamponade also causes tachypnea, tachycardia, and other signs of cardiovascular collapse. If there is a slower accumulating tamponade, right-sided heart failure manifestations will be present with dyspnea, tachycardia, jugular vein distention, ascites, hepatomegaly, and edema. The manifestations in constrictive pericarditis are similar (e.g., dyspnea, fatigue, edema) to pericarditis with or without tamponade but are slower in onset.

Diagnosis and Treatment

Diagnosis of pericarditis is accomplished through a history and physical examination. Some EKG changes in acute pericarditis include inflammatory changes with diffuse ST segment elevation with no Q waves or reciprocal changes as seen in myocardial infarction (MI). Echocardiogram and/or CT may demonstrate an effusion, wall thickening, and constriction. Chest X-rays, complete blood count (CBC), and magnetic resonance imaging (MRI) or other tests such as a pericardial biopsy may be necessary to aid in diagnosis. Treatment focuses on the underlying cause (e.g., antibiotics for infection) and reducing the inflammation (e.g., nonsteroidal anti-inflammatory medications and colchicine are effective in reducing the development of fibrosis). Steroidal anti-inflammatory drugs can be considered if nonsteroidal anti-inflammatory medications are contraindicated. Analgesics may be administered to manage pain. Additionally, bed rest is important to reduce metabolic needs and cardiac workload. Oxygen therapy can increase available oxygen. Pericardiocentesis may be performed to withdraw excess fluid from pericardium, or a pericardiectomy (a surgical procedure in which a window is created in the pericardium) may be performed to release constriction and allow excess fluid to drain into the pleural cavity.

Infective Endocarditis

Infective endocarditis (IE) (previously called *bacterial endocarditis*) is an infection of the endocardium. Infections are more common on or near the heart valves but can occur anywhere on the endocardium. The organisms commonly involved will vary depending on whether the valve is native or prosthetic and whether the infection is community acquired or nosocomial. *Staphylococcus aureus* commonly found on the skin and the gastrointestinal tract is the most common causative organism in IE. *S. aureus* is an organism that often causes infection due to healthcare contact such as surgery, hospitalization, or procedures (American Heart Association, 2015). Injection drug users have a higher incidence of IE from *S. aureus*. Viridans streptococci, commonly found in the mouth, account for many cases of community-acquired IE. *Enterococcus* species—bacteria commonly found in the gastrointestinal tract—are another frequent causative organism. Less common causes include other bacterial species, viruses, fungi, rickettsia, and parasites.

IE is more common in adults as there is a higher incidence of valvular disease, implanted cardiac devices, exposure to healthcare-related procedures (e.g., intravenous catheters), and injection drug use. Advances in health care have increased survival among children with congenital heart disease leading to a subsequent higher risk of developing IE. Neonatal and pediatric disease management in intensive care units has become more complex, involving more invasive procedures such as central line placements. As a consequence, nosocomial infections are a common cause of IE in children, even in those with no heart disease. Rheumatic heart disease, which is not as prevalent in the United States, is more of a predisposing factor for IE in developing countries.

The pathogenesis of IE involves endothelial damage, which attracts platelets and stimulates thrombus formation. Bacteria start adhering to the linings and go into the thrombus where the bacteria are protected by the fibrin clots. Vegetation (including platelets, fibrin, microorganisms, inflammatory cells, and granulomatous tissue) collects on the internal structures because of damage from the infection, much like the process that occurs when a boat's anchor is placed in a body of water for an extended length of time and barnacles develop. With each heart contraction, some of this vegetation is dislodged and ejected from the heart. These small thrombi move throughout the body, collecting in the microcirculation and creating microhemorrhages (e.g., petechiae and hematuria). The thrombi can also travel to other locations, in which case they are known as embolisms, and become lodged there. These emboli can cause serious and often life-threatening complications such as myocardial infarction, stroke, seizures, and pulmonary embolism. In addition, the heart valves can become scarred and perforated (FIGURE 4-15). If untreated, infective endocarditis is usually fatal, especially when it involves the valvular structures.

Clinical Manifestations

Clinical manifestations of infective endocarditis will depend on whether IE presents acutely or subacutely. Acute signs and symptoms tend to be worse (e.g., higher fever) than subacute. IE may infect different valves and to different degrees, which also influences presentation. Systemic involvement varies and may include the

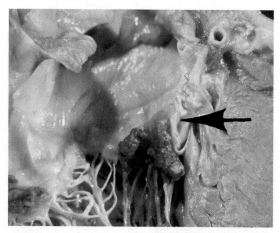

FIGURE 4-15 Infective endocarditis.
Courtesy of Leonard V. Crowley, MD, Century College.

lungs, kidneys, eyes, musculoskeletal system, and neurologic alterations. Infectious and inflammatory manifestations include fever, chills, myalgias, arthralgias, and malaise. A heart murmur may be new or worsened. Heart failure may be present. Skin and mucous membranes findings may include petechiae (bleeding capillaries), painful red nodules on the finger and toe (Osler nodes), nonpainful hemorrhages on the palms and soles (Janeway lesions), and splinter hemorrhages under the nailbed. Arterial emboli can occur in up to 50% of patients and symptoms will vary depending on which organ has the emboli. Renal dysfunction and hematuria may occur with kidney involvement.

Diagnosis and Treatment

Due to the high variability in disease presentation and challenges in diagnosis, criteria were developed to define and aid clinicians. This schema is known as the modified Duke criteria and incorporates clinical, laboratory, and echocardiogram findings. Some of the criteria include bacteremia such as positive blood cultures, echocardiogram findings such as a new regurgitant valve or a mass on valve, and predisposing risks or fever. Several exclusion criteria for IE include a likelihood of an alternative diagnosis or resolution and nonrecurrence of symptoms with ≤ 4 days of antibiotics. Other diagnostic procedures for IE include a CBC, erythrocyte sedimentation rate, C-reactive protein, immune complex titers, urinalysis, serum rheumatoid factor, EKG, and chest X-ray. Treatment is based on management of the identified causative agent (e.g., antibiotics for bacteria or antifungal agents for fungi). The anti-infective therapy for IE is often long-term (a minimum of 4 weeks). Other treatments are initiated to maintain cardiac function and treat other symptoms and include bed rest, oxygen therapy, and antipyretic agents. Repair or replacement of cardiac valves may be indicated when there is heart failure, uncontrolled infection, or higher mortality with medical treatment only (e.g., *S. aureus* with vegetations and septicemia). Antibiotic prophylaxis prior to certain dental procedures may be necessary in certain high-risk patients such as those with prosthetic cardiac valves or congenital heart disease to prevent IE.

Diagnostic Link

Echocardiogram

Echocardiograms are noninvasive tests frequently used to evaluate the structure and function of the heart. An echocardiogram produces images and recordings through ultrasound (high-frequency sound waves). The echocardiogram can be used to evaluate the pericardium (for effusion); ventricles (for hypertrophy, dilatation, wall motion, and thrombi); valves (for stenosis and regurgitation); great vessels (for aortic dissection); and septal areas (for trauma or congenital disease). The echocardiogram generates anatomic images in different modes: one-dimensional (M mode), two-dimensional, and three-dimensional. The test can be a transthoracic echocardiogram (TTE) where the transducer is on the chest wall or a transesophageal echocardiogram (TEE), where the transducer is placed in the esophagus. There are no contraindications for the TTE, but evaluation limitations exist when the patient has a thick chest wall like in an obese patient or rib crowding like in an underweight patient. The TEE requires intravenous and local anesthesia and, therefore, is a bit more complex to perform. The TEE is a useful adjunct when the TTE evaluation is inconclusive or limited and more detailed information is needed. **Doppler** While the different modes generate anatomic images in echocardiogram, the addition of Doppler-ultrasound provides hemodynamic data of the velocity and direction of blood flow through the valves, pulmonary artery, and veins. An echocardiogram can be done with contrast to evaluate shunts (e.g., patent foramen ovale) and many other additions and enhancements can be done. Technologic advances are being evaluated to enhance the capacities of the frequently used echocardiogram.

Myocarditis

Myocarditis is an inflammation of the myocardium. The incidence of this disease is difficult to determine as the pathophysiology is poorly understood, there are many clinical presentations making diagnosis difficult, and at least several weeks (in some cases a decade) lapse between exposure of the causative agent and the development of symptoms. Myocarditis can be caused by infectious and noninfectious agents. Infectious causes are usually due to a virus (e.g., influenza, coxsackie, cytomegalovirus, adenovirus, hepatitis C, herpes, HIV, or parvovirus).

Other organisms causing myocarditis are bacterial (e.g., Lyme disease, *Chlamydia*, *Mycoplasma*, or *Streptococcus*), or fungal (e.g., *Aspergillus*, *Candida*, *Cryptococcus*, or *Histoplasma*). A common origin is Chagas disease in developing countries, particularly Latin America (Mexico, Central America, and South America), which is caused by a parasite, *Trypanosoma cruzi*. Noninfectious causes may include allergic reactions, chemical exposure, radiation, or inflammatory disorders (e.g., rheumatoid arthritis or sarcoidosis). With myocarditis, organisms, blood cells, toxins, and immune substances penetrate the myocardium and can result in muscle fiber dysfunction and degeneration that impairs contractility and conduction. Most cases of myocarditis are benign, but some cases result in heart failure, dilated cardiomyopathy, dysrhythmias, and thrombi development. The term *inflammatory cardiomyopathy* is sometimes used instead of myocarditis when there is cardiac muscle dysfunction.

Clinical Manifestations

The patient may be asymptomatic or present with flulike symptoms, chest pain usually from pericarditis, syncope, palpitations, and joint pain/swelling. Physical exam findings will also vary and can include fever, a pericardial rub, tachyarrhythmias, and less commonly, bradyarrhythmias. Signs of heart failure or cardiogenic shock will be present in severe cases.

Diagnosis and Treatment

Diagnosis of myocarditis is accomplished through a history, physical examination, and blood cultures. EKG may reveal sinus tachycardia, pericarditis, or myocardial infarction changes. The cardiac enzyme troponin is more commonly elevated than creatinine kinase. Endomyocardial biopsy is considered a gold standard for diagnosis but is a risky procedure and not necessary in every case. Other tests can include a CBC, erythrocyte sedimentation rate, chest X-rays, and echocardiogram. Management centers on treating the causative agent (e.g., antibiotics for bacteria and antifungals for fungi). Antipyretics, anticoagulants, antidysrhythmics, diuretics, and immunosuppressants (e.g., corticosteroids or nonsteroidal anti-inflammatory drugs) may be used to treat symptoms or complications. Increasing bed rest, restricting activity, and limiting fluids can reduce cardiac workload.

Valvular Disorders

Valvular disorders cause disruption of normal blood flow through the heart. These disorders

BOX 4-1 Application to Practice

Mrs. Fulcher is a 58-year-old married homemaker who was recently discharged from the hospital because of recurrent infective endocarditis. Her most recent episodes were a *S. aureus* infection of the mitral valve 12 months ago and a *Streptococcus mutans* infection of the aortic valve 1 month ago. During her most recent hospitalization, an echocardiogram showed aortic stenosis, moderate aortic insufficiency, chronic valvular vegetation, and moderate atrial enlargement. In addition, Mrs. Fulcher has a history of chronic joint pain.

After being home for 1 week, Mrs. Fulcher was readmitted to the telemetry floor with endocarditis. She reports chills, fever, fatigue, joint pain, malaise, and a headache for the last 24 hours. At admission, Mrs. Fulcher's blood pressure was 172/48 mmHg (supine) and 100/40 mmHg (sitting), her pulse was 116, respirations were 20, and her temperature was 101.9°F. She was oriented to person, place, and time but was drowsy. Physical exam further revealed a murmur; clear and bilaterally equal lung sounds; extremities with 2+ pitting tibial edema; no peripheral cyanosis; and multiple petechiae on the skin of her arms, legs, and chest. She also has hematuria.

Upon admission, IV infusion of normal saline at 125 mL/hr and vancomycin IV every 8 hours was ordered to be continued over the next 4 weeks. Other routine medications ordered included furosemide (Lasix), amlodipine (Norvasc), and metoprolol (Lopressor).

1. What is the significance of the orthostatic hypotension, the wide pulse pressure, and tachycardia?
2. What is the significance of the hematuria, joint pain, and petechiae?
3. For which complications of embolization should Mrs. Fulcher be assessed?

Modified from Story, L. (2017). *Pathophysiology: A Practical Approach* (3rd ed.). Burlington, MA: Jones & Bartlett Learning.

---

are distinguished based on the valve affected and the type of alteration. Valvular disorders can be congenital or acquired. Two types of alterations are stenosis and regurgitation. Aortic and mitral valve disease are more common due to the higher pressures and workload on the left side of the heart.

Stenosis is a narrowing of a structure—in this discussion, heart valves. When the valves are stenosed, blood moving through the valve is reduced, causing blood to back up in the chamber just before the valve. Atresia refers to a lack of the valve opening (e.g., the valve cusps may be fused together) that would otherwise allow blood flow. Pressures in the overfilled chambers increase to pump against the resistance of the stenosed valve. Because the heart (specifically the chamber) is working harder, hypertrophy of the chamber develops. Hypertrophy and increased workload escalate the heart's oxygen demands, but the decreased cardiac output resulting from the stenosis makes it difficult to meet these increased demands. The cardiac output ultimately decreases, leading to clinical deterioration. Other heart disorders such as cardiomyopathy and heart failure can develop. Aortic stenosis is one of the most common valvular diseases in the United States.

Regurgitation, also called *insufficiency or incompetence*, occurs when the valve leaflets do not completely close, so blood continuously leaks. Additionally, heart valves normally allow blood to flow in one direction; incompetent valves, however, allow blood to flow in both directions. This regurgitation of blood increases the amount of blood that must be pumped and, in turn, increases the cardiac workload. The increased workload contributes to hypertrophy developing in the affected chambers. Additionally, the increased blood volume in the heart causes the chambers to dilate to accommodate the larger volume. Valves can also be both stenotic and incompetent such as when the mitral valve annulus (fibrous ring around valve) becomes calcified. Valve calcification can occur secondary to degenerative changes, atherosclerosis, and other diseases. Due to the calcifications, the mitral valve is unable to close properly (regurgitation) leading to an ineffective contraction and the calcifications cause a narrower opening (stenosis).

Valvular disorders may have a number of causes such as congenital defects, infections, endocarditis, rheumatic fever, hypertension, myocardial infarction, cardiomyopathy, and heart failure. Some diseases affect more than one valve, such as in Marfan syndrome where the aortic and mitral valve can become regurgitant. One valve disorder may be the cause of another valve disorder such as in mitral valve stenosis. Mitral stenosis causes backup of blood into the lungs, causing a rise in pulmonary pressures, and, ultimately, right-sided heart issues develop with tricuspid and pulmonic valve changes. When considering valvular disease, it is important to identify the affected valve as well as think of the blood flow consequences, whether forward or backward, caused by the diseased valve.

Learning Points

Mitral Valve Prolapse

Mitral valve prolapse (MVP) is caused by structural abnormalities in the leaflets, chordae, or annulus of the valve. MVP is a common valve disorder and is the most common cause of mitral regurgitation; however, MVP does not always result in regurgitation. The structural abnormalities can occur due to many disorders such as connective tissue disease (e.g., Marfan syndrome), myocardial infarction, von Willebrand disease, and skeletal abnormalities. MVP causes the valve leaflets to billow into the left ventricle or flail and prolapse into the left atrium during systole (**FIGURE 4-16**).

Clinical Manifestations

Clinical manifestations are the consequences of the flow alterations, the valve involved, the nature of the alteration, and the severity (**TABLE 4-1**). As an example, aortic stenosis causes classic manifestations such as syncope, angina, and heart failure. Angina occurs because oxygen supply is reduced as the heart is

working hard to eject blood through a stenotic aortic valve and is unable to meet the demands. Angina even occurs with normal coronary arteries. Ventricular hypertrophy, which is compensatory at first, will lead to heart failure. Syncope, which is usually exertional, can be caused by a decreased cardiac output. Aortic stenosis may exist for many years without symptoms or with minimal symptoms until it becomes notably stenotic (e.g., 1 cm^2).

Diagnosis and Treatment

Valvular heart disease can be diagnosed with a history and physical examination and evaluation with an echocardiogram. Other diagnostic tests are ordered to evaluate causes or consequences of the valve disease and can include heart catheterization, chest X-rays, EKG, or MRI. Management is geared toward the actual or potential consequences of the valve disease such as heart failure, cardiomyopathy, and symptomatology. Medications often used to treat valvular disorders include diuretics, antidysrhythmics, vasodilators, angiotensin-converting enzyme (ACE) inhibitors, beta-adrenergic blocking agents, and anticoagulants that decrease the workload on the heart and prevent thrombi. Additional strategies may include oxygen administration and a low-sodium diet. Valve replacement may be with a mechanical valve or a biologic valve (pig, cow, or human). Mechanical valves generally have a longer duration, but patients will

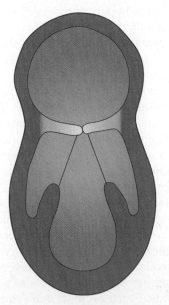

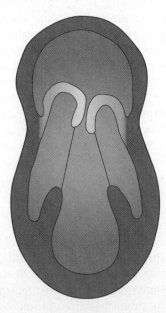

Normal   Prolapse

FIGURE 4-16 Normal mitral valve leaflets (left) compared with prolapsing mitral leaflets associated with mild mitral insufficiency (right).

TABLE 4-1	Clinical Manifestations of Valvular Stenosis and Regurgitation				
Manifestation	**Aortic stenosis**	**Aortic regurgitation**	**Mitral stenosis**	**Mitral regurgitation**	**Tricuspid regurgitation**
Cardiovascular effects	Left ventricular hypertrophy, angina	Left heart hypertrophy, angina	Right ventricular hypertrophy, angina	Left heart hypertrophy, angina	Right heart hypertrophy, angina
General symptoms	Fatigue	Fatigue	Fatigue, edema	Fatigue, dizziness, peripheral edema	Peripheral edema
Respiratory effects	Dyspnea on exertion	Dyspnea on exertion	Dyspnea on exertion, orthopnea, paroxysmal nocturnal dyspnea, predisposition to respiratory infections, hemoptysis, pulmonary hypertension	Dyspnea; occasional hemoptysis	Dyspnea
Central nervous system effects	Syncope, especially on exertion	Syncope	Neural deficits only associated with emboli	None	None
Gastrointestinal effects	None	None	Ascites, hepatic angina with hepatomegaly	None	Ascites, hepatomegaly (with heart failure)
Heart rate, rhythm	Bradycardia, variety of dysrhythmias	Palpitations, water hammer pulse	Palpitations	Palpitations	Atrial fibrillation
Heart sounds	Systolic murmur	Diastolic and systolic murmurs	Diastolic murmur, accentuated first heart sound	Murmur throughout systole	Murmur throughout systole
Most common cause	Congenital, rheumatic fever	Bacterial endocarditis; aortic root disease	Rheumatic fever	Insufficient valve, coronary artery disease	Congenital

Modified from Huether, S., & McCance, K. (2000). *Understanding pathophysiology* (2nd ed.). St. Louis, MO: C. V. Mosby.

need to be on lifelong anticoagulation while those with biologics do not need to be on anticoagulation. Factors determining the use of a particular valve include anticoagulation risk and age as biologics deteriorate fast and are not the best for the young. Aortic stenosis or regurgitation can be medically managed, but most patients will ultimately need valve repair or replacement. Mitral stenosis and regurgitation can be treated medically first, but there are circumstances when repair or replacement is necessary urgently (e.g., acute mitral regurgitation caused by an MI or chest trauma). In addition to replacement valve repair can include techniques such as valvotomy. This technique involves percutaneously introducing a catheter with a balloon that goes through the stenotic valve and is inflated to clear the calcifications.

Cardiomyopathy

Cardiomyopathies are disease of the heart muscle that can lead to several types of structural (e.g., hypertrophy) and functional (e.g., systolic/diastolic dysfunction) changes. The structural and functional changes in cardiomyopathy can cause heart failure. Most cardiomyopathies are classified into three groups—dilated cardiomyopathy (DCM), hypertrophic cardiomyopathy (HCM), and restrictive cardiomyopathy (FIGURE 4-17). These three groups are descriptive of the morphology (structure), function, and phenotype (observable characteristics) of the cardiomyopathy. Many cardiomyopathies develop due to genetic abnormalities. The type of genetic abnormalities is not incorporated in the three-group scheme. Several newer classifications also incorporate genetic information

Normal heart

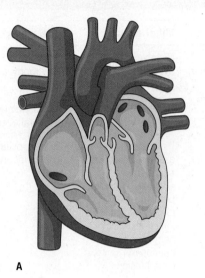

A

Dilated cardiomyopathy

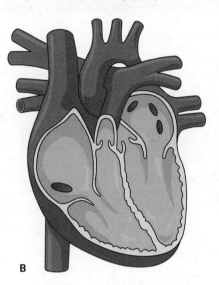

B

Hypertrophic cardiomyopathy

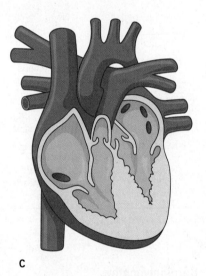

C

Restrictive cardiomyopathy

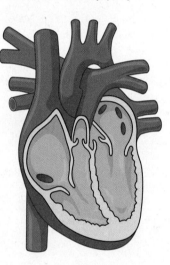

D

FIGURE 4-17 Comparing cardiomyopathies.

(e.g., MOGE(S)). Genetic testing can provide information pertaining to the etiology and used to identify patients at risk before structural and functional changes occur. Other diseases such as myocardial infarction and hypertension cause heart muscle damage. However, newer definitions of cardiomyopathies have been proposed by major societies such as the World Health Organization and the American Heart Association and these definitions exclude cases of heart muscle damage as a result of coronary artery disease, valvular disease, hypertension, or congenital heart disease. In the literature, often cardiomyopathies may still be described as hypertensive

Learning Points

Cardiomyopathy Classification

MOGE(S) stands for:

M	**m**orphofunctional phenotype
O	**o**rgan involvement
G	**g**enetic or family inheritance pattern
E	**e**tiologic description
S	functional **s**tatus.

MOGE(S) is one example of a cardiomyopathy classification incorporating genetic information. Descriptors are listed under each heading much like the concept of the tumor size, nodal involvement, and metastatic progress cancer staging system.

cardiomyopathy or ischemic cardiomyopathy. The classification of *ischemic* and *nonischemic* cardiomyopathy is also not preferred.

Over 100 genes are linked or may be linked with cardiomyopathy. Although cardiomyopathies may be nongenetic, most are inherited, and most are autosomal dominant with some recessive and X-linked inheritance pattern. The gene mutations associated with cardiomyopathy cause a wide variety of clinical presentations and disease severity. In addition to the mutation, other factors such as lifestyle and genomic variation can influence clinical presentations. There have been many advancements in identifying which genomic variations are benign or pathologic. People with the identical mutations may have different clinical presentations. Some individuals have the genotype but never develop cardiomyopathy as a result of incomplete or reduced penetrance. Within each of the three categories of cardiomyopathy, there are heterogenous structural and functional changes and risk. For example, a person with hypertrophic cardiomyopathy can have a dilated or restrictive

pattern. Some cardiomyopathies are associated with lethal cardiac rhythms that cause sudden cardiac death, but some people with the same type of cardiomyopathy are not at risk. Through genetic testing, identifying those at risk for lethal arrhythmias is possible. Individuals known to be at risk could prophylactically get an implantable cardioverter-defibrillator to manage the lethal arrhythmias. A person with a genetic mutation associated with cardiomyopathy may be asymptomatic or have minor symptoms for many years (e.g., until age > 50 years) before manifestation of the disease. Identifying people before the disease starts underscores the importance of genetic testing. The delayed manifestation described is an example of the genetic concept of age-dependent penetrance. This type of penetrance is similar to a man becoming bald as he gets older.

While new classifications exist, the three groups (hypertrophic, restrictive, dilated) will be used to discuss cardiomyopathy clinical manifestations. Treatment protocols are also based on this classification (see **TABLE 4-2**).

TABLE 4-2 Cardiomyopathy Classification

Type	DCM	HCM	Restrictive
Etiology: broad categories	Systemic disorders and genetic mutations (up to 50%)	Genetic mutations (most)	Systemic disorders and genetic mutations
Key heart changes	Dilated hypertrophied ventricle but normal wall thickness / Systolic dysfunction	Hypertrophied/thick-walled ventricle (usually interventricular septum) / Diastolic dysfunction	Rigid ventricle walls/but normal wall thickness / Diastolic dysfunction
Age variations	Age range 20–60 yrs / Most common type in pediatrics	Avg. age 40 yrs / Common cause of sudden cardiac death (SCD) in young	Varies
Early symptoms	Exertional intolerance	Exertional intolerance, chest pain, syncope with or after exertion or sudden cardiac death (SCD) in young athletes	Exertional intolerance
Signs and symptoms	Reduced ejection fraction (EF) / Mitral/tricuspid regurgitation / Left heart failure (HF): Dyspnea, orthopnea, paroxysmal nocturnal dyspnea	Normal EF / Mitral regurgitation / Left HF (see *DCM* column)	Normal or reduced EF / Mitral/tricuspid regurgitation / Right HF: Edema, splenomegaly, hepatomegaly, ascites
Complications	Atrial fibrillation / Ventricular tachyarrhythmias / Heart failure	Atrial fibrillation / Ventricular tachyarrhythmias—SCD / Heart failure	Atrial fibrillation / Ventricular tachyarrhythmias / Heart failure

Dilated cardiomyopathy develops when the ventricles become enlarged (dilated) and there is systolic dysfunction. Usually this condition starts in the left ventricle and eventually affects the right ventricle. Although the ventricles are enlarged, the wall thickness is normal. As systolic function worsens, there is backflow with increasing pulmonary vascular resistance and development of pulmonary hypertension. Myocardial fibrosis contributes to the development of arrhythmias and heart failure. Risk for developing DCM increases with age. The incidence is higher in Black men, and they have a higher mortality rate. DCM due to nonischemic events has a higher prevalence rate than DCM due to ischemic causes. Most patients who receive heart transplants have dilated cardiomyopathy.

Many noncardiac causes of DCM are due to genetic and systemic abnormalities. Systemic abnormalities include cardiotoxic substances; infections; and autoimmune, metabolic, and hormonal disorders. Heavy alcohol use (> 10 years) is a common cause of DCM in the United States. Other cardiotoxins include long-term cocaine use even without coronary disease and stimulants such as methamphetamine and 3,4-methylenedioxymethamphetamine (known as *MDMA* and *ecstasy*). Chemotherapeutic anthracycline-based agents (e.g., doxorubicin and daunorubicin) are also cardiotoxic and cause DCM. Many other drugs (e.g., decongestant pseudoephedrine, attention-deficit/hyperactivity disorder medications) can lead to DCM when abused or taken in large quantities.

Up to 50% of DCM cases are caused by genetic abnormalities. Mutations affect sarcomere and cellular mechanisms. One example is peripartum-related DCM (PPCM), which is thought to be caused by chromosomal abnormalities. In addition to chromosomal abnormalities, inflammation and autoimmunity may also cause PPCM, but most often the cause is unknown. The incidence of PPCM is increasing as a result of more frequent recognition, older age in pregnancy, and multiple births (e.g., twins, triplets). Black women have a higher incidence of PPCM. The risk of death due to PPCM is extremely low overall but is higher in Black women in comparison to other ethnic groups. In women with DCM, recurrence is substantial in subsequent pregnancies.

Human immunodeficiency syndrome (HIV) can lead to DCM. Some theories of pathogenesis of HIV and DCM include viral invasion (HIV or other viral coinfection) of myocardial cells, long-term immunosuppression, cardiotoxicity from HIV drugs, or substance abuse.

Autoimmune disorders (e.g., SLE, scleroderma, rheumatoid arthritis), although rare, can cause restrictive and dilated cardiomyopathy. Obesity (particularly severe) causes ventricular dysfunction and structural changes (i.e., dilation, hypertrophy). Obese individuals often have cardiovascular disorders, such as hypertension and atherosclerosis, that also affect the myocardium. The comorbidities of obesity and the obesity-related myocardial changes lead to an increased risk of DCM. Long-term thyroid disorders can cause myocardial injury and lead to DCM, although rare. Some other disorders associated with DCM, which often present at first as restrictive or with dilated and restrictive features, include sarcoidosis (granulomas on various organs), amyloidosis (abnormal protein deposits in the heart and other organs), and hemochromatosis (increased iron). Intense emotions or stress can cause an interestingly named DCM called *takotsubo*, which is a Japanese octopus-trapping jar. Other terms for takotsubo DCM are stress cardiomyopathy, broken heart syndrome, and apical ballooning syndrome. The overall incidence of takotsubo DCM is not known but can be present in up to 2% of individuals who present with some ischemic syndromes. Takotsubo DCM is more common with aging, and women have a much higher incidence. In the pediatric population, most cardiomyopathies are DCM and familial. Other causes of DCM in the pediatric populations are similar to some adult causes already discussed.

Unlike dilated cardiomyopathy, which mainly affects systolic function, **hypertrophic cardiomyopathy** mainly affects diastolic function. HCM is common, affecting 1 out of 500 people (NIH, 2016). HCM is a common cause of sudden cardiac death in young people, especially young athletes. In HCM, the hypertrophied ventricular wall becomes stiff and unable to relax during ventricular filling. With a reduction in ventricular filling, cardiac output decreases while atrial and pulmonary pressures increase. The septum between the ventricles is the most common place of hypertrophy (FIGURE 4-18). In addition to hypertrophy, the myocardium becomes fibrotic and forms scars. These scarred areas can incite arrhythmias such as ventricular tachycardia and atrial fibrillation. The blood vessel lumens are compressed due to the thick walls, which reduces

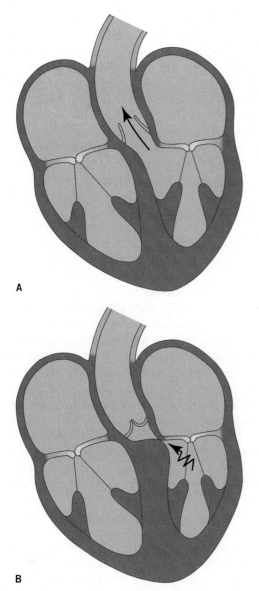

A

B

FIGURE 4-18 A comparison of normal cardiac function with malfunction characteristic of hypertrophic cardiomyopathy. **A** Normal heart, illustrating unobstructed flow of blood from left ventricle into aorta during ventricular systole. **B** Hypertrophic cardiomyopathy, illustrating obstruction to outflow of blood from left ventricle by hypertrophied septum, which impinges on anterior leaflet of mitral valve.

blood flow and causes ischemia. Hypertrophic cardiomyopathy occurs with or without outflow obstruction.

HCM is the most common familial heart disease and is inherited through an autosomal dominant pattern. Mutations of the sarcomere (functional unit in the heart muscle) gene occur. Like DCM, age dependence and incomplete penetrance is present. The average age of disease development in HCM is 40. Despite having the genotype, some people remain without disease development, and many different disease expressions are possible with the same mutation.

Restrictive cardiomyopathy is the least common of the cardiomyopathies but is more common in parts of South and Central America, India, Asia, and Africa. This type of cardiomyopathy is characterized by rigidity of the myocardium and diastolic dysfunction. The ventricular rigidity does not allow for proper filling, and pressure in the ventricle increases. The atrium enlarges as a consequence. Wall thickness is usually normal, and systolic function is unaffected or mildly affected; therefore, cardiac output is maintained until worsening of the disease. In restrictive cardiomyopathy, fibrosis and myocyte damage are usually due to infiltrative disorders. The various disorders include amyloidosis, hemochromatosis, sarcoidosis, connective tissue disorders, and radiation exposure. As with the other cardiomyopathies, genetic mutations are implicated in the development.

Clinical Manifestations

Patients with cardiomyopathy can be asymptomatic for years. The clinical manifestations will also vary greatly depending on the type of dysfunction and the stage of disease presentation (e.g., early, late). General symptoms for cardiomyopathies are due to the structural and functional changes. The underlying disorder may also affect different parts of the heart directly. For example, the valves may be affected by the infiltrative disorders in restrictive cardiomyopathy. In all the cardiomyopathies, backflow pressures and volume eventually lead to atrial enlargement. Right- and/or left-sided heart dysfunction will lead to symptoms depending on the predominant side affected.

Diagnosis and Treatment

Obtaining a detailed family history is important in identifying hereditary patterns. Any history of sudden cardiac death or early death from cardiac disease should be questioned extensively because often people just assume the death was due to a heart attack. In addition to a complete history and physical, an echocardiogram will be done. Cardiac imaging may include nuclear studies. An EKG may be done to evaluate for arrhythmias and conduction abnormalities. A myocardial biopsy may be necessary, particularly in restrictive cardiomyopathy.

Treatment varies depending on the type and cause. Treatment may be supportive with a focus on relieving heart failure symptoms by decreasing afterload and enhancing contractility. General pharmacologic treatments usually include ACE inhibitors, diuretics, digoxin, beta-adrenergic blocking agents, and antidysrhythmic agents to decrease the cardiac workload. Other treatment strategies include an implantable cardioverter-defibrillator, pacemaker, valve repair, and heart transplant. Anticoagulation may be necessary to prevent stroke in those with atrial fibrillation. Additionally, lifestyle modification includes a low-fat, low-sodium diet, tobacco cessation, regular physical activity, and abstinence from alcohol or other cardiotoxins.

In HCM, surgical removal or ablation of excess myocardium may be necessary for those patients who do not respond well to medications. If there is obstruction with HCM, controlling the heart rate and decreasing contractility is important as uncontrolled heart rate and increased contractility may worsen the obstruction and lead to sudden cardiac death. Pharmacologic agents with negative inotropic effects such beta-adrenergic blocking agents and calcium channel blockers are often used. Hypovolemia amid HCM with obstruction can worsen symptoms. Additionally, strenuous activity (e.g., running) or competitive sports should be avoided as most cases of sudden death associated with HCM have occurred with these types of activities.

Electrical Alterations

The normal myocardium rhythmically contracts (depolarization) and relaxes (repolarization), and there is synchronization between the atria and ventricles. An electrical stimulus (i.e., action potential) precedes this cycle. An action potential is caused by electrically charged particles (e.g., Na^+, K^+, Ca^+) that flow in and out of the cardiac cell membrane. Normally, the electric impulses originate in the SA node, the natural pacemaker of the heart. This impulse follows a predictable, consistent path. While cardiac cells can create their own impulses without external stimuli, the rate is mostly regulated by the autonomic nervous system. Sympathetic stimulation increases the rate while parasympathetic (vagal) stimulation decreases the rate. Normal electric conduction is referred to as *sinus rhythm*, whereas deviations from normal are referred to as *dysrhythmias* or *arrhythmias*.

Dysrhythmias are usually categorized as slow (bradyarrhythmias) or fast (tachyarrhythmias) and occur due to problems with impulse formation, conduction, or both. Abnormal impulses can be generated at an abnormal rate from the SA node or from an ectopic site (an area that is not the SA node). Impulses can also be conducted abnormally. Conduction can be slowed or blocked. When the block is at the AV node, the impulse cannot get through despite the SA firing, and another, slower pacemaker site (e.g., AV junction) takes over. When the bundle of His or both bundle branches are blocked, SA impulses will also be blocked. If only one bundle is blocked, the impulse from the SA node is transmitted and goes through the bundle that is not blocked. The path of conduction continues through a modified route, resulting in a longer time for the ventricles to depolarize (QRS $\geq$ 0.12 sec) and a change in the QRS shape.

Bradyarrhythmias are usually caused by problems in the SA node or in the AV conduction system. Most tachyarrhythmias occur due to firing from multiple ectopic foci and/or reentry mechanisms. With reentry, an impulse becomes its own circuit, firing continuously and at a fast rate. The various areas of reentry can include the atria (e.g., atrial flutter, atrial fibrillation), ventricles (e.g., ventricular tachycardia), and AV node (e.g., supraventricular tachycardia). Impulse conduction can deviate from the normal path through abnormal accessory pathways between the atria and ventricle that develop congenitally. These accessory pathways are in different locations and can conduct impulses faster and bypass normal pathways. Impulses can travel through these fast pathways in different manners depending on their locations (e.g., from atria to the ventricle and then back through the AV node to the atria) in a circuitlike manner. The accessory pathway can cause tachyarrhythmias.

Dysrhythmias vary in severity and are classified according to their origin (FIGURE 4-19). The most common dysrhythmia in adults is atrial fibrillation, and the most common in children is supraventricular tachycardia. The effects of dysrhythmias on cardiac output and blood pressure are partially influenced by their site of origin, which also determines the dysrhythmias' clinical significance. Causes of dysrhythmias are numerous and can include the following conditions: acid–base imbalances, hypoxia, congenital heart defects, connective tissue disorders, degenerative changes (e.g., aging), drug toxicity, electrolyte imbalances (especially K^+, Ca^+); stress, myocardial hypertrophy, ischemia, or infarction.

Clinical Manifestations

Clinical manifestations may vary according to the specific dysrhythmia. Some dysrhythmias may be asymptomatic, whereas others can cause sudden death. The danger and symptoms depend on the extent they reduce cardiac output. Some general manifestations of dysrhythmias include palpitations, fluttering sensation, skipped beats, fatigue, confusion, syncope, and dyspnea. Physical exam will reveal an abnormal heart rate and/or rhythm. Other findings will be dependent on the cause (e.g., myocardial infarction) and/or the consequences (e.g., heart failure, shock).

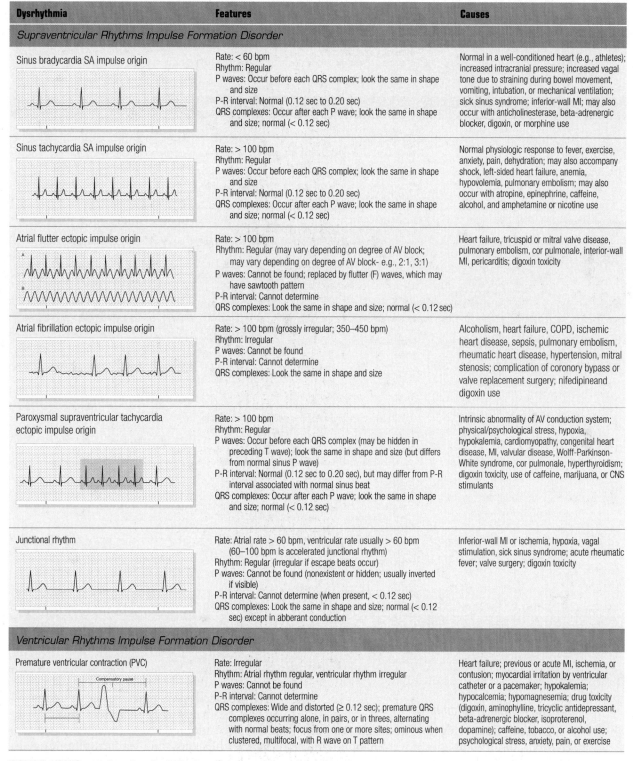

Dysrhythmia	Features	Causes
Supraventricular Rhythms Impulse Formation Disorder		
Sinus bradycardia SA impulse origin	Rate: < 60 bpm Rhythm: Regular P waves: Occur before each QRS complex; look the same in shape and size P-R interval: Normal (0.12 sec to 0.20 sec) QRS complexes: Occur after each P wave; look the same in shape and size; normal (< 0.12 sec)	Normal in a well-conditioned heart (e.g., athletes); increased intracranial pressure; increased vagal tone due to straining during bowel movement, vomiting, intubation, or mechanical ventilation; sick sinus syndrome; inferior-wall MI; may also occur with anticholinesterase, beta-adrenergic blocker, digoxin, or morphine use
Sinus tachycardia SA impulse origin	Rate: > 100 bpm Rhythm: Regular P waves: Occur before each QRS complex; look the same in shape and size P-R interval: Normal (0.12 sec to 0.20 sec) QRS complexes: Occur after each P wave; look the same in shape and size; normal (< 0.12 sec)	Normal physiologic response to fever, exercise, anxiety, pain, dehydration; may also accompany shock, left-sided heart failure, anemia, hypovolemia, pulmonary embolism; may also occur with atropine, epinephrine, caffeine, alcohol, and amphetamine or nicotine use
Atrial flutter ectopic impulse origin	Rate: > 100 bpm Rhythm: Regular (may vary depending on degree of AV block; may vary depending on degree of AV block- e.g., 2:1, 3:1) P waves: Cannot be found; replaced by flutter (F) waves, which may have sawtooth pattern P-R interval: Cannot determine QRS complexes: Look the same in shape and size; normal (< 0.12 sec)	Heart failure, tricuspid or mitral valve disease, pulmonary embolism, cor pulmonale, interior-wall MI, pericarditis; digoxin toxicity
Atrial fibrillation ectopic impulse origin	Rate: > 100 bpm (grossly irregular; 350–450 bpm) Rhythm: Irregular P waves: Cannot be found P-R interval: Cannot determine QRS complexes: Look the same in shape and size	Alcoholism, heart failure, COPD, ischemic heart disease, sepsis, pulmonary embolism, rheumatic heart disease, hypertension, mitral stenosis; complication of coronary bypass or valve replacement surgery; nifedipineand digoxin use
Paroxysmal supraventricular tachycardia ectopic impulse origin	Rate: > 100 bpm Rhythm: Regular P waves: Occur before each QRS complex (may be hidden in preceding T wave); look the same in shape and size (but differs from normal sinus P wave) P-R interval: Normal (0.12 sec to 0.20 sec), but may differ from P-R interval associated with normal sinus beat QRS complexes: Occur after each P wave; look the same in shape and size; normal (< 0.12 sec)	Intrinsic abnormality of AV conduction system; physical/psychological stress, hypoxia, hypokalemia, cardiomyopathy, congenital heart disease, MI, valvular disease, Wolff-Parkinson-White syndrome, cor pulmonale, hyperthyroidism; digoxin toxicity, use of caffeine, marijuana, or CNS stimulants
Junctional rhythm	Rate: Atrial rate > 60 bpm, ventricular rate usually > 60 bpm (60–100 bpm is accelerated junctional rhythm) Rhythm: Regular (irregular if escape beats occur) P waves: Cannot be found (nonexistent or hidden; usually inverted if visible) P-R interval: Cannot determine (when present, < 0.12 sec) QRS complexes: Look the same in shape and size; normal (< 0.12 sec) except in abberant conduction	Inferior-wall MI or ischemia, hypoxia, vagal stimulation, sick sinus syndrome; acute rheumatic fever; valve surgery; digoxin toxicity
Ventricular Rhythms Impulse Formation Disorder		
Premature ventricular contraction (PVC)	Rate: Irregular Rhythm: Atrial rhythm regular, ventricular rhythm irregular P waves: Cannot be found P-R interval: Cannot determine QRS complexes: Wide and distorted (≥ 0.12 sec); premature QRS complexes occurring alone, in pairs, or in threes, alternating with normal beats; focus from one or more sites; ominous when clustered, multifocal, with R wave on T pattern	Heart failure; previous or acute MI, ischemia, or contusion; myocardial irritation by ventricular catheter or a pacemaker; hypokalemia; hypocalcemia; hypomagnesemia; drug toxicity (digoxin, aminophylline, tricyclic antidepressant, beta-adrenergic blocker, isoproterenol, dopamine); caffeine, tobacco, or alcohol use; psychological stress, anxiety, pain, or exercise

FIGURE 4-19 Types of cardiac dysrhythmias.

Reproduced from *Arrhythmia recognition: The art of interpretation*, courtesy of Tomas B. Garcia, MD.

Rhythm descriptions and appearances may vary particularly when there are multiple abnormalities (e.g., atrial flutter with a left bundle branch block produces a wide QRS).

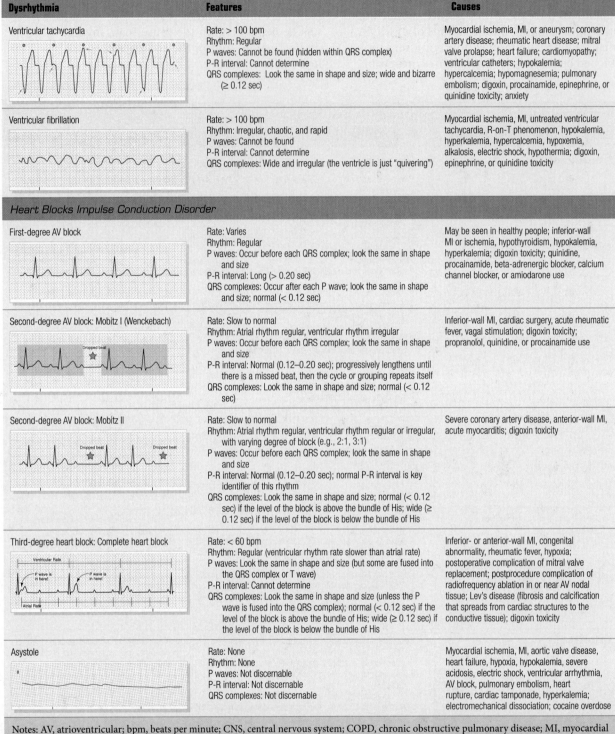

Dysrhythmia	Features	Causes
Ventricular tachycardia	Rate: > 100 bpm Rhythm: Regular P waves: Cannot be found (hidden within QRS complex) P-R interval: Cannot determine QRS complexes: Look the same in shape and size; wide and bizarre (≥ 0.12 sec)	Myocardial ischemia, MI, or aneurysm; coronary artery disease; rheumatic heart disease; mitral valve prolapse; heart failure; cardiomyopathy; ventricular catheters; hypokalemia; hypercalcemia; hypomagnesemia; pulmonary embolism; digoxin, procainamide, epinephrine, or quinidine toxicity; anxiety
Ventricular fibrillation	Rate: > 100 bpm Rhythm: Irregular, chaotic, and rapid P waves: Cannot be found P-R interval: Cannot determine QRS complexes: Wide and irregular (the ventricle is just "quivering")	Myocardial ischemia, MI, untreated ventricular tachycardia, R-on-T phenomenon, hypokalemia, hyperkalemia, hypercalcemia, hypoxemia, alkalosis, electric shock, hypothermia; digoxin, epinephrine, or quinidine toxicity

Heart Blocks Impulse Conduction Disorder

Dysrhythmia	Features	Causes
First-degree AV block	Rate: Varies Rhythm: Regular P waves: Occur before each QRS complex; look the same in shape and size P-R interval: Long (> 0.20 sec) QRS complexes: Occur after each P wave; look the same in shape and size; normal (< 0.12 sec)	May be seen in healthy people; inferior-wall MI or ischemia, hypothyroidism, hypokalemia, hyperkalemia; digoxin toxicity; quinidine, procainamide, beta-adrenergic blocker, calcium channel blocker, or amiodarone use
Second-degree AV block: Mobitz I (Wenckebach)	Rate: Slow to normal Rhythm: Atrial rhythm regular, ventricular rhythm irregular P waves: Occur before each QRS complex; look the same in shape and size P-R interval: Normal (0.12–0.20 sec); progressively lengthens until there is a missed beat, then the cycle or grouping repeats itself QRS complexes: Look the same in shape and size; normal (< 0.12 sec)	Inferior-wall MI, cardiac surgery, acute rheumatic fever, vagal stimulation; digoxin toxicity; propranolol, quinidine, or procainamide use
Second-degree AV block: Mobitz II	Rate: Slow to normal Rhythm: Atrial rhythm regular, ventricular rhythm regular or irregular, with varying degree of block (e.g., 2:1, 3:1) P waves: Occur before each QRS complex; look the same in shape and size P-R interval: Normal (0.12–0.20 sec); normal P-R interval is key identifier of this rhythm QRS complexes: Look the same in shape and size; normal (< 0.12 sec) if the level of the block is above the bundle of His; wide (≥ 0.12 sec) if the level of the block is below the bundle of His	Severe coronary artery disease, anterior-wall MI, acute myocarditis; digoxin toxicity
Third-degree heart block: Complete heart block	Rate: < 60 bpm Rhythm: Regular (ventricular rhythm rate slower than atrial rate) P waves: Look the same in shape and size (but some are fused into the QRS complex or T wave) P-R interval: Cannot determine QRS complexes: Look the same in shape and size (unless the P wave is fused into the QRS complex); normal (< 0.12 sec) if the level of the block is above the bundle of His; wide (≥ 0.12 sec) if the level of the block is below the bundle of His	Inferior- or anterior-wall MI, congenital abnormality, rheumatic fever, hypoxia; postoperative complication of mitral valve replacement; postprocedure complication of radiofrequency ablation in or near AV nodal tissue; Lev's disease (fibrosis and calcification that spreads from cardiac structures to the conductive tissue); digoxin toxicity
Asystole	Rate: None Rhythm: None P waves: Not discernable P-R interval: Not discernable QRS complexes: Not discernable	Myocardial ischemia, MI, aortic valve disease, heart failure, hypoxia, hypokalemia, severe acidosis, electric shock, ventricular arrhythmia, AV block, pulmonary embolism, heart rupture, cardiac tamponade, hyperkalemia; electromechanical dissociation; cocaine overdose

Notes: AV, atrioventricular; bpm, beats per minute; CNS, central nervous system; COPD, chronic obstructive pulmonary disease; MI, myocardial infarction. Rhythm descriptions and appearances may vary particularly when there are multiple abnormalities (e.g., atrial flutter with a left bundle branch block produces a wide QRS).

FIGURE 4-19 *Continued.*

Diagnosis and Treatment

Diagnostic procedures for dysrhythmias include a history, physical examination, and EKG. Additional tests may be performed to identify the underlying cause and may include invasive electrophysiologic studies. Pharmacology is the mainstay of treatment and may include beta-adrenergic blocking agents, calcium channel blockers, and antiarrhythmics (e.g., amiodarone). Other interventions may include an internal cardiac defibrillator, pacemaker, cardioversion, defibrillation, and ablation. Avoiding triggers such as caffeine, tobacco, and stress can decrease the occurrence and severity of some dysrhythmias.

Atrial Fibrillation

Atrial fibrillation (AF) is one of the most common supraventricular tachyarrhythmias in adults and the incidence increases significantly over the age 60. AF significantly increases the risk of stroke (fivefold), heart failure (threefold), dementia, and mortality (twofold). When a patient with AF has a stroke, it is likely to be worse than a stroke due to other causes. AF is characterized by rapid, chaotic, ectopic atrial impulse formation (over 400 impulses a minute) causing an ineffective quivering atrial contraction (Figure 4-19). The AV node normally acts as a gatekeeper and prevents most of these impulses generated in AF from traveling to the ventricles. However, the AV node can become less effective, allowing too many impulses to get through, resulting in a dangerously high ventricular rate (e.g., 200 impulses per minute). The number of impulses that are conducted is usually variable, causing the classic description of AF being irregularly irregular. The ineffective atrial quivering type contraction causes blood to pool, promoting clot formation (usually in the left atrium). The ventricles do not fill adequately, which leads to an insufficient volume being ejected. The fluctuating heart rate (usually fast) also contributes to variations in ventricle filling/ejection. These factors can cause a decrease in cardiac output and potential embolization—most commonly to the brain (stroke).

AF can be classified by the duration: paroxysmal ($\leq$ 7 days), persistent ($>$ 7 days), long persistent ($>$ 12 months), and permanent. In permanent AF, normal sinus rhythm (NSR) does not seem achievable, or efforts at restoration are no longer being attempted. *Chronic* is often used to describe AF clinically, but this term has varying definitions. Since AF can be asymptomatic at times, the duration can be hard to determine. However, the duration can be a clue to the cause when known and can guide therapeutic decisions. Paroxysmal and persistent AF usually occur due to an area in the atria that is generating impulses ectopically or through reentry mechanisms. Once AF becomes persistent or permanent, structural and/or electrophysiologic changes are likely to exist.

Structural changes in the atrial tissue and/or electrical system can trigger AF and cause it to recur or be sustained. AF is often associated with heart diseases and may be a cause of the disease or due to the disease. Common diseases such as hypertension, coronary artery disease, heart failure, and valvular disorders can lead to structural changes such as atrial dilation, hypertrophy, inflammation, and fibrosis. Atrial inflammatory changes and fibrosis occur with aging or cardiac surgery and can be present even when there is no heart disease. The rapid heart rate of AF causes cell necrosis and apoptosis, which further affects impulse response and conduction. These changes create an environment for more arrhythmias. Infiltrative diseases cause the deposition of substances such as amyloid fibrils or intracellular iron that infiltrate cardiac tissue and promote AF. Noncardiac disorders such as hyperthyroidism, sleep apnea, obesity, alcohol, and other drugs promote AF. Electrophysiologic alterations leading to AF include ectopic impulse formation, reentry abnormalities, and autonomic nervous system stimulation. RAAS stimulation causes structural and electrical changes that can lead to AF.

Clinical Manifestations

Patients with AF may be asymptomatic or have variable symptoms depending on the ventricular rate and other comorbid diseases causing or associated with AF. Patients may complain of tiring easily and may struggle with exercise. Patients may experience palpitations, dizziness, or syncopal episodes. When the heart rate is high, hemodynamic compromise can occur, particularly in people with heart failure or those who already have cardiovascular impairment.

Diagnosis and Treatment

Diagnosis will be made with a history, physical, and an EKG, which confirms the presence of AF. An echocardiogram is also important to evaluate cardiac structure and function. Labs will include electrolyte, renal, and hepatic analysis; thyroid panel; and a CBC. Additional tests can include additional rhythm monitoring (e.g., telemetry or Holter monitoring), and a chest X-ray to reveal pulmonary disease (e.g., pulmonary edema) or cardiac disease (e.g., enlargement). A transesophageal echocardiogram is ordered to evaluate for left atrial (LA) thrombi or to determine risk of LA thrombi development. Exercise testing is done to evaluate rate control. Electrophysiologic studies may be conducted to evaluate for other arrhythmias that occur with AF such as atrial tachycardia or to determine sites for ablation.

Management of AF involves rate control and/ or rhythm control as well as anticoagulation for stroke prevention. Rate control can be achieved with beta adrenergic blocking agents, calcium channel blockers, and cardiac glycoside (e.g., digoxin). Amiodarone can be considered in those who do not respond to the other agents. Rhythm control involves cardioversion, AV nodal blocking agents (e.g., calcium channel blockers), and ablation. Antiarrhythmics can be used to attempt to convert AF to sinus rhythm. The CHA_2DS_2-VASc score can be calculated to evaluate the risk of ischemic stroke in patients with AF. CHA_2DS_2-VASc stands for congestive heart failure, hypertension, age, diabetes mellitus, sex, and vascular disease history. Each criterion is given a point value, and the higher the score, the more likely the risk of thromboembolism. The score can be used to determine the need for anticoagulation. Most patients will need anticoagulation. A direct thrombin inhibitor (e.g., dabigatran) or factor Xa inhibitor (e.g., rivaroxaban or apixaban) is used if they have nonvalvular AF. Warfarin can be used as an alternate and in those with valvular AF. Aspirin combined with clopidogrel is not as efficacious but is another option. Stroke prevention can also be accomplished with percutaneous occlusion or surgical excision of the left atrial appendage. Pacemakers and implantable cardioverter-defibrillators can be implanted to prevent AF. Treatment strategies will include avoidance of factors that caused or contribute to AF such as alcohol cessation and weight loss.

Heart Failure

Heart failure is a condition in which the heart has a problem with ventricular filling or ejection, which then leads to a decreased cardiac output and inadequate perfusion. These problems occur due to structural or functional impairment. Heart failure is the consequence of many disorders, but the most common risk factors include hypertension, metabolic syndrome, diabetes mellitus, and atherosclerotic disease. One of the top causes of death from cardiovascular disease is heart failure, with a 50% death rate usually occurring within 5 years of diagnosis (American Heart Association, 2017). Heart failure incidence increases dramatically after the age of 65. Heart failure is more prevalent in men, but women live longer so half of heart failure cases are in women. Both non-Hispanic Black men and women have a higher incidence and mortality from heart failure than non-Hispanic Whites, which correlates with the higher incidence of hypertension, diabetes mellitus,

and obesity seen in this population. More people are surviving and living longer with heart disease such as MI or valve disease because therapies are better. These diseases, however, can lead to heart failure, so the incidence of heart failure is rising.

Heart failure is often called *congestive heart failure*; however, this term has become less commonly used as many patients with heart failure do not exhibit manifestations of volume overload (congestion). Heart failure is often categorized as systolic or diastolic heart failure, but many patients have normal ejection fraction (EF), meaning there is no systolic dysfunction. Therefore, two categorizations for heart failure are preferred—heart failure with reduced EF (HFrEF) for systolic dysfunction and heart failure with preserved EF (HFpEF) for diastolic dysfunction. These two categories are used for left-sided heart disease. Right-sided heart failure is a result of right ventricle impairment and is most often a consequence of left-sided heart failure. Right ventricle impairment can also occur with pulmonary diseases that cause pulmonary hypertension and this is termed *cor pulmonale* (i.e., pulmonary heart disease). The term *cor pulmonale* is generally not used when the right-side dysfunction is due to left-sided heart failure. Right-sided heart failure can also be the result of other disorders that cause pulmonary hypertension such as, pulmonic and tricuspid valve stenosis. Most people with heart failure will present with clinical manifestations due to dysfunction on the left and right, and many people also have elements of systolic and diastolic dysfunction.

Causes of HFrEF and HFpEF are different but often overlap. The most common causes of either type of heart failure are coronary artery disease (60–75%) and hypertension (75%). Valvular disorders, cardiomyopathy, myocarditis, fibrosis (e.g., sarcoidosis and amyloidosis), and chronic dysrhythmias are other cardiac causes of heart failure. Noncardiac causes include drug effects such as anticancer drugs, antidiabetics, and appetite suppressants, chronic lung diseases, anemia, thyroid disorders, and thiamine deficiency (beriberi). Rheumatic heart disease and Chagas disease are frequent causes of heart failure in other countries. HFpEF is more prevalent in older women with hypertension. Other common risks more frequently seen in patients with HFpEF are diabetes, obesity, coronary artery disease, and dyslipidemia.

Several compensatory mechanisms are activated in times of decreased cardiac output (**FIGURE 4-20**). Initially, the SNS is stimulated

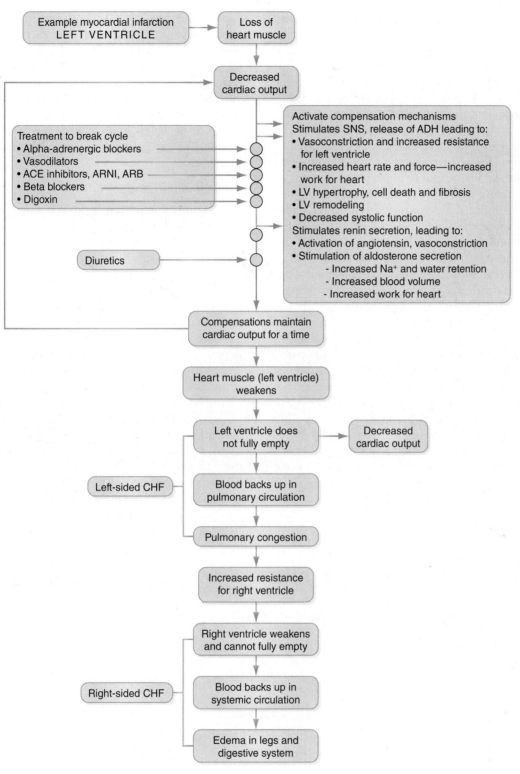

FIGURE 4-20 Course of heart failure.

ACE- angiotensin converting enzyme
ADH- antidiuretic hormone
ARNI- angiotensin receptor-neprilysin inhibitor
ARBS- take off the S and then it stands for angiotensin receptor blocker
CHF- change both to HF and then it stands for heart failure
LV- left ventricle
SNS- sympathetic nervous system

with catecholamine release (epinephrine and norepinephrine), which causes vasoconstriction, increases heart rate, contractility, and antidiuretic hormone secretion. With SNS stimulation and decreasing cardiac output, renal perfusion decreases, which activates RAAS. Renin, angiotensin, and aldosterone are released, which leads to fluid retention, vasoconstriction, cell hypertrophy, cell death, and myocardial fibrosis. These compensatory mechanisms increase cardiac output in the beginning, but they eventually lead to excessive preload and afterload. The compensatory mechanisms eventually become inadequate to meet the body's metabolic needs, and excessive myocardial oxygen demand and an increased preload result in decreased contractility and decompensation. Left ventricle (LV) remodeling refers to changes in the mass, volume, and shape of the heart and occurs in response to decompensation and injury. The remodeling includes myocyte loss, decreased contractility, loss of support structure, LV dilation, and hypertrophy. Beta-adrenergic desensitization (so there is less response) occurs and cellular metabolic processes are affected. In addition to the SNS and RAAS stimulation causing remodeling, other contributors of remodeling include inflammatory cytokines such as endothelin (vasoconstrictor), tumor necrosis factor, and reactive oxygen species. Systolic function is impaired, and EF declines to ≤ 40% (HFrEF), making heart failure clinical manifestations more evident.

In patients with HFpEF, systolic function is mildly impaired to normal (i.e., preserved) and stroke volume and cardiac output are maintained, and so the EF is > 40%. The dysfunction in HFpEF is during diastole with decreased ventricle filling from abnormal myocardial relaxation and decreased compliance (stiffness). Up to 50% of left heart failure is categorized as HFpEF. Most patients have a combination of both.

Clinical Manifestations

Heart failure can present as an acute or chronic problem. Acute heart failure can be new onset of HF or an exacerbation of worsening chronic heart failure. Acute heart failure may be related to a temporary condition and can resolve with treatment of that condition. Chronic heart failure, in contrast, is a progressive condition with exacerbations.

The clinical manifestations of heart failure depend on the side affected and on the severity. The manifestations of right-sided failure reflect systemic fluid accumulation , while left-sided failure is characterized by pulmonary fluid accumulation (**TABLE 4-3**). Left-sided symptoms are a result of ineffective left ventricular contractility. As cardiac output falls, blood that is not being pumped into the body backs up first in the left atrium and then in the pulmonary circulation, leading to pulmonary congestion. Main complaints are dyspnea with exertion and fatigue. As the disease worsens, symptoms start to

TABLE 4-3	Clinical Manifestations of Left- and Right-Sided Heart Failure	
	Left-sided heart failure	**Right-sided heart failure**
Basic effects	Decreased cardiac output and pulmonary congestion	Decreased cardiac output and systemic congestion
Key manifestations	Pulmonary congestion, dyspnea, and activity intolerance	Edema and weight gain
Forward effects (decreased output)	Fatigue, weakness, dyspnea, exercise intolerance, and cold intolerance	Fatigue, weakness, dyspnea, exercise intolerance, and cold intolerance
Compensations	Tachycardia, pallor, secondary polycythemia, and daytime oliguria	Tachycardia, pallor, secondary polycythemia, and daytime oliguria
Backup effects	Symptoms: orthopnea, cough, shortness of breath, paroxysmal nocturnal dyspnea, hemoptysis Signs: inspiratory crackles, wheezing, hypertension or hypotension, S3 gallop, cyanosis, mitral/tricuspid murmur	Symptoms: anorexia, early satiety, nocturia, headache Signs: dependent edema in feet/ankles, sacral area, hepatomegaly, splenomegaly, ascites, distended neck veins, S4 gallop

Modified from Story, L. (2017). *Pathophysiology: A practical approach* (3rd ed). Burlington, MA: Jones & Bartlett Learning.

occur with less activity and even at rest. Orthopnea (shortness of breath when supine) is a late symptom and occurs due to fluid shifts from the peripheral to the central circulation. The fluid shifts occur while in a supine position and results in increased pulmonary pressure. Increased pressure around bronchial vessels and the increased airway resistance causes paroxysmal nocturnal dyspnea. Paroxysmal nocturnal dyspnea symptoms include coughing and wheezing that wake patients up at night. If blood continues to accumulate, pulmonary edema and right-sided heart failure will develop. Right-sided heart failure is a result of ineffective right ventricular contraction. Because of this condition, blood does not move appropriately out of the right ventricle. Blood backs up first in the right atrium, and then the peripheral circulation, causing increased pressures in the peripheral capillary bed. The patient begins to gain weight, as fluid is not excreted by the kidneys. Tissue becomes edematous, as pressures in the capillaries push fluid out of the circulatory system. Most patients have a combination of left- and right-sided heart failure and therefore manifestations will reflect a combination of both.

Diagnosis and Treatment

The American College of Cardiology and the American Heart Association have a classification system based on stages (A–D) to determine the severity of the heart failure and identify treatment strategies. Patients at stage A are at risk, and patients at B have structural disease but no symptoms yet. Patients in stage C and D have clinical heart failure. Once patients are staged, they cannot go backwards. For example, they can go from A to B but never back to A. Another common classification system is for patients who already have heart failure symptoms (i.e., stage C or D). This system—New York Heart Association classes (I–IV)—is used to evaluate functional capacity symptoms of heart failure with activity. Patients can go back and forth with New York Heart Association classes (i.e., III–II or I–II).

Diagnosis, staging, and class determination are based on a history and physical and diagnostic tests. These diagnostic tests will include an echocardiogram to evaluate function and causes. A brain natriuretic peptide or N-terminal pro brain natriuretic peptide, which is a hormone released by the ventricles in response to overstretching, will be measured. A chest X-ray may reveal signs of fluid retention such as pleural effusions and

vascular congestion. Thoracic ultrasonography can be used at the bedside in those who are critically ill and in life threatening situations where imaging is needed immediately. Thoracic ultrasonography can be used to evaluate for acute cardiopulmonary respiratory failure, pleural effusion, and pneumothorax. A 12-lead EKG may expose causes and coexisting disorders that occur with heart failure such as atrial fibrillation and myocardial infarction, but no finding is specific to heart failure. Other routine labs include urinalysis, CBC, a chemistry profile with calcium and magnesium, lipid panel, liver function, and thyroid-stimulating hormone evaluation. Other additional blood work may be ordered if there is suspicion of certain causes of the heart failure (e.g., HIV, hemochromatosis). With patients who are hospitalized, additional tests may include a troponin test, arterial blood gases, cardiac catheterization, and myocardial biopsy depending on causes and status.

Management of heart failure begins with identifying and treating the underlying causes and managing comorbidities that contribute to worsening heart failure. Additional strategies include lifestyle modification (e.g., weight reduction, tobacco cessation, reduced salt consumption, fluid restriction, and exercise). Pharmacotherapeutic agents that are mainstays for HFrEF are angiotensin-converting enzyme (ACE) inhibitors (to stop the renin–angiotensin–aldosterone cycle), angiotensin receptor blockers (ARBs), or an angiotensin receptor neprilysin inhibitors (ARNIs). The latest pharmacologic addition, ARNIs, are a combination of an ARB with an inhibitor of the enzyme neprilysin. Neprilysin causes the breakdown of beneficial natriuretic peptides, which help to maintain fluid homeostasis; by inhibiting the breakdown, natriuresis can occur. All patients with heart failure should be on either an ACE, ARB, or ARNI and a selective beta-1–adrenergic blocking agent or an alpha-1, beta-1, beta-2 receptor blocker (to slow the heart rate and thereby increase diastolic filling). Not all beta blockers are effective (e.g., short-acting metropolol) and reviewing the latest guidelines is important. Ivabradine, which blocks I_f (one of the current systems in the SA node), can be used with a beta blocker to reduce the heart rate. Additional medications can be added depending on circumstances and can include diuretics (preferably loop diuretics, which act at the loop of Henle to prevent sodium or chloride reabsorption), which are used for patients with volume overload. For those patients with persistent symptoms, hydral-nitrates hydralazine and isosorbide dinitrate (vasodilators) can be added and are particularly useful in Blacks with heart failure. Aldosterone receptor agonists such as spironolactone can be considered in select patients (e.g., New York Heart Association stage II–IV with EF < 35%). Aldosterone agonists act at distal tubules as opposed to the loop diuretics, but the results are the same with diuretic effects through Na$^+$, Cl$^-$, and water excretion. Inotropic agents (increase myocardial contractility) such as digoxin can be used. Milrinone (phosphodiesterase inhibitor) and dobutamine (adrenergic agonist) are examples of two inotropic agents that can be administered as an intravenous continuous infusion for heart failure. These medications can be for short- or long-term use. Certain categories of pharmacotherapeutics are often used in cardiovascular diseases or other disorders that have no benefit or can even worsen heart failure. These medications include calcium channel blockers, which can depress contractility. Nonsteroidal anti-inflammatory drugs (NSAIDs), which are sold over the counter and often prescribed for pain, can cause Na+ and water retention. Unfortunately, treatment guidelines for HFrEF have not been as effective or adequately evaluated in patients diagnosed with HFpEF. Treatment of HFpEF is mainly

focused on managing blood pressure, symptoms, and risk factors.

Device therapy for HF can include implantable cardioverter-defibrillators and a biventricular pacemaker (i.e., cardiac resynchronization therapy). As patients worsen and/or decompensate, additional therapy may include advanced therapies such as ultrafiltration (volume overload), potent vasoconstrictors (e.g., vasopressin antagonists), intra-aortic balloon pump, and other methods to support cardiovascular decompensation. Mechanical circulatory support can be achieved with the use of ventricular assist devices (**FIGURE 4-21**), which act as a pump to circulate blood and can be used temporarily while the patient recovers and/or awaits a heart transplant. Ventricular assist devices can be used as destination therapy (until removal or death) for those who cannot get a transplant, and they can live long-term with the device.

Congenital Heart Defects

Congenital heart defects (CHD) include a number of structural issues that may be present at birth, affecting 1% of live births in the United States (NIH, 2011). CHDs are the most common type of birth defects and a leading cause of infant death and illness (CDC, 2019b). Some CHDs will not be present until adulthood. Some defects are asymptomatic and found only during routine examination. Due to advances in treatment, adults with CHD now outnumber children with CHD (Triedman & Newburger, 2016). The structural and functional impairments can range from simple to complex and involve the myocardium, heart valves, and vessels near the heart. According to the AHA (2017), there are 18 recognized distinct CHDs. Ventricular septal defects are the most common type, accounting for up to 34% of all CHD. Examples of congenital heart defects include the following conditions (**TABLE 4-4**):

- Septal defects—holes in the wall that separates the atria (ASD) and ventricles (VSD), including patent foramen ovale (PFO), an opening between atria fails to close (**FIGURE 4-22**)
- Patent ductus arteriosus (PDA)—failure of the ductus arteriosus, the vessel between the aorta and the pulmonary artery, to close after birth
- Valve disorders (e.g., stenosis, atresia, regurgitation)
- Coarctation of the aorta—narrowing of the aorta

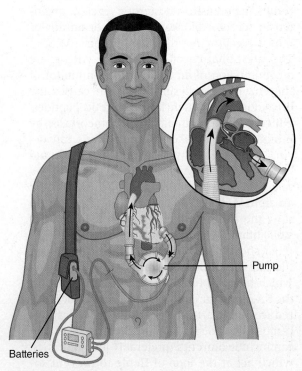

FIGURE 4-21 Left ventricular assist device.

TABLE 4-4	Congenital Heart Defects			
Disorder*	**Problem**	**Shunting or obstruction**	**Manifestations**	**Associated defects**
Ventricular septal defect: (most common—approx. 1/3 of all defects)	Opening between ventricles	LV-to-RV shunt ↑ Pulmonary flow	Absence of cyanosis Murmur—↑ flow across VSD (systolic murmur) and ↑ flow across mitral valve (diastolic murmur) Smaller VSD—asymptomatic Large VSD—heart failure	Larger VSD/lower PVR = ↑ shunting and eventual increase in PVR and subsequent pulmonary htn If PVR becomes greater than SVR leads, irreversible pulmonary htn and shunt reverses (RV to LV) leading to Eisenmenger syndrome with cyanosis
Atrial septal defect: one common type—PFO	Opening between atria PFO—failure of closure of normal fetal channel between RA and LA	LA-to-RA shunt ↑ Pulmonary flow	Absence of cyanosis Murmur—↑ flow across pulmonary valve (systolic murmur) Asymptomatic until older	Due to less pressure in atria vs. ventricles; ASD less often causes or takes longer to lead to ↑ PVR Eisenmenger—(see above) except shunt RA to LA
Patent ductus arteriosus	Failure of closure of normal fetal channel—between PA and aorta	Left- (aorta) to-right (PA) shunt ↑ Pulmonary flow	Absence of cyanosis Murmur—continuous; Bounding pulses Smaller PDA—asymptomatic Larger PDA—difficulty breathing, poor feeding and weight gain, fatigue	Eisenmenger—(see above) except shunt PA to aorta
Pulmonary stenosis: Severe type Pulmonary atresia—complete closure, no flow through pulmonary valve	Narrow valve	Obstructed flow RV to PA ↓ Pulmonary flow	Cyanosis (if severe) Murmur—pulmonary valve (systolic murmur) Dyspnea Fatigue	If severe, blood backs up into RV and RA causing high right side pressure; PFO opens and get RA-to-LA shunt with ↑ pulmonary flow/PVR, cyanosis Pulmonary atresia—complete closure, no flow through pulmonary valve
Transposition of great arteries	Abnormal attachment Aorta to RV and PA to LV	Unoxygenated blood to systemic—PA to LV Oxygenated blood to pulmonary—RV to aorta	Cyanosis Murmur (only with VSD) Hypoxemia, HF	Survival until treated is via circulation through the ductus arteriosus and the foramen ovale and VSD (if present)
Tetralogy of Fallot	Four abnormalities: VSD; PS causes; RV hypertrophy; overriding aorta over VSD	RV-to-LV shunt (PS/ ↑ PVR) ↓ Pulmonary flow	Cyanosis with right-to-left shunt (more common) Murmur—across obstructed outflow (systolic) If the patient is hypoxic: polycythemia, clubbing, poor feeding	Absence of cyanosis with left-to-right shunt if large VSD

(*continues*)

TABLE 4-4	Congenital Heart Defects (*Continued*)			
Disorder*	Problem	Shunting or obstruction	Manifestations	Associated defects
Coarctation of the aorta	Narrow aorta	Obstructed flow through aorta (usually at arch) Shunt if with a PDA	Murmur—across aorta (systolic) Milder: asymptomatic until older—htn, decreased pulses in lower extremities Severe: heart failure, hypotension, shock	May also have a bicuspid aortic valve
Aortic stenosis	Narrow valve	Obstructed flow LV to aorta	Murmur—aortic valve systolic murmur Mild to moderate stenosis—lack of symptoms Severe stenosis—syncope, chest pain, dyspnea	
Atrioventricular canal defect: complete, partial, or transitional	Failure of fusion of the septa and AV valves	LA/LV-to-RA/RV shunt	Absence of cyanosis If complete: HF VSD-type symptoms also with mitral valve systolic murmur	

*Disorder from most to less common (all ≥ 5% incidence). Incidence statistics vary slightly depending on source.
LA, left atrium; RA, right atrium; PVR, pulmonary vascular resistance; SVR, systemic vascular resistance; PA, pulmonary artery; RV, right ventricle; LV, left ventricle; VSD, ventricular septal defect; htn, hypertension; AV, atrioventricular; PFO, patent foramen ovale; ASD, atrial septum defect; ↓, decreased; ↑, increased.

- Transposition of the great arteries—the aorta and the pulmonary artery are switched in position
- Tetralogy of Fallot—a combination of pulmonary valve stenosis, a large ventricular septal defect, misplacement of the aorta directly over the ventricular septal defect, and right ventricular hypertrophy

Heredity may play a role in some heart defects. Genetic abnormalities are presumed to be present in most congenital heart disease. In addition, some genetic disorders (e.g., Down syndrome), fetal exposure to tobacco and certain medications (e.g., oral retinoid for acne), and maternal health status (e.g., preexisting diabetes, obesity) can cause and increase the risk of congenital heart disease.

The defects can cause alterations in blood flow with abnormal shunting of blood (FIGURE 4-23) through abnormal opening (e.g., septal defects) or through normal fetal openings that did not close. Some defects do not shunt blood but alter blood flow due to obstructions (e.g., stenotic valves, aortic narrowing). Abnormal flow can occur due to large vessel defects or abnormal attachments (e.g., transposition of great vessels). Some defects

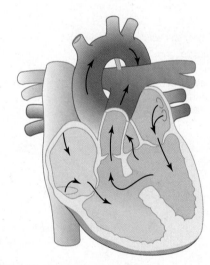

FIGURE 4-22 Ventricular septal defect.

cause cyanosis while others are acyanotic. Some defects are a mixture of shunting and obstructions (e.g., tetralogy of Fallot).

Clinical Manifestations

Various clinical manifestations may be present and are dependent on the type and severity of the defect (Table 4-4). General manifestations may include a heart murmur, dyspnea,

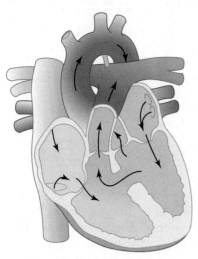

Blood flow patterns in common congenital abnormalities.
Patent ductus arteriosus.

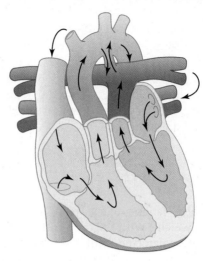

Transposition of the great arteries.

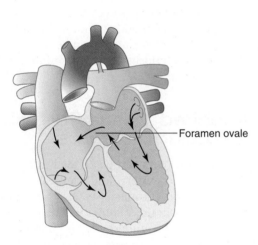

Atrial septal defect; foramen ovale.

Foramen ovale

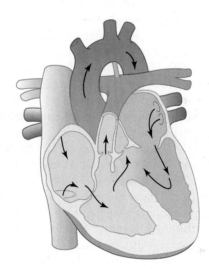

Tetralogy of Fallot.

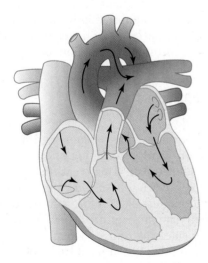

Blood flow patterns in common congenital abnormalities.
Patent ductus arteriosus.

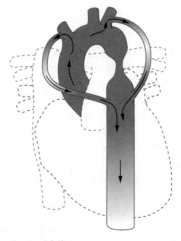

Thoracic aorta constriction.

FIGURE 4-23 Blood flow patterns in common congenital abnormalities. The patent ductus arteriosus is a description for the image which it is under.

BOX 4-2 Application to Practice

You are examining a 5-week-old infant and hear a systolic murmur at the lower left sternal border. You suspect a ventricular septal defect. The parents are concerned and have several questions.

1. What is the cause of a ventricular septal defect?
2. What problems will our baby have due to his VSD?
3. How does the defect create these problems?
4. What diagnostic tests will be ordered?
5. What treatment will our baby need?

tachypnea, fatigue, chest pain, or difficulty gaining weight. With VSD and ASD, a murmur may not be detected until 2 weeks after birth when the pulmonary vascular resistance (PVR) normally decreases. The ventricular and atrial chamber pressures are higher than the PVR, and a murmur from shunting through the defect can be heard. Some defects cause shunting of oxygenated blood to deoxygenated blood (left to right side shunt) and an increase in pulmonary blood flow; these defects are generally considered acyanotic (e.g., VSD, ASD, PDA). Some defects cause a shunting of deoxygenated blood to oxygenated blood (right to left side shunt) and a decrease in pulmonary blood flow; these defects are considered cyanotic (e.g., tetralogy of Fallot). Obstructive lesions (e.g., coarctation of the aorta, pulmonary stenosis, aortic stenosis) do not generally cause shunting but rather flow is decreased to the respective outflow tract. Obstructive defects often lead to heart failure, hypotension, and if on the right side (e.g., pulmonary stenosis) pulmonary congestion and cyanosis can be present. Murmurs in obstructions are created by the turbulent flow through the narrowed valve or vessel.

Diagnosis and Treatment

Diagnostic procedures for congenital heart defects include a history, physical examination, fetal ultrasound, echocardiogram, EKG, chest X-ray, cardiac catheterization, or cardiac magnetic resonance imaging (MRI). Treatment depends on the type and severity of the defect. Strategies may include repair with a heart catheterization or with surgery. Surgeries may include dilating narrowed openings (e.g., valve stenosis), closing defective openings (e.g., VSD/ASD), cutting away defective areas (e.g., coarctation of the aorta, PDA), reattaching vessels (e.g., transposition of the great arteries), or heart transplant. Medications are used to manage symptoms and complications

(e.g., diuretics, antidysrhythmic agents, antihypertensives). Additional measures such as mechanical ventilation and inotropic support may be necessary to support cardiovascular function. The ductus arteriosus normally closes completely by 21 days or less. In some CHD cases, it may be preferable to close the ductus arteriosus sooner; however, it is preferable that the ductus remain open for longer in other circumstances. Prostaglandin can be used to keep the ductus arteriosus open, and inhibition will lead to closure.

Impaired Tissue Perfusion: Vascular Disorders

Vascular disorders can be divided into arterial and venous disorders, and they can occur in peripheral or coronary vessels. Categorizing the disorders in this manner will help with understanding the underlying mechanisms and consequences of the vascular injury. Dyslipidemia is a common culprit, causing arterial disease and subsequent atherosclerosis. Arterial and venous abnormalities can significantly impair tissue perfusion and create an environment for thrombus formation and potential embolization.

Arterial Disorders

Aneurysms

Walls of arteries can weaken, and areas can balloon outward, a condition known as aneurysm (FIGURE 4-24). This weakening happens much like a worn spot on a tire or a bulge in an old balloon. Just like the tire and the balloon, an aneurysm can rupture when the pressure builds inside the wall or when the wall becomes too thin. When it ruptures, blood spills out of the circulatory system, also known as exsanguination. Aneurysms may also develop slow leaks as opposed to rupturing. Aneurysms can occur in any artery, but some common

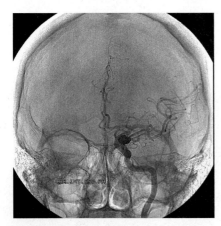

FIGURE 4-24 Aneurysm. This X-ray shows a ballooning of one of the arteries in the brain. If untreated, an aneurysm can rupture, causing a stroke.

© wenht/iStock/Getty Images.

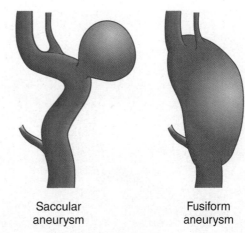

Saccular aneurysm   Fusiform aneurysm

FIGURE 4-25 Types of aneurysms.

locations include the aorta, particularly the abdominal and thoracic areas, and intracranial vessels. Other areas are the femoral and popliteal arteries. Intracranial aneurysms will be discussed in chapter 11.

The most common causes of aneurysms are atherosclerosis and hypertension. Atherosclerosis and subsequent plaque formation reduce elasticity and cause erosion. Blood traveling through narrowed arteries, like in hypertension, causes a lot of force on the arterial walls, leading to weakening and potential aneurysm development. Other factors that increase the risk of developing an aneurysm include genetic predispositions and congenital disorders (e.g., Marfan syndrome). Disorders that damage the arterial walls such as dyslipidemia and tobacco usage can lead to aneurysms. Diabetes mellitus, although associated with atherosclerosis, in epidemiologic studies has been inversely associated with the risk of aneurysm development. The reason for this inverse relation is unclear but theories include possible protective effects from antidiabetic agents (e.g., metformin). Injury (e.g., trauma) and infections (e.g., syphilis) can also cause aneurysms. The incidence of aortic aneurysms increases with age (> 65 years), and prevalence is higher in men.

True aneurysms are those that affect all three layers of the vessel. Two major types of true aneurysms exist—saccular and fusiform (**FIGURE 4-25**). The most common site of true aneurysms is the abdominal aorta. A saccular aneurysm is a bulge on the side of the vessel. A fusiform aneurysm affects the entire circumference of the vessel. A false aneurysm,

in contrast to true aneurysm, does not affect all three layers of the vessel but occurs when there is vessel damage. The damaged vessel causes blood to leak into the surrounding area (e.g., hematoma) or the injury leads to blood traveling and splitting the media layer. This splitting is known as a dissection (**FIGURE 4-26**). The larger the aneurysm, the greater the likelihood of rupture.

Clinical Manifestations

Clinical manifestations of aneurysms may vary based on their location. Most aneurysms are asymptomatic until they rupture. Before rupture, thoracic aorta aneurysms can cause pressure around surrounding areas such as the lungs and esophagus. This pressure causes dysphagia, chest pain, dyspnea, and cough. Abdominal aorta aneurysms may cause a pulsating abdominal mass as well as flank and back pain. Once an aneurysm rupture occurs, symptoms intensify (e.g., severe pain, worsening dyspnea) and cardiovascular collapse can occur due to life-threatening bleeding.

Diagnosis and Treatment

Diagnosis of aneurysms often occurs incidentally during a routine physical examination or during imaging studies (e.g., X-ray) done for other purposes. If clinical manifestations are present, diagnostic procedures are necessary to confirm the diagnosis and can include an echocardiogram, CT, MRI, and arteriography (i.e., angiography). The goal of treatment is to prevent rupture or limit expansion by eliminating or treating causes (e.g., controlling blood pressure). Management of cardiovascular risk factors can include statin and antiplatelet therapy. Smoking cessation is crucial as there is a

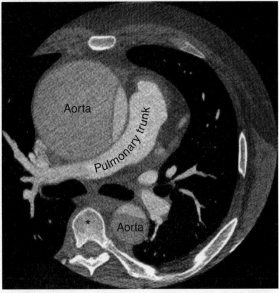
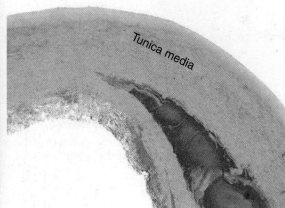

FIGURE 4-26 Aortic dissection.

Courtesy of Dr. Donald Yandow, Department of Radiology, University of Wisconsin School of Medicine and Public Health.

high association of rupture with continuation of smoking. The presence of symptoms with an aneurysm increases the chance of rupture and surgical repair is often indicated. Even in the absence of symptoms surgical repair may be indicated. As an example, if an aortic aneurysm has a diameter greater than 5 cm, surgery may be done to prevent rupture even in an asymptomatic patient. The larger the aortic aneurysm, the higher the risk of rupture. There is a high mortality once rupture occurs, and immediate surgery is required. Screening for abdominal aortic aneurysm is recommended for men ages 65–75 years who have smoked or have a family history.

Dyslipidemia

Dyslipidemia, or hyperlipidemia, refers to an elevated level of lipids in the blood. These lipids include cholesterol and triglycerides (fats) and phospholipids. While cholesterol and fats are different types of lipids, the term *cholesterol* is often used in place of lipids and/or used interchangeably with fats. High lipid levels are associated with an increased risk and severity of cardiovascular diseases such as atherosclerosis, coronary artery disease, hypertension, and stroke. In the United States from 2013 to 2016, a total of 27% of people over the age of 20 had high cholesterol levels (i.e., ≥ 240 mg/dL) or were taking a cholesterol-lowering medication (CDC, 2017). Of the 27% total, approximately 29% were males and 25% were females. The prevalence of high cholesterol among those

6–19 years of age in the United States from 2011 to 2014 was 7.4% (CDC, 2019). In the younger age group, girls had a higher incidence than boys. In both the young and old, obesity is associated with a higher cholesterol level.

Lipids are not soluble in water or plasma, and while some lipids are hydrophobic, others have a hydrophilic component (e.g., phospholipid). For the lipids to be transported around the body, they have to be bound to a carrier protein such as an apolipoprotein. The bound lipids are termed *lipoproteins*. Lipids are important in providing and storing energy, cellular membrane composition, steroid hormone production (e.g., testosterone, estradiol), and production of bile acids.

Lipids are introduced into the bloodstream in two ways—diet and liver production (**FIGURE 4-27**). Dietary cholesterol is found in animal products, and dietary triglycerides are found in saturated fats (e.g., fried foods and cakes). Often the foods high in fats are also high in cholesterol. The human liver makes more cholesterol than the body could possibly use, so even though cholesterol is necessary for survival, eating it is not necessary. When dietary fats and cholesterol are ingested, they are transported around by chylomicrons (bundles of lipoproteins). These chylomicrons are found in the small intestine. The chylomicrons consist primarily of triglycerides (> 80%), and the remainder are phospholipids, cholesterol, and protein. Chylomicrons' role, therefore, is to supply the tissues with fat

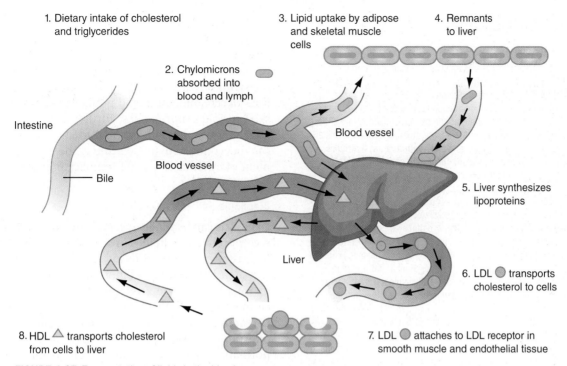

1. Dietary intake of cholesterol and triglycerides

2. Chylomicrons absorbed into blood and lymph

3. Lipid uptake by adipose and skeletal muscle cells

4. Remnants to liver

Intestine

Blood vessel

Bile

Blood vessel

Liver

5. Liver synthesizes lipoproteins

6. LDL ● transports cholesterol to cells

7. LDL ● attaches to LDL receptor in smooth muscle and endothelial tissue

8. HDL △ transports cholesterol from cells to liver

FIGURE 4-27 Transportation of lipids in the blood.

FIGURE 4-28 Low-density lipoprotein and key protein, cholesterol, phospholipid, and triglyceride.

FIGURE 4-29 High-density lipoprotein and key protein, cholesterol, phospholipid, and triglyceride.

from dietary ingestion. Remnants of chylomicrons are transported to the liver. In the liver, several lipoproteins are synthesized. Lipoproteins are classified according to their density. This density is based on the number of triglycerides, which are low in density, versus the number of proteins, which are highly dense (**FIGURE 4-28** and **FIGURE 4-29**). In other words, triglyceride number and degree of density are inversely proportional. The main classes of lipoproteins are chylomicrons, very-low-density lipoproteins (VLDLs), low-density lipoproteins (LDLs), intermediate-density lipoproteins (IDLs), and high-density lipoproteins (HDLs). The highest triglyceride level (i.e., low density) starts with the chylomicrons and the level of triglyceride diminishes in the following order:

VLDL, LDL, IDL, HDL. The most significant of these lipoproteins in terms of cardiovascular injury and protection are LDL and HDL.

There are primary and acquired dyslipidemias. Acquired dyslipidemia is more common and development is usually polygenic and influenced by environmental factors (e.g., diet, obesity). Primary dyslipidemia is inherited and monogenic, and is often not related to external factors such as diet and it is not as common as acquired dyslipidemia. The primary dyslipidemias include disorders of triglycerides, apolipoproteins, cholesterol, or a combination. The most common primary dyslipidemia is hypercholesteremia, which is usually a result of LDL receptor mutation and defects in breakdown.

Triglycerides

Triglycerides are fats in blood. Fat is mainly stored in adipose tissue. Triglycerides are made of glycerol and three fatty acid chains. The fats can be saturated (have more hydrogen bonds) or unsaturated (have fewer hydrogen bonds). An unsaturated fat can be further divided into either monounsaturated and polyunsaturated. So what does this all mean in terms of lipids and diet? Saturated fat molecules are tightly packed, making them solid at room temperature. So think of butter, cooking lard, and cheese. Saturated fats are also high in animal products (meat and dairy) and plant-based oils such as coconut and palm kernel oil. Saturated fats have been associated with higher cholesterol levels, heart disease, stroke, and diabetes. Healthier types of fats are those that are monounsaturated or polyunsaturated. Examples of monosaturated fat sources include olive, canola, peanut, and sesame oils (nontropical oils) that are all in liquid form at room temperature. Monounsaturated fats are also found in avocados, peanut butter, and other nuts and seeds. Polyunsaturated fats are found in walnuts, soybeans, corn oil, sunflower, and tofu. Omega-3 and omega-6 fatty acids are types of polyunsaturated fats that can only come from dietary sources (i.e., essential fatty acids) and are found in sources such as salmon, chia, and flaxseed. Trans fats are actually unsaturated fats that are naturally found in small amounts in some food products (e.g., meats and dairy), and when consumed in small quantities, do not have negative health effects. However, trans fats have been produced artificially to make liquid vegetable oils more solid, resulting in a high quantity of trans fats in many food products (e.g., fried foods, doughnuts, cookies, icings, and processed snacks). Foods made with trans fats can be stored longer and are inexpensive to use, and trans fats add flavor and texture to food. Trans fats have a more negative impact on health than saturated fats, but both raise cholesterol levels as well as increase risk for heart disease, stroke, and diabetes. Trans fats are banned in cooking products in several parts of the United States. All fats, regardless of type, contain approximately 9 calories per gram. While there are many diets proposing a high fat consumption, recommendations from the American Heart Association (2014) are to reduce and replace saturated and trans fats for healthier monounsaturated and polyunsaturated fats.

Cholesterol

LDL is known as the" bad" cholesterol. because the small, dense molecules of LDL are damaging. Most serum cholesterol is made up of LDL. You can remember LDL as the *"lousy"* cholesterol. Because it is the bad cholesterol, you want the LDL level as low as you can get it. Ways to decrease LDL through lifestyle modifications include dietary changes such as avoiding high-cholesterol, high-fat foods.

HDL is known as the good cholesterol because it assists in removing some of the cholesterol from the bloodstream. You can remember this point by considering it the *happy* cholesterol. Because it is the "good" cholesterol, you want the HDL level as high as you can get it. Ways to increase HDL through lifestyle modifications include tobacco cessation and exercise.

Clinical Manifestations

Dyslipidemia is often asymptomatic until it develops into other diseases (e.g., atherosclerosis, coronary artery disease, or stroke). At that point, the symptoms are related to those diseases. Cholesterol screening and lipid profiles can identify specific lipid abnormalities. Further testing (e.g., angiography, ultrasound, and nuclear scanning) can be conducted to determine the development of other diseases and complications.

Diagnosis and Treatment

Diagnosis can be made by laboratory analysis of a comprehensive lipid panel. Other diagnostic tests that can be used to aid in cardiovascular risk identification or in determining treatment options include the ankle brachial index, calcium score, and inflammatory markers such as C-reactive protein and lipoprotein-associated phospholipase-A_2. The goal of treatment is to normalize lipid levels and prevent complications. The commonly used clinical guideline for cholesterol management has been developed and updated by multiple organizations such as the American College of Cardiology and the American Heart Association (Grundy et al., 2018). Treatment regimens to lower lipid levels include lifestyle modifications such as consumption of low-cholesterol, low-fat foods, routine exercise, and weight reduction. Pharmacologic treatment is predominantly based on LDL levels and other clinical criteria (e.g., cardiovascular disease or risk). Pharmacologic agents should be initiated in all patients over 21 years old with clinical atherosclerotic cardiovascular disease (ASCVD) and in those with LDL levels $\geq$ 190 mg/dL. Examples of ASCVD include angina, myocardial infarction, peripheral artery disease, stroke, or transient ischemic attack. For those between the ages of 40 and 75 years who have diabetes mellitus and/or atherosclerotic risk (i.e., > 5%), pharmacologic therapy may be necessary in addition to lifestyle modifications. Atherosclerotic risk can be calculated using age, sex, race, blood pressure, total cholesterol, LDL and HDL levels, history of diabetes, and hypertension. Online calculators (e.g., www.cvriskcalculator.com/) and mobile applications can be used to provide a risk calculation. In patients under 21 years old and in those over 75 years, risk of cardiovascular disease and pharmacologic versus benefits must be individually evaluated.

While a wide range of lipid-lowering pharmacologic agents exists, pharmacologic treatment

BOX 4-3 Application to Practice

Mr. Delano comes in to discuss the results of cardiovascular diagnostic tests. He is a 61-year-old White man with no complaints.

Past medical history: left hip osteoarthritis and gout.
Past surgical history: none.
Allergies: none known.
Medications: allopurinol 100 mg by mouth once a day.

Social history: one to two alcoholic drinks three times a week; smokes one cigar every other month; exercises for 1 hour six times a week; retired nurse—works per diem at hospital once a week.
Family history: mother, father, and one brother with hypertension; one brother with dyslipidemia.

Physical exam: vital signs: temperature 98.5°F, pulse 60 beats per minute, respiration rate 20 per minute, and blood pressure 134/67 mmHg; height 180 cm; weight; 85.5 kg; body mass index 26.3; physical exam unremarkable.
Cardiovascular diagnostics:

Lipid panel	Results	Optimal values
Cholesterol, total	239 mg/dL	< 200
HDL cholesterol	57 mg/dL	≥ 40
Triglycerides	128 mg/dL	< 150
LDL cholesterol	156 mg/dL	< 100
Cholesterol-to-HDLC ratio	4.2 calculated	≤ 3.5
Non-HDL cholesterol	182 mg/dL	< 130
Lipoprotein subfractions		
LDL particle number	1,722 nmol/L	< 1,260
LDL small	258 nmol/L	< 162
LDL medium	511 nmol/L	< 201
HDL large	6,091 nmol/L	> 9,386
Apolipoproteins		
Apolipoprotein B	120 mg/dL	< 80
Lipoprotein (a)	33 nmol/L	< 75
Inflammatory markers		
HS CRP	0.5 mg/L	< 1.0
Lp-PLA$_2$ activity	93 nmol/min/mL	< 75
CT cardiac scoring screen	23 (mild amount)	< 99

Lp-PLA$_2$, lipoprotein-associated phospholipase-A$_2$.

Answer the following questions based on this scenario:

1. Which of the cardiovascular diagnostic values demonstrate dyslipidemia and risk for atherogenesis?
2. Interpret and describe lipoprotein subfractions and apolipoproteins results.
3. Which of the cardiovascular diagnostic values are in the cardioprotective range?
4. What lifestyle recommendations, such as diet and exercise will be made based on these results?
5. What is his ASCVD risk score? What parameters (e.g., blood pressure) are used to calculate the risk score?
6. In addition to lifestyle recommendations, what pharmacotherapeutics are recommended? Choose all that apply.
   a. None
   b. Aspirin
   c. Statin
   d. Nicotinic acid

primarily focuses on use of HMG-CoA reductase inhibitors (also known as *statins*). HMG-CoA reductase is an enzyme used by the liver during the manufacture of cholesterol and inhibition will therefore decrease production. Statins also facilitate breakdown of LDL so that cholesterol can be reabsorbed. Statin therapy is either moderate or high intensity. Moderate-intensity therapy refers to lowering LDL levels by $\geq$ 50% (e.g., atorvastatin 10–20 mg or rosuvastatin 5-10 mg), while high-intensity therapy refers to lowering LDL by 30–50% (e.g., atorvastatin 40–80 mg or rosuvastatin 20-40 mg). Other pharmacologic agents are not commonly prescribed but include bile acid sequestrants, cholesterol absorption inhibitors, nicotinic acid, fibrates, and omega-3 fatty acids. In 2017, the Food and Drug Administration approved a new medication, evolocumab, that works by increasing liver clearance of LDL by inhibiting the protein PCSK9. This protein usually decreases the number of receptors involved in LDL clearance, and thereby inhibition will increase the number of receptors available for LDL clearance.

Atherosclerosis

Atherosclerosis is a chronic inflammatory disease characterized by thickening and hardening of the arterial wall. The result is decreased perfusion, ischemia, and infarct. Atherosclerosis can occur in any part of the vascular system but most commonly occurs in coronary arteries, the thoracic and abdominal aorta, popliteal and femoral arteries, and carotid and cerebral arteries (**FIGURE 4-30**).

Many causes contribute to atherosclerosis development, such as dyslipidemia and smoking (**TABLE 4-5**). Some causes are modifiable (e.g., diet, obesity) while others are not (e.g., aging, gender, family history). The innermost protective vessel wall layer, the endothelium, is injured and becomes dysfunctional, initiating the atherosclerotic process regardless of the cause. The development of atherosclerosis proceeds through various stages (**FIGURE 4-31**). Endothelial injury begins early in life, progresses over time, and worsens with aging. Endothelial injury triggers the immune and inflammatory system, and the endothelial

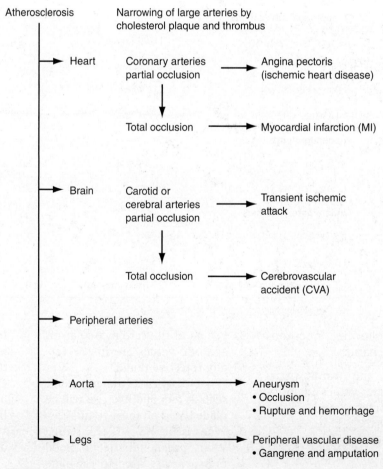

FIGURE 4-30 Possible complications of atherosclerosis.

TABLE 4-5	Risk Factors for Atherosclerosis and Coronary Artery Disease		
Nonmodifiable risk factors	**Modifiable risk factors**	**Negative risk factors**	**Emerging risk factors**
Age: men > 45 years; women > 55 years or premature menopause Family history: history of premature coronary artery disease in first-degree male relatives > 55 years or first-degree female relatives > 65 years	Tobacco use Obesity Physical inactivity Atherogenic diet Stress Diabetes mellitus Hyperlipidemia Hypertension	High HDL cholesterol	Elevated C-reactive protein and homocysteine levels Decreased adiponectin; increased leptin Medications: nonsteroidal anti-inflammatory drugs

Modified from Story, L. (2017). *Pathophysiology: A practical approach* (3rd ed.). Burlington, MA: Jones & Bartlett Learning.

lining that is normally a protective barrier becomes dysfunctional.

Nitric oxide, a vasodilator produced by the endothelial cells, is diminished, leading to an inability to maintain vascular tone and antithrombotic activity (i.e., prevention of platelet adhesion). Reductions in nitric oxide additionally allow for cellular proliferation and leukocyte adhesion. LDL enters the intimal layer and becomes oxidized. Oxidation results in a change in LDL which facilitates accelerated LDL uptake by macrophages. Inflammatory cytokines and the oxidized LDL stimulate endothelial cells to release molecules (e.g., vascular cell adhesion molecule-1 and P-selectin) that lead to monocyte binding. Monocytes enter the endothelial lining and travel to the intima and become macrophages. These macrophages start ingesting LDL. The macrophages full of oxidized LDL look like foam from the sea and are termed *foam cells*. The foam cells are considered the early stage of the atheroma (i.e., plaque). The foam cells release cytokines (e.g., tumor necrosis factor and interleukins) and growth factors as well as leukocytes, such as T lymphocytes, are recruited. Lipid continues to accumulate in the intimal layer, forming a fatty streak. These fatty streaks develop and are evident at a young age, such as at 15 years of age. Cytokines induce more endothelial activation, and the smooth muscle proliferates into the intima. The smooth muscle cells, sensing the damage, start to form a fibrous cap made of proteins such as collagen and elastin around the fatty streak. The fibrous cap and fatty streak are what make up a fibrous plaque. Eventually, calcium and a necrotic lipid core become part of the plaque. The plaque bulges into the lumen of the artery, resulting in a smaller vessel radius, and resistance to flow is increased. The arterial walls become stiff and not as compliant. A fragile microvascular network begins supplying the plaque as it continues to grow.

The plaque may slowly cause narrowing and be stable. However, plaques can also be prone to rupturing and cause an acute obstruction, and these plaques are considered unstable. Generally, atherosclerosis and the resulting obstruction are a clinically silent disease, meaning no symptoms are apparent. When obstruction becomes significant (e.g., 70% lumen stenosis), symptoms of ischemia, such as angina or claudication, can begin to occur, particularly during increased myocardial demand (e.g., exercise). Unstable plaques can rupture without significant stenosis and blood flow impairment. Acute vascular events, such as myocardial infarction or stroke, are usually due to plaque rupture as opposed to vessel narrowing. Platelets aggregate, the clotting cascade is stimulated, and a thrombus forms when the plaque ruptures (Figure 4-31).

Clinical Manifestations

Much like dyslipidemia, atherosclerosis is often asymptomatic until complications develop. At that point, clinical manifestations will be related to those specific disorders. The various disorders are discussed elsewhere in this chapter (e.g., angina in *Coronary Artery Disease* section).

Diagnosis and Treatment

Diagnostic procedures for atherosclerosis include tests that identify contributing factors (e.g., lipid panel, C-reactive protein, and homocysteine levels). Increased C-reactive protein levels indicate the presence of inflammation and are considered a risk factor for atherosclerosis. Other diagnostic procedures are used to

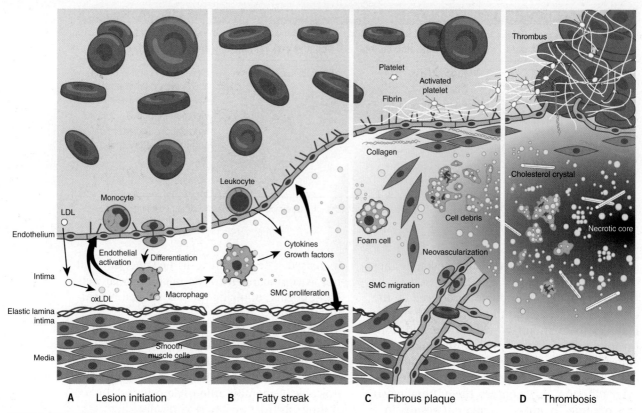

FIGURE 4-31 Pathogenesis of atherosclerosis.

Pathogenesis of atherosclerosis. **A** In the first stage, low density lipoprotein-cholesterol (LDL) is deposited in the endothelium and undergoes oxidative modification, resulting in oxidized LDL (oxLDL). OxLDL stimulates endothelial cells to express adhesion molecules (vascular cell adhesion molecule-1 [VCAM-1], P-Selectin) and various chemokines (e.g., Monocyte Chemoattractant Protein-1 (MCP-1), Interleukin 8 [IL-8]). This leads to a recruitment of monocytes, which transmigrate into the intima and differentiate to pro-atherogenic macrophages; **B** Macrophages harvest residual oxLDL via their scavenger receptors and add to the endothelial activation and, subsequently, leukocyte recruitment with the secretion of Tumor Necrosis Factor α (TNF-α) and IL-6; **C** The increasing plaque volume promotes neovascularization. Proliferating smooth muscle cells (SMCs) stabilize the nascent fibrous plaque. With deposition of fibrin and activated platelets on the dysfunctional endothelium that expresses tissue factor (TF) and von Willebrand factor (vWF), a pro-thrombotic milieu is formed; **D** Foam cells can undergo apoptosis and release cell-debris and lipids, which will result in the formation of a necrotic core. In addition, proteases secreted from foam cells can destabilize the plaque. This can lead to plaque rupture, in which case extracellular matrix molecules (e.g., collagens, elastin, TF, vWF) catalyze thrombotic events.

Steinl, D., & Kaufmann, B. (2015). Ultrasound imaging for risk assessment in atherosclerosis. *International journal of molecular sciences, 16*(5), 9749-9769.

determine whether complications have developed (e.g., angiography, ultrasound, and nuclear scanning).

Treatment for atherosclerosis is like that for dyslipidemia. In addition, angioplasty opens occluded arteries (**FIGURE 4-32**), bypass procedures detour blood around the occlusions, laser procedures disintegrate the plaque, and atherectomy removes the plaque. B-complex vitamins can help lower homocysteine levels if warranted.

Peripheral Artery Disease

Atherosclerosis can cause injury to any part of the vascular system, but the extremities are often affected. When the upper or lower extremities are affected, it is commonly termed *peripheral artery disease*. Peripheral artery disease is also the designation used to include arterial occlusive disorders due to other non-atherosclerotic disorders. Risk factors for peripheral artery disease development are similar to those for atherosclerosis, particularly factors

Diagnostic Link

Diagnostic Link-Homocysteine

Homocysteine is an amino acid commonly obtained from eating meat. High levels in the serum are associated with development of cardiovascular and cerebrovascular disorders such as development of atherosclerosis and thromboembolic disorders. The mechanism by which high levels causes vascular disorders is unclear. Vitamins, particularly folate, vitamin B6, and vitamin B12, are necessary for homocysteine metabolism, and deficiencies can result in increased levels. Other causes of increased levels include chronic kidney disease (reduced clearance and metabolism), smoking, and certain medications such as metformin (for type 2 diabetes mellitus), methotrexate (for rheumatic disorders). Levels can be reduced with vitamin supplementation and eating a healthier diet (e.g., increased vegetables, fruit, and low fat diet). However, most research has found that reducing levels does not prevent or reduce the incidence of vascular disorders.

that also affect the coronary circulation (e.g., dyslipidemia, smoking). Peripheral artery disease is a risk equivalent for the development or presence of coronary artery disease. The

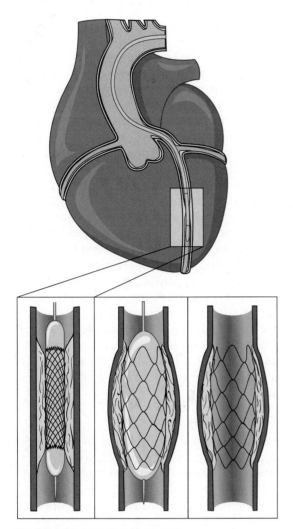

FIGURE 4-32 Principles of angioplasty.

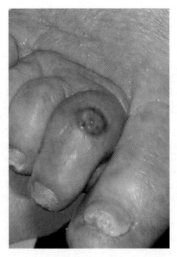

FIGURE 4-33 Arterial insufficiency ulcer; arterial wound.

risk factors for peripheral artery disease include advanced age (i.e., > 70), diabetes mellitus, dyslipidemia, smoking, or other factors that increase risk for atherosclerosis, such as hypertension.

Clinical Manifestation

Extremity peripheral artery disease is often asymptomatic. Manifestations will be present once the stenosis is sufficient to cause a decreased perfusion. Manifestations will include extremity pain (upper and lower), particularly pain that is present during physical activity and relieved with rest. This pain is termed *intermittent claudication*. The pain worsens with elevation of the extremity as blood is diverted away from the distal tissue. The pain improves with extremity dependence as blood then flows down to the extremity. Lower extremity peripheral artery disease pain can be in the calf (popliteal artery), thigh (femoral artery), or buttock/hip (aortoiliac artery). The pain may be unilateral or bilateral. If the aortoiliac artery is affected, the femoral pulses may be diminished, and erectile dysfunction may present. If the popliteal or femoral arteries are affected, distal pulses (i.e., pedal, posterior tibialis) will be diminished. Foot claudication may be present and indicates disease of the tibial or peroneal arteries. As occlusion worsens, manifestations may include signs of poor perfusion such as lower extremities that are dry, cool, shiny, and hairless. Nonhealing ulcers (i.e., ischemic ulcer) may be present over bony areas and look "punched out" (FIGURE 4-33). Necrotic areas may be evident as the severity of occlusion worsens. The skin may appear whitish or bluish when elevated due to decreased blood flow and reddish when dependent due to increased blood flow. Once an occlusion becomes severe, pain may be present even at rest and cause limb pain that is diffuse rather than focal. The diffuse, acute, and, severe pain is the result of obstruction due to thrombosis. The sudden presence of the six *Ps*—**p**allor, **p**ulselessness, **p**aresthesia, **p**aralysis, **p**oikilothermia (i.e., cold), and **p**ain are ominous findings. Urgent recognition and action, such as surgical revascularization, are necessary to save the limb.

Most commonly, upper extremity peripheral artery disease presents as unequal blood pressure readings in the arms (> 15 mmHg). The collateral circulation in the upper arms often compensates for upper arm stenosis or occlusions, and manifestations are not as common. If present, upper extremity peripheral artery disease can have similar manifestations to lower extremity peripheral artery disease (e.g., pain that increases with activity and resolves with rest). Patients with upper extremity peripheral artery disease often have lower extremity peripheral artery disease.

Diagnosis and Treatment

Diagnosis is accomplished with a history and physical examination. The initial diagnostic test for upper extremity peripheral artery disease will be duplex ultrasound. Duplex ultrasound (combination of doppler—checks blood flow—and regular ultrasound—creates images) will reveal stenosis or occlusion. Blood pressure measurements in different arteries (i.e., segmental blood pressures) can be evaluated and used to calculate the ankle brachial index (ABI) for lower extremity peripheral artery disease or the wrist brachial index for upper extremity peripheral artery disease. The ABI is the initial diagnostic exam and is often done with a dupplex doppler ultrasound for lower extremity peripheral artery disease. The ABI is calculated by measuring the systolic pressure in the right and left brachial artery and dorsalis pedis as well as posterior tibial in a supine position. The highest foot pressure is then divided by the highest arm pressure. Doppler or plethysmographic waveforms are often done with the ABI to localize what part of the artery is affected. The ABI measurements can be accomplished at the bedside but is preferably conducted in a diagnostic center; it can be done at rest and/or after exercise. An ABI of ≤ 0.90 is diagnostic for peripheral artery disease. Angiography with computed tomography (CTA) or magnetic resonance (MRA) may be

indicated depending on the severity of symptoms or if findings from other diagnostic tests are questionable. Laboratory evaluation will be the same as those for atherosclerosis and dyslipidemia (e.g., lipid panel, homocysteine, C-reactive protein).

Treatment focuses on risk reduction strategies as in atherosclerosis and dyslipidemia such as smoking cessation, weight loss, diabetes mellitus, and hypertension management. For those with symptomatic peripheral artery disease, antiplatelet therapy with aspirin or clopidogrel are recommended to reduce other cardiovascular events (e.g., MI, stroke). Cilostazol is an antiplatelet medication but is often not tolerated due to side effects (e.g., headache, diarrhea, palpitations). Treatment will include an exercise program that consists of activities such as warm up and cool down as well as gradual increase in walking. The exercise program is efficacious when done under supervision or with guidance. Treatments may also include revascularization, angioplasty, and stenting.

Coronary Artery Disease

When atherosclerosis develops in the arteries supplying the myocardium, coronary artery disease develops. Despite great advancements in treatment, cardiovascular disease (including coronary artery disease) remains the leading cause of death in the United States for men and women. Coronary artery disease accounts for most of the cardiovascular deaths (AHA, 2017). In coronary artery disease, often termed *coronary heart disease*, blood flow diminishes in the coronary arteries, causing subsequent oxygen reduction (i.e., ischemia) to the cardiac muscle. Coronary artery disease due to atherosclerosis is the most common cause of ischemia. Coronary vasospasm (i.e., Prinzmetal angina) is another cause of myocardial ischemia and may occur with or without atherosclerosis. Myocardial ischemia can occur under any circumstance where myocardial oxygen demand supersedes coronary supply. Normal coronary arteries are usually able to compensate when demand is increased. With coronary artery disease, the vessels may not be able to compensate, and increases in demand (e.g., hypotension, anemia, or valve disease) can cause ischemia. Myocardial ischemia is usually due to a combination of both increased demand and inadequate supply. Myocardial ischemia may or may not cause permanent damage, or infarction, to the myocardium. Coronary artery disease can also cause heart failure, dysrhythmias, and sudden death. Additional contributing factors for coronary artery disease—some modifiable and some not—are the same as those for atherosclerosis (e.g., diabetes mellitus, hypertension, and tobacco) (Table 4-5).

Clinical Manifestations

Coronary artery disease clinical manifestations are a result of myocardial ischemia and are a common cause of chest pain. The term used for ischemic chest pain is *angina pectoris* or simply *angina*. Ischemia causes the sensation of angina due to an accumulation of lactic acid and metabolic waste products (e.g., reactive oxygen species, adenosine). This accumulation can stimulate nerves that correspond to the same dermatome as the heart, causing the pain to radiate to other parts of the body such as the lower jaw, neck, left arm (uncommonly right), epigastrium, and rarely, the back. The chest pain with angina is often described as pressure, heaviness, or tightness in the center or left side of the chest. Some patients who have angina may say they do not have pain but rather discomfort or indigestion. The chest pain is often diffuse, as opposed to localized in a particular area, and often starts gradually. Angina may be accompanied by cool, clammy extremities, diaphoresis, exertional shortness of breath, lightheadedness, and fatigue. Gastrointestinal symptoms may include nausea and vomiting, belching, and indigestion. Angina is not usually described as sharp, knifelike, or aching. The pain does not increase with movement or palpation and does not worsen with breathing like with pleuritis. Physical examination may reveal no findings or increased heart rate, blood pressure, extra heart sounds (e.g., S_3, S_4), or murmurs.

New onset of angina (< 2 months) may present as stable or unstable. **Stable angina** refers to ischemia that is initiated by increased demand (e.g., activity) and relieved with the reduction of that demand (e.g., rest). In addition to activity, situations that can increase demand include a cold environment, sexual intercourse, stress, or stimulants such as cocaine. The duration of angina is often less than 5 minutes.

The angina is considered unstable when it becomes unpredictable, occurs at rest, or increases in frequency or duration (e.g., > 20 minutes). **Unstable angina** is considered a preinfarction state and, along with myocardial infarction, is considered an acute coronary syndrome. However, unstable angina ischemia is reversible, but once there is an infarction the tissue death is irreversible.

Prinzmetal angina (i.e., vasospastic angina or variant angina) is a type of angina that occurs due to vasospasm in the coronary arteries without atherosclerosis. The incidence is rare (2 in 100 angina cases) (AHA, 2015), and patients are likely to be younger (i.e., < 50 years). Risk factors are not the same as in other forms of angina except for smoking; however, Prinzmetal angina can occur in those with atherosclerosis. The vasospasm is a result of arterial smooth muscle hypercontractility. The vasospasm often occurs at night (e.g., midnight to early morning) due to increased vagal tone and increased sympathetic activity that occurs at night. Endothelial dysfunction such as increased oxidative stress or increased vasoconstriction from endothelin contributes to vasospasms. Manifestations are similar to other types of angina except the pain is mainly at rest and occurs at night.

Microvascular angina is caused by dysfunction in the coronary microvasculature (i.e., prearterioles and arterioles). Patients are usually younger and more often women in comparison to patients with angina from coronary artery disease. Various mechanisms are thought to cause dysfunction in these small vessels, and many mechanisms are similar to other causes of angina development such as endothelial dysfunction from smoking, hyperlipidemia, and diabetes. The small vessels have an imbalance in vasomotor tone with an increase in vasoconstriction and a decrease in vasodilation. The vessels normally affected by coronary artery disease may be normal with microvascular angina. Manifestations are similar to other types of angina, but pain can occur at rest or exertion and the duration of pain is at times longer.

Diagnosis and Treatment

Diagnosis of coronary artery disease is often made clinically with a history consistent with angina manifestations and risk factors. Diagnostic procedures for coronary artery disease, particularly if angina is present, is an EKG. The EKG is often normal, but chronic ischemia can cause EKG changes (usually ST-segment depression). An ambulatory EKG (monitoring done over an extended period of time) can be done. Other diagnostic tests can include a stress test, which will further confirm the diagnosis

BOX 4-4 Application to Practice

Mrs. Jameson, a 60-year-old woman, comes into the clinic complaining of chest pain, which has occurred three to four times since her last visit 4 months ago. She describes the pain as a squeezing, substernal pressure that is worse after climbing stairs in her home. The pressure resolves after 2 minutes of rest. During the last two episodes, she felt like she had indigestion and became a bit nauseous. The last episode of chest pressure was 2 days ago.

Medications:
- Metformin 1,000 mg by mouth once daily
- Lisinopril 30 mg by mouth once daily

Allergies: none known.

Social history: quit smoking 2 years ago; smoked 1 pack per day for 30 years (30 pack years); diet high in saturated fats; says she eats whatever she wants; attempts to exercise, walks one to two times a week; widowed for 2 years.

Past medical history: htn for 10 years; type 2 diabetes mellitus for 5 years.

Past surgical history: appendectomy as a child.

Family history: mother died of breast cancer age 60; father died of MI age 57; no siblings.

Physical examination: vital signs: temperature 98.0°F, pulse 76 per minute, respirations 20 per minute, BP 130/76 mmHg.

Answer the following questions:

1. What is the likely diagnosis?
2. What are the most common causes of this disease and which one is the most likely in Mrs. Jameson?
3. Describe the risk factors for coronary artery disease and the mechanism by which atherosclerotic plaque develops.
4. How does coronary artery disease lead to the symptoms Mrs. Jameson is experiencing?
5. How is coronary artery disease different in women in comparison to men?

---

of coronary artery disease and is useful in evaluating severity. Evaluating for associated risk factors includes diagnostic tests similar to those for atherosclerosis such as a lipid panel and metabolic panel. Cardiac biomarkers such as troponin will be normal if the angina is transient and intermittent. Coronary arteriography is indicated in some cases of angina to confirm and evaluate the severity of an obstruction.

Treatment focuses on preventing myocardial infarction by reducing modifiable risk factors through the same strategies used to treat dyslipidemia and atherosclerosis (e.g., dietary changes, tobacco cessation, physical activity, weight reduction, stress reduction, diabetes management, hypertension control, angioplasty, bypass procedures, laser procedures, antiplatelet agents, anticoagulants, thrombolytics, and lipid-lowering medications). Medications to specifically treat the angina include nitrates, beta-adrenergic blocking agents, and calcium channel blockers to vasodilate the coronary arteries and increase the oxygen supply. Nitrates and calcium channel blockers are first-line therapy for Prinzmetal angina. Nitrates may not be as effective in patients with microvascular angina. Oxygen therapy may also be used to increase oxygen supply. Ranolazine, a sodium channel blocker, is one of a newer class of medication for angina that reduces angina and increases exercise capacity.

Myocardial Infarction

Myocardial infarction (MI) is death of the myocardium from a sudden blockage of coronary artery blood flow (FIGURE 4-34). MI, like unstable angina, is an acute coronary syndrome. The acute coronary syndromes are usually the result of the sequelae of atherosclerosis—coronary artery disease whether silent or symptomatic, and persistent ischemia or obstruction (FIGURE 4-35). Risk factors for such an event include those for atherosclerosis, including dyslipidemia, diabetes mellitus, hypertension, stress, and tobacco. Death from cardiovascular disease is usually a result of cardiac damage after an MI. Every 40 seconds, a person dies of an MI (AHA, 2017). Myocardial infarction, while usually associated with coronary artery disease and plaque thrombus formation, can also occur in circumstances without coronary artery disease. Any circumstance when oxygen supply and demand are imbalanced can cause a myocardial infarction. Procedures meant to

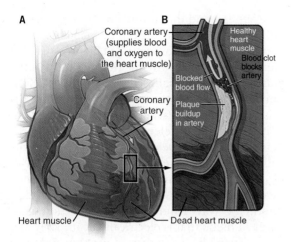

FIGURE 4-34 Myocardial infarction. **A** An overview of a heart and coronary artery showing damage (dead heart muscle) caused by a heart attack. **B** A cross-section of the coronary artery with plaque buildup and a blood clot.

Reproduced from National Heart, Lung, and Blood Institute. (2015). What is a heart attack? Retrieved from http://www.nhlbi.nih.gov/health/health-topics/topics/heartattack/

be therapeutic such as percutaneous coronary intervention, stents, and coronary artery bypass carry risks of a MI.

In most cases of MI, an unstable plaque tears or ruptures, triggering platelet aggregation, the coagulation cascade, and thrombus formation (Figure 4-31). As a result, the vessel becomes occluded, and the myocardial oxygen supply cannot meet the body's demand for oxygen. An MI occurs in progressive stages as the blood flow to the myocardium decreases. Cells can become ischemic within 10 seconds and die in about 20 minutes as the coronary blood and oxygen supplies dwindle. Cellular death proceeds from the subendocardial layer all the way through to the full heart muscle thickness (i.e., transmural). The degree and location of the infarct is dependent on several factors and includes the severity and duration of the ischemia, the artery affected, and the amount of

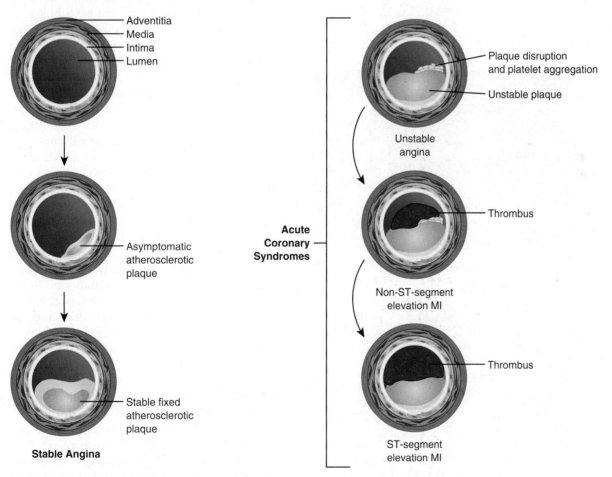

FIGURE 4-35 Stable angina and acute coronary syndromes.

collateral circulation. Most infarcts occur in the left ventricle, resulting in acute pump failure and risk for heart failure, cardiogenic shock, and death. With an infarction, the electrical system is also affected; therefore, dysrhythmias often develop. Just as muscle tissue is supplied by certain coronary arteries, the electrical system components, such the SA or AV node, are supplied by certain arteries (e.g., right coronary artery or left circumflex). The trigger for the MI is not always known but may be similar to those precipitating unstable angina such as physical exertion, outside activity in cold weather, and severe emotional stress. An MI can also occur during sleep or rest.

MIs are categorized into two groups—non–ST elevation MI (NSTEMI) or ST elevation MI (STEMI) (Figure 4-34 and **FIGURE 4-36**). The ST segment is normally isoelectric (goes to baseline on an EKG). With myocardial ischemia with no ST elevation, there is most likely an unstable plaque that may or may not develop a thrombus. In these circumstances, partial obstruction is present, and these patients either have unstable angina or an NSTEMI. The manifestations

are similar, and the distinction between unstable angina and NSTEMI can be made by evaluating cardiac biomarkers (**TABLE 4-6**). Unstable angina biomarkers are not elevated until hours after the onset of pain, while with an NSTEMI, myocardial damage is more severe, and necrosis occurs and biomarker elevations are quicker. The ST segment is elevated as well as biomarkers with STEMI. The occlusion in STEMI is usually complete. Some NSTEMIs and STEMIs lead to the development of a pathologic Q wave. Pathologic Q waves are wider and deeper than normal Q waves and they are a reflection of an area of tissue that is electrically dead. They can take several hours to days to develop and once present they rarely disappear. MIs can be referred to as *Q wave MI* (usually STEMI) or *non–Q wave MI*.

Clinical Manifestations

Some people do not experience symptoms of MI or the symptoms are atypical and not perceived as harmful to the patient and care is not sought. Such an asymptomatic MI is known as a silent MI. The risk for a silent MI is higher in those with known coronary heart disease but the risk is even higher in persons who have diabetes mellitus, neurologic dysfunction such as neuropathy, or history of a prior MI because of decreased pain innervations. Women and the elderly are also more likely to have silent MIs. When clinical manifestations of an MI are present, they are similar to those with unstable angina. Patients who are having an MI often voice a sense an impending doom. The intensity of the pain is high, and the duration can be longer than angina (e.g., 30 minutes). MI pain does not respond to pain relief measures such as rest or sublingual nitroglycerin. The elderly who are having an MI are more likely to present with atypical symptoms such as dyspnea, weakness, syncope, palpitations, altered mental status, and confusion. Physical examination may reveal cool, moist skin, and the patient may be restless and agitated. Signs of increased sympathetic tone will be tachycardia and hypertension, and the reverse occurs with increased vagal tone—bradycardia and hypotension. Other signs will be dependent on the artery occluded, such as left ventricle dysfunction with left coronary artery occlusion. Right ventricular infarction will cause blood flow backup signs including jugular vein distention and edema. Dysrhythmias and EKG changes (Figure 4-19; **FIGURE 4-37**) can manifest. These changes might include bundle branch block,

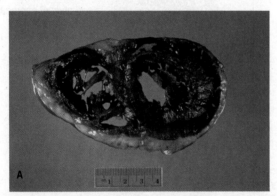

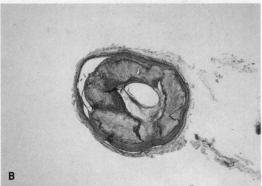

FIGURE 4-36 Myocardial infarction. **A** Sectioned heart showing myocardial infarction of the posterior left ventricle. **B** Severely occluded coronary artery with calcification from an elderly woman with a fatal myocardial infarction.

TABLE 4-6	Cardiac Biomarkers		
Biomarker	**Onset**	**Advantages**	**Disadvantages**
CK-MB (creatine kinase-muscle/ brain)	4–6 hours	Rapid Cost-effective Detected early in infarction	Loss of specificity with skeletal muscle damage Detected after 6 hours of myocardial necrosis
Myoglobin	1 hour	Highly sensitive Early detection of MI, within 2 hours Detects reperfusion Most useful in ruling out MI	Low specificity with skeletal muscle injury Rapid return to normal
Troponins	2–6 hours	Powerful tool for risk stratification Greater sensitivity and specificity than CK-MB Detects recent MI, up to 2 weeks prior to testing Helpful to determine therapy Detection of reperfusion	Low sensitivity to MI of less than 6 hours Require repeat measures at 8–12 hours if first result is negative Less able to detect late, minor MIs

Reproduced from Story, L. (2017). *Pathophysiology: A practical approach* (3rd ed.). Burlington, MA: Jones & Bartlett Learning.

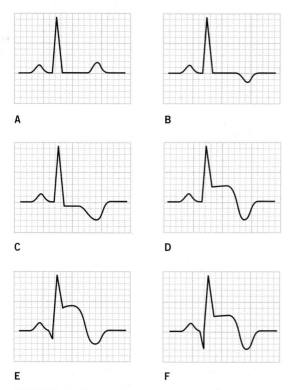

FIGURE 4-37 EKG ischemia and infarction patterns. **A** Normal EKG for comparison. **B** Mild ischemia demonstrated by inverted T wave. **C** Moderate ischemia demonstrated by slight ST-segment depression and inverted T wave. **D** and **E** ST-segment elevation myocardial infarction. **F** ST-segment myocardial infarction with prominent Q wave indicating more severe myocardial damage.

Modified from *Introduction to 12-Lead ECG: The Art of Interpretation,* courtesy of Tomas B. Garcia, MD.

ventricular tachycardia, ventricular fibrillation, and asystole.

Diagnosis and Treatment

Diagnosis of an MI is based on a history, physical examination, EKG (Figure 4-36), and cardiac biomarker result (Table 4-6). Other diagnostic tests may include stress testing, nuclear imaging, and angiography. Treatment is complex and depends on when the individual sought treatment (FIGURE 4-38).

Complications are more likely to occur when MIs are not treated early and aggressively. Prognosis hinges on early identification and treatment—ideally within 90 minutes of symptom onset. Early interventions will include pain management with the use of morphine and nitrates. Antiplatelet therapy with aspirin is administered at initial presentation. Immediate reperfusion therapy (e.g., thrombolytics, percutaneous coronary intervention) should be accomplished within 30 minutes of presentation for those who meet criteria and have no contraindications. Percutaneous coronary intervention is preferred but if there is a long anticipated delay then thrombolytic therapy should be instituted. Thrombolytic therapy involves the use of agents that stimulate the activation of plasminogen to plasmin (i.e., plasminogen activators). Therapeutic fibrinolytic agents used in MI include recombinant agents

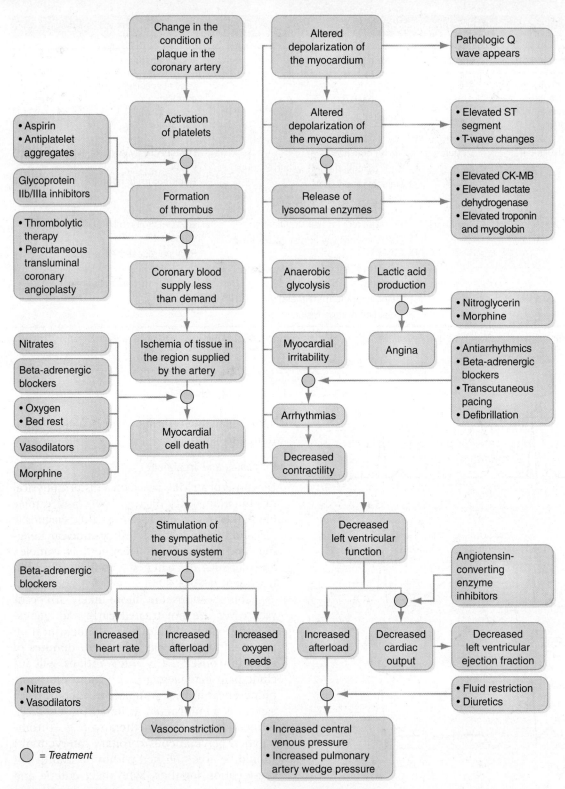

FIGURE 4-38 Treating an MI.

such as TNK-tPA (tenecteplase), and t-PA (alteplase) and streptokinase (derived from beta-hemolytic streptococcus cultures) (Figure 4-31). Percutaneous coronary interventions include procedures such as balloon angioplasty (opens the occlusion) and stent placement (prevent abrupt artery closure) The two types of stents include drug-eluting and bare metal stents. Laser procedures (e.g., laser atherectomy) may be indicated. In certain clinical situations coronary artery bypass graft may be necessary (e.g., multivessel coronary artery disease with complex anatomy).

Antiplatelet therapy with platelet $P2Y_{12}$ receptor blockers (e.g., clopidogrel)or a glycoprotein IIb/IIIa receptor inhibitor (e.g., abciximab) and other agents is indicated if angiography or percutaneous coronary intervention is undertaken. Beta blockers should be initiated within 24 hours. After that point, treatment options and ability to reverse damage become limited. After an MI, taking steps to prevent another MI through lifestyle modifications (e.g., dietary changes, tobacco cessation, physical activity, weight reduction, stress reduction, diabetes management, and hypertension control) is vital. Long-term pharmacologic treatment will include antiplatelet agents, anticoagulants, beta blockers, lipid-lowering medications, and an annual influenza vaccine. Contracting the flu can cause another MI, therefore an influenza vaccine is highly recommended.

Learning Points

Myocardial Infarction (MI) Treatment

Initial treatment of an MI can be remembered using the acronym MONA:

M	morphine
O	oxygen
N	nitroglycerin
A	aspirin

Initiating these strategies during the triage and assessment period is critical to achieve optimal patient outcomes.

Reproduced from Story, L. (2017). *Pathophysiology: A practical approach* (3rd ed.). Burlington, MA: Jones & Bartlett Learning.

Kawasaki Disease

Kawasaki disease, previously known as mucocutaneous lymph node syndrome, is a systemic vasculitis (i.e., vascular inflammation) that affects children. While considered rare, it is one of the most common types of vasculitis in children. Kawasaki disease incidence is highest in children of Asian and Pacific Islander descent; however, other races and ethnicities can be affected. Boys are more likely to be affected, and the incidence is highest in children under the age of 5.

Arteries are usually the affected blood vessels. The cause of the vessel inflammation and vascular damage is unknown but thought to be a response to a stimulus such as an infection or toxin. Since the disorder is prevalent in a specific population and in family members, genetic factors may contribute to disease development. Most cases are self-limiting and resolve within 12 days; however, serious cardiovascular complications such as coronary artery aneurysm, myocardial infarction, and heart failure can occur.

Clinical Manifestations

Fever is one of the key manifestations in children with Kawasaki disease. Characteristically, the fever has a longer duration (> 5 days) than fever from other disorders. The fever is usually above 101.3°F (38.5°C) and remains high despite administration of antipyretics. Diagnostic criteria are based on fever and a combination of at least four of five criteria that may be present during this acute febrile period. These diagnostic criteria include various mucocutaneous inflammatory signs, including 1) bilateral conjunctivitis (no exudates); 2) oral mucositis with dry, cracked lips, and a strawberry tongue; 3) rash in trunk, extremities, and perineal area that is erythematous and desquamates; 4) hands/palm and feet/sole edema and erythema; or 5) cervical lymphadenopathy with one node that is at least > 1.5 cm.

Manifestations that are not part of the diagnostic criteria but may be present include arthritic joint pain usually of the knee, ankle, or hip. Cardiovascular findings may present in the acute phase (i.e., < 10 days) or after and may include abnormal heart sounds such as a gallop or muffled tones; coronary artery dilation; aneurysms of the brachial artery or the coronary artery; and reduced perfusion signs including cool, cyanotic extremities. Other nonspecific manifestations can include gastrointestinal complaints such as diarrhea, vomiting, and decreased intake. Irritability or lethargy, cough, and rhinorrhea are other manifestations.

Diagnosis and Treatment

The diagnosis of Kawasaki disease is based on fever (≥ 5 days) and the presences of four out of five diagnostic criteria previously described. Laboratory findings that support the diagnosis include elevated acute-phase reactants such as estimated sedimentation rate and C-reactive protein; leukocytosis such as immature neutrophils, thrombocytosis (i.e., increased platelets), and elevated liver enzymes. An echocardiogram is done at diagnosis to evaluate cardiac status. Echocardiograms should be done routinely (e.g., at 2 and 6 weeks) to monitor for cardiovascular complications.

Initial treatment involves the administration of a single infusion of intravenous immunoglobulin and several days of aspirin to reduce the risk of cardiovascular complications. Intravenous immune globulin is most effective if administered within 10 days. Concerns about Reye syndrome with aspirin use in children must be considered. Reye syndrome, however, is usually associated with aspirin use for treatment of varicella or influenza. Recovery from Kawasaki disease is usually complete, particularly with treatment, and cardiovascular effects into adulthood are rare. Live vaccine administration should be postponed until approximately 11 months after receiving immune globulin as antibodies formed may affect the effectiveness of the vaccine.

Raynaud Disease

Raynaud disease is a peripheral vascular disease not associated with atherosclerosis as with peripheral artery disease. Raynaud disease is a result of vasospasm of the small arteries and arterioles, most often of the hands, that occurs because of sympathetic (alpha-2 adrenergic) stimulation (FIGURE 4-39). The vasospasms are triggered by cold exposure and stress. The disease is more common in women and those with a family history. Smoking, vascular disorders (e.g., cardiac disorders), and migraines increase risk for development. The age of onset is in adolescence and young adulthood. Raynaud phenomenon describes the state in which

such vasospasm occurs in association with an autoimmune disease (e.g., systemic lupus erythematosus and scleroderma). During episodes of vasospasms, the patient will have a "white attack," characterized by demarcated skin pallor due to constricted blood flow. Following the pallor, the patient will have a "blue attack," reflecting cyanosis from tissue hypoxia. The attack can last up to 20 minutes. With resolution of the attack, reperfusion causes skin color to return to normal. In addition to hand pain, patients can complain of numbness, clumsiness, and aching. Diagnosis for Raynaud disease and phenomenon is confirmed by a history and physical examination. Diagnostic tests will include nail fold capillaroscopy (performed by placing oil on periungual area and examining under an opthalmoscope) to distinguish between the disease and the phenomenon. Other diagnostic tests (e.g., thermography, angiography) can be used to evaluate vascular responses in the distal extremities. Treatment involves minimizing cold exposure and keeping the body warm with exposure. Stress management will reduce attacks. To abort an attack, the hands can be warmed with moving or rubbing the hands or placing them under warm water. Smoking and sympathomimetics such as decongestants or amphetamines should be avoided. If nonpharmacologic agents are ineffective, calcium channel blockers can be used.

Arterial and Venous Disorders
Buerger Disease

Thromboangiitis obliterans, or Buerger disease, is a peripheral vascular disease not associated with atherosclerosis as with peripheral artery disease. Buerger disease can affect arteries and veins. Buerger disease is an inflammatory condition of the blood vessels in the extremities caused by smoking (FIGURE 4-40). Tobacco, particularly

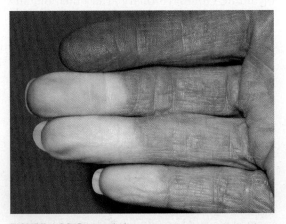

FIGURE 4-39 Raynaud phenomenon.
© Twinschoice/iStock/Getty Images.

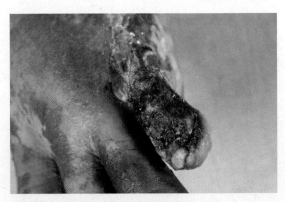

FIGURE 4-40 Thromboangiitis obliterans.
© Medicimage/Visuals Unlimited, Inc.

TABLE 4-7	Comparison of Venous and Arterial Thrombi	
Manifestation	**Venous thrombus**	**Arterial thrombus**
Pulse	Present	Weak or absent
Skin color	Erythema	Cyanosis/pallor
Skin temperature	Warm	Cool
Edema	Present	Minimal or absent

Venous thrombus

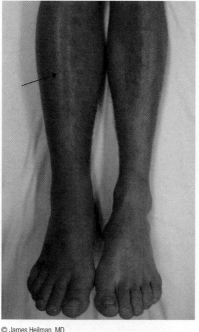

© James Heilman, MD.

Arterial thrombus

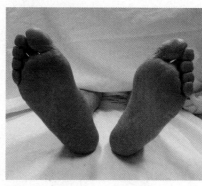

© James Heilman, MD.

Venous thrombus and arterial thrombus images © James Heilman, MD.
Reproduced from Story, L. (2017). *Pathophysiology: A practical approach* (3rd ed.). Burlington, MA: Jones & Bartlett Learning.

homemade cigarettes using raw tobacco, causes inflammation in the vessel lumen with thrombus formation. Smoking cigars or marijuana and chewing tobacco have also been implicated in the development of Buerger disease. The incidence is more prevalent in men (up to 90%) than women (up to 30%), and the onset is around 40 years old. Clinical manifestations include ischemic pain in the distal vessels, particularly in the toes and fingers. As time progresses, proximal arteries are affected and become occluded. Usually more than one extremity is affected. Often phlebitis with nodules along an affected vein are present. Patients can have pale extremities when exposed to cold as in Raynaud disease. The extremities can develop ulcerations and gangrene from the ischemia. Diagnosis is predominantly based on history of smoking, younger age, and clinical presentation. Biopsy is only necessary in unusual presentations, but it is the only way to confirm a diagnosis. Discontinuation of all forms of tobacco use is necessary to stop the progression of the disease and significantly reduce pain. Other treatments provide symptom relief and can include vasodilators, spinal cord stimulation, and sympathectomy.

Thrombi and Emboli

A thrombus is a blood clot that consists of platelets, fibrin, erythrocytes, and leukocytes. Such clots can form anywhere in the circulatory system (**TABLE 4-7**). Three conditions—endothelial injury, sluggish blood flow, and increased coagulopathy (collectively referred to as *Virchow triad*)—promote thrombus formation (**FIGURE 4-41**). When a vessel wall is injured, the endothelial damage attracts platelets and inflammatory mediators to the site, thereby stimulating clot formation. Stagnant blood flow allows platelets and clotting factors

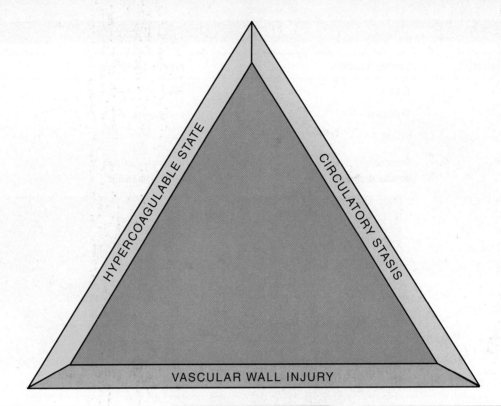

FIGURE 4-41 Virchow triad.

to accumulate and adhere to the vessel wall. Hypercoagulopathy states promote clot formation inappropriately. (See chapter 3 for a discussion of hematopoietic function.)

The consequences of thrombus formation may include occlusion of a blood vessel or embolus development. An embolus occurs when a portion or all of the thrombus breaks loose and travels through the circulatory system, eventually becoming embedded in a smaller vessel. In addition to thrombi, any other bodies (e.g., air, fat, tissue, bacteria, amniotic fluid, tumor cells, and foreign substances) traveling through the circulatory system can become emboli.

Emboli that originate in the venous circulation, such as with deep vein thrombus, travel to the right side of the heart and then on to the pulmonary circulation, creating a pulmonary embolism (**FIGURE 4-42**). Superficial venous thrombosis can extend into the deeper veins and lead to pulmonary embolism. Venous thrombi

are more common than arterial thrombi due to the presence of valves and a lower pressure blood-flow environment. Most emboli in the arterial system originate in the left side of the heart and travel to other organs such as the brain and heart, causing an infarction.

Clinical Manifestations

Clinical manifestations of thrombi and emboli depend on whether they are arterial or venous as well as their location (Table 4-7). Many patients with deep vein thrombosis are asymptomatic. When manifestations are present, they include pain, edema (usually unilateral), warmth, erythema, and possibly dilated veins. Arterial thrombi can lead to ischemia of varying degrees. Manifestations of arterial thrombi will include decreased pulse and cyanosis/pallor, and edema is minimal to absent. Critical obstruction will be manifested as the six *P*s (see *Peripheral Artery Disease* section).

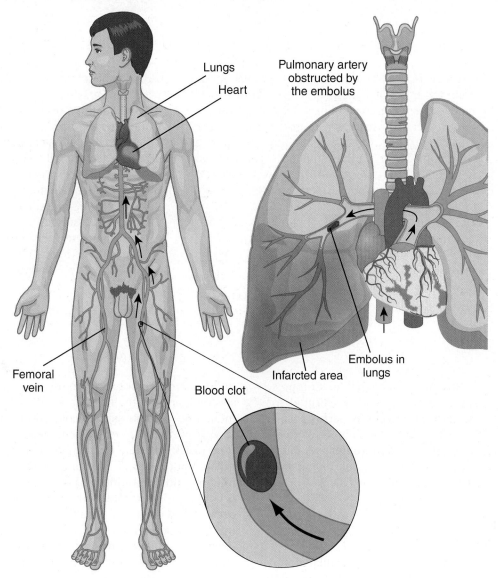

Lungs

Heart

Pulmonary artery
obstructed by
the embolus

Femoral
vein

Blood clot

Infarcted area

Embolus in
lungs

FIGURE 4-42 Pulmonary embolism.

Diagnosis and Treatment

Diagnostic procedures will initially include Doppler ultrasound. Photoplethysmography is a noninvasive test that involves the use of an optical technique (e.g., infrared light) to measure blood flow. Other noninvasive tests can include arterial or venous angiography (CT or MRI). If there is critical ischemia, evaluation can be done with a catheter-based arteriogram or in a surgical suite.

Treatment of thrombi and emboli centers on prevention. Venous emboli require anticoagulation urgently during the first 10 days, which is the most likely time for development of recurrent thrombi. Then, patients usually require anywhere from 3 to 12 months of continuing anticoagulation, and some patients are on anticoagulation indefinitely.

Choice of anticoagulation (e.g., low molecular weight heparin, factor Xa inhibitors) are weighed against the risks of bleeding. Other therapies can include the insertion of an intravenous catheter filter or direct administration of thrombolytics into the blood clot or thrombus removal (e.g., extraction, thrombectomy). When the patient has received anticoagulation, nonpharmacologic therapy can commence and includes increasing mobility, hydration, antiembolism hosiery, and sequential compression devices. These measures are the key to preventing thrombus formation. Arterial thrombi treatment includes anticoagulation, thrombolysis, and embolectomy. However, emergency revascularization is warranted in those with limb-threatening ischemia, which can occur within 4 hours. An amputation is indicated

BOX 4-5 Application to Practice

Compare the following two scenarios.

Scenario 1: Mr. Fernandez is a 62-year-old man who comes into the clinic complaining of left lower leg swelling that started 5 days ago. He says the leg hurts but mainly when he walks and does not get better after rest. He denies any trauma or fever. He returned from an international trip 2 days before the swelling started. He is healthy except for hypertension, which is well controlled with a daily thiazide diuretic.

Scenario 2: Mr. Kraft is a 65-year-old man who comes in complaining of lower leg pain that he has had for the past 3 months. He says both his legs cramp up in his calves when walking. He sits down to rest and the cramps go away. He denies any trauma or fever. He has smoked 1 pack of cigarettes a day for the past 35 years. He has type 2 diabetes for which he takes metformin twice a day.

Answer the following questions based on these two scenarios:

1. In which scenario are the history findings consistent with a venous disorder and which is consistent with an arterial disorder?
2. What are the most likely venous and arterial disorder diagnoses?
3. Describe the pathogenesis of these venous and arterial disorders.
4. What would be expected physical examination findings with a venous disorder and which with an arterial disorder?
5. Which diagnostic tests and treatment are indicated for a venous disorder? For an arterial disorder?

---

when the extremity is not viable. Compression therapy is generally contraindicated for patients with arterial disease as perfusion can worsen. Once the patient is stable and treatment has been initiated, a thorough evaluation of the etiology for the thrombus or embolus should then become the focus.

Venous Disorders

Varicose Veins

Varicose veins or varicosities, are dilated, tortuous, engorged veins (3 mm), that develop because of improper venous valve function (FIGURE 4-43). Telangiectasias (< 1 mm) and reticular veins (1–3 mm) describe the dilation of smaller veins that can develop from venous dysfunction. The enlarged veins are most commonly found in the legs, but they can also occur in the esophagus (esophageal varices), the rectum (hemorrhoids), and the vulva (usually during pregnancy). Increased venous pressure and blood pooling cause the veins to enlarge, stretching the valves. The valves become incompetent, blood flow is reversed, and venous pressure and distention are further increased. Venous pressure that is prolonged and persistent results in another venous disorder known as **chronic venous insufficiency**. The increased venous pressure causes the capillary pressure to increase, causing fluid and pigment to leak out, leading to edema and skin discoloration. The edema is usually pitting; it can be in the ankle area or extend to the knees and, in severe cases, the thighs. As a result, stasis pigmentation (brown skin discoloration referred to as *hemosiderin stains*), subcutaneous induration (thick, hardened skin), dermatitis (skin inflammation), and thrombophlebitis (vein inflammation resulting from a thrombus) can occur. The pressure caused by the edema can decrease circulation, resulting in metabolic needs not being met. Failure to meet cellular oxygen and nutrient needs can lead to necrosis and **venous stasis ulcers** (FIGURE 4-44).

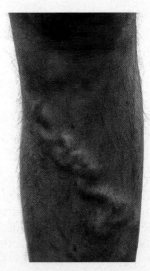

FIGURE 4-43 Varicose vein.
© Audie/Shutterstock.

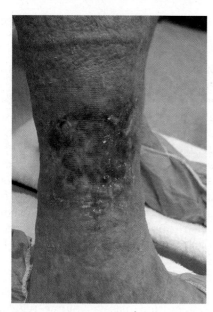

FIGURE 4-44 Venous leg ulcer.

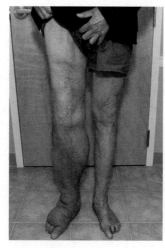

FIGURE 4-45 Lymphedema.
© Anthony Ricci/ShutterStock.

The following factors increase a person's risk for developing varicosities:

- Genetic predisposition
- Pregnancy (lower extremity and vulvar)
- Obesity
- Prolonged sitting or standing
- Alcohol abuse and liver disorders (esophageal varices)
- Constipation (hemorrhoids)

Clinical Manifestations

Varicose veins may be asymptomatic or are usually minor and include the following signs and symptoms: irregular, purplish, and bulging veins, edema, and fatigue as well as aching, numbness, and tingling in the legs. Manifestations may worsen with development of chronic venous insufficiency, which results in shiny, pigmented, hairless skin on the legs and feet, as well as ulcer formation. The telangiectasia and reticular veins that appear like a web of red and blue veins are commonly called *spider veins*.

Diagnosis and Treatment

Diagnosis of varicosities is usually accomplished through visualization during physical examination. Additional tests may initially include a duplex Doppler ultrasound. Photoplethysmography and venogram are other diagnostic tests. Treatment ranges from conservative to invasive and includes the following measures:

- Rest with the affected leg elevated
- Compression stockings
- Avoiding prolonged standing or sitting

- Exercise
- Sclerotherapy (injection of a sclerosing agent that produces fibrosis inside the vessel)
- Surgical removal
- Endovenous ablation (use of radiofrequency or laser energy to cauterize the vein)

Other venous varicosities (esophageal) manifestations and treatment are discussed in chapter 9.

Lymphedema

Lymphedema refers to swelling, usually in the arms and legs, because of lymph obstruction (**FIGURE 4-45**). This swelling can occur on its own (primary) or because of another disease or condition (secondary). Primary lymphedema is rare and related to a congenital absence or decreased number of lymphatics. Secondary lymphedema is usually related to one of the following events:

- Surgery (when lymph nodes and lymph vessels are removed or severed, as with a mastectomy)
- Radiation (causes scarring and inflammation of lymph nodes or lymph vessels, restricting the flow of lymph fluid)
- Cancer (occludes lymphatic vessels)
- Infection (can infiltrate lymph vessels and lymph nodes, restricting the flow of lymph fluid)
- Injury (damages lymph nodes or lymph vessels)

Clinical Manifestations

Clinical manifestations may not appear for months to years before edema and skin changes are evident. Patients complain of heaviness in their legs. Edema is usually pitting and improves with limb elevation. The edema may be unilateral or bilateral, and it usually occurs in the extremities. As the disorder progresses, elevation becomes ineffective in reduction of edema, and pitting is not as pronounced as the underlying tissue becomes fibrotic and fatty. Later stages include skin changes such as hyperpigmentation, ulceration, and thickening (referred to as *brawny edema*). The skin begins to appear thick and rough like elephant skin (elephantiasis). Lymphedema and chronic venous insufficiency may have similar presentations and often coexist.

Diagnosis and Treatment

Diagnostic procedures consist of a physical examination, MRI, CT, Doppler ultrasound, and nuclear imaging. Diagnostic testing is geared toward looking for a cause (e.g., neoplasm). Treatment of lymphedema includes the following measures:

- Sequential compression devices
- Compression stockings
- Exercise
- Massage therapy (complex decongestive physiotherapy)
- Antibiotics (to treat existing infections)
- Benzopyrone agents (to increase lymphatic flow)
- Diuretics (to remove excess fluid as it returns to the circulatory system)
- Surgery (to remove excess skin)

Conditions Resulting in Decreased Cardiac Output and Altered Perfusion

Hypertension

Hypertension is a prolonged elevation in blood pressure. It is one of the most prevalent chronic health conditions in the United States, affecting 45.6% of U.S. adults (AHA, 2017); hypertension is prevalent worldwide. Hypertension is the leading risk factor for cardiovascular disease (e.g., coronary artery disease, myocardial infarction, heart failure, and stroke). The incidence of hypertension in U.S. youth age 12–19 years is 4%, which is a decline from previous statistics (CDC, 2018). The young with hypertension are more likely to be obese. Cardiovascular risk (e.g., hypertension, obesity, and diabetes) in the young often continues into adulthood. In adults and the young, hypertension is higher in non-Hispanic Blacks

and Hispanics in comparison to non-Hispanic Whites. Men and boys have a higher incidence; however, the incidence in women after menopause (e.g., around 55 years old) is similar to men.

Determinants of blood pressure are cardiac output (i.e., HR × SV) and systemic vascular resistance (see Figure 4-11). These variables will change in an attempt to maintain a blood pressure adequate to perfuse tissues. Changes in any of these variables, whether transient or sustained, can result in an increase in blood pressure. In hypertension, arterial systemic vasoconstriction is sustained. The sustained vasoconstriction occurs due to a complex interaction between dysfunctional cardiovascular and renal systems, specifically the sympathetic nervous system, renin–angiotensin–aldosterone system, and plasma volume regulation. These systems become dysfunctional as a result of polygenic (i.e., multiple genetic variants) and epigenetic abnormalities as well as environmental factors including obesity and diet. Over 100 genes are involved in blood pressure regulation.

In hypertension, the cardiovascular system dysfunction includes SNS overreactivity resulting in an increased heart rate and vasoconstriction (**FIGURE 4-46**). The SNS overreactivity is due to catecholamine increases and/or catecholamine receptor sensitivity. Vascular changes such as remodeling and increased insulin resistance occur as a response to the SNS overreactivity, but, in turn, these changes further stimulate the SNS. Vascular remodeling refers to changes in lumen size due to inflammation, apoptosis, and fibrosis, which causes an increase in resistance. The vascular changes also include endothelial dysfunction with imbalances in nitric oxide (vasodilator) and endothelin (vasoconstrictor). Insulin is a hormone that can have a protective or detrimental effect on the vascular system. Protective influences include such responses as vasodilation and anti-inflammatory actions. Detrimental effects include vasoconstriction, proinflammatory effects, and Na^+ retention. These insulin effects are altered in hypertension.

In the renal system, the RAAS is also overreactive. This overreactivity and a decreased renal perfusion from the SNS effects lead to renin release. Renin release causes angiotensin II production, which is a powerful vasoconstrictor. Na^+ and water are reabsorbed. Aldosterone is released, which further promotes Na^+ and water retention (Figure 4-12). Overall, blood volume increases. The increased volume

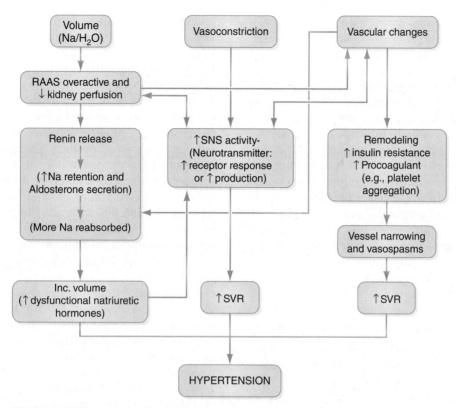

FIGURE 4-46 Development of hypertension.

stimulates the release of natriuretic hormones that normally act to reduce Na^+ retention and promote water excretion while causing vasodilation. These natriuretic hormones, however, are dysfunctional in hypertension, leading to worsening of vasoconstriction. The RAAS dysfunction also causes vascular changes. In addition to the dysfunction described, several risk factors cause or exacerbate hypertension.

The risk factors for developing hypertension include the following:

- **Age:** Vessel compliance decreases with aging.
- **Race:** Hypertension is more prevalent in Blacks, and the possible reasons include higher incidence of low birthweight infants (possible impaired renal growth), less nocturnal blood pressure decline, diet higher in sodium and low in potassium, and higher genetic susceptibility
- **Family history:** Genetic factors.
- **Overweight or obesity:** Increased RAAS and SNS activity, inflammation, insulin resistance, endothelial dysfunction, and vascular remodeling. Adipokines (cytokines released by adipose tissue) are changed with obesity and may cause vascular dysfunction.
- **Physical inactivity:** Increases heart rate, which increases cardiac workload;

increased insulin resistance; and possible vascular and endothelial dysfunction.
- **Tobacco use:** Nicotine immediately raises blood pressure temporarily, and the chemicals in tobacco can cause vascular dysfunction.
- **High-sodium diet:** Too much sodium causes fluid retention, which increases blood pressure. Some patients are salt sensitive while for others salt intake does not have as much of an influence on blood pressure. There are no practical tests to determine who falls into which category.
- **Low-potassium, -calcium, and -magnesium diet:** These elements help balance the amount of sodium in cells; without enough, too much sodium accumulates in the blood.
- **High vitamin D intake:** This factor has an uncertain effect, though vitamin D may affect the RAAS.
- **Excessive alcohol consumption:** Over time, heavy drinking—that is, more than two to three drinks in one sitting—can cause hypertension via several mechanisms such as SNS and RAAS dysfunction.
- **Stress:** High levels of stress can lead to a temporary, but dramatic, increase in blood pressure.

Hypertension is divided into two major forms—primary and secondary. In most hypertension cases (95%) in adults, there is no identifiable cause. This type of hypertension, called *primary hypertension* or *essential hypertension*, tends to develop gradually over many years. The other cases of hypertension (5%) are caused by an underlying condition. This type of hypertension, called *secondary hypertension*, tends to appear suddenly or manifests as stable blood pressure that becomes labile. In secondary hypertension, blood pressure levels are higher than in primary hypertension. Secondary hypertension tends to be resistant to antihypertensive agents in recommended doses and with multiple agents. Those patients with secondary hypertension tend to be younger (e.g., < 30), may not be obese, or have a family history. A variety of conditions and medications can lead to secondary hypertension, such as:

- Renal disease (e.g., renal artery stenosis, polycystic kidney disease, and diabetic nephropathy)
- Adrenal gland disorders (e.g., primary aldosteronism, pheochromocytoma)
- Sleep apnea syndrome
- Certain congenital heart defects (e.g., coarctation of the aorta)
- Endocrine disorders (e.g., Cushing syndrome, hypothyroidism, hyperparathyroidism)
- Certain medications (e.g., birth control pills, hormone replacement therapy, antihistamines, decongestants, and glucocorticoid steroids)
- Illegal drugs (e.g., cocaine and amphetamines)

Occasionally, hypertension is classified as isolated systolic hypertension or isolated diastolic hypertension, depending on which measurement is elevated. Often, elderly persons have higher systolic readings and lower diastolic readings (i.e., increased pulse pressure) because of aging changes (e.g., decreased vascular compliance). Isolated systolic hypertension with an increased pulse pressure is associated with an increased risk for cardiovascular diseases (e.g., stroke, MI, and renal dysfunction). Isolated diastolic hypertension is associated with increased risk for cardiovascular events in younger people.

Hypertension can also occur during pregnancy, posing a serious health threat as one of the top causes of maternal death. A spectrum of hypertension disorders can occur in pregnancy, including gestational hypertension and preeclampsia/eclampsia. **Gestational hypertension** (i.e., ≥ 140 mmHg systolic or ≥ 90 mmHg diastolic) is defined as the onset of hypertension at ≥ 20 weeks with resolution 12 weeks after birth. If the hypertension does not resolve, the diagnosis becomes chronic hypertension. If proteinuria is present with gestational hypertension, then the diagnosis is **preeclampsia** (formerly known as toxemia). If there is no proteinuria, other diagnostic criteria for preeclampsia can include thrombocytopenia (< 100,000 cells/μL), impaired liver function tests, renal insufficiency (elevated serum creatinine), pulmonary edema, or cerebral/visual disorders. Preeclampsia can be further classified as severe when there are several diagnostic criteria present and/or a systolic blood pressure that is ≥ 160 mmHg and/or a diastolic that is ≥ 90 mmHg. The diagnosis of preeclampsia with grand mal seizures is termed **eclampsia**. A woman may have had hypertension prior to pregnancy and develop what is termed *superimposed preeclampsia/eclampsia*.

Multiple factors increase the risk for developing preeclampsia; some of these include hypertension, renal disease, diabetes mellitus (type 1 or 2), multiple fetuses, maternal age younger than 18 years or older than 35 years, obesity, and autoimmune disorders (e.g., SLE). Preeclampsia develops as a result of placental vascular alterations that cause placental decreased perfusion, hypoxia, and ischemia. The maternal inflammatory reaction is activated in response to the placental alterations with resulting endothelial dysfunction, systemic inflammation, and a thrombotic state. The kidneys and liver are particularly affected by the placental hypoperfusion, so alterations are included in the diagnostic criteria (e.g., increased creatinine, proteinuria, and abnormal liver function tests). The cardiovascular system and brain are also damaged by the endothelial dysfunction, causing fluid shifts and vasospasm (e.g., pulmonary edema, headaches). The hematologic changes occur as a result of fluid shifts and the inflammatory response (e.g., thrombocytopenia, increased prothrombin time [PT] or partial thromboplastin time [PTT]). Poor fetal development and placental abruption may result.

Management of hypertension in pregnancy focuses on early identification and frequent evaluation for complications such as preeclampsia (e.g., liver enzymes, proteinuria). Fetal well-being will be monitored regularly with ultrasounds and nonstress tests.

Early delivery, such as at 37–38 weeks, may be necessary. Preeclampsia is managed similarly with frequent evaluation and early delivery. Prevention and nonpharmacologic measures are geared toward protecting the mother and the fetus. If preeclampsia has severe features or eclampsia is present, treatment measures include bed rest and magnesium sulfate (to prevent and treat seizures). Severe hypertension can be managed with hydralazine, labetalol, or nifedipine.

Clinical Manifestations

Hypertension, particularly primary hypertension, is called the *silent killer* because many people do not have symptoms. Often by the time symptoms become evident, the hypertension is advanced, or the blood pressure is remarkably high. When present, clinical manifestations include fatigue, headache, malaise, and dizziness.

During a history and physical examination, clinical manifestations may reveal target end-organ damage (e.g., left ventricular hypertrophy, retinal hemorrhages). The higher the blood pressure and the longer it goes uncontrolled, the greater the damage. Uncontrolled high blood pressure can lead to numerous target end-organ complications:

- **Cardiovascular system**: Atherosclerosis, left ventricle hypertrophy, ischemia, infarction, aneurysms, heart failure, sudden death, and peripheral artery diseases
- **Kidneys**: Decreased glomerular filtration rate, glomerulosclerosis, and renal failure
- **Brain**: Transient ischemic attacks, stroke, and aneurysm
- **Eyes**: Exudate, hemorrhage, retinopathy, and vision loss

Hypertension can be part of a cluster of disorders known as metabolic syndrome that is associated with increased cardiovascular risks. Other components of the cluster include increased waist circumference, high triglycerides, low HDL, impaired fasting glucose, and insulin resistance.

Diagnosis and Treatment

Diagnosis of hypertension is based on accurate measurement of blood pressure and repeated high readings (i.e., during more than two visits with or without out-of-office confirmation). The values defining hypertension vary per national guidelines and organizations. The Joint National Committee on Prevention, Detection, Evaluation, and Treatment of High Blood Pressure (JNC 8) (James et al., 2014) defines hypertension as a systolic $\geq$ 140 mmHg and/or diastolic $\geq$ 90 mmHg. Therapeutic target goals are $\leq$ 150/90 mmHg for those over 60 years of age and goals for all others is $\leq$ 140/90 mmHg. In 2017, the American Heart Association and the American College of Cardiology (AHA/ACC) redefined hypertension as systolic $\geq$ 130 mmHg and/or diastolic $\geq$80 mmHg. Diagnostic criteria are dependent on which guideline is used; however, clinical judgment remains paramount in choosing a course of action (e.g., risk of cardiovascular disease, therapy risk/benefits). Additionally, target goal recommendations from the American Diabetes Association and the National Kidney Foundation vary slightly in their therapeutic target goals for those with diabetes and chronic kidney disease (e.g., < 140/80 mmHg).

Accuracy of blood pressure measurement is important in diagnosis. The following should be done while measuring the blood pressure:

- Seat the patient in a chair with feet on floor and back supported for a few minutes.
- The patient should avoid caffeine, exercise, and smoking 30 minutes prior to measurement.
- Do not engage the patient in conversation during measurement.
- Support the arm at the right atrium level (i.e., sternum midpoint).
- Use calibrated sphygmomanometer with appropriate cuff size (e.g., encircles 80% of the arm).
- Repeat measures should be separated minimally by 1 minute.

If readings are high in the office or the patient describes normal levels outside the office, a patient may have "white coat hypertension." In these circumstances, home measurement or ambulatory monitoring should be conducted. The cutoff for hypertension with home/ambulatory monitoring varies again based on guidelines interpreted but is generally less than clinical measurements (e.g., $\geq$ 125/75 mmHg). Normally, the blood pressure dips by 10% at night, and the patient is diagnosed with nocturnal hypertension if dipping does not occur. Cardiovascular risk may be higher with nocturnal hypertension than in those whose pressure dips at night.

Hypertension can be diagnosed at initial screening (i.e., one reading) if blood pressure is high (e.g., systolic $\geq$ 160 mmHg and/or diastolic

≥ 100 mmHg) with target end-organ damage, or blood pressure is systolic ≥ 180 mmHg and/or diastolic ≥ 120 mmHg. **Hypertensive urgency**, which can be at an initial visit or subsequent encounters, is defined as a blood pressure systolic ≥ 180 and/or diastolic ≥120 mmHg in a patient who is relatively asymptomatic (e.g., mild headache) and there is no evidence of acute target end-organ damage (e.g., ischemia). A **hypertensive emergency** (i.e., malignant hypertension) is defined as the same blood pressure as an urgency but the patient is symptomatic and/or with evidence of acute/ongoing target organ damage.

In addition to blood pressure measurement, diagnostic evaluation will center on identifying a cause and determining the presence of any complications and cardiovascular risks. Diagnostic testing for those newly diagnosed will include an EKG and laboratory tests (e.g., urinalysis, CBC, lipid panel, and chemistry panel for glucose, calcium, creatinine, potassium, and thyroid profile). Other exams are

dependent on presence or suspicion of other disorders such as an albumin creatinine ratio for chronic kidney disease or an echocardiogram for heart failure. In primary hypertension, these results may all be normal.

The prognosis for persons with hypertension depends on treating any underlying causes and maintaining blood pressure control. Early detection and treatment are crucial to prevent or minimize cardiovascular risks and complications. Treatment of hypertension is based on ACC/AHA 2017 standards (**FIGURE 4-47**) with recognition that other guidelines (JNC 8 standards) exist. Adhering to a protocol will increase the likelihood of successful blood pressure control. Lifestyle changes are the mainstay of prevention and treatment. These changes can be implemented in those individuals who have or are at risk for developing hypertension. Dietary changes are the cornerstone to these lifestyle changes and include adequate potassium intake and the Dietary Approaches to Stop Hypertension (DASH) diet

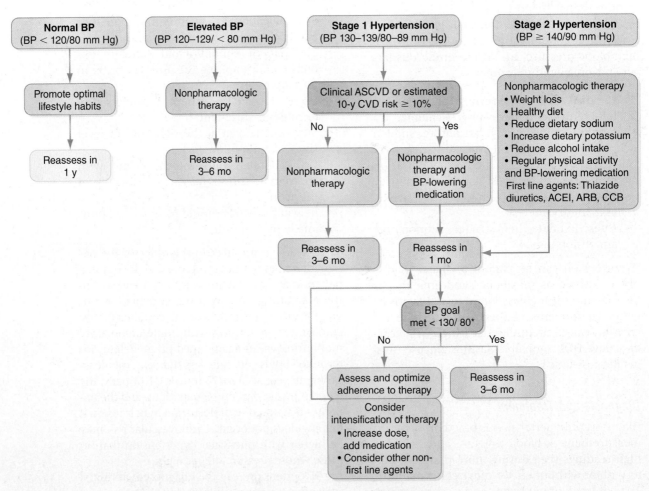

FIGURE 4-47 Blood pressure threshold and recommendations for treatment and follow-up.
ASCVD = arteriosclerotic cardiovascular disease

(NIH, 2015). The research-driven DASH diet includes the following recommendations:

- Limiting saturated fat, cholesterol, total fat, and salt
- Focusing on fruits, vegetables, and fat-free or low-fat dairy products
- Increasing whole grains, fish, poultry, beans, seeds, and nuts
- Minimizing sweets, added sugar and sugary beverages, and red meats

Limiting salt consumption to 2,300 mg (less than a teaspoon) per day has been shown to lower blood pressure. Further restricting salt intake to 1,500 mg per day can lower blood pressure to an even greater extent. The 1,500 mg restriction is advised for individuals diagnosed with hypertension, diabetes, and chronic kidney disease as well as Blacks, middle-aged individuals, and older adults. Following these guidelines, particularly the salt recommendations, can significantly decrease the risk for developing hypertension.

Other lifestyle changes that can help prevent or treat hypertension include being active, maintaining a healthy weight, smoking cessation, stress management, and alcohol consumption (if used) in moderation. Additionally, individuals should have their blood pressure measured regularly with a home monitor and by healthcare professionals. These readings should be documented in a blood pressure journal (including the blood pressure reading, date, time of day, activities just before the reading, and any symptoms) and brought to visits with the healthcare provider. Home care monitoring devices should be periodically brought into the office to compare measurements.

Numerous pharmacologic agents are used to treat hypertension. Based on ACC/AHA 2017 guidelines, the initial choice of therapy should be a thiazide or thiazide-type diuretic, an angiotensin-converting enzyme inhibitor (ACEI) or an angiotensin receptor blocker (ARB) or a calcium channel blocker. These pharmacologic

agents can be prescribed either as a single agent or in combination depending on blood pressure level and goal. ACEI, ARB, and direct renin inhibitors, however, should never be administered together due to potential serious harm. Other antihypertensive pharmacotherapeutic categories include diuretics (e.g., loop, potassium sparing), beta blockers (e.g., cardioselective, alpha/beta receptor combined), alpha-1 blockers, centrally acting drugs, and direct vasodilators (i.e., direct renin inhibitors).

Shock

Shock is a clinical syndrome resulting from inadequate tissue and organ oxygenation because of decreased perfusion, decreased oxygen delivery, increased oxygen use, or abnormal oxygen use. Shock occurs due to a problem with the heart (pump), the vasculature (vessel), or volume, or a combination. Any changes in the variables that affect blood pressure (e.g., tissue perfusion), which are determined by cardiac output (i.e., stroke volume × heart rate) and systemic vascular resistance, can cause shock. Shock can be classified into three categories—distributive, cardiogenic, and hypovolemic—based on its precipitating factors. Distributive shock is also known as *vasogenic* (e.g., neurogenic, septic, and anaphylactic), and examples of hypovolemic shock include hemorrhagic shock and burn shock. Septic shock is the most common type of shock and is the leading cause of death in the intensive care unit, while hemorrhagic shock is the most common type of shock in trauma patients. Some patients have more than one type of shock.

Shock progresses through three stages that are common to all types of shock—compensatory (i.e., pre-shock), progressive (i.e., decompensated), and irreversible (i.e., refractory). **Compensatory** mechanisms are bodily responses that become activated when arterial pressure and tissue perfusion decrease and that represent an effort to maintain cardiac and cerebral function. Early signs of decreased perfusion may be simply tachycardia, modest changes in blood pressure (low or high), and an elevated lactate level due to anaerobic metabolism. These compensatory mechanisms include the activation of the SNS and RAAS. The pituitary and adrenal medulla release hormones in response to decreased perfusion. The compensatory mechanism responses overlap and, while described separately, work together to maintain heart and brain function. Reversal is possible at this stage with restoration of tissue and organ oxygenation. In general, cardiac output is diminished and a compensatory increase in systemic vascular resistance is present with hypovolemic and cardiogenic shock (i.e., there are volume and pump issues). In distributive shock (i.e., there is a vessel issue), systemic vascular resistance is diminished with a compensatory increase in cardiac output.

The **progressive** stage of shock begins when these compensatory mechanisms fail to maintain cardiac output. Tissues continue becoming hypoxic, lactic acid continues to build up, and metabolic acidosis develops. This acidotic state further impairs cardiac functioning, causing sluggish blood flow and increasing the risk for disseminated intravascular coagulation. **Irreversible** end-organ damage occurs as the shock progresses, leading to respiratory and cardiac failure (**FIGURE 4-48**).

In **distributive shock**, vasodilation causes the inappropriate distribution of plasma/blood (volume) from the vasculature into the tissue. The primary problem, therefore, is with the vasculature, while in general, the volume is adequate and the pump is unaffected. The inappropriate volume distribution ultimately leads to poor perfusion as with other types of shock.

Three types of distributive shock are distinguished—neurogenic, septic, and anaphylactic. **Neurogenic shock** occurs as a result of central nervous system injury (e.g., severe brain injury, thoracic spinal cord level 6 or higher/cervical cord injuries). Below the level of the injury (e.g., below T6), sympathetic tone is impaired or blocked, resulting in a loss of sympathetic tone in vascular smooth muscle and massive vasodilation. The vasodilation causes blood to pool in the venous system, leading to decreased venous return, cardiac output, and blood pressure. The compensatory mechanisms of tachycardia and vasoconstriction from the SNS are not present in response to hypotension. However, the parasympathetic response remains intact and is unopposed, so the patient will have bradycardia. In neurogenic shock, the patient will have a triad of bradycardia, vasodilation, and hypotension.

Learning Points

Spinal Shock

Spinal shock and neurogenic shock are two different disorders although both can be due to spinal cord injury and can occur together. Spinal shock is not considered a true shock but rather is an altered physiologic state in response to spinal cord injury (the cord is shocked by injury). This causes the loss of motor and sensory function such as flaccid paralysis, anesthesia, or loss of reflexes below the level of injury. The manifestations usually occur immediately after the injury. Recovery can occur in hours to weeks.

In **septic shock**, an organism's endotoxin or exotoxins activate an immune reaction. Septic shock is on a continuum that starts off with a systemic inflammatory immune response syndrome (SIRS). SIRS can be a response to any inflammatory or clinical insult that is infectious or noninfectious (e.g., pancreatitis, ARDS). SIRS can progress to septicemia (blood infection), then sepsis (systemic response to infection), and at the end of the continuum is septic shock. In comparison to neurogenic shock, the inappropriate distribution of volume in septic shock is a result of inflammatory mediators causing increased capillary permeability, capillary pooling, and fluid shifts from the vascular compartment to the tissue. This inappropriate distribution of volume leads to a falling cardiac output and multiple organ dysfunction syndrome (MODS). Common causes of septic shock are bacterial species, specifically gram-negative bacteria (e.g., *Escherichia coli*, *Pseudomonas aeruginosa*, *Klebsiella*, *Acinetobacter*). Gram-positive bacteria (e.g., staphylococci, streptococci) infection causes sepsis but not necessarily shock in comparison to gram-negative infections. Other less frequent organisms are fungal (e.g., *Candida albicans*, *Candida glabrata*, *Aspergillus*), and these infections are more likely to progress from sepsis to shock. Viruses (e.g., *Cytomegalovirus*, influenza A and B) are organisms that can also cause shock.

Learning Points

SIRS Diagnostic Criteria

SIRS diagnostic criteria include two or more of the following findings: tachypnea (> 20/minute), tachycardia (> 90/minute), $PaCO_2$ of less than 32 mmHg, and temperature decrease ($< 38°C$) or increase ($> 38°C$) *and* a white blood cell count that is either low ($< 4,000$ cell/mm^3) or high ($> 12,000$ cell/mm^3) or higher than 10% bands.

Anaphylactic shock is a widespread, immediate systemic reaction resulting from a sudden release of mast cells and basophil mediators. Most causes of anaphylaxis are immune mediated with immunoglobulin E as the most likely type of response. Food (e.g., peanuts, shellfish, milk, eggs) is a common cause of anaphylaxis in children, while insect venom (e.g., wasps, bees), and medications (e.g., antibiotics) are the most likely immunoglobulin E–mediated anaphylactic triggers in adults. Other immunologic mechanisms can cause IgG mediated anaphylaxis. Non-immunologic agents can also cause anaphylaxis (i.e., they are anaphylactoid) where triggers such as radiocontrast agents directly activate mast cells

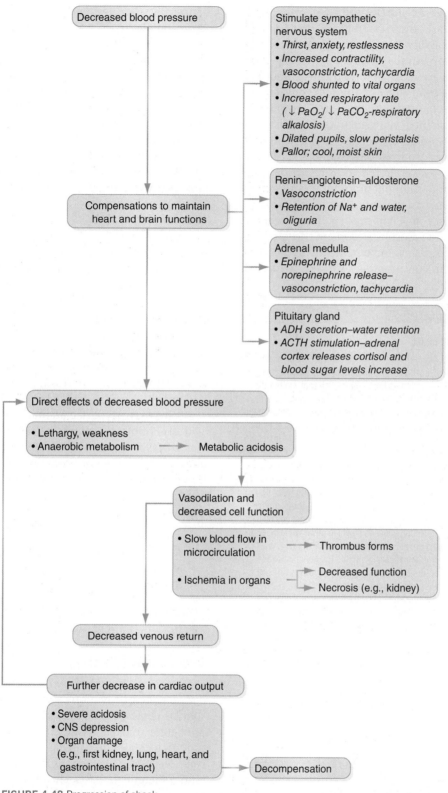

FIGURE 4-48 Progression of shock.

ACTH = adrenocorticotropic hormone

and basophils. Additionally, anaphylaxis causes can be idiopathic. Anaphylactic shock leads to a cascade of events similar to that of septic shock, except that the mediators differ. Bronchospasm and laryngeal edema occur that can impair respiratory status. Early detection of anaphylaxis is critical to prevent anaphylactic shock. (See chapter 2 for a discussion of immunity.)

Cardiogenic shock results when the pump fails. The heart cannot contract, fill, or eject, leading to an inability to maintain adequate cardiac output. A myocardial infarction (usually anterior wall) is the most common cause, and usually greater than 40% of the left ventricle has been affected. Cardiomyopathies, arrhythmias such as sustained ventricular tachycardia, and other intracardiac disorders such as a dissecting aorta can lead to cardiogenic shock. Noncoronary causes are referred to as *obstructive shock* and include tension pneumothorax, pulmonary embolism, and tamponade. As with other shock, compensatory mechanisms such as increased heart rate and vasoconstriction are triggered, but these mechanisms increase cardiac workload and oxygen consumption, further worsening

Learning Points

Lowering Salt Intake

Cutting back on salt intake can be challenging on many levels. First, eating large amounts of salt over time decreases taste sensation on the tongue, such that foods without it will lack flavor initially. Those taste buds will wake up again with a little time. Gradually decreasing salt intake may help with this transition. For instance, have patients start by not adding salt to food once it is prepared, and then begin changing how food is prepared.

Second, salt is used in many foods of convenience as a preservative. In today's fast-paced society, these foods have become commonplace and almost a necessity. Unfortunately, processed foods (e.g., canned food, boxed meals, frozen dinners, and sandwich meats) usually contain large amounts of salt. Additionally, salt is often added to meats to preserve them, even when those meats are already naturally high in salt (e.g., pork).

Third, the practice of eating outside the home in a wide range of restaurants has increased. Salt content is difficult to control when others are preparing the food.

Finally, salt is hidden in many seasonings and condiments. As people attempt to move away from salt, they may turn to these seasonings and condiments to enhance flavor—but these items may be just as bad as using salt. Seasonings that have *salt* in their name have salt in their contents (e.g., seasoning salt, garlic salt, and onion salt). Condiments such as hot sauce and mustard also have high salt content.

The following recommendations can help people cut back on salt and avoid foods with hidden salt content:

- Eat at home using fresh foods as much as possible.
- Attempt to purchase foods on the perimeter of the grocery store (where the fresh foods can be found) and avoid items in the center (where most of the processed foods can be found).
- Limit consumption of pork and cured meats.
- Use seasonings that are salt free or MSG free (e.g., garlic powder, onion powder).
- Read the labels of all products, paying attention to the sodium (salt) content and serving sizes.

Reproduced from Story, L. (2017). *Pathophysiology: A practical approach* (3rd ed.). Burlington, MA: Jones & Bartlett Learning.

contractility. Consequently, tissue and organ perfusion decreases, leading to MODS.

In **hypovolemic shock**, venous return declines because of intravascular volume losses that are hemorrhagic (e.g., penetrating trauma bleeding) or nonhemorrhagic (e.g., burns). In hemorrhagic hypovolemic shock, the patient loses blood; in nonhemorrhagic hypovolemic shock, he or she loses other fluids. In hypovolemic shock, preload drops, decreasing ventricular filling and stroke volume. As cardiac output falls, tissue and organ perfusion decreases.

Clinical Manifestations

Clinical manifestations of shock vary based on the stage, type, and cause of the shock. Ultimately, all manifestations reflect the impaired tissue perfusion and poor oxygenation. General manifestations include the following signs and symptoms: tachycardia (except neurogenic); hypotension; tachypnea with increased work of breathing; changes in level of consciousness such as restlessness, agitation, confusion; cold, clammy skin progressing to mottled skin and cyanosis; and decreased urine output (i.e., < 30 mL/hr). Hyperlactatemia and metabolic acidosis are often present in shock.

MODS is a complication of shock that starts during the progressive stage and can result in multiple organ failure and death. Clinical manifestations of MODS are multiple and system wide. Dysfunction and failure of these organs is discussed in corresponding chapters as listed next.

- Acute respiratory distress syndrome (chapter 5)
- Renal disease (chapter 7)
- Disseminated intravascular coagulation (chapter 3)
- Encephalopathy (chapter 11)

Diagnosis and Treatment

Diagnosis of shock is based on the underlying disorder (e.g., hemorrhage or hypovolemic shock), clinical findings, including hypotension or oliguria, and diagnostic exams. Diagnostic procedures for shock are varied but will often include basic diagnostic evaluations consisting of a CBC with differential, basic chemistry panels (e.g., blood glucose), renal and liver function tests, cardiac biomarker testing, natriuretic peptide testing, coagulation studies, D-dimer serum levels, and a chest X-ray. EKG, echocardiogram, ultrasounds, and CT scans are some other diagnostic tests. If infection is suspected then diagnostic testing may include cultures of blood culture, urine, and lungs.

BOX 4-6 Application to Practice

Mr. Jones, a 70-year-old professor, is 7 days post–laparoscopic cholecystectomy. He denies any pain at the surgical site, but he is complaining of fatigue, heart palpitations, and some shortness of breath. He says the palpitations started 2 days ago and last a few minutes.

He denies fever, chest pain, nausea, vomiting, and diaphoresis.

Past medical history: anterior wall MI 3 years prior.

Social history: drinks three to four glasses of liquor a day, which he has done for 20 years; quit smoking after MI 3 years ago.

Medications: metoprolol 50 mg once daily; simvastatin 40 mg once daily; aspirin 81 mg once daily. He forgets to take his aspirin often and misses a dose of other medications about once a week.

Allergies: no known drug allergies.

Physical examination: vital signs—temperature 97.5°F; pulse 118/minute and irregular; respirations 20/minute; blood pressure 126/74 mmHg.

General: alert and oriented.

Neck: no jugular vein distention, no bruits.

Cardiovascular system: irregular rhythm, no gallops or murmurs.

Lungs: bibasilar, fine crackles.

Skin: warm and dry with no edema, cyanosis.

Other: 12-lead EKG with evidence of anterior wall MI and atrial fibrillation with a ventricular rate of 118.

Answer the following questions:

1. What are possible reasons for Mr. Jones's new-onset atrial fibrillation?
2. Describe atrial fibrillation.
3. What are risks associated with atrial fibrillation?
4. What is Mr. Jones's CHA_2DS_2-VASc score? What are treatment recommendations based on this score?

Modified from Story, L. (2017). *Pathophysiology: A practical approach* (3rd ed.). Burlington, MA: Jones & Bartlett Learning.

Diagnostic Link

Point-of-Care Ultrasonography

The use of bedside ultrasonography allows for the rapid examination of many organs (e.g., heart, lung, abdomen) in order to identify a possible cause for shock. Ultrasonography is portable, relatively inexpensive, and there is no exposure to radiation. Ultrasonography can also be used as a guide to therapy (e.g., peritoneal drainage) and to determine the effectiveness of treatment (e.g., after pericardiocentesis). The key disadvantage of bedside ultrasonography is the decreased sensitivity in comparison to other definitive diagnostic modalities. As an example, an echocardiogram is preferred over a bedside sonogram if cardiac effusions are complex.

Prompt treatment is crucial for positive patient outcomes. Management of shock includes the identification and treatment of the underlying cause. Goals are to restore and maintain tissue perfusion. Rapid fluid resuscitation is the mainstay of therapy in shock. Crystalloids are preferred unless the shock is from hemorrhaging; then blood products are best. Treatment will include cardiovascular monitoring and respiratory maintenance with therapies such as oxygen or mechanical ventilation. Pharmacologic agents often used are vasopressors such as norepinephrine or dobutamine. Other pharmacologic agents are dependent on the type of shock and can include vasodilators, beta blockers, alpha agonists, phosphodiesterase inhibitors, steroids, antihistamines, and anticoagulants. Infections will be treated with antibiotics or antifungals depending on the organism. Patients may require an intra-aortic balloon pump, ventricular assist device, or extracorporeal membrane oxygenation. (See chapter 5 for more on pulmonary function.)

Learning Points

One-Hour Sepsis Bundle

The sepsis bundle, as other bundles, is a set evidenced-based practices that have been proven to improve outcomes when provided collectively (Resar et al., 2005). The Surviving Sepsis Campaign was started in 2002 by the Society of Critical Care Medicine and the European Society of Intensive Care Medicine. The sepsis bundle's latest update was 2018 (www.survivingsepsis.org). The 1-hour sepsis bundle begins once sepsis or septic shock elements are identified. The bundle consists of the following five steps:

1. Measure lactate level. Remeasure if initial lactate is > 2 mmol/L.
2. Obtain blood cultures prior to administration of antibiotics.
3. Administer broad-spectrum antibiotics.
4. Begin rapid administration of 30 mL/kg crystalloid for hypotension or lactate ≥ 4 mmol/L.
5. Apply vasopressors if the patient is hypotensive during or after fluid resuscitation to maintain mean arterial pressure ≥ 65 mmHg.

CHAPTER SUMMARY

The cardiovascular system is responsible for transporting the body's life fluids to maintain a delicate internal balance. This system has a reciprocal relationship with all the other systems—one in which problems in one system create problems in another system. Problems in the cardiovascular system are highly prevalent and most likely will be encountered in any setting. Understanding these issues is vital to provide appropriate care. Prevention of cardiovascular issues often includes lifestyle changes. Early identification and treatment of these conditions are crucial to improve outcomes.

REFERENCES AND RESOURCES

AAOS. (2004). *Paramedic: Anatomy and physiology*. Sudbury, MA: Jones and Bartlett Publishers.

American Heart Association (AHA). (2014). Dietary fats. Retrieved from https://www.heart.org/en/healthy-living /healthy-eating/eat-smart/fats/dietary-fats

American Heart Association (AHA). (2015). Prinzmetal's or prinzmetal angina, variant angina, or angina inversa. Retrieved from https://www.heart.org/en/health -topics/heart-attack/angina-chest-pain/prinzmetals-or -prinzmetal-angina-variant-angina-and-angina-inversa

American Heart Association (AHA). (2017, January 25). Heart disease and stroke statistics—2017 update: A report from the American Heart Association. *Circulation*. Epub ahead of print. Retrieved from https://www.ahajournals .org/doi/full/10.1161/CIR.0000000000000485

American Heart Association. (2017). Understanding blood pressure readings. Retrieved from https://www.heart.org /en/health-topics/high-blood-pressure/understanding -blood-pressure-readings

Arbustini, E., Narula, N., Tavazzi, L., Serio, A., Grasso, M. Favalli, V., . . . Narula, J. (2014). The MOGE(S) classification of cardiomyopathy for clinicians. *Journal of the American College of Cardiology, 64*(3), 304–318. https://doi .org/10.1016/j.jacc.2014.05.027

Baddour, L., Wilson, W., Bayoer, A., Fowler, V., Tleyjeh, I., . . . Taubert, K. (2015). Infective endocarditis in adults: Diagnosis, antimicrobial therapy, and management of complications: A scientific statement for healthcare professionals from the American Heart Association. *Circulation, 132,* 1435-1486. https://www.ahajournals.org/doi/full/10.1161/cir .0000000000000296

Baltimore, R. S., Gewitz, M., Baddour, L. M., Beerman, L. B., Jackson, M. A., Lockhart, P. B., . . . Willoughby, R. (2015). Infective endocarditis in childhood: A scientific statement from the American Heart Association [2015 update; originally published September 15, 2015]. *Circulation, 132,* 1487–1515. https://doi.org/10.1161/CIR.0000000000000298

Banga, S., & Chalfoun, N. T. (n.d.). Arrhythmias and antiarrhythmic drugs. In A. Elmoselhi (Ed.). *Cardiology: An integrated approach*. New York, NY: McGraw-Hill. Retrieved from http://accessmedicine.mhmedical.com.ezproxy.fiu .edu/content.aspx?bookid=2224&sectionid=171660848

Bejar, D., Colombo, P. C., Latif, F., & Yuzefpolskaya, M. (2015). Infiltrative cardiomyopathies. *Clinical Medicine Insights. Cardiology, 9*(Suppl 2), 29–38. http://doi.org/10.4137/CMC .S19706

Burke, M. A., Cook, S. A., Seidman, J. G., & Seidman, C. E. (2016). Clinical and mechanistic insights into the genetics of cardiomyopathy. *Journal of the American College of Cardiology, 68*(25). http://dx.doi.org/10.1016/j.jacc.2016.08.079

Centers for Disease Control and Prevention (CDC). (2015). Deaths: Final data for 2013. *National vital statistics report*. Retrieved from http://www.cdc.gov/nchs/data/nvsr /nvsr64/nvsr64_02.pdf

Centers for Disease Control and Prevention (CDC). (2016). High blood pressure. Retrieved from http://www.cdc .gov/bloodpressure/

Centers for Disease Control and Prevention (CDC). (2017). Cholesterol. Retrieved from https://www.cdc.gov/nchs /fastats/cholesterol.htm

Centers for Disease Control and Prevention (CDC). (2018). High blood pressure during childhood and adolescence. Retrieved from https://www.cdc.gov/bloodpressure/youth.htm

Centers for Disease Control and Prevention (CDC). (2019a). High cholesterol facts. Retrieved from https://www.cdc .gov/cholesterol/facts.htm

Centers for Disease Control and Prevention (CDC). (2019b). Congenital heart defects (CHDs). Retrieved from https:// www.cdc.gov/ncbddd/heartdefects/index.html

Chiras, D. (2013). *Human biology* (8th ed.). Burlington, MA: Jones & Bartlett Learning.

Crowley, L. V. (2016). *An introduction to human disease* (10th ed.). Burlington, MA: Jones & Bartlett Learning.

Elling, B., Elling, K., & Rothenberg, M. (2004). *Anatomy and physiology*. Sudbury, MA: Jones and Bartlett Publishers.

Farrow, W. (2010). Phlebolymphedema—a common underdiagnosed and undertreated problem in the wound care clinic. *Journal of the American College of Certified Wound Specialists, 2*(1), 14–23. Retrieved from https://www.ncbi .nlm.nih.gov/pubmed/24527138

Garcia, T. B., & Holtz, N. E. (2003). *Introduction to 12-lead ECG*. Sudbury, MA: Jones and Bartlett Publishers.

Gerhard-Herman, M. D., Gornik, H. L., Barrett, C., Barshes, N. R., Corriere, M. A., Drachman, D. E., . . . Walsh, M. E. (2016). 2016 AHA/ACC guideline on the management of patients with lower extremity peripheral artery disease: Executive summary: A report of the American College of Cardiology/American Heart Association Task Force on Clinical Practice Guidelines. *Circulation*, 135, e686–e725.

Grundy, S. M., Stone, M. J., Bailey, A. L., Beam, C., Bircher, K., Blumenthal, R. S. . . . Braun, L. T. (2018). 2018 AHA/ ACC/AACVPR/AAPA/ABC/ACPM/ADA/AGS/APhA/ ASPC/NLA/PCNA Guideline on the management of blood cholesterol: A Report of the American College of Cardiology/American Heart Association Task Force on Clinical Practice Guidelines. *Journal of the American*

College of Cardiology, November, 2018. 25709; doi:10.1016/j.jacc.2018.11.003

James, P. A., Oparil, S., Carter, B. L., Cushman, W. C., Dennison-Himmelfarb, C., Handler, J., . . . Ortiz, E. (2014). 2014 Evidence-based guidelines for the management of high blood pressure in adults: Report from the panel members appointed to the Eight Joint National Committee (JNC 8). *Journal of the American Medical Association, 311*(5), 507–520.

Jameson, J., Fauci, A. S., Kasper, D. L., Hauser, S. L., Longo, D. L, & Loscalzo J. (Eds.). *Harrison's Principles of Internal Medicine* (20th ed.). New York, NY: McGraw-Hill.

January, C. T., Wann, L. S., Calkins, H., Chen, L. Y., Cigarroa, J. E., Cleveland, J. C.,. . . Ellinor, P. T. (2019). 2019 AHA/ ACC/HRS Focused update of the 2014 AHA/ ACC/ HRS guideline for the management of patients with atrial fibrillation: A report of the American College of Cardiology/ American Heart Association task force on clinical practice guidelines and the Heart Rhythm Society. *Circulation, 0.* https://doi.org/10.1161/CIR.0000000000000665

Long, T. L., Brucker, M. C., Osborne, K., I., & Jevitt, C. M. (Eds.). (2019). *Varney's Midwifery* (6th ed.). Sudbury, MA: Jones and Bartlett Publishers.

Madara, B., & Pomarico-Denino, V. (2008). *Pathophysiology* (2nd ed.). Sudbury, MA: Jones and Bartlett Publishers.

Maron, B. J., Maron, M. S., & Semsarian, C. (2012). Genetics of hypertrophic cardiomyopathy after 20 years. *Journal of the American College of Cardiology, 60*(8), 705–715; doi: 10.1016/j.jacc.2012.02.068

Morton, P. G., & Fontaine, D. K. (2018). *Critical care nursing: A holistic approach* (8th ed.). Philadephia, PA: Wolters Kluwer.

National Institutes of Health (NIH). (2010). What is endocarditis? Retrieved from https://www.nhlbi.nih.gov/health/health-topics/topics/endo

National Institutes of Health (NIH). (2011). What are congenital heart defects? Retrieved from https://www.nhlbi.nih.gov/health/health-topics/topics/chd

National Institutes of Health (NIH). (2015). What is the DASH eating plan? Retrieved from http://www.nhlbi.nih.gov/health/health-topics/topics/dash/

National Institutes of Health (NIH). (2016). What is cardiomyopathy? Retrieved from http://www.nhlbi.nih.gov/health/health-topics/topics/cm/

Professional guide to pathophysiology (3rd ed.). (2010). Philadelphia, PA: Lippincott Williams & Wilkins.

Resar, R., Pronovost, P., Haraden, C., Simmonds, T., Rainey, T., & Nolan, T. (2005). Using a bundle approach to improve ventilator care processes and reduce ventilator-associated pneumonia. *Joint Commission Journal on Quality and Patient Safety, 31*(5), 243–248.

Savoy, M. L. (2017). Differences between the AAFP atrial fibrillation guideline and the AHA/ACC/HRS guideline. *American Family Physician, 96*(5), 284–285.

Selby, V. N. (2017). Myocarditis, toxic cardiomyopathy, and stress cardiomyopathy. In M. H. Crawford (Ed.). *CURRENT diagnosis & treatment: Cardiology* (5th ed.). New York, NY: McGraw-Hill. Retrieved from http://accessmedicine.mhmedical.com.ezproxy.fiu.edu/content.aspx?bookid=2040&sectionid=152996032

Semsarian, C., Ingles, J., Maron, M. S., & Maron, B. J. (2015). New perspectives on the prevalence of hypertrophic cardiomyopathy. *Journal of the American College of Cardiology, 65*(12), 1249–1254. doi: 10.1016/j.jacc.2015.01.019

Society of Critical Care Medicine (2016). Surviving sepsis campaign guidelines. Retrieved from http://www.survivingsepsis.org/Guidelines/Pages/default.aspx

Triedman, J. K., & Newburger, J. W. (2016). Trends in congenital heart disease: The next decade. *Circulation, 133*(25), 2716-2733.

Whelton, P. K., Carey, R. M., Aronow, W. S., Casey, D. E., Collins, K. J., Dennison Himmelfarb, C. . . . Wright, J. T. (2017). 2017 Guideline for the prevention, detection, evaluation, and management of high blood pressure in adults. *Journal of the American College of Cardiology, 71*(19), e127–e248. doi: 10.1016/j.jacc.2017.11.006

Zulfiqar, S., & Veerasamy, M. (n.d.). Pericardial diseases. In A. Elmoselhi (Ed.). *Cardiology: An integrated approach* New York, NY: McGraw-Hill. Retrieved from http://accessmedicine.mhmedical.com.ezproxy.fiu.edu/content.aspx?bookid=2224&sectionid=171662157

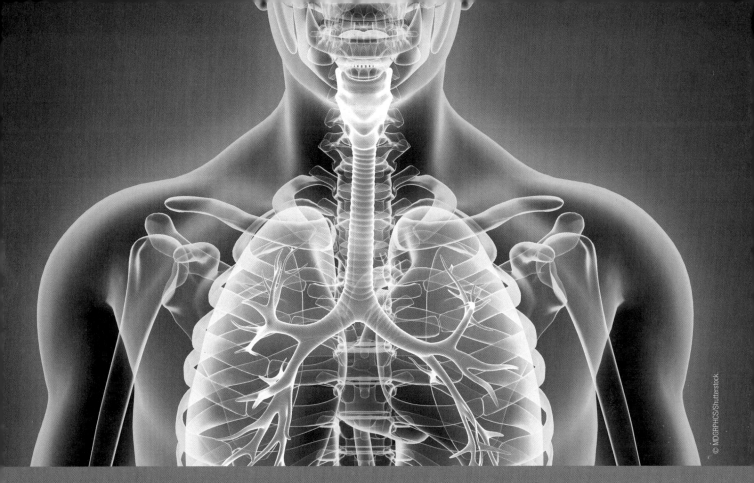

CHAPTER 5
Pulmonary Function

LEARNING OBJECTIVES

- Discuss normal pulmonary anatomy and physiology.
- Differentiate upper and lower respiratory infectious disorders.
- Differentiate restrictive and obstructive disorders.
- Differentiate pleural disorders.
- Describe the major types of lung cancer.
- Summarize how various disorders cause impaired ventilation and perfusion.

- Describe the clinical consequences of impaired ventilation and perfusion.
- Apply understanding of alterations in the pulmonary system when describing various common disorders such as respiratory infections, pleural disorders, malignancy, obstructive disorders, and restrictive disorders.
- Develop diagnostic and treatment considerations for various pulmonary disorders.

The pulmonary system includes the organs and structures associated with breathing and gas exchange. The structures of the pulmonary system are grouped into two branches—the upper respiratory tract (oral cavity, nasal cavity, paranasal sinuses, pharynx, and larynx) (**FIGURE 5-1**) and the lower respiratory tract (trachea, bronchi, bronchioles, and alveoli). This chapter focuses on normal and abnormal states of the pulmonary system. The respiratory tract functions automatically to provide cells with oxygen and to remove carbon dioxide waste. Disorders of the pulmonary system can become serious quickly because of the body's critical need for oxygen.

Anatomy and Physiology

The pulmonary system provides vital oxygen and removes toxic carbon dioxide through the act of breathing. The respiratory tract allows a person to breathe in and out approximately 23,000 times each day or over half a million times a month. The act of breathing allows for gas exchange of oxygen and carbon dioxide. Oxygen is necessary for cells to produce energy through cellular metabolism; carbon dioxide is the waste product of this process. Through its gas exchange functions, the pulmonary system plays a pivotal role in maintaining homeostasis.

The pulmonary system consists of two basic functional divisions—an air-conducting portion and a gas-exchanging portion (**TABLE 5-1**). The air-conducting portion delivers air to the lungs, while the gas-exchanging portion allows gas exchange to occur between the air and the blood (Figure 5-1). The gas-exchanging portion of the respiratory tract includes the lungs with their millions of alveoli and capillaries (**FIGURE 5-2**).

Air enters the respiratory tract through the nose and mouth, then travels to the pharynx. Infants up to the age of 3 months primarily

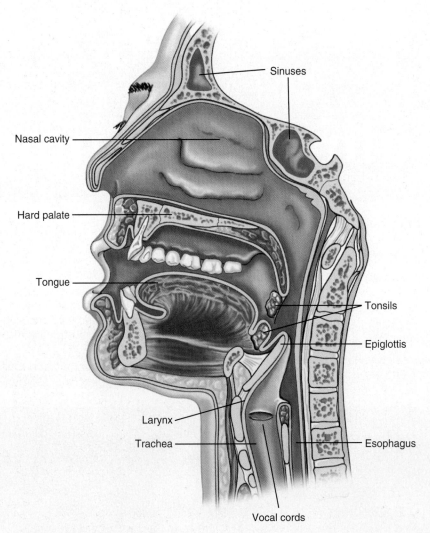

FIGURE 5-1 The upper respiratory tract.

TABLE 5-1	Summary of the Pulmonary System

Organ	Function
Air Conducting	
Nasal cavity	Filters, warms, and moistens air; also transports air to pharynx
Oral cavity	Transports air to pharynx; warms and moistens air; helps produce sounds
Paranasal sinuses: Frontal, maxillary, ethmoid, sphenoid	Warms and moistens air
Pharynx	Transports air to larynx
Epiglottis	Covers the opening to the trachea during swallowing
Larynx	Produces sounds; transports air to trachea; helps filter incoming air; warms and moistens incoming air
Trachea and bronchi	Warms and moistens air; transport air to lungs; filter incoming air
Bronchioles	Control air flow in the lungs; transport air to alveoli
Gas Exchange	
Alveoli	Provide area for exchange of oxygen and carbon dioxide

Modified from Story, L. (2017). *Pathophysiology: A practical approach* (3rd ed.). Burlington, MA: Jones & Bartlett Learning.

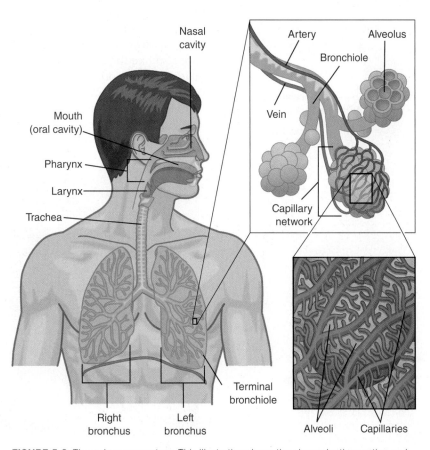

FIGURE 5-2 The pulmonary system. This illustration shows the air-conducting portion and the gas-exchange portion of the human respiratory system. The insert shows a higher magnification of the alveoli where oxygen and carbon dioxide exchange occurs.

breathe through their nose as opposed to the mouth. Nasal congestion in an infant, therefore, can significantly impair breathing. The paranasal sinuses are four air-filled extensions of the nasal cavity that act to warm and moisten the air. The anterior ethmoid sinus consists of an ostiomeatal complex, which opens into the middle turbinate located on lateral wall of the nose. The complex is a drainage pathway for the frontal, maxillary, and ethmoid sinuses. The pharynx joins the larynx, or voice box (FIGURE 5-3). The larynx is made of cartilage and plays a central role in swallowing and talking. When food is swallowed, the larynx rises

so that it is closed by the epiglottis. This process prevents food and liquids from entering the lungs, where they would cause severe irritation. Even so, food does occasionally enter the lungs, often triggering the cough reflex (a primitive protective reflex). The larynx works much like the strings of a guitar or violin to produce sound—tightening and loosening to change pitch. It opens up into the trachea, or windpipe. From the trachea, the air travels to the mainstem bronchi, where it branches into the right and left bronchi, for each lung (FIGURE 5-4). The left bronchus is narrow and positioned more horizontally than the right bronchus; the right bronchus is shorter and wider than the left bronchus and extends downward more vertically. Because of the difference in size between the two bronchi, objects are more easily inhaled (aspirated) into the right bronchus.

Inside the lungs, the bronchi branch extensively into a series of smaller and smaller tubes, or bronchioles, until they reach the alveoli. This branching from larger to smaller tubes mimics the vessels in the cardiovascular system. Children's airways are much smaller than those of adults, making them more vulnerable to obstructions. With advanced aging, the airway diameter also decreases, leading to increased airflow resistance. The walls of the bronchioles are also like the vessel walls in that they mostly consist of smooth muscle. The smooth muscle allows for constriction and dilation of the bronchioles to control air flow. When oxygen needs are higher (e.g., during exercise or stress), the airways dilate more to allow more air to enter

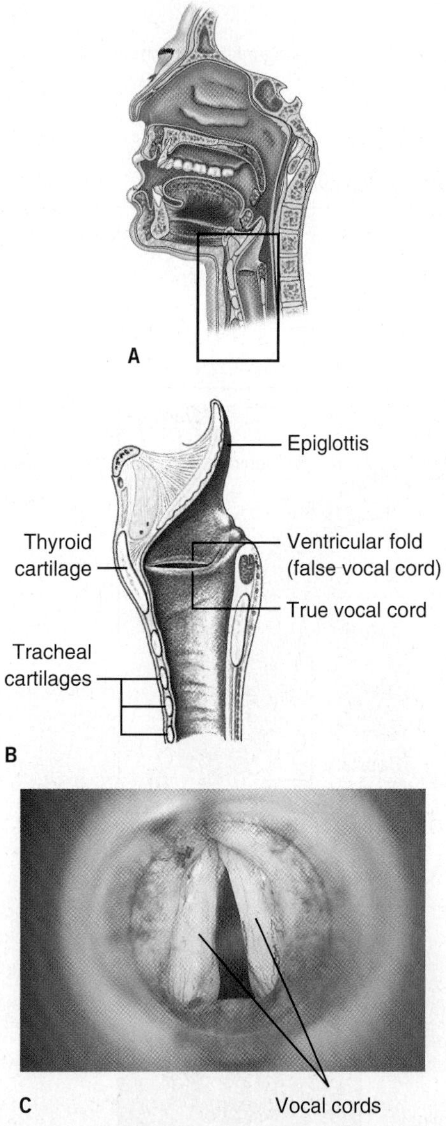

A

Epiglottis

Thyroid cartilage

Ventricular fold (false vocal cord)

True vocal cord

Tracheal cartilages

B

C   Vocal cords

FIGURE 5-3 The vocal cords. **A** Uppermost portion of the respiratory system showing the location of the vocal cords. **B** Longitudinal section of the larynx showing the location of the vocal cords. Note the presence of the false vocal cord, so named because it does not function in phonation. **C** View into the larynx showing the true vocal cords from above.

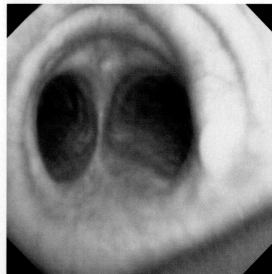

FIGURE 5-4 The bifurcation of the trachea at the carina into the right and left mainstem bronchi.

the lungs. In times of normal or decreased oxygen needs (e.g., during sleep), the airways may narrow (constrict) slightly. Disease processes may cause constriction to the point of impeding air flow—a dangerous development.

The air entering the respiratory tract often contains particles that can be harmful. These particles may include infectious organisms such as bacteria, viruses, and fungi, as well as environmental agents like dust, pollen, and pollutants. The pulmonary system, as part of the innate immune defense, is equipped to filter out some of these particles as well as to protect the body against those that gain entry. The air-conducting portion of the respiratory tract filters many particles by trapping them in the mucous layer (FIGURE 5-5). Mucus is a thick,

sticky substance produced by the goblet cells in the epithelial lining of the nose, trachea, and bronchi. This epithelial lining also contains many cilia, or hairlike projections, that move in a wavelike motion to propel the mucus and trapped particles upward to the mouth, where they can be removed through coughing, sneezing, and expectorating (spitting out). Cigarette smoking and air pollution can decrease mucus production and destroy cilia, increasing the risk of respiratory infections. Alcohol consumption can paralyze cilia, also increasing infection risk.

Additionally, the immune system is outfitted with immunoglobulin A (IgA) cells in the pulmonary system; these cells prevent the attachment and invasion of bacteria and viruses on mucous membranes. Macrophages are also present around the alveoli in the lungs; they keep the lungs clean by phagocytizing particles that gain access to this area (FIGURE 5-6). Once the macrophages fill with particulates, they move into the surrounding connective tissue. When an unusually large number of particulates are present (e.g., with cigarette or marijuana smoking and when breathing in heavy pollution), the lungs become blackened by the accumulation of the particles.

The air-conducting portion of the respiratory system also moistens and warms incoming air. An extensive network of capillaries lies beneath the epithelium of the respiratory tract. These capillaries release moisture into the incoming air, humidifying it to prevent drying of the respiratory tract. The warm blood circulating through the capillaries heats this air prior to entering the lungs, protecting the lungs from cold temperatures. As the air leaves the respiratory tract, much of the water that has been added to the air condenses onto the slightly cooler lining of the nasal passages. The condensation is recycled for the next inhalation to conserve water and contributes to runny noses on cold days.

Alveoli are the site for gas exchange with the bloodstream (FIGURE 5-7). Oxygen is delivered to the alveoli by the air-conducting portion of the pulmonary system, and carbon dioxide is brought to the lungs by the circulatory system. During childhood, the alveoli increase in size and number, and they continue to mature for several years. By adulthood, each human lung contains approximately 150 million alveoli, which collectively create a surface area approximately the size of a tennis court for gas exchange. The alveoli and capillaries are often a single cell layer thick, which

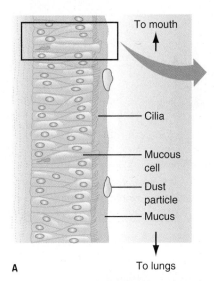

To mouth

Cilia

Mucous cell

Dust particle

Mucus

To lungs

A

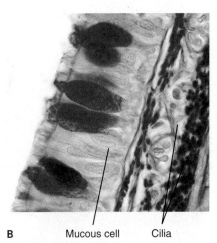

B   Mucous cell   Cilia

FIGURE 5-5 Mucus trap. **A** Drawing of the lining of the trachea. Mucus produced by the mucous cells of the lining of much of the pulmonary system traps organisms and other particulates in the air. The cilia transport the mucus toward the mouth. **B** Higher magnification of the lining showing a mucous cell and ciliated epithelial cells.

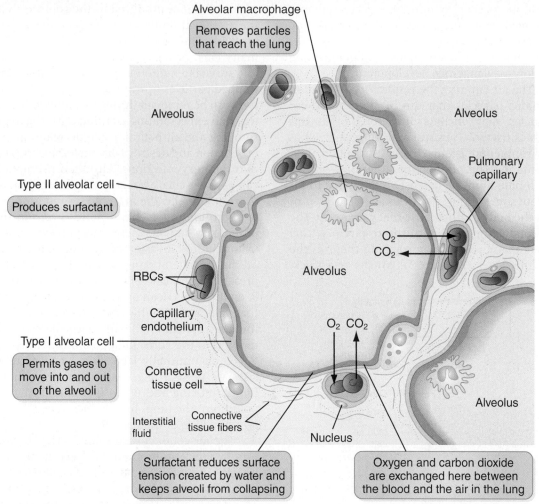

Alveolar macrophage

Removes particles that reach the lung

Alveolus

Alveolus

Pulmonary capillary

Type II alveolar cell

Produces surfactant

O_2

CO_2

RBCs

Alveolus

Capillary endothelium

Type I alveolar cell

Permits gases to move into and out of the alveoli

O_2 CO_2

Connective tissue cell

Alveolus

Interstitial fluid

Connective tissue fibers

Nucleus

Surfactant reduces surface tension created by water and keeps alveoli from collapsing

Oxygen and carbon dioxide are exchanged here between the blood and the air in the lung

FIGURE 5-6 The alveolar macrophages.

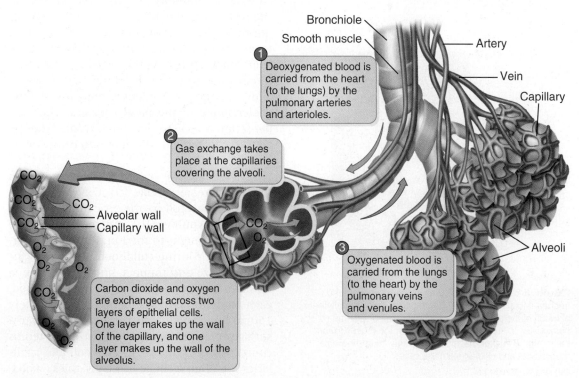

Bronchiole

Smooth muscle

Artery

Vein

Capillary

1 Deoxygenated blood is carried from the heart (to the lungs) by the pulmonary arteries and arterioles.

2 Gas exchange takes place at the capillaries covering the alveoli.

CO_2
CO_2 CO_2
CO_2 Alveolar wall
CO_2 Capillary wall
O_2
O_2 O_2
CO_2

CO_2
O_2

Alveoli

3 Oxygenated blood is carried from the lungs (to the heart) by the pulmonary veins and venules.

O_2
O_2

Carbon dioxide and oxygen are exchanged across two layers of epithelial cells. One layer makes up the wall of the capillary, and one layer makes up the wall of the alveolus.

FIGURE 5-7 Gas exchange in the lungs.

further facilitates gas exchange. Interstitial connective tissue supports the capillaries. The amount of gas exchanged depends on the total surface area available and the thickness of the alveoli and capillary walls. The more surface area and the thinner the layers, the more rapidly gas diffuses. With normal aging, the alveolar ducts degenerate and become dilated, causing the alveolar sacs to enlarge, resulting in a decreased surface area.

Gas exchange in the alveoli requires adequate ventilation, which is the process of air reaching the alveoli, and sufficient perfusion of blood to the alveoli. The ventilation-to-perfusion ratio, or VQ ratio, is a measurement of the efficacy and adequacy of these two processes. In the ideal lung, inspired air reaches all the alveoli and all the alveoli have the same blood supply. In reality, neither alveolar ventilation nor capillary blood flow is uniform. The supply of air and blood never match perfectly, even in healthy persons. Because of gravity, the lower parts of the lungs have greater blood flow than the upper parts. Distribution of alveolar ventilation from the top to the bottom of the lungs is also uneven. Normal ventilation is 4 liters of air per minute, and normal perfusion is 5 liters of blood per minute. This difference makes the expected VQ ratio 4:5, or 0.8. A VQ ratio higher than 0.8 indicates that ventilation exceeds perfusion, and a VQ ratio less than 0.8 indicates poor ventilation. Some respiratory disorders involve ventilation problems, whereas others result from perfusion issues. In any event, the result is impaired gas exchange. A VQ lung scan is a nuclear medicine scan where radioactive particles are inhaled to assess airflow, and particles are also given intravenously to assess blood flow. A VQ scan can be used to evaluate for pulmonary emboli, which would cause decreased or absent perfusion in areas of the lung.

When air is inhaled, gases are exchanged between the alveoli and the capillaries; carbon dioxide is removed through expiration, and oxygen is delivered to cells by the cardiovascular system. Various gases (oxygen, carbon dioxide, nitrogen) and water are in atmospheric air, the alveoli, and blood. These gases diffuse between the alveoli, blood, and tissues because they each exert different pressures. For example, oxygen's partial pressure is high in the alveoli in comparison to oxygen's partial pressure in the pulmonary capillaries, so oxygen will diffuse into the pulmonary capillaries. In contrast, the partial pressure of carbon dioxide is low in the alveoli and high in the pulmonary

capillaries, so carbon dioxide will diffuse into the alveoli. The delivery of oxygen to the tissues is dependent on the amount of oxygen content in the blood, the amount of oxygen saturated to hemoglobin, and the partial pressure of oxygen. Oxyhemoglobin, which forms in the lungs, is the combination of oxygen and hemoglobin (i.e., hemoglobin saturation with oxygen—SaO_2). Oxyhemoglobin travels to the cells where oxygen is released and hemoglobin is reduced (i.e., hemoglobin desaturation). The rate at which hemoglobin binds and releases oxygen (i.e., affinity of hemoglobin for oxygen) is affected by several factors such as temperature and pH and is graphically described in the oxyhemoglobin dissociation curve (FIGURE 5-8).

Learning Points

Partial Pressure

How are pressures determined? The atmospheric pressure is the total of all the pressure exerted by the different gases in the air. At sea level, this pressure is 760 mmHg. Each gas has a different concentration in the atmosphere and, therefore, will exert a different pressure. The pressure each gas exerts is known as *partial pressure* and is designated by a capital P before the gas (e.g., PO_2, PCO_2). Atmospheric air consists of 21% oxygen and the PO_2 is, therefore, 160 mmHg (e.g., 760 mmHg $\times$ 0.21 = 160 mmHg). When you see PaO_2, the *a* refers to *arterial*.

Learning Points

Carbon Monoxide Poisoning

Carbon monoxide is a gas that is the byproduct of pollutants in the air. A high percentage is in motor vehicle exhaust and in faulty heating systems. Smoke from fire, generator exhaust, and paint thinner are some other sources of carbon monoxide. This colorless, odorless gas is readily inhaled. Carbon monoxide has a high affinity for hemoglobin (200–250 times more than oxygen), and the result is an abnormal hemoglobin called *carboxyhemoglobin*. Carboxyhemoglobin does not transport oxygen. The result is hypoxemia. Carbon monoxide poisoning causes hundreds of deaths a year; > 400 unintentional deaths (CDC, 2018a). The amount of exposure and how quickly it is recognized and treated will determine the outcome.

The distensibility of the lungs is resisted by fluids in the alveoli that create surface tension. This tension is created by the attraction of water molecules on the surface of the alveoli, and this tension acts to collapse and increase pressure in the alveoli. However, the surface of the alveoli contains a substance called *surfactant*. Surfactant is a lipoprotein produced by alveoli cells (type II pneumocytes) that has a detergent-like quality. This watery substance

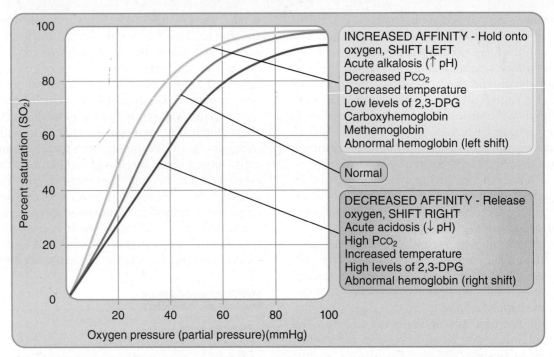

FIGURE 5-8 Oxyhemoglobin dissociation curve. The lower portion of the normal (purple) line represents the body's tissue, and the upper half of the normal (purple) line represents the lungs. Diseases and other conditions will change the affinity. At a PO_2 of 80, saturation minimally changes. Decreased oxygen affinity, when hemoglobin releases more oxygen, occurs when tissue needs more oxygen and causes a shift to the right. Increased oxygen affinity, when hemoglobin holds on to oxygen, causes a shift to the left.

reduces surface tension on the alveoli, which enhances pulmonary compliance (elasticity) and prevents the alveoli from collapsing. Because pressure in the lungs is negative compared with atmospheric pressure, walls of the alveoli tend to draw inward, making them collapse. This pressure is much like that seen with a vacuum-sealed pack of coffee. The pressure and the risk of collapse further increase at the end of expiration. Surfactant promotes reinflation of the alveoli during inspiration. Disease states and other conditions can decrease surfactant, leading to the collapse of the alveoli (a condition called *atelectasis*). For example, premature infants lack surfactant as it is not produced until about 20 weeks' gestation, and airway secretions start at around 30 weeks. Synthetic surfactant may be administered to overcome any inadequacies in production.

The process of breathing is largely involuntary and controlled by the medulla oblongata in the brain. This center is located in the brainstem, which controls many vital body functions (e.g., heart rate, blood pressure, and temperature). Breathing includes two phases: inspiration (inhalation) and expiration (exhalation).

Inspiration is an active neural process that begins when nerve impulses travel from the

brain to the diaphragm, the dome-shaped muscle that separates the thoracic and abdominal cavities (FIGURE 5-9). These impulses cause the diaphragm to contract, lower, and flatten, which draws air into the lungs. Inspiration also involves the intercostal muscles between the ribs. Nerve impulses cause intercostal muscles to contract, lifting the ribs up and out. Contraction of the diaphragm and intercostal muscles changes intrapulmonary pressure, causing air to naturally flow into the lungs. With aging, the chest wall becomes less compliant as the intercostal and diaphragmatic muscles lose mass. In aging, the bone and joints are affected by calcifications and structural changes due to osteoporosis (e.g., kyphosis). Elastic recoil of lung tissue is reduced. These normal physiologic changes can lead to alterations in activity tolerance. However, the effect of these normal changes is influenced by the presence of pulmonary disease and prior fitness levels. Normal pulmonary changes of aging effects such as decreased activity tolerance must also be distinguished from pathologic changes that are more prevalent with aging and present with similar symptoms. (e.g., chronic lung disease, heart failure).

In contrast to inspiration, expiration is passive—not requiring muscle contraction. As

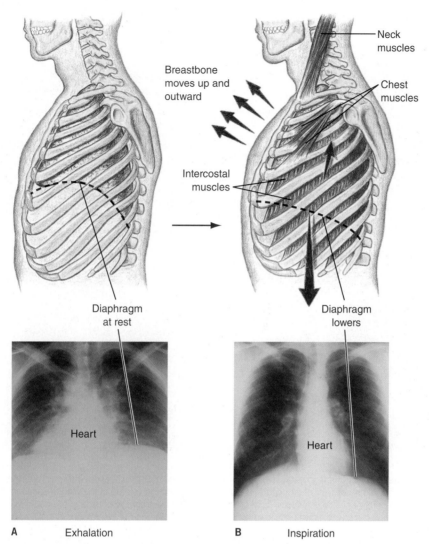

Neck muscles

Breastbone moves up and outward

Chest muscles

Intercostal muscles

Diaphragm at rest

Diaphragm lowers

Heart

Heart

A   Exhalation

B   Inspiration

FIGURE 5-9 Breathing. The rising and falling of the chest wall through the contraction of intercostal muscles (muscles between the ribs), illustrating the bellows effect. Inspiration is assisted by the diaphragm, which assumes a lower position in the chest. Like pulling a plunger back on a syringe, the rising of the chest wall and the lowering of the diaphragm draw air into the lungs. Illustrations and X-rays showing the lungs in **A** full exhalation and **B** full inspiration.

© S IU/Visuals Unlimited, Inc.

the lungs fill with air, the diaphragm and intercostal muscles relax, returning to their previous position. Returning to their natural position decreases thoracic volume and increases intrapulmonary pressure. This greater pressure forces air out of the lungs. Elastic fibers in the lungs aid in passive expiration by causing the lungs to recoil. Expiration can also be active—that is, created by contracting the chest and abdominal muscles.

Muscle contraction and nerve impulses are not the only factors involved in air movement. Pressure gradients between the atmosphere and lungs must exist to facilitate air movement

in and out of lungs and prevent collapse of the alveoli and lungs (**FIGURE 5-10**). Air moves from areas of high pressure to low pressure. There are three pressures that are important concerning breathing and maintenance of expanded lungs—atmospheric, intrapulmonary, and intrapleural. Atmospheric pressure is created by a mixture of gases, and at sea level, these gases exert a pressure of 760 mmHg. Intrapulmonary (within the lungs) pressure is created by the gases in the lungs and is influenced by lung volume (space). Pressure and volume are inversely proportional (e.g., when one goes up, the other goes down and vice versa).

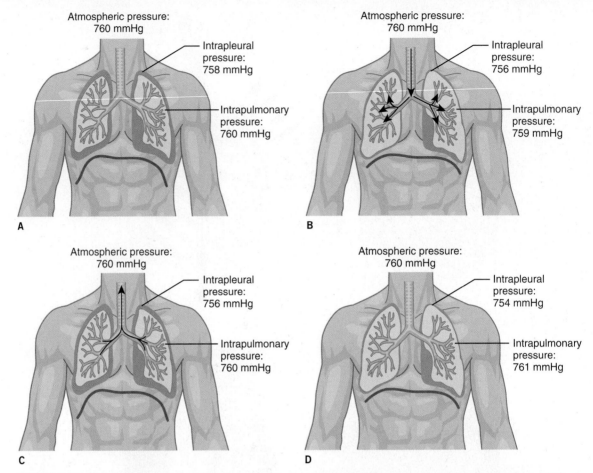

FIGURE 5-10 Pressure changes during inspiration and expiration. **A** At the end of expiration, intrapulmonary pressure equals atmospheric pressure, and no movement of air occurs. **B** During inspiration, the volume of the pleural space increases, causing the pressure in the intrapulmonary spaces (alveoli) to decrease. Air then flows from the outside of the body, where the pressure is greater (760 mmHg), into the alveoli, where it is lower (759 mmHg). **C** At the end of inspiration, intrapulmonary pressure again equals atmospheric pressure, and no movement of air occurs. **D** During expiration, the volume of the pleural spaces decreases, causing the intrapulmonary pressure to increase (761 mmHg). Because the intrapulmonary pressure exceeds the atmospheric pressure (760 mmHg), air flows out of the lungs.

As we **inhale**, lung volume expands, gases move in and have more space, so the pressure decreases slightly (e.g., -3 to 757 mmHg) in the lung. This decreased pressure is often referred to as *negative pressure* because some pressure is lost and not necessarily that there is a negative number (i.e., the 757 is not negative). Then, air from the atmosphere (higher pressure) comes into the lower pressure lungs. This air movement causes pressure in lung to go up because there are more gases (e.g., 760 mmHg) now in the lung.

Then we **exhale** and volume decreases, but we still have the gases in the lungs with less space for a moment, causing the pressure in the lungs to go up even a bit higher (e.g., 763 mmHg). This increase is often referred to as *positive pressure*. Air then goes from the lung (higher pressure) back to the atmosphere, which at the time is lower,

and then lung pressure drops to 760 mmHg. Inhalation occurs and the inspiratory–expiratory cycle starts all over.

One more pressure is the pressure between the lung and chest wall, which is known as the *intrapleural pressure*. The intrapulmonary pressure is greater than the intrapleural pressure, and this pressure keeps the parietal and visceral pleura clinging together and the lungs expanded. The pleura is the thin, serous membrane surrounding the lungs, which also lines the thoracic cavity. The pleura folds back onto itself to form the two-layered pleural sac. The pleural sac is filled with a watery fluid that protects the lungs and minimizes friction during breathing.

Air flow, both inspiratory and expiratory, can be measured to aid in diagnosis of respiratory

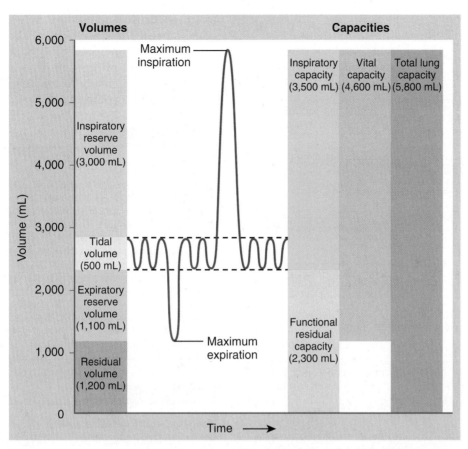

FIGURE 5-11 Illustration of lung volumes and capacities. Tidal volume during resting conditions.

disorders. Pulmonary function tests evaluate lung volumes and capacities (**FIGURE 5-11**). Tidal volume is the amount of air involved in one normal inhalation and exhalation. The average tidal volume is 500 milliliters but is smaller in shallow breathing. Minute respiratory volume is the amount inhaled and exhaled in 1 minute. This volume is calculated by multiplying the tidal volume by the number of respirations per minute; the average is 6 liters per minute. Inspiratory reserve volume is the amount of air beyond the tidal volume that can be taken in with the deepest inhalation. Inspiratory reserve volume averages 2–3 liters. Expiratory reserve volume is the amount of air beyond tidal volume that can be forcibly exhaled beyond the normal passive exhalation. The average expiratory reserve volume is 1–1.5 liters. Vital capacity is the sum of the tidal volume and reserves. Some air is always present in the lungs, and this amount is called *residual volume*. Even after the most forceful exhalation, 1–1.5 liters of air remain in the lungs, which ensures efficient and consistent gas exchange. Forced expiratory volume in 1 second (FEV_1) is compared to forced vital capacity to diagnose pulmonary disease (e.g., asthma).

The medulla controls breathing through nerve cells that generate nerve impulses to the respiratory muscles. These impulses cease when the lungs are full, allowing the muscles to relax. Chemoreceptors inside the brain and arteries also regulate breathing. These receptors detect carbon dioxide levels and send messages to the medulla. Carbon dioxide levels, not oxygen levels, normally drive breathing (**FIGURE 5-12**). When these levels go up, respiration depth and rate increase to excrete the excess carbon dioxide, and vice versa. In some disease states, this drive becomes altered, and then oxygen levels drive breathing. Additionally, stretch receptors in the lungs aid in breathing by detecting when the lungs are full. In such a case, stretch receptors in the lungs send a message to the medulla to cease firing. This effect, which is called the *Hering-Breuer reflex*, prevents overinflation of the lungs. The body also has oxygen receptors, but they are not sensitive. These receptors do not generate impulses until oxygen levels fall to a critical

Normal cycle

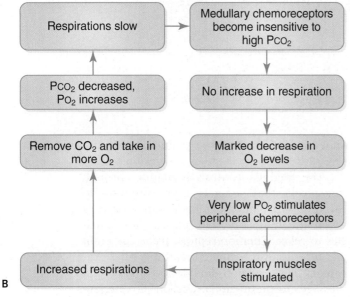

A

Hypoxic drive with chronic elevated P_{CO_2} levels
(e.g., emphysema)

B

FIGURE 5-12 **A** Normal respiratory control and **B** hypoxic drive.

point. With aging, the chemoreceptors become less sensitive, further contributing to decreased activity tolerance.

In addition to regulating oxygen and carbon dioxide levels, the lungs aid in regulating pH by altering breathing rate and depth. Carbon dioxide is a source of acid in the body. Increasing the respiratory rate and depth will lead to excretion of more carbon dioxide, making the blood less acidic (increasing pH). Conversely, decreasing the respiratory rate and

depth will cause retention of more carbon dioxide, making the blood more acidic (decreasing pH). This compensatory mechanism allows for a quick fix of pH imbalances to reestablish homeostasis (see chapter 6 for further discussion of acid–base homeostasis).

Pulse Oximetry

Pulse oximetry is a noninvasive method to measure arterial oxygen saturation (SaO_2). A pulse oximeter is a sensor that is placed on a person's finger that can rapidly detect the percentage of a person's hemoglobin that is carrying oxygen. Normal pulse oximetry readings of oxygen saturation is > 90%, which means 90% of the person's hemoglobin is carrying oxygen. This reading is dependent on adequate circulation to the individual's fingers. This reading can look high in times of decreased hemoglobin (e.g., anemia). In such cases, the reading may read 90–100% indicating 90–100% of that person's hemoglobin is carrying oxygen, but the individual may not have enough hemoglobin to meet his or her needs.

End-Tidal Carbon Dioxide Monitoring

End-tidal carbon dioxide ($ETCO_2$) monitoring is a quick, noninvasive method to measure the amount of carbon dioxide (CO_2) produced and exhaled during breathing. Various types of devices can be used in intubated and nonintubated patients. The results can be numeric (capnometry) or waveforms (capnography). High $ETCO_2$ values indicate effective ventilations, while lower numbers occur with poor ventilation and poor perfusion (there is less blood passing through the alveoli, so there is less gas exchange). Operating rooms and intensive care units have been the main areas using $ETCO_2$ monitoring, but use now encompasses prehospital areas, outpatient surgical centers, and so forth. Clinical scenarios for use include verification of endotracheal placement, during sedation for procedures, or evaluating cardiopulmonary resuscitation.

Pregnancy Changes

Pregnancy alters pulmonary function in several ways. Estrogen changes and increased blood volume stimulate the nasal passages to increase mucus secretion and become edematous and hyperemic. These changes cause an increased feeling of nasal congestion and rhinitis. Dyspnea even at rest is common. The cause of the dyspnea is not well understood but may be due to an increased sensitivity to carbon dioxide and oxygen levels and increased progesterone levels. In response, minute ventilation increases, causing a sensation of dyspnea. Respiratory rate, however, is not significantly higher, and tachypnea may be a sign of a pulmonary disorder.

Understanding Conditions That Affect the Pulmonary System

When considering alterations in the pulmonary system, it is best to organize them based on their basic underlying pathophysiology to increase understanding. Those pathophysiologic concepts include conditions that are infectious in nature, problems with ventilation, and issues with perfusion. Infectious conditions may involve either the upper respiratory tract or the lower respiratory tract. The pulmonary system requires both ventilation and perfusion to function properly. Problems in either of these areas will impair the pulmonary system's ability to meet the body's needs. Ventilation conditions result from problems with moving air into or out of the lungs. Ventilation disorders can further be described as obstructive or restrictive. Obstructive disorders are characterized by difficulty with exhaling, and restrictive disorders are characterized by difficulty with inhalation. Perfusion conditions result from problems that prevent gas exchange; many of these conditions are cardiovascular in nature (e.g., pulmonary embolism).

While this organization is intended to increase understanding, many of the alterations overlap and/or have other causes in addition to the causes under which they are categorized. For example, pneumonia is listed under infections; however, there are also noninfectious causes such as irritants. Additionally, pneumonias lead to problems with gas exchange.

Infectious Disorders

Upper Respiratory Tract Infections

The upper respiratory tract includes the mouth, nasal cavity, sinuses, pharynx, and larynx. Infections of these structures trigger the inflammatory response, which explains many of the symptoms associated with these conditions. Most of the upper respiratory tract infections (URIs) are interrelated and usually occur together, or one condition may lead to another. Viruses are frequently the causative organisms and the specific pathogen cannot be identified in most cases. Primary bacterial infections are the cause in approximately 25% of cases. In a small percentage of individuals, the breach in the physical and chemical barriers from a virus can lead to secondary bacterial infections.

Infectious Rhinitis

Infectious rhinitis, also referred to as *nasopharyngitis* or the *common cold*, is a viral upper respiratory infection. Infectious rhinitis is a significant contributor to work and school absences, with adults averaging two to three colds per year and children having even more such infections (Centers for Disease Control and Prevention [CDC], 2016b). As with other infections, individuals who are younger or elderly or immunocompromised are at higher risk.

The most frequent causative organism is a rhinovirus, but many other viruses (e.g., parainfluenza, adenovirus, and coronavirus) can cause this illness. More than 200 organisms can cause infectious rhinitis, making it difficult to develop immunity. In infectious rhinitis, the infectious organism invades the epithelial lining of the nasal mucosa. Mild cellular inflammation leads to nasal discharge, mucus production, and shedding of the epithelial cells. The virus is highly contagious because it is shed in large numbers from the nasal mucosa and can survive for several hours outside the body. Close physical contact with the virus transmits the infection through exchanges with other people (e.g., shaking hands) and surfaces (e.g., doorknobs and telephones). Transmission may occur through inhalation. Despite popular misconceptions, wet and cold conditions do not cause or increase occurrences of infectious rhinitis. The apparent increase in occurrence of the infectious rhinitis during rainy and cold weather is due to increased congregation in confined spaces. Those persons in more frequent, closer contact with other people, such as children in day care centers, healthcare providers, and teachers, will be at higher risk for developing the infection. There are several other causes of rhinitis as allergens (allergic rhinitis), and nonallergic causes such as medications (rhinitis medicamentosa), hormonal changes, and aging changes.

Clinical Manifestations

An individual who contracts infectious rhinitis usually experiences an incubation period between the invasion of the virus and the onset of symptoms, which is approximately 1–3 days. Clinical manifestations include clear nasal discharge that can become white, yellow, or green and causes rhinorrhea (runny nose). This discharge leads to sneezing and nasal congestion. The mucus drips down the pharynx, causing a pharyngitis, a subsequent sore throat, and usually a nonproductive cough. The virus can also affect the larynx and cause hoarseness (laryngitis). Due to the activation of the immune response, other systemic symptoms such as low-grade fever, chills, myalgia (muscle aching), and malaise may be present. A headache can be caused by inflammation of the mucus in the sinus cavities. During physical examination, nasal passages may be inflamed and erythematous, and mucus may be visualized. An external crease from a repeated upward wiping of the nose (nasal salute) may be present. The back of the throat may reveal mild increased erythema and increased lymphatic tissue (along the oropharynx) caused by the virus and mucus running down the back of the throat. Palatine and pharyngeal tonsils may be enlarged, along with lymph nodes in the neck. Conjunctivitis may be present with lacrimation (see chapter 14).

Diagnosis and Treatment

Diagnosis of infectious rhinitis is primarily made based on the presence of signs and symptoms. URIs such as infectious rhinitis, pharyngitis, sinusitis, and bronchitis often have similar and at times nonspecific clinical manifestations, making it more challenging to determine if an etiology is viral or bacterial. In general, the diagnosis of infectious rhinitis is usually made when there is a lack of a localized or focused complaint or infection on one anatomic location such as the throat. The presence of purulence and fever is often considered bacterial; however, these manifestations can be present with viral infections.

Treatment is symptomatic. Most over-the-counter cold preparations are ineffective in shortening the course of the infection, but they can relieve symptoms. Cold preparations should be avoided in children younger than 4 years. Pharmacologic therapies that may be used include antipyretics (for fever), analgesics (for discomfort), decongestants (for nasal symptoms), cough suppressants, or expectorants. Humidifiers can liquefy secretions to aid in expectoration. Maintaining adequate hydration can also liquefy secretions and help manage fevers. Nasal saline can ease nasal discomfort. The benefit of vitamin C, echinacea, and zinc in prevention and treatment remains controversial. Most symptoms resolve within 7–10 days, although cough may take longer to resolve in pregnant women.

Proper hand washing remains the longstanding cornerstone of prevention because the hands are a significant source of transmission. Additional prevention measures include covering one's mouth when coughing and sneezing, using tissue or the upper sleeve of one's shirt, and disposing of tissue immediately after use.

Infectious rhinitis generally leads to no significant sequelae. However, the breach in the physical and chemical barriers of the respiratory tract increases vulnerability of other parts of the head and/or respiratory system and may lead to secondary bacterial invasions. Infectious rhinitis can lead to otitis media, rhinosinusitis, bronchitis, and pneumonia, or secondary bacterial infections may be present in these same areas. The risk for secondary bacterial infections is increased in individuals who smoke because of the chronic damage done by smoke to the mucosa and cilia. Pregnant women have an increased risk for sinusitis and bronchitis because of normal hormonal changes that increase vascularity and swelling in the respiratory lining. As with viruses, the very young, elderly, and immunocompromised are at higher risk. Suspicions of secondary bacterial infection should occur when the illness is prolonged, the presentation is more severe, or when manifestations become more localized like in the sinuses.

Rhinosinusitis

Sinusitis is an inflammation of one or more of the four paranasal sinuses. The maxillary is the most commonly affected, followed by the ethmoid. In children, the maxillary and ethmoid sinuses are present at birth, but the sphenoid sinus does open until the age of 5. The frontal sinus starts appearing at 7 and continues developing into adolescence. Sinusitis rarely occurs without concurrent rhinitis; therefore, rhinosinusitis is the more appropriate term. Rhinosinusitis affects all genders and ages and ethnicities equally.

Rhinosinusitis is most often caused by viruses that also produce infectious rhinitis (e.g., rhinovirus [30%], influenza, or adenovirus). Noninfectious causes include allergies, barotrauma, nasal/sinus tumors, and irritant exposure. Acute bacterial rhinosinusitis occurs in 2% of cases and is often preceded by a viral infection. Most common bacterial infections are caused by *Streptococcus pneumoniae* or *Haemophilus influenzae* in adults and *Moraxella catarrhalis* in children. In immunocompromised patients or those with diabetes, fungi (e.g., *Aspergillus* or Mucorales) may be the causative organisms. Fungal infection from molds and aspergilli are also implicated in atopic individuals who develop a type I hypersensitivity. In patients with cystic fibrosis or nosocomial sinus infections, the most common organisms are *Staphylococcus aureus* and *Pseudomonas aeruginosa*. Nosocomial infections are usually polymicrobial, resistant to therapies, and can also include *Klebsiella pneumoniae*, *Serratia marcescens*, and *Enterobacter* types. Increased risk for rhinosinusitis development includes environmental temperature changes or irritants such as smoke exposure and air pollutants; immunocompromised status such as HIV positivity; conditions that increase inflammation or mucus production such as cystic fibrosis, asthma, sarcoidosis, and Wegener granulomatosis; nasal structural abnormalities such as nasal polyps; and dental abscesses with fistula development into the sinuses.

In rhinosinusitis, the inflammation and increased mucus prevents outflow of nasal secretions. These infectious secretions proliferate and cause damage to the ciliated pseudostratified lining in the sinus. The lack of secretion clearance and inflammation provide an environment for microbial growth. The basic underlying problem in all the etiologic and/or predisposing risk factors for sinusitis consists of the blockage of the sinus to nasal cavity openings and/or ciliary damage (**FIGURE 5-13**).

Sinusitis can present as several different types:

- Acute, which lasts up to 4 weeks
- Subacute, which lasts 4–12 weeks

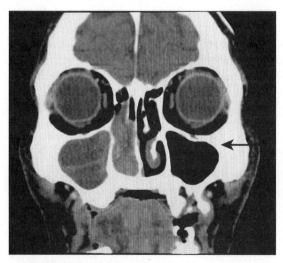

FIGURE 5-13 Blocked sinus.
© Karan Bunjean/Shutterstock.

- Chronic, which lasts more than 12 weeks and can continue for months or even years
- Recurrent, with several (four or more) attacks occurring within a year with remissions in between episodes.

Clinical Manifestations

As exudate accumulates, pressure builds in the sinus cavity, which causes facial bone pain and headache usually of a throbbing and/or pressurelike quality. The location of pain can indicate which sinus is affected (**FIGURE 5-14**). Coughing, sudden movements, or anything that increases head pressure intensifies the pain. Lying down or bending forward increases pain in frontal sinusitis, while standing worsens maxillary sinus pain. Toothache may be present with maxillary sinusitis. Retro-orbital pressure and eye pain may be present with ethmoid sinusitis. Other clinical manifestations of rhinosinusitis include nasal congestion, purulent nasal discharge, hyposmia (reduced ability to smell), halitosis (foul-smelling breath), mouth breathing, fever, sore throat, nonproductive cough, and malaise. Facial pain without purulent discharge or vice versa are not consistent with rhinosinusitis. Objective findings include an edematous, erythematous nasal mucosa with purulent drainage from the middle meatus. If transillumination (shining a light) of the sinus is diminished, it may indicate sinusitis, although there are other reasons for a decrease. Ethmoid sinusitis will cause eye problems such as a conjunctival erythema, eyelid mucous membrane swelling (chemosis), eye protrusion (proptosis), and fixation, and eye muscle weakness and tremors. Palpation over an affected sinus may cause pain. Children often have accompanying otitis media (middle ear infection). Nosocomial sinusitis may often occur in the critically ill, particularly in those who are intubated without typical manifestations; therefore, this diagnosis should be considered when a fever is present in intubated patients.

Diagnoses and Treatment

Diagnostic procedures for rhinosinusitis are not necessary initially, and clinical manifestations will usually point to the diagnosis. Most cases of rhinosinusitis are viral, but bacterial infections are suspected when symptoms persist and do not improve after 10 days or when symptoms worsen when a person was improving. Complicated presentations such as fungal infections, intracranial extension, subacute/chronic cases, and complicated acute

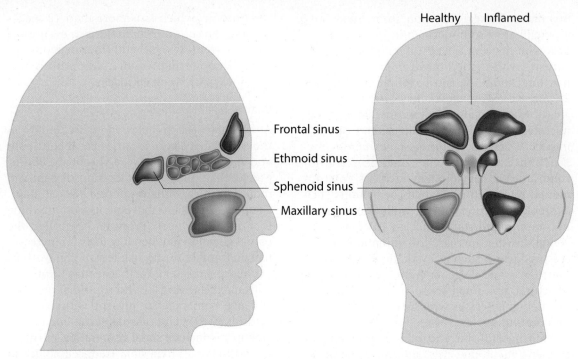

Healthy | Inflamed

Frontal sinus

Ethmoid sinus

Sphenoid sinus

Maxillary sinus

FIGURE 5-14 Sinusitis.
© Alila Medical Media/Shutterstock.

bacterial rhinosinusitis warrant further evaluation. Diagnostic tests may include nasal cultures and/or biopsies, sinus X-ray, and sinus CT, which is the radiography of choice. Treatment usually includes decongestants or nasal corticosteroid spray to shrink swollen nasal membranes; analgesics; and nasal irrigation with salt water until the sinuses begin draining. Bacterial infections require antibiotic therapy to resolve. Other measures may include humidifiers (to liquefy secretions and aid in drainage), warm compresses, adequate hydration, and avoidance of irritants (e.g., smoke, chemicals, and other allergens). Endoscopic sinus surgery or balloon sinuplasty may be necessary for chronic or recurrent rhinosinusitis. In children with recurrent sinusitis or other frequent upper respiratory infections, removing the adenoids may resolve the issue.

While not common, complications of acute bacterial sinusitis can include orbital abscess and cellulitis, meningitis, and brain abscess. Children are at higher risk for these complications than adults. Sinusitis from fungal infection are usually invasive and cause life-threatening illness. Individuals with diabetes or who are immunocompromised (e.g., transplant, chronic steroid use) are at most risk. Acute cases can become subacute, and chronic cases are often thought to be caused by repeated infections (rather than persistent)

that damage the mucociliary lining and ability for secretions to clear.

Pharyngitis/Tonsillitis

Pharyngitis is an inflammation of the pharynx, which is simply known as a *sore throat*. Tonsillitis is an inflammation of the palatine tonsils. If the tonsils are predominantly affected, the diagnosis of tonsillitis is given; however, pharyngitis and tonsillitis often occur together, and the term *pharyngitis* will be used in reference to both. Pharyngitis is common among adults and children, and it is a frequent reason for seeking health care. Various infectious and noninfectious causes result in pharyngitis/tonsillitis. While many commonalities exist among the varying causes of pharyngitis, certain age groups have a higher prevalence of certain organisms. There are differences in pathogenesis, clinical manifestations, and treatments; therefore, viral pharyngitis, infectious mononucleosis, enterovirus oral infections (herpangina and hand-foot-and-mouth disease), and bacterial pharyngitis will be discussed individually.

Viral Pharyngitis

As with other URIs, most cases of pharyngitis cases are infectious and caused by viruses (e.g., rhinovirus, coronavirus, influenza A and B, parainfluenza, respiratory syncytial virus (RSV). Pharyngitis is more prevalent in children overall.

Most of these viruses create an inflammatory response, leading to erythema and edema. The main complaint is a sore throat described as soreness, irritation, or scratchiness. Since viral pharyngitis is often a part of a URI, clinical manifestations and treatment are similar.

Infectious Mononucleosis

In about 2% of cases, pharyngitis is caused by the **Epstein-Barr virus** (also known as *human herpesvirus 4*). Epstein-Barr virus (EBV) is the most common cause of infectious mononucleosis. Many children contract EBV in childhood and remain asymptomatic, usually resulting in lifelong immunity. Adults can also get infected with EBV, have a mild disease, and never get diagnosed with mononucleosis. One in four adolescents and young adults infected with EBV, however, will get infectious mononucleosis. Other causes of infectious mononucleosis include cytomegalovirus (CMV), which is more common in adults between the age of 30 and 60. Once infected, the virus remains inactive (dormant), and while rare, it can be reactivated in immunocompromised states. Transmission occurs via saliva and less frequently with other body fluids such as blood and semen.

EBV causes a lymphocytosis, and cytotoxic (CD8+) lymphocytes infect B lymphocytes. Lymphoid tissue in the throat, lymph nodes, and spleen can all be affected. In CMV mononucleosis, the macrophages are infected as opposed to the B cell. Both B lymphocyte and macrophage infection lead to T-lymphocyte reactivity.

EBV and CMV infection may be clinically silent. The incubation period is between 4 and 6 weeks. If symptomology occurs, both usually cause a fever, sore throat, myalgia, and malaise. Physical examination may reveal lymphadenopathy and an exudative pharyngitis, which is more severe with EBV. Splenomegaly and hepatomegaly are more common in EBV infection, although overall this finding is not common. EBV infection can cause hepatitis due to T lymphocytes releasing cytokines in the liver, which get trapped. Jaundice is more likely in adults over 30 with EBV or CMV infection. The classic EBV mononucleosis presentation is more common in the 12–25 age group and consists of fever, sore throat, and neck lymphadenopathy. CMV is usually associated with more severe fatigue, and duration is longer than EBV mononucleosis. Symptoms last about 2–4 weeks but fatigue can last much longer.

Diagnosis and Treatment

Diagnosis is made based on the clinical presentation. EBV infection can be confirmed with several lab tests. A common, quick test is the monospot blood test. A complete blood count (CBC) may reveal increased bands, neutrophils, lymphocytes, reactive lymphocytes, and thrombocytopenia.

Diagnostic Link

Monospot

Antibody testing for EBV is commonly evaluated with the monospot. This tests evaluates proteins in the blood known as *heterophile antibodies* produced in response to EBV. These antibodies peak around 2 to 6 weeks after infection and can present in low levels for about a year. This test does have a 25% false negative rate because children (usually < 2 years old) do not produce heterophile antibodies, and some people do not produce them at any age. The test may be negative if EBV is not the cause or if it is done too early. Other EBV antibody testing (e.g., viral capsid antigen) testing is available.

Treatment of infectious mononucleosis is focused on symptom management. Analgesics can be used for fever and myalgias. Short-term oral glucocorticoids may be useful in cases of grossly enlarged tonsils or if airway obstruction is a concern. Antivirals are not usually necessary as the symptoms are a result of the immune response as opposed to viral replications, but they can be considered in some situations like chronic EBV. Contact sports are to be avoided due to the risk of splenic rupture and should not be resumed until splenomegaly is resolved, which occurs in a few weeks. Fatigue is common for up to two months but can continue for up to 6 months.

Complications of EBV mononucleosis can include splenic rupture. EBV infection is also a risk factor for the development of B cell lymphoma. Some complications of EBV and CMV infections include hemolytic anemia, thrombocytopenia, meningitis, myelitis, and Guillain-Barré syndrome and reactivation with immunosuppressive states. Prior CMV infection leads to the virus remaining latent in the body. The latent CMV is present in all solid organs, and the CMV infection can be reactivated when a transplantation occurs with subsequent immunosuppressive therapy.

Herpangina and Hand-Foot-and-Mouth Disease

Enteroviruses, particularly the **coxsackievirus**, are implicated in two conditions known as *herpangina* and *hand-foot-and-mouth disease*, which are more common in children. Transmission occurs from contaminated hands, respiratory secretions, and fecal matter. The incubation period is 4–6 days. In hand-foot-and-mouth disease, vesicles (small blisters) that can ulcerate appear mainly on the buccal mucosa and tongue. The vesicles can also be on the palate, tonsils, hands, and feet. In herpangina, the lesions are more toward the back of the mouth on the soft palate, uvula, and tonsils. The lesions are grayish-white papulovesicular (raised and blistery) sores that ulcerate. Usually fever, malaise, and odynophagia (painful swallowing) is present. Treatment is geared toward symptom relief, and both diseases are self-limiting and resolve in 7–10 days.

Bacterial Pharyngitis

Bacteria are another common cause of pharyngitis and usually result in an exudate on the tonsils and oropharynx. *Streptococcus pyogenes* is a group A beta-hemolytic (GABHS) bacteria that is responsible for up to 30% of pharyngitis cases in children and up to 15% in adults (CDC, 2016b). Other organisms such as *Mycoplasma* and *Chlamydia* species are also implicated in bacterial pharyngitis but are not as common. The peak prevalence is between the ages of 5 and 15 years. GABHS has an M protein on its cell surface, which resists phagocytosis. GABHS also has a polysaccharide capsule made of hyaluronic acid, which protects it from phagocytosis. Pharyngeal epithelial cells have $CD4_+$, which is a hyaluronic acid-binding protein, and this protein is one reason why GABHS infections manifest on the throat. The GABHS capsule binds with CD44, leading to colonization (the presence of an organism without evidence of infection). Transmission occurs through saliva and nasal secretions from person to person. The highest risk for infection is close contact with someone who is infected. Some people can be carriers and not have symptoms. Carriers can still transmit the infection but not as commonly as those with symptoms.

Clinical Manifestations

The incubation period for GABHS pharyngitis is 2–5 days. Clinical manifestations include a sudden sore throat, painful swallowing, and fever (> 100.4°F). Cough is usually absent. Physical exam will reveal cervical lymphadenopathy (anterior more common); tonsillar erythema, hypertrophy, and exudates (may also

be absent); and petechiae on the palate. A scarlatiniform rash can develop starting in the neck and chest and spreading throughout the body. The rash consists of numerous red papules.

The other less common causes of bacterial pharyngitis include *Chlamydia trachomatis*, *Neisseria gonorrhoeae*, and *Treponema pallidum* (syphilis), which are all sexually transmitted. Unvaccinated individuals can get pharyngitis from *Corynebacterium diphtheriae*. These bacteria will may cause different presentations. Diphtheria, for example, may cause the development of an adherent pseudomembrane that may appear grayish-green and bleeds when removal is attempted.

The diagnosis of bacterial pharyngitis is made clinically and can be confirmed with a rapid antigen detection test (RADT) or throat culture. These tests involve swabbing the throat. The results take about 20 minutes, and the cultures can take up to 48 hours. A throat culture should be completed if the results are negative, especially in children, because they have a higher likelihood of developing complications such as rheumatic fever and glomerulonephritis from GABHS.

Antibiotics are the mainstay of treatment in bacterial pharyngitis, and the choice is dependent on the organism (e.g., GABHS vs. gonorrhea). Infection can be self-limiting in GABHS, but antibiotics shorten the length of disease, reducing transmission and preventing complications from developing. Penicillin or amoxicillin is the first choice in GABHS. Other treatments are supportive (e.g., antipyretics, salt water gargles).

Epiglottitis

Epiglottitis is a life-threatening condition of the epiglottis, the protective cartilage lid covering the trachea opening. Epiglottitis is also known as *supraglottitis*. In the past, *Haemophilus influenzae* type b (Hib) was the most common cause in the United States, but widespread use of the Hib vaccine has dramatically decreased the rate of Hib infections in recent years. Common culprits now include group A beta-hemolytic *Streptococcus*, *Streptococcus pneumoniae*, and *Staphylococcus aureus*. Other noninfectious causes include throat trauma from events such as drinking hot liquids, swallowing a foreign object, a direct blow to the throat, or smoking crack or heroin.

Regardless of the cause, the inflammatory response is triggered, causing, the epiglottis (particularly the supraglottis) to quickly swell and block the air entering the trachea. The swelling and obstruction can lead to respiratory failure. The bacteria can also travel to the bloodstream, leading to life-threatening sepsis. Adults have an upper airway that is wider and more rigid than that of children and is, therefore, less predisposed to getting an obstruction with epiglottitis; however, obstruction can occur in adults and should not be overlooked.

Clinical Manifestations

The onset of clinical manifestations is typically rapid in children, developing in a matter of hours, but it occurs more slowly in adults, over a few days. The manifestations include high fever, sore throat, muffled quality speech ("hot potato voice"), dysphagia (swallowing difficulty), drooling with an open mouth, inspiratory stridor, and subsequent hypoxemic signs such as central cyanosis, pallor, irritability, anxiety, and restlessness. A child may assume a forward-leaning sitting position in an attempt to facilitate breathing (tripod position). Respiratory distress and failure can follow. The throat should not be examined as it may precipitate laryngospasm and worsen the obstruction.

Diagnosis and Treatment

If epiglottitis is suspected, maintaining the airway and stabilizing respiratory status is the priority before diagnostic procedures are performed. Efforts to preserve respiratory function include humidified oxygen therapy (likely delivered via mask), endotracheal intubation with mechanical ventilation, and tracheotomy. Additional efforts to minimize oxygen consumption should include keeping the patient calm and controlling fever (e.g., with antipyretics and hydration). Aerosolized epinephrine and systemic steroids (often treatments for croup) should be avoided because they may worsen the condition. Once the patient is stabilized, diagnostic procedures include visualization of the epiglottis through a fiber-optic camera, X-rays (neck and chest), cultures (throat and blood), arterial blood gases (ABGs), and a CBC. The neck X-ray on lateral view may have a "thumbprint sign," which is created by the edematous epiglottis.

Intravenous antibiotics will be used to treat infections quickly. Hib vaccinations should be encouraged for children, the elderly, and immunocompromised persons so transmission rates will continue to be low. Other prevention strategies include proper hand washing, avoiding crowds, cleaning objects such as toys, and not sharing objects like pacifiers and bottles.

Peritonsillar Abscess

One of the complications of a tonsillitis or pharyngeal infection is the development of an abscess (accumulation of pus). The abscesses can be in the peritonsillar, retropharyngeal, and lateral pharyngeal areas. The infections are often polymicrobial (e.g., *Staphylococcus aureus*, *Streptococcus pyogenes*). Noninfectious causes include trauma from foreign body or procedures (e.g., intubation, endoscopy). Clinical manifestations are similar to other pharyngeal infections in the beginning with dysphagia (may be one side), odynophagia, drooling, fever, and voice quality changes. Airway obstruction is possible, and evaluating the respiratory status is a priority as an abscess can be difficult to distinguish from epiglottitis. Physical examination may be difficult due to trismus (jaw locking). If the throat can be examined, there will usually be a unilateral (rarely bilateral) swelling of the tonsil with exudate, asymmetry of the soft palate, and uvula displacement to the opposite side. If there is any concern that epiglottitis may be present, examination should not be conducted. Radiographic imaging or CT with contrast can aid in diagnosis. A CBC, electrolytes to evaluate hydration status, blood cultures, and ABG may be necessary.

In patients with airway compromise, management focuses on stabilizing the airway and may include intubation or tracheotomy. Intravenous antibiotics, hydration, and pain control are other treatment strategies. Incision and drainage of the abscess results in resolution in most cases. Drainage can be accomplished with topical anesthesia and a needle aspiration or with an incision. Either procedure should be done by an experienced clinician or otolaryngologist as hemorrhage and pus may accumulate in the airway, leading to respiratory compromise. Some patients such as young children may require drainage under general anesthesia. Tonsillectomy is another surgical alternative.

Laryngitis

Laryngitis is an inflammation of the larynx. With laryngitis, the vocal cords become irritated and edematous and vibrate irregularly because of the inflammatory process. This inflammation distorts sounds, leading to hoarseness that is harsh and voice quality changes or aphonia (voice loss). Acute laryngitis is the most common cause of hoarseness and is usually the result of the same viral organisms (e.g., rhinovirus) that also cause other URIs.

BOX 5-1 Application to Practice

Review the pharyngitis cases and answer the questions.

Case 1: Susan is a 16-year-old with sudden onset of severe sore throat for the past day. She feels like she had a fever but did not check her temperature (i.e., subjective fever). She states it is very painful to swallow, and she thinks she sees white spots on her throat. She denies cough, rhinorrhea, nausea, otalgia, shortness of breath, or headache. She reports no exposure to sick individuals.

Medications: none
Allergies: none
Social history: nonsmoker and drinks alcohol (two to three beers) one to two times a month.

Physical exam:
Vital signs: temperature 101.0°F, pulse 100 per minute, respiration rate 18 per minute; blood pressure 110/66 mmHg.
General: ill and tired appearance.
Head, Eyes, Ears, Nose, and Throat unremarkable except for erythematous oropharynx with small petechiae and white tonsillar exudates.
Neck: anterior cervical lymphadenopathy; two on right, three on left; all small (< 0.5 cm) and tender.
Cardiovascular, lungs, abdomen are unremarkable.

What is the most likely diagnosis and pathogen causing this disorder and mode of transmission?
Discuss data that support your decision.
What diagnostic test, if any, should be done?
Develop a treatment plan for this patient.

Case 2: Mr. Jones is a 54-year-old man with complaints of a scratchy, raw sore throat and painful swallowing, mild productive cough, and runny nose for the past 2 days. He says his sputum is whitish-yellow. His ears feel full, and he feels like he is getting a achy. He reports taking throat lozenges and denies nausea, fever, shortness of breath, chest pain, or headache. He states he teaches in a high school and a lot of his students have had colds.

Medications: none.
Allergies: none.

Social history: nonsmoker and does not drink alcohol.

Physical exam:
Vital signs: temperature 99.0°F, pulse 84 per minute; respiratory rate 18 per minute; blood pressure 120/70 mmHg.
General: cough during exam.
HEENT: unremarkable except for mild erythematous oropharynx with no exudates; nares with mild erythema and scant yellowish discharge.
Neck, CV, lungs, abdomen are unremarkable.

What is the most likely diagnosis and pathogen causing this disorder and mode of transmission?
Discuss data that support your decision.
What diagnostic test, if any, should be done?
Develop a treatment plan for this patient.
Compare the causes, clinical manifestations, diagnosis and treatment of pharyngitis in these two cases.

Occasionally, the airway can become blocked. Bacteria such as *Streptococcus pneumoniae*, *Haemophilus influenzae*, and *Moraxella catarrhalis* can also cause laryngitis. Laryngitis can also be associated with croup and epiglottitis. Noninfectious causes of laryngitis include irritants (e.g., stomach acid, inhaled smoke, excessive alcohol use, or chemicals) or overuse (e.g., screaming, singing). These noninfectious causes can cause acute or chronic laryngitis.

Clinical Manifestations

Clinical manifestations of laryngitis can include hoarseness, a weak voice or aphonia, and a tickling sensation and raw feeling in the throat. The throat may feel dry and other symptoms of URI manifestations such as rhinorrhea and cough may be present. Laryngitis symptoms usually persist about a week longer than other URI symptoms.

Diagnosis and Treatment

Diagnosis of acute laryngitis is based on clinical presentation, and diagnostic testing is not indicated. Treatment strategies aim to increase comfort or decrease the duration of the inflammation and includes resting the voice and warm humidification. Decongestants, antihistamines, and corticosteroids can dry out the mucous membranes and may lead to worsening of symptoms.

Acute laryngitis from viral infections or overuse is usually self-limiting. Lack of proper voice rest and shouting/singing; however, may lead to trauma and hemorrhage in the vocal cords or to the development of cysts and polyps during cases of laryngitis. Persistent laryngitis, usually beyond 2 weeks, or chronic hoarseness or voice quality changes may be indicative other disorders such as vocal cord cysts, polyps, granulomas, or ulcers. Smoking is a cause of laryngeal disorders and squamous cell laryngeal cancer and should be considered in evaluating laryngitis. Nodules on the vocal cords can develop in singers or with frequent screaming. The vocal cords can become paralyzed either unilaterally or bilaterally due to many causes such as vagal or laryngeal nerve damage from neck surgery. The cause of the paralysis could also be idiopathic. Laryngopharyngeal reflux caused by gastric acid can cause hoarseness, and it may be present with or without signs of gastroesophageal reflux (e.g., heartburn). All of these diseases require laryngoscopic evaluation. Management is based on the cause.

Laryngotracheobronchitis

Laryngotracheobronchitis, or croup, is a common viral infection in children 3 months to 3 years of age, but it can occur in older children and adults. The most common causes are parainfluenza viruses. Other viruses include adenoviruses and respiratory syncytial virus, and bacterial causes include *Mycoplasma pneumoniae*. Noninfectious causes include allergens and irritants (e.g., stomach acid, inhaled smoke, or chemicals). Outbreaks and epidemics occur in autumn and early winter coinciding with increased viral syndromes, but cases can occur sporadically year-round. Croup was once a deadly disease caused by diphtheria bacteria, but the introduction of antibiotics and immunizations have improved its prevention and treatment. Today, most cases of croup are mild. Nevertheless, this disease can still be dangerous as severe upper airway obstruction can occur.

Croup generally affects the larynx and trachea and leads to edema of the subglottic area and may extend to the bronchi. The subglottic tissue, as with other areas of the larynx, is looser, allowing for edema to develop readily. This edema leads to airway narrowing and obstruction.

Clinical Manifestations

Croup usually begins as an upper respiratory infection with rhinorrhea, fever, and sore throat. Signs and symptoms, 1 to 2 days later, progress to hoarseness and a seallike barking cough because of laryngeal swelling. Inspiratory stridor, cyanosis, altered level of consciousness, impaired air entry, and retractions may be present. These five symptoms form part of the Westley score to determine the severity of croup. The worse these symptoms (e.g., stridor at rest, decreased air entry, severe retractions), the higher the score. Noninfectious causes of croup can present with similar symptoms but occur more suddenly, resolve quickly, and occur more often in older children.

Diagnosis and Treatment

Diagnosis is usually made on clinical evaluation, and diagnostic tests are usually not necessary. If diagnostic testing is done, it may include a nasopharyngeal swab to determine viral antigen. Depending on presentation, other diagnostic tests may include a CBC, ABGs, and neck X-ray, which may reveal a narrowing of the upper trachea (often referred to as the *steeple sign* because the narrowing looks like a church steeple) in 50% of cases (FIGURE 5-15).

Croup is usually self-limiting, but if severe, cases can be life threatening without supportive therapy. Treatment strategies include cool humidity, corticosteroids to decrease edema, humidified oxygen (which can be administered via an oxygen tent over an infant's crib), and hydration to combat fever, moisten the airway, and liquefy secretions. Aerosolized epinephrine's (alpha and beta) adrenergic effects can reduce secretions and edema but epinephrine is usually reserved for severe cases. Heliox (a mixture of helium and oxygen) can also be used for cases of severe airway narrowing. Heliox

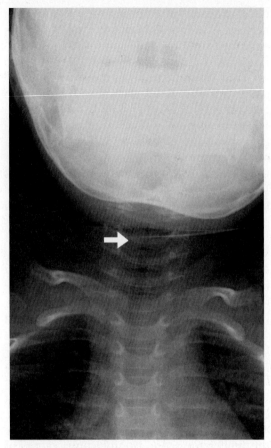

FIGURE 5-15 Steeple sign.
Courtesy of Hugh Dainer, MD, PhD.

decreases airway resistance, which reduces the work of breathing. Cool humidity may decrease edema, but no studies have supported this treatment. This intervention should be avoided in patients with asthma because it may trigger bronchial constriction. Cool humidity can be accomplished with a cool-mist humidifier, exposure to cool outside air especially at night, and exposure to a cold shower mist in a closed bathroom. Strategies to decrease oxygen consumption include keeping the patient calm and avoiding unnecessary procedures. Additionally, educating the public regarding diphtheria vaccination compliance is critical to manage this once life-threatening condition.

Influenza

Influenza, or flu, is a viral infection that may affect the upper and lower respiratory tract. Influenza viruses are known as *orthomyxoviruses*, and three types are distinguished—A, B, and C.

- Type A influenza, which includes several subtypes, is the most common type of influenza virus. This type is usually responsible for the most serious epidemics and global

pandemics (worldwide epidemics), such as those that occurred in the United States in 1918, 1957, 1968, and 2009. A subgroup of type A is H1N1, colloquially referred to as the *swine flu*, which was responsible for a serious pandemic that started in the United States and Mexico in 2009. Type A influenza goes through continual antigenic changes. These changes make type A highly adaptive and constantly mutating, which in turn prevents the development of any long-term immune defense.

- Type B influenza outbreaks can also cause regional epidemics, but the disease is generally milder than that caused by type A. Type B can have antigenic change at times but to a lesser degree than A.
- Type C influenza causes sporadic cases and minor, local outbreaks. Type C has never been connected with a large epidemic. Type C is antigenically stable.

Type A influenza viruses are found in humans and many animals (e.g., ducks, chickens, pigs, and whales). Type B is isolated primarily in humans, whereas type C is found in humans, pigs, and dogs. Type A influenza has been found in aquatic birds for years without causing harm to them, but recently this frequently mutating flu virus has shown that it can jump the species barrier from wild birds to domesticated poultry and swine. Pigs can be infected by avian and human flu, especially in areas where human contact is frequent. If a pig becomes infected with the avian and human flu simultaneously, the two types may exchange genes. This exchange leads to a reassortment and what is termed an *antigenic shift*, which is abrupt and causes severe outbreaks. When infectivity occurs in the body, it does not recognize the animal component, so antibodies are not produced and immunity does not develop. The other human component allows replication. Immunity, therefore, does not occur. This lack of immunity development is usually how pandemics start. Since influenza B and C are primarily in humans, reassortment between species (e.g., humans and animals) does not occur, so the antigenic changes (i.e., antigenic drift) lead to new strains and spread occurs slowly. Reassorted flu can sometimes spread from pigs to humans and may cause a more or less severe strain. In 1997, scientists found that a form of avian H5N1 flu skipped the pig step and infected humans directly for the first time. Alarmed health officials feared a pandemic.

Fortunately, the virus could not pass from person to person, so it did not spark an epidemic. As of July 2018, 860 human cases of the avian flu virus have been confirmed worldwide, which resulted in 454 deaths (World Health Organization [WHO], 2018a).

Millions of Americans contract the flu each year. The flu season (i.e., when the incidence is the highest) in the United States is typically between October and March. The virus is transmitted through the inhalation of or contact with respiratory droplets. Children are two to three times more likely than adults to contract the flu, and children frequently spread the virus to others. The 2015–2016 U.S. flu season saw mostly influenza type A (H1N1 and H3N2) (CDC, 2016a). The 2017–2018 flu season was less severe and did not reach the pandemic levels of the 2009–2010 season (CDC, 2018). The 2017–2018 season was the first season to be classified as high severity with mostly cases of type A (H3N2). The 2017–2018 flu season peaked close to levels seen in 2009, and the duration was longer than in other seasons (≥ 19 weeks). The 2017–2018 saw high levels of outpatient visits for influenza-like illness and rates of hospitalization. The number of reported deaths attributed to pneumonia and influenza was at or above epidemic levels compared with recent years, and the number of pediatric deaths was higher than in other years. Persons at greater risk for having negative outcomes because of the flu include children; elderly people; pregnant women; individual who are immunocompromised; those who are severely obese (with a body mass index of 40 or higher); and those with preexisting chronic diseases such as asthma, cardiovascular disease, diabetes mellitus, or kidney disease.

The antigen changes that occur with influenza and lead to the development of various subtypes of type A are categorized by two surface glycoproteins hemagglutinin (HA) and neuraminidase (NA). Antibodies are directed mainly toward the HA, which is a protein continually evolving into new strains. On the surface of the virus, HA has large globules, and on these globules is a pocket, which is the viral attachment site. Antibodies are unable to penetrate this pocket. The NA glycoprotein is involved in the viral replication cycle by helping to release viral particles. NA may also help the virus penetrate the mucin in the respiratory tract, so it could then reach the epithelial cells.

The influenza virus is unique because of the continual antigenic changes of HA and NA.

Other respiratory viruses do not display significant antigenic changes. The virus changes due to gene mutations that accumulate. The immune system allows these new antigen variants to flourish. This process eventually leads to a new strain.

Once a person is infected by the virus, replication occurs quickly as the virus shuts down the host cell protein synthesis for 3 hours. This short shutdown allows for viral proliferation. The influenza virus has an incubation period of 1–4 days, with peak transmission risk starting at approximately 1 day before onset of symptoms and lasting 4–7 days afterward in adults. The innate immune system releases interferon, which has an antiviral effect and is part of the recovery process. Acquired immunity (humoral/antibody and cell mediated) responses are not seen until 7–14 days after infection. Cytotoxic T lymphocytes attack the viral internal proteins and external glycoproteins. Children can be infectious for more than 10 days, and young children can spread the virus for 6 days before the onset of symptoms. Severely immunocompromised persons can spread the virus for weeks or months. Flu differs from infectious rhinitis (common cold) in that the flu usually has a sudden onset of symptoms (**TABLE 5-2**).

TABLE 5-2	Comparison of Infectious Rhinitis and Influenza Manifestations	
Symptoms	Infectious rhinitis	Influenza
Fever	Rare	Usual; high (100°F to 102°F, but occasionally higher, especially in young children); lasts 3–4 days
Headache	Rare	Common
Myalgia	Slight	Usual; often severe
Malaise	Sometimes	Usual; can last up to 3 weeks
Exhaustion	Never	Usual; at the beginning of the illness
Stuffy nose	Common	Sometimes
Sneezing	Usual	Sometimes
Sore throat	Common	Sometimes
Chest discomfort, cough	Mild to moderate, nonproductive cough	Common; can be severe

Modified from National Institutes of Allergy and Infectious Disease. (2008). Is it the cold or the flu? Retrieved from http://www.niaid.nih.gov/topics/Flu/Documents/sick.pdf

Clinical Manifestations

Clinical manifestations occur as a result of the immune response (e.g., mononuclear infiltration, cytokine release). The signs and symptoms common with the flu include fever, chills, headache, myalgia, malaise, exhaustion, and a nonproductive cough with chest discomfort. Other clinical manifestations are similar to those found in infectious viral rhinitis but are not as common and include nasal congestion, sore throat, and watery rhinorrhea. Vomiting and diarrhea occur more often in children than adults. Typically, fever and body aches last 3–5 days, while rhinitis, cough, and fatigue may last for 2 or more weeks. Physical examination findings are usually similar to those in viral URIs (e.g., cervical lymphadenopathy and erythematous oropharynx and nasal passages).

Diagnosis and Treatment

Diagnosis is usually made clinically, particularly if a patient has manifestations during the flu season and when there are known outbreaks. However, diagnostic tests may be important if diagnosis is questionable or if a patient is immunocompromised or has signs of a severe respiratory illness. There are several diagnostic tests used to evaluate for the influenza virus. These influenza tests can detect parts of the virus (i.e., antigen), or genetic testing of the virus (e.g., viral RNA, nucleic acid testing) can be done. Some tests can distinguish between types such as A or B. The test results can be ready within 30 minutes. Viral culture results can be obtained anywhere from 1–10 days after collection. Treatment is symptomatic and supportive unless a secondary bacterial infection is present. Antiviral medications such as amantadine or rimantadine are known as *M2 ion inhibitors* and are useful for type A influenza; however, these drugs are not recommended unless similar strains that were responsive return due to drug resistance. Zanamivir, oseltamivir (Tamiflu), and peramivir are NA inhibitors that can be used for type A or B to reduce the severity and duration of the symptoms. Resistance can occur and is more common in children. Baloxavir marboxil (Xofluza) is a newer category of medication for the flu that inhibits polymerase acidic endonuclease, which is necessary for viral reproduction. It prevents replication while NA inhibitors stop the release of the virus. Only one dose is necessary in comparison to oseltamivir, which requires at least 10 days of administration. Both are only effective if taken within 48 hours of exposure. Antivirals can be given on a post-exposure basis as a preventive measure to decrease the likelihood of developing the flu. Other treatment strategies include increased fluid intake, adequate rest, antipyretics, and analgesics.

Complications can occur from the flu. The damaged respiratory epithelium is vulnerable to secondary bacterial pathogens such as staphylococci, streptococci, and *Haemophilus influenzae* as well as other viral pathogens. These pathogens invade the lower respiratory system, causing pneumonia. More commonly, the pneumonia is caused by a combination of a virus and bacteria. The staphylococcal bacteria split the HA glycoprotein, allowing for high levels of virus to infect the lungs. Deaths associated with the flu are often a result of secondary bacterial pneumonia. Although rare, influenza A and B can cause acute encephalopathy (Reye syndrome) in children and adolescents.

Prevention strategies are similar to those used to prevent the common cold (e.g., hand washing and avoiding crowds) but also include vaccinations. Currently, vaccinations exist for the seasonal flu and H1N1 flu (if warranted). Four types of seasonal flu vaccinations are produced—regular seasonal flu vaccine (the form most commonly administered to people 6 months and older), high-dose vaccine (for people age 65 and older), intradermal vaccine (for people age 18–64), and intranasal flu vaccine, which is approved for healthy, nonpregnant people age 2–49. The intranasal vaccine is attenuated (live), and the other types are inactivated. Prior to each flu season (usually before the previous season is over), the CDC develops a seasonal flu vaccine based on predictions of the likely strain to be encountered. In the United States, the seasonal flu vaccine should be administered each year in October, but it may be recommended to be administered again in February. The vaccine is recommended to everyone age 6 months and older, especially those in high-risk groups (e.g., persons with a chronic medical condition or who are immunocompromised persons age 50 years or older or those between 6 months to less than 5 years, those who are pregnant, persons living in a community setting, and those who are caregivers or have contact with anyone in any of these groups). When outbreaks of other types of the flu occur, as with the H1N1 influenza in 2009, the CDC develops vaccinations specific for those strains.

Myth Busters

A common misconception is that you can get the flu from the flu vaccine. What fuels this myth is that some people may experience very mild flulike symptoms (e.g., low-grade fever, aches, malaise) after receiving the vaccination. These symptoms do not occur because the individual has a mild case of the flu; rather, they are due to the process through which the immune system develops antibodies against the virus. An additional factor fueling this myth is the possibility that people may still have the flu even after receiving the vaccination. This infection is not caused by the flu vaccine; rather, it occurs because the person encountered a strain of the flu that was not covered by the vaccination. Remember, the vaccination is based on predictions. Negative outcomes from the flu vaccine are rare and minimal. So get vaccinated and encourage others to do the same!

Reproduced from Story, L. (2017). *Pathophysiology: A practical approach* (3rd ed.). Burlington, MA: Jones & Bartlett Learning.

Vaccine development can be a lengthy process. In many cases, the vaccines are grown in fertilized chicken eggs for approximately 10 months. Therefore, flu vaccines should not be administered to persons with egg allergies. Additionally, children younger than 6 months and people with a history of Guillain-Barré syndrome should not be vaccinated. People with an active febrile illness should wait to be vaccinated until after the illness resolves.

Lower Respiratory Tract Infections

The lower respiratory tract includes the trachea, bronchi, bronchioles, and alveoli. Infections can have similar manifestations to upper respiratory tract infections. URIs can progress to lower respiratory tract infections. Lower respiratory tract infections can be life threatening such as with pneumonia. Laryngotracheobronchitis spans across the upper and lower tracts but is discussed in the *Upper Respiratory Tract Infections* section.

Acute Bronchitis

Acute bronchitis is an inflammation of the tracheobronchial tree or large bronchi. This inflammation is most commonly caused by a wide range of viruses (e.g., influenza, rhinovirus, respiratory syncytial virus, and adenovirus). Bacterial invasions, which are not as common, can include *Chlamydiae pneumoniae*, *Mycoplasma pneumoniae*, and *Bordetella pertussis*. Secondary bacterial infections can occur after a viral infection and are usually caused by *Streptococcus pneumoniae* and *Haemophilus influenzae*. Secondary bacterial infections are more likely to occur in those with chronic obstructive pulmonary disease (COPD). In most cases, a pathogen cannot be identified. Noninfectious causes of acute bronchitis are less frequent and include irritant inhalation (e.g., smoke, marijuana, pollution, and ammonia) and allergic reactions. Young children, the elderly, and smokers are at the highest risk for developing acute bronchitis. In acute bronchitis, the bronchial lining becomes irritated, and the airways become narrowed due to the results of the inflammatory process (e.g., capillary dilation, edema, and exudate).

Clinical Manifestations

Clinical manifestations of acute bronchitis are usually mild and resolve in 7–10 days, but coughing may linger for several weeks after the infection is resolved. Acute bronchitis often begins with a nonproductive cough as the key complaint, but the cough can become productive. The cough is paroxysmal (sudden outburst), and musculoskeletal chest pain often occurs due to the coughing. The chest pain is usually retrosternal. Due to the inflammation, the airways may narrow and cause wheezing, which may be intermittent. Patients can have other symptoms similar to pneumonia such as fever, chills, malaise, and shortness of breath. Physical exam may reveal oropharynx erythema and neck lymphadenopathy. Wheezing may be present along with rhonchi and crackles; however, pulmonary consolidation signs (e.g., dullness to percussion) are absent. If consolidation signs are present, pneumonia is the probable diagnosis.

Diagnosis and Treatment

Diagnosis of acute bronchitis is usually made based on clinical evaluation. Diagnostic tests such as a CBC and cultures (e.g., nasal secretions, sputum, blood) may be considered but are not necessary to confirm diagnosis. Chest X-ray findings will be normal and without evidence of an infiltrate or consolidation.

Acute bronchitis is generally self-limiting; therefore, treatment is supportive. Pharmacologic treatment may include antipyretics, analgesics, antihistamines, decongestants, cough suppressants, bronchodilators, and antibiotics in cases of bacterial infection. Cough suppressants should be used cautiously, as coughing mobilizes secretions and can prevent pneumonia. Other strategies include increasing fluid intake, avoiding smoke, and breathing humidified air.

Bronchiolitis

Bronchiolitis refers to a common acute inflammation of the bronchioles that usually results from a viral infection. The most common virus is the respiratory syncytial virus (RSV). Other viruses include parainfluenza, influenza, adenoviruses, and metapneumoviruses (an emerging paramyxovirus). Bronchiolitis often occurs in children younger than 1 year of age, and the incidence increases in the fall and winter months. According to the CDC (2017c), 2.1 million children younger than the age of 5 years seek medical attention annually for RSV infection, and nearly all children will have an RSV infection by the time they are 2 years old.

When the virus infects the bronchioles, these small airways become inflamed and swollen. The cell mediated response to the antigens results in the mobilization of eosinophils, neutrophils, monocytes, and lymphokines (e.g., interleukin, interferon), which initiate the inflammatory process. As a result of the inflammatory process, cellular debris from destroyed epithelial cells and mucus collects in these small airways. Bronchospasm may further occlude the airways. The airway obstruction leads to trapping of air and hyperinflation. Atelectasis (collapse of the alveoli) and ventilation problems occur as expiration is impaired, all leading to increasing breathing difficulties. Transmission of RSV occurs through contact with or inhalation of infected respiratory droplets. Factors contributing to the development of bronchiolitis include neonatal prematurity, asthma family history, and cigarette smoke exposure.

Clinical Manifestations

Clinical manifestations of bronchiolitis vary in severity and include the following: rhinorrhea, cough, decreased appetite, malaise, and fever.

Varying degrees of respiratory distress such as dyspnea, tachypnea, tachycardia, expiratory wheezing, rales or rhonchi, rapid shallow respirations, and labored breathing (e.g., retractions, nasal flaring, and grunting) may be present. Severe cases may alter chest structure by increasing the anterior–posterior diameter (like a barrel), and if there is significant swallowing of air, the abdomen can become distended.

Diagnosis and Treatment

Diagnosis is usually made by clinical evaluation. Other diagnostic procedures may include a CBC and ABGs. Nasal specimens may be evaluated for RSV. A routine chest X-ray is also not necessary unless complications or comorbidities are suspected. Depending on the severity, the chest X-ray may reveal hyperexpansion (air gets trapped in lungs and they get overinflated) and infiltrates (accumulation of abnormal substances in interstitium or alveoli). Treatment strategies are geared towards symptoms as no specific therapy exists. These strategies include oxygen therapy, cool humidity, suctioning secretions, increased fluids (either by mouth or intravenously), keeping the patient calm, bronchodilators, and corticosteroids. Mild cases can be managed on an outpatient basis. Patients with severe cases or children at risk for decompensation (e.g., lung or heart disease, immunocompromise) will need to be hospitalized. Atelectasis and respiratory failure require more aggressive treatment and possible intubation with ventilator support.

Prevention strategies are the same as those previously discussed for other infectious respiratory conditions (e.g., hand washing). RSV has two glycoproteins—F glycoprotein, which attaches to the membrane of the target cell, and G glycoprotein, which targets the cilia in the airway. The vaccine palivizumab is a monoclonal antibody that binds to the F glycoprotein on RSV, preventing the virus from infecting the cells. This vaccine can be given to at-risk infants during RSV season to prevent and minimize infection. Other vaccines for RSV are in development but are not yet commercially available. Bronchiolitis may be linked to asthma development.

Pneumonia

Pneumonia is an inflammatory process of the lung parenchyma. The parenchyma is the portion of the lungs where gas transfer occurs and includes the respiratory bronchioles, alveolar ducts, and alveoli. Pneumonia is usually caused by infectious agents (e.g., bacteria, viruses, and fungi), but parenchymal injury with inflammation can occur through inhalation of chemicals such as smoke or from aspiration (e.g., stomach contents). According to the CDC (2017b), pneumonia accounts for 1.1 million hospitalizations and nearly 52,000 deaths in the United States annually.

Treatment decisions and prognosis are based on identification of the cause of pneumonia. The identification of specific causative pathogens in pneumonia can be challenging, and several categorizations of pneumonia exist. These categorizations include individual risk characteristics (e.g., immunocompromise, advanced age, underlying lung diseases, and alcoholism) and anatomic lung distribution involvement (e.g., lobar, bronchopneumonia, and interstitial pneumonia). Other categories include location of acquisition such as **community-acquired pneumonia** and **hospital-acquired pneumonia** [HAP]). The pathogen prevalent for each location, individual risks, and anatomic location can vary.

The gram-positive bacteria, *Streptococcus pneumoniae* (i.e., pneumococcal pneumonia) is responsible for most cases of community-acquired pneumonia. Other gram-positive organisms are *Haemophilus influenzae* and *Staphylococcus aureus*. Gram-negative bacilli include *Klebsiella pneumoniae* and *Pseudomonas aeruginosa*. **Atypical pneumonia** refers to infections with atypical organisms, which includes *Mycoplasma pneumoniae*, *Chlamydia pneumoniae*, and *Legionella* species. The term *atypical* is used clinically as the pneumonia from these pathogens may not respond to usual antibiotics, and symptoms and X-ray findings may be slightly different than pneumonia from typical pathogens. HAP is a pneumonia that occurs 48 hours after admission to a hospital, and another group is **ventilator-associated pneumonia** which develops 48 hours after intubation. HAP and ventilator-associated pneumonia causes are numerous and can be polymicrobial; the causes include organisms such *S. aureus, P. aeruginosa, Klebsiella,* and *Enterobacter*. Viruses can also be a common cause of pneumonia. Immunocompromised patients are at high risk for pneumonia from fungal infections.

Pathogens can enter the lung parenchyma as a result of aspirating oropharyngeal secretions or inhaling particles in the air through coughing, sneezing, or particles that have been aerosolized from equipment such as a respiratory mask. The introduction of devices such as endotracheal tubes and suction catheters can be a portal of entry for pathogens. Contiguous (adjacent) spread occurs when a site close to the lung is infected and causes a direct spread of the pathogen to the lung (e.g., amebic liver abscess). Another route for pathogens to enter the lungs is hematogenously (via bloodstream). The hematogenous mechanism is not as common but can occur with central line infection, urinary tract infection, endocarditis, or from any other bacteremic process.

Once the pathogen has entered the lungs, the innate immune defenses are activated. The first line of defense can become overwhelmed if the pathogen is sufficiently virulent, is present in large numbers, and/or the person has risk factors such as smoking or pre-existing lung disease (e.g., cystic fibrosis). The spongy character of the lung facilitates movement of pathogens. Some epithelial cells in the airway can recognize pathogens such as *Pseudomonas aeruginosa* or *Staphylococcus* and continue to mount a defense. The key defense cells, however, are the alveolar macrophages. These macrophages have pattern recognition receptors that can recognize a limited number of pathogens. This early detection leads to the activation of neutrophils, lymphocytes, platelets, and fibrinogen that travel to the site of infection. Macrophages, mast cells, and other cells release cytokines and chemokines (e.g., tumor necrosis factor-alpha, IL-1). Antigens are presented to the adaptive immune system

Diagnostic Link

Chest X-Ray: Consolidation

An X-ray involves the use of electromagnetic waves to create images. Different tissues absorb different amounts of radiation, and therefore the images are in shades of black and white. Tissue density refers to the amount of radiation absorption, and objects with higher density are termed *radiopaque* and appear white while objects with lower density are radiolucent and appear black. In between are various shades of gray. Bones absorb more radiation and are dense and appear white (radiopaque). Fat and soft tissue are less dense and absorb less and have a gray appearance. Air absorbs the least amount of radiation and appears black (radiolucent). A consolidation on a chest X-ray refers to alveoli that have fluid, blood, pus, or other substances. Consolidations are dense and cause opacities (white areas). The opacities can be focal (lobar), diffuse, or multifocal. Pneumonia is the most common cause of consolidation, and different pathogens can produce different patterns (e.g., streptococcal pneumonia is lobar).

(B and T cells) to further fight the infection. Neutrophils phagocytize pathogens and create a proteinlike mesh called a *neutrophil extracellular trap* in an attempt to trap bacteria. The inflammatory process ensues; bronchial, alveolar, and capillary membranes become damaged, and fluid goes into the interstitial space. A high-protein content exudate develops. The exudate and cell debris accumulate in the alveoli and bronchioles, impairing gas exchange and causing dyspnea and hypoxemia. The mixture of white blood cells, red blood cells, and fibrin fill areas of the lung affected by the infection and lead to a consolidation (inflamed, solid area). The consolidated area may be detected through physical exam (e.g., dullness to percussion) or chest X-ray.

Legionnaires' disease is a specific type of pneumonia that is caused by *Legionella pneumophilia*. These bacteria thrive in warm, moist environments (e.g., air-conditioning systems, standing fresh water, respiratory therapy equipment, and whirlpools), and most people acquire this type of pneumonia from inhaling the bacteria. Persons with a weakened immune system are at highest risk for developing legionnaires' disease. Although most people with this type of pneumonia recover without incident, the disease can be fatal if untreated. Symptoms are similar to other types of pneumonia and usually appear 10–14 days postexposure. Additional symptoms may include nausea, vomiting, and diarrhea. In addition to the usual pneumonia diagnostic procedures, a urine test can be performed to identify the presence of *Legionella* antigens. Legionnaires' disease treatment is similar to that of other pneumonias.

Viral pneumonias can be caused directly by influenza virus, adenoviruses, paramyxovirus (e.g., metapneumovirus, RSV). Having other viral diseases such as varicella (chickenpox) or rubeola (measles) can lead to the development of viral pneumonia. **Severe acute respiratory syndrome** (SARS) is a respiratory illness that presents similarly to atypical pneumonia. SARS is caused by a coronavirus, SARS-CoV. First identified in China, its prevalence rates remain higher in Asian countries. Transmission occurs through inhalation of respiratory droplets or close contact, although oral–fecal contact may also be a mechanism of transmission. SARS has high mortality and morbidity rates. The incubation period for this disease is 2–7 days. The first stage presents as a flulike syndrome (e.g., fever, chills, headache, myalgia, anorexia, and diarrhea) that lasts 3–7 days. Several days later, a dry cough and dyspnea develop as the lungs become damaged and the patient moves into the second stage of the disease. Interstitial congestion and hypoxia progress rapidly. Additionally, liver damage can occur. If the patient continues to the third stage, severe and sometimes fatal respiratory distress can develop. Diagnostic procedures for SARS consist of a history, physical examination, and chest X-ray. Treatment focuses on maintaining oxygenation and respiratory status, with strategies including oxygen therapy, bronchodilators, and antiviral drugs. Endotracheal intubation with mechanical ventilation support may be required as hypoxia worsens.

An emerging illness in the same coronavirus family is **Middle East respiratory syndrome** (MERS-CoV). It was first reported in Saudi Arabia in 2012 and has since spread to several other countries, including the United States (CDC, 2017a). Between its discovery in April 2012 and May 2018, 2,200 cases and 790 deaths from this disease were reported worldwide (WHO, 2018b). The virus is currently isolated to four countries in the Arabian Peninsula. Dromedary camels are hosts, and there can be camel-to-human transmission and human-to-human transmission, but the CDC is still working on better understanding the virus (CDC, 2017c).

Most healthy people do not develop pneumonia from fungal exposure. Instead, many of these illnesses occur as opportunistic infections, which can be fatal in immunocompromised individuals (e.g., children and persons with AIDS or cancer). *Pneumocystis jiroveci* pneumonia, formerly known as *Pneumocystis carinii* pneumonia, is a specific type of pneumonia that is caused by yeastlike fungus. Diagnosis is accomplished through identification of the fungus through a sputum culture. Aggressive and early treatment will improve outcomes in these vulnerable patients. Other fungal-related pneumonias include histoplasmosis, coccidioidomycosis, and cryptococcal pneumonia.

In addition to previously discussed risk factors, persons at risk for developing pneumonia from any cause and having serious complications include children, the elderly, immunocompromised individuals, those with existing chronic disease conditions, smokers, and alcoholics. Otherwise-healthy patients usually recover completely from pneumonia when treated properly. By comparison, high-risk persons are more likely to develop complications including septicemia, pulmonary edema, lung abscess, pleural effusion, and acute respiratory distress syndrome.

Irritating agents or events can also lead to pneumonia—for example, aspiration of gastric contents and inhalation of smoke or chemicals. Aspiration pneumonia frequently occurs when the gag reflex is impaired because of a brain injury or anesthesia. Aspiration can also occur because of impaired lower esophageal sphincter closure secondary to nasogastric tube placement or disease (e.g., gastroesophageal reflux disease). Additionally, inappropriate gastric tube placement can lead to tube-feeding formulas entering the lungs rather than the stomach. Gastric contents and tube-feeding formulas irritate the lung tissue, triggering the inflammatory response. The inflammatory response increases mucus production, which can in turn lead to atelectasis and pneumonia. Tube-feeding formulas also contain sugar and protein, creating a superior medium in which bacteria can grow and flourish. Finally, pneumonia can develop from stasis of pulmonary secretions. When these secretions become thick and stagnate, ciliary action cannot remove the bacteria-laden mucus, leading to pneumonia. Activities such as movement, talking, and coughing normally keep pulmonary secretions moving, and adequate hydrations keep secretions thin.

Pneumonia is classified based on the causative agents or events previously discussed and its location in the lung (**TABLE 5-3**). Lobar pneumonia is confined to a single lobe and is described based on the affected lobe (e.g., right upper lobe). Bronchopneumonia is the most frequent type and is a patchy pneumonia spread throughout several lobes. Interstitial pneumonia, or atypical pneumonia, occurs in the areas between the alveoli. Interstitial pneumonia is routinely caused by viruses (e.g., influenza type A and B) or by atypical bacteria (e.g., *Legionella pneumophilia* and *Mycoplasma pneumoniae*).

Clinical Manifestations

Clinical manifestations of pneumonia may vary depending on type. General signs and symptoms include the following: productive or nonproductive cough, fatigue, pleuritic pain, dyspnea, fever, chills, crackles, consolidation signs (e.g., dullness to percussion), decreased breath sounds, pleural rub, tachypnea, and mental status changes (especially in the elderly). Viral pneumonia and bacterial pneumonia have some notable differences (**TABLE 5-4**). Viral pneumonia is usually mild and heals without intervention, but it can lead to virulent bacterial pneumonia.

Diagnosis and Treatment

Early diagnosis and treatment of pneumonia are paramount to have positive outcomes. A history and physical may be sufficient to diagnose pneumonia; however, a chest X-ray is an important diagnostic test as findings may aid in determining the pathogen, identifying

TABLE 5-3	Types of Pneumonia		
	Lobar pneumonia	**Bronchopneumonia**	**Interstitial pneumonia**
Distribution	All of one or two lobes	Scattered small patches	Scattered small patches
Cause	*Streptococcus pneumoniae*	Multiple bacteria	Influenza virus; *Mycoplasma*
Pathophysiology	Inflammation of the alveolar wall and leakage of cells, fibrin, and fluid into alveoli, causing consolidation	Inflammation and purulent exudates in alveoli, often developing from pooled secretions or irritation	Interstitial inflammation around alveoli Necrosis of bronchial epithelium
Onset	Sudden and acute	Insidious	Variable
Signs	High fever Chills Productive cough of rusty sputum Crackles progressing to absent breath sounds in affected lobes	Mild fever Productive cough of yellow-green sputum Dyspnea	Variable fever Nonproductive hacking cough Headache Myalgia

Reproduced from Story, L. (2017). *Pathophysiology: A practical approach* (3rd ed.). Burlington, MA: Jones & Bartlett Learning.

TABLE 5-4 Comparison of Viral and Bacterial Pneumonia

	Viral	Bacterial
Cough	Nonproductive	Productive
Fever	Low grade	Higher
WBC	Normal (low)	Elevated
X-ray	Minimal change	Infiltrates
Severity	Less	More
Antibiotics	No	Yes

Reproduced from Story, L. (2017). *Pathophysiology: A practical approach* (3rd ed.). Burlington, MA: Jones & Bartlett Learning.

pleural effusions, or detecting the development of cavities (walled hollow structures in the lungs). The information from the chest X-ray can then be used to choose efficacious treatments to expeditiously treat the pneumonia. Community-acquired pneumonia can be managed on an outpatient basis. Hospitalization (e.g., general or intensive care unit) may be necessary if illness is severe as manifested in degree of respiratory distress or septicemia. When deciding on place of treatment, either home or hospital, other factors that should be taken into consideration are ability to take and adhere to a medication regimen, self-care and cognitive abilities, and living situation (e.g., homelessness, distance from a hospital). Two clinical prediction scores can be used to determine need for admission—evaluation of confusion, blood urea nitrogen, respiratory rate, blood pressure, and age and this is commonly known by the acronym CURB-65. The second prediction score—the pneumonia severity index—uses multiple clinical data input such as age, gender, neoplastic disease, and congestive heart failure; a score is assigned for the multiple variables.

Additional diagnostic testing for pneumonia can include sputum cultures and gram staining, CBC, ABGs, and bronchoscopy. Managing respiratory distress is a priority, and endotracheal intubation may be necessary to provide ventilation support and maintain oxygenation. Antibiotics are required if bacterial infection is present. If treatment is empiric, antibiograms should be used to determine the most appropriate antibiotic. Antibiograms are created as part of infection control measures in an effort to promote antibiotic stewardship. Antibiograms are developed from institutional culture results to identify antibiotic susceptibility and resistance patterns. Additional treatment may include bronchodilators, corticosteroids, antipyretics, analgesics, humidified oxygen therapy, chest physiotherapy, increased fluids (either by mouth or intravenously), and rest. If aspiration is the cause of the pneumonia, additional treatment includes eliminating the causes and not giving the patient anything by mouth until swallowing studies can be performed. Pneumonia prevention strategies include hand washing, avoiding crowds, vaccinations (e.g., for pneumococcus, influenza, and Hib), mobilizing secretions (e.g., turning, coughing, deep breathing), and smoking cessation.

Tuberculosis

Tuberculosis (TB), an ancient disease, is one of the world's deadliest conditions. Although on the decline, TB remains a major cause of illness, with one-third of the world's population being infected. According to the World Health Organization, TB was responsible for approximately 1.3 million deaths worldwide in 2017, and it is the leading cause of death for persons infected with HIV (WHO, 2018c). An additional 1.7 billion people are thought to have latent TB infection and are at risk for developing active TB (WHO, 2018c). In the United States, TB rates are highest among Asians at 18.0 per 100,000 persons, and the lowest rate is in White, non–Hispanic persons at 0.6 per 100,000 (CDC, 2018b).

TB is caused by *Mycobacterium tuberculosis*, a slow-growing aerobic bacillus that is somewhat resistant to the body's immune efforts because it has a capsule composed of waxes and fatty substances. Other mycobacteria (e.g., *M. bovis* and *M. africanum*) are rare in the United States. Person-to-person transmission occurs through the inhalation of tiny infected aerosol droplets. Only people with active TB can spread the disease to others. The bacillus is capable of surviving in dried sputum for weeks, but ultraviolet light, heat, alcohol, glutaraldehyde, and formaldehyde destroy it. Many people contract TB but do not develop the disease because of an intact, healthy immune system or early treatment. Multidrug-resistant TB strains are relatively rare but account for 78 cases annually in the United States (CDC, 2018b); there are over 558,000 diagnosed cases worldwide (WHO, 2018c). Extensively drug-resistant TB is

BOX 5-2 Application to Practice

Review the pulmonary infection cases and discuss whether the diagnosis is infectious rhinitis, influenza, acute bronchitis, acute bronchiolitis, or pneumonia.

Case 1: Jack is a 21-year-old complaining of a sudden onset of myalgia with his body aching all over and headache for the past day. He feels tired and has the chills, and his temperature was 100°F. He has a mild nonproductive cough. He denies rhinorrhea, sinus pain, nausea, otalgia, or shortness of breath. He reports exposure to sick contacts in his dorm, stating, "Everyone seems to be coughing and catching a cold or the flu."

Medications: none.
Allergies: penicillin.
Past medical history: healthy.
Social history: college student, lives in a dormitory. Nonsmoker and drinks alcohol once a week, about two or three beers.

Physical exam:
Vital signs: temperature 100.5°F, pulse 98 per minute, respiratory rate 18 per minute, blood pressure 110/70 mmHg pulse oximeter 98%.
General: ill and tired appearance.
Head, Eyes, Ears, Neck, Throat: unremarkable.
Neck: no lymphadenopathy; negative Kernig sign, negative Brudzinski sign.
Cardiovascular: lungs, abdomen are unremarkable.

What is the most likely diagnosis and pathogen causing this disorder? Discuss the mode of transmission and discuss the data that supports your decision.
What diagnostic test, if any, should be done?

Develop a treatment plan for this patient.

Case 2: Mr. Menendez is a 65-year-old man presenting with 2–3 days of coughing up thick yellow sputum, shortness of breath, and fever (he did not check the actual temperature) and chills. He states his chest hurts when he breathes. He denies headache, rhinorrhea, sinus pain, and nausea. He reports no exposure to sick individuals.

Medications: lisinopril 10 mg a day by mouth.
Allergies: no known drug allergies.
Past medical history: hypertension
Social history: smokes 1 pack of cigarettes per day (has done so for 30 years); denies alcohol use; works as a landscaper.

Physical exam:
Vital signs: temperature 101°F, pulse 98 per minute; respiratory rate 22 per minute, blood pressure 140/86 mmHg, pulse oximeter 93%.
General: ill and tired appearance, coughing during visit with thick yellow sputum noted.
HEENT: unremarkable.
Neck: small anterior and posterior cervical nodes.
CV: unremarkable.
Lungs: right basilar crackles with dullness to percussion in right lower lobe.
Abdomen: unremarkable.
What is the most likely diagnosis and pathogen causing this disorder? Discuss the mode of transmission. Discuss the data that support your decision.
What diagnostic test, if any, should be done?

Develop a treatment plan for this patient.

Case 3: Jamie is a 1- year-old girl who is coughing and has had rhinorrhea with yellowish discharge for the past day. Her father says today he felt like she had a fever and has not been eating or playing; she has been mostly sleeping. Her 5-year-old sibling has had a cold for a week.

Medications: none.
Allergies: no known drug allergies.
Vaccinations: up to date for age.
Social history: in day care; lives with mother and father and 5-year-old sibling.

Physical exam:
Vital signs: temperature 101.5°F, pulse 120 per minute, respiratory rate 34 per minute; blood pressure 100/60 mmHg, pulse oximeter 92%.
General: sitting in father's lap; ill, lethargic appearance, and coughing.
HEENT: nasal flaring, nasal mucus yellowish bilaterally; oropharynx with mild erythema.
Neck: small anterior and posterior cervical nodes.
CV: unremarkable.
Lungs: intercostal retractions, expiratory wheezing.
Abdomen: unremarkable.
What is the most likely diagnosis and pathogen causing this disorder? Discuss the mode of transmission and discuss data that supports your decision.
What diagnostic test, if any, should be done?
Develop a treatment plan for this patient.

Influenza
Rapid flu test
Tamiflu /APAP 10TC
prevent transmission

PNA

extremely rare in the United States, with only one known case occurring in 2016; in contrast, extensively drug-resistant TB is a global threat that has been linked to cases in more than 100 countries. TB is often considered an opportunistic infection because it is more likely to become active in someone with a weakened immune system. At-risk persons include those with immune deficiency (e.g., AIDS and cancer), malnutrition, diabetes mellitus, and alcoholism. Poverty, overcrowding, homelessness, and drug abuse also increase the risk for acquiring TB. Young children (less than 2 years old) and adolescents are also at greater risk than adults.

There are two stages of TB pathogenesis—primary and secondary infection. Primary TB infection occurs when the bacillus first enters the body. In this phase, macrophages engulf the microbe, causing a local inflammatory response that is different from the usual inflammatory response. The macrophages are unable to phagocytize the bacteria. Some bacilli are carried to the lymph nodes and around the lungs, activating the type IV hypersensitivity reaction. Cell mediated immunity is the main mechanism by which the body fights the tubercle bacillus and starts a few weeks after infection. Lymphocytes (helper T and cytotoxic T) and macrophages congregate to form a granuloma (an epithelial nodule). The granuloma contains some live bacilli, forming a tubercle. Caseous necrosis, a cottage cheese–like material, develops in the center of the tubercle. This complex of cells and necrosis is called a *caseating granuloma*, which stimulates a granulomatous inflammation. An intact immune system can resist this development, so the lesions—referred to as *Ghon complexes* (**FIGURE 5-16**)—remain small, become walled off by fibrous tissue, and calcify. The bacilli can remain dormant and viable in the tubercle for years as long as the immune system is intact. In this phase, the individual has been infected by the bacilli and remains asymptomatic. At this time, the person is said to have latent tuberculosis infection (LTBI). Transmission to others does not occur even though there are organisms in the granuloma. However, any time the immune system is compromised the disease may reactivate and cause pulmonary TB disease.

In about 10% of infected people, the initial exposure leads to active primary tuberculosis. In other words, upon initial infection 90% develop LTBI and 10% go on to develop active

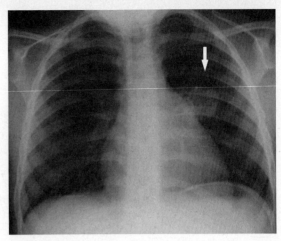

FIGURE 5-16 Ghon complexes.
Courtesy of Benjamin M. Marais.

primary tuberculosis. Primary active tuberculosis development after initial exposure is more likely if there is a large inhalation of the tubercle or if the person is immunocompromised. The remaining 90% of cases of active pulmonary tuberculosis occurs because of reactivation of latent TB, and at this point, the TB is a secondary infection. The reactivation can occur at any time, even years after the infection occurred. Reinfection with TB can also occur. During the active phase, whether from primary infection at initial exposure or reactivation of latent TB, the bacillus spreads throughout the lungs, and hematogenous spread can infect other organs and tissues (e.g., kidney, brain, and bone marrow). The infected solid organs look like millet seeds due to the multiple foci, and, hence, disseminated TB is called *miliary tuberculosis*. Even when the pulmonary infection has healed, progression to extrapulmonary organs can proceed.

Clinical Manifestations

Latent TB does not produce any symptoms and is not considered infectious. With development of the disease, whether from primary active infection (i.e., disease after first exposure) or latent infection that reactivates, the manifestations tend to appear gradually. Manifestations are a result of chronic infection and the immune process and include productive cough, night sweats, fever, chills, fatigue, unexplained weight loss, and anorexia. Hemoptysis may occur when granulomas erode into the pulmonary vasculature. Other symptomatology may be present depending on other organ involvement (e.g., bone pain, neurologic symptoms).

Diagnosis and Treatment

Diagnostic procedures for TB are multifaceted, usually beginning with a tuberculin skin test (TST) (also known as the *Mantoux test*) or a blood test called *interferon gamma release assays* (IGRAs). For the TST, a small amount of a purified protein-derivative tuberculin is injected just below the dermis. If the person has been infected by the bacilli, a local reaction (e.g., redness and induration) will occur. The degree of induration is measured to determine if the person is positive or negative (see **TABLE 5-5**). Persons will test positive once the bacilli trigger the inflammatory response. A history of bacillus Calmette-Guérin (BCG) vaccination will produce a false-positive reaction. Additionally, previously treated TB will generate a false-positive reaction. Conversely, persons with immature immune systems (e.g., children) or immunocompromise may not generate enough of a response to test positive. The two IGRAs include the QuantiFERON TB Gold in-tube and the T-SPOT, which measure CD4+ T cells' interferon gamma concentration in response. The IGRAs are not affected by the BCG vaccine, and, therefore, are more accurate in those previously vaccinated. The TST or the IGRAs do not help to differentiate between latent and active TB. Because of the uncertainty that the TB skin test creates, chest X-rays and sputum for stained smears and cultures (most definitive) are used after a positive TST is noted (either to confirm an original case or to assess reinfection). A computed tomography (CT) scan can also be used to visualize TB lesions, as this imaging modality is more sensitive than an X-ray. Nucleic acid amplification may be performed on the sputum to detect the presence of resistant strains. Extrapulmonary manifestations will require collection of specimens from the areas of infection (e.g., pericardium, bone).

TB is often successfully treated in the home setting; however, it takes diligence to eradicate the disease. Treatment requires an average of 6–9 months of antimicrobial therapy. The goal of treatment is to cure the patient and prevent transmission. Combination therapy (consisting of two or more drugs) is recommended to prevent the emergence of resistant strains. The slow-growing bacilli have a high mutation rate, with those mutations often appearing when the pathogen is exposed to monotherapy. Because TB is a public health risk, antituberculin medications are provided free of charge by the U.S. Public Health Service. In some states, therapy noncompliance is unlawful, and imprisonment may be used to ensure adherence when other measures (e.g., direct observed therapy) fail. Compliance is a common problem in treating TB because of the length of therapy and the medication side effects (e.g., nausea, paresthesias, discolored bodily secretions). Patient education, including an emphasis on taking the entire regimen of drugs as ordered, is crucial to maximize therapy success and prevent resistance. People with LTBI should also be treated as they still have organisms even though they do not spread the infection. Treating LTBI reduces the probability of having TB reactivate and cause a secondary infection in the future.

Strategies to prevent the transmission of TB include respiratory precautions (e.g., TB-approved masks, covering one's mouth when coughing, and disposing of tissues), adequate ventilation (if the patient is at home), and placing the patient in a negative-pressure isolation room (if hospitalized). The bacillus

TABLE 5-5	Classification of the Tuberculin Skin Test Reaction

An induration of **5 or more millimeters** is considered positive in:

- HIV-infected persons
- A recent contact of a person with TB disease
- Persons with fibrotic changes on chest radiograph consistent with prior TB
- Patients with organ transplants
- Persons who are immunosuppressed for other reasons (e.g., taking high dose prednisone for 1 month)

An induration of **10 or more millimeters** is considered positive in:

- Recent immigrants (< 5 years) from high-prevalence countries
- Injection drug users
- Residents and employees of high-risk congregate settings
- Mycobacteriology laboratory personnel
- Persons with clinical conditions that place them at high risk
- Children < 4 years of age
- Infants, children, and adolescents exposed to adults in high-risk categories

An induration of **15 or more millimeters** is considered positive in:

- Any person, including person with no known risk factors for TB

Centers for Disease Control and Prevention, October 2011.

BOX 5-3 Application to Practice

The CDC (2018b) recommends that certain people who are at higher risk for becoming infected with tuberculosis (TB) get tested. Those individuals include:

- Those who have had exposure/time spent with someone who has TB disease
- Infants, children, and adolescents exposed to adults who are at increased risk for latent tuberculosis infection or TB disease
- Persons who are living or traveling from a country where TB disease is more common (most countries in Latin America, the Caribbean, Africa, Asia, Eastern Europe, and Russia)
- Persons who are living or working in high-risk settings such as correctional facilities, long-term care facilities or nursing homes, and homeless shelters)
- Healthcare workers who care for patients at increased risk for TB disease

The recommended frequency of testing for healthcare workers varies on the risk of exposure classification (e.g., low, medium, or ongoing). The TST may also be conducted using two-step testing. The two steps occur as follows:

First step: TST administered

If positive, the person probably has TB infection

If negative, retest done 1–3 weeks later

Second step: TST administered 1–3 weeks after initial test

If positive, it is considered a boosted reaction from latent infection that occurred at some time prior (usually years)

If negative, the person probably does not have TB

Review the following TB testing cases. Interpret the findings and identify a diagnosis. Develop a management plan.

Case 1: 45-year-old registered nurse who works on a medical surgical unit. TST is 10 mm.

Case 2: 35-year-old man with HIV. TST is 4 mm.

Case 3: 25-year-old woman who is an international student (from Peru, South America) who has been studying in the United States for the past year. TST is 11 mm.

Case 4: 3-year-old boy who just moved from Asia to the United States. TST is 10 mm.

Case 5: 20-year-old-woman. TST is 11 mm.

Case 6: 50-year-old man with a history of BCG vaccination. TST 11 mm.

Calmette-Guérin vaccination is primarily used in children in countries with a high rate of *Mycobacterium tuberculosis*.

Alterations in Ventilation

Asthma—Obstructive

Asthma is a chronic pulmonary disease that is characterized by chronic airway inflammation and bronchial hyperresponsiveness (FIGURE 5-17). Asthma is one of the most common noncommunicable chronic illnesses globally and in children in the United States. Most cases (approximately 50%) of asthma are diagnosed in childhood with a peak prevalence at the age of 3 years old. Adults who develop asthma (about 33%) are usually diagnosed by the age of 40 years. Women are more likely to have asthma than men, but in children, boys are more likely to have asthma than girls. Persons of multiple races/ethnicities and Black adults and children are more likely to have asthma than White adults and children.

Many mechanisms underlie asthma development, and there is increasing recognition that asthma may be a syndrome rather than one disease entity. Over 100 genes are implicated in the development of asthma. The genetic predisposition coupled with environmental factors further enhance the likelihood of asthma development. Asthma development is thought to be polygenic with multiple genes interacting to then cause the variable phenotype (observable expression) of asthma. Genetic alterations are not only implicated in disease development but also in modifying asthma severity and response to treatment.

Various theoretical propositions explain the development of asthma. The most well-known

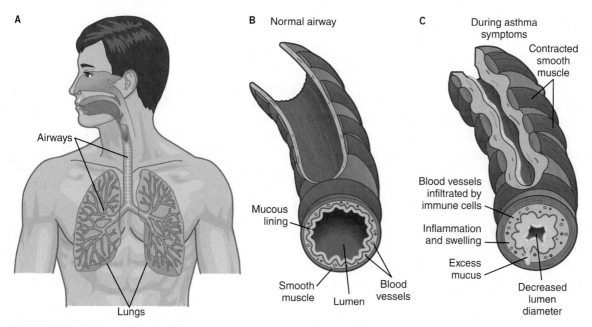

FIGURE 5-17 Asthma. **A** Location of the lungs and airways in the body. **B** Cross-section of a normal airway. **C** Cross-section of an airway during asthma symptoms.

and clear association is between asthma and atopy. Atopy is a genetic predisposition to producing a usually exaggerated IgE response to allergens or irritants. Determining if atopic and asthma genetic alterations are the same or different is difficult. For example, people with asthma often have other atopic diseases such as allergic rhinitis and eczema; however, not all people with atopic diseases develop asthma. Atopic diseases and asthma share genetic alterations that lead to genetic immune dysregulation. Other factors such as smoking, pollen, and other environmental factors also contribute to this immune dysregulation.

Key characteristics of asthma are chronic airway inflammation and bronchial hyperresponsiveness with intermittent, reversible airway obstruction. Exposure to an antigen or irritant in a sensitized individual triggers a cascade of innate and adaptive immune responses. The result is bronchoconstriction, bronchospasm, bronchiole edema, and mucus production.

An episode of asthma (asthma flare-up or attack) is characterized by two phases—an early response and a late response. The early response phase is primarily related to bronchospasm and bronchoconstriction and is usually signaled by coughing. Peaking within 30 minutes and resolving usually in less than 3 hours, the inflammatory mediators released as a result of mast cell degranulation include leukotrienes, histamine, and prostaglandins. Mast

cell degranulation also results in release of tumor necrosis factor, which causes recruitment and activation of inflammatory cells.

The dendritic cells present the antigen, and Th2 (T helper) lymphocytes release several cytokines (interleukin: 3, 4, 5, 8, 9, 13, 17, 22 and granulocyte macrophage-stimulating factor). The cytokines cause B cell activation, mast cell proliferation, eosinophil production and survival, neutrophil release, basophil survival, and T cell recruitment and differentiation into Th2 cells. The cytokine effects and/or specific interleukins cause tissue injury, release of toxic chemicals, an enhanced inflammatory response, an impaired mucociliary response, increased fibroblasts, and airway remodeling.

A few hours after the acute event a late response can occur. Neutrophils, lymphocytes, and eosinophils can further release many of the same mediators from the acute phase. The late response peaks within 6 hours of symptom onset. This phase is a result of airway edema and mucus production. Leukotrienes are synthesized, causing smooth muscle contraction. The alveolar hyperinflation causes air trapping. The airways start scarring, and bronchial hyperresponsiveness continues, leading to impaired clearing of mucus and the formation of mucous plugs (glycoproteins). The mucous plugs are secreted by goblet cells in the airways. Leaky bronchial vessels also release plasma proteins contributing to mucous plug development. Without treatment, irreversible changes develop, which include fibrosis under the epithelial layer and hypertrophy of smooth muscle and mucous glands. These changes are termed *airway remodeling*.

The polygenic and environmentally mediated nature of asthma is evident in the various phenotypes. Asthma genetics is complex. For example, different people can have different genes and yet have one type of asthma expression. Genetic alterations cause development of asthma but also influence severity and response to treatment. In addition to the atopic asthma (i.e., eosinophilic asthma), several other phenotypes include exercise-induced asthma, aspirin-induced asthma, and intrinsic asthma. Asthma may occur independent of atopy.

In general, asthma severity remains relatively constant within an individual. This consistency means that a person with mild asthma will usually continue to have mild asthma throughout their life, and those who develop severe asthma were likely to have had severe asthma around the time of diagnosis and will continue to have a severe disease expression.

The onset of asthma during childhood is usually due to atopy and allergies. Adult-onset asthma is highly variable. Atopy is a more common cause in those with mild-to-moderate disease (approximately 50%); however, atopy is not a likely cause in adult-onset asthma in patients who have severe disease (**TABLE 5-6**).

Nonatopic asthma, which is more common in adults, has been linked to individuals with high eosinophil levels. Eosinophils are often associated with atopy (production of IgE in response to allergens) but those individuals with eosinophilic asthma do not necessarily have allergies. Another nonatopic asthma is that associated with chronic rhinosinusitis, nasal polyposis, and reaction to aspirin. The asthma is called *aspirin-exacerbated respiratory disease*. These nonatopic disorders can coexist, and both are considered severe asthma phenotypes. The mechanism of aspirin sensitivity occurs because under normal circumstances aspirin and other drugs such as nonsteroidal anti-inflammatory drugs block enzymes called *cyclooxygenase* that lead to arachidonic acid conversion to prostaglandins, which stimulates leukotriene release—a powerful bronchoconstrictor. Consequently, there is arachidonic dysregulation and an overproduction of leukotrienes with subsequent bronchoconstriction and promotion of airway inflammation in cases of aspirin sensitivity. Other types of asthma phenotypes include exposure to occupational allergens such as plant proteins or animal proteins (e.g., farmers) or other chemicals (e.g., plastic or formaldehyde), which has been implicated in the development of asthma independent of atopy. Symptoms develop over time, worsen with each exposure, and improve when away from work (e.g., on weekends or during vacations).

In individuals with severe adult-onset asthma, there is variability in response to glucocorticoids. Some individuals have little to no response (resistance) while others require high doses (dependence). Children with severe asthma have also demonstrated resistance to glucocorticoids. Another example of genetic

TABLE 5-6	Classification of Asthma Severity			
Step/classification*	Daytime symptoms	Nighttime symptoms	PEF or FEV₁**	PEF variability
Step 1: Intermittent	≤ 2 times/week	≤ 2 times/week	≥ 80%	< 20%
Step 2: Mild persistent	> 2 times/week, but < daily	> 2 nights/month	> 80%	20–30%
Step 3: Moderate persistent	Daily	>1 night/week, but < daily	60–80%	> 30%
Step 4: Severe persistent	Continual	Frequent	≤ 60%	> 30%

* Classification is based on symptoms and lung function before treatment. Patients should be assigned to the most severe step in which any feature occurs.

** Percentage of predicted function.

PEF = peak expiratory flow (rate); FEV₁ = forced expiratory volume in 1 second.

Modified from National Heart, Lung, and Blood Institute. (2007). *National Asthma Education and Prevention Program, Expert Panel Report 3: Guidelines for the diagnosis and management of asthma.* NIH Publication Number 08-5846. Retrieved from https://www.nhlbi.nih .gov/files/docs/guidelines/asthsumm.pdf variations and medication response in asthma is evident in those with a polymorphism of the beta-adrenergic receptor gene, which is known as the *Arg16Arg genotype*. Long-acting beta agonists (LABA) often used in the management of asthma increase bronchospasm in those with the genetic polymorphism.

Exercise-induced asthma is more common in childhood. The hyperventilation that occurs with exercise is thought to lead to airway fluid lining changes and mast cell mediator release. With exercise-induced asthma, the attack usually occurs 10–15 minutes after physical activity ends. Symptoms can linger for an hour with this type of asthma. The airways can become cool and dry during exercise, and asthmatic symptoms may be a compensatory mechanism to warm and moisten the airways. Following each episode of exercise-induced asthma, a refractory (symptom-free) period begins within 30 minutes and can last 90 minutes. During this time, little or no bronchospasm can be induced even if the person is rechallenged with vigorous exercise. Athletes often take advantage of this fact by warming up vigorously to induce a refractory period prior to competition. Weather changes such as cold air or hot weather can trigger asthma symptoms in the same manner as exercise.

Several other factors trigger or influence asthma manifestations. Some women report a premenstrual worsening of their asthma, demonstrating that hormonal changes can be a trigger. Stress can induce asthma symptoms through a cholinergic reflex pathway. In addition to aspirin and nonsteroidal anti-inflammatory drugs previously discussed, medications such as beta blockers can trigger asthma. Some people with asthma have worsening symptoms at night. This nocturnal trigger usually occurs between 3:00 and 7:00 a.m. and is thought to be related to circadian rhythms. At night, cortisol and epinephrine levels decrease, while histamine levels increase. Changes in these naturally occurring substances lead to bronchoconstriction. Individuals who are obese (body mass index $\geq$ 30 kg/m^2) have a higher incidence of asthma, and this increased risk is possibly related to fat stores having adipokines (cytokines secreted by adipose tissues) that are proinflammatory and have less anti-inflammatory capacity. The roles of obesity and asthma, however, are still not clear. Several other factors such as diet, in utero smoke exposure, acetaminophen ingestion in childhood, and so forth continue to be evaluated for association and causality.

Learning Points

Hygiene Hypothesis and Asthma

Another theory, referred to as the *hygiene hypothesis*, suggests that the modern Western lifestyle's focus on hygiene and sanitation limits early childhood allergen and infection exposure. Childhood microbial exposure normally leads to a proinflammatory Th1 response, which does not involve IgE production and confers immune protection in a different manner. The lack of exposure, however, leads instead to a Th2 immune response with interleukin release and an IgE and eosinophil activation. This Th2 response renders individuals more vulnerable to the development of asthma. Another way to think of the hygiene hypothesis is that the lack of exposure to microbes does not allow the immune system to develop and teach the immune system how to react. The hygiene theory has been disputed as there are several instances where asthma incidence is high in less hygienic environments.

Clinical Manifestations

Asthma is usually classified by its severity (intermittent, mild persistent, moderate persistent, and severe persistent) (Table 5-5). Clinical manifestations of asthma include expiratory wheezing, dyspnea, chest tightness, cough, anxiety, tachypnea, and tachycardia. The expiratory phase is prolonged. The work of breathing will increase, wheezing may be heard during inspiration but is commonly heard on expiration, and accessory muscles use becomes evident if the asthma attack is not treated or not responding to treatment. The increased work of breathing leads to hypoxemia.

Status asthmaticus is a life-threatening, prolonged asthma attack that does not respond to usual treatment. Maintaining a patent airway is critical in such cases, and endotracheal intubation with ventilation support may be necessary. In addition, acid–base imbalances—specifically respiratory alkalosis from expelling too much carbon dioxide because of tachypnea and hypoxemia, can develop early in the attack. Eventually, respiratory muscles fatigue as the obstruction of airflow and hyperinflation continues, causing CO_2 retention and respiratory acidosis.

Diagnosis and Treatment

Diagnosis is made with a thorough history and physical examination along with pulmonary function tests (Figure 5-11). Pulmonary function findings consistent with asthma include FEV_1 decreases, which are reversible. Other tests include chest X-ray, ABGs, CBC, challenge testing (i.e., bronchoprovocation), and allergen testing to search for underlying causes and triggers. Although airflow obstruction is usually reversible, some individuals can develop irreversible airflow limitation.

Asthma cannot be cured, but its symptoms can be controlled. Unless treated promptly, asthma attacks can lead to impaired gas exchange and death. Left untreated, long-term asthma can result in bronchial damage and scarring. The goals of treatment are to minimize the occurrence and severity of asthma attacks. Pharmacologic treatment for all patients with asthma at any classification includes a short-acting beta agonist (SABA), which relaxes bronchial smooth muscle and causes bronchodilation. These SABAs are commonly called *rescue inhalers*. Other medications for acute attacks can include anticholinergics and corticosteroids. Long-term management is guided by the use of the stepwise approach from the 2007 National Heart, Lung, and Blood Institute and National Institutes of Health expert panel report. Medication choice is dependent on the frequency of symptoms, SABA use, nighttime awakenings, interference with normal daily activities, and peak flow measurements. The step a person is deemed to be at and the level of control will guide the use of various other

pharmacotherapeutics such as inhaled and systemic corticosteroids, long-acting beta-2 agonists (LABA), leukotriene modifiers, mast cell stabilizers, methylxanthines, anticholinergics, and immunotherapy. These agents can be delivered orally, by inhalation, and/or intravenously. Biologics are the newest category of medications approved for severe asthma. These medications are humanized monoclonal antibodies that are categorized as anti-IgE antibodies (e.g., omalizumab) or interleukin-5 antagonists (e.g., reslizumab, mepolizumab). Additional strategies include developing an asthma plan and teaching it to all caregivers. This plan will include the avoidance of triggers, environmental cleanliness such as air filters and hypoallergenic sheets and pillowcases, maintaining a healthy immune system by exercising, proper nutrition, and receiving vaccines.

Chronic Obstructive Pulmonary Disease

Chronic obstructive pulmonary disease (COPD) describes a group of chronic respiratory disorders characterized by recurrent respiratory symptoms and airway obstruction that are attributed to irreversible airway and/or alveolar abnormalities (**FIGURE 5-18**). The irreversible nature of COPD is in contrast to asthma, where airway obstruction is reversible despite underlying chronic inflammation. Asthma is predominantly viewed as an allergic IgE phenomenon with different mediators and inflammatory cells (e.g., more eosinophils) while COPD is caused by smoking with a subsequent different inflammatory response and damage. Individuals, however, can have coexisting asthma and COPD. The limitation in airflow with COPD causes persistent respiratory symptoms (e.g., dyspnea, cough, and sputum production). COPD can impair an individual's ability to work and function independently and leads to premature death. Severe hypoxia and hypercapnia can lead to respiratory failure. The chronic hypercapnia shifts the normal breathing drive from the need to expel excess carbon dioxide to the need to raise oxygen levels (Figure 5-12).

Prevalence rates for COPD are likely underestimated because this disease is often asymptomatic in its early stages, is masked by smoking symptoms, or is underreported. According to the CDC (2015a), COPD was the third leading cause of death in the United States in 2011 and the fourth leading cause of death worldwide. Fifteen million Americans are currently diagnosed with COPD. Symptoms usually present

---

Learning Points

Cough Diagnostic Tips

Cough is an important protective mechanism but can become a bother and harmful. Coughing occurs because of irritation of cough receptors (afferent) located in the respiratory tract (larynx, trachea, bronchi, pleura), ear canal and eardrum, pericardium, esophagus, stomach, and diaphragm. The receptor stimulation travels through the vagus nerve to the cough center in the medulla. The result is a corresponding spinal, phrenic, and vagus effector response of cough. Coughing is a common symptom for which people seek health care. Clinicians, at some point in time, will care for someone with a cough. Classifying cough by duration can be useful in determining likely diagnostic possibilities. Acute cough is defined as one that exists for less than 3 weeks. Acute coughs are usually due to a respiratory tract infection. Subacute cough exists for 3–8 weeks. Subacute cough is often postinfectious even with resolution of other infectious symptoms (e.g., myalgia, fever) or due to upper airway cough syndrome (i.e., postnasal drip cough). Chronic cough is one that exists for greater than 8 weeks. The three most common causes (up to 90% of cases of nonsmokers or those not taking angiotensin-converting enzymes) of chronic cough are postnasal drip cough, asthma, or gastroesophageal reflux. Postnasal drip cough is most likely due to allergic and nonallergic rhinitis or sinusitis. While patients may complain of heartburn or sour taste in the mouth with reflux disease, cough may be the only symptom in up to 40% of cases.

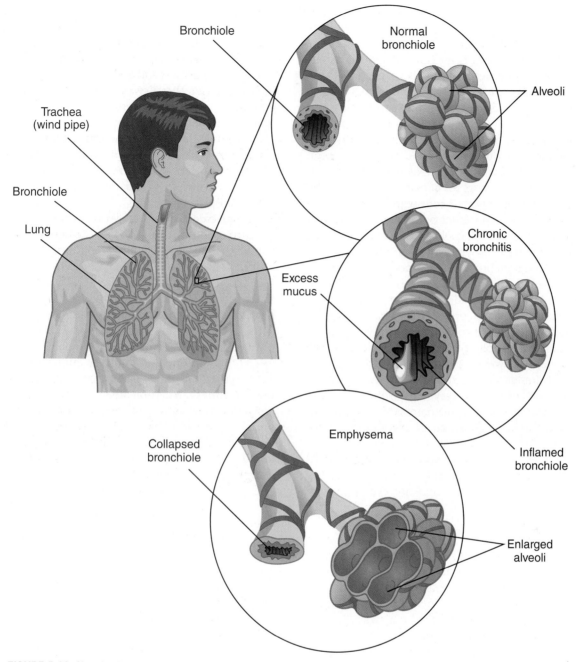

FIGURE 5-18 Chronic obstructive pulmonary disease (COPD) is often one disease or a mixture of two diseases—chronic bronchitis and emphysema.

around 60 years of age. A rare familial type of COPD (emphysema only) is due to alpha-1 antitrypsin deficiency (AATD). AATD presents much earlier—in the 30s or 40s. Groups at higher risk of developing COPD include Whites, individuals of lower socioeconomic status, and persons with a history of asthma. It was considered that men had a higher incidence, but the incidence of smoking has increased in women making the disease equally prevalent in men and women (Global Initiative for Chronic Obstructive Lung Disease, 2019).

The most significant contributing factor to developing COPD is cigarette smoking. Other contributing factors include the inhalation of pollution and chemical irritants as well as a variety of host factors. The chronic inflammation from smoking affects the large airways, small airways (e.g. bronchioles), and parenchyma. Emphysema is a destruction of the alveoli, and although it is often used as a clinical diagnosis, it is just reflective of one of the pathologic changes that occurs in COPD. Chronic bronchitis, conversely, is a clinical diagnosis as opposed to the description of a structural lung change as in emphysema. COPD is often a mixture of two diseases—chronic bronchitis and emphysema (FIGURE 5-18). Chronic bronchitis is defined as an obstructive respiratory disorder characterized by inflammation of the bronchi, a productive cough, and excessive mucus production that occurs for at least 3 months of the year and for at least 2 consecutive years.

Smoking and other pollutant sources, such as using wood to cook and burning garbage, cause chronic airway irritation and trigger the inflammatory process. Large airway changes due to smoking include an increase in size and number of goblet cells and submucosal glands, which increases mucus production. These changes lead to a chronic productive cough, which characterizes chronic bronchitis. The large airway changes, however, are not reasons for the airflow limitation in COPD. The airflow limitation is caused by small airway (e.g., bronchioles) and alveolar or alveolar duct damage (emphysema). COPD as a combination of chronic bronchitis and emphysema has variability in presentations. As an example, not everyone with chronic bronchitis has airflow limitation (e.g., small airway and alveolar damage), and not everyone with COPD has increased mucus secretion (e.g., large airway damage).

The inflammatory response that is triggered during COPD is heightened in comparison to other inflammatory responses to insults. Neutrophils, macrophages, and lymphocytes release inflammatory mediators and oxidants, which infiltrate the airway. The inflammatory mediators attract more inflammatory cells from the circulation, enhance the inflammatory response, and start the process of structural lung changes. Fibrosis then ensues, leading to small airway damage and subsequent airflow limitation.

Normally, a balance between proteases (enzymes like elastase) and antiproteases (alpha antitrypsin) keeps elastin in lung connective tissue from being destroyed. Inflammatory and epithelial cells increase the level of the destructive proteases, causing parenchymal damage. The alveoli turn into large, irregular pockets with gaping holes with air spaces (termed *bullae*). Gas exchange becomes ineffective. Blebs (smaller than bullae)—air spaces near the pleura—also develop and contribute

to the reduced gas exchange. The result is a limitation of oxygen entering the bloodstream. The elastic fibers and surfactant that normally keep the alveoli open are slowly destroyed. The loss of elastic recoil and small airway limitations causes the airway to collapse during expiration, causing trapping of gas during expiration. Hyperinflation from this gas trapping leads to respiratory muscle impairment and increased work of breathing during inspiration and expiration. Hypercapnia and hypoxemia occur due to ventilation and perfusion abnormalities.

Emphysema (i.e., alveolar damage) can occur throughout the lung. When the destruction is in the upper lobes, with alveoli distal to the bronchioles remaining intact, the term is *centriacinar* (centrilobular) *emphysema*. When the lower lobe (distal) alveoli are involved, the term is *panacinar* (panlobular) *emphysema*. The latter is more common in older adults and those individuals with AATD. Genetics also plays a role in COPD development. Alpha-1 antitrypsin is an enzyme that prevents elastase from attacking the lungs' structural fibers; therefore, the enzyme acts as an antielastase. With AATD, alveolar destruction ensues in smokers as well as nonsmokers. Symptoms of AATD appear at a younger age (e.g., early 30s–40s) and accounts for about 3% of COPD cases. Other genes are being evaluated in relation to COPD.

Lung underdevelopment, whether due to gestational issues (e.g., maternal smoking during pregnancy), birth issues such as low birthweight, or environmental exposure such as secondhand smoke, can also influence the development of COPD in adult life. Older age is also associated with COPD development. The normal aging lung demonstrates evidence of structural airway and alveolar changes similar to those seen in COPD. These normal aging changes include a decrease in total lung capacity (TLC) and an increase in residual volume (RV) (Figure 5-11). FEV_1 can slowly decrease every year. In addition to normal aging structural changes, older adults have a lifetime of environmental exposure to substances that can affect the lungs. These factors contribute to COPD development. People with asthma or airway hyperresponsiveness (without asthma) have an increased risk of developing COPD.

Clinical Manifestations

Patients with COPD typically first start complaining of a cough, which is often referred to as a *smoker's cough*. The cough may be productive or nonproductive and varies greatly. At times, patients may swallow the mucus rather than expectorate it. Chest tightness and wheezing is another complaint. Wheezing, cough, and sputum production can be intermittent. Airflow limitation may be present without cough. Dyspnea is a key clinical complaint in those with COPD. At first, the dyspnea manifests with activity and patients will complain of decreased activity tolerance, and as the disease progresses, the dyspnea occurs at rest. The description of dyspnea is subjective, and objective findings may not be present. The description of dyspnea varies among patients and can be described as a sense of gasping for air or chest heaviness.

Airway resistance results in hypoventilation, hypoxemia, and hypercapnia. In response to the hypoxemia, erythropoietin stimulates increased red blood cell production leading to secondary polycythemia, clubbing of fingers, cyanosis, and dyspnea at rest. Patients will complain of malaise, fatigue, and lack of appetite with weight loss. Anxiety and depression may be present. Physical abnormalities early in the course of the disease may not be present. As the disease progresses, findings may include intermittent inspiratory and expiratory wheezing as well as prolonged expiration (longer than 3 seconds). A barrel chest occasionally is evident, although it is more common when there is emphysematous damage. Hypoxemia eventually leads to pulmonary hypertension, which increases right-sided heart filling pressures, leading to right ventricular structural changes (e.g., hypertrophy) and right-sided heart failure (cor pulmonale). Cor pulmonale may manifest as weight gain and edema. See chapter 4 for a discussion of cor pulmonale.

Acute exacerbations of COPD are common and manifest as worsening respiratory status. Exacerbations can be triggered by various stimuli such as pollutant exposure or viral and bacterial infections. With COPD, the impaired pulmonary defenses (e.g., cilia damage and decreased phagocytic activity) result in frequent respiratory infections, further injuring the airway. In some cases, respiratory failure occurs. Exacerbations worsen the inflammation and heighten respiratory symptoms (e.g., dyspnea, hypoxemia). Infections can also present with fever, increased sputum volume, and purulent sputum, which are more consistent with a bacterial infection. The most common reason for an exacerbation, however, is a rhinovirus infection (i.e., common cold). Patients who recover slowly from their exacerbations (requiring more than 10 days) and/or have more frequent episodes tend to have a worse prognosis. Common comorbidities with COPD are usually due to smoking and aging and include cardiovascular disease (e.g., hypertension, ischemic heart disease), diabetes mellitus, normocytic anemia, and osteoporosis.

Diagnosis and Treatment

Spirometry is the diagnostic test used to evaluate COPD. Confirmatory diagnostic criteria include a postbronchodilator FEV_1/Forced Vital Capacity of $< 0.70\%$, which is evidence of airflow limitation (Figure 5-11) and presence of risk for COPD (e.g., smoking, poor lung development). COPD should be suspected in anyone with persistent and progressive dyspnea and dyspnea associated with activity, chronic cough with or without sputum or wheezing, or chronic sputum production.

Bronchodilators used for testing include a short-acting beta-2 agonist (SABA) and/or a short-acting anticholinergic. Patients with COPD may be evaluated for AATD even if they are older as the diagnosis may have been missed when they were younger. Chest X-rays are used to evaluate for other diagnoses that may present with similar symptoms. Findings on X-ray that are caused by COPD include a flat diaphragm, more air retrosternally due to hyperinflation, and hyperlucency (increased air, decreased density). Pulse oximetry and ABGs can be used to evaluate oxygenation status. During exacerbations, sputum cultures may be helpful, but waiting for results should not delay treatment for those suspected of bacterial infections (e.g., purulent sputum with dyspnea and/or increased sputum volume). Procalcitonin, if available, is a peptide biomarker that is released during bacterial infections and may be used to guide antibiotic administration.

Management strategies include smoking cessation, which is paramount in changing the course of COPD. Common medications for COPD include bronchodilators that are short- and long-acting beta-2 agonists (i.e., SABA and LABA) and short- and long-acting anticholinergic inhalers. Anticholinergic agents are also known as *antimuscarinic* (muscarine is a type of acetylcholine receptor). These agents act by relaxing bronchial smooth muscle. Other medications that can be considered are methylxanthines, which cause bronchodilation. Inhaled corticosteroids for maintenance and oral glucocorticoids have anti-inflammatory effects and can be used for acute exacerbations. Phosphodiesterase 4 inhibitors (e.g., roflumilast) reduce inflammation without bronchodilation and can decrease exacerbations as well as improve lung function. Mucolytics can be used to help with mucus clearance. Alpha-1 antitrypsin augmentation therapy is useful for those with deficiencies. Pulmonary rehabilitation, which includes exercise and self-management education, is beneficial for reducing dyspnea, enhancing exercise tolerance, and improving overall health status. Oxygen therapy can increase survival in patients with hypoxemia and is used during exercise for others. Ventilation support can be provided noninvasively with a variety of devices such as nasal, face, or mouth mask during exacerbations and respiratory failure. Invasive and surgical interventions for COPD can include bullectomy, lung volume reduction surgery, or lung transplantation.

Antibiotics are used during bacterial infections. Common pathogens include *Streptococcus pneumoniae* and *Haemophilus influenzae*; therefore, prescribed antibiotics should provide coverage for these organisms. Antibiotic selection is also guided by local resistance patterns and susceptibility to *Pseudomonas aeruginosa*. Hospitalization is indicated when hypoxemia and dyspnea are worsening, respiratory rate is high, and signs of altered mental status such as confusion and lethargy are present. These signs may be manifestations of acute respiratory failure or an exacerbation that is nonresponsive to treatment. Patients with heart failure, arrhythmias, or other serious comorbidities, as well as those who are not in environments where they can receive support may need to be hospitalized. Management in the hospital will be similar to the therapies previously described, such as increasing short-acting bronchodilator frequency and dose and short-term oral steroids. Oxygen therapy is administered while monitoring saturation with arterial or venous blood gases. Caution should be taken not give too much oxygen and knock out the newly oxygen-centered respiratory drive. Intubation or tracheostomy may be necessary for unstable patients (e.g., those with PaO_2 40 mmHg, respiratory acidosis, tachycardia, tachypnea, or hypotension). Patients with COPD should receive pneumococcal and influenza vaccines.

Sleep Apnea—Obstructive

Sleep apnea is characterized by the recurrent cessation or limitation of airflow through the mouth and nose despite continuing breathing efforts. The result is hypercapnia, hypoxemia, and fragmented sleep. Sleep apnea, a sleep-related breathing disorder, is categorized as obstructive (OSA) or central (CSA) in origin. OSA is associated with episodes of hypopnea (decreased depth and rate of breathing)—not solely apnea—and is also termed *OSA-hypopnea*. Of the two types, OSA is common and CSA is rare. OSA affects approximately 25 million Americans adults (Peppard et al., 2013). The incidence of OSA is on the rise due to the association and higher rates of obesity; men are affected at twice the rate of women. Risk factors include older age, obesity, and craniofacial or upper airway abnormalities. A higher prevalence of OSA is seen in people with chronic disorders such as heart failure, end-stage renal disease, and chronic lung disorders. OSA is more likely in smokers, during pregnancy, and in menopausal women. Asthma and prematurity are additional risk factors noted in children.

During sleep, there is a normal loss of muscle tone and reduced muscle activity in the upper airways, particularly during the phase of rapid eye movement. Usually there are no consequences to these physiologic changes; however, upper airway collapse, obstruction, and narrowing can occur in those predisposed to OSA. Anatomic or neuromuscular factors are associated with the predisposition to develop OSA. This collapse and the obstruction are recurrent. The obstruction is usually at the level of the soft palate/nasopharynx (i.e., velopharyngeal) or the tongue (i.e., oropharynx). (**FIGURE 5-19**).

Anatomic variations, specifically those involving craniofacial, soft tissue, and vascular factors, can cause a decrease in size of the upper airway and an increase in pressure. Enlargement of the tonsils, tongue, or oral structures (e.g., soft tissue, pharyngeal wall, long soft palate or long uvula) contribute to OSA

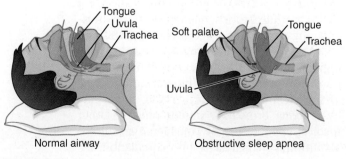

FIGURE 5-19 Apnea.

development. Enlargement of these structures often occurs with obesity; however, they can also be independent of body mass index. Enlarged tonsils and adenoids are a particular risk factor and cause of OSA in children. Craniofacial and upper airway variations that contribute to OSA can include abnormal maxillary size, short mandible size, or a lower jaw that is set farther back than the upper jaw (like an overbite). Some of these structural variations are a cause in Asians who have OSA independent of obesity. Increased vascular volume in the neck may also contribute to OSA, and this increase is more likely in patients with volume overload states such as heart failure and end-stage renal disease. Although risk factors are known, there are many instances when the exact pathophysiologic mechanism is unclear.

CSA is not as common as OSA and is more likely the result of input from inhibitory respiratory center in the brain exceeding excitatory signals. The result is a lack or decreased respiratory effort and subsequent episodes of cessation or decreased airflow (i.e., apnea-hypopnea). CSA is often associated with heart or brain abnormalities. Cheyne-Stokes respirations, which occur with stroke and heart failure, are associated with CSA. Cheyne-Stokes is a pattern of breathing characterized by deep and fast breathing followed a decrease and slow or absent breathing, so Cheyne-Stokes breathing includes cycles of hyperpnea and apnea. Drug abuse, particularly opioids, can also cause CSA.

Learning Points

Snoring

Snoring is created by vibration of tissue in the upper airway during sleep. Snoring occurs during inhalation. Almost everyone snores at some time, but some people snore habitually. Men do so more than women. Snoring is more likely with aging. Habitual snoring is a sign of airway resistance and collapse. Snoring is caused by many of the same factors that lead to OSA, such as obesity, craniofacial abnormalities, and tonsillar hypertrophy. Snoring may be associated with sleep disruption or without sleep disruption. If airway resistance increases secondary to weight gain or other factors, respiratory effort increases as a compensatory mechanism and may start to cause sleep disturbances. Persistent airway resistance can then lead to OSA. In summary, snoring may or may not be associated with OSA. The main reason for evaluating causes of snoring, in addition to sleep alteration, is to identify OSA. Treatment of snoring is similar to OSA and includes weight loss, smoking cessation, reduction of alcohol consumption particularly just prior to bedtime, and sleeping on one's side; and several devices such as nasal dilators can be beneficial.

Clinical Manifestations

Clinical manifestations include:

- Snoring that is habitual, often loud, and frequent
- Periods of silence in breathing or apnea (witnessed by bed partner or another person)
- Sleep characterized by nighttime choking, gasping, or breath holding
- Nonrestorative sleep with daytime sleepiness, fatigue, poor concentration, and irritability

Other symptoms that are nonspecific and may be present include nocturia and morning headaches.

Diagnosis and Treatment

Diagnosis is based on history and physical examination and a sleep study (i.e., polysomnography) as the first-line diagnostic study. Criteria for diagnosis includes:

- Five or more obstructive respiratory events (e.g., apnea, hypopnea, increased respiratory effort) per hour of sleep with one or more of the bulleted clinical manifestations discussed and/or a diagnosis of hypertension, mood disorder, cognitive dysfunction, coronary artery disease, stroke, heart failure, atrial fibrillation, or type 2 diabetes mellitus
- Fifteen or more obstructive respiratory events per hour of sleep regardless of the presence of comorbidities

The sleep study can be done in a laboratory or home setting. The laboratory setting is preferred if there are comorbidities as additional parameters such as seizure activity or limb movement can be measured.

The treatments for sleep apnea include weight loss, behavioral measures, and the delivery of continuous positive airway pressure (CPAP). Behavioral modification includes non-supine sleeping position and avoidance of alcohol or sedating medications, particularly at night. Daytime reduction of alcohol and sedating medications may also decrease the incidence, improve sleep, and promote weight loss. Various oral and nasal appliances such as a nasal splint or tongue retaining apparatuses may be beneficial. CPAP is the cornerstone of therapy; however, there are other modes of positive pressure administration such as bilevel positive airway pressure and auto-titrating positive airway pressure. CPAP is the simplest as well as the most clinically studied and used. The principle of CPAP therapy involves the delivery of pharyngeal pressure so that it exceeds surrounding pressure, which in turn prevents collapse.

Cystic Fibrosis—Obstructive

Cystic fibrosis (CF) is a common inherited respiratory disorder that causes severe lung damage and nutritional deficits. Approximately 1,000 new patients are diagnosed each year in the United States (Cystic Fibrosis Foundation, n.d.). Whites are more likely to develop cystic fibrosis than other ethnic groups, followed by Latinos and American Indians. Most children (66%) are diagnosed by the age of 1 year and of newly diagnosed patients 58% are detected by newborn screening. (CF Registry, 2017).

The genetic defect that leads to cystic fibrosis is a mutation in the gene that makes transmembrane conductance regulator (CFTR) protein. In CF, there are CFTR defects in production, processing, regulation, or conduction. The mutated gene has been isolated to chromosome 7, and transmission follows an autosomal recessive pattern. Over 1,700 mutations in the defective CFTR gene are possible, but only some of the mutations are disease causing. One mutation known as the *F508del* is a common cause of many CF symptoms. Out of the 1,480 amino acids that make up the CFTR protein, the F508del mutation causes one single amino acid to develop into an abnormal shape and an inability for the CFTR protein to function properly. More than 10 million Americans (1 in 31) are carriers of this faulty gene, and many do not know they are carriers.

CFTR defects cause problems with chloride movement across the cell membrane, also causing imbalances in sodium and water transport. Cystic fibrosis changes the cells that produce mucus, sweat, saliva, and digestive secretions. The number and size of goblet cells increases resulting in more mucus production. The lungs and pancreas are primarily affected, but other organs can also be involved (e.g., liver, intestines, sinuses, and reproductive organs). In CF, normally thin secretions become thick and tenacious as a result of defects in chloride secretion and excess sodium reabsorption. In the respiratory tract, the secretions occlude airways, ducts, and passageways instead of providing normal lubrication. Occlusions also occur in cilia fluid layer is reduced and the cilia become ineffective in clearing the excess mucus.

Neutrophils are abundant in the airways of those with CF and contribute to the lung damage by releasing various oxidants. Neutrophil elastase damages elastin, promotes inflammation, and further stimulates mucus secretion. Antioxidants, as part of the defense mechanisms, are not able to cross the defective channels, rendering defense mechanisms ineffective. Immunoglobulin G is also destroyed by neutrophil elastase, further insulting the immune system. Atelectasis develops as airways are obstructed, leading to permanent damage (FIGURE 5-20). Mucus stagnates, becoming a prime medium for bacterial growth. *Pseudomonas aeruginosa* is commonly present in the airway of those with CF. Infections are recurrent and, combined with the cycle of impaired mucus clearance and chronic airway inflammation, progressive lung destruction ensues. Bronchiectasis (permanent abnormal dilatation and destruction of bronchial walls) and emphysema-like changes are common as fibrosis and obstructions advance. Abscesses and bullae may develop. The bullae can burst and lead to pneumothorax. The vascular changes in the lung lead to pulmonary hypertension and cor pulmonale. Respiratory failure is the most common cause of death in people who have cystic fibrosis.

In the digestive tract, the mucus blocks the intestines, producing a meconium ileus in the newborn. Mucus also blocks pancreatic ducts, leading to damaged acinar cells that are not able to produce and transport pancreatic enzymes. Without these digestive enzymes, malabsorption and malnutrition develop. The trapped digestive enzymes damage pancreatic tissue by causing autodigestion. Additionally, the acinar cells become atrophic. These changes contribute to the development of diabetes mellitus and osteoporosis. Blocked bile ducts add to the malabsorption issues and increase risk for developing cirrhosis.

Salivary glands are only mildly affected by blockages. Sweat glands produce sweat high in sodium chloride, which can cause electrolyte imbalances in times of excessive loss (e.g., during exercise or hot weather). Obstructions in the reproductive system can lead to sterility and infertility.

Clinical Manifestations

Clinical manifestations of cystic fibrosis may appear at birth and progressively worsen throughout the life span. Lung function often starts declining in early childhood. The severity

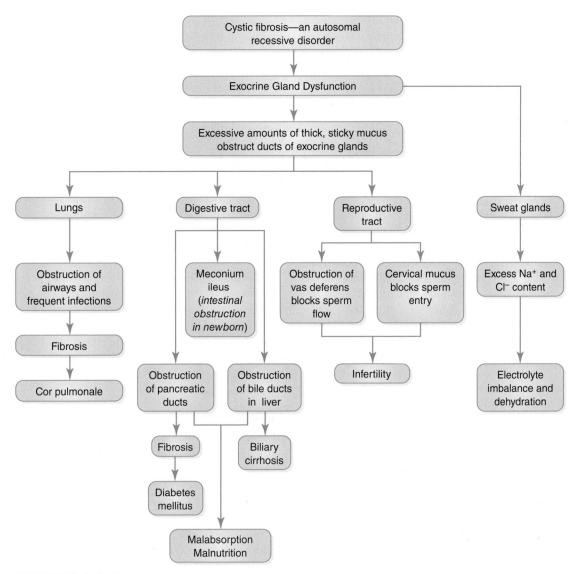

FIGURE 5-20 Cystic fibrosis.

of the disease varies even with the same mutations, and genetic variants also influence disease progression and survival. Some mutations are more commonly associated with gastrointestinal instead of lung symptoms, but awareness of the type of mutation is not always consistent with presentation or severity.

Meconium ileus in the newborn may occur. Parents may notice their baby's skin tastes salty when they kiss their child. Respiratory manifestations include frequent respiratory infections, chronic cough with tenacious sputum, dyspnea, fatigue, and activity intolerance. Digital clubbing, wheezing, rhonchi, chronic sinus infections, and nasal polyps may also be present. Thoracic changes such as a barrel chest appear later in the disease. Hemoptysis is a sign of damage to the vascular system due

to bronchiectasis. Gastrointestinal manifestations include steatorrhea (fatty, foul-smelling stools) and fat-soluble vitamin deficiency (vitamins A, D, E, and K). Despite a voracious appetite, weight is difficult to maintain, and growth may be delayed or impaired. Various complications can develop, and manifestations will vary for each. Manifestations could include chronic bronchitis, failure to thrive, cardiomegaly, diabetes mellitus, pancreatitis, rectal prolapse, liver disease, cholelithiasis, osteoporosis, hyponatremia, metabolic alkalosis, and infertility.

Diagnosis and Treatment

Diagnosis of cystic fibrosis can be accomplished prenatally when family history warrants testing. In the United States, all newborns are screened for cystic fibrosis regardless of family history.

This screening involves analysis of the newborn's blood for higher than normal levels of immunoreactive trypsinogen (IRT), a chemical released by the pancreas. IRT level may be elevated because of prematurity or a stressful delivery; therefore, other tests are used to confirm the diagnosis. Sweat analysis (i.e., sweat chloride test) is the standard for diagnosing CF. The test can be conducted as soon as the infant is 48 hours old or as long as enough sweat can be produced. Sweat analysis is used to detect sweat chloride concentration. A level of greater than 60 mmol/L is diagnostic. The delta F508 test can identify the chromosome 7 mutation, and it is often used if a false-negative sweat test is suspected or to identify carrier status of siblings. Genotyping for the CFTR mutation is done to evaluate for CF. Stool can be evaluated for the presence of pancreatic (e.g., fecal elastase) content. Other tests that assess lung function include chest X-rays, pulmonary function tests, and ABGs.

Cystic fibrosis treatment requires diligent family involvement and an interdisciplinary approach because of the progressive, multisystem nature of the disease. Treatment regimens have improved the life expectancy for patients who have cystic fibrosis, with some people living into their 40s or 50s. Treatment often requires a multidisciplinary team including cystic fibrosis specialists, respiratory therapists, dietitians, and psychological counselors. Strategies are focused on respiratory care and infection control. Airway clearance therapy is important to facilitate the expectoration of mucus. These therapies include intensive chest physiotherapy either manually or with a mechanical percussor, postural drainage, and coughing and breathing exercises. Regular, moderate aerobic exercises can improve pulmonary health. Adequate hydration, humidified air, and avoidance of respiratory irritants such as smoke, pollution, and allergens or contact with infectious people are also part of respiratory care. Good hand washing and maintaining clean respiratory equipment can reduce infections. Categories of medications for pulmonary health include aerosol therapy, antibiotics, anti-inflammatory drugs, and CFTR modulators. Aerosol therapies can include beta-2 agonists and anticholinergics. Mucolytics, such as dornase alfa or hypertonic saline, improve mucociliary clearance. Inhaled or oral corticosteroids are not recommended and are considered harmful, but other anti-inflammatories such as ibuprofen, glutathione, N-acetyl cysteine, leukotriene modifiers or azithromycin may be beneficial in reducing inflammation. Antibiotics can be considered for maintenance and treatment of pulmonary infections. Various studies are underway to evaluate the best choice of antibiotics, method of delivery, and duration of treatment. CFTR modulators are medications that target the underlying genetic mutation and correct the malfunctioning protein. These medications are categorized as potentiators, correctors, and amplifiers and include such medications as ivacaftor or ivacaftor/lumacaftor. Gene therapy is under investigation.

Nutritional and gastrointestinal guidelines include pancreatic enzyme, bile salt, and fat-soluble vitamin replacement. A well-balanced, high-protein, low-fat, high-sodium diet is recommended. Enteral tube feedings may be necessary if a patient has an inadequate oral intake. Lung transplantation may be considered for severe lung disease. Even if the transplant is successful, other areas (e.g., gastrointestinal) are still affected by CF. Management of comorbidities is essential.

Lung Cancer

Lung cancer is the second most often diagnosed cancer in men and women and the leading cause of cancer in the United States (American Cancer Society, 2018). Primary lung cancers (e.g., bronchogenic carcinoma) arise from the epithelial cells that line the bronchi or bronchioles. After increasing for decades, lung cancer incidence and mortality rates are now decreasing in parallel with decreases in rates of cigarette smoking in this country. Frequently, other cancers—such as breast, bladder, and colon—metastasize to the lung tissue causing secondary lung cancer.

Smoking contributes to the majority (80–90%) of lung cancer cases. The more than 4,000 chemicals in cigarette smoke include carcinogens and chemicals that paralyze cilia. The risk for developing lung cancer is directly related to the length of time a person smokes and the number of cigarettes smoked. Secondhand smoke can also be a significant contributing factor. Smoking cessation or removing the smoke exposure will gradually decrease risk. Inhalation of other chemicals (e.g., asbestos, radon gas, tar, and pollution) and chronic lung disease can also increase risk (FIGURE 5-21).

The lungs provide an optimal environment for tumor development and growth. Carcinogens can seek refuge in the many nooks and crannies of the air passages. Upon exposure to the carcinogen, irreversible oncogene DNA mutations and inactivation of tumor suppressor genes occur in the epithelial stem cells. The cells are unable to grow or differentiate

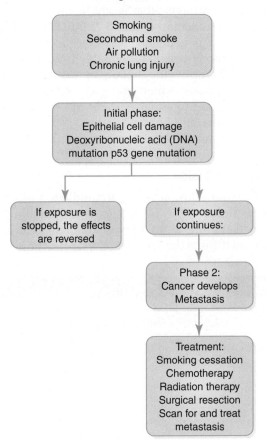

FIGURE 5-21 Lung cancer.

properly and rather become metaplastic and eventually progress to invasive carcinoma. Inherited genetic predispositions contribute to lung cancer development. Epidermal growth factor and inflammatory mediators promote tumor growth. The scores of blood vessels supplying the lungs serve as entrance points for distant cancer cells to gain access, and those vessels furnish the cancer with a rich blood source to facilitate its growth.

There are different categorizations of lung cancers, but generally, they can be divided into two types—small cell and non–small cell carcinomas (FIGURE 5-22). Small cell carcinoma is often referred to as *oat cell carcinoma* and is considered a neuroendocrine tumor. Other neuroendocrine tumors include large cell neuroendocrine and typical and atypical carcinoid tumors. Small cell carcinoma occurs almost exclusively in heavy smokers and is less frequent than non–small cell cancers. Prognosis is poor as the tumors grow rapidly and metastasis occurs early in the disease. Non–small cell carcinoma is the most common type of malignant lung cancer, accounting for 85% of all cases of lung cancer. Non–small cell carcinoma is classified into several subgroups—squamous cell carcinoma, adenocarcinoma, and large cell undifferentiated carcinoma. Adenocarcinoma is the most prevalent of all lung tumors. Other lung cancer tumors (e.g., mesothelioma) exist, but they are considered to be rare.

Tumors in the lungs lead to several issues including airway obstruction and inflammatory changes, which cause a cough and contribute to infections. Fluid can accumulate in the pleural

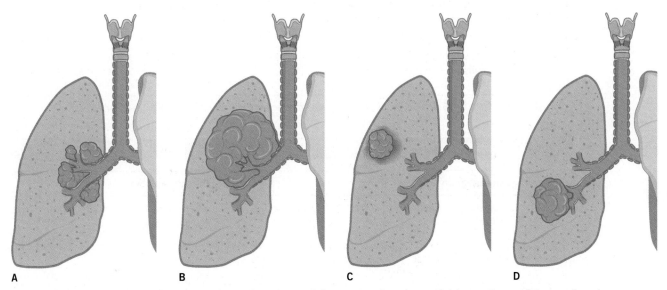

FIGURE 5-22 Cancer of the lung. A Small cell (oat cell) carcinoma. B Squamous cell carcinoma. C Adenocarcinoma. D Large cell carcinoma.

space, leading to an effusion, hemothorax, or pneumothorax. Some tumors cause an endocrine dysfunction associated with secretion of hormones and cause a paraneoplastic syndrome.

Clinical Manifestations

Clinical manifestations of lung cancer are insidious because they mimic signs of smoking (e.g., cough). Manifestations can include a persistent cough or a change in usual cough, dyspnea, hemoptysis, and frequent respiratory infections. Chest pain and hoarseness may be present. Anorexia, anemia, and weight loss accompany symptoms. Other symptoms specific to the site(s) of metastasis, such as bone pain, should be evaluated. Paraneoplastic syndromes can be manifested in multiple systems (e.g., endocrine, neurologic, dermatologic). Syndrome of inappropriate antidiuretic hormone and hypercalcemia are some common signs (see chapter 10 for more on endocrine function and chapter 6 for more on fluid and electrolyte homeostasis).

Diagnosis and Treatment

Diagnostic procedures for lung cancer include a history, physical examination, chest X-ray, CT, MRI, bronchoscopy, sputum studies, biopsy, positron emission tomography, bone scans, and pulmonary function tests. Treatment is based on staging and can include usual cancer treatment—that is, chemotherapy, surgery, and radiation (**TABLE 5-7**; **TABLE 5-8**). The treatment is generally palliative because the tumor rarely responds favorably to treatment. Early diagnosis and treatment may improve this prognosis. Other strategies include those to maintain optimal respiratory function—oxygen therapy, bronchodilators, and antibiotics (if bacterial infections are present).

Pleural Effusion

A pleural effusion is the accumulation of excess fluid in the pleural cavity. Normally, a small amount of fluid (approximately 20 mL.) drained from the lymphatic system is present

TABLE 5-7	Staging and Treatment of Non–Small Cell Lung Cancer	
Stage	**Description**	**Usual treatment plan**
Stage I	Cancer has invaded the underlying lung tissue but has not spread to the lymph nodes.	Surgery
Stage II	Cancer has spread to neighboring lymph nodes or invaded the chest wall.	Surgery, radiation, and chemotherapy
Stage IIIA	Cancer has spread from the lung to lymph nodes in the center of the chest.	Combined chemotherapy and radiation, sometimes surgery based on results of treatment
Stage IIIB	Cancer has spread locally to areas such as the heart, blood vessels, trachea, and esophagus—all within the chest—or to lymph nodes in the area of the collarbone or to the tissue that surrounds the lungs within the rib cage (pleura).	Chemotherapy, sometimes radiation
Stage IV	Cancer has spread to other parts of the body, such as the liver, bones, or brain.	Chemotherapy, targeted drug therapy, clinical trials, supportive care

Reproduced from Story, L. (2017). *Pathophysiology: A practical approach* (3rd ed.). Burlington, MA: Jones & Bartlett Learning.

TABLE 5-8	Staging and Treatment of Small Cell Lung Cancer	
Stage	**Description**	**Usual treatment plan**
Limited	Cancer is confined to one lung and to its neighboring lymph nodes.	Combined chemotherapy and radiation, sometimes surgery
Extensive	Cancer has spread beyond one lung and nearby lymph nodes and may have invaded both lungs, more remote lymph nodes, or other organs.	Chemotherapy, clinical trials, supportive care

Reproduced from Story, L. (2017). *Pathophysiology: A practical approach* (3rd ed.). Burlington, MA: Jones & Bartlett Learning.

in this space to lubricate the constantly moving lungs. Effusions develop because there is either excess pleural fluid formed or decreased lymphatic removal. Excessive fluid in the pleural cavity can compress the lung and limit expansion during inhalation. Effusions vary in nature and may affect both lungs or one lung.

Effusions are categorized by whether they are transudative or exudative. Identifying the cause of the effusion is facilitated by categorization. **Transudative effusions** are caused by systemic processes, such as heart failure, cirrhosis, or kidney disease. Transudates result because of changes in hydrostatic and osmotic pressure that shift fluid into the pleural space. In heart failure, the excess fluid in the interstitial space increases hydrostatic pressure, causing fluid to enter the pleural space. Hypoproteinemia, which can occur with cirrhosis or kidney disease, causes a reduction in oncotic pressure drawing water out of the capillaries and into the pleural space. **Exudative effusions** can be more difficult to diagnose as there are a variety of mechanisms. In general, exudative effusions occur when there is a localized lung or pleural alteration such as inflammation or decreased lymphatic drainage. The inflammatory process occurs in disorders such as pneumonia, lung abscesses, or bronchiectasis that increase capillary membrane permeability causing shifting of fluid into the pleural space. Impairment in lymphatic drainage results in an accumulation of pleural fluid due to decreased removal. Some exudates have observable characteristics. Grossly purulent effusions are termed **empyema**. An effusion

known as a **hemothorax** (blood in the pleural space) is usually due to trauma. Another type of effusion is a **chylothorax** (an accumulation of a milky white fluid composed of fat droplets and lymph) that can also occur due to trauma or alterations in the lymph system. Lymphoma, lung, and breast cancers are the three most common tumors (75%) that cause a malignancy-associated pleural effusion, and the type is usually exudative.

Pleurisy, or pleuritis, can precede or follow the effusion, or it may occur independently. Pleurisy comprises inflammation of the pleural membranes, which leads to swollen and irregular tissue. This inflammation is often associated with pneumonia and creates friction in the pleural membranes.

Clinical Manifestations

Clinical manifestations and consequences of pleural effusion depends on its type, location, amount, and fluid accumulation rate. Patients may have few to no symptoms with small effusions and/or complain of dyspnea and chest pain (usually sharp and worsens with inhalation). Physical examination findings can include tachypnea, tachycardia, pleural friction rub (pleurisy), and diminished or absent lung sounds over the effusion. Dullness to percussion may be elicited over the effusion. Large effusions can cause the pleural membranes to separate, preventing their cohesion during inhalation (**FIGURE 5-23; FIGURE 5-24**). This lack of cohesion impedes full expansion, leading to

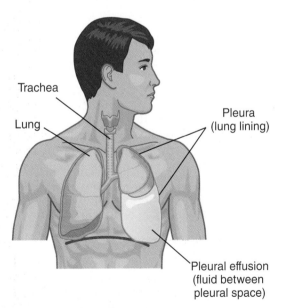

FIGURE 5-23 Pleural effusion is a buildup of fluid in the lining of the lungs.

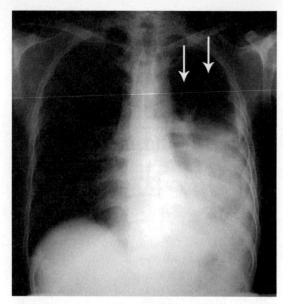

FIGURE 5-24 X-ray of pleural effusion.

Courtesy of Michael-Joseph F. Agbayani.

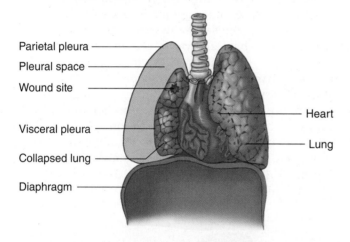

Parietal pleura

Pleural space

Wound site

Visceral pleura

Collapsed lung

Diaphragm

Heart

Lung

FIGURE 5-25 Serous membranes showing how a pneumothorax occurs when air leaks into the pleural space between the parietal and visceral pleura. The lung collapses as air fills the pleural space and the two pleural membranes are no longer in contact with each other.

atelectasis and a pneumothorax. Large effusions can impair venous return in the inferior vena cava and cardiac filling by exerting pressure on those structures, causing a mediastinal shift (heart, esophagus, trachea) to the unaffected side. A shift can cause cardiopulmonary compromise, which can be life threatening.

Diagnosis and Treatment

Diagnostic procedures for pleural effusion include a history, physical examination, chest X-ray, CT, ABGs, and CBC. Thoracentesis (needle aspiration of fluid) with subsequent examination to distinguish between transudative

versus exudative effusions is indicated when there is a new pleural effusion. If the effusion is small or the diagnosis is clear, such as heart failure, thoracentesis may be postponed. Pleural fluid analysis starts with gross appearance (e.g., hemothorax) and evaluation of cells (e.g., eosinophils, lymphocytes), pH, protein (e.g., levels are low in transudative effusion), lactic dehydrogenase, and glucose levels. Additional tests of the fluid, such as acid-fast bacillus staining for tuberculosis, may be warranted depending on clinical suspicion.

Treatment focuses on addressing the underlying cause. Regardless of etiology, removal of the fluid is necessary to promote full expansion of the lungs. Strategies to do so may include thoracentesis, placement of a chest drainage tube, and antibiotics. However, small effusions can cause minimal symptoms and resolve with just the correction of the underlying problem (e.g., heart failure).

Pneumothorax

Pneumothorax refers to air in the pleural cavity. The presence of atmospheric air in the pleural cavity and the separation of pleural membranes can lead to a partial or complete collapse of a lung (**FIGURE 5-25** and **FIGURE 5-26**). The air enters in one of two ways. Damage to the visceral pleura surrounding the lung causes air to escape from the lungs to the intrapleural space. The visceral pleura can be damaged due to pulmonary disease or lung injury. Air can also enter when the parietal pleura that lines the chest wall or the chest wall itself is injured and atmospheric air enters the intrapleural space. A small pneumothorax causes mild symptoms and may heal on its own. A larger pneumothorax generally requires aggressive treatment to remove the air and reestablish pulmonary negative pressure. Risk factors for developing pneumothorax include smoking, tall stature, and history of lung disease or previous pneumothorax.

Several types of pneumothoraces are distinguished, based on their cause. Pneumothoraces can be categorized as spontaneous or traumatic. A **spontaneous (nontraumatic) pneumothorax** occurs in the absence of trauma. The pneumothorax develops when air enters the pleural cavity from an opening in the internal airways. Primary spontaneous pneumothorax occurs when a small air blister on the top of the lung (bleb) ruptures. Blebs cause a weakness in the lung tissue. Bleb development without other lung disease is more

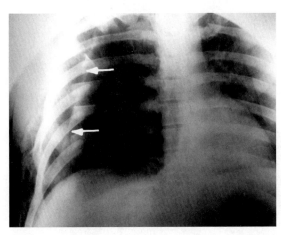

FIGURE 5-26 X-ray of a pneumothorax.

Courtesy of Leonard V. Crowley, MD, Century College.

common in tall, thin healthy men between the ages of 20 and 40 years. The bleb may rupture, often for no apparent reason, and cause a spontaneous pneumothorax. Mutations in the folliculin gene have been linked to the incidence of spontaneous pneumothorax in families. Rupture can also occur from changes in air pressure, such as occur when scuba diving, flying, mountain climbing, or listening to extremely loud music. Additionally, a spontaneous pneumothorax may happen while smoking marijuana—a deep inhalation, followed by slowly breathing out against partially closed lips, forces the smoke deeper into the lungs. Primary spontaneous pneumothoraces tend to be milder with less serious consequences than other types of pneumothoraces.

Spontaneous pneumothoraces can develop in people with preexisting lung disease (e.g., emphysema, pneumonia, cystic fibrosis, or lung cancer). A pneumothorax from prior lung disease can also be termed *secondary pneumothorax*. In these cases, the pneumothorax occurs because the diseased lung tissue is weakened, and usually air blisters within the lung tissue (bullae) and/or on top (blebs) rupture (similar to primary pneumothoraces). A pneumothorax from preexisting disease can be more severe and even life threatening because diseased tissue can create a larger opening in the lung, allowing more air to enter the pleural space. Additionally, pulmonary disease reduces lung reserves, making any further reduction in lung function more serious. Chronic obstructive lung disease is a common cause of spontaneous pneumothorax.

A **traumatic pneumothorax** defines the mechanism by which a pneumothorax occurs (i.e., traumatically) and can stem from

blunt trauma (e.g., vehicle air bag deployment) or penetrating injury (e.g., knife or gunshot wounds) to the chest. Traumatic pneumothoraces can inadvertently occur during certain medical procedures, such as chest tube insertion or removal, cardiopulmonary resuscitation, and lung or liver biopsy; this is termed *iatrogenic pneumothorax*. Mechanical ventilation is another cause of traumatic pneumothorax. Mechanical ventilation can increase alveolar pressures and cause alveolar rupture (barotrauma), leading to air escaping outside the alveolar space. Overdistention of the lungs from mechanical ventilation (volutrauma) can cause a pneumothorax. Using high levels of positive end-expiratory pressure (PEEP) and tidal volume during mechanical ventilation increases the risk of pneumothorax. Pneumothorax can also be categorized as open or closed. When the chest wall is intact, the term used is *closed pneumothorax;* causes include traumatic nonpenetrating injuries such as blunt trauma, rib fractures, or spontaneous bleb rupture from COPD. An open pneumothorax involves a breach in the chest wall whether iatrogenic or traumatic.

Learning Points

PEEP

One of the settings on a mechanical ventilator is PEEP. Mechanical ventilation causes inactivation of the normal surfactant that keeps alveoli from collapsing. During mechanical ventilation, alveolar capillary membrane permeability is increased, causing frequent alveolar opening and collapsing with resulting increased pressure to reopen the alveoli. The use of applied PEEP from the ventilator provides an external pressure to avoid alveoli collapse at the end of expiration so that more alveoli (recruitment) remain available for gas exchange. While PEEP can be used therapeutically such as with acute respiratory distress syndrome (ARDS), there are negative consequences with high delivered pressures (e.g., pneumothorax, decreased cardiac output, increased intracranial pressure).

A **tension pneumothorax** is the most serious consequence of a pneumothorax; it occurs when the pressure in the pleural space is greater than the atmospheric pressure (Figure 5-10). The increased pressure rises due to air getting trapped in the pleural space during inspiration, but the air cannot escape during expiration. The force of the trapped air can cause the affected lung to collapse completely and shift the heart toward the uncollapsed lung (called *mediastinal shift*), compressing the unaffected lung and the heart (**FIGURE 5-27**).

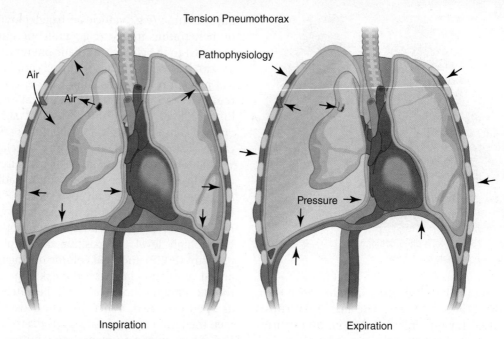

FIGURE 5-27 Tension pneumothorax. A one-way valve from a penetrating injury allows air into the pleural space during inspiration, but not out during expiration.

Tension pneumothorax progresses rapidly and is fatal if not treated quickly. Tension pneumothorax can occur from open penetrating trauma or even if the chest is closed, as with positive pressure mechanical ventilation or after chest tube removal.

Clinical Manifestations

Clinical manifestations vary in severity depending on the type of pneumothorax. These manifestations include the following signs and symptoms: sudden chest pain over the affected lung, chest tightness, anxiety, and dyspnea. Physical findings can include tachypnea, tachycardia, and decreased breath sounds as well as hyperresonance over the affected area. Chest expansion may be asymmetrical. A pneumothorax, particularly a tension pneumothorax, can lead to a deviated trachea and mediastinal shift, hypotension, and rapid deterioration and cardiovascular collapse if not corrected.

Diagnostic procedures for pneumothorax consist of a history, physical examination, chest X-ray, CT, and ABGs. Treatment usually involves removal of the air and reestablishment of negative pressure, allowing for full expansion of the lungs. Such strategies may include thoracentesis and placement of a chest drainage tube with suction, which removes fluid and reestablishes negative pressure. Surgery may be required in some cases

to correct and prevent future episodes. During surgery, the leak is repaired, and a chemical may be used to scar the area (pleurodesis). Blebs can be removed when there is recurrence or other situations. To reduce the incidence of mechanical ventilation–induced pneumothorax, pressures and volumes should be titrated (usually lowered), taking into consideration therapeutic benefit versus risk of pulmonary compromise.

Acute Respiratory Distress Syndrome—Restrictive

Acute respiratory distress syndrome (ARDS) is a sudden failure of the respiratory system due to massive alveolar capillary membrane injury and acute lung inflammation. ARDS has many other names, such as shock lung, wet lung, stiff lung, and noncardiogenic pulmonary edema. Multiple conditions can precipitate ARDS, including prolonged shock, burns, aspiration, and smoke inhalation. This condition involves an acute hypoxemic event that is cardiac in origin resulting from an indirect systemic event, a direct pulmonary event, or a combination. An indirect systemic event could be a trauma, septicemia, acute pancreatitis, a drug overdose, a cardiopulmonary bypass, or a transfusion reaction. A direct pulmonary event could involve illicit drug and toxic gas inhalation, pneumonia, RSV infection, gastric acid aspiration, near drowning, or fat embolism. Pneumonia with sepsis would be an example of both. ARDS develops rapidly, often within 90 minutes of a systemic inflammatory response or within 48 hours of a lung injury. Risk factors include the presence of a chronic lung disease (e.g., emphysema, chronic bronchitis, and asthma), alcoholism, age greater than 65 years, and severe illness on presentation.

Multiple blood transfusions can cause a type of ARDS known as *transfusion-related acute lung injury*, which is one of the main causes of death due to transfusion. Sepsis is a common cause of ARDS. Varying criteria and definition of ARDS over the years and advances in management have led to various statistics pertaining to incidence and mortality. In general, ARDS is fatal in approximately one-third of cases. Individuals who survive will fully recover; however, it may take as long as a year for them to regain complete lung function, and they can have neurocognitive changes for up to 5 years.

ARDS progresses through phases that have varying and overlapping clinical and pathologic changes. These three phases are the exudative, proliferative, and fibrotic phases. The exudative phase is early in the course of ARDS and begins within 4 hours of the causative event and can last up to 7 days. Injury to the alveolar epithelial cell (i.e., type I pneumocytes) and the capillary endothelial cell membranes leads to the release of chemical inflammatory mediators (e.g., interleukin 1 and 8, tumor necrosis factor) (**FIGURE 5-28**; **FIGURE 5-29**). These mediators increase capillary permeability, promote fluid and protein accumulation in the alveoli and interstitial spaces, and damage surfactant-producing cells (type II pneumocytes). Lung damage progresses as neutrophils migrate to the site, releasing proteases and other mediators, further damaging the alveolar capillary membrane and causing further leaking of fluid, proteins, and blood into the interstitium and alveoli. A hyaline membrane (a thin layer of tissue) forms in the alveoli and causes them to become stiff. Increased platelet aggregation and complement activation promotes microemboli development, further injuring the pulmonary vasculature. These events result in decreased gas exchange with severe hypoxemia and hypercapnia, reduced pulmonary blood flow, and limited lung expansion. Diffuse atelectasis and reduced lung capacity ensue.

Acute Respiratory Distress Syndrome (ARDS)

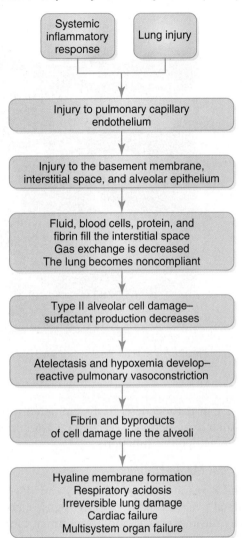

FIGURE 5-28 Acute respiratory distress syndrome pathogenesis.

The proliferative phase lasts up to 21 days, and signs of resolution begin with pulmonary edema resolving. Type II pneumocytes begin making more surfactant along the alveolar wall and become type I pneumocytes for gas exchange. While some people recover during this phase, others continue to have lung injury and begin to develop fibrosis. During the fibrotic phase, the alveoli and interstitium are fibrotic with emphysematous changes and bullae development. The fibrotic processes damage pulmonary circulation leading to pulmonary hypertension. Pneumothorax can occur along with acute respiratory failure. If the patient survives, scattered necrosis and fibrosis are apparent throughout the lungs. ARDS is

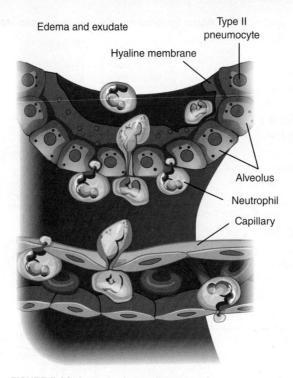

Edema and exudate

Type II pneumocyte

Hyaline membrane

Alveolus

Neutrophil

Capillary

Acute respiratory distress syndrome:

In ARDS, type I cells die as a result of diffuse alveolar damage.

Intra-alveolar edema follows, after which there is formation of hyaline membrane composed of proteinaceous axudate and cell debris.

In the acute phase, the lungs are markedly congested and heavy.

Type II cells multiply to line the alveolar surface.

Interstitial inflammation is characteristic.

The lesion may heal completely or progress to interstitial fibrosis.

FIGURE 5-29 Acute respiratory distress syndrome.

similar in pathogenesis to disseminated intravascular coagulation (see chapter 3 for more on hematopoietic function).

Clinical Manifestations

Clinical manifestations of ARDS can develop suddenly or insidiously. Early signs such as tachypnea, dyspnea, and tachycardia can be subtle or a sign of many other illnesses. As lung injury continues, respiratory efforts worsen with evident accessory muscle use, anxiety, restlessness, and hypoxemia. Lung sounds, which are initially normal, begin to reflect the edema, and coarse crackles can be heard. In ARDS, supplemental oxygen delivery is usually not effective, and arterial oxygen saturation (SaO_2) decreases. If damage continues, mental status becomes altered. Bowel sounds decrease, generalized edema sets in, and progression continues with symptoms of multiple organ dysfunction syndrome. Other systemic changes are often occurring simultaneously with ARDS as the chemical mediators affect more than just the lung. The inflammatory activation is initially protective but becomes detrimental and leads to what is termed *systemic inflammatory response syndrome*. This syndrome occurs often with ARDS and also leads to multiple organ dysfunction syndrome. Systemic inflammatory response syndrome criteria include tachypnea (> 20 breaths/minute), tachycardia (> 90 beats/minute), $PaCO_2$ of less than 32 mmHg, and temperature decrease (< 38°C) or increase (> 38°C) with a white blood cell count that is either low (< 4,000 cell/mm³) or high (> 12,000 cell/mm³) or higher than 10% bands.

Diagnosis and Treatment

Diagnostic procedures for ARDS consist of ABGs, chest X-ray, CT, and CBC and other tests such as blood cultures to identify the cause. Chest X-rays in the early stages may be normal, and blood gases may reveal a respiratory alkalosis. As time progresses, chest X-rays may reveal bilateral infiltrates and fluid in the alveoli (air bronchogram). Respiratory and metabolic acidosis become evident. The Berlin criteria were developed to predict ARDS prognosis and to define diagnostic criteria. For ARDS to be diagnosed respiratory symptoms must have begun within 1 week of injury/insult. To diagnose ARDS, opacities on chest X-ray or CT scanning and clinical findings must not be explained by other diseases (e.g., lung collapse or pleural effusion), and oxygenation must be low with three categories (i.e., mild, moderate, or severe) determined by PaO_2/FiO_2 and PEEP or CPAP settings (e.g., moderate is $100 < PaO_2/FiO_2 \leq 200$ with PEEP ≥ 5 cm H_2O). The *mild Berlin category* is now the term used instead of *acute lung injury*.

The main goal of treatment is to maintain adequate oxygenation and respiratory status. Such strategies include mechanical ventilation. To prevent ventilator-induced lung injury, recommendations are to use low tidal volumes ($<$ 6 mL/kg of predicted body weight) with PEEP (10–15 cm H_2O) to counterbalance the use of high oxygen administration (FiO_2). Extracorporeal membrane oxygenation, which is useful in neonatal respiratory distress might be beneficial in certain cases. Extracorporeal membrane oxygenation, as opposed to a ventilator, facilitates the process of gas exchange through an artificial membrane lung. Pharmacologic therapy may include antibiotics empirically (not prophylactically), bronchodilators, mucolytics, and sedatives. Cardiovascular status must be carefully monitored. Other strategies include nutritional support (e.g., enteral feedings), conservative fluid therapy, and stress ulcer and deep vein thrombosis prophylaxis and other supportive therapies in critically ill patients. Appropriate treatment of underlying causes is key to treating ARDS.

Alterations in Ventilation and Perfusion

Atelectasis—Restrictive

Atelectasis refers to incomplete alveolar expansion or collapse of the alveoli. It occurs when the walls of the alveoli stick together. Atelectasis may be caused by the following conditions:

- Surfactant deficiencies
- Bronchus obstruction (e.g., foreign objects, mucous plugs, and tumors)
- Lung tissue compression (e.g., tumor, pneumothorax, pleural effusion, and abdominal distention)
- Increased surface tension (e.g., pulmonary edema)
- Lung fibrosis (e.g., emphysema)

When alveoli are not filled with air, they shrivel—much like raisins. This ventilation issue can, in turn, impair blood flow through the lung. The ineffective ventilation and perfusion then impair gas exchange. Surgery and immobility increase the risk for developing atelectasis for this reason.

Atelectasis can occur in either small or large areas. If only a small area is affected, the respiratory rate will increase to improve the excretion of carbon dioxide and control the carbon dioxide levels. The larger the area affected,

the more severe the symptoms experienced. Necrosis, infection (e.g., pneumonia), and permanent lung damage can occur if the alveoli are not reinflated quickly.

Clinical Manifestations

The clinical manifestations of atelectasis are due to impaired ventilation and perfusion and include dyspnea, cough, anxiety, and restlessness. Physical exam findings include diminished breath sounds, asymmetrical chest expansion, tachypnea, tachycardia, and fever.

Diagnosis and Treatment

Diagnostic procedures for atelectasis include determining a cause and may include a chest X-ray (FIGURE 5-30), CT, bronchoscopy, ABGs, and CBC. A high white blood cell count can occur with atelectasis. Treatment focuses on remedying the underlying causes (e.g., antibiotics for infections, thoracentesis for fluid accumulation) and reinflating the alveoli. Incentive spirometry (a device to promote ventilation) is effective in reinflating the alveoli. For severe cases, noninvasive ventilation with use of various modes such as continuous positive airway pressure or endotracheal intubation may be necessary for ventilation support. Prevention strategies include increasing mobility (e.g., turning and ambulating), coughing, and deep breathing exercises (e.g., incentive spirometry) every 1 to 2 hours. Effective pain management and postoperative incisional splinting increase the likelihood that these interventions will be performed adequately.

Acute Respiratory Failure

Acute respiratory failure (ARF) is a life-threatening condition that can result from a variety of disorders, including COPD, asthma, ARDS, amyotrophic lateral sclerosis, alcohol or drug overdose, and spinal cord injury. Normally, oxygen levels are in the range of 80–100 mmHg, and carbon dioxide levels are in the range of 35–45 mmHg. In ARF, oxygen levels (PaO_2) become dangerously low (less than 50 mmHg) or carbon dioxide levels ($PaCO_2$) become dangerously high (greater than 50 mmHg). The low oxygen levels observed in ARF are not sufficient to meet the body's metabolic needs, and the nervous system quickly becomes affected by the shortage of oxygen. The oxygen level becomes progressively worse as the patient's condition worsens. Respiratory acidosis develops as the carbon dioxide levels rise. The hypoxia and acidosis trigger a reflex

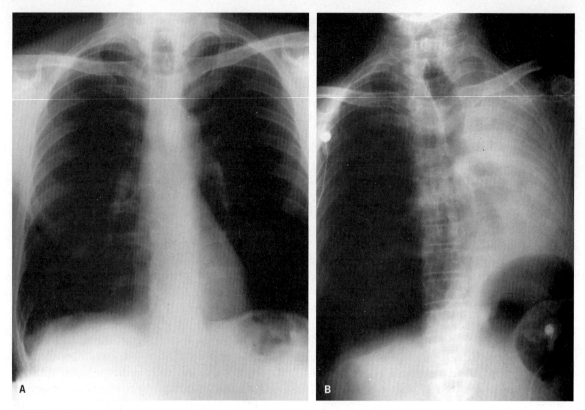

FIGURE 5-30 X-ray of atelectasis. **A** Normal lung. **B** Lung with atelectasis (whiter area on right).

Courtesy of Leonard V. Crowley, MD, Century College.

pulmonary vasoconstriction, further impairing gas exchange and increasing cardiac workload. The heart decompensates from the lack of oxygen, which could lead to cardiac arrest. Respiratory arrest may occur as the respiratory system ceases all activity from the strain. See chapter 6 for discussion of respiratory acidosis.

Clinical Manifestations

Clinical manifestations are usually evident and result from the impaired gas exchange. Shallow respirations, tachycardia, dysrhythmias, altered mental status, and other signs of hypoxemia may be present with ARF.

BOX 5-4 Application to Practice

Now that we have learned what can go wrong in the pulmonary system, let us put that knowledge into practice. While working in the emergency department, the following patients need to be triaged.

- A 2-year-old with a history of asthma with a fever, lethargy, and multiple uses of short-acting beta agonist treatments prior to arrival

- A 25-year-old male with nasal drainage and hoarseness *Rhinitis*
- A 40-year-old female with fever, severe body aches, and nasal congestion *Influenza*
- A 59-year-old male with stage III bronchogenic carcinoma who reports increased shortness of breath *acute or alt progression*

Which patient would have the highest priority? Explain why.

What are possible diagnoses in each scenario? What clinical manifestations would be consistent with each possible diagnosis?

Modified from Story, L. (2017). *Pathophysiology: A practical approach* (3rd ed.). Burlington, MA: Jones & Bartlett Learning.

BOX 5-5 Application to Practice

Case 1: A 25-year-man was playing basketball and develops sudden chest pain and shortness of breath. He is healthy. His body mass index is 20. History is negative for smoking and drug use. He presents to the emergency department and a chest X-ray reveals a pneumothorax. He asks why this happened. Explain the cause of pneumothorax in this young man.

Case 2: Thomas Jones, a 15-year-old who has a history of asthma, is complaining of increasing asthma symptoms (wheezing, shortness of breath) for the past 3–4 months. He states he has been using his short-acting bronchodilator <u>3–4 times a week</u> and feels his symptoms have been flaring up. He has been waking up at <u>night about 2 times a month</u>. His vital signs are temperature: 98.6°F, pulse 84 beats per minute, respiratory rate 18 per minute, and blood pressure 110/70 mmHg. His pulse oximeter reading is 96%.

Upon examination, he is awake, alert, talking in full sentences, and is in no acute distress. Lung auscultation reveals <u>mild expiratory wheezing throughout</u>. The remainder of the clinical examination reveals no other abnormalities.

1. What asthma step/classification would Thomas fall into?
   a. Intermittent
   b. Mild persistent *(circled)*
   c. Moderate persistent
   d. Severe persistent
2. A pulmonary function test is conducted. What two results would be consistent with the classification Thomas is in?
   a. Increased peak expiratory flow *(circled)*
   b. Decreased residual volume
   c. Increased total lung capacity
   d. Decreased forced expiratory volume in 1 second *(circled)*
3. An inhaled corticosteroid is prescribed for Thomas. Describe the effects of a corticosteroid on asthma pathophysiology and symptomatology.

Case 3: Mrs. Garcia brings her 5-year-old, Manuel, to the emergency department with high fever, irritability, sore throat, and inspiratory stridor. She reports that he has had croup several times in the past and has required hospitalization for treatment twice. You see that Manuel is anxious and is sitting on his mother's lap leaning forward. She says he has had trouble swallowing because of his sore throat, and he is drooling a lot. She is concerned he has croup again, but he is not coughing like before.

The healthcare provider suspects acute epiglottitis. Describe epiglottitis causes and compare to croup causes.

Which of the manifestations in this case are consistent with epiglottitis in comparison to croup?

Modified from Story, L. (2017). *Pathophysiology: A practical approach* (3rd ed.). Burlington, MA: Jones & Bartlett Learning.

Diagnosis and Treatment

Diagnostic procedures for ARF consist of ABGs, chest X-ray, electrocardiogram, and CBC. Treatment focuses on resolving the cause and maintaining adequate respiratory status. Strategies include oxygen therapy, support of ventilation with a noninvasive positive pressure ventilation, or invasive mechanical ventilation. Treatment for underlying causes may include bronchodilators, antibiotics (if bacterial infection is present), corticosteroids, and treatment of emboli (e.g., embolectomy and anticoagulants). Cardiac support such as cardiopulmonary resuscitation, sympathomimetic medications, or inotropic agents are usually inevitable as the heart arrests under the strain.

CHAPTER SUMMARY

The pulmonary system plays a crucial role by supplying the oxygen essential for cellular metabolism and excreting the carbon dioxide waste product of that metabolism. Because of this vital function, pulmonary disorders can cause extensive and devastating problems throughout the body. Often the healthcare team has a limited amount of time to identify and respond to some of these pulmonary disorders to control their negative consequences. Additionally, many of these diseases are preventable; therefore, identifying those persons at increased risk and implementing prevention strategies can limit the severity or halt the development of these debilitating conditions. Prevention, early detection, early diagnosis, and prompt treatment will improve outcomes of patients with these conditions.

REFERENCES AND RESOURCES

American Cancer Society. (2018). *Cancer facts & figures 2018.* Atlanta, GA: American Cancer Society.

American Lung Association (2013). Trends in COPD (chronic bronchitis and emphysema) morbidity and mortality. Retrieved from https://www.lung.org/our-initiatives/research /monitoring-trends-in-lung-disease/

Bauman, M. & Cosgrove, C. (2012). Understanding end-tidal CO2 monitoring. *American Nurse Today, 7*(11).

Centers for Disease Control and Prevention (CDC). (2015a). Chronic obstructive pulmonary disease. Retrieved from http://www.cdc.gov/copd/index.html

Centers for Disease Control and Prevention (CDC). (2015b). Trends in asthma prevalence, health care use, and mortality in the U.S., 2001–2010. Retrieved from https://www .ncbi.nlm.nih.gov/pubmed/22617340

Centers for Disease Control and Prevention (CDC). (2016a). 2015–2016 influenza season week 39 ending October 1, 2016. Retrieved from https://www.cdc.gov/flu/weekly /pdf/External_F1641.pdf

Centers for Disease Control and Prevention (CDC). (2016b). Common cold. Retrieved from http://www.cdc.gov/dotw /common-cold/index.html

Centers for Disease Control and Prevention (CDC). (2017a). Middle East respiratory syndrome. Retrieved from http:// www.cdc.gov/coronavirus/mers/index.html

Centers for Disease Control and Prevention (CDC). (2017b). Pneumonia. Retrieved from http://www.cdc.gov/nchs /fastats/pneumonia.htm

Centers for Disease Control and Prevention (CDC). (2017c). Respiratory syncytial virus infection. Retrieved from http://www.cdc.gov/rsv/research/us-surveillance.html

Centers for Disease Control and Prevention (CDC). (2018). Carbon monoxide poisoning. Retrieved from

Centers for Disease Control and Prevention (CDC). (2018). Tuberculosis—2017. Retrieved from https://www.cdc .gov/mmwr/volumes/67/wr/mm6711a2.htm?s_cid =mm6711a2_e

Chiras, D. (2015). *Human biology* (8th ed.). Burlington, MA: Jones & Bartlett Learning.

Crowley, L. V. (2016). *An introduction to human disease* (10th ed.). Burlington, MA: Jones & Bartlett Learning.

Cystic Fibrosis Foundation. (n.d.). About cystic fibrosis. Retrieved from http://www.cff.org/AboutCF/

Cystic Fibrosis Foundation. (2017). Patient registry. Retrieved from https://www.cff.org/Research/Researcher -Resources/Patient-Registry/

Elling, B., Elling, K., & Rothenberg, M. (2004). *Anatomy and physiology.* Sudbury, MA: Jones and Bartlett Publishers.

Fan, E., Del Sorbo, L., Goligher, E. C., Hodgson, C. L., Munshi, L., Walkey, A. J., . . . Brochard, L. J., on behalf of the American Thoracic Society, European Society of Intensive Care Medicine, and Society of Critical Care Medicine. (2017). An official American Thoracic Society/European Society of Intensive Care Medicine/ Society of Critical Care Medicine clinical practice guideline: Mechanical ventilation in adult patients with acute respiratory distress syndrome. *American Journal of Respiratory and Critical Care Medicine, 195*(9). https://doi.org /10.1164/rccm.201703-0548ST

Flume, P. A., Robinson, K. A., O'Sullivan, B. P., Finder, J. D., Vender, R. L., Willey-Courand, D. B., . . . Marshall, B. C., for the Clinical Practice Guidelines for Pulmonary Therapies Committee. (2009). Cystic fibrosis pulmonary guidelines: Airway clearance therapies. *Respiratory Care, 54*(4), 522–537.

Global Initiative for Chronic Obstructive Lung Disease. Global strategy for the diagnosis, management, and prevention of chronic obstructive pulmonary disease: 2019 report. Retrieved from https://goldcopd.org/wp-content /uploads/2018/11/GOLD-2019-v1.7-FINAL-14Nov2018 -WMS.pdf

Gould, B. (2015). *Pathophysiology for the health professions* (5th ed.). Philadelphia, PA: Elsevier.

Kanaji, N., Watanabe, N., Kita, N., Bandoh, S., Tadokoro, A., Ishii, T., . . . Matsunaga, T. (2014). Paraneoplastic syndromes associated with lung cancer. *World Journal of Clinical Oncology, 5*(3) 197–223. doi: 10.5306/wjco.v5.i3.197

LeGrys, V. A., Yankaskas, J. R., Quittell, L. M., Marshall, B. C., & Mogayzel, P. J., for the Cystic Fibrosis Foundation. (2007). Diagnostic sweat testing: The Cystic Fibrosis Foundation guidelines. *Journal of Pediatrics, 151*(1), 85–89.

Madara, B., & Pomarico-Denino, V. (2008). *Pathophysiology* (2nd ed.). Sudbury, MA: Jones and Bartlett Publishers.

Mogayzel, P. J., Jr., Naureckas, E. T., Robinson, K. A., Mueller, G., Hadjiliadis, D., Hoag, J. B., . . . Marshall, B., for the Pulmonary Clinical Practice Guidelines Committee. (2013). Cystic fibrosis pulmonary guidelines: Chronic medications for maintenance of lung health. *American Journal of Respiratory Critical Care Medicine, 187*(7), 680–689.

Morton, P. G., & Fontaine, D. K. (2018). *Critical care nursing: A holistic approach* (11th ed.). Philadelphia, PA: Wolters Kluwer.

National Asthma Education and Prevention Program, Third Expert Panel on the Diagnosis and Management of Asthma. (2007). Expert panel report 3: Guidelines for the diagnosis and management of asthma. Bethesda, MD: National Heart, Lung, and Blood Institute. Available from: https://www.ncbi.nlm.nih.gov/books/NBK7232/

National Institutes of Allergy and Infectious Disease. (2016). Cold versus flu. Retrieved from http://www.cdc.gov/flu /about/qa/coldflu.htm

The National Lung Screening Trial Research Team. (2011). Reduced lung-cancer mortality with low-dose computed tomographic screening. *New England Journal of Medicine, 365*, 395–409.

Peppard, P. E., Young, T., Barnet, J. H., Palta, M., Hagen, E. W., & Hla, K. M. (2013). Increased prevalence of sleep-disordered breathing in adults. *American Journal of Epidemiology, 177*(9), 1006–1014.

Professional guide to pathophysiology (3rd ed.). (2010). Philadelphia, PA: Lippincott Williams & Wilkins.

Ralston, S., Lieberthal, A., Meissner, H., Alverson, B., Baley, J., Gadomski, A., & Hernandez-Cancio, S. (2014). Clinical practice guideline: The diagnosis, management, and prevention of bronchiolitis. *Pediatrics, 134*(5), e1474–e1502.

Reilly, J. P., Christie, J. D. (2015). Acute lung injury and the acute respiratory distress syndrome: Clinical features, management, and outcomes. In M. A. Grippi, J. A. Elias, J. A. Fishman, R. M. Kotloff, A. I. Pack, R. M. Senior, & M. D. Siegel (Eds.). *Fishman's pulmonary diseases and disorders* (5th ed.). New York, NY: McGraw-Hill. Retrieved from http://accessmedicine.mhmedical.com.ezproxy.fiu.edu/content.aspx?bookid=1344&sectionid=81206199

Saiman, L., Siegel, J. D., LiPuma, J. J., Brown, R. F., Bryson, E. A., Chambers, M. J., . . . Weber, D. J. (2014). Infection prevention and control guideline for cystic fibrosis: 2013 update. *Infection Control and Hospital Epidemiology,* (35, Suppl 1), S1–S67.

Sanders, D. B., Solomon, G. M., Beckett, V. V., West, N. E., Daines, C. L., Heltshe, S. L., . . . Goss, H. L. (2017). Standardized Treatment of Pulmonary Exacerbations (STOP) study: Observations at the initiation of intravenous antibiotics for cystic fibrosis pulmonary exacerbations. *Journal of Cystic Fibrosis, 16*(5), 592–599. doi: 0.1016/j.jcf.2017.04.005

Shulman, S. T., Bisno, A. L., Clegg, H. W., Gerber, M. A., Kaplan, E. L., Lee, G., . . . Van Beneden, C. (2012); Clinical practice guideline for the diagnosis and management of group A streptococcal pharyngitis: 2012 update by the Infectious Diseases Society of America. *Clinical Infectious Diseases, 55*(10), e86–e102. https://doi.org/10.1093/cid/cis629

Silvestri, R. C. (2017). Evaluation of subacute and chronic cough in adults. T. W. Post (Ed.). *Uptodate.* Waltham, MA: UpToDate, Inc. Retrieved from https://uptodate.com

U.S. Cancer Statistics Working Group. (2012). *U.S. cancer statistics: 1999–2008 incidence and mortality web-based report.* Atlanta, GA: Department of Health and Human Services, Centers for Disease Control and Prevention and National Cancer Institute.

VanDevanter, D. R., Heltshe, S. L., Spahr, J., Beckett, V. V., Daines, C. L., Dasenbrook, E. C., . . . Flume, P. A. (2017). Rationalizing endpoints for prospective studies of pulmonary exacerbation treatment response in cystic fibrosis. *Journal of Cystic Fibrosis, 16*(5), 607–615. doi: 10.1016/j.jcf.2017.04.004

West, N. E., Beckett, V. V., Jain, R., Sanders, D. B., Nick, J. A., Heltshe, S. L . . . Flume, P. A. (2017). Standardized Treatment of Pulmonary exacerbations (STOP) study: Physician treatment practices and outcomes for individuals with cystic fibrosis with pulmonary exacerbations. *Journal of Cystic Fibrosis, 16*(5), 600–606. doi: 10.1016/j.jcf.2017.04.003

World Health Organization (WHO). (2018a, May 28). Cumulative number of confirmed human cases for avian influenza A(H5N1) reported to WHO, 2003-2018. Retrieved from http://www.who.int/influenza/human_animal_interface/2018_05_28_tableH5N1.pdf?ua=1

World Health Organization (WHO). (2018b). Middle East respiratory syndrome coronavirus. Retrieved from http://www.who.int/emergencies/mers-cov/en/

World Health Organization (WHO). (2018c). Tuberculosis. Retrieved from https://www.who.int/tb/publications/global_report/tb18_ExecSum_web_4Oct18.pdf?ua=1

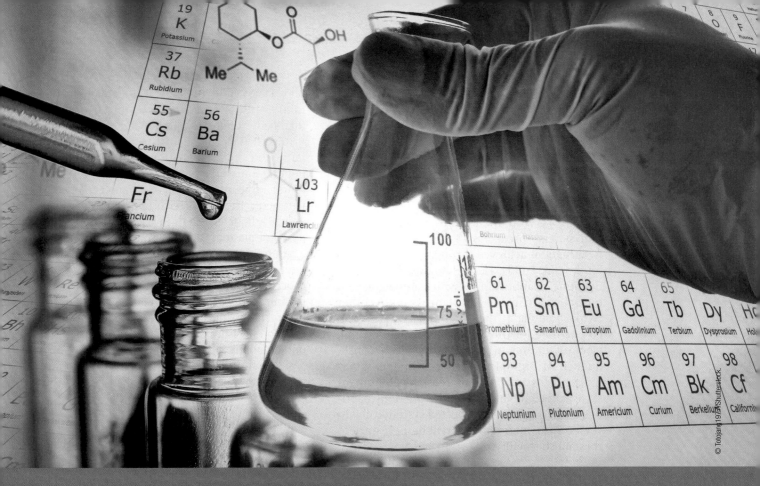

CHAPTER 6
Fluid, Electrolyte, and Acid–Base Homeostasis

LEARNING OBJECTIVES

- Discuss normal fluid composition and distribution.
- Discuss fluid and electrolyte movement and regulation.
- Discuss acid–base regulation and compensatory mechanisms.
- Analyze arterial blood gases.
- Determine cause and effect of fluid, electrolyte, and acid–base imbalances.

- Summarize the interrelationship of electrolytes and components in fluids.
- Apply understanding of fluid, electrolyte, and acid–base imbalances when describing various disorders associated with imbalances.
- Develop diagnostic and treatment considerations for various fluid, electrolyte, and acid–base imbalances.

The human body requires a delicate balance, or homeostasis, to function optimally. The body continuously employs strategies to maintain this balance. Fluids, electrolytes, and pH all play critical roles in sustaining homeostasis. Fluids are distributed in various body compartments and move among these compartments to preserve equilibrium. Electrolytes are vital for cellular function, and they work with the various fluids to maintain stability. Acid–base balance is critical for health and is achieved through a complex buffer system. Fluids, electrolytes, and pH have a dynamic relationship in which imbalances in one area can cause imbalances in the other two. Additionally, the other areas can serve to compensate for those imbalances. Often fluid, electrolyte, and pH imbalances are a consequence of multiple disorders. Compensatory mechanisms may fail to reestablish homeostasis affecting many bodily functions. Serious consequences are reflected systemically. In such a case, interventions will be necessary to reestablish stability.

Fluid and Electrolyte Balance

Distribution

Body fluid is made of water (i.e., solvent) and solutes (e.g., Na^+, Cl^-). Water is the medium within which metabolic reactions and other processes occur. Water carries nutrients into the cells, waste products out of the cells, enzymes in digestive secretions, and blood cells around the body. Fluid also facilitates movement of body parts (e.g., the joints, lungs, and heart). Fluid found inside the cells is referred to as intracellular fluid (ICF) and fluid found outside the cells is referred to as extracellular fluid (ECF) ECF is further divided into interstitial (between the cells), intravascular (inside the blood vessels), and transcellular (between epithelial lined spaces) compartments. The transcellular compartment includes fluid in the peritoneal, pleural, and pericardial cavities, cerebrospinal fluid, and fluid in the joint spaces, lymph system, eyes and gastrointestinal tract. The cell membrane serves as a barrier that substances and water must pass through to move to or from the intracellular compartment (i.e., between ECF and ICF. Collectively, the ICF accounts for approximately two-thirds of the body's water (weight 40% of total body weight).

The ICF is rich in potassium, magnesium, phosphates, and proteins. The remaining one third of the body fluid makes up the ECF (20% of total body weight). Approximately three fourths of the ECF (i.e., 15% of total body weight) is found in the interstitial compartment, and the remaining one fourth (i.e., 5% of total body weight) is found in the intravascular and transcellular compartment. The ECF is rich in sodium, chloride, and bicarbonate. The intravascular space is composed of plasma. Blood (serum) electrolyte tests examine only intravascular electrolytes, but inferences from these tests can be made as to what is occurring in the other compartments. Despite the intravascular fluid only being a small portion of total body fluids, it is this fluid that contributes to blood pressure. See chapter 3 for a discussion of hematopoietic function.

The summary of body weight (adult man) is as follows:

- Body weight: 100% = Solids 40% + total body fluids 60%
- Total body fluids Weight: 60% = intracellular 40% + extracellular 20% (15% interstitial + 5% intravascular/transcellular)

The distribution of fluid varies based on gender and age. The weight and percentages discussed describe a healthy adult male (FIGURE 6-1). A newborn and infant have less body fat and, therefore, the amount of water in the body is higher (i.e., 70–80%). As a child matures, the body water amount decreases until puberty, when adult ratios are reached. Men have more muscle and less fat and, therefore, have a higher amount of body water than women. Women have higher body fat (adipose cells do not store water) and, therefore, a lower total body water than men. Regardless of the gender, the higher the muscle mass, the more body water, and the higher the fat composition, the lower the body water. Obesity, whether in childhood or adulthood (male or female), results in lower body water. Those who are obese, very young, or very old are more susceptible to the effects of fluid imbalances such as dehydration and hypovolemia when body water is lost. Even though newborns and infants have a high amount of body water, it is a significantly large amount in comparison to their total body size. Infants' compensatory mechanism to manage imbalances are less mature. Due to these factors, body water loss such as from diarrhea in or vomiting by newborns and infants can result in serious consequences. With aging, muscle mass decreases and fat increases resulting in

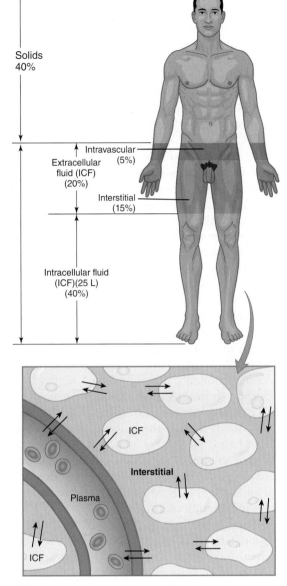

FIGURE 6-1 Fluid compartments of the body.

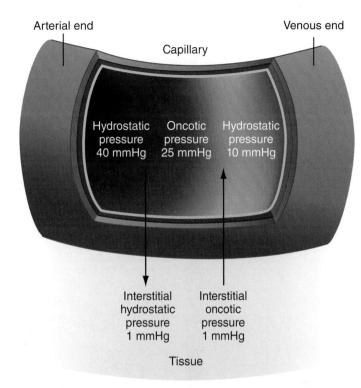

FIGURE 6-2 Pressures that control fluid balance.

decreased body water. The elderly are also prone to severe consequences due to fluid losses because their compensatory mechanisms (e.g., kidneys), while mature, decline in function with age.

Fluid Movement

Fluids are constantly circulating throughout the body and moving among compartments to maintain homeostasis. The body exchanges solutes (e.g., ions) and water between compartments to compensate for conditions that increase or decrease losses. This movement between compartments is primarily accomplished through osmosis, the movement of fluid (specifically water) across a semipermeable membrane

from an area of lower solute concentration to an area of higher solute concentration. Water moves across the semipermeable membrane until equilibrium is achieved, at which point there is an equal ECF and ICF osmolality. See chapter 1 for a discussion of cellular function.

Because water moves freely across cell membranes, this equilibrium is usually easy to achieve. The movement of water depends on hydrostatic (push) and osmotic (pull) pressures (FIGURE 6-2). The ability of the solutes, proteins, and electrolytes to attract water is what determines the osmotic pressure of a fluid (FIGURE 6-3). In other words, solute concentration is what determines osmotic pressure. Sodium (Na^+), chloride (Cl^-), and bicarbonate (HCO_3^-) are the main (95%) determinants of osmotic pressure in the ECF with minor (5%) contributions from urea and glucose. Potassium (K^+), adenosine triphosphate (ATP), phosphate (PO_4^-), and phospholipids are key determinants of osmotic pressure in the ICF. A pressure opposing osmotic pressure is hydrostatic pressure which is created by the water pushing against the cell membrane. Colloid osmotic pressure, which is known as oncotic pressure, is created mainly by the protein albumin. Water is pulled in with higher oncotic pressures. To summarize, the osmotic pressure created by solute

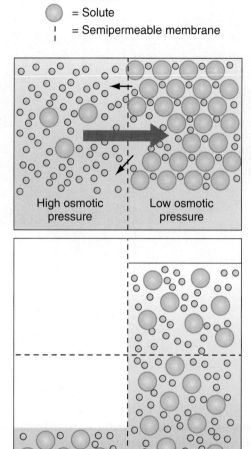

○ = Solvent
◯ = Solute
| = Semipermeable membrane

High osmotic pressure | Low osmotic pressure

FIGURE 6-3 Osmotic pressure.

concentration and oncotic pressure created by albumin pull or attract water to the compartments of highest concentration. Hydrostatic pressure created by water pushes water away. These pressures are usually in balance.

Pressures (e.g., hydrostatic, oncotic) vary along the capillary. At the arteriolar end of the capillary, the blood net hydrostatic pressure (blood pressure) is higher than the net oncotic pressure, moving (pushing) fluid out of the intravascular compartment and into the interstitial compartment to meet cellular needs. At the venous end of the capillary, the net oncotic (colloid osmotic) pressure is higher than hydrostatic pressure, moving (pulling) fluid from the interstitial compartment to the intravascular compartment to aid in the exchange of waste products to be excreted. The higher pressure at the venous end is due to the hydrostatic pressure decreasing rather than the oncotic pressure increasing because the proteins,

such as albumin, do not cross the semipermeable membrane. Most of the movement of water is dependent on the pressures intravascularly as interstitial pressures are very low. To be an effective osmole (i.e., create pressure/attract water), the solute must not be able to pass passively through a semipermeable membrane (e.g., Na^+, protein). Urea can create pressure, but urea moves freely across the membrane and is, therefore, an ineffective osmole.

The effect of the osmotic pressure or tension on the cell is termed *tonicity*. Tonicity is determined by the osmotic pressure of two solutions (i.e., solvent and solute) separated by a semipermeable membrane and the concentration relative to one and other on each side of the membrane (i.e., intracellular and extracellular). These two terms can be complex to understand, so it is helpful to review differences between the two. Osmotic pressure is created by several solutes such as sodium, which is an effective osmole, and ineffective osmoles, such as urea or other toxins. Osmotic activity is described as the osmolarity or osmolality of a solution. Osmolality is the preferred term when referring to fluids inside the body. Osmolarity (e.g., intravenous fluids) is best used to describe fluids outside the body. Tonicity, on the other hand, only takes into account osmotic pressure created by effective osmoles (e.g., sodium, glucose) and not the ineffective ones. Tonicity is always discussed in reference to two sides of a membrane.

Tonicity is often used to describe the cell's response to an external solution (**FIGURE 6-4**). In health care, the external solution described in relation to tonicity consists of intravenous (IV) solutions, specifically those containing electrolytes (e.g., Na^+, K^+) and nonelectrolytes (e.g., glucose). These solutions are termed *crystalloids* and are used to treat a variety of patient conditions (e.g., dehydration and shock). These solutions are classified based on their tonicity prior to infusion and in relationship to the intravascular plasma and there are three categories—isotonic, hypotonic, and hypertonic. IV solutions are administered with the intention to therapeutically alter the fluid dynamics between the ECF and ICF. **Isotonic solutions** (e.g., 0.9% saline, lactated Ringer's solution, 5% dextrose in water solution) have concentrations of solutes equal to those in the intravascular compartment. As a result of these equivalent solute concentrations (i.e., equal in the IV solution and plasma), isotonic solutions allow

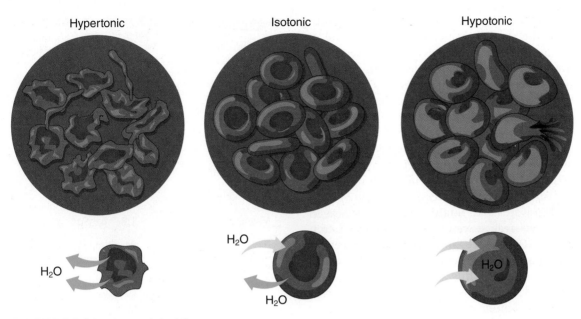

FIGURE 6-4 Cellular response to tonicity.

Courtesy of Mariana Ruiz Villarreal.

fluid to move equally between compartments and do not cause notable shifts in fluid volume. **Hypotonic solutions** (e.g., 0.45% saline) have a lower concentration of solutes (i.e., lower osmotic pressure) than those in the intravascular compartment. Hypotonic solutions cause fluid to shift from the intravascular compartment to the intracellular space. **Hypertonic solutions** (e.g., 5% dextrose in 0.9% saline, 3% saline, 10% dextrose in water) have a higher concentration of solutes (i.e., higher osmotic pressure) than those in the intravascular compartment. Hypertonic solutions cause fluid to shift from the intracellular compartment to the intravascular space.

Tonicity is also a way to classify sodium and water imbalances. For example, these imbalances can be isotonic, hypotonic, and hypertonic. When discussing tonicity from this perspective, the imbalance is between the various fluid compartments.

In addition to fluid moving between compartments, fluid is added to the body through the ingestion of food and fluids, and a small amount is replenished as an internal cellular by-product. Approximately 100 mL of water is needed per 100 calories (i.e., energy) ingested to help with metabolism (i.e., the bodily processes of catabolism and anabolism) and waste elimination. As an example, a person who expends 1,500 calories in a day will require 1,500 mL of water for proper metabolism. Water ingestion is, therefore, critical for proper metabolism. Fluid is primarily lost in the urine and feces, but additional insensible (immeasurable) losses occur through the skin (e.g., perspiration) and the respiratory tract (e.g., breathing, coughing, talking, and mechanical ventilation). A small amount is even lost in vaginal secretions. The minimum urine output for proper elimination of waste products is termed the *obligatory urine output,* and in adults this is approximately 500 mL. Formulas that incorporate kilograms are used to calculate the minimum in adults and children (see chapter 7 for a discussion of urinary function).

Fluid Regulation

Body fluid intake and output balance is maintained through several mechanisms. Water balance is closely related to sodium balance. Sodium is responsible for most of the osmotic force in the ECF and serum sodium concentration is determined by water balance (ECF volume). Water balance (volume) is determined by the serum sodium concentration (osmolality). For purposes of simplicity and understanding fluid regulation, water balance is equated with volume and sodium serum concentration is equated with osmolality or tonicity.

Many of the compensatory mechanisms that maintain fluid balance involve the suppression or excretion of hormones that influence sodium and water. The osmoreceptor cells, for example, sense intravascular osmolality. Increased osmolality triggers the thirst mechanism in the hypothalamus to increase oral intake. The thirst sensation occurs with even the smallest water losses and is one of the best regulators to prevent water loss. This thirst sensation can decrease with aging (a phenomenon called *hypodipsia*). Changes in osmolality will also trigger antidiuretic hormone (ADH), also known as vasopressin which is the primary regulator of water excretion. Released from the pituitary gland in times of increased osmolality, ADH promotes reabsorption of water into the blood from the renal tubules. ADH suppression will conversely lead to water loss. So thirst is the mechanism to protect against water loss through ingestion while ADH suppression is the mechanism to regulate water through excretion (increased or decreased). While water balance changes occurred in response to osmolality (i.e., created by sodium concentration), the sodium balance changes occur in response to volume. Changes in volume activate kidney, heart, and vascular receptors to then increase or decrease sodium excretion. Decreased volume leads to decreased perfusion to the kidneys causing activation of the renin-angiotensin-aldosterone- system (see chapter 4 for more on cardiovascular function). Renin ultimately leads to development of angiotensin II which directly stimulates aldosterone and causes aldosterone release from the adrenal cortex. The hormone aldosterone when stimulated increases reabsorption of sodium, and subsequently water in the renal tubules. There are also volume sensors in the heart. Atrial natriuretic peptide from the atria, and brain natriuretic peptide from the ventricles, are released when the chambers of the myocardium become overstretched, indicating increased fluid volume. This peptide stimulates renal vasodilation, thereby increasing urinary excretion of urinary sodium. Additionally, natriuretic peptides suppress aldosterone secretion, further increasing urinary output. Pressure receptors in the vascular system, particularly the aorta and carotids sense changes in volume. Decreases in volume activate the receptors which activate the sympathetic nervous system leading to renin activation, norepinephrine release and vasoconstriction and sodium retention.

Electrolytes

Electrolytes play a crucial role in homeostasis. Electrolytes are minerals with electrical charges found in the blood, urine, and other body fluids. Electrolytes in the body include

TABLE 6-1	Normal Serum Values of the Major Electrolytes*
Electrolyte	**Normal range**
Sodium (Na$^+$)	135–145 mEq/L
Chloride (Cl$^-$)	98–108 mEq/L
Potassium (K$^+$)	3.5–5 mEq/L
Calcium (Ca^{++})	8.8–10.3 mg/dL
Phosphorus (P)	2.5–4.5 mg/dL
Magnesium (Mg^{++})	1.8–2.4 mEq/L
Bicarbonate (HCO$_3^-$)	24–31 mEq/L

*Values may vary slightly.
Modified from Story, L. (2017). *Pathophysiology: A practical approach* (3rd ed.). Burlington, MA: Jones & Bartlett Learning.

sodium, chloride, potassium, calcium, magnesium, and phosphorus (**TABLE 6-1**). Cations are positively charged, whereas anions are negatively charged. Cations and anions are attracted to each other, so a cation like sodium will be attracted to an anion like chloride or bicarbonate (i.e., NaCl, NaHCO$_3$). The main extracellular electrolytes are sodium, chloride, and bicarbonate. The intracellular electrolytes are potassium, calcium, and magnesium. The charge on each side of the membrane is relatively neutral, so cation and anion charges are equal. Electrolytes are important in muscle and neural activity and in acid–base and fluid balance. The purpose and regulation of each electrolyte are discussed with each respective imbalance. Bicarbonate plays an important role in acid–base balance and is discussed in the *Acid–Base Balance* section.

Fluid and Electrolyte Imbalances

Imbalances in fluid and electrolytes are usually related to disorders of intake (excessive or inadequate) or impairment in elimination (increased or decreased). Disorders often occur when an imbalances exceed the body's ability to compensate for them. The kidney is the primary organ regulating electrolyte and fluid balance. Despite the kidneys' key role, the catalyst for the imbalance can be another system. These systems can include disorders in the neurologic system (e.g., pituitary issues), cardiovascular system (e.g., heart failure), or the liver (e.g., cirrhosis). Fluid and electrolyte imbalances are a reflection of an underlying disorder and require further investigation to identify the cause. A fluid or electrolyte imbalance rarely occurs in isolation and is often just one piece of the puzzle in determining a disorder. Imbalances constantly fluctuate, meaning an imbalance is a reflection of a certain point in time in the trajectory of a disorder, so repeat measurements and evaluations may reveal a different result. While some imbalances are transient and inconsequential, some, such as potassium and sodium shifts, can be life threatening.

Water, Sodium, and Chloride Relationship

Water and sodium balances are intricately linked. Chloride is attracted to sodium, so changes in sodium cause the same changes in chloride (e.g., decreased sodium, decreased chloride). The body is made up of approximately 60% fluids (this varies by weight, age, and gender), and most of that fluid is water with sodium as the most abundant solute in the ECF. Serum sodium concentration is the major determinant of the volume (i.e., water) of the ECF. Whenever an imbalance occurs there is either a problem with sodium, water or both. Imbalances in sodium (an effective osmole) will alter the tonicity (i.e., change in concentration between two cell membranes) within the ECF and between the ECF and ICF. These alterations in tonicity may cause intravascular water shifting. These changes in tonicity are classified as isotonic, hypertonic, or hypotonic (see Figure 6-4). Isotonic fluid shifts occur when water and sodium are lost proportionately (i.e., relatively equal amounts). No changes in osmolality occur with isotonic shifts, so the fluid between the ICF and ECF does not move and the cell is not affected. The shifts occur in the ECF compartments between interstitial and intravascular. Hypertonic shifts are mainly due to excess sodium (i.e., hypernatremia) with insufficient water. Osmolality increases due to the hypernatremia, so water shifts from the ICF to the high-sodium ECF. Because water leaves the cells, hypertonic shifts cause the cells to shrivel. Hypotonic shifts are mainly due to inadequate sodium (i.e., hyponatremia) with excessive water. Osmolality decreases due to the hyponatremia, so water shifts from the ECF to the ICF. Hypotonic water shifts are opposite of hypertonic shifts because water enters the

cell with hypotonic shifts and causes the cell to burst (i.e., lysis).

To review, isotonic imbalances are water shifts from the intravascular to interstitial spaces (both ECF compartments), while hypertonic imbalances are water shifts from ICF to the ECF. Hypotonic imbalances cause shifts from the ECF to the ICF. Volume (i.e., water) imbalances are generally in reference to the intravascular compartment. Volumes may shift as a result of changes in tonicity as just described. These volume shifts may be categorized as euvolemic (normal intravascular volume), hypervolemia (increased intravascular volume), and hypovolemia (decreased intravascular volume). Hypervolemia is at times used interchangeably with edema; however, edema is a result of fluid shifts from interstitial and intracellular and may also occur with hypovolemia.

Several disorders can cause sodium and/or water imbalances, which can present challenges in determining the cause. In general, volume disorders (excess or deficits) are due to altered sodium control, and ECF sodium concentration disorders are usually due to altered water control. Some imbalances are rare or unlikely which can also help in determining the cause. As an example, hypernatremia with hypervolemia is rare. Likewise, sodium excess from too much intake (oral or IV) is not too common. People do not usually ingest salts in amounts sufficient to cause hypernatremia because they would usually become thirsty and drink water to counterbalance. Some other disorders that cause sodium and water imbalances, such as Cushing syndrome, are rare in the overall population. Determining the cause of imbalances will guide treatment decisions. Imbalances are managed with fluid replacement, which involves determining the type of fluid (e.g., isotonic, hypertonic, or hypotonic crystalloids), the amount, the rate, and the route. Fluid management can also include withholding of fluids or removal of fluids and electrolytes with pharmacotherapeutics (e.g., diuretics) or dialysis.

Fluid Excess

Ideally, fluid intake should be equal to the amount of loss. As previously discussed, fluid excesses are usually due to problems with sodium control as opposed to water control. A common issue with fluid excesses is too much sodium with water being retained, specifically in the ECF. The excess usually occurs because

TABLE 6-2	Disorders of Fluid Excess and Deficit

Fluid excess—hypervolemia/edema; hyponatremia or hypernatremia	Fluid deficit—hypovolemia/dehydration- hyponatremia or hypernatremia
Excessive sodium*—excessive intake or decreased elimination • Excess hypertonic solutions: D10W, Hypertonic 3% saline, enteral feedings • Excess dietary intake (e.g., processed foods, sodas, and certain seasonings)—a rare cause in a healthy person • Corticosteroid disorders • Cushing syndrome (glucocorticoid disorder)—e.g., adrenal gland or medication • Hyperaldosteronism (mineralocorticoid disorder)—increase sodium retention • Near-drowning in salt water	***Deficient sodium*—decreased intake or increased elimination*** • Inadequate intake • Excessive diuretic use (e.g., thiazide) • Low aldosterone—hypoaldosteronism, Addison disease
Excessive water*—excessive intake or decreased elimination • Psychogenic polydipsia (excessive water ingestion) • Free water (pure) intake • Syndrome of inappropriate antidiuretic hormone (excessive ADH levels, which increases water retention) • Hypotonic intravenous saline (0.45% saline) • Cardiac disorders (e.g., heart failure) (see chapter 4) • Renal disorders (e.g., renal water retention) can cause excess or deficit (see chapter 7)	***Deficient water*—inadequate intake or excessive elimination*** • Inadequate intake—impaired ability to communicate (e.g., confusion, stroke, dementia); altered thirst (hypodipsia, adipsia) • Inadequate replacement • Gastrointestinal losses—watery diarrhea, vomiting, nasogastric suctioning • Excessive insensible losses—excessive diaphoresis, prolonged hyperventilation • Excessive diuresis—diuretics • Diabetes insipidus—insufficient ADH (an inability to concentrate urine, leading to excess water loss) • Hyperglycemia (e.g., uncontrolled diabetes mellitus, mannitol infusion) leads to glucose excretion and, in turn, water losses • Massive fluid losses—burns, hemorrhaging, open wounds • Renal disorders (e.g., nephrosis, which causes excess protein and water loss) can cause excess or deficit (see chapter 7)

* Excessive and deficient states are not necessarily reflected in serum plasma as several factors, particularly the underlying disorder, degree of alteration, and other losses that affect fluid balance such as potassium and glucose, which are not reflected in this table, can contribute to imbalances.

of inadequate water and sodium elimination and less commonly due to an excessive amount of sodium or water intake. Various disorders lead to fluid excess (**TABLE 6-2**). The fluid excess causes hypervolemia and edema. Usually hypernatremia or hyponatremia results depending on the causes of the fluid excess. As previously discussed, *hypervolemia* is the term used for shifts into the intravascular space rather than edema. Edema describes fluid shifts into the interstitial or intracellular spaces. The concepts of hypervolemia and edema are often used interchangeably by clinicians. Clinicians often refer to hypervolemia also as "fluid

overload" and edema is considered the clinical manifestation of the overload. While hypervolemia can cause edema, hypervolemia can also occur without edema. Likewise, edema can occur without hypervolemia.

Fluid excesses in the interstitial compartment is edema. Intracellular fluid excesses are a result of water intoxication. Significant daily gains or losses do not usually occur in the transcellular compartments. Transcellular increases may occur with certain physiologic conditions or traumatic events such as pericarditis, pleurisy, and ascites. Significant fluid increases in the transcellular compartment are often referred to as *third spacing* because fluid is not easily exchanged among the other extracellular fluids. The concept of third spacing can also refer to the massive movement of fluid from the intravascular into the interstitial space, as occurs with burns.

Edema is a problem of fluid distribution. In other words, the fluids are in the wrong place. Edema occurs when hydrostatic forces are greater than osmotic forces, causing the movement of fluid from the intravascular compartment to the interstitial space. The lymphatic system, which normally removes fluid, is unable to keep up with the excess. The venous system usually transports about 80% of fluid from the interstitial spaces while the lymphatic system accounts for approximately 20%. The arterial end of the capillary can tolerate changes in pressure, but the venous end of the capillary does not tolerate pressure changes well. Any increase in volume or obstruction in the venous system can increase capillary hydrostatic pressure and lead to edema. Disorders that cause sodium and water retention under circumstances that the body is unable to accommodate such volume increases, such as heart or renal failure, will lead to increased venous pressure and edema. Although the sodium is retained, the sodium plasma levels may actually be low (dilutional hyponatremia) as there is a proportionate amount of water retained. Venous pressure can also increase when the fluid return system is affected, which occurs with cardiac pump failure. Other causes of increased venous pressure not related to sodium or water imbalances are venous insufficiency (the veins are unable to return blood), being in a prolonged or chronic dependent position such as lying, and inadequate calf muscle pump activity that can occur with paralysis or gait issues. Deep vein thrombosis causes venous obstruction, increasing venous pressure. Medications can also cause edema. Medications, such as calcium channel blockers or pregabalin (e.g., Lyrica), cause edema through a slightly different mechanism. These medications cause arteriolar dilatation with subsequent increased capillary pressure with fluid extravasation. The edema that occurs with calcium channel blockers and pregabalin is usually in the lower extremities and mild. Some patients will discontinue the medication due to edema development. The edema from calcium channel blockers is an effect of dihydropyridines (e.g., amlodipine, nifedipine) and does not occur with nondihydropyridines (e.g., verapamil, diltiazem). Therefore, evaluating possible medications as the cause of the edema is an important component of diagnosis.

Learning Points

Albumin-Related Edema

Edema can occur due to a decreased colloid osmotic pressure (i.e., oncotic pressure). Hypoalbuminemia leads to a decrease in plasma oncotic pressure (pulling force) and fluid shifts from the intravascular to the interstitial space. Proteins (e.g., albumin), in a sense, attract water. Low albumin levels can occur with nephrotic syndrome or gastrointestinal disorders (excess loss) or liver disease (decreased production). Vascular injury can cause increased capillary permeability, resulting in a loss of albumin and a shift of fluid into the interstitial space. Vascular injury can occur with many conditions such as burns, trauma, and infection.

Fluid excess can also occur in the intracellular space, a condition known as water intoxication. Water intoxication occurs as a result of ingesting large amounts of water faster than it can be eliminated. The high intravascular water concentration and dilutional hyponatremia (hypotonic) causes water to shift into ICF causing the cells to burst. Water intoxication can occur if someone drinks an excessive amount of water in a short period of time. Thirst triggers increased water ingestion, but healthy kidneys can only excrete up to 1 liter of fluid per hour. During rehydration, individuals should keep this in mind. Men on average need 3 liters of fluid per day while women need 2 liters per day. However, many factors influence the actual fluid needs such as climate, exercise, age, and health status. Psychogenic polydipsia is a disorder characterized by compulsive water drinking and occurs in patients with mental health disorders such as schizophrenia. Patients with this disorder can drink up to 10 liters per day, which can lead to water intoxication. ICF excess can lead to the rupture, or lysis, of the cells. Cerebral cells are the most sensitive to lysis, and cerebral edema can also be present.

Edema may be localized to one area (e.g., the feet, around the eye, or scrotum) and can be unilateral or bilateral. Edema can be acute or chronic, as with nephrotic syndrome or chronic venous insufficiency, respectively. Edema may be in dependent or nondependent areas. Dependent refers to areas most affected by gravity (e.g., the lower body).

Nondependent refers to areas less affected by gravity (e.g., upper body). Bilateral edema in dependent areas (e.g., feet, legs, sacrum) is often due to systemic problems such as heart failure. Nondependent edema such as that in the face or arms can be caused by albumin disorders, as this fluid is throughout the body. The most common cause of unilateral edema is deep vein thrombosis. Weeks to months after the the thrombus is resolved the affected extremity can develop intermittent or persistent edema. This edema after a blood clot is known as **post-thrombotic syndrome**. The disorder occurs as a result of damage to the venous valves leading to valvular incompetence and increased venous pressure as a result of the clot. Unilateral edema can also be due to infections like cellulitis or muscular injury like an ankle sprain. Edema that is pitting (**FIGURE 6-5**) is caused by excess interstitial fluid. Nonpitting edema is usually either caused by a lymphatic disorder or a thyroid disorder. Generalized severe edema throughout the body, referred to as *anasarca*, is usually the result of liver cirrhosis or renal failure.

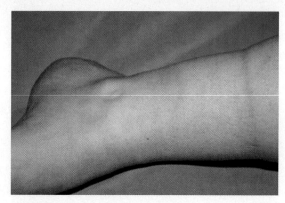

FIGURE 6-5 Pitting edema.
© Jones & Bartlett Learning. Photographed by Kimberly Potvin.

Learning Points

Lymphedema, Lipoedema, and Myxedema

Lymphedema is a type of edema that occurs when there is a blockage in lymphatic channels (e.g., tumor) or removal of lymph nodes (e.g., breast cancer). Lymphedema differs from other causes of edema (e.g., sodium imbalances) as the lymphatic system is structurally altered. Lymphedema is thought to occur due to a combination of increased capillary protein permeability and polysaccharides binding to excess proteins, preventing the lymphatics from effective removal of fluids.

Lipoedema is a type of edema caused by excess deposition of fat cells in an irregular and disproportional manner and not fluid shifts. The fat deposition is usually in the legs, thighs, and buttocks but can go to the arms. The legs will look like block columns. Lipoedema occurs mostly in women and rarely in men. It can occur with or without obesity. Eventually, lipoedema can cause venous and lymphatic problems.

Myxedema is another type of edema not related to fluid shifts. Myxedema refers to a thick nonpitting edema caused by deposits of mucopolysaccharides in the skin as a consequence of thyroid disorders.

Clinical Manifestations

Clinical manifestations of fluid excess can include edema. If the disorder causing the edema is a systemic problem (e.g., heart failure), then the edema is more likely to be peripheral, bilateral, dependent (e.g., ankle, feet, sacrum), and pitting (Figure 6-5). Edema can be generalized (anasarca) or localized periorbital (e.g., nephrotic syndrome). Cerebral edema can cause headache, confusion, irritability, anxiety, nausea, and vomiting. Other signs of fluid excess include dyspnea, bounding pulse, tachycardia, hypertension, jugular vein distention, crackles, and bulging fontanelles in infants. Fluid excesses can also be manifested as pleural effusions, pulmonary edema, or ascites. Rapid weight gain (3 pounds in a week or 1–2 pounds in a day; 1 pound approximately equals 500 mL of fluid) may be noted. Localized edema from disorders such as cellulitis or focal trauma (e.g., sprained ankle) will generally not cause systemic manifestations.

Diagnosis and Treatment

Diagnosis of fluid excess is based on physical examination. The diagnostic procedures for fluid excess are focused on determining the cause, and the history and physical findings are the starting point. The choice of procedures will be determined by clinical suspicion. As an example, suspected deep vein thrombosis will require evaluation with a venous duplex Doppler ultrasound. Suspicion for heart failure will warrant a chest X-ray, echocardiogram, and other tests. The appropriate and recommended diagnostic procedures are discussed in other chapters in the text for each respective disorder—cardiovascular, endocrine, urinary, and so forth.

Management of fluid excess focuses on identifying and treating the underlying cause. Strategies may consist of wearing compression stockings and administering diuretics, as well as restricting sodium and fluids. Fluid administration, although counterintuitive, may be necessary and include the administration of colloids or crystalloids to shift fluids from the interstitial to intravascular space. Any fluid

BOX 6-1 Application to Practice

The following activity includes several case presentations of edema. Make a diagnosis for each case, remembering the following questions:

Is the edema acute/sudden or chronic (e.g., duration, progression)? Is it unilateral or bilateral? Is the edema generalized or localized? Is it pitting or nonpitting? Is it dependent? In addition to edema, what other characteristics are associated with the edema (e.g., redness, pain)? What is the pertinent past or coexisting medical history? What medications is the patient taking? You may want to refer to chapter 3 and chapter 4 to help determine the diagnosis.

Activity: Identify the probable diagnosis and what data support your decision. Describe the pathogenesis for the diagnosis. What data are inconsistent with your diagnosis? What diagnostic tests would you order, if any, and how would you treat this patient? Note: Assume history and exam is normal if not listed.

Case 1: 45-year-old Mrs. Rodriguez is complaining of intermittent mild bilateral feet/ankle swelling for the past 2 months, but it is worse on her right leg. She denies leg pain, but she does describe her legs as feeling heavy at times and reports standing for long periods worsens the swelling. She notes her veins are getting larger in her legs. For the past 8 months, she has been experiencing intermittent numbness in her feet and reports her left knee has been achy. She is a server at a busy restaurant and sometimes works 10-hour days. She denies any fever, warmth, erythema, or trauma.

  Past medical history: obesity (BMI 31); type 2 diabetes mellitus.
  Medications: metformin.

Physical examination: vital signs are within normal limits; exam is unremarkable except for bilateral tortuous veins in both lower extremities, which are worse on the right leg, and decreased sensation in both feet.

Case 2: 68-year-old Mr. Quincy is complaining of left leg swelling for the past 2 weeks. The swelling started while he was on a cruise. The swelling is intermittent and below the knee to his foot. He describes a cramplike pain in his left calf. Lately, both legs have been cramping while walking, but it resolves when he sits. He denies any fever, warmth, erythema, or trauma.

  Past medical history: iliofemoral deep vein thrombosis of his left leg after he had left hip replacement for osteoarthritis 9 months ago; treated with rivaroxaban for 6 months; stable angina; obesity (BMI 31); dyslipidemia.
  Social history: quit smoking 4 years ago but resumed one-fourth pack per day 1 year ago.
  Medications: simvastatin; aspirin; metoprolol.
  Physical examination: vital signs are within normal limits; right leg is within normal limits except hairless, shiny skin; left leg has 1+ pitting edema in the pretibial area and foot; mild pain with left calf compression and one small tortuous vein on the medial aspect of his calf; left leg is also hairless and shiny.
  A venous duplex Doppler ultrasound of his left leg was done and reveals no deep vein thrombosis.

Case 3: 85-year-old Mrs. Delaney has bilateral ankle and foot swelling for the past 3 weeks; she states her feet hurt and her shoes feel tight and describes this swelling as the first occurrence; she denies fever, erythema, warmth, or trauma.

  Past medical history: aortic valve replacement; hypertension; dyslipidemia; osteoporosis.
  Medications: amlodipine; benazepril; atorvastatin; alendronate sodium; aspirin.
  Physical examination: vital signs within normal limits; exam unremarkable except for grade 1 systolic ejection murmur at the left sternal border, second intercostal space with no radiation, and mild ($< 1+$) pitting edema bilateral ankles and feet.

Case 4: 78-year-old Mr. Smith is complaining of increased swelling in his lower legs for the past 3 weeks. He states it worsens when his legs are hanging down and gets a bit better when he elevates them. The swelling started about a week after he left the hospital for an episode of pneumonia. He states his legs occasionally swell, especially when he eats too much salt, and the last time it happened was about 8 months ago. He reports taking a water pill for a while but not lately. He noted that he feels like he has put on a few pounds this week and feels a bit more tired and short of breath. He has had to sleep propped up with two pillows. He denies leg pain, fever, warmth, or trauma.

  Past medical history: anterior wall myocardial infarction 2 years ago; hypertension; heart failure with reduced ejection fraction; dyslipidemia.

(continues)

BOX 6-1 Application to Practice (Continued)

Social history: one pack a day smoker for 30 years—quit 2 years ago.

Medications: sacubitril/valsartan; metoprolol; rosuvastatin; aspirin (which he forgets to take).

Physical examination: temperature 98.5°F, pulse 70 beats/minute, respirations 22 breaths/minute, blood pressure 150/80 mmHg; pulse oximeter 96%; weight increase of 5 pounds in 1 month; cardiovascular exam remarkable for an S3 gallop; lungs with bibasilar fine inspiratory crackles;

bilateral lower extremities pretibial to feet with 2+ pitting edema and mild pain when depressing skin.

Case 5: 40-year-old Mr. Jason is complaining of right leg swelling, pain, erythema, and warmth for the past 2 days. The swelling started after he accidentally cut the front of his leg with a pocket knife while fishing.

Past medical history: hypertension.

Medications: amlodipine.

Social history: drinks four to five beers on the weekends and has smoked one or two

cigarettes a day for the last 15 years (he states he is trying to quit).

Physical examination: temperature 100°F, pulse 88 beats/minute, respirations 18 breaths/minute; blood pressure 140/92 mmHg; exam unremarkable except for edematous anterior right leg with open linear wound approximately 1-inch long; wound with scant purulent drainage; area is warm and tender with blanching erythema that extends 3 inches around the wound.

administration must be monitored carefully as use of fluids may worsen the excess, causing further compromise.

Fluid Deficit

Fluid deficit occurs when total body fluid levels are insufficient to meet the body's needs. As with excesses, fluid deficits are usually due to problems with sodium control as opposed to water control. The most common issue in fluid deficit is too little sodium with an inability to retain water (see Table 6-2). The deficits usually occur because of excessive water and sodium elimination, but inadequate water and sodium intake can also be present. Fluid deficit may be referred to as *dehydration* or *hypovolemia*. Hypovolemia is a fluid deficit in the intravascular compartment as a result of total volume loss (sodium and water). Dehydration refers to water loss alone, which results in hypernatremia. The terms are often used interchangeably. Dehydration causes a hypertonic state which leads cell shriveling (Figure 6-4) as fluid shifts from the ICF to ECF. This ICF cell dehydration often affects brain (neurons) cells (edema also affects neurons) with subsequent neurologic manifestations. Fluid deficit

can occur independently or with electrolyte imbalances, such as hypernatremia or hyponatremia. Sodium alterations are dependent on how much sodium is in the fluid that is lost. As an example, diarrhea or vomiting may cause a significant loss in relation to the water. If sodium loss is greater than water loss (e.g., as with thiazide diuretics), then plasma sodium levels fall. Sodium, along with levels of other blood solutes (e.g., blood cells and electrolytes), increases if water loss is greater than sodium losses because of hemoconcentration. If sodium loss and water loss are relatively equal, plasma sodium levels may not be altered. Fluid volume deficits can cause hypotension and orthostasis.

Learning Points

Rule of Threes: Survival

Fluid deficits can happen in healthy people; however, deficits are usually due to lack of water being accessible. The rule of threes is a good way to remember how long a person can survive without water and other basics of life. A person can survive approximately 3 minutes without oxygen, 3 days without water, 9 days without sleep (multiple of 3), and 3 weeks without food. Water ranks high in the basic needs.

BOX 6-2 Application to Practice

An example of osmotic diuresis can be seen in a tragic case in which a newborn was fed concentrated formula by mistake. Often, tube feeding and baby formulas are high in glucose and other electrolytes. Many times, these formulas come concentrated for shipping purposes. The newborn's father was unaware that the formula required dilution prior to feeding it to his child. The high concentrations of glucose caused excessive urination, and the baby died because of hypertonic dehydration.

Reproduced from Story, L. (2017). *Pathophysiology: A practical approach* (3rd ed.). Burlington, MA: Jones & Bartlett Learning.

Learning Points

Fluid Balance: Elimination

While imbalances can occur due to excessive or inadequate intake of sodium or water, the usual culprit is elimination (i.e., loss). Intake issues are not as likely to occur. For example, excessive water intake to the point of illness is not likely. Decreased water intake issues are probably more prevalent in comparison to excess water intake, but the balance can be restored with an intact thirst mechanism unless a person has no access (e.g., running out of water in extreme conditions). Likewise, excessive salt intake causing imbalance by itself is not too common as salt alone is not very palatable. Even drinks with electrolytes are often more sugar and, therefore, water retaining, so they balance out the excess salt. There are situations where even reasonable amounts of salt intake can be an issue, such as with heart failure and other disorders. Even under those circumstances, the issue is the that salt intake causes water retention (problem with elimination). Inadequate pumping decreases renal perfusion and decreased elimination. Clinicians should be aware of the side effects of hypotonic or hypertonic administrations, whether parenteral or gastric, and adjustments should be made (e.g., enteral feeds with water boluses or continuously). Even disorders that cause retention of water or sodium or both are not common in the general population, so elimination is the most common issue with either too much sodium or water eliminated or too much sodium or water retained (see chapter 7 for further details on urinary function).

Clinical Manifestations

Clinical manifestations of fluid deficits include thirst and altered level of consciousness. Hypovolemia may cause hypotension or orthostatic symptoms (e.g., dizziness) with compensatory tachycardia. As volume continues to decrease, the pulses become weak and thready. Signs opposite of edema (fluid excess) such as flat jugular veins, sunken fontanelles in infants, decreased skin turgor, dry mucous membranes, oliguria, and weight loss can occur.

Diagnosis and Treatment

Diagnosis of fluid deficit is based on physical examination. The diagnostic procedures for fluid deficit are focused on determining the cause, and the history and physical findings are the starting point. The choice of procedures will be determined by clinical suspicion. As an example, diagnostic tests may include a complete blood count (CBC), chemistry profile, stool samples (to test for *Clostridium difficile*), and others if a person has hypotension with excessive vomiting and diarrhea. The appropriate and recommended diagnostic procedures are discussed in other chapters in the text for each respective disorder—gastrointestinal, urinary, and so forth.

Management focuses on identifying and treating the underlying cause of the fluid deficit. Strategies include fluid replacement—oral fluids for mild losses and intravenous fluids (IVFs) for greater losses, usually isotonic. Prompt management and awareness of fluid deficits are aimed at avoiding hypovolemic shock (see chapter 4).

Learning Points

Glucose and Fluid Balance

Glucose normally has a minor contribution to osmotic pressure in comparison to sodium. Glucose, like sodium, is an effective osmole as it does not freely cross the cell membrane and needs to be transported by insulin. So, excess glucose (hyperglycemia) in the ECF, specifically intravascular fluid, increases osmotic pressure and hypertonicity, causing water to be drawn out of the ICF (cells). The cells become dehydrated. The kidneys compensate by eliminating the excess glucose and water, causing what is termed an *osmotic diuresis*. Potassium follows glucose out of the cell with resulting hyperkalemia (in the intravascular compartment). However, other electrolytes like sodium get diluted due to the excess water. For every 100 mg/dL of serum glucose above normal, sodium decreases about 1.6 mEq/L. Hyperglycemia can cause a fluid deficit due to water being pulled out of the cell and compensatory diuresis. A high glucose solution like mannitol is used for cerebral edema or increased intracranial pressure with the intent that water moves out of the cells.

Sodium

Sodium is considered the most significant cation. The most prevalent electrolyte within the

ECF, sodium's primary function is to control serum osmolality and water balance. Sodium accounts for most of the extracellular osmolality, so sodium changes, in turn, alter osmolality. There are negligible amounts of sodium in the ICF and the sodium in the interstitial space is bound and osmotically inactive. Sodium has an affinity for chloride and helps maintain acid–base balance when combined with another anion, bicarbonate (HCO_3^-).

Sodium concentration is determined by the volume (i.e., water) status. Mechanisms to increase or decrease sodium are regulated by the kidneys as well as aldosterone produced by the adrenal cortex. When aldosterone is released the kidneys retain sodium. The sympathetic nervous system assists the kidneys in sodium regulation by changing the glomerular filtration rate, which is a reflection of renal blood flow. Increasing the glomerular filtration rate increases sodium excretion; decreasing the glomerular filtration rate decreases sodium excretion. The renin–angiotensin–aldosterone mechanism also manipulates sodium in the kidneys; this mechanism is triggered in times of decreased renal perfusion (e.g., hypovolemia and hypotension). Renin, a protein, converts angiotensinogen to angiotensin I; subsequently, angiotensin I is converted to angiotensin II in the lungs. Angiotensin II causes the kidneys to retain sodium (also causes release of aldosterone) and, in turn, water. Volume and pressure receptor activation can lead to sodium retention or excretion.

The cellular membrane is permeable to sodium, but it is dependent on the sodium–potassium pump to transport these ions. Sodium facilitates muscle and nerve impulses through the pump. As sodium moves into the cell, potassium shifts out of the cell, resulting in depolarization (increasing the membrane potential or excitability) of the cell membrane. When sodium shifts out of the cell, potassium moves back into the cell, resulting in repolarization (restoring the resting potential) of the cell membrane.

Sodium is primarily brought into the body through dietary intake and a common type ingested is sodium chloride (i.e., table salt). Many other types of sodium are in food products such as sodium bicarbonate (i.e., baking soda). The key is to look for the word *sodium* in the ingredients (e.g., monosodium glutamate, sodium phosphate). The recommended dietary allowance (RDA) of sodium is 2–4 grams. This electrolyte can be found in many sources, such as table salt (1 teaspoon contains more than 2 grams of sodium), processed or prepackaged foods (e.g., canned foods and deli meats), snack foods (e.g., chips), condiments (e.g., ketchup and hot sauce), and certain cooking seasonings (e.g., garlic salt and seasoned salt).

Normally, sodium losses occur in the kidneys. Excessive losses can occur through the gastrointestinal tract through vomiting, diarrhea, and nasogastric suctioning. Extensive burns can also cause sodium losses through the skin. Finally, sodium losses can occur with excessive sweating (e.g., fever and strenuous exercise).

Hypernatremia is defined as a high serum sodium levels (greater than 145 mEq/L). The excessive sodium levels generally lead to high serum osmolality (greater than 295 mOsm/kg) because of the imbalance between sodium and water. As sodium levels rise, hypertonicity occurs, and water shifts out of the intracellular space and into the intravascular compartment. This shift leads to intracellular dehydration, shrinking the cells (Figure 6-4). Hypernatremia usually results from water imbalances due to excessive loss without adequate replacement as opposed to actual sodium excess issues (e.g., rapid ingestion without water or hypertonic solution administration). Inadequate water replacement occurs as a result of impairment in thirst or lack of access to water. Excessive water losses can be categorized as extrarenal or renal losses. Extrarenal losses can occur as a result of gastrointestinal losses (e.g., severe diarrhea, vomiting) or profuse sweating and insensible losses from mechanical ventilation. Renal water loss is a result of the kidneys' inability to retain water. Conditions that cause an osmotic diuresis such as hyperglycemia from poorly controlled diabetes mellitus or mannitol infusion will initially lead to hyponatremia with hypertonicity but water losses become progressive and ultimately hypernatremia ensues. Administration of hyperalimentation whether enteral or parenteral with high protein (causes increased urea) can also cause an osmotic diuresis. Diabetes insipidus is a disorder that results in ADH deficiency or an unresponsiveness of the kidneys to ADH (see chapter 10 for more on endocrine function). Diabetes insipidus will cause water loss. Usually two clinical scenarios occur with hypernatremia—either 1) a loss of sodium with even greater amounts of water loss causing hypovolemia, or 2) excessive water loss relative to sodium loss (i.e., hemoconcentration) (Table 6-2).

Hyponatremia is defined as low serum sodium levels (less than 135 mEq/L). Serum osmolality levels also fall below 280 mOsm. As sodium levels decrease, hypotonicity occurs and water shifts from the ECF into the ICF. The cells swell with water, causing intracellular edema. The brain is particularly susceptible to hyponatremia as water moves into brain cells, causing cerebral edema. Additionally, nerve conduction becomes impaired as the sodium levels fall. Hyponatremia occurs due to excessive water usually from inadequate renal water excretion (water intake must still be present). Therefore, to determine the cause of hyponatremia, it is important to figure out why the kidneys are unable to excrete the water and also determine all the water sources (is there an excess taken in beyond the kidney capacity). Often there is impaired ADH suppression; but there can also be increased ADH secretion both situations will lead to with water retention. ADH suppression may however be intact. Hyponatremia is generally associated with hypotonic states. Disorders that lead to decreased water excretion and therefore hyponatremia include:

- Renal failure—the lack of ability of the kidneys to filter causes an inability to excrete.
- Severe volume depletion—usually from gastric losses (e.g., vomiting and diarrhea) leads to ADH release (water retained with hyponatremia).
- Diuretics—particularly thiazides impair water excretion and increased sodium excretion.
- Syndrome of inappropriate antidiuretic hormone—abnormal ADH secretion (see chapter 10 for more on endocrine function).
- Adrenal insufficiency or failure—impaired adrenocorticotropic hormone leads to inability to suppress ADH (water retained) and aldosterone deficiency leads to release of ADH (water retained).
- Lack of sodium intake or too much water ingestion—such as can occur with psychogenic polydipsia, excessive beer drinking (beer is dilute and has little solute), dietary sodium restriction, prolonged exercise can increase ADH secretion (water retained).
- Decompensated heart failure, liver failure, or nephrotic syndrome—leads to water retention.

Hyponatremia can be associated with hypertonic states although this is not as common. As an example, there is hyponatremia with hyperglycemia, as the glucose creates a hypertonic state and water shifts from the ICF to the ECF. Mannitol, a type of glucose infusion, will create a hyponatremia with hypertonic state. Extremely high triglycerides (generally in the 1000s when normal range is less than 150 mg/dL) or high proteins as can occur with multiple myeloma can also act as effective osmoles. These are other circumstances causing hyponatremia with hypertonicity.

Clinical Manifestations

Sodium imbalances generally result in neuromuscular clinical manifestations. Manifestations of hypernatremia can range from subtle to serious, depending on the severity of the hypernatremia itself. Manifestations include lethargy, headache, confusion and irritability, seizures, and coma (i.e., usually greater than 158 mEq/L). Hypernatremia usually causes hypovolemia, and manifestations can include hypotension, dry mucous membranes, thirst, and decreased urine output.

Manifestations of hyponatremia can also cause similar neuromuscular manifestations (e.g., headache, lethargy, confusion, seizures, and coma) and are likely to be present with extremely low levels (i.e., less than 125 mEq/L). Levels of 130 mEq/L generally cause gastrointestinal symptoms such as nausea, vomiting, and diarrhea. Signs of hyponatremia with hypovolemia will be similar to fluid deficits such as hypotension. Hyponatremia with hypervolemia will cause fluid excess signs such as edema.

Diagnosis and Treatment

Diagnoses of sodium imbalances are made based on serum levels. Diagnostic procedures for hypernatremia and hyponatremia include a history, physical examination, blood chemistry, and urine analysis. Other diagnostic tests are conducted to identify the cause. Generally, serum osmolality will be increased with hypernatremia and decreased with hyponatremia Urine sodium and osmolality evaluation can aid in determining the underlying disorder.

Management of hypernatremia focuses on treating the underlying cause. If the cause is related to water loss, treatment begins with replacing water and remedying any electrolyte deficits. Glucose-electrolyte solutions (e.g., sports drinks) are given orally for less severe cases. Electrolyte solutions are also available for infants and young children. More severe cases can be corrected with IV hypotonic (e.g., 5% dextrose in water or 0.45% saline) solutions. The healthcare professional must use caution to avoid correcting the hypernatremia too rapidly. The brain can become accustomed to the high levels of sodium; as the levels drop with the treatment of hypernatremia, water moves into cerebral cells, causing cerebral edema. Generally, hypernatremia should initially be reduced no faster than 1 mEq/L per hour, however, the total reduction in 24 hours should be no greater than 12 mEq/L. Additionally, seizure precautions (e.g., low lighting and decreased stimuli) and neurologic checks should be part of the patient's plan of care.

Management of hyponatremia focuses on treating the underlying cause (e.g., administering corticosteroids for Addison disease; discontinue medication if it is causing syndrome of inappropriate antidiuretic hormone). In cases caused by excessive water, intake may be limited, whether orally or IV (i.e., avoid hypotonic solutions). Diuretics or dialysis may be necessary to remove excess free water. In cases caused by deficient sodium, intake may be increased either orally or with hypertonic solutions. Correction of sodium levels should be done slowly as with hypernatremia. Rapid correction can cause fluid to shift into the intravascular space and overload the heart. Rapid correction may also cause cerebral cellular volume changes with serious neurologic consequences and death. With hyponatremia, patients should be on seizure precaution (e.g., low lighting and decreased stimuli) and neurologic checks should be part of the patient's plan of care.

Diagnostic Link

Urine: Specific Gravity and Urine Osmolality

Urine osmolality and specific gravity are reflections of urine concentration and reflect hydration (volume) status and kidney functioning. These tests are used in conjunction with serum values (i.e., electrolytes, osmolality) to identify causes of alterations in urine output or serum electrolyte imbalances. Specific gravity is determined by the number and size of the solutes in the urine as opposed to urine osmolality witch is determined by the number of solutes in the urine. Specific gravity, therefore can be less accurate. Osmolality in urine is determined by the same solutes as in serum such as sodium, chloride, urea, potassium, and glucose. The higher the solutes, the higher the urine osmolality. The osmolality is considered more accurate than urine specific gravity as large molecules (e.g., glucose, proteins) invalidate results with specific gravity. A high urine osmolality means there are increased solutes with decreased water in the urine (e.g., dehydration). A low urine osmolality means there are decreased solutes with increased water in the urine (e.g., diabetes insipidus indicates inadequate ADH). The normal urine-to-serum osmolality ratio is 3:1. As an example, if urine osmolality is 855, then serum osmolality is 285 under normal circumstances. Alterations in the ratio can occur with concentrated urine (increased solutes, inadequate water), which will cause a high ratio. Poorly concentrated urine (decreased solutes, too much water), which will cause a low ratio.

Chloride

Chloride is a mineral electrolyte and the major extracellular anion. Chloride assists in fluid distribution by attaching to sodium or water. Because of its negative charge, chloride can bind and travel with positively charged ions such as sodium, potassium, or calcium. This electrolyte is found in gastric secretions, pancreatic juices, and bile. In the stomach, it unites with hydrogen to form hydrochloric acid. Chloride is abundant in cerebrospinal fluid, where it binds with sodium. When bound to sodium, it behaves just like sodium in regard to water balance. When bound to hydrogen, chloride plays an important role in acid–base balance.

Diet is the main source of chloride. The chloride RDA is 3–9 grams. Chloride is easily obtained through consumption of a balanced diet. Common sources of chloride include table salt, fruits, vegetables, cheese, milk, eggs, fish, canned foods, and processed meats. The kidneys are primarily responsible for chloride excretion, but some chloride is also lost through sweating. **Hyperchloremia** is an excess amount of chloride in the blood (greater than 108 mEq/L). Hyperchloremia is usually a result of an underlying condition; it does not have its own clinical manifestations, but the companion condition may cause signs and symptoms (e.g., metabolic acidosis). **Hypochloremia** occurs when chloride levels fall below 98 mEq/L. Hypochloremia rarely occurs in the absence of other abnormalities (e.g., metabolic alkalosis), so as with hyperchloremia, it does not have its own set of clinical manifestations. Cystic fibrosis is caused by a mutation in the gene that makes transmembrane conductance regulator protein, and defects in this protein cause problems with chloride movement across the cell membrane, which, in turn, causes imbalances in sodium and water transport. Chloride imbalances are often due to the same disorders that affect sodium and water balance (Table 6-2). Metabolic acidosis and hyperparathyroidism can cause hyperchloremia (excess calcium attracts chloride), and metabolic alkalosis and hypothyroidism cause hypochloremia.

Diagnostic procedures include a history, physical examination, blood chemistry, urine analysis, and measurement of arterial blood gases (ABGs). Management of hyperchloremia and hypochloremia focuses on treating the underlying cause. With hyperchloremia, administering diuretics to assist in eliminating sodium will, in turn, assist in the removal of chloride.

Administering bicarbonate can correct acidosis if present. Some strategies for treating hypochloremia include increasing oral sodium intake and administering sodium-containing IV solutions. Additionally, ammonium chloride can be given with caution to raise chloride levels. Saline solutions can also be used to irrigate gastric tubes.

Potassium

Potassium is the primary intracellular cation. It plays a crucial role in electrical conduction throughout the body (e.g., nerves, skeletal system, and cardiac system), acid–base balance, and metabolism of carbohydrate, protein, and glucose. Potassium is present in huge quantities in the intracellular space (98% of total body potassium)—a store that can be utilized if serum levels drop. However, certain circumstances such as lysis cause excessive amounts of potassium to shift to the intravascular space, which can be dangerous (especially within the heart). Serum potassium cannot fluctuate much—either up or down—without causing serious issues. The sodium–potassium pump regulates ICF and ECF potassium exchange and the exchange ratio is 3 sodium ions for 2 potassium ions. The kidneys regulate levels through retention or elimination. Potassium along with ATP, phosphate, and phospholipids maintain intracellular osmotic pressure. Potassium levels in the ICF, which are not measured clinically, are approximately 140–150 mEq/L. Serum potassium, which is clinically measured, is 3.5–5.0 mEq/L. Insulin and catecholamines, particularly beta-2 adrenergic receptors, cause activation of the sodium–potassium pump with potassium shifting back into cells. Acid–base balance through hydrogen also influences shifts. Hydrogen and potassium exchanges occur between the ICF and ECF when pH is altered. For example, hydrogen increases in the blood with metabolic alkalosis (increased pH); therefore, potassium does not shift out of the cell, resulting in hypokalemia (low potassium levels in the serum). Aldosterone promotes retention of sodium but regulates potassium by promoting excretion (see chapter 7 for more on urinary function).

Dietary intake (e.g., cantaloupes, raisins, bananas, oranges, green leafy vegetables, and lentils) is the primary source of potassium. The RDA for potassium is 40–60 mEq as the average adult stores are about 50 mEq/kg (the amount varies with weight and muscle mass). Most potassium (about 90%) is excreted in the kidneys, but some potassium is lost through the gastrointestinal tract (i.e., in the stool) and some in sweat.

Hyperkalemia refers to serum potassium levels greater than 5 mEq/L. Hyperkalemia is unusual in the healthy individual. Hyperkalemia may be a medical emergency. Generally, the most common causes of hyperkalemia are conditions that decrease excretion. Conditions that increase intake or release potassium out of the cells can cause hyperkalemia. **Hypokalemia** occurs when potassium levels drop below 3.5 mEq/L. Hypokalemia typically results from opposite causes of hyperkalemia; this includes excessive loss, decreased intake, or increased potassium cellular uptake (**TABLE 6-3**).

Diagnostic Link

Pseudohyperkalemia

Many reports of hyperkalemia are not due to actual body imbalances but rather occur due to errors in the handling of the serum sample prior to the analysis. The factors leading to a pseudohyperkalemia include errors in obtaining a sample that include applying the tourniquet too tightly, leaving the tourniquet on for longer than 1 minute, fist clenching, traumatic venipuncture, the wrong needle diameter, or excessive force when withdrawing. After the sample is obtained, errors that can cause pseudohyperkalemia include excessive force with transferring to the vacutainer and vigorous mixing, whether by hand or by centrifuge. Delays in processing and cold temperature storage are other considerations. When hyperkalemia is seen on a report, go back to your patient to evaluate if the result makes sense—a potassium of 6.5 mEq/L in a person who is awake, alert, and has no concerns does not make sense. Even in the critically ill, go back and evaluate the likelihood that potassium would go up so high. Evaluate the patient first, then treat while keeping in mind the possibility of pseudohyperkalemia due to serum sample errors.

Clinical Manifestations

Hyperkalemia and hypokalemia can affect several body systems in which potassium plays key functions, including the nervous, cardiac, respiratory, and gastrointestinal systems (**TABLE 6-4**; **FIGURE 6-6**; **FIGURE 6-7**). The severity of these effects depends on the extent of the hyperkalemia and hypokalemia. A bit of an oversimplified way to remember differences between manifestations is: *Hyperkalemia makes things excitable, while hypokalemia depresses or slows things down.*

Diagnosis and Treatment

A chemistry panel, which includes potassium levels, is a common diagnostic test in most clinical settings. Potassium imbalance is

TABLE 6-3	Hyperkalemia and Hypokalemia Causes and Mechanisms

Hyperkalemia causes and mechanisms	Hypokalemia causes and mechanisms
Decreased excretion—renal • Renal failure • Addison disease—decreased aldosterone (reducing excretion) • Medications: potassium-sparing diuretics (e.g., spironolactone), nonsteroidal anti-inflammatory drugs, angiotensin-converting enzyme, angiotensin receptor blockers decrease response or production of aldosterone • Gordon syndrome—rare genetic disorder in which the kidneys are unable to respond to aldosterone	**Excessive loss—renal and gastrointestinal** • Renal losses • Potassium-losing diuretics (e.g., thiazide, loop) • Renal failure—diuretic phase • Corticosteroid elevations—decreases sodium excretion and increases potassium excretion (e.g., in hyperaldosteronism, Cushing syndrome, medications, stress-related trauma, surgery) • Gastrointestinal losses • Vomiting and diarrhea (e.g., with illness, excessive laxative use) • Nasogastric suctioning • Gastrointestinal fistula
Increased intake • Oral/enteral—excessive supplements, salt substitutes (potassium chloride) more common with renal disease • Rapid intravenous administration—undiluted potassium can be lethal even with normal kidney function	**Decreased intake** • Deficient diet (e.g., malnutrition, extreme dieting, alcoholism) • Intake inability/difficulties—chewing, swallowing (e.g., in the elderly) • Inadequate potassium replacement with intravenous solution
Release from cells to ECF • Acidosis—increased hydrogen-potassium shifts out • Deficient insulin (diabetic ketoacidosis)—potassium not transported back into cell • Blood transfusions—can cause blood lysis with increased potassium • Burns, tissue trauma, extreme activity or seizures	**Increased cellular uptake from ECF** • Alkalosis—decreased hydrogen-potassium shifts into cell • Insulin excesses—transports potassium back into the cell (e.g., used during diabetic ketoacidosis)

TABLE 6-4	Clinical Manifestations of Hyperkalemia and Hypokalemia

	Hyperkalemia*	Hypokalemia*
Neuromuscular	Paresthesias Muscle cramps Weakness/fatigue **Hyperreflexia** Flaccid paralysis (later) **Anxiety**	Paresthesias Muscle cramps Weakness/fatigue **Hyporeflexia** Flaccid paralysis **Confusion/depression**
Cardiovascular	Electrocardiogram (EKG) changes and dysrhythmias (delayed conduction—bradyarrhythmias/asystole) Cardiac arrest	**Hypotension** Weak, irregular pulse EKG changes and dysrhythmias (Ventricular fibrillation) Cardiac arrest
Respiratory	**Respiratory depression/arrest—diaphragm weakness**	
Gastrointestinal	Nausea/vomiting **Diarrhea** **Cramping**	Nausea/vomiting **Constipation** **Distention and ileus**

* Bold indicates differential manifestations

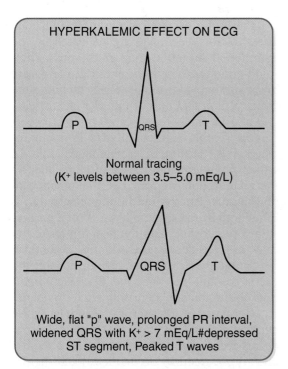

FIGURE 6-6 Hyperkalemic effects on the electrocardiogram.

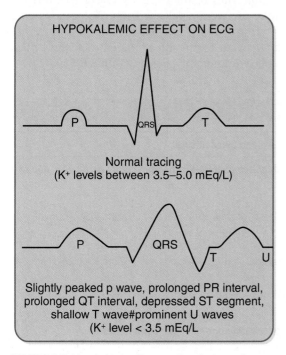

FIGURE 6-7 Hypokalemic effects on the electrocardiogram.

considered an emergency. When looking for a cause, the most common reasons should be evaluated initially, such as renal disease for hyperkalemia. A 12-lead EKG is a common diagnostic test conducted to identify the potential cardiac disturbances (e.g., dysrhythmias, slowed conduction). An ABG is done to check for acid–base imbalances.

Emergent management of hyperkalemia includes methods to increase excretion. These methods include dialysis, sodium polystyrene sulfonate (Kayexalate), and insulin with IV dextrose to prevent hypoglycemia. Sodium polystyrene sulfonate induces gastrointestinal potassium excretion. Acidosis, if present, is treated prior to the hyperkalemia so that potassium can shift back into the cells and a true potassium level can be obtained. Calcium gluconate may be administered to minimize dysrhythmias. Hyperkalemia due to excess dietary intake will necessitate discussing reduction of foods high in potassium. Medications such as angiotensin-converting enzymes that can cause hyperkalemia may have to be discontinued, or if the elevation is minor, close serial potassium evaluation will be necessary.

Management strategies of hypokalemia are directed at increasing the amount of potassium available to the body. Oral potassium is administered for mild cases, while IV potassium that is diluted is administered for more severe deficits. For rapid replacement, patients will usually be in an intensive care unit to monitor for potentially life-threatening cardiac side effects (e.g., ventricular tachycardia, asystole). Rapid infusions need to be delivered using a central line as the amounts that can be safely administered peripherally are lower. Administering potassium IV can be caustic to the veins, which is another reason that potassium must be given diluted and slowly. Once the potassium gets to a safe level with IV infusion, then a transition to oral replacement over days is done.

Calcium

Most of the body's calcium is found in the bones and teeth (99%). Most of the remaining amount (1%) is found in the blood. Ionized (unbound or free) can be used for several physiologic processes—for example, blood clotting, hormone secretion, receptor functions, nerve transmission, and muscular (e.g., skeletal and cardiac) contraction. The other form of calcium in the blood is mostly bound to albumin, and a small amount is bound (chelated) with phosphate,

determined by serum levels (remember laboratory errors). The next step is determining the reason for the alteration by conducting a history and physical examination. Imbalances can cause severe consequences, so the evaluation should be conducted rapidly, with the extreme values (e.g., 2.5 mEq/L or 6.0 mEq/L) citrate, and sulfur. Calcium has an inverse relationship with phosphorus and a synergistic relationship with magnesium. When calcium levels go up, phosphorus goes down, and vice versa. Calcium needs magnesium to fully function as well as balance its effects.

Calcium is brought into the body through the absorption of dietary sources in the gastrointestinal tract, specifically the small intestines; therefore, conditions affecting intestinal absorption or surgical procedures that change the gastrointestinal tract (e.g., gastric bypass) can alter calcium absorption. Vitamin D aids in calcium absorption; it is primarily obtained through sun exposure and from fortified dairy products. Vitamin K also plays an important role in calcium regulation and bone formation (vitamin K binds to calcium in the bone); it is primarily found in green leafy vegetables. Calcium is found in large amounts in dairy products, salmon, sardines, green leafy vegetables, pinto beans, almonds, and figs, among other sources. The RDA of calcium is 800–1,200 mg/day; however, individuals' daily needs vary with certain conditions (e.g., pregnancy, childhood, and osteoporosis). The RDA of vitamin D is 400–600 international units/day up to the age of 70 and then 800 international units/day after 70 years of age.

Calcium is excreted in the urine and stool. Levels of this electrolyte are regulated by the parathyroid hormones and calcitonin (a thyroid hormone). When serum calcium levels are low, parathyroid hormone quickly mobilizes the bone calcium and pulls it into the bloodstream and also increases renal reabsorption. To compensate for this shift, parathyroid hormone replaces this calcium by activating vitamin D, which promotes intestinal absorption and renal reabsorption, and increases elimination of phosphorus. Parathyroid hormone secretion is influenced by magnesium levels. When magnesium levels are low, parathyroid is inhibited, and calcium levels decrease. Calcitonin, in contrast, regulates elevated calcium levels by pushing the excess calcium into the bone, decreasing intestinal absorption and increasing renal excretion.

Normal total adult serum calcium levels are between 8.8 and 10.3 mg/dL. **Hypercalcemia** occurs with levels that are above 10.3 mg/dL, and **hypocalcemia** occurs below 8.8 mg/dL. Values vary slightly for children. Hypercalcemia may result from excessive calcium intake or calcium release from the bone as well as from inadequate excretion. Hypocalcemia may occur as a result of increased losses or decreased intake of calcium (**TABLE 6-5**).

TABLE 6-5	Hypercalcemia and Hypocalcemia Causes and Mechanisms

Hypercalcemia causes and mechanisms	Hypocalcemia causes and mechanisms
Decreased excretion—renal • Renal failure • Thiazide diuretics—increase renal reabsorption	***Excessive loss—renal and gastrointestinal and serum active loss due to increased binding*** • Renal failure • Alkalosis—serum hydrogen decreases and unbinds from albumin leading to more albumin bound to calcium (i.e., less free) • Medications (e.g., diuretics, calcitonin, and gentamicin) • Hyperphosphatemia—phosphate binds the calcium (i.e., less free) • Diarrhea • Pancreatitis (decreases intestinal absorption of fat; calcium binds to fat and is excreted)
Increased intake/absorption (gastrointestinal) or increased bone resorption • Cancer (e.g., breast, lung, multiple myeloma) • Excess intake—diet, antacids (e.g., Tums), supplements • Excess vitamin D • Parathyroid hormone abnormalities (e.g., hyperparathyroidism) • Prolonged immobility • Medications (e.g., corticosteroids) • Hypophosphatemia	***Decreased intake/absorption or decreased bone release*** • Deficient diet (e.g., malnutrition, extreme dieting, alcoholism) • Absorption disorders (e.g., Crohn disease) • Vitamin D deficiency (e.g., kidney disease) • Excessive laxative use (e.g., increased phosphate causing decreased absorption) • Parathyroid hormone abnormalities (e.g., hypomagnesemia, hypoparathyroidism) impair release from bone

Vitamin D

When vitamin D is absorbed from the sun and small amounts from food, it must undergo processes in the liver and kidney to become activated. Serum measures include 25-hydroxyvitamin D_2 and 25-hydroxyvitamin D_3, and these two metabolites are part of 25-hydroxyvitamin D [25(OH)D], which is clinically used when evaluating overall body status. The two measures of 25-hydroxyvitamin D include nanomoles per liter (nmol/L) or nanograms per milliliter (ng/mL). Levels consistent with deficiency are < 30 nmol/L (i.e., < 12 ng/mL). These low levels can be associated with bone diseases such as rickets and osteomalacia. Optimal levels are > 50 nmol/L (> 20 ng/mL); however, controversy exists regarding appropriate levels due varied laboratory measurement standards. Efforts are being made to adopt an international gold standard for measurement.

Calcium and Albumin Levels

Serum calcium measurements are often done to evaluate several disorders such as kidney disease and parathyroid disorders. Total serum calcium levels consist of the three stores: 1) active (free, unbound, ionized), 2) bound mainly to albumin, and 3) bound to anions such as phosphate. The bound forms are metabolically inactive. The active ionized level is regulated by hormones such as parathyroid hormone and is the more clinically relevant value. The report may only contain the total serum calcium levels; however, the total levels can be misleading as they also reflect inactive bound levels. Therefore, the total is affected by albumin levels (high or low). In cases where the calcium and albumin are abnormal, a corrected level should be calculated or an active ionized calcium serum level should be obtained to get a real reflection of the active calcium level. For example, the total calcium may be abnormal, but it might be because there is hypo- or hyperalbuminemia where the active ionized level is normal. Before a clinical decision is made about a high or low total calcium, take a look at the albumin level. The most common unit of measure for calcium in the United States are mg/dL, and other units of measure include mEq/L and mmol/L.

Clinical Manifestations

Calcium is involved in cell membrane depolarization and repolarization, and imbalances are often a reflection of increased or decreased cell excitability. Clinical manifestations of hypercalcemia reflect decreased cell membrane excitability and renal effects. Hypocalcemia increases cell membrane excitability (TABLE 6-6). Manifestations are often nonspecific. The cardiac, nervous, musculoskeletal, gastrointestinal systems, can all be affected by high or low calcium levels. Hypercalcemia can also affect the renal system while hypocalcemia can affect the respiratory and hematologic systems. Tetany describes spasms of the skeletal muscle that are specific to hypocalcemia. Two clinical examinations can be used to evaluate hypocalcemia facial and carpopedal spasms—Trousseau and Chvostek signs. To test for Trousseau sign, arterial blood flow is occluded by using an inflated blood pressure cuff. The cuff is placed on the upper arm and inflated above the individual's usual systolic pressure measurement. The inflated cuff is left in place for approximately 3 minutes. The test is considered positive for increased neuromuscular irritability if it elicits a carpal spasm (flexed wrist and metacarpophalangeal joints, extended interphalangeal joints, and adducted thumb) (FIGURE 6-8). To test the Chvostek sign, the patient's facial nerve in front of the ear is tapped. A spasm or brief contraction of the corner of the mouth, nose, eye, and muscles in the cheek is considered a positive sign and indicates increased neuromuscular irritability (FIGURE 6-9).

Diagnosis and Treatment

Diagnostic procedures include a history, physical examination, blood chemistry, and 12-lead EKG. Management focuses on identification (e.g., renal failure, parathyroid disorders) and treatment of the underlying cause (e.g., dialysis). For hypercalcemia, several medications, including oral bisphosphonate preparations and calcitonin, can inhibit osteoclastic activity, reducing the amount of calcium released from the bone. Increasing mobility can also prevent resorption. Other medications, such as corticosteroids or mithramycin (antineoplastic), reduce resorption and are used with cancer-associated hypercalcemia. Increasing hydration with IVF administration can increase renal excretion of calcium. Loop diuretics may be necessary to enhance this excretion further. Thiazide diuretics are usually avoided as they can increase calcium levels.

Hypocalcemia is often treated with oral supplements in mild deficiencies and IV calcium gluconate or calcium chloride in moderate to severe deficiencies. Vitamin D supplements can increase intestinal calcium absorption. Additionally, phosphorus intake may be decreased to bring calcium levels up. Supplemental parathyroid hormone can be administered for hypoparathyroidism.

TABLE 6-6	Clinical Manifestations of Hypercalcemia and Hypocalcemia	
System	**Hypercalcemia**	**Hypocalcemia**
Neuromuscular	Personality changes and behavior changes: confusion, memory changes, psychosis Headache Lethargy/stupor/coma Muscle weakness/atrophy Decreased deep tendon reflexes Osteopenia/osteoporosis	Anxiety Confusion Depression Irritability Fatigue Lethargy Paresthesia Muscle spasms/tetany—positive Chvostek and/or Trousseau signs Laryngeal spasms Tremors/seizures Increased deep tendon reflexes
Cardiovascular	EKG changes and dysrhythmias—short QT interval; atrioventricular blocks Hypertension Cardiac arrest—hypercalcemic crisis (acute increase)	EKG changes and dysrhythmias—prolonged QT interval with risk for ventricular dysrhythmias; heart blocks Hypotension
Renal	Renal calculi Renal insufficiency Polyuria/polydipsia (hypercalcemia interferes with ADH, resulting in increased water excretion) Dehydration	
Gastrointestinal	Anorexia Nausea/vomiting Constipation Abdominal pain Pancreatitis (e.g., stones in pancreatic duct)	Increased bowel sounds Abdominal cramping/spasms
Hematologic		Increased bleeding tendency (e.g., bruising, petechiae)

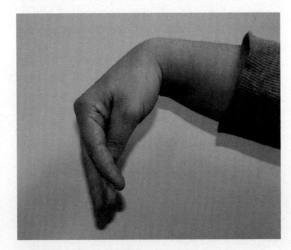

FIGURE 6-8 Trousseau sign.
© Jones & Bartlett Learning. Photographed by Carolyn Arcabascio.

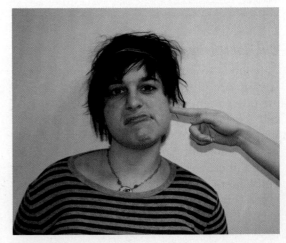

FIGURE 6-9 Chvostek sign.
© Jones & Bartlett Learning. Photographed by Carolyn Arcabascio.

Phosphorus

Most of the body's phosphorus, or phosphate, is found in the bones, with smaller quantities in the cells (organic phosphate) and in even smaller amounts circulating in the intravascular space (inorganic phosphate). Serum levels are slightly higher in children due to the higher levels of growth hormone. As previously mentioned, phosphorus has an inverse relationship with calcium. Phosphorus plays a key role in bone and tooth mineralization, cellular metabolism, acid–base balance, and cell membrane formation, among other functions.

Phosphorus primarily enters the body through dietary sources, and its elimination mainly occurs in the urine. Foods with high phosphorus concentrations include dairy products, protein sources (e.g., chicken, beef, fish, and nuts), grains, and carbonated sodas. The RDA of phosphorus is approximately 1,000 mg/day. Absorption of phosphorus is decreased when it is ingested with foods containing calcium, magnesium, and aluminum—all of which bind with phosphorus. Phosphate levels are regulated by the kidneys. When serum levels are high, more is excreted, and when levels are low, more is reabsorbed by the kidneys. Parathyroid hormone influences renal reabsorption.

Hyperphosphatemia in adults occurs when phosphorus levels are above 4.5 mg/dL. It usually results from decreased excretion, increased intake, or redistribution from ICF to ECF phosphorus (**TABLE 6-7**). **Hypophosphatemia** occurs when phosphorus levels drop below 2.5 mg/dL. This imbalance is usually caused by increased excretion or decreased intake, decreased absorption, or redistribution of phosphorus. More than one mechanism can be causing phosphorus imbalances, such as increased excretion with intracellular shifting (hypophosphatemia).

Clinical Manifestations

Clinical manifestations of hyperphosphatemia are similar to those observed with hypocalcemia and are rarely seen alone. Clinical manifestations for hypophosphatemia are similar to those associated with hypercalcemia (Table 6-6).

Diagnosis and Treatment

Diagnostic procedures for phosphate imbalances consist of a history, physical examination, and blood chemistry. Management includes identification and treatment of the underlying cause (e.g., dialysis for renal failure). Aluminum hydroxide and aluminum carbonate can bind to phosphorus and increase intestinal excretion and, therefore, is used as a treatment for hyperphosphatemia. Additionally, treatment of hypocalcemia may be necessary.

Hypophosphatemia can be treated with the administration of oral supplements (in mild deficiencies) and IV potassium phosphate (in moderate to severe deficiencies). However, supplementation with phosphate in certain

TABLE 6-7	Hyperphosphatemia and Hypophosphatemia Cause and Mechanism

Hyperphosphatemia causes and mechanisms	Hypophosphatemia causes and mechanisms
Decreased excretion—renal • Renal failure • Hypoparathyroidism (decreases renal excretion) • Adrenal insufficiency • Hypothyroidism	**Increased excretion** • Renal failure/renal tubular defects • Hyperparathyroidism (increases renal excretion)
Increased intake/absorption and ICF to ECF shifts • Laxatives, especially those containing phosphorus (decrease calcium levels, which increases phosphorus levels) • Cellular damage (e.g., burn, trauma, rhabdomyolysis, and chemotherapy) • Seizures • Potassium deficiency • Hypocalcemia • Acidosis (increased phosphorus shifts from the intracellular compartment to the intravascular compartment)	**Decreased intake/absorption and ECF to ICF shifts** • Malabsorption • Vitamin D deficiency • Magnesium, aluminum, and calcium antacids • Alcoholism • Decreased dietary intake (rare) • Alkalosis (increased amounts of phosphorus shift from the intravascular compartment to the intracellular compartment as well as increased renal excretion)

disorders causing hypophosphatemia (e.g., hyperparathyroidism) can increase the risk for development of extracellular calcifications.

Magnesium

Magnesium is an intracellular cation (second most abundant) that is mostly stored in the bone and muscle (approximately 50% in bone and muscle and 50% in cells). Only small amounts (e.g., 1%) of magnesium are in the intravascular space, and it is protein bound. This electrolyte helps maintain normal muscle and nerve function, regular cardiac rhythm, a healthy immune system, bone strength, blood glucose levels, and normal blood pressure; it is also involved in energy metabolism (i.e., ATP from ADP) and protein synthesis (i.e., DNA and RNA processes). Magnesium has a direct relationship with calcium and an inverse relationship with phosphorus. Parathyroid hormone requires magnesium, and calcium levels will not be balanced without it. Magnesium also blocks potassium movement out of cells, and potassium can leave the cell if magnesium is low, decreasing intracellular potassium.

Magnesium is obtained through dietary intake, absorbed in the intestines, and excreted through the kidneys. Foods with a high magnesium content include green vegetables, legumes, nuts, seeds, and whole grains. The RDA for magnesium is approximately 400 mg per day. Magnesium balance is regulated by the kidneys excreting more or less magnesium in response to serum magnesium levels. Various hormones (e.g., parathyroid hormone and calcitonin) may also alter magnesium balances, and their roles in homeostasis are unclear.

Hypermagnesemia occurs when magnesium levels increase above 2.4 mEq/L. This imbalance is rare. It usually results from renal failure, as the kidneys are the only regulators of magnesium levels, or from excessive intake as with parenteral administration for eclampsia or excessive ingestion of magnesium-containing preparations (e.g., enemas, laxatives, Epsom salts). Because of magnesium's synergistic relationship with calcium, hypercalcemia is often seen with hypermagnesemia, and hypophosphatemia may be present due to calcium's inverse relationship with phosphorous.

Hypomagnesemia results when magnesium levels drop below 1.8 mEq/L. Hypomagnesemia is more common than hypermagnesemia because the levels can fall quickly as bone magnesium does not rapidly exchange in the circulation. Mobilization from the bone can take many weeks. Low levels can result from inadequate intake (e.g., chronic alcoholism, malnutrition) or decreased absorption. More commonly, the cause is increased loss from the gastrointestinal or renal systems (e.g., diuretics, diarrhea, renal tubular disorders). Because of magnesium's synergistic relationship with calcium, hypocalcemia is often seen with hypomagnesemia, and hyperphosphatemia may be present due to calcium's inverse relationship with phosphorous. Additionally, low levels of magnesium may increase potassium renal excretion, so hypokalemia may be present.

Clinical Manifestations

Clinical manifestations of magnesium imbalances are due to the neuromuscular and cardiovascular system effects. Hypermagnesemia causes decreased neuromuscular function with resulting decreased deep tendon reflexes, confusion, and lethargy. The cardiovascular effects of hypermagnesemia are due to magnesium-blocking calcium channels, causing a shortened QT interval. Hypermagnesemia manifestations are often masked by the manifestations of hypercalcemia. Because hypomagnesemia is usually accompanied by hypocalcemia and hypokalemia, clinical manifestations are similar to those imbalances such as neuromuscular excitability with tremor, tetany, and QRS widening.

Diagnosis and Treatment

Diagnostic procedures include a history, physical examination, and blood chemistry. Treatment strategies for hypermagnesemia consist of diuretics and IVF administration to promote renal excretion and dialysis if magnesium levels do not decrease. Additionally, administering IV calcium can be used to directly antagonize the neuromuscular and cardiac effects of magnesium. Treatment strategies for hypomagnesemia include magnesium oral supplements for mild deficits and IV magnesium for more severe cases.

Acid–Base Balance

Acid–base stability is crucial to sustain life and maintain health. Acid–base balance is achieved through a variety of buffer systems and compensatory mechanisms. Body fluids, the kidneys, and the lungs all play pivotal roles in maintaining this balance. Acid–base balance is measured by examining pH, which is the concentration of hydrogen (H^+) ions and has a narrow safety margin (serum pH of 7.35–7.45). Acid–base imbalances can vary in severity based on the degree of pH change. Death can occur if serum pH levels fall below 6.8 or rise above 7.8. Changes in pH may be caused by a variety of conditions, including infection, organ failure, or trauma. In many cases, the acid–base fluctuations can cause more negative effects than the causative condition; therefore, the resulting acid–base imbalance is often corrected before treating the underlying condition.

pH Regulation

One way to measure serum hydrogen is by pH, which reflects acid–base status. The pH measure is a negative logarithm that reflects the hydrogen (H^+) concentration; the higher the H^+ concentration, the lower the pH number (**FIGURE 6-10**). Hydrogen is necessary for maintaining the cellular membranes and for enzyme activities. Acids are produced as a by-product of protein, carbohydrate, and fat metabolism. Three key types of acids in the body

are critical to be balanced: 1) CO_2 and carbonic acid, 2) organic acids, and 3) nonvolatile acids. The acidic by-products are found in body fluids as volatile acids, such as carbonic acid (H_2CO_3), and nonvolatile acids, such as hydrochloric, sulfuric, lactic, and phosphoric acids. Carbonic acid breaks down into H^+ and bicarbonate HCO_3^- (base). Additionally, an acidic volatile gas is produced as a by-product of cellular respiration, such as carbon dioxide (CO_2). Carbon dioxide combines with water to become carbonic acid (**FIGURE 6-11**). There are two acids, carbonic acid and carbon dioxide, in the extracellular space that must remain in balance. The balance is maintained because carbon dioxide is expelled through breathing, regulating carbonic acid level. The nonvolatile acids, such as sulfuric acids (by-products of amino acids containing sulfur), are managed by the kidneys by excreting it in urine or the kidneys adding more bicarbonate to the extracellular supply. Several organic nonvolatile acids, such as lactic acid and citric acid, are the result of normal metabolic reactions and are neutralized into other substances such as glucose and water. Balance of the body's acids is maintained by three systems that work together—the buffers, respiratory system, and renal system.

Buffers

Buffers are the chemicals that combine with an acid or a base to change pH. Buffering is an immediate reaction to counteract pH variations until compensation is initiated. Acids and bases are paired together just like cations and anions are paired together. During buffering processes, acid and bases are exchanging with other acids and bases (e.g., weak acid/conjugate base

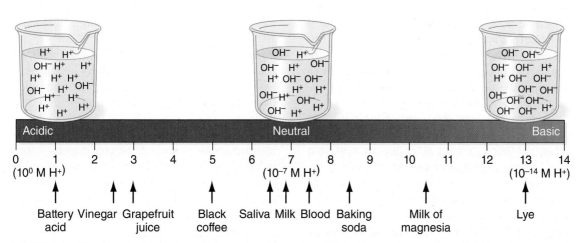

FIGURE 6-10 The pH scale. Acids release hydrogen ions (lower pH), while bases accept or combine with hydrogen ions (higher pH).

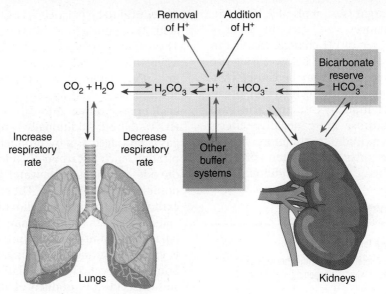

FIGURE 6-11 Acid–base balance.

for a strong acid/conjugate base). The body has several chemical buffer mechanisms—the bicarbonate–carbonic acid system, the protein system, the phosphate system, and hydrogen-potassium exchange.

The bicarbonate–carbonic acid system is the most significant buffering mechanism in the extracellular fluid. Carbonic acid and bicarbonate (base) are the key players in this system. Carbon dioxide (acid) is a by-product of cellular metabolism. Once produced, it diffuses into the interstitial fluid and blood, where it reacts with water to form carbonic acid. The carbonic acid decomposes immediately, because of the presence of the enzyme carbonic anhydrase, to form hydrogen ions and bicarbonate (Figure 6-11). Carbonic anhydrase is present at many sites in the body, including the lungs and kidneys. In the lungs, this reaction is reversed so that carbon dioxide can be expired along with water—a process that decreases the amount of carbonic acid. In the kidneys, the reaction forms hydrogen ions that are then excreted in the urine and bicarbonate that is returned to the blood.

Several proteins, both intracellular and extracellular, form part of a large buffering mechanism. Proteins can act as either an acid or a base by binding to or releasing hydrogen, respectively. Proteins exist in the intracellular and extracellular fluids but are most abundant inside the cells. Albumin and other plasma proteins are the primary buffers in the intravascular space. Hydrogen and carbon dioxide diffuse across the cell membrane to bind with proteins inside the cells. The protein hemoglobin, found in the erythrocytes, works as a buffer by binding to or releasing hydrogen and carbon dioxide. When combined with oxygen, hemoglobin tends to release hydrogen. Exposing hemoglobin to acid and lower oxygen concentrations in the capillaries causes it to release the oxygen that is bound to it. Hemoglobin then becomes a weaker acid, taking up extra hydrogen. This change maintains the pH in the capillaries. The opposite change occurs when hemoglobin is exposed to the higher oxygen concentrations found in the lungs. As hemoglobin binds with oxygen, it becomes more acidic (more prone to release hydrogen). Hydrogen reacts with bicarbonate to form carbonic acid, which is then converted to carbon dioxide and released into the alveoli.

The phosphate system acts much like the bicarbonate–carbonic acid system. Phosphates are found in high concentrations in the intracellular fluid. Some of these phosphates act as weak acids, whereas others act as weak bases. Buffering in this system primarily takes place in the kidneys by accepting or donating hydrogen.

In addition to these systems, two positively charged ions—potassium and hydrogen—move in opposite directions in and out of the cell to maintain the pH balance. With extracellular excess of hydrogen, hydrogen moves inside the cell for buffering purposes; in exchange, potassium moves out of the cell. With extracellular deficit of hydrogen, these ions move in the opposite directions. As previously mentioned, potassium imbalances can lead to acid–base imbalances, and acid–base imbalances can lead to potassium imbalances.

Respiratory Regulation

The respiratory system manages pH deviations by changing carbon dioxide (acid) excretion. Increasing ventilation will lead to excretion of more carbon dioxide, thereby decreasing acidity (increasing pH). Decreasing ventilation will lead to excretion of less carbon dioxide, thereby increasing acidity (decreasing pH). Chemoreceptors that sense pH and PCO_2 fluctuations trigger this change in breathing pattern. The only way the lungs can remove acids is through the elimination of carbon dioxide from carbonic acid—the lungs cannot remove other acids. The respiratory system is also a mechanism that can respond quickly to pH imbalances, although it cannot bring it back a normal baseline. The quick action of the respiratory system is generally short lived. The respiratory system reaches its maximum response in 12–24 hours but can maintain the changes in breathing pattern for only a limited time before becoming fatigued.

Renal Regulation

The renal system is the slowest mechanism to react to pH changes, taking hours to days to achieve its buffering effect, but it is the longest lasting. The kidneys respond to alterations in pH by changing the excretion or retention of hydrogen (acid) or bicarbonate (base). The renal system acts to balance pH levels by permanently removing hydrogen from the body. The kidneys are the only organs that can remove hydrogen ions. When carbonic acid is catalyzed into hydrogen and bicarbonate, the hydrogen combines with urinary buffers to be excreted. These buffers are necessary for the kidneys to eliminate hydrogen. Two important urinary buffers are phosphate and ammonia. These buffers attach to the hydrogen ions, which are then excreted in the urine. The kidneys maintain pH balance by reabsorbing bicarbonate. The kidneys correct pH imbalances by regenerating bicarbonate from the reabsorbed carbon dioxide. The kidneys also excrete nonvolatile acids like sulfate, phosphate, and chloride that are buffered (e.g., body proteins or bicarbonate).

Compensation

To maintain homeostasis, the body will take actions to compensate for the pH changes. The body never overcompensates; rather, the pH is adjusted so that it remains just within the normal range. The pH is a ratio of bicarbonate and carbon dioxide. There is an attempt to maintain the ratio with imbalances, and the cause of the imbalance often determines the compensatory change FIGURE 6-12. For instance, the renal system will kick in to compensate if the pH is becoming more acidic because of lung disease that limits gas exchange, such as emphysema, by releasing more bicarbonate and excreting more hydrogen. The kidneys will compensate if a lung disease is increasing carbon dioxide excretion (e.g., it is causing hyperventilation), which will increase pH, by decreasing bicarbonate production and decreasing hydrogen excretion. In contrast, the lungs can compensate for problems that originate outside the lungs. For example, the lungs will decrease the rate and depth of respirations to retain more carbon dioxide (acid) when a condition increases the loss of acids such as by vomiting. The lungs will increase the rate and depth of respirations to excrete more carbon dioxide (acid) if a condition increases the loss of bases, perhaps from diarrhea, and, in turn. If the kidneys and lungs cannot compensate to restore the pH levels to normal range, cellular activities are affected, leading to disease states. The degree of compensation is determined by the severity of the imbalance. The expected compensatory responses have been derived from experimental studies. The expected responses are most accurate when a baseline of the patient's acid–base balance is known prior to the imbalance occurring (TABLE 6-8). If compensatory mechanisms are not appropriate (e.g., more or less of a response) the compensating system may be affected. As an example, if a patient is in metabolic acidosis, lack of a respiratory response may indicate disorder in the respiratory system. Compensation mechanisms for respiratory alkalosis or mild to moderate respiratory acidosis may be sufficient to return the pH to normal. However, compensatory mechanisms are generally inadequate to return the pH to normal for metabolic acidosis or alkalosis or severe respiratory acidosis. As previously discussed, pulmonary system compensation for metabolic derangements is not as effective as kidney compensation.

Metabolic Acidosis

Metabolic acidosis results from a deficiency of bicarbonate (base) or an excess of hydrogen

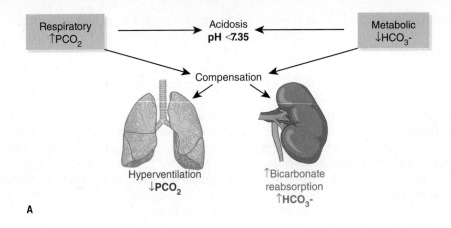

A

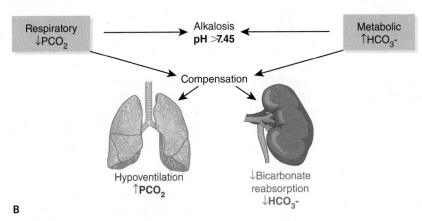

B

FIGURE 6-12 A. Acidosis and compensatory mechanisms. **B.** Alkalosis and compensatory mechanisms.

TABLE 6-8	Compensatory Responses in Acid–Base Imbalances

Acid–base imbalance	Duration of imbalance	Compensatory response	Initiation and duration of response
Metabolic acidosis	Acute or chronic	Respiratory PaCO$_2$ ↓ 1.2 mmHg per 1 mEq/L ↓ HCO$_3^-$ Lowest drop of PaCO$_2$ 8–12 mmHg	Within 30 minutes, with completion within 12–24 hours; duration may be limited by respiratory fatigue
Metabolic alkalosis	Acute or chronic	Respiratory PaCO$_2$ ↓ 0.7 mmHg per 1 mEq/L ↓ HCO$_3^-$ Highest increase of PaCO$_2$ 55 mmHg	Within 30 minutes, with completion within 12–24 hours
Respiratory acidosis	Acute Chronic	Kidneys HCO$_3^-$ ↓ 1 mEq/L per 10 mmHg ↓ PaCO$_2$ HCO$_3^-$ ↓ 3.5–5 mEq/L per 10 mmHg ↓ PaCO$_2$	Up to 5 days for completion
Respiratory alkalosis	Acute Chronic	Kidneys HCO$_3^-$ ↓ 2 mEq/L per 10 mmHg ↓ PaCO$_2$ HCO$_3^-$ ↓ 4-5 mEq/L per 10 mmHg ↓ PaCO$_2$	Up to 5 days for completion

↓ = decreases; ↑ = increases.

TABLE 6-9	Acid–Base Imbalances	
	Acidosis	**Alkalosis**
Respiratory System		
Causes	Slow, shallow respirations Respiratory congestion	Hyperventilation
Effect	Increased $PaCO_2$	Decreased $PaCO_2$
Compensatory mechanism	Kidneys excrete more hydrogen and reabsorb more bicarbonate	Kidneys excrete less hydrogen and reabsorb less bicarbonate
Diagnostic findings	High $PaCO_2$ High bicarbonate Compensated: pH = 7.35–7.4 Decompensated: pH < 7.33	Low $PaCO_2$ Low bicarbonate Compensated: pH = 7.4–7.45 Decompensated: pH > 7.47
Metabolic System		
Causes	Diarrhea Renal failure Diabetic ketoacidosis Tissue hypoxia	Vomiting Excessive antacid use
Effect	Decreased bicarbonate	Increased bicarbonate
Compensatory mechanism	Rapid, deep respirations (Kussmal) Kidneys excrete more hydrogen and increase bicarbonate absorption (when not involved)	Slow, shallow respirations Kidneys excrete less hydrogen and decrease bicarbonate absorption (when not involved)
Diagnostic findings	Low bicarbonate Low $PaCO_2$ Compensated: pH = 7.35 – 7.4 Decompensated: pH < 7.33	High bicarbonate High $PaCO_2$ Compensated: pH = 7.4–7.45 Decompensated: pH > 7.47

$PaCO_2$ = partial pressure of carbon dioxide; PO_2 = partial pressure of oxygen.
Modified from Story, L. (2017). *Pathophysiology: A practical approach* (3rd ed.). Burlington, MA: Jones & Bartlett Learning.

(acid) due to increased production or decreased excretion (**TABLE 6-9**). These conditions drop the pH below 7.35. Causes of metabolic acidosis include the following:

- Bicarbonate deficit, including that caused by the following:
  - Intestinal losses (e.g., diarrhea and fistulas)
  - Renal losses (e.g., those caused by early renal failure, renal tubular acidosis)
- Acid excess (i.e., increased production or decreased renal excretion), including that caused by the following:
  - Tissue hypoxia resulting in lactic acid accumulation (e.g., shock and cardiac arrest)
  - Ketoacidosis (caused by uncontrolled diabetes, excessive alcohol consumption, starvation, and extreme dieting)

- Drugs and toxins (e.g., antifreeze, aspirin, and hyperalimentation)
- Renal retention—uremia (e.g., renal failure)

Clinical Manifestations

Metabolic acidosis occurs when the bicarbonate and pH levels are lower than normal (**TABLE 6-10**). Metabolic acidosis results from an existing problem; therefore, the characteristics of that condition are manifested along with the acidosis. Clinical manifestations of metabolic acidosis are often neurologic in nature, but the gastrointestinal, cardiac, and respiratory systems can also be affected. These manifestations include the following signs and symptoms: headache, malaise, weakness, fatigue that progresses to lethargy, confusion, and coma. The severity of the manifestations

TABLE 6-10	Normal Serum Arterial Blood Gas Values*
Blood gas	**Normal range**
pH	7.35–7.45
PaO_2	95–100 mmHg
$PaCO_2$	35–45 mmHg
Bicarbonate (HCO_3^-)	22–26 mEq/L
Base excess	−2.4 to +2.5 mEq/L
Arterial O_2 saturation	96–98%

*Values may vary slightly. PaO_2 = partial pressure of oxygen; $PaCO_2$ = partial pressure of carbon dioxide.
Modified from Story, L. (2017). *Pathophysiology: A practical approach* (3rd ed.). Burlington, MA: Jones & Bartlett Learning.

reflects the severity of the acidosis. Gastrointestinal symptoms include nausea, vomiting, and anorexia. Cardiovascular symptoms include hypotension, dysrhythmias, and shock. Kussmaul respirations are deep, rapid respirations that develop in an attempt to eliminate excess acid by exhaling more carbon dioxide.

Diagnostic Link

Blood Gases: Arterial and Venous

Arterial blood gases sampling can be difficult and painful to obtain unless the patient has an arterial line. Venous blood gases are an alternative way of evaluating carbon dioxide and pH. Venous samples can be obtained peripherally or via a central venous catheter. Blood gases from a central venous catheter are the most understood and correlated with arterial blood gases, so they are preferred over peripheral venous sampling. The venous sample measures all the same components as arterial sampling (e.g., oxygen, carbon dioxide). The values are labeled with a subscript *v* for venous (e.g., P_vCO_2). The oxygen value is not useful as most of the oxygen has been extracted. The venous sampling does provide one additional measure, which is the oxyhemoglobin saturation (S_vO_2). The S_vO_2 is a reflection of the amount of oxygen actually used by the tissue. Arterial and venous blood gas values are slightly different; therefore, for interpretation correlation and reference ranges need to be used.

Learning Points

Acid-Base Compensation

Compensation can be a challenge to understand. First, make sure you understand acids and bases. Carbon dioxide and hydrogen are acids; bicarbonate is a base. The body will increase or decrease the excretion of these substances in an attempt to restore pH balance. If the body excretes more acid or produces more base, then the pH will become more alkaline. If the body retains more acid or produces less base, then the pH will become more acidic.

Two body systems can compensate for pH imbalances—the renal and respiratory systems. If the cause of the imbalance originates within one of those systems, then the other system will have to perform the role of the primary compensatory mechanism. The system that is the source of the pH imbalance will not be able to resolve its own problem. Thus, the kidneys will manage problems that originate in the lungs. If the problem originates outside the lungs, the lungs will manage it.

Reproduced from Story, L. (2017). *Pathophysiology: A practical approach* (3rd ed.). Burlington, MA: Jones & Bartlett Learning.

Diagnosis and Treatment

Diagnostic procedures for metabolic acidosis include a history, physical examination, ABGs, blood chemistry, and CBC. As previously mentioned, the pH will be low and bicarbonate from the blood gas or serum will be low with metabolic acidosis. Evaluation of the anion gap is often used to determine the cause of the metabolic acidosis (**FIGURE 6-13**). The anion gap is used to identify the anions that are not usually measured, such as albumin, sulfates, and phosphates. Conditions that cause metabolic acidosis because of excess acid, whether from increased production or decreased excretion, will increase the anion gap; otherwise, the anion gap will remain normal. These disorders of acid are termed *high anion gap metabolic acidoses*. With metabolic acidosis caused by loss of bicarbonate, anion gap will remain normal and this is also termed *nonanion gap metabolic acidosis*. Chloride is retained when bicarbonate is lost as a way of maintaining balance, so normal anion gap acidosis is also called *hyperchloremic metabolic acidosis*. Under normal conditions, the sum of cations is approximately equal to the sum of anions in the extracellular fluid. Sodium is the most plentiful cation in the extracellular fluid, while bicarbonate and chloride are the most abundant anions. To determine the anion gap, the bicarbonate and chloride results are added together and subtracted from the sodium (sodium−[bicarbonate + chloride]). A normal anion gap is 3–10 mEq/L. Each laboratory may have a different range for an anion gap, and clinically, it is best to follow trends rather than ranges. As an example, if an anion gap is 3 mEq/L at first, and subsequent measurement is 10 mEq/L, this is considered significant even though the anion gap is within the normal range. Different anion gap formulas that include potassium with sodium are available. Albumin is a key anion that affects the gap, and

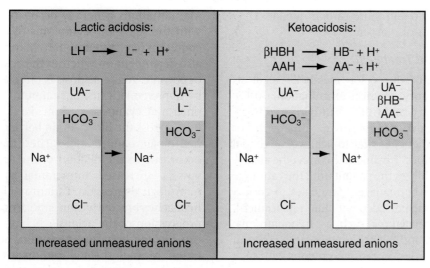

FIGURE 6-13 Anion gap with metabolic acidosis.

UA^- = unmeasured anion
$HCO3$ = Bicarbonate
Cl^- = Chloride
Na^+ = sodium
H^+ = hydrogen

a corrected measure must be calculated if the albumin is low. Electrolyte imbalances such as hyperkalemia, hypercalcemia, and hypermagnesemia will reduce an anion gap by approximately 2 mEq/L.

Identifying and treating the causative condition (e.g., antidiarrheal agents or dialysis) is vital to achieve successful patient outcomes. Treatment to correct the acidosis merely stabilizes the patient until the causative condition can be managed. Strategies to correct the acidosis may include the administration of IV sodium bicarbonate, particularly when the pH is below 7.1. Indications for sodium bicarbonate administration are controversial. Other strategies include correcting electrolyte disturbances such as hyperkalemia (e.g., administering IV insulin for diabetic ketoacidosis) and improving oxygenation (e.g., oxygen therapy, mechanical ventilation).

Metabolic Alkalosis

Metabolic alkalosis results from excess bicarbonate because of increased intake or retention, deficient acid, or both (Table 6-9). These conditions cause the pH to rise above 7.45. The most common causes are due to the loss of acids, usually from the gastrointestinal tract. Causes of metabolic alkalosis include the following:

- Excess bicarbonate, such as that caused by the following:
  - Excessive antacid use
  - Use of bicarbonate-containing fluids (e.g., lactated Ringer's solution)

- Hypochloremia (increases bicarbonate reabsorption)
- Deficient acid, such as that caused by the following:
  - Gastrointestinal loss (e.g., vomiting or nasogastric suction)
  - Hypokalemia (low potassium levels cause hydrogen to shift inside the cells)
  - Renal loss (e.g., renal failure or diuretics)
  - Hypovolemia (decreases renal perfusion)
  - Hyperaldosteronism (excessive aldosterone increases renal excretion of hydrogen)

Clinical Manifestations

Metabolic alkalosis exists when the bicarbonate and the pH levels rise to greater than normal (Table 6-10). Much like metabolic acidosis, metabolic alkalosis manifestations generally occur in combination with the manifestations of the causative conditions (e.g., hypovolemia, hypokalemia). Patients can also be asymptomatic. Clinical manifestations of metabolic alkalosis are mostly neuromuscular in nature. Alkalosis causes calcium to bind, so manifestations are similar to hypocalcemia (e.g., paresthesias, tetany, seizures, mental confusion, and increased deep tendon reflexes). Bicarbonate alterations causes fewer alterations in pH in the intracellular compartment and blood–brain barrier, so symptoms do not occur as quickly as with other acid–base imbalances (e.g., such as in respiratory alkalosis where CO_2 shifts are transmitted immediately). With metabolic alkalosis, respirations will decrease in an attempt to retain more carbon dioxide. Dysrhythmias may also occur.

Diagnosis and Treatment

Diagnostic procedures for metabolic alkalosis include a history, physical examination, ABGs, blood chemistry, and CBC. Identifying and treating the causative condition (e.g., antiemetics or fluid replacement) is vital to achieve successful patient outcomes. Treatment to correct the alkalosis merely stabilizes the patient until the causative condition can be managed. Strategies to correct the alkalosis include adequate fluid replacement. Electrolyte imbalances such as hyponatremia, hypokalemia, and hypochloremia can be present as they are also lost in gastric secretions with such as occurs with vomiting and suctioning. Chloride can be replaced by administering arginine hydrochloride or a weak hydrochloric acid solution. Potassium chloride will correct two deficits.

Respiratory Acidosis

Respiratory acidosis results from carbon dioxide retention, which increases the amount of carbonic acid present and, in turn, decreases the pH level (Table 6-9). This increase in carbon dioxide usually follows a state of hypoventilation or decreased gas exchange in the lungs. Many conditions can cause hypoventilation and/or impair gas exchange, including:

- Respiratory center depression (e.g., brain trauma, oversedation, drug overdose)
- Thoracic cage/muscle disorders (e.g., flail chest, respiratory muscle paralysis)
- Lung parenchyma disorders (e.g., chronic obstructive pulmonary disease, pneumonia, pulmonary edema)

Respiratory acidosis can occur acutely, such as in narcotic overdose, or it can be chronic, such as occurs in patients with chronic obstructive lung disease. The medullary center usually responds to carbon dioxide levels to control breathing. In patients with chronic obstructive lung disease, the chronic high carbon dioxide level causes the medullary center to adapt. The stimulus to breathe becomes low oxygen levels as opposed to the high carbon dioxide levels. The chronically high carbon dioxide also causes bicarbonate reabsorption to maintain the pH balance.

Clinical Manifestations

Respiratory acidosis exists when the carbon dioxide levels rise (i.e., hypercapnia occurs) and the pH levels fall below normal (Table 6-10).

Manifestations generally occur in combination with the signs and symptoms of the causative condition (e.g., pneumonia). Manifestations are also dependent on whether the acidosis is acute or chronic. Acute acidosis is often accompanied by hypoxemia, causing symptoms such as dyspnea and cyanosis. Carbon dioxide easily diffuses across the blood–brain barrier, causing the neurologic manifestations. These manifestations occur due to the dilation of the cerebral blood vessels, increased intracranial pressure, and neurologic depression. Patients will complain of headache, blurred vision, and irritability. With progression of the acidosis, behavioral changes can include lethargy, confusion, and disorientation. Musculoskeletal tremors, twitching, and paralysis may occur. Cerebrospinal pressure and coma can ensue in severe cases. Cardiovascular depression can occur with arrhythmias, hypotension, or fluctuations in blood pressure. The elevated carbon dioxide levels may cause warm and flushed skin with diaphoresis unless hypoxemia is present.

Diagnosis and Treatment

Diagnostic procedures for respiratory acidosis include a history, physical examination, ABGs, blood chemistry, CBC, and chest X-ray. Treatment centers on improving respiratory status by relieving hypoxia and hypercapnia. Strategies may include oxygen therapy, optimizing ventilation with positioning, and bronchial hygiene measures (e.g., coughing, deep breathing, and chest physiotherapy). Mechanical ventilation may be necessary. Other strategies center on treatment of causative conditions such as antibiotics for pneumonia. Some patients with chronic obstructive lung disease may develop worsening hypercapnia with the administration of oxygen, so the patient should be monitored for respiratory depression.

Respiratory Alkalosis

Respiratory alkalosis results from excess exhalation of carbon dioxide, which leads to carbonic acid deficits and increased pH (Table 6-9). Respiratory alkalosis generally occurs because of conditions that cause hyperventilation and/or stimulation of the medullary respiratory center, including:

- Acute anxiety
- Pain
- Fever (which causes excessive oxygen utilization, increasing respirations)
- Hypoxia (e.g., oxygen deprivation and high altitudes)

- Gram-negative septicemia (which triggers the respiratory centers in the brain to increase respirations)
- Aspirin overdose (also triggers the medulla to increase respirations)
- Excessive mechanical ventilation
- Hypermetabolic states such as hyperthyroidism (which causes excessive oxygen utilization, increasing respirations)

Clinical Manifestations

Respiratory alkalosis exists when the carbon dioxide levels fall and the pH levels rise above normal (Table 6-10). Clinical manifestations reflect central nervous system irritability and decreased cerebral blood flow. Manifestations of hypocalcemia may be present secondary to calcium binding to protein as a result of alkalosis. Clinical manifestations of respiratory alkalosis include paresthesia, dizziness, syncope, and neuronal hyperexcitability causing twitching, tetany, and seizures. The patient may complain of dyspnea, dry mouth, and feelings of panic and anxiety.

Diagnosis and Treatment

Diagnostic procedures for respiratory alkalosis include a history, physical examination, ABGs, blood chemistry, CBC, and chest X-ray. Treatment of the underlying cause and increasing carbon dioxide levels is crucial to improve patient outcomes. Often the solution is as simple as breathing into a paper bag—an intervention that allows carbon dioxide to be recirculated back to the lungs. Strategies that are more aggressive may be needed if the patient is unable to follow directions or is unconscious. They may include controlled mechanical ventilation and anxiety-reduction interventions (e.g., sedatives and therapeutic communication).

Mixed Disorders

Mixed disorders occur when respiratory and metabolic disorders result in an acidotic or alkalotic state. Such an outcome occurs when both the respiratory and renal systems demonstrate an imbalance of acid or base. The severity of the pH imbalance depends on the degree of acid and base disturbances. Suspicion of a mixed acid–base disorder can be evaluated by the history and determination of whether the compensatory response of the kidneys and respiratory system are not as expected (e.g., too high or too low). Many conditions can create this synergistic effect (FIGURE 6-14). Such mixed disorders are common in patients with comorbid conditions (e.g., renal and respiratory

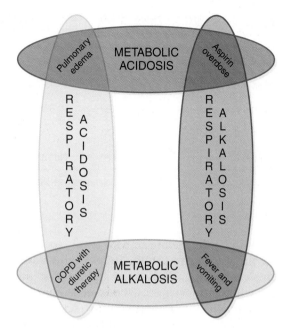

FIGURE 6-14 Mixed acid–base disorders.

disease) and in those who are critically ill. Mixed disorders can be complex to manage.

Arterial Blood Gas Interpretation

Arterial blood gases (ABGs) have traditionally been, and remain today, the principal diagnostic tool for evaluating acid–base balance (Table 6-9). ABG interpretation can be confusing particularly in determining whether the values are due to compensation or a mixed disorder. Additionally, it is important to keep in mind that an ABG is a single point in time, and serial measurements must often be undertaken to determine what is occurring. Through simple steps, the ABG riddle can be solved and interpreted in context of the clinical evaluation so the patient can receive appropriate care. First, the following descriptions of the results found on an ABG, some of which have already been discussed, should be reviewed again:

- The pH measures the hydrogen concentration in the plasma.
- $PaCO_2$ (the partial pressure of carbon dioxide) indicates the adequacy of pulmonary ventilation.
- HCO_3^- (bicarbonate) indicates the activity in the kidneys to retain or excrete bicarbonate.
- PaO_2 (the partial pressure of oxygen) indicates the concentration of oxygen in the arterial blood.
- Base excess/deficit indicates the concentration of buffer—in particular, bicarbonate. Positive values indicate an excess of base or a deficit of acid. Negative values indicate a deficit of base or an excess of acid.

TABLE 6-11	Arterial Blood Gas Interpretation			
Acid–base disorder	Ph	PaCO$_2$	HCO$_3$	Compensation
Respiratory acidosis	< 7.4 (A)	> 45 mmHg (A)	Normal	HCO$_3$ > 26 mEq/L (B)
Respiratory alkalosis	> 7.4 (B)	< 35 mmHg (B)	Normal	HCO$_3$ < 22 mEq/L (A)
Metabolic acidosis	< 7.4 (A)	Normal HCO$_3$	< 22 mEq/L (A)	PaCO$_2$ > 35 mmHg (B)
Metabolic alkalosis	> 7.4 (B)	Normal HCO$_3$	> 26 mEq/L (B)	PaCO$_2$ > 45 mmHg (A)

Reproduced from Story, L. (2017). Pathophysiology: A Practical Approach, 3rd Edition. Burlington, MA: Jones & Bartlett Learning.

When interpreting an ABG result, focus on the pH, PaCO$_2$, and HCO$_3^-$. Interpreting ABGs involves looking for patterns and understanding what those patterns indicate, keeping in mind the patient's total clinical picture. Recall that PaCO$_2$ is an acid and HCO$_3^-$ is a base. More acid will lower the pH, whereas less acid will raise the pH. More base will raise the pH, whereas less base will lower the pH.

Turning to the ABG results, use a systematic approach when examining them (**TABLE 6-11**). Make note of the patient's pH, PaCO$_2$, and HCO$_3^-$ on a piece of paper. Start by examining the pH. Is it high, low, or normal? The pH is half of the puzzle. The pH will identify whether the condition is acidosis or alkalosis. If it is high, write a *B* for *basic* beside it. If the pH is low, write an *A* for *acidic*. If it is normal, which side of normal is it? For results less than 7.4, write an *A*; for results greater than 7.4, write a *B*.

Next, check the PaCO$_2$. Is it high, low, or normal? In respiratory disturbances, pH and CO$_2$ move in opposite directions. If the CO$_2$ goes up, the pH goes down, and vice versa. Because CO$_2$ is an acidic influence, write an *A* if it is high and a *B* if it is low. If it is within normal range, write an *N* beside it.

Next, examine the HCO$_3$. Is it high, low, or normal? With metabolic disturbances, the pH and HCO$_3^-$ move in the same direction. Because HCO$_3^-$ is a base influence, write a *B* if it is high and an *A* if it is low. If it is within normal range, write an *N* beside it.

At this point, you should have three letters written down beside your patient's ABG results. Now you just match up the *A*s and *B*s you have written down to the disturbance. Finally, determine if the body has been able to compensate. The results with the paired *A* or *B* are the primary changes. The third unpaired result indicates the compensation. If the unpaired result is still normal, then it is uncompensated. If the unpaired result has changed to the opposite letter of the pairs and the pH is still abnormal, then it is partially compensated; if the pH has returned to normal, then it is fully compensated.

To review, these are the steps in ABGs interpretation:

1. Is the pH high, low, or normal?
   a. If pH > 7.4, write a *B* beside it for *basic*.
   b. If pH < 7.4, write an *A* beside it for *acidic*.
   c. Make note if pH is within normal limits (7.35–7.45).
2. Is the PaCO$_2$ high, low, or normal?
   a. If PaCO$_2$ is between 35 and 45 mmHg, write an *N* beside it for *normal*.
   b. If PaCO$_2$ > 45 mmHg, write an *A* beside it for *acidic*.
   c. If PaCO$_2$ < 35 mmHg, write a *B* beside it for *basic*.
3. Is the HCO$_3$ high, low, or normal?
   a. If HCO$_3$ is between 22 and 26, write an *N* beside it for *normal*.
   b. If HCO$_3$ > 26 mEq/L, write a *B* beside it for *basic*.
   c. If HCO$_3$ < 22 mEq/L, write an *A* beside it for *acidic*.
4. Look for patterns:
   a. Two *A*s indicate acidosis. If one of the *A*s is CO$_2$, then the disorder is respiratory. If one of the *A*s is HCO$_3^-$, then the disorder is metabolic. In both cases, the other *A* is the pH.
   b. Two *B*s indicate alkalosis. If one of the *B*s is CO$_2$, then the disorder is respiratory. If one of the *B*s is HCO$_3$, then the disorder is metabolic. In both cases, the other *B* is the pH.
   c. Three *A*s or *B*s indicate a mixed disorder. All *A*s indicate mixed respiratory and metabolic acidosis. All *B*s indicate mixed respiratory and metabolic alkalosis.

5. Determine compensation and whether the compensation is appropriate:
   a. If the unpaired result is within normal range, then the disturbance is uncompensated.
   b. If the unpaired result is the opposite letter of the pairs but the pH is still abnormal, then the disturbance is partially compensated.
   c. If the unpaired result is the opposite letter and the pH has returned to normal range, then the disturbance is fully compensated.
6. Determine the anion gap, particularly for metabolic acidosis.
7. Determine a cause or causes of the disorder.

Practice Arterial Blood Gas Interpretation

Practice 1

pH:	7.32	**A**
PaCO₂:	37 mmHg	**N**ormal
HCO₃⁻:	14 mEq/L	**A**

Practice 2

pH:	7.50	**B**
PaCO₂:	30 mmHg	**B**
HCO₃⁻:	24 mEq/L	**N**ormal

Practice 3

pH:	7.33	**A**
PaCO₂:	55 mmHg	**A**
HCO₃⁻:	28 mEq/L	**B**

Practice 4

pH:	7.47	**B**
PaCO₂:	48 mmHg	**A**
HCO₃⁻:	29 mEq/L	**B**

Practice 5

pH:	7.38	**A** (but within normal limits)
PaCO₂:	48 mmHg	**A**
HCO₃⁻:	29 mEq/L	**B**

Practice 6

pH:	7.44	**B** (but within normal limits)
PaCO₂:	49 mmHg	**A**
HCO₃⁻:	29 mEq/L	**B**

Practice 7

pH:	7.30	**A**
PaCO₂:	50 mmHg	**A**
HCO₃⁻:	19 mEq/L	**A**

Practice 8

pH:	7.49	**B**
PaCO₂:	32 mmHg	**B**
HCO₃⁻:	30 mEq/L	**B**

Reproduced from Story, L. (2017). *Pathophysiology: A practical approach* (3rd ed.). Burlington, MA: Jones & Bartlett Learning.

BOX 6-3 Application to Practice

A 70-year-old woman was recently treated for pneumonia with antibiotics. After 1 week on antibiotics, she started developing severe diarrhea of 6–7 loose, watery stools per day. The diarrhea has been present for 3 days. She also has a decreased appetite, feels nauseous, and has not been drinking a lot of fluids. She feels very weak and dizzy. She lives alone, so she called 911 and was brought to the emergency department. She is diagnosed with diarrhea, presumptive *Clostridium difficile*.

Patient medical history: *Clostridium difficile* 2 years prior.

Physical exam: temperature 99.0°F, pulse 100 beats/minute, respirations 24 breaths/minute, and blood pressure 90/50 mmHg, which dropped to 70/40 when seated.

Exam unremarkable except for dry mucous membranes and generalized mild abdominal tenderness with palpation.

Laboratory findings reveal:

Chemistry panel: sodium 135 mEq/L; potassium 3.4 mEq/L; chloride 100 mmol/L; HCO₃⁻ 12 mEq/L; blood urea nitrogen 40 mg/dL.

Creatinine: 1.2 mg/dL.

ABG: pH 7.22, PaO₂ 85 mmHg, PaCO₂ 20 mmHg, HCO₃⁻ 12 mEq/L.

Analyze the ABG and determine the acid–base disturbance. Calculate the compensation response and determine if it is appropriate. Calculate and interpret the anion gap. Discuss the diagnosis and reasons for the acid-base disturbance. Develop a treatment plan.

CHAPTER SUMMARY

Fluid, electrolytes, bases, and acids are constantly moving among body compartments. This movement is influenced by intake, output, cellular metabolism, and pathologic states. The body is equipped with numerous mechanisms to maintain fluid, electrolyte, and pH homeostasis among these compartments. When these mechanisms fail, conditions that threaten the individual's well-being arise. Imbalances are generally a reflection of an underlying disorder and early identification and action are crucial to improve the prognosis of the person encountering these conditions.

REFERENCES AND RESOURCES

Baumberger-Henry, M. (2008). *Fluid and electrolytes* (2nd ed.). Sudbury, MA: Jones and Bartlett Publishers.

Chiras, D. (2015). *Human biology* (8th ed.). Burlington, MA: Jones & Bartlett Learning.

Clark, R. K. (2006). *Anatomy and physiology: Understanding the human body*. Sudbury, MA: Jones and Bartlett Publishers.

Crawford, A., & Harris, H. (2011). I.V. fluids: What nurses need to know. *Nursing2015, 41*(5), 30–38. doi: 10.1097/01.NURSE.0000396282.43928.40

Elling, B., Elling, K., & Rothenberg, M. (2004). *Anatomy and physiology*. Sudbury, MA: Jones and Bartlett Publishers.

Emmett, M., & Palmer, B. F. (2019). Simple and mixed acid–base disorders. T. W. Post (Ed.). *Uptodate*. Waltham, MA: UpToDate, Inc. Retrieved from https://uptodate.com

Gould, B. (2015). *Pathophysiology for the health professions* (5th ed.). Philadelphia, PA: Elsevier.

Madara, B., & Pomarico-Denino, V. (2008). *Pathophysiology* (2nd ed.). Sudbury, MA: Jones and Bartlett Publishers.

Preston, R. A. (2018). *Acid-base, fluids, and electrolytes made ridiculously simple* (3rd ed.). Miami, FL: MedMaster, Inc.

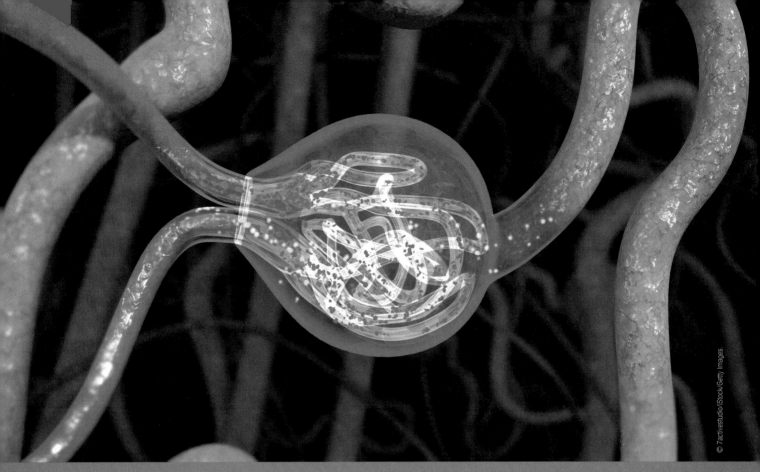

CHAPTER 7
Urinary Function

The urinary system plays a pivotal role in homeostasis. Structures of the urinary system include the kidneys, ureters, bladder, and urethra (FIGURE 7-1). This system regulates fluid volume, blood pressure, metabolic waste and drug excretion, vitamin D conversion, pH regulation, and hormone synthesis. This chapter focuses on normal and abnormal states of the urinary system. Disorders of this system can create imbalances in homeostasis quickly. Hence, these disorders require a prompt response to restore the body's delicate balance.

Anatomy and Physiology

Structure and Function

The urinary system regulates fluid volume, blood pressure, metabolic waste and drug excretion, vitamin D conversion, pH balance, and hormone synthesis. It includes the kidneys, ureters, bladder, and urethra. See chapter 6 for a discussion of fluids and pH balance.

The kidneys are bean-shaped organs about the size of a person's fists; they are positioned on either side of the vertebrae in the retroperitoneal space. Connective tissue called the *renal capsule* surrounds each kidney. The area immediately beneath the capsule is known as the *renal cortex*; it contains the functional units of the kidney, the nephrons, and blood vessels. The inner layer is called the *medulla*, which contains the renal pyramid. The renal artery supplies each kidney with blood. The renal hilum is the opening in the kidney through which the renal artery and nerves enter and the renal vein and ureter exit. The hilum opens medially into a cavity called the *renal sinus*. The central portions of the renal sinuses enlarge to form the *renal pelvis*. Urine drains in a manner similarly to a funnel into the renal pelvis through tubes called *calyces*. The calyces drain urine into the ureters, which transport the urine using peristaltic actions to the bladder for storage. Urine then

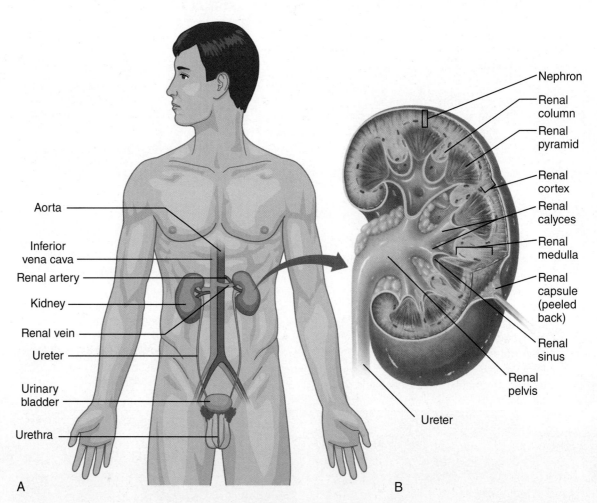

Aorta
Inferior vena cava
Renal artery
Kidney
Renal vein
Ureter
Urinary bladder
Urethra

Nephron
Renal column
Renal pyramid
Renal cortex
Renal calyces
Renal medulla
Renal capsule (peeled back)
Renal sinus
Renal pelvis
Ureter

A   B

FIGURE 7-1 The urinary system. **A** Anterior view showing the relationship of the kidneys, ureters, urinary bladder, and urethra. **B** A cross-section of the human kidney showing the cortex, medulla, and renal pelvis.

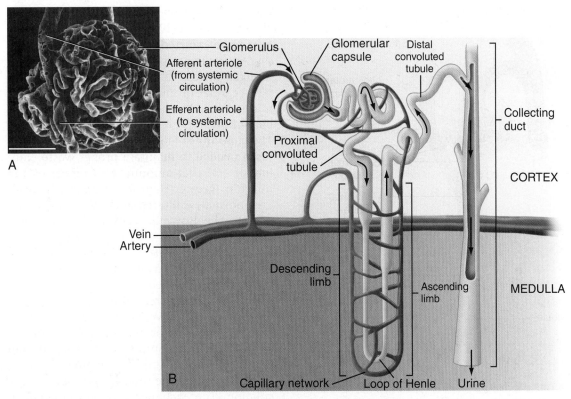

Glomerulus

Afferent arteriole (from systemic circulation)

Efferent arteriole (to systemic circulation)

Glomerular capsule

Distal convoluted tubule

Proximal convoluted tubule

Collecting duct

CORTEX

Vein
Artery

Descending limb

Ascending limb

MEDULLA

A

B

Capillary network   Loop of Henle   Urine

FIGURE 7-2 Nephrons of the kidney. Part of the nephron is located in the cortex, and part is located in the medulla. The electron micrograph to the left of the illustration is of a glomerulus from a human nephron.

Courtesy of Kenjiro Kimura, MD, PhD.

leaves the body through the urethra and urinary meatus.

The kidneys are the primary site for carrying out the urinary system's functions. One kidney contains 1 million to 2 million microscopic filtering units, or *nephrons*, to accomplish its functions (Figure 7-1 and **FIGURE 7-2**). Each nephron is similar to a funnel with a long stem (i.e., renal tubules). The tubules are connected to the circulatory and the urinary systems. The tubules contain multiple sections including the loop of Henle, proximal convoluted tubule, and distal convoluted tubule, and each of these sections is responsible for secreting substances from the blood into the filtrate or reabsorbing specific substances from the filtrate back into the blood (**TABLE 7-1**). The proximal convoluted tubule of the kidney enlarges into a double-membrane chamber called the *Bowman capsule* (i.e., glomerular capsule). The capsule contains an inner visceral layer and an outer parietal layer, and the space in between these two layers, called the *Bowman space*, is where the filtrate that will become urine is created. Most of the nephron structures are in the

TABLE 7-1	Components of the Nephron and Their Functions
Component	**Function**
Glomerulus	Mechanically filters the blood
Bowman capsule	Mechanically filters the blood
Proximal convoluted tubule	Reabsorbs 75%* of the water, sodium,** glucose, potassium, bicarbonate, phosphate, urea, and amino acids
	Secretion of hydrogen, other substances (e.g., medications)
Loop of Henle	Participates in countercurrent exchange, which maintains the concentration gradient
	Reabsorption of water and sodium
	Secretion of urea
Distal convoluted tubule	Reabsorption of sodium, water, and bicarbonate
	Secretion of hydrogen, potassium, urea, ammonia and certain drugs

* approximate; % varies by molecule. **chloride follows sodium.

Modified from Story, L. (2017). *Pathophysiology: A Practical Approach* (3rd ed.). Burlington, MA: Jones & Bartlett Learning.

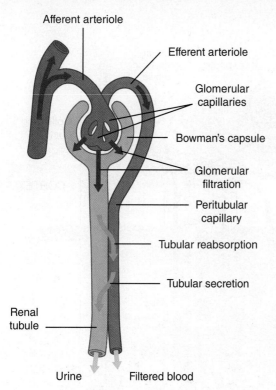

Afferent arteriole

Efferent arteriole

Glomerular capillaries

Bowman's capsule

Glomerular filtration

Peritubular capillary

Tubular reabsorption

Tubular secretion

Renal tubule

Urine   Filtered blood

FIGURE 7-3 The glomerulus of the kidneys. The nephron carries out three processes: glomerular filtration, tubular reabsorption, and tubular secretion. All three processes contribute to the filtering of the blood.

cortex with parts of the loops dipping into the medulla, and these nephrons are termed *cortical nephrons*. About 20% of the nephrons are in the cortex, but their tubules' longer lengths go through the entire medulla, and these nephrons are termed *juxtamedullary nephrons* (i.e., they are in the cortex but next to the medulla). The juxtamedullary nephrons have a key role in concentrating urine. The Bowman capsule surrounds a cluster of capillaries referred to as the *glomerulus*. Blood enters the glomerulus through an afferent arteriole and exits through an efferent arteriole (**FIGURE 7-3**). The efferent arteriole connects to peritubular capillaries that are found throughout the cortex and medulla and bring reabsorbed substances back to the blood through the renal vein.

Urine Formation and Elimination

The human body can excrete waste through the kidneys, skin, liver, and intestines, with the kidneys being the primary site for excretion. Urine formation is dependent on renal blood flow, tubular reabsorption, and secretion functions. Blood goes to the glomerulus (afferent arteriole) where a protein-free filtrate (i.e., ultrafiltrate) is created, and the filtrate goes

through the tubules where substances are reabsorbed into the blood or secreted into the filtrate to be excreted (i.e., urine).

Approximately 25% of cardiac output is directed toward kidney perfusion. For example, a cardiac output of 5 liters (5,000 mL) per minute would translate into 1,250 mL/min of blood flow to the kidneys (25% of 5,000 mL). This amount of blood supply to the glomerulus is needed to maintain proper waste elimination. Of that amount, an average of 125 mL/min (greater than 90 mL/min is considered normal) is filtered in the glomerulus and goes to the Bowman capsule. The speed at which the blood moves through the glomerulus is called the *glomerular filtration rate* (GFR). GFR is the best measure of renal functioning and can be calculated using a formula that incorporates serum creatinine levels, age, gender, and ethnicity. While an average 125 mL/min of filtrate is produced, that is not the amount of urine output. Only 1–2 mL/min ends up in urine, and the remainder is reabsorbed back into the tubules and then the circulation. The exchange mechanism between the glomerulus and the Bowman capsule is influenced by the same factors influencing capillary exchange such as oncotic pressure and capillary permeability. Approximately 90% of blood flowing through the kidney goes through the cortex, while the remaining 10% passes through the medulla. During times of decreased renal perfusion (e.g., decreased cardiac output, shock), blood is shunted to the medulla so that urine concentration is maintained.

Renal blood flow is affected by the same factors affecting blood pressure. The renin–angiotensin–aldosterone system is a key regulator of renal blood flow. The mechanisms that cause vasoconstriction and a decrease in renal blood flow include sympathetic nervous system stimulation with release of catecholamines, angiotensin II, antidiuretic hormone (ADH), and endothelins. Substances causing vasodilation include dopamine, prostaglandins, and nitric oxide. Natriuretic peptides (e.g., atrial, brain) respond to increases in blood volume (e.g., heart failure) and cause afferent arteriole dilation and efferent arteriole constriction, both which increase urine formation. Urodilatin, a natriuretic peptide, is produced in the distal tubule and collecting duct. Urodilatin also responds to volume increases by inhibiting water and sodium reabsorption and causing vasodilation and diuresis.

TABLE 7-2	Important Metabolic Wastes and Substances Excreted from the Body	
Chemical	**Source**	**Organ of excretion**
Ammonia	Deamination (removal of amine group) of amino acids in liver	Kidneys
Urea	Derived from ammonia	Kidneys and skin
Uric acid	Nucleotide breakdown in the liver	Kidneys
Bile pigments	Hemoglobin breakdown in the liver	Liver (into the small intestine)
Urochrome	Hemoglobin breakdown in the liver	Kidneys
Carbon dioxide	Breakdown of glucose in cells	Lungs
Water	Food and water; breakdown of glucose	Kidneys, skin, and lungs
Inorganic ions*	Food and water	Kidneys and sweat glands

* Ions are not a metabolic waste product like the other substances shown in this table. Nonetheless, ions are excreted to maintain constant levels in the body.
Modified from Story, L. (2017). *Pathophysiology: A Practical Approach* (3rd ed.). Burlington, MA: Jones & Bartlett Learning.

See chapter 4 for a discussion of cardiovascular function.

In addition to the neural and hormonal mechanisms, intrinsic renal mechanisms maintain renal blood flow. One of these intrinsic mechanisms is known as the juxtaglomerular complex (i.e., juxtaglomerular apparatus). The complex is a group of specialized cells located next to the blood vessels (afferent and efferent arterioles) and the distal tubule that regulate blood flow and produce renin. This complex senses systemic arterial blood pressure changes, particularly sodium levels in the distal tubule, and pressure changes in the afferent arteriole. Decreases in GFR and sodium stimulate the complex, leading to dilation of the afferent arteriole and renin release, which causes efferent arteriole vasoconstriction with a resulting increased GFR. If there is an increase in GFR and sodium, then the reverse happens with afferent arteriole constriction and efferent arteriole dilation, which results in a decreased GFR. Several renal vascular disorders can affect renal blood flow, such as renal artery stenosis and renal vein thrombosis. The renal vasculature serves as another intrinsic mechanism by directly dilating and constricting in response to solute, water, and blood volume changes. This vasoactive capacity can maintain renal blood flow independent of systemic blood pressure changes.

Cells continuously produce waste products as they carry out their internal processes (**TABLE 7-2**). The body removes these waste products to maintain homeostasis through urine formation. The tubules of the kidneys are the site of reabsorption and secretion of water, electrolytes, and nutrients (Table 7-1; **FIGURE 7-4**). The kidneys regulate the concentration of water and electrolytes by increasing or decreasing their excretion to maintain stability within the body. Mechanisms of exchange of water, electrolytes, and other substances in the tubular structure are similar to other exchange mechanisms throughout the body (e.g., active and passive transport, osmosis). The ultrafiltrate, which is protein free, enters the **proximal**

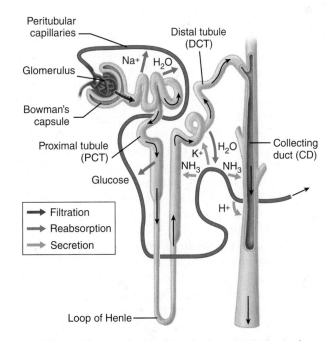

FIGURE 7-4 The steps in urine formation in successive parts of a nephron are filtration, reabsorption, and secretion.

convoluted tubule and contains plasma substances such as sodium, potassium, creatinine, urea, glucose, and amino acids. The proximal convoluted tubule reabsorbs (back into the blood) most of the filtrate components and is also a site of secretion (blood to filtrate). In addition to water, urea is a significant component of urine. Approximately 50% of **urea** is reabsorbed in the proximal convoluted tubule, and the remainder moves through the tubule and is excreted in the urine. Urea is derived from **ammonia**, which is a highly toxic chemical that results from the breakdown of amino acids in the liver. Amino acid breakdown generally occurs in the presence of an excess of protein or a deficit of carbohydrates in the diet; however, carbohydrate deficits are rare in industrialized countries except in persons on high-protein diets. When amino acids are broken down, the amino groups are stripped from the molecules in a process called *deamination*. These amino groups are converted to ammonia following deamination. Most of this ammonia is then converted to urea in the liver, which is then excreted in the urine. Liver disease can impair this process, leading to extremely high levels of ammonia. **Uric acid** is another metabolism by-product produced by the liver. Uric acid results from the breakdown of nucleotides, the building blocks of deoxyribonucleic acid (DNA). Excess uric acid levels in the serum can lead to gout, which results in uric acid crystal deposits in the joints. See chapter 6 for a discussion of fluid, electrolyte, and acid–base homeostasis. See chapter 9 for a discussion of gastrointestinal function. See chapter 12 for a discussion of musculoskeletal function.

Some molecules (e.g., glucose, creatinine) need a carrier molecule to cross the membrane. A limited number of carriers is available, and the excess molecules get excreted in urine (i.e., transport maximum). A classic example is the glycosuria that occurs when serum glucose levels are high (e.g., 180 mg/dL).

The filtrate passes from the proximal convoluted tubule to the **loop of Henle**, which is the site of countercurrent exchange and urine concentration. The cortical nephron loops dip into the medulla, but the juxtamedullary nephrons are longer and dip further into the medulla. The further into the medulla, the greater the concentration gradient and fluid exchanges between the vasa recta (i.e., capillaries around loops in the medulla) and the loop. Sodium, along with chloride, potassium, and water move back and forth as osmolality

between the tubule and interstitium varies. The epithelial lining of the loop of Henle produces a protein known as uromodulin (i.e., Tamm-Horsfall protein). This protein is thought to have protective functions against uropathogens by binding and sequestering organisms as well as preventing kidney stone formation, but the role in kidney injury is unclear. Uromodulin is being evaluated as a potential marker of kidney function in addition to GFR.

The filtrate entering the **distal convoluted tubule** is more dilute (hypotonic). Hormones, such as ADH and aldosterone, alter this rate of excretion of sodium and water in the distal convoluted tubule (**FIGURE 7-5**). In part, this mechanism of water and electrolyte regulation aids in blood pressure management and, simultaneously, renal blood flow. The kidneys regulate acid–base balance through the secretion of hydrogen ions, which bind with base buffers, such as ammonia and phosphate, and are excreted in the urine. See chapter 6 for more on acid–base balance.

The kidneys have two other important functions with systemic effects—vitamin D conversion into its active form and erythropoietin production. The inactive form of vitamin D is produced by the action of ultraviolet rays on cholesterol in the skin or is ingested. The active form of vitamin D created by conversion aids in calcium and phosphorus absorption. The reabsorption of calcium and phosphorus occurs mainly in the proximal convoluted tubule. People with renal disease will have issues converting vitamin D into its active form. Most (95%) of the hormone erythropoietin is produced by the kidneys and is released in response to decreased oxygen delivery to the kidneys. Erythropoietin increases red blood cell production in the bone marrow. See chapter 3 for a discussion of hematopoietic function.

Urine is mainly composed of water (approximately 95%) and dissolved waste products by the time it is excreted. The next most abundant component is urea (approximately 2%), then sodium chloride (approximately 1%), and the remainder includes many other dissolved organic wastes (e.g., creatinine and uric acid). Ions in urine include potassium, calcium, magnesium, ammonia, sulfates, and phosphates. Many other substances are present in urine including carbohydrates, hormones, and enzymes.

Urine leaves the collecting duct once it is formed, traveling to the renal pelvis and funneling into the ureters to the bladder. The uroepithelium is the protective lining from the

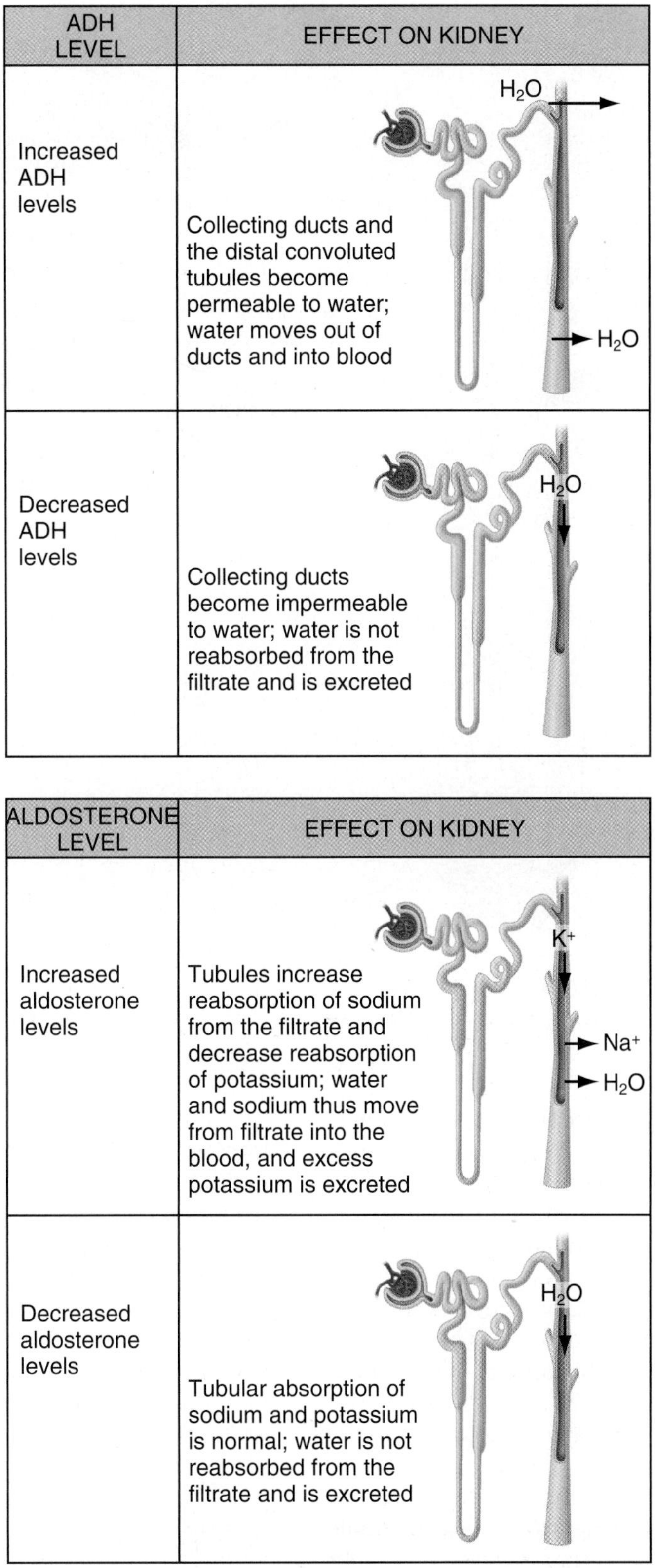

ADH LEVEL	EFFECT ON KIDNEY
Increased ADH levels	Collecting ducts and the distal convoluted tubules become permeable to water; water moves out of ducts and into blood
Decreased ADH levels	Collecting ducts become impermeable to water; water is not reabsorbed from the filtrate and is excreted

ALDOSTERONE LEVEL	EFFECT ON KIDNEY
Increased aldosterone levels	Tubules increase reabsorption of sodium from the filtrate and decrease reabsorption of potassium; water and sodium thus move from filtrate into the blood, and excess potassium is excreted
Decreased aldosterone levels	Tubular absorption of sodium and potassium is normal; water is not reabsorbed from the filtrate and is excreted

FIGURE 7-5 Effects of antidiuretic hormone and aldosterone on the kidneys.

renal pelvis to the urethra. The ureters enter the bladder at an angle, and the bladder pushes against the ureters when it contracts to prevent urine backflow (**FIGURE 7-6**). The muscular bladder serves as a reservoir for urine until it can be excreted. As the volume of urine in the bladder increases, the urine exerts pressure on the two bladder sphincters (internal and

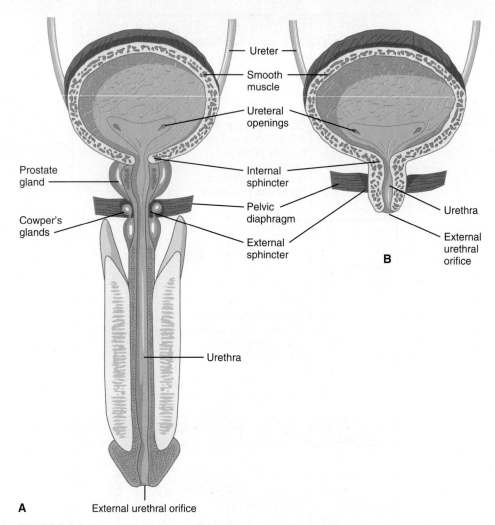

Prostate gland

Cowper's glands

Ureter

Smooth muscle

Ureteral openings

Internal sphincter

Pelvic diaphragm

External sphincter

Urethra

External urethral orifice

Urethra

External urethral orifice

A

B

FIGURE 7-6 **A** Male urinary bladder and **B** female urinary bladder and related structures.

external) and stretch receptors in the bladder. A pressure of 200 to 300 mL on the sphincters and receptors sends nerve impulses to the brain, triggering the urge to urinate (FIGURE 7-7). The amount of urine the bladder can store varies depending on age. An adult can store approximately 300–600 mL of urine. In children between the ages of 2 and 16 years old, the formula is estimated bladder capacity (mL) = (age of the patient in years + 2) × (30 mL).

Urination, or micturition, is a voluntary act. When urination is initiated, the bladder contracts and the internal and external sphincter relax, forcing urine out through the urethra. The external sphincter is able to stay closed despite high pressures and is able to close to stop urination once initiated. The urethra is approximately 1.5 inches long in women and 6–8 inches long in men. The shorter urethra in women, in combination with use of a sitting position for urination,

increases women's risk for developing urinary tract infections. The muscles of the pelvic floor maintain bladder placement and contribute to urination control.

The minimum urine output for proper elimination of waste products is termed the *obligatory urine output*, and this output is approximately 500 mL/day in adults. Formulas incorporate kilograms of body weight to calculate the minimum urine output in adults and children, including:

- Adult: 0.5 mL/kg/hr
- Child (> 1 year old): 1.0 mL/kg/hr
- Neonate/infant (< 1 year old): 2.0 mL/kg/hr

With aging, the kidneys begin functioning less efficiently. Renal blood flow decreases due to decreased arterial elasticity and increased stiffness. The decreased blood flow results in decreased number of nephrons, and the glomeruli enlarge as a compensatory mechanism.

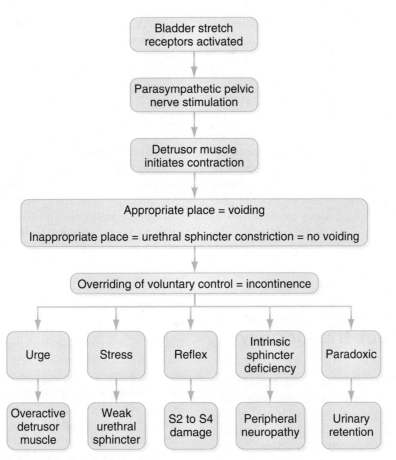

FIGURE 7-7 Urination.

Diagnostic Link

Blood Urea Nitrogen and Serum Creatinine

Various diagnostic serum laboratory tests are commonly used to evaluate renal function. The most common are blood urea nitrogen (BUN), serum creatinine, and GFR. Ammonia is converted in the liver to urea, which is the end product of protein metabolism. Urea is excreted entirely by the kidneys; therefore, **BUN** is an indication of liver and kidney function. Creatinine forms when creatine phosphate is used in skeletal muscle contractions and from dietary meat intake. The serum **creatinine** level is also an indication of renal function because it is entirely excreted by the kidneys. The creatinine level is not affected by hepatic function, so it is a more precise indication of renal function than is BUN. Creatinine levels double when there is a 50% reduction in GFR. However, creatinine fluctuates with dietary protein intake or supplements and decreases with malnutrition, muscle wasting, and amputation.

Diagnostic Link

Estimating GFR

The **glomerular filtration rate (GFR)** is the best measure of renal function, but it can only be estimated and not measured directly. There are two common methods to estimate GFR. One calculation uses the serum creatinine and incorporates age, sex, and race; this calculation is reported as estimated GFR (eGFR). Another calculation uses the serum creatinine and a 24-hour urine sample; this calculation is reported as the creatinine clearance. The creatinine clearance is the rate that creatinine is cleared from the blood by the kidneys in 24 hours.

Diagnostic Link

Urinalysis Components

The urinalysis is a commonly used laboratory test to evaluate for many disorders (e.g., urinary tract infections, kidney stones). The test consists of three parts: 1) a visual examination for color and clarity; 2) a chemical examination for variables such as pH, specific gravity, blood, protein, glucose, bilirubin, urobilinogen, nitrite, leukocyte esterase, and ketones; and 3) a microscopic examination for red blood cells, white blood cells, epithelial cells, casts, crystals, and organisms (e.g., bacteria). Electrolytes such as sodium, potassium, and calcium can be measured but are not part of a routine urinalysis. The urine sample can also be used to screen for substances such as cocaine, marijuana, and amphetamines.

The glomeruli become hypertrophic and sclerosed. The nephrons cannot regenerate. Every decade after 40 an average of 10% of nephrons are lost, which means by age 80 up to 40% of nephrons may be lost. The kidneys, however, despite the decreased number of nephrons are able to function adequately. The tubular structures shorten, lose mass, and atrophy. These tubular changes result in concentration difficulties, fluid imbalances, and acid–base and electrolyte imbalances. This decreased functioning can be further exacerbated by the presence of chronic conditions (e.g., diabetes mellitus, hypertension, and arteriosclerosis). Additionally, renal-related complications are common with aging changes (e.g., anemia, hypertension, and osteoporosis). Aging persons may require alternative medication dosing (usually a smaller dose or doses spaced farther apart) to prevent drug toxicity because of this impaired filtration. Also, several micturition issues such as incontinence from menopause or obstruction from an enlarged prostate can occur with aging.

Understanding Conditions That Affect the Urinary System

When considering alterations in the urinary system, organize them based on their basic underlying pathophysiology to increase understanding. Those pathophysiologic concepts include those conditions that alter urinary elimination and impair renal function. Conditions that alter urination may include infections, structural barriers, or problems with the act of urination). Infections could include cystitis or pyelonephritis; a structural barrier might be nephrolithiasis, a congenital disorder, or a tumor; and a problem with the act of urination could be incontinence. These conditions require interventions to promote urination (e.g., antibiotics, catheterization, bladder training, or surgery). Conditions that impair renal function can be life threatening (e.g., acute kidney injury) and include those disorders that prevent the kidneys from regulating fluid and electrolytes as well as excreting waste products and other substances. These conditions require prompt recognition and treatment (e.g., dialysis) to restore and maintain homeostasis and avoid progressive kidney disease.

Conditions Resulting in Altered Urinary Elimination

The act of urination requires 1) a functioning bladder with stretch receptors that can sense the filling of the bladder with urine, 2) an intact parasympathetic pelvic nerve to transmit the signal for emptying, and 3) working detrusor muscles to initiate bladder contractions to expel the urine (Figure 7-7). The sympathetic nerve innervations to the detrusor muscle cause detrusor relaxation and internal urethral sphincter contraction, which then lead to urine storage (see Figure 7-6). Somatic neurons (which provide voluntary control) cause external sphincter relaxation when inhibited and contraction when stimulated. Upper motor impulses can delay voiding by tightening the urethral sphincter. Although urination is mostly a voluntary act, voiding can be delayed only to a certain point. If the urge to void is ignored too long, bladder contractions take over the neural delaying mechanism and involuntary urination occurs.

Incontinence

Urination is a reflex in very young children, but it is controlled consciously in older children and adults. In children up to 3 years of age, urination is completely reflexive. Once the bladder expands, it empties. As children grow older, they learn to control urination. In older children and adults, the external sphincter is under conscious control—it will not relax until deliberately allowed to do so.

Older children and adults sometimes lose control over urination, resulting in a condition referred to as *urinary incontinence* (Figure 7-7). Urinary incontinence is a common and often embarrassing problem that has many causes. Incontinence is more common with aging, and women are more affected than men. There are four main types of incontinence—stress, urge/overactive bladder, overflow, and mixed (**FIGURE 7-8**). Other terms to describe incontinence include *functional*, *gross total*, and *transient* incontinence. In children, incontinence is divided into nighttime incontinence (i.e., enuresis) or daytime incontinence.

Stress incontinence describes loss of urine from increased intraabdominal pressure (stress)

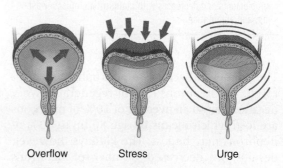

Overflow   Stress   Urge

FIGURE 7-8 Types of incontinence.

exerted on the bladder by coughing, sneezing, laughing, exercising, or lifting something heavy without any bladder contraction. Stress incontinence occurs when the urethra becomes hypermobile. The pelvic floor muscles and vaginal connective tissue normally support the urethra and bladder neck, and when support is lost, the urethra and bladder shift and no longer close by pushing against the anterior vaginal wall. The lack of connective and muscular support usually occurs in women due to physical changes resulting from pregnancy, childbirth, and obesity. Another cause of stress incontinence is intrinsic sphincter deficiency, causing an inability of the sphincter to close properly. Additionally, women may develop a cystocele (bulging of the bladder through the vaginal wall) because of these physical changes (lack of support), which can also increase their risk for stress incontinence. In men, prostate removal is the most common cause of stress incontinence. Other causes in men can include pelvic or neurologic trauma. Additional factors contributing to stress incontinence in both genders include obesity and chronic coughing. Chronic coughing such as that caused by smoking and lung disease can increase stress on the urinary sphincter. Congenital (e.g., meningomyelocele) and neurologic disorders can also cause stress incontinence due to structural abnormalities or deficits. See chapter 8 for a discussion of reproductive function.

Urge incontinence is a sudden, intense urge to urinate, preceding or occurring simultaneously with an involuntary loss of urine. *Overactive bladder* is a term that is often used interchangeably with *urge incontinence* as they often coexist. Overactive bladder is involuntary contractions with dysuria, urgency, and nocturia with or without incontinence. In urge incontinence, the detrusor muscle contracts involuntarily while the bladder is filling and may give the individual only a few seconds' to a minute's warning before voiding. With urge incontinence, the need to urinate is felt often, including throughout the night. The causes can be due central nervous system disorders altering inhibition of voiding, thereby, resulting in overactivity. Central nervous system disorders causing urge incontinence include stroke, Parkinson disease, and multiple sclerosis. Urge incontinence can also be the result of muscle changes in the bladder due to nerve-ending damage or detrusor muscle changes from aging. Urinary tract infections, bladder irritants, bowel conditions, and smoking may all cause urge incontinence.

Overflow incontinence is the result of an inability to empty the bladder, or retention. The bladder does not empty properly because the detrusor contractility is impaired due to aging, muscle damage and fibrosis, neuropathy, spinal detrusor efferent nerve disorders (e.g., multiple sclerosis), or low estrogen (e.g., menopause). Retention is usually due to an obstruction of the urethra, such as in prostate enlargement or a uterine fibroid compressing the urethra. Indications of overflow incontinence include dribbling urine and a weak urine stream. Chronic overdistention, also colloquially called *nurse's bladder* and *teacher's bladder*, occurs because of a perceived inability to interrupt work to void. This chronic avoidance of emptying the bladder results in detrusor muscle areflexia and overflow incontinence.

Mixed incontinence occurs when symptoms of more than one type of urinary incontinence are experienced. With **functional** incontinence, there are no urinary system disorders, but rather a physical or mental impairment prevents toileting in time. Functional incontinence occurs in many older adults, especially in people in nursing homes. For example, a person with severe arthritis may not be able to undress quickly enough to prevent incontinence.

Gross total incontinence refers to a continuous leaking of urine, day and night, or the periodic uncontrollable leaking of large volumes of urine. In these cases, the bladder has no storage capacity. This type of incontinence can occur because of anatomic defects, spinal cord or urinary system injuries, or a fistula (abnormal opening) between the bladder and an adjacent structure, such as the vagina.

Transient incontinence refers to urinary incontinence resulting from a temporary condition. Such conditions include delirium, infection, atrophic vaginitis, use of certain medications (e.g., diuretics and sedatives), psychological factors (e.g., depression and anxiety), high urine output (e.g., from overhydration), restricted mobility, fecal impaction, alcohol, and caffeine.

Incontinence in children can be divided into daytime or nighttime incontinence (i.e., enuresis). Incontinence in children is the involuntary urination by a child after 4–5 years of age, when bladder control is expected; however, nighttime bladder control may be achieved later (by 5–7 years old) than daytime control. Most children have only nocturnal enuresis, or bed-wetting, and no other symptoms (i.e., monosymptomatic enuresis). If a child never achieved nighttime dryness, then the enuresis is primary, but if they were not bedwetting for greater than 6 months and then start wetting, it is termed *secondary enuresis*. Enuresis is more common in boys than girls. Possible causes of primary enuresis include nighttime polyuria due to increased fluids taken at night or reduced ADH response or decreased ADH secretion (ADH follows a circadian pattern and normally increases at night), detrusor overactivity, and sleeping disorders. The relationship of ADH and enuresis are unclear. There may even be a genetic predisposition to enuresis as children who are bed wetters often have parents who were bed wetters. Enuresis may be due to a delay in the normal maturation of the central nervous system or small bladder capacity. Secondary enuresis may occur with an impactful event occurring in a child's life, such as parental divorce, and can be associated with poor bowel and voiding habits (e.g., constipation, holding urine). Most cases of enuresis resolve spontaneously.

If a child has enuresis as well as other urinary tract symptoms such as urgency, hesitance, or daytime incontinence, the condition is termed *nonmonosymptomatic enuresis*. Those children with enuresis and daytime incontinence are more likely to have urinary tract dysfunction, such as frequent urinary tract infections or neurologic disorders. Daytime incontinence can also occur without enuresis and can be caused by various disorders such as an overactive bladder or spinal cord disorders (e.g., spina bifida). Daytime incontinence can occur because children hold their urine. Over time, holding urine causes the bladder to become distended, and the detrusor muscle overstretches and becomes hypoactive. Bladder contractions become ineffective.

Generally, risk factors for developing urinary incontinence include the following conditions:

- **Being female:** Women are more likely than men are to have stress incontinence. Pregnancy, childbirth (particularly vaginal delivery), menopause, and normal female anatomy account for this difference. However, men with prostate conditions are at increased risk for urge and overflow incontinence.
- **Advancing age:** The muscles of the bladder and urethra lose some of their strength with age. Changes with age may also reduce bladder capacity and increase the risk

of involuntary urination. However, incontinence is not inevitable with age, and incontinence is not normal at any age, except during infancy.

- **Being overweight:** Being obese or overweight increases the pressure on the bladder and surrounding muscles, weakening them and allowing urine to leak out under stress (e.g., stress caused by coughing or sneezing).
- **Smoking:** Chronic coughing associated with smoking can cause episodes of incontinence or aggravate incontinence that has other causes. Constant coughing puts stress on the urinary sphincter, leading to stress incontinence. Smokers are also at risk of developing overactive bladder.
- **Other diseases:** Renal disease or diabetes mellitus may increase the risk for incontinence because of changes in renal function and nerve innervations.

Urinary incontinence can lead to complications ranging from minor to severe in nature. Skin problems (e.g., rashes, skin infections, and ulcers) can result from the presence of constant moisture. Recurrent urinary tract infections can develop from incomplete emptying of the bladder. Additionally, urinary incontinence can negatively affect psychological health and quality of life (e.g., it can cause poor self-image, embarrassment, sexual dysfunction, anxiety, and depression), and changes can occur in the individual's usual activities (e.g., work and exercise).

Diagnosis and Treatment

Diagnostic procedures for urinary incontinence include a history, physical examination, urinalysis, and urine cultures, if indicated. Bladder diaries (e.g., kept for 24–72 hours) can be completed to establish how often and when the incontinence occurs. Bladder stress testing in women can be done to evaluate for stress incontinence. This test involves having the patient vigorously cough or perform a Valsalva maneuver (i.e., forced exhalation with nose pinched and mouth closed) in a lithotomy and/ or standing position while the examiner visualizes the urethra for urine leakage. Postvoid residual measurement can assess for bladder and bladder outlet activity and can be evaluated with a bladder ultrasound or catheterization. A normal postvoid residual is usually less than 50 mL and up to 100 mL in older adults, but norms vary by age. Postvoid residuals are particularly useful for evaluating retention and overflow issues but can be used for other concerns. Other urinary system diagnostic tests include a cystourethrogram (X-ray of the bladder and urethra while the bladder is full and during urination), cystoscopy (visualization of the bladder with a small, lighted instrument), pelvic ultrasound, and urodynamic testing (which measures pressures and flow rate in the bladder). A prostate specific antigen test should be done for men. If there is suspicion of spinal cord disorder, then neurologic imaging (e.g., magnetic resonance imaging [MRI]) is indicated. Treatment for urinary incontinence depends on the type, underlying cause, and severity. Treatment and management strategies range from conservative to aggressive and include:

- Bladder training
- Scheduled toileting
- Fluid and diet management (e.g., avoiding alcohol, caffeine, or acidic foods; reducing liquid consumption; losing weight; or increasing physical activity)
- Pelvic floor muscle exercises (e.g., Kegel exercises)
- Electric stimulation (electrodes are temporarily inserted into the rectum or vagina to strengthen pelvic floor muscles through gentle electric stimulation)
- Medications (e.g., anticholinergics or estrogen replacement)
- Urethral inserts (small, tampon-like disposable devices or plugs inserted into the urethra)
- Pessary (a stiff ring inserted into the vagina to hold up the bladder)
- Radiofrequency therapy (a nonsurgical procedure that uses radiofrequency energy to heat tissue in the lower urinary tract, causing it to become firmer)
- Botulinum toxin type A (BOTOX) injections into the bladder muscle
- Bulking material injections (e.g., collagen, carbon-coated zirconium beads, Coaptite) into tissue surrounding the urethra
- Sacral nerve stimulator (an implanted device that emits painless electrical impulses that stimulate the sacral nerve)
- Artificial urinary sphincter (a fluid-filled ring implanted around the neck of the bladder that is controlled by a manual subcutaneous valve)
- Sling procedures (a surgically constructed pelvic sling or hammock around the bladder neck and urethra created by using strips of tissue, synthetic material, or mesh)
- Bladder neck suspension (a surgical procedure to raise and support the bladder in a more normal anatomic position)
- Absorbent pads and protective garments
- Urinary catheter (usually as an intermittent self-catheterization)
- Increased perineal hygiene
- Skin barrier creams
- Safety measures (e.g., moving any rugs or furniture out of path to the restroom, providing adequate lighting, widening the bathroom doorway, and installing an elevated toilet seat)
- Acupuncture
- Hypnotherapy
- Herbal remedies (e.g., *Crataeva nurvala*, horsetail [*Equisetum*], aloe vera extract)
- Coping strategies and support

For children with enuresis, additional strategies and treatments are available (e.g., motivation, support, and alarm systems). Desmopressin is a synthetic version of ADH that can be used for children with enuresis who have not responded to behavioral strategies. Other treatment strategies are centered on the cause, if known. Incontinence can resolve with time with or without treatment.

Neurogenic Bladder

Neurogenic bladder (FIGURE 7-9) refers to all bladder dysfunction caused by an interruption of normal bladder nerve innervation along any part of the peripheral or central nervous system. The bladder either becomes spastic and incapable of urine storage or flaccid with an inability to empty properly. A combined dysfunction in storage and emptying may also be present. Spastic issues generally occur with upper motor lesions that alter central nervous system control (i.e., brain or spinal cord) centers. Under these circumstances, micturition reflexes continue to function and control the bladder. With a spastic bladder, detrusor hyperreflexia with or without sphincter dyssynergia (uncoordinated) may be presented. If the disease is above the micturition center in the pons, then the bladder and the external urinary sphincter function in coordination (i.e., the bladder fills, the sphincter relaxes, and the bladder empties). Examples of disorders associated with a spastic bladder with detrusor hyperreflexia are brain injury, stroke, and multiple sclerosis. If the injury is below the micturition center of the pons but above the micturition center of the sacral area (between cervical level 2 and sacral level 1), then coordination between the

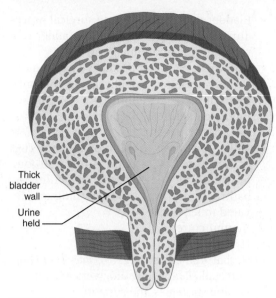

Thick
bladder
wall

Urine
held

FIGURE 7-9 Neurogenic bladder.

bladder contraction and the external sphincter is absent, and they both contract together, leading to an obstructive problem. The result is hyperactive bladder that does not relax (i.e., it is spastic) and cannot store much urine, bladder pressures rise easily, and symptoms of an overactive bladder occur. Disorders causing this detrusor-sphincter dyssynergia include Guillain-Barré syndrome, multiple sclerosis, and intervertebral disc problems.

Flaccid bladder issues are a result of interruption in sacral area or peripheral nerve conduction (sensory or motor) from the bladder and the spinal cord (i.e., the lower motor neuron) while the central nervous system remains intact. This results in detrusor areflexia with a hypotonic or atonic bladder with a loss of sensation. Examples of disorders associated with a flaccid bladder are congenital anomalies such as meningomyelocele, cauda equina syndrome

---

Learning Points

Urinary Incontinence

Here is an easy acronym to remember the causes of acute urinary incontinence.

DRIPS

D delirium, dehydration, diapers
R retention, restricted mobility
I impaction, infection, inflammation
P pharmaceuticals (opiates and calcium antagonists cause urinary retention and constipation; anticholinergics cause retention; alpha-adrenergic antagonists cause reduced urethral resistance in women; diuretics increase urine production), psychological problems (e.g., depression, neurosis, or anxiety)
S stool impaction (constipation) (Resnick & Yalla, 1998, p. 1045)

(damage to the bundle of nerves in the lumbosacral area), and peripheral nerve neuropathies (e.g., those involving the pelvic nerve or herpes zoster).

Clinical Manifestations

Clinical manifestations of neurogenic bladder include symptoms of a spastic overactive bladder such as frequency, urgency, and urge incontinence. Symptoms of a flaccid underactive bladder include urinary retention as well as distention with stress and overflow incontinence. If sensation is intact, the patient may feel a full bladder but contractions for emptying will not occur.

Diagnosis and Treatment

Diagnostic procedures for neurogenic bladder consist of a history, physical examination, bladder diary, urinalysis, urine cultures, cystourethrogram, cystoscopy, pelvic ultrasound, postvoid residual measurement, and urodynamic testing. Additional procedures (e.g., computed tomography [CT], MRI) may be performed to determine the underlying cause. Treatment strategies depend on the etiology and include those therapies previously discussed for incontinence.

Painful Bladder Syndrome/Interstitial Cystitis

Painful bladder syndrome, often referred to as *interstitial cystitis,* is a syndrome manifested by chronic bladder pain without an apparent cause for the pain. Despite the term *cystitis,* bladder inflammation is usually absent; however, the term continues to be used in the literature and by clinicians. The syndrome is five times more prevalent in women than men, and the highest incidence occurs in the 30s and 40s. Psychosocial factors and quality of life are often impacted with painful bladder syndrome due to difficulty with sleep and sexual dysfunction. The urinary symptoms can also impact work and social life.

The pathogenesis is poorly understood, but the diagnosis is often associated with other pain syndromes such as fibromyalgia, vulvodynia (vulvar pain of an unknown cause), and irritable bowel syndrome. Painful bladder syndrome is considered part of a group of hypersensitivity disorders that affect multiple organ systems because of the association with other pain syndromes. The disorder was originally associated with the development of visible ulcers known as Hunner lesions on cystoscopy. However, the lesions are only present in a small number (i.e., < 10%) of those with the disorder. In these patients, evidence of inflammation with accompanying mast cells and development of fibrosis is present. These findings are not present in the remainder of patients. Theories that continue to be explored are related to changes in the urothelial lining of the bladder and altered nerve sensitivity noted in those with painful bladder syndrome. A loss of integrity in the glycosaminoglycan (GAG) lining (a coating of urothelial cells) allows for increased permeability to irritants. The loss of urothelial integrity leads to activation of nerve and muscle tissue in the bladder, further perpetuating damage. Autoimmunity has been proposed as a mechanism. Bladder neuron sensitivity and central sensitization are increased, which is a result of abnormal brain processing of sensory input. Central sensitization results in more pain with less stimuli.

Clinical Manifestations

The key characteristic of painful bladder syndrome is suprapubic bladder pain, pressure, or discomfort with bladder fullness. The pain improves with urination. The pain is also usually in the pelvis but can be in the lower back and abdomen. Pain can worsen with ingestion of certain foods (e.g., tomatoes, spicy foods) or fluids (e.g., caffeine, alcohol). Frequency and urgency are common, but these manifestations are also present in other disorders such as overactive bladder or urinary tract infections. The symptoms must be present for more than six weeks with no other causes that explain the symptoms (e.g., urinary tract infection, malignancy).

Diagnosis and Treatment

Painful bladder syndrome diagnosis is made by conducting a history and physical examination. Diagnostic tests are done to exclude other disorders causing the symptoms. Cystoscopy and urodynamic evaluation are recommended when diagnosis is in doubt or complications are present. Treatment is geared toward symptom control. Treatment should be initiated in a stepwise approach, starting with conservative measures. Treatment should also be instituted individually so that an evaluation can be made regarding the effectiveness. Treatments initially include measures such as relaxation, behavioral modification like bladder training and avoiding bladder irritants, and urinary pain analgesics (e.g., phenazopyridine). Other treatments include physical therapy, oral medications (e.g., amitriptyline, instillation of medications in the bladder [e.g., glycosaminoglycan]), intradetrusor botulinum toxin, sacral neuromodulation, and surgical urinary diversion, in this order.

Congenital Disorders

Abnormalities of the urinary and reproductive systems are the most common congenital defects. Because of these systems' close proximity and intertwined structure, an abnormality in one system will often lead to an abnormality in the other. Numerous congenital disorders of the urinary system are possible, most of which are structural problems. Some defects cause no symptoms (e.g., both ureters draining one kidney and abnormal kidney positioning), whereas others are life threatening (e.g., renal agenesis [failure of an organ to develop in utero]). Problems with kidney development can be the most severe. The kidneys begin to develop in approximately the fifth week of gestation. Urine formation begins at 9–12 weeks' gestation. Urine is the main component of amniotic fluid, which is vital for normal fetal development.

Urinary Tract Infections—Cystitis and Pyelonephritis

Urinary tract infections (UTIs) are very common and include any infections that begin in the urinary tract. Infections can be categorized as upper urinary tract, which include the kidneys (i.e., pyelonephritis), or lower urinary tract, which include the bladder (i.e., cystitis) and the urethra (i.e., urethritis). The lower urinary tract is the most frequent site for infection. UTIs can be further divided into acute uncomplicated (e.g., simple cystitis) and acute complicated (e.g., pyelonephritis). UTIs can also be recurrent or chronic.

UTIs are caused by a direct invasion of the urinary tract by bacteria. Urine is an excellent medium for microorganism growth because of its protein content. Most bacteria that enter the urinary tract are quickly removed by the body before they cause symptoms. Notably, the urinary system contains several mechanisms to prevent infection, including one-way valves where the ureters attach to the bladder; urination, which washes microbes out of the body; the bladder lining, which has a barrier against bacteria; prostate secretions that slow bacterial growth in men; periurethral flora of *Lactobacillus* that prevents colonization in women; and the general functions of the immune system. Occasionally, the bacteria resist the body's defenses and cause infection. Due to the high concentration of bacteria, most infections invade the urethra from the meatus from microorganisms in the perineal area. The microorganism can then ascend through the urethra to the bladder, causing a cystitis, and then can move along the ureters to the kidneys, causing a pyelonephritis. Occasionally, microorganisms may invade the kidneys from the blood (hematogenous spread); this pathogenesis is more likely in the very young or immunocompromised. Pyelonephritis is more common in those persons who require frequent medical attention, experience recurrent UTIs, or have contracted an antibiotic-resistant bacterial strain.

UTIs are most often caused by *Escherichia coli*, which is part of the normal intestinal flora. Virulent forms of *E. coli* can avoid being washed away during urination by attaching to the mucosa along the urinary tract. *E. coli* can gain access to the urinary tract due to the anus' proximity to the urinary meatus, especially in women. In addition to this proximity, women are more vulnerable to developing UTIs for the following reasons:

- Women have shorter urethras, so the microorganisms have a shorter distance to travel.
- Women usually urinate in a sitting position, which prevents full emptying of the bladder.
- Women may experience increased perineal tissue irritation from sexual activity, tampons, bubble baths, bathing suits, tight-fitting pants, and deodorants as well as nylon, lace, and thong underwear.
- Women who are postmenopausal have a change in the periurethral flora, which increases the risk of urethral colonization.
- Women are more predisposed to urethrovesical reflux when doing any activities that involve bearing down, such as coughing and squatting. The pressure from bearing down pushes urine into the urethra, and it flows backwards in the bladder when pressure decreases.

Other organisms implicated in UTIs are Enterobacteriaceae species (e.g., *Klebsiella pneumoniae, Proteus mirabilis*) and *Staphylococcus saprophyticus*. Healthcare-associated urinary infections (whether from exposure or instrumentation), the recent use of antibiotics, and travel to areas with multidrug-resistant organisms may reveal the presence of other UTI-causing organisms. These other causes include species such as *Pseudomonas* or methicillin-sensitive or -resistant *Staphylococcus aureus*.

Although men are less likely than women to experience a UTI, when they do develop a UTI they are likely to have a recurrent UTI because the bacteria can hide deep inside prostate tissue. Recurrence in men is uncommon and defined as the return of symptoms within a few weeks after treatment. Recurrence in men is suspect for underlying disorders such as prostatitis or anatomic abnormalities. Urologic evaluation is usually warranted in men with recurrent UTI. In contrast to men, recurrent simple cystitis in women is defined as more than two infections in 6 months or more than three infections in 1 year. Most of the recurrences are due to reinfection rather than relapse. Relapses are considered when an infection occurs shortly after completion of a treatment (e.g., < 2 weeks) and the organism is the same. Relapses may require further evaluation or different management option such as long-term antibiotics.

Children with recurrent UTIs need to be evaluated for vesicoureteral reflux (VUR), which is the backward flow of urine from the bladder into the upper urinary tract. The most common cause of VUR is a defect in the closure of ureterovesical junction (**FIGURE 7-10**). In VUR, the ureter is congenitally short, and part of the ureter is embedded abnormally into the bladder wall. High bladder pressures as a result of anatomic defects or obstruction (e.g., neurogenic bladder) may also cause recurrent UTIs in children, and the condition can also be hereditary. Because the urine is flowing backwards, there is incomplete emptying with a predisposition to infections. The infected urine can then travel to the kidneys, causing pyelonephritis. The recurrent infections can lead to renal scarring and kidney failure. VUR can be detected by ultrasound prenatally when hydronephrosis is present. A child will usually have fever along with recurrent UTIs. There can be spontaneous resolution of a VUR depending on the characteristic of the reflux (e.g., whether it is unilateral or less severe).

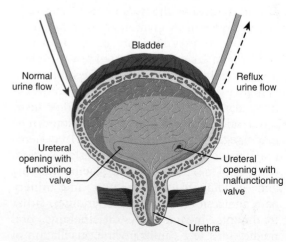

FIGURE 7-10 Primary vesicoureteral reflux.

Vesicoureteral Reflux (VUR), National Institute of Diabetes and Digestive and Kidney Diseases, Retrieved from https://www.niddk.nih.gov/health-information/urologic -diseases/urine-blockage-newborns/vesicoureteral-reflux.

Other risk factors for developing UTIs include the following:

- Benign prostatic hypertrophy (causes urinary obstruction/retention or decreased bactericidal prostatic activity with aging)
- Congenital urinary tract abnormalities (can alter urinary flow)
- Immobility (prevents complete bladder emptying, leading to urinary stasis)
- Urinary or bowel incontinence (can increase the potential for contamination of the urinary meatus)
- Renal calculi (obstruct urine output, leading to urinary stasis)
- Decreased cognition (increases the risk for incontinence and toileting issues)
- Pregnancy (the growing uterus puts pressure on the bladder, impairing urinary flow)
- Impaired immune response (e.g., diabetes mellitus)
- Impaired nerve innervations or neurogenic bladder (e.g., spinal cord injuries)
- Urinary catheterization and instrumentation (provides a direct pathway to the urinary system; the most common source of nosocomial infections, particularly gram-negative septicemia)
- Improper personal hygiene (increases the number of microorganisms)
- Using a diaphragm or spermicide for birth control (increases bacterial growth)
- Using unlubricated condoms (increases irritation)

Clinical Manifestations

For acute simple cystitis, clinical manifestations include urgency, dysuria, frequency, suprapubic pain, hematuria, bacteriuria, and cloudy, foul-smelling urine. Acute UTI symptoms when accompanied by fever (> 99.9° F/37.7° C), systemic manifestations (e.g., significant fatigue, chills, rigor), flank pain, and costovertebral angle tenderness more likely indicate pyelonephritis or an infection beyond the bladder (i.e., prostatitis). In men, the presence of pelvic or perineal pain is suggestive of a complicated UTI (i.e., prostatitis). In the elderly and frail, a UTI may present with nonspecific findings such as confusion or change in mental status, falls, or other functional impairments. Systemic infectious manifestations in the elderly tend to be subtle (e.g., less fever). Most instances of simple acute cystitis resolve without sequelae.

With pyelonephritis, the kidneys become grossly edematous, and structures fill with exudate and can compress the renal artery. Abscesses (e.g., corticomedullary, perinephric) and necrosis can develop, impairing renal function and causing permanent damage.

Diagnosis and Treatment

A diagnosis of UTI can often be made by history and physical examination. A urinalysis can be done to confirm the diagnosis or is useful when manifestations are not classic or questionable. A urinalysis and urine culture and sensitivity should be done in men even with a simple case of cystitis. The urinalysis can be done with a urine dipstick or by microscopy. Urinalysis will reveal pyuria (white blood cells in the urine). Leukocyte esterase is an enzyme in the urine that is released by white blood cells; the presence of leukocyte esterase in the urine reflects pyuria and is consistent with the presence of a UTI. Nitrites in urine are reflective of infection with Enterobacteriaceae (e.g., E. coli). These organisms convert nitrate to nitrite. A positive nitrite test suggests significant bacteriuria. However, urine dipsticks can yield false-negative nitrite results when the urine has not been in the bladder long enough to allow the conversion of nitrate to nitrite. Some organisms do not cause nitrate conversion (e.g., Enterococcus faecalis). A low urine pH (e.g., such as with cranberry juice ingestion) may cause a false-negative nitrite reading. Despite a negative nitrite reading, treatment should be provided if the history is suggestive of a UTI. Substances that make the urine turn red, such as beets or the use of phenazopyridine (e.g., bladder analgesic), will cause a false-positive nitrite test. White blood cell casts indicate kidney inflammation and are present in acute pyelonephritis.

A UTI is usually treated by targeting the most common causative organism (e.g., E. coli). A urine culture and sensitivity test can further provide information regarding the organism and antibiotic susceptibility (i.e., sensitivity). A culture and sensitivity test should be done on those patients with complicated infection (e.g., pyelonephritis, urosepsis), atypical presentation, failure to respond to therapy, and recurrent symptoms. Blood cultures are necessary for those patients with urosepsis.

Asymptomatic bacteriuria is the term used when urine contains bacteria (i.e., $\geq 10^5$ colony-forming units/mL, with or without pyuria and without symptoms of a UTI. The reasons for the lack of symptoms may be related to the pathogen (e.g., less virulent strains) or patient factors. Most cases of asymptomatic bacteriuria will not progress, so treatment is not necessary. Potential for an adverse drug event

BOX 7-1 Application to Practice

Review the following urinary infection cases and determine the most likely cause, including pathogen and mode of transmission. Discuss data that supports your decision and treatment strategies.

Case 1: A 50-year-old woman presented complaining of burning sensation when urinating and feeling like she has to go every hour for the last day. She denies fever and suprapubic or back pain.

> Past medical history: dyslipidemia and hypertension.
> Medications: atorvastatin.
> Allergies: sulfa.
> Physical examination: temperature 98.5° F; pulse 80 beats per minute; respiration rate 18 breaths per min; blood pressure 110/66 mmHg; examination unremarkable; no suprapubic or costovertebral angle tenderness; urine dipstick reveals moderate leukocytes and positive nitrites, with all other values within normal limits.

1. What is the most likely diagnosis and pathogen causing this disorder and mode of transmission? Discuss data that support your decision.
2. What diagnostic test, if any, should be done? What diagnostic test findings would support your diagnosis?
3. Develop a treatment plan for this patient.

Case 2: A 65-year-old woman with no urinary system complaints had a routine urinalysis with the results shown in the table.

1. What is the most likely diagnosis and pathogen causing this disorder and mode of transmission?
2. Discuss data that support your decision.
3. What diagnostic test, if any, should be done?
4. Develop a treatment plan for this patient.

Case 3: A 45-year-old woman is complaining of urgency and dysuria for the past 2 days. Yesterday, she started getting chills, feels she is getting a fever, and her back hurts.

> Past medical history: UTI 1 year ago.
> Medications: none.
> Allergies: no known drug allergy (NKDA).
> Physical examination: temperature 100° F, pulse 86; respiration rate 18 per min; blood pressure 110/70 mmHg; positive costovertebral angle and suprapubic tenderness, otherwise unremarkable; urine dipstick reveals positive leukocytes but negative for nitrites and blood.

1. What is the most likely diagnosis and pathogen causing this disorder and mode of transmission?
2. Discuss data that support your decision.
3. What diagnostic test, if any, should be done? What diagnostic test findings would support your diagnosis?
4. Develop a treatment plan for this patient.

Urinalysis, complete	Result	Reference range
Color	Dark yellow	Yellow
Appearance	Cloudy	Clear
Specific gravity	1.022	1.001–1.035
pH	≤ 5.0	5.0–8.0
Glucose	Negative	Negative
Bilirubin	Negative	Negative
Ketones	Negative	Negative
Occult blood	Negative	Negative
Protein	Negative	Negative
Nitrite	Negative	Negative
Leukocyte esterase	Moderate	Negative
White blood cells	5–10 WBC/HPF	≤ 5 /HPF
Red blood cells	0–2 RBC/HPF	≤ 2 /HPF
Squamous epithelial cells	6–10 HPF	≤ 5 /HPF
Bacteria	None seen	None seen/HPF
Hyaline casts	None seen	None seen/HPF

HPF = high-power field.

with antibiotics is considered riskier in comparison to the presence of benign bacteriuria. Treatment may also cause a higher chance of antibiotic resistance. In certain groups, however, treatment of asymptomatic bacteriuria is warranted, including pregnant women, those undergoing urologic intervention (e.g., prostate resection), and renal transplant patients.

Diagnostic Link

Urine Culture and Sensitivity

A urine culture can confirm the presence of bacteriuria and provide antibiotic susceptibility information. The optimal urine sample should be a clean-catch midstream specimen (i.e., discard initial urine). When obtaining a specimen, females should spread the labia and uncircumcised males should retract their foreskin. A positive culture is defined as $\geq 10^5$ colony-forming units/mL. However, lower bacterial counts with pyuria and symptoms of UTI may still be diagnostic for a UTI. A lower bacterial count with a UTI is more common in men (contamination is rare), with organisms other than *E. coli*, or with concurrent antibiotic therapy. Lower bacterial counts without pyuria may be indicative of contamination. Sensitivity reports will include information classifying the organism's expected antibiotic effect into one of the three categories—susceptible, intermediate, or resistant.

Other diagnostic tests can evaluate for causes, particularly if a UTI is recurrent, relapsing, chronic, or complicated and include a cystoscopy, cystourethrogram, and imaging of the kidneys, ureters, and bladder (e.g., ultrasound, X-ray, CT, MRI). Not all complicated UTIs require imaging, particularly if there is a prompt response and improvement with antibiotic treatment. UTI treatment focuses on eradicating the microorganism with antibiotics. Length of antibiotic therapy can vary from 3 days for acute, simple cystitis to 14 days for pyelonephritis. Patients with pyelonephritis may need to be treated in a hospital if there are manifestations of critical illness (e.g., septicemia), an inability to remain hydrated, or an intolerance of oral medications. Additional strategies concentrate on prevention of UTIs:

- Increasing hydration, especially consumption of water and juices (increases flushing of the urinary tract)
- Avoiding irritants (e.g., bubble bath and deodorants)
- Performing proper perineal hygiene (women should clean from front to back, and uncircumcised men should retract the foreskin to clean the penis)

- Wearing cotton underwear
- Wearing loose-fitting clothing
- Not delaying urination
- Adequately emptying the bladder, especially after intercourse
- Providing appropriate catheter care (when present)
- Probiotics (reestablish normal flora)

Urinary Tract Obstructions

The urinary system is similar to the basic plumbing in any house. Blockages in any part of the plumbing system prevent the flow of the liquid, causing the system to back up. Many opportunities for blockages to occur exist throughout the urinary system, making urinary obstructions common (FIGURE 7-11). These blockages may stem from functional and/or anatomic abnormalities and be as simple as particulates collecting and forming stones to being as complex as the growth of tumors. Areas proximal to the obstruction are affected as pressure builds up and structures dilate (e.g., hydroureter, hydronephrosis). Urinary tract obstructions can cause urinary infections, and unless the obstruction is resolved, renal scarring and damage can occur. Obstructions can be acute or chronic as well as cause a complete or partial blockage. The blockage can be unilateral or bilateral (e.g., enlarged prostate).

Nephrolithiasis

Nephrolithiasis refers to the presence of renal calculi (kidney stones). Calculi are hard masses of crystals composed of minerals that the kidneys normally excrete (FIGURE 7-12). These stones, which can vary in size from as small as a grain of sand to as large as a golf ball, are the most common cause of urinary obstruction. Nephrolithiasis is more common in men and Whites. Adults are more commonly affected than children. Generally, the calculi form in the renal pelvis, ureters, and bladder. *Urolithiasis* is a general term used for a stone located or formed anywhere in the urinary system such as the bladder, while nephrolithiasis refers to those stones located or formed in the kidneys. The renal medullary interstitium is probably the site of most stone formation.

Calculi may contain various combinations of chemicals (**TABLE 7-3**). The most frequently encountered type of calculi (about 80%) contains calcium in combination with either oxalate (80% of calcium stones) or phosphate (5% of calcium stones). Other types of calculi

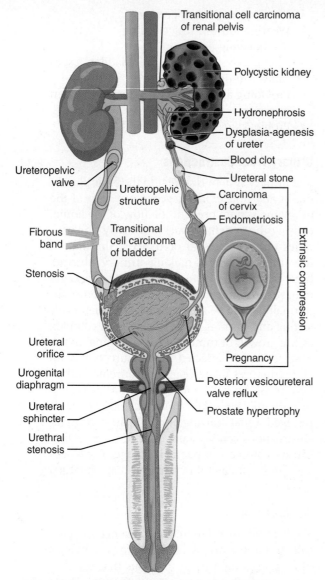

FIGURE 7-11 Urinary tract obstruction and hydronephrosis. (**a**) Causes of urinary tract obstruction. (**b**) Hydronephrosis, marked dilation of renal pelvis and calyces with thinning of parenchyma.

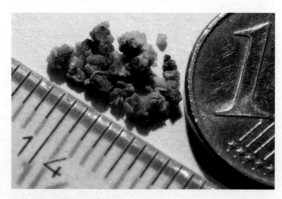

FIGURE 7-12 Renal calculi.
© Eskimo71/Dreamstime.com.

include struvite or infection stones, uric acid stones, and cystine or xanthine stones. The calculi may be smooth or jagged, and they are usually yellow or brown.

In a healthy individual, urine contains chemicals that prevent crystals from forming. Once the minerals begin to precipitate, they grow like a snowball being rolled in the snow. Calcium crystals can form in the interstitium of the kidney and cause a small plaque (i.e., Randall plaque). Subsequently, crystal deposition occurs in this plaque with stone formation. Conditions that increase the likelihood of the crystals forming include urine pH changes (whether alkaline or acidic), excessive concentration (e.g., as with dehydration, bone disease, gout, renal disease, and dietary increases) of insoluble salts in the urine in relation to volume, and urinary stasis (e.g., from immobility or anatomic abnormalities). Several inhibitors of stone formation act as natural protectors, such as citrate, magnesium, and pyrophosphate. Low levels of these inhibitors can increase risk for nephrolithiasis. Citrate is considered one of the key inhibitors and acts by forming a complex with calcium in the urine. A reduction in urine citrate (i.e., hypocitraturia) can be due to factors such as high animal protein diet or chronic metabolic acidosis. Additional risk factors for developing nephrolithiasis include family history, obesity, hypertension, and diet (high-protein, high-sodium, or low-calcium diet). A low calcium diet may contribute to stone formation. Usually calcium binds to oxalate and when there is insufficient calcium there is less binding. Therefore, the increased oxalate results increased tendency to stone formation.

Clinical Manifestations

Calculi usually cause symptoms only when they obstruct urine flow. This obstruction can lead to hydronephrosis (enlargement of renal pelvis and calyces). The movement of calculi through the urinary system (i.e., renal pelvis to the ureter) can be quite painful and cause irritation of the urinary mucosa, increasing the risk for a UTI. Clinical manifestations of nephrolithiasis include the following signs and symptoms:

- Colicky pain (pain that fluctuates in intensity, with periods of pain lasting 20–60 minutes; often severe, this pain is due to the calculi scraping the ureter wall, and it is colicky due to ureter spasms that occur in an attempt to move the calculi along; the pain is located in the flank area for upper

TABLE 7-3	Types of Renal Calculi	
Type	**Causes**	**Treatment**
Calcium	Increased absorption of calcium from the small bowel Hyperparathyroidism Inability of renal tubules to reabsorb calcium Dietary excess of calcium Chronic bowel disease that results in steatorrhea; fat then combines with calcium and renders the calcium unable to bind to oxalate, causing stone formation Alkaline urine High urine calcium, high urine oxalate, or low urine citrate Low urine volume	Cellulose phosphate or thiazide diuretics to decrease dietary absorption of calcium Surgical resection of the parathyroid gland to reduce hyperparathyroidism Thiazide diuretic therapy to correct renal tubular defects, resulting in the inability to reabsorb calcium Purine dietary restrictions to reduce uric acid production Increased fluid intake and treatment of chronic diarrhea
Struvite (magnesium ammonium phosphate)	Urase-producing bacteria Urinary pH around 7.2 Usually large in size (e.g., staghorn calculi) Texture is relatively soft Associated with frequent UTI More common in women (due to increased UTI) UTI is a common cause in children	Prevention of UTI Percutaneous nephrolithotomy
Uric acid	Excess uric acid excretion (e.g., gout) Urine pH lower than 5.5 encourages insoluble urate salt formation Rapid and dramatic weight loss Some malignancies	Dissolution of large calculi by increasing the urine pH above 6.5 with potassium citrate (the solubility of urate salt is then increased) Purine dietary restrictions to reduce uric acid production
Cystine or xanthine	Genetic disorder causing abnormal excretion of cystine or xanthine (amino acids), ornithine lysine, and arginine	Prevention: increase fluid intake and increase urine pH above 7.5

Modified from Story, L. (2017). *Pathophysiology: A Practical Approach* (3rd ed.). Burlington, MA: Jones & Bartlett Learning.

ureteral or renal pelvic obstruction while pain with radiation to the lower abdomen and groin area (ipsilateral testicle or the labia) occurs with lower ureteral obstruction

- Hematuria, gross or microscopic (at least three RBCs per HPF; almost always present)
- Dysuria, frequency, and urgency with calculi in the distal ureter
- Nausea and vomiting
- Fever and chills (if an infection is present)

Some patients have asymptomatic nephrolithiasis, and stones are found incidentally when imaging is done for another purpose.

Diagnosis and Treatment

Diagnosis of nephrolithiasis is accomplished with a history and physical examination along with a urinalysis. The urinalysis may reveal hematuria. The stone should be analyzed at least one time to determine the type and/or if treatments are not effective. A noncontrast, low-dose CT scan of the abdomen and pelvis (standard contrast dose can be alternative) is the preferred diagnostic exam. The CT can detect stone size, location, and presence of hydronephrosis. The second option is an ultrasound of the kidneys and bladder (i.e., renal ultrasound) if CT technology is not available or if there is concern regarding radiation exposure (e.g., pregnancy). The ultrasound detects hydronephrosis but is less reliable in detecting stones and less accurate in stone measurement or location. Other procedures may include an abdominal X-ray, which detects stones but with less accuracy and does not detect hydronephrosis. An MRI is rarely used as stones are relatively invisible.

If hyperparathyroidism is suspected as a cause of stone formation, then a parathyroid hormone level should be evaluated. Serum studies can include calcium, uric acid, and phosphate levels.

The acute treatment of nephrolithiasis often includes pain management. Nonsteroidal anti-inflammatory agents (e.g., ketorolac) will help with pain reduction and decrease ureteral spasms. Opioids are another pharmacologic pain management option. Treatment of nephrolithiasis is specific to the type of calculi present (Table 7-3); therefore, determining the type of calculi is crucial to resolve the current calculi and prevent future calculus development. To determine the type of calculi, all urine is strained to capture any passed calculi. Small stones (< 5 mm) can pass through the urinary system, and the likelihood of spontaneous passage decreases as stones get larger (e.g., those stones > 4 mm). Stones ≥ 10 mm rarely pass. If there is underlying ureteral dilation, some larger stones may pass. Patients with uric acid stones may report passing gravel rather than a stone. Strategies to assist the passing of these calculi include engaging in physical activity (if possible) and increasing fluid intake to 2.5–3.5 L throughout the day to achieve a urine output of 2.5 L per day. The increased presence of fluid in the urinary system will expand the diameter of the ureters and urethra, easing the passage of the calculi. Two pharmacotherapeutic agents can be used as medical expulsive therapy—tamsulosin (alpha blocker) and nifedipine (calcium channel blocker)—particularly if the stone is within the 5–10-mm range. Larger calculi can be broken up to allow for passing of the smaller pieces. Procedures to disintegrate these calculi include extracorporeal shock wave lithotripsy (high-frequency sound waves are directed at the calculi to pulverize them), percutaneous nephrolithotomy (a laser is directed at a calculus with a fiber-optic scope), and ureteroscopy (a forceps is used to grab a calculus and remove it through a fiber-optic scope). Surgical removal of the calculi may be indicated in the following situations:

- The calculi do not pass after a reasonable period of time and cause constant pain.
- A calculus is too large to pass on its own or is lodged in a difficult location.
- The calculi obstruct urinary flow.
- The calculi cause ongoing UTIs, renal damage, or constant bleeding.
- The calculi have enlarged.

Treating the underlying cause (e.g., with antibiotics, antigout agents, or urine pH–modifying agents) of the calculi and pain management will also be necessary.

Recurrence is common with nephrolithiasis. However, the lapse between episodes can be years (e.g., 15% incidence 1 year after passage of the first stone and 50% incidence 10 years after passage of the first stone), so prevention strategies are essential. Dietary changes are the mainstay of prevention, with the changes implemented being specific to the type of calculi (Table 7-3). Additional prevention strategies include adequate fluid intake (2–2.5 L per day) and physical activity.

Diagnostic Link

Urinary Imaging

Renal ultrasound (US) is useful in evaluation of urinary tract obstruction and hydronephrosis. Kidney stones may be obscured by the bowel in the lower abdomen/pelvis; therefore, a pelvic ultrasound may also be necessary. Due to its safety (no contrast media or invasiveness), renal US is commonly recommended and used for renal disorders of unknown cause. A renal US may identify renal masses (e.g., tumors or simple or complex cysts); however, CT is more sensitive. Doppler US can be used to evaluate renal flow and is indicated in disorders such as renal artery stenosis, renal vein thrombosis, and renal infarction. The renal US can be used to guide placement of needles or catheters. Abdominal and pelvis CT is the test of choice for nephrolithiasis (noncontrast low dose). The CT is more useful than renal US for location of obstruction and stone size. The CT with contrast is best for evaluation of masses and for identifying abscesses. The concern with a CT is the exposure to radiation. The intravenous pyelogram is infrequently used due to the need to administer intravenous contrast, high-radiation exposure, and other tests such as the US and CT that are safer and can provide the same information.

Hydronephrosis

Hydronephrosis is an abnormal dilation of the renal pelvis and the calyces of one or both kidneys that occurs secondary to a disease (FIGURE 7-13). Diseases that obstruct urine flow are commonly associated with this condition, including nephrolithiasis, tumors, benign prostatic hyperplasia, strictures, and stenosis. Congenital urologic defects can also cause hydronephrosis, including reflux nephropathy, a congenital condition that causes backflow of urine into the kidneys. Unilateral renal involvement indicates an obstruction in one of the ureters, and bilateral renal involvement indicates an obstruction in the urethra.

Because urine is continuously forming, the presence and severity of clinical manifestations depend on the degree of urinary obstruction. Partial obstructions with mild hydronephrosis may not produce any initial symptoms. Complete obstruction with severe hydronephrosis, by comparison, applies direct pressure and compresses tissue and blood vessels, leading to atrophy, necrosis, and glomerular filtration

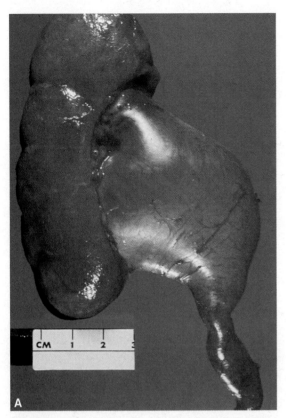

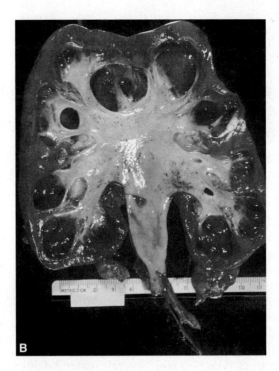

FIGURE 7-13 Hydronephrosis.
Courtesy of Leonard V. Crowley, MD, Century College.

cessation. When present, clinical manifestations include the following signs and symptoms:

- Colicky flank pain or pressure
- Bloody, cloudy, or foul-smelling urine
- Dysuria
- Decreased urine output
- Frequency
- Urgency
- Nausea and vomiting
- Abdominal distention
- UTIs

Diagnostic procedures for hydronephrosis include a history, physical examination, urinalysis, renal ultrasound, CT, intravenous pyelogram, and MRI. Prognosis depends on the severity of the hydronephrosis and early treatment. Treatment focuses on resolving the underlying cause, and facilitating urine flow will be necessary if UTIs develop. If the hydronephrosis is prolonged, permanent renal damage can occur to one or both kidneys.

Tumors and Cysts

Bladder or renal masses can be cystic or solid (i.e., tumor). The masses can also be benign (adenomas, papillomas) or malignant (e.g., renal cell carcinoma). Cysts are the most common type of masses found on the kidneys. Most cysts are benign; however, most urinary tumors are malignant. These tumors can occur at any point along the urinary system. Regardless of their location, tumors can obstruct urine flow and impair renal function in addition to leading to the consequences of cancer (e.g., metastasis, pain, and weight loss).

Wilms Tumor

Wilms tumor, or nephroblastoma, is a rare kidney cancer that primarily affects children. According to the National Cancer Institute (2016), 500 new cases of Wilms tumor are diagnosed each year. The peak incidence of Wilms tumor occurs around the age of 3–4 years (American Cancer Society, 2016). This tumor usually occurs in one kidney, but it can affect both (in 4–5% of cases). A second tumor may appear later in the remaining kidney. Wilms tumor usually grows as a solitary mass that can become quite large (**FIGURE 7-14**). In some cases (10%), there are multiple tumors in one kidney.

The exact cause of Wilms tumor is unknown, but it is thought to arise in utero when the cells that normally form the kidneys fail to develop properly. This development issue

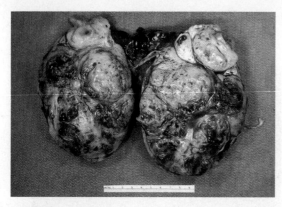

FIGURE 7-14 Wilms tumor.

© University of Alabama at Birmingham Department of Pathology PEIR Digital Library (http://peir.net).

usually occurs due to spontaneous and sporadic genetic mutations. Notably, Wilms tumor has been associated with genetic mutations, such as tumor suppressor loss of function on chromosome 11 (e.g., *WT1*, *WT2* genes), chromosome 17 (p53), as well as on the X chromosome. Despite awareness of various genetic mutations, the correlation and development of Wilms tumor is still unclear. Wilms tumors occur in conjunction with several congenital defects (about 10% of cases) and is termed *WAGR syndrome*. The defects include aniridia (absence of the iris of the eye), genitourinary anomalies (e.g., cryptorchidism and hypospadias), and intellectual disability. Disorders such as Denys-Drash syndrome includes hemihypertrophy, renal disease, and Wilms tumor. Wilms tumor is rarely familial, with only up to 2% of cases having a family history. The mode of transmission is autosomal dominant. The risk of developing this tumor also seems to be higher in females and Blacks. In contrast, Asian Americans have a lower risk of developing Wilms tumor than other ethnic groups.

Clinical Manifestations

Because of improved diagnostic procedures, Wilms tumor can now be detected early, leading to an improved prognosis for children affected by this disease. The long-term survival rate is excellent with early detection and treatment. Unfortunately, Wilms tumor may sometimes go undetected early because the tumor can grow quite large without causing pain; nevertheless, most of these tumors are diagnosed before they have metastasized.

Patients with Wilms tumor usually present with an abdominal mass or swelling with pain (up to 40%) or without pain. Accompanying manifestations include hematuria in up to 25%

of cases with fever and hypertension in another 25% of cases. Other manifestations may be present if Wilms tumor is associated with other congenital syndromes, such as in Denys-Drash syndrome (e.g., hemihypertrophy) or WAGR syndrome (e.g., genitourinary anomalies). On physical examination, the abdominal mass is usually firm and nontender, and it does not usually cross the midline.

Diagnosis and Treatment

Diagnostic procedures for Wilms tumor include a history and physical examination, as well as an abdominal ultrasound as the usual first diagnostic test. The renal tumor will then be further evaluated with doppler ultrasound and abdominal CT with contrast or abdominal MRI. A biopsy is necessary for histologic confirmation. Evaluation of the chest (e.g., chest CT and X-ray) will be conducted to evaluate for metastasis. Laboratory analysis will include a BUN, creatinine, creatinine clearance, complete blood count, liver function tests, serum calcium, coagulation studies, and urinalysis. Once diagnosed, two staging systems guide treatment. One staging system, used prior to chemotherapy, is the National Wilms Tumor Study (NWTS) system. The NWTS system includes the following stages:

- **Stage I:** The cancer is in only one kidney and generally can be completely removed with surgery.
- **Stage II:** The cancer has metastasized to the tissues and structures near the kidney, but it can still be completely removed by surgery.
- **Stage III:** The cancer has metastasized beyond the kidney area to nearby lymph nodes or other structures within the abdomen and may not be completely removed by surgery.
- **Stage IV:** The cancer has metastasized to distant structures, such as the lungs, liver, or brain.
- **Stage V:** Cancer cells are found in both kidneys.

The standard treatment for Wilms tumor is surgery (e.g., simple, partial, or radical nephrectomy) and chemotherapy, but radiation therapy may be used if warranted by tumor histology. The 5-year survival rate can be as high as 90% with the administration of multiple treatments. Recurrence is dependent of the type of tumor histology, and rates can be as low

TABLE 7-4	Bosniak Classification for Renal Cysts	

Bosniak classification	Description	Treatment/malignancy potential
Type I	Benign simple cyst—imperceptible cell wall, round	Further evaluation and treatment not necessary; repeat US (e.g., 6–12 months) may be done to confirm stability Malignancy potential: < 1%
Type II	Minimally complex, benign cysts that are well marginated and with a few thin septa, thin calcifications, and nonenhancement	Further evaluation and treatment not necessary; repeat US (e.g., 6–12 months) may be done to confirm stability Malignancy potential: < 1%
Type IIF	Minimally complex cysts that have suspicious features in comparison to II such as thicker calcification, multiple septa, and perceived enhancement	Further evaluation with CT or MRI with contrast (preferred) Malignancy potential 5%
Type III	Indeterminate are thick, nodular septa and show enhancement	Further evaluation and treatment include fine-needle biopsy, partial nephrectomy, and radiofrequency ablation Malignancy potential 55%
Type IV	Malignant cysts that are solid mass with necrosis	Further evaluation and treatment include partial or total nephrectomy Malignancy potential 85–100%

as 15% and as high as 50%. Coping strategies and support interventions (e.g., allowing play time and local support groups) will be beneficial for the family and child. Additionally, once the patient is diagnosed, subsequent palpation of the abdomen should be avoided because the renal capsule may rupture, and the cancer may spread.

Renal Cysts

Cystic masses, particularly simple cysts, are found in normal kidneys and increased incidence occurs with aging. Simple renal cysts, which are considered benign, are the most common type of masses found in the kidneys. Cysts on kidneys are often found incidentally on imaging (e.g., ultrasound, CT) done for other purposes. Most cysts cause no symptoms, result in no sequalae, and require no treatment. However, some cysts are complex and associated with the risk of malignancy. If a cyst is detected on ultrasound, then a CT scan is generally indicated. The radiologic system known as the Bosniak classification uses contrast CT scan findings to evaluate cysts and categorize them from I to IV based on the cyst appearance. The Bosniak classification is useful in determining the diagnosis, treatment, and follow-up for renal cysts (**TABLE 7-4**).

In additional to the incidental finding of renal cysts, there are several diseases associated with the development of cysts such as

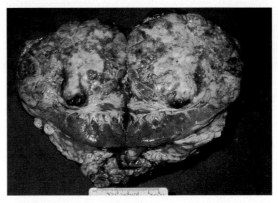

FIGURE 7-15 Renal cell carcinoma.
Courtesy of Dr. Edwin P. Ewing, Jr./CDC.

polycystic kidney disease, as well as medullary and cortical kidney diseases. Cysts can form as a consequence of chronic kidney disease. A few of these disorders will be discussed elsewhere.

Renal Cell Carcinoma

Renal cell carcinoma is the most frequently occurring kidney cancer in adults (most common in those 50–70 years of age). The National Cancer Institute (2018b) estimated that nearly 65,340 new cases of renal cancer would be diagnosed in 2018, with more than 14,000 deaths attributed to this cancer. Most cases (approximately 85%) of renal cell carcinoma are primary tumors arising from the renal cortex (**FIGURE 7-15**). The remaining renal cell carcinomas (approximately 8%) arise from the renal pelvis (i.e., transitional or urothelial cell carcinoma). Other tumors, such as renal sarcoma and renal medullary carcinoma, occur infrequently. Its exact cause is unknown. Risk factors for developing this type of cancer include being male, obesity, advanced kidney disease particularly those requiring dialysis treatment, family history, hypertension, other kidney disease (e.g., horseshoe kidney and polycystic kidney disease), toxin exposure (e.g., asbestos), prolonged analgesic use (e.g., aspirin, acetaminophen), chronic hepatitis C infection, kidney stones, and smoking. Metastasis to the liver, lungs, bone, or nervous system is common at the time of diagnosis.

Clinical Manifestations

Renal cell carcinoma (i.e., renal adenocarcinoma) is typically asymptomatic in its early stages. When present, the most common clinical manifestations include the following signs and symptoms: hematuria, an abdominal renal mass that is firm, abdominal flank pain described as dull and achy, and unexplained weight loss. Other symptoms may include scrotal varicoceles. If the inferior vena cava is affected, then manifestations can include edema, ascites, and hepatic problems. Patients can present with manifestations of metastasis. Patients can develop paraneoplastic syndromes, such as anemia with erythropoietin suppression or polycythemia with tumors that secrete erythropoietin or erythropoietin-like substances. Fever is usually intermittent with night sweats and fatigue. Hypertension may occur due to high renin levels. Hypercalcemia (due to ectopic parathyroid hormone production by the tumor or bone metastasis) or Cushing syndrome (increased adrenocorticotropic hormone) are other paraneoplastic syndromes.

Diagnosis and Treatment

Diagnosis is often made incidentally, but unexplained hematuria should be evaluated for possible renal cell carcinoma. Renal cell carcinoma should be considered with the presence of clinical manifestations. Initial imaging evaluation is usually with an abdominal CT; however, an abdominal ultrasound can be used. Further diagnostic procedures will include a biopsy, and the abdominal CT can be used for staging. Other diagnostic procedures are to determine whether metastasis has occurred and can include a bone scan, MRI, positron emission tomography scan, and chest CT. Laboratory analysis will include a liver function panel, complete blood count, and blood chemistry. The tumor, node, metastasis staging system is used for staging renal cell carcinoma.

Interestingly, renal cell carcinoma is one of the few tumors where the tumor can regress spontaneously in the absence of therapy, but this is very rare and may not lead to long-term survival (National Cancer Institute, 2018b). Partial or complete surgical nephrectomy is recommended because the cancer is generally unresponsive to radiation or chemotherapy, although some newer chemotherapy agents (e.g., multikinase inhibitors) have shown promise in this indication. Surgery is considered curative if there is no metastasis. Hormone therapy and immunotherapy may have modest effects in shrinking the tumor. Prognosis is better when the condition is diagnosed prior to metastasis of the cancer.

Bladder Cancer

Bladder cancer refers to any cancer that forms in the tissue of the bladder. Most bladder cancers (90%) are urothelial (transitional)) cell carcinomas (cancer beginning in the cells that make up the inner bladder lining). The urothelial cells also line the ureters, urethra, and renal pelvis, but the cancerous cells usually arise from the bladder. Urothelial bladder cancer is most commonly caused by chemical carcinogenesis, particularly smoking. Other less common types of bladder cancer are termed *nonurothelial* and include squamous cell carcinoma (cancer beginning in thin, flat cells), adenocarcinoma (cancer beginning in the cells that make and release mucus and other fluids), and small cell tumors. The cells that form squamous cell carcinoma and adenocarcinoma develop in the inner lining of the bladder because of chronic irritation and inflammation usually from infection. This type of cancer usually evolves as multiple invasive tumors that extend through the bladder wall and surrounding structures. Metastasis to the pelvic lymph nodes, liver, and bone is common. Benign tumors can arise in the bladder (e.g., urothelial papilloma, inverted papilloma) and usually have a low rate of recurrence and progression.

The National Cancer Institute (2018a) estimated that nearly 81,190 new cases of bladder cancer would be diagnosed in 2018, with more than 17,000 deaths being attributed to this cancer. Although bladder cancer most frequently occurs in older adults, it can occur at any age, and it is more common in men and Whites. The median age at diagnosis is 69–71 years.

Smoking is the most common risk factor and is associated with almost half of all bladder cancers. Other persons at increased risk include those who work with chemicals (e.g., dye, rubber, hairdressing chemicals, and aluminum), have excessive use of analgesics, experience recurrent UTIs, have long-term catheter placement, family history, and received chemotherapy or radiation. Genetic mutations of the RAS and tumor suppressor genes are associated with bladder cancer. See chapter 1 for more about cellular function.

Clinical Manifestations

The initial clinical manifestation of bladder cancer is painless hematuria that is gross (i.e., visible) or microscopic. The hematuria is intermittent and occurs throughout all of micturition as opposed to just the beginning. Irritative symptoms such as frequency, urgency, and dysuria may be present and occur due to detrusor overactivity, obstruction, or decrease in bladder capacity. Flank or abdominal pain (e.g., suprapubic) are usually signs of more advanced cancer. Other general symptoms such as fatigue, weight loss, or anorexia are also manifestations of more advanced disease. Physical examination findings may reveal the presence of a pelvic or abdominal mass (if advanced) and prostate induration.

Diagnosis and Treatment

As with renal cell carcinoma, unexplained hematuria (e.g., not from renal calculi or UTI) needs an evaluation for possible bladder cancer particularly in individuals over the age of 40. A urine evaluation can be conducted with a dipstick and microscopy, which will confirm the presence of blood. Urine dipsticks can sometimes be positive for blood even when there are no red blood cells (RBCs) upon microscopy. This finding may be caused by myoglobin (muscle injury) rather than hemoglobin. Clinically significant hematuria consists of more than three RBCs/HPF on microscopic examination. The morphology of RBCs in bladder cancer is usually normal, and the presence of abnormal shapes or RBC casts usually indicates intrinsic (intrarenal) renal disease. A cystoscopy is the diagnostic test of choice for diagnosing and staging bladder cancer. A urinalysis, urine cytology, and urine-based markers that identify tumor-related proteins can supplement cystoscopy findings. After cystoscopy, staging is also done with a transurethral resection of bladder tumor that is performed under anesthesia. The resected tumor histology and depth of invasion are then determined. Stage I lesions are confined to the submucosa; stage II includes invasion into the muscle; stage III is beyond the muscle and into the fat, possibly beyond the bladder; and stage IV lesions have metastasized. A CT scan with and without contrast of the abdomen and pelvis or an MRI are diagnostic procedures that can further evaluate metastatic disease. Other procedures to evaluate for metastasis can include a chest X-ray, chest CT scan, bone scan, and positron emission tomography scan. Even with early diagnosis and treatment, bladder cancer often reoccurs. Treatment strategies are based on staging and include surgical removal of the tumor, generally for nonmuscle invasive bladder cancer. Intravesical chemotherapy is infused during the resection and administered for maintenance therapy. Patients with stage II disease generally require a cystectomy, and those with muscle-invasive disease (stage III

Diagnostic Link

Cystoscopy and Ureteroscopy

A cystoscopy is a common diagnostic test used for evaluating the lower urinary tract. The procedure can be done in an office. A flexible or rigid scope is inserted in the urethra after application of local anesthesia. Either water or saline is infused into the bladder for better visualization. A ureteroscopy can also be performed through insertion of a flexible or rigid scope to view the ureters and kidneys. Renal calculi can be removed during ureteroscopy, and ureter stents can be placed.

Diagnostic Link

Hematuria

Hematuria is the presence of urine in the blood. Gross hematuria is visible to the naked eye, and the urine may be brown or red. As little as 1 mL of blood per 1 L of urine can cause a change in color. Hematuria with clots is more likely with a lower urinary tract disorder. Hematuria may only be detected microscopically with a urinalysis or a urine dipstick. Urine dipsticks can detect 1–2 RBCs per HPF. Myoglobin (e.g., seen with rhabdomyolysis) and hemoglobin (e.g., with hemolytic disorders) will cause a false positive on the urine dipstick, and there will be few to no RBCs. Additionally, menstrual blood may contaminate a urine specimen (i.e., dipstick or urinalysis). Drugs such as phenazopyridine (a urinary analgesic) or phenytoin can cause a false urine blood result. When a urinalysis report is positive for blood, the next step is evaluation of the number of RBCs present. Abnormal hematuria is defined as the presence of three or more RBCs per HPF. The presence abnormal RBC morphology or red blood cell casts is generally indicative of an upper urinary tract disorder (i.e., kidney) as opposed to the bladder.

BOX 7-2 Application to Practice

Review the following case and urinalysis report.

A 46-year-old woman is asymptomatic and has a routine urinalysis as part of her annual physical. The urinalysis with microscopy report is shown in the table.

Describe the urinalysis findings and determine possible reasons for the findings and follow-up, if necessary.

Urinalysis, complete	Result	Reference range
Color	Dark yellow	Yellow
Appearance	Cloudy	Clear
Specific gravity	1.022	1.001–1.035
PH	≤ 5.0	5.0–8.0
Glucose	Negative	Negative
Bilirubin	Negative	Negative
Ketones	Negative	Negative
Occult blood	1+	Negative
Protein	Negative	Negative
Nitrite	Negative	Negative
Leukocyte esterase	Negative	Negative
White blood cells	None seen	≤ 5 /HPF
Red blood cells	0–2	≤ 2 /HPF
Squamous epithelial cells	6–10	≤ 5 /HPF
Bacteria	None seen	None seen/HPF
Hyaline casts	0–5	None seen/HPF

HPF = high-power field.

and above) will have a radical cystectomy which includes removal of adjacent organs and lymph nodes. A patient with a cystectomy will need to undergo a urinary diversion procedure. The diversion procedure may include the creation of an ileal conduit (in which urine flows from the ureter through the ileum and then a skin stoma) or creation of an orthoptic neobladder where a piece of intestine is created into a new bladder. The new bladder is attached to the ureters and urethra allowing for a normal urine flow pattern. Other therapies can include radiation and immunologic agents.

Benign Prostatic Hyperplasia

Although the prostate is a structure of the male reproductive system, diseases of the prostate can cause significant issues in the lower urinary system because of its close proximity to those structures (FIGURE 7-16). Benign prostatic hyperplasia (BPH), also called *benign prostatic hypertrophy*, is a common, nonmalignant enlargement of the prostate gland that occurs as men age, usually appearing by age 50. Its exact cause is unknown, but multiple factors that cause prostatic stromal cell proliferation are implicated. This increase in proliferation enlarges the prostate gland. Hormones such as testosterone, dihydrotestosterone (DHT), and estrogen seem to be involved in BPH development, but their contribution is not clear. Testosterone levels decrease with aging; however, DHT (the active form of testosterone) remains at a relatively normal amount in the stromal

FRONT VIEW

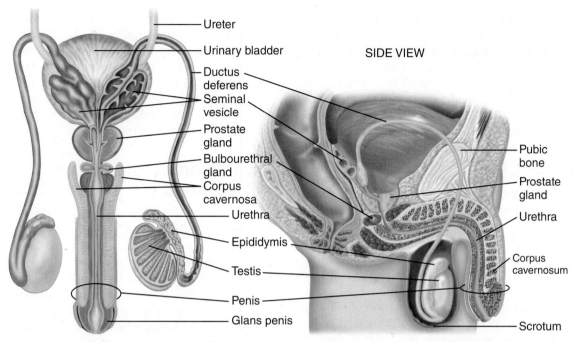

SIDE VIEW

- Ureter
- Urinary bladder
- Ductus deferens
- Seminal vesicle
- Prostate gland
- Bulbourethral gland
- Corpus cavernosa
- Urethra
- Epididymis
- Testis
- Penis
- Glans penis

- Pubic bone
- Prostate gland
- Urethra
- Corpus cavernosum
- Scrotum

FIGURE 7-16 Urethra and prostate gland.

tissue of the prostate. DHT, which is reduced by the enzyme 5α-reductase from testosterone, is one of the hormones necessary for normal prostatic growth. Inhibitors of 5α-reductase are used to treat BPH. With aging, there is an increased ratio of estrogen to androgen. Estrogen may contribute to BPH development by making the prostate tissue susceptible to hypertrophy. A second theory postulates that stem cells in the prostate do not mature and die as they are programmed to do (apoptosis). The resulting imbalance between dying cells and reproducing cells enlarges the prostate over time. As the prostate expands, it presses against the urethra like a clamp on a hose. Clamping the urethra obstructs urine flow, leading to urinary stasis and UTIs. The bladder wall becomes thick and irritated as urine overfills this organ. The bladder begins to contract with even small amounts of urine, and, over time, it loses its ability to empty completely.

Clinical Manifestations

Lower urinary tract symptoms (LUTS) are the clinical manifestations of BPH. By age 50, approximately half of men with BPH will have symptoms, and by age 80, the incidence of LUTS increases to 80% of men with BPH. Manifestations are usually slow and insidious. The size of the prostate is not correlated with the presence and severity of symptoms. LUTS can

be divided into storage symptoms and voiding symptoms.

Storage symptoms are also known as irritative symptoms and include daytime frequency, nocturia, urgency, and incontinence. Voiding symptoms are also known as obstructive symptoms and include changes in urine stream such as slowing or spraying of stream. The stream can be intermittent, and there may be hesitance, straining to void, and dribbling at the end of the void. Complications are more common in untreated men and can include urinary retention, overflow incontinence, recurrent UTIs, and kidney failure.

Some men have BPH and remain asymptomatic. BPH does not increase prostate cancer risk, but the clinical presentation is similar to that of prostate cancer. When manifestations of prostate cancer appear, the disease is usually advanced. Physical examination findings consistent with BPH include a large (> 17 grams or bigger than a walnut; normal is 7-16 grams), palpable prostate that is smooth, symmetrical, and rubbery. Asymmetry or nodules are consistent with prostate cancer while an exquisitely tender prostate is associated with prostatitis. See chapter 8 for discussion of reproductive function.

Diagnosis and Treatment

Diagnosis of BPH is accomplished with a history, physical examination, and measurement of the prostate-specific antigen (PSA). Other diagnostic tests are conducted to evaluate for other possible causes of LUTS. Urinalysis and renal function exams (e.g., BUN, creatinine) are usually normal with BPH. While hematuria may occur with BPH, evaluation for other causes should be conducted as hematuria is also associated with urinary tract cancers. Other diagnostic procedures for BPH diagnosis are usually not necessary unless there is concern or risk for other urinary disorders such as cancer, urinary retention, or kidney disease. In men with moderate to severe LUTS and diagnosed BPH, other diagnostic procedures can include uroflowmetry, postvoid residual measurements, cystoscopy, and rectal ultrasound.

Treatment centers on relieving the urinary obstruction. Pharmacologic strategies to improve urine flow include alpha-1 blockers and 5α-reductase inhibitors. Alpha-1–adrenergic blocking agents cause relaxation of bladder neck and urethra, leading to decreased resistance while 5α-reductase inhibitors shrink or limit growth of the prostate. Anticholinergics can be used for men with irritative symptoms. Phosphodiesterase type 5 inhibitors can be used for men with BPH (relaxes smooth muscle in bladder neck, urethra, and prostate) and erectile dysfunction (relaxes smooth muscle in penis, improving blood flow). Herbal remedies (e.g., saw palmetto) have also been used, although only limited evidence supports their effectiveness. Behavioral modifications include limitation of fluids around bedtime, reducing diuretic type drinks (e.g., caffeine, alcohol), and making sure the bladder empties completely (i.e., double voiding). Men with BPH who sit to urinate have a reduction in LUTS as the pelvic and hip muscles are more relaxed, allowing for faster and stronger force of urination and better bladder emptying. Other strategies to improve BPH symptoms include minimally invasive procedures such as laser therapy, transurethral needle ablation, transurethral electrovaporization of the prostate, hyperthermia, high-density forced ultrasound, intraurethral stents, and transurethral balloon dilation. Partial or complete surgical removal of the prostate gland may be necessary. Additionally, use of alcohol should be avoided because it can make symptoms worse.

Conditions Resulting in Impaired Renal Function

Kidney disorders and injury, specifically the nephron (i.e., glomerulus, tubules, and arteriole), will lead to alteration in the formation of urine. While other structures are considered as part of the kidneys (e.g., renal calyx and pelvis), usually disorders that stem from this area (e.g., nephrolithiasis and pyelonephritis) result in problems of elimination. Problems of elimination, whether or not from the lower tract (i.e., bladder or prostate), can result from kidney insult and subsequent impairment in urine formation. Glomerular disorders are a common cause of kidney failure.

Polycystic Kidney Disease

Polycystic kidney disease (PKD) is an inherited disorder characterized by numerous, grape-like clusters of fluid-filled cysts in both kidneys (FIGURE 7-17). These cysts enlarge the kidneys while compressing and eventually replacing the functional kidney tissue. The exact trigger for the formation of the cysts is unknown, but genetic defects result in abnormal tubular epithelium.

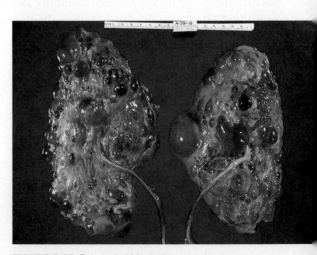

FIGURE 7-17 Polycystic kidney disease.
Courtesy of Dr. Edwin P. Ewing, Jr./CDC.

BOX 7-3 Application to Practice

Hematuria is common and can be due to benign conditions (e.g., strenuous exercise) or serious disorders (e.g., renal cell carcinoma).

Review the following cases and determine the most likely cause of the hematuria. Discuss data that support your decision as well as diagnostic and treatment strategies.

Case 1: A 50-year-old White man is complaining of left-sided flank pain that started about 3 hours ago. He describes the pain as sharp and intermittent. He notes that his urine is a bit darker, but he denies seeing blood. The pain started after he finished mowing a client's lawn (he is a gardener). He denies dysuria, urgency, or fever.

Past medical history: gout.
Medications: allopurinol 100 mg orally every day.
Allergies: no known drug allergies (NKDA).
Social history: denies smoking, alcohol use, or drug misuse.
Physical examination: temperature 98.5° F, pulse 96 beats/minute, respiration rate 20 per min, blood pressure 138/88 mmHg.
General: anxious, holding left side, and moving around; otherwise exam is unremarkable.
Urinalysis: positive for blood with 15 RBCs per HPF; remainder unremarkable.

Case 2: An 8-year-old Black girl is complaining of burning when urinating for the past day. She reports wetting herself at school because she was unable to hold it until she was able to get to the bathroom. When she toileted, she voided only small amounts. She denies fever, back, or suprapubic pain. The child is accompanied by her mother.

No past medical history or medications.
Allergies: penicillin (hives).
Vaccines: up to date.
Physical examination: vital signs and exam are within normal limits.
Urine dipstick: positive for leukocytes, nitrites, and blood

Case 3: A 68-year-old White man is concerned because he thinks he is peeing blood. He noticed it about 1 month ago, and he thought it was related to sex as he noticed it right after intercourse. However, he has had two other episodes within the past two weeks not related to sexual intercourse. He denies fever, dysuria, frequency, abdominal, back, or pelvic pain. He states he used to have a weak stream and have to urinate at night, but these symptoms have improved since starting finasteride (5α-reductase inhibitor).

Past medical history: BPH.
Medications: finasteride.
Allergies: no known drug allergy (NKDA).
Social history: has smoked 1 pack of cigarettes per day for the past 40 years; drinks two to three beers on the weekends.
Physical examination: body mass index 32; vital signs and exam are within normal limits.
Urinalysis with microscopic evaluation: positive for blood with 40 RBCs/HPF; no casts or dysmorphic cells noted.

Prognosis and progression of the disease vary widely, depending on the type of PKD. Autosomal dominant PKD is the most common type; it has been mapped to mutations on the short arm of chromosomes 4 (for PKD2) and 16 (for PKD1). Both these genes encode for polycystin-1 and polycystin-2, and these proteins are involved in cellular growth, differentiation, and calcium signaling in the kidneys. This form of PKD occurs in both children and adults, but it is much more common in adults, with symptoms often emerging in middle age. Autosomal recessive PKD, like most recessive conditions, is far less common. This type can be detected prenatally or soon after birth, but it can appear in infancy or childhood. The recessive PKD occurs due to mutations on *PKHD1* gene which causes decreased or absent fibrocystin. This protein's role is not clear; however, fibrocystin seems to be involved in kidney development. Recessive PKD tends to be extremely serious and progresses rapidly, resulting in renal failure and generally causing death in infancy or childhood. PKD affects males and females equally regardless of age.

Learning Points

The Urinary System

The urinary system is a basic human septic system. The kidneys remove waste and unneeded substances from the blood to have them excreted. The kidneys collect these products in the form of urine much like a toilet, and flushing the toilet is much like what the kidneys do in sending the urine to the bladder. The bladder acts like a septic tank, holding the waste until the tank is full. When full, the bladder (and the septic tank) must be emptied.

When obstructions occur at any point in the urinary system, urine backs up, much like the septic system would do if it were obstructed. This backflow can cause severe damage in both cases: in the urinary system, the kidneys become damaged by the irritation and pressure of the excess urine; in the septic system, the house becomes damaged from the corrosive septic contents.

Clinical Manifestations

Clinical manifestations depend on the individual's age and the type of PKD. These manifestations reflect the structural changes associated with the disease and the resulting renal impairment. In neonates, manifestations include the following signs and symptoms:

- Potter facies, which are pronounced epicanthic folds (skin folds at the corner of the eyes on either side of the nose), pointed nose, small chin, and floppy, low-set ears
- Large, bilateral, symmetrical masses on the flanks
- Respiratory distress (caused by fluid accumulation from renal impairment)
- Hyponatremia (due to dilution from fluid accumulation)

In adults, manifestations include the following signs and symptoms:

- Lumbar or flank pain
- Increased abdominal girth
- Swollen, tender abdomen
- Grossly enlarged, palpable kidneys

Some other symptoms may affect both groups:

- Hypertension (due to activation of the renin–angiotensin–aldosterone system)
- Hematuria (due to impaired glomerular filtration)
- Nocturia (related to an inability to concentrate urine)
- Uremia (waste accumulation due to renal impairment) with symptoms such as drowsiness

Other conditions that may occur in conjunction with PKD include brain aneurysms, cysts in other organs (especially the liver), and colon diverticula. Because of the renal impairment associated with this condition, PKD can lead to critical complications such as renal insufficiency, pyelonephritis, cyst rupture, retroperitoneal bleeding, and chronic kidney disease. Other, less serious complications include anemia, hypertension, and renal calculi (kidney stones).

Diagnosis and Treatment

Diagnosis of PKD consists of a history, physical examination, and imaging of the kidneys, usually with a renal ultrasound. Other imaging modalities can include a CT or MRI. Genetic testing confirms the diagnosis. Screening of patients with a family history usually involves renal ultrasound and genetic testing. Genetic testing for screening purposes in asymptomatic individuals with a positive family history should be completed by clinicians experienced in providing counseling. Information pertaining to the benefits and consequences of testing should be discussed, such as family planning and awareness of symptoms.

PKD often progresses slowly, leading to end-stage renal disease. The following treatment strategies focus on controlling symptoms and preventing complications:

- Pharmacology, including the following agents:
  - Antibiotics (when infections are present)
  - Analgesics (for pain)
  - Antihypertensive agents for stringent blood pressure control
  - Diuretics
  - Statins for cardiovascular risk reduction
- Adequate hydration
- Low-salt and low-protein diet
- Surgically draining cystic abscesses or retroperitoneal bleeding
- Dialysis
- Kidney transplant

Glomerular Disorders

Within the kidney are millions of filtering units composed of tufts of capillaries in between the afferent and efferent arterioles. The glomerulus sits inside the Bowman capsule (Figure 7-2). An in-depth look at the glomerulus is necessary as disorders are categorized or described based on the glomerular structure (e.g., membranous glomerulonephritis) (FIGURE 7-18). There are three layers of the glomerulus. The inner layer is the endothelial lining that is fenestrated. The middle layer is the glomerular basement membrane. The basement membrane acts as a barrier to large molecules. Surrounding these two layers are the outer layer of parietal epithelial cells that transition to the tubular structures or podocytes. The podocytes are footlike structures that connect the outer layer to the basement membrane and cover the capillaries. The podocytes are another important barrier in the filtration of large molecules. The inside of the glomerulus is surrounded and supported by an interglomerular matrix, mesangium, which consists of mesangial cells.

Several possible injuries can occur to the various microcomponents of the glomerulus and cause various types of disease. These disorders are grouped into clinical syndromes. Additionally, glomerular disorders are termed based on the cellular (i.e., histologic) changes, the affected glomerular layer in the capillary

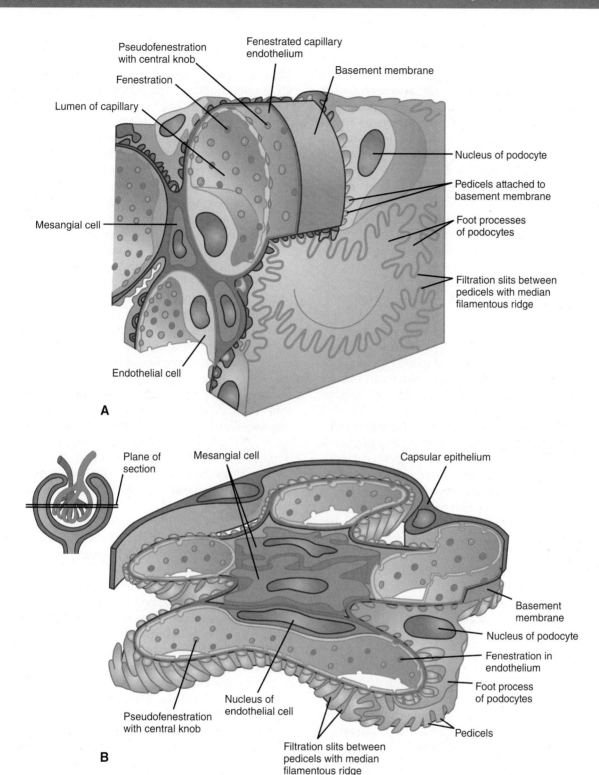

Pseudofenestration
with central knob

Fenestration

Lumen of capillary

Fenestrated capillary
endothelium

Basement membrane

Mesangial cell

Endothelial cell

Nucleus of podocyte

Pedicels attached to
basement membrane

Foot processes
of podocytes

Filtration slits between
pedicels with median
filamentous ridge

A

Plane of
section

Mesangial cell

Capsular epithelium

Basement
membrane

Nucleus of podocyte

Fenestration in
endothelium

Foot process
of podocytes

Pedicels

Nucleus of
endothelial cell

Pseudofenestration
with central knob

Filtration slits between
pedicels with median
filamentous ridge

B

FIGURE 7-18 A schematic representation of fine structure of glomerular filter as visualized by electron microscopy. **A** Segment of glomerular capillaries. **B** Cross-section through the center of the glomerulus, including part of the Bowman capsule.

membrane or supporting structure, the location and extent of the glomerular lesions, and underlying dysfunction. The following terminology is used to describe glomerular injury:

Diffuse and focal: Lesions that involve all or most (> 50%) of the glomeruli (plural) are termed *diffuse*, and lesions that involve some (< 50%) of the glomeruli are termed *focal* (e.g., focal segmental glomerulonephritis).

Global and segmental: When a whole glomerulus (singular) is affected, the lesion is termed *global*, and the lesion is considered segmental if only a portion (< 50%) of the glomerulus is affected.

Proliferative, sclerosing, and necrotizing: These terms are structural (histologic) descriptors. *Proliferative* refers to an increase in glomerular cells (e.g., mesangial, endothelial, basement membrane). Proliferation in the extracapillary space forms specific lesions that are termed *crescents*, which are made of macrophages, fibroblasts, and other cells. These crescent cells accumulate in the Bowman space and represent a rupture of the capsule. *Sclerosing* refers to glomerular scar formation, and when the scarring is between the glomerulus and tubules, it is referred to as *interstitial fibrosis*. *Necrotizing* refers to cellular death.

Multiple causes and mechanisms of glomerular disorders can lead to dysfunction. The pathogenesis of glomerular injury can include immunologic and nonimmunologic mechanisms (e.g., hypertension, diabetes) and most often a combination of both. Hereditary diseases are due to many different types of genetic mutations. The inciting cause of glomerular disorders can include infections (e.g., streptococcus), toxin exposure (e.g., drugs, chemicals), autoimmune diseases (e.g., systemic lupus erythematosus), and vascular disorders (e.g., hypertension). The cause of glomerular disorders can also be idiopathic. Glomerular disorders manifest as a variety of clinical syndromes and includes asymptomatic hematuria and/or proteinuria, nephritic, and nephrotic syndromes. The two broad categories of glomerular disease are glomerulonephritis and glomerulosclerosis.

Glomerulonephritis

Glomerulonephritis is an inflammatory disorder of the glomeruli, and most forms occur as a result of activation of immune mechanisms (FIGURE 7-19). The triggering antigens can be endogenous, such as in systemic lupus erythematosus, or exogenous, such as in infections from streptococci or hepatitis C. The trigger, however, is often unknown. Glomerulonephritis may occur when there is a genetic predisposition to develop an immune response to triggering antigens.

Glomerulonephritis involves a humoral and cellular mediated immune response. The humoral response is a key mechanism of injury as many glomerular disorders (up to 90%) involve the development of immune complexes that are composed of immunoglobulins and complement components. The antigens can be nonrenal, such as in the DNA nucleosome complexes in lupus, or abnormal IgA, as in IgA nephropathy. These antigens can be passively trapped, can bind to receptors on mesangial cells, or can be planted in the glomerulus and then bound to antibodies. In any situation, the depositions of these complexes activate the complement system and stimulate an immunologic response with release of multiple substances (e.g., cytokines and nitrous oxide). The result is capillary wall injury with increased permeability. The basement membrane, which acts as a charge-selective contact, loses its negative charge. Large proteins, such as albumin and red blood cells, are able to pass through into the filtrate and manifest as hematuria and proteinuria. Platelets and T cells play a role in the development of glomerular disease even in the absence of antibodies being deposited (e.g., as in focal segmental glomerulosclerosis). Platelets aggregate and lead to thrombosis and release of vasoactive substances that cause vasodilation and contribute to worsening capillary permeability. The cellular mediated T cell response results in macrophages and lymphocyte release, which each contribute to proliferation into the extracapillary space and crescent formation. The damaged glomerular cells and macrophage proliferation lead to obstruction to blood flow, which reduces glomerular blood flow and, in turn, GFR. Sclerosis and fibrosis continue, and ultimately, renal failure develops.

Antigens are usually nonrenal in origin; however, some antigens can be a normal (or intrinsic) part of the glomerular basement membrane. In **anti–glomerular basement membrane (anti-GBM) glomerulonephritis**, usually immunoglobulin G (IgG) and, at times, IgA or IgD target type IV collagen in the membrane. This type of immune response (type II hypersensitivity) often results in rapid and progressive renal failure. The anti-GBM antibodies also react with pulmonary alveolar basement membrane and cause pulmonary hemorrhage. Anti-GBM is often referred to as **Goodpasture disease** or **Goodpasture syndrome**, and the terms are sometimes used synonymously. Anti-GBM is rare but aggressive. Causes are generally unknown but may be due to infection (e.g., influenza), toxin, or drug exposure. Treatment centers on removal of antibodies through plasmapheresis and inhibiting antibody production (e.g., with corticosteroids).

Glomerulonephritis is associated with two clinical syndromes—nephritic syndrome and

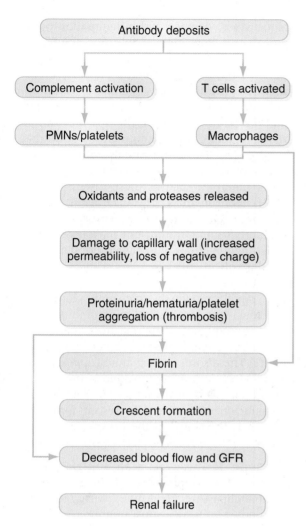

FIGURE 7-19 Immune mechanisms of glomerular injury.

nephrotic syndrome. Nephritic syndrome is associated with an immune response that is inflammatory. Nephrotic syndrome is associated with an immune response that is noninflammatory. The location of the injury in the glomerulus can be a determinant of whether the patient will have a nephritic or nephrotic clinical presentation. These two clinical syndromes can both be present in some disorders and some disorders progress from one to another.

Nephritic Syndrome

A key feature of nephritic syndrome is the passage of leukocytes, red blood cells, and plasma proteins which occur as a result of inflammation. Glomerular disorders that affect endothelial and mesangial cells (Figure 7-18) are exposed to all the factors activated during the immune response such as neutrophils, macrophages, and complement proteins. The result is glomerular inflammation, cellular proliferation, and capillary damage with red blood cells

and white blood cells escaping into the urine (i.e., hematuria and leukocyturia). Proteins, usually albumin, will also be present in the urine but in much smaller amounts than in nephrotic syndrome. Glomerulonephritis with nephritic syndrome can occur after an infection (i.e., acute postinfectious glomerulonephritis) and with other disorders such as lupus nephritis. Nephritic syndrome can also present clinically as rapidly progressive glomerulonephritis.

Acute postinfectious glomerulonephritis usually occurs after an infection with group A beta-hemolytic streptococci. The disorder is the most common cause of acute glomerulonephritis in children, particularly in developing countries. The incidence has decreased in countries such as the United States due to treatment of streptococcal infections of the throat (e.g., pharyngitis) or skin (e.g., impetigo). The risk is highest in children between the ages of 5 and 12. The incidence in adults is greater after age 60, and adults are more likely to be infected with staphylococcus. Adults with diabetes, alcoholism, cancer, or intravenous drug addiction are at higher risk for developing acute postinfectious glomerulonephritis. Other organisms causing acute glomerulonephritis can include viruses such as hepatitis or parasites. The mechanism of acute postinfectious glomerulonephritis includes the formation of immune complexes, which are composed of the antigenic organism streptococcus with IgG and C3 complement. Infection with staphylococcus reacts more with IgA in addition to IgG. The immune complexes are either circulating in the blood or formed within the glomerulus. The complexes activate the immune system, resulting in proliferation of cells in the endothelial and mesangial cells. The capillary membrane becomes permeable.

Up to 50% of patients with acute poststreptococcal glomerulonephritis can be asymptomatic or have mild hematuria. Symptoms usually occur 1–2 weeks after a throat infection and up to 6 weeks after impetigo. In patients infected with staphylococcus, the infection can be from the skin, heart, bone, and other areas but not usually the throat as in streptococcus. Some patients with acute poststreptococcal glomerulonephritis can present with a more severe complete acute nephritic syndrome, which is characterized by sudden hematuria. Patients may describe their urine color as a tea or cola. The urine usually has dysmorphic cells with or without red blood cell casts. Pyuria is also present. Proteinuria levels can vary and are usually not in the nephrotic range (i.e., $\geq$ 3.5 grams per day). The thickened membrane decreases blood flow and GFR, leading to sodium and water retention as well as oliguria. The retention causes generalized edema and hypertension, which can range from mild to severe. Manifestations may also include malaise, irritability, and fever. Acute hypertension can cause central nervous system manifestations (e.g., headache, vomiting, and seizures). Other complications can include fluid overload with pulmonary edema, acute renal failure, and rarely hypertensive encephalopathy. Adults who are more likely to have staphylococcal infection may have cutaneous vasculitis, which imitates other vasculitis causing glomerulonephritis such as IgA vasculitis (Henoch-Schönlein purpura) and antineutrophil cytoplasmic antibody (ANCA) vasculitis.

Diagnosis is usually made based on clinical findings with a history of recent streptococcal or staphylococcal infection (e.g., positive culture or serologic antistreptolysin titers). In addition to the abnormal urine findings, complement levels (C3 and CH50 total complement) levels are low. Renal biopsy to diagnose streptococcal infection is usually not indicated as resolution of the disorder usually begins within 1 month. With staphylococcal infections, a kidney biopsy is usually necessary to confirm diagnosis due to the multiple differential diagnoses. Treatment includes antibiotics and supportive care that includes managing fluid overload with salt and water restriction and diuretics. Dialysis may be necessary with fluid overload, hyperkalemia, and uremia (elevated BUN) that are not responding to other therapies. Adults with staphylococcal infection can have resolution but often have persistent proteinuria and can progress to end-stage renal disease.

IgA vasculitis (i.e., Henoch-Schönlein purpura) is a systemic immune vasculitis that affects mainly small vessels throughout the body. The vessels affected are usually in the skin and cause palpable purpura. Affected vessels in the gastrointestinal tract will cause abdominal pain, and affected vessels in the musculoskeletal system will cause arthralgia and arthritis. The disease is mostly seen in children between the ages of 3 and 15 with a higher prevalence in boys than girls. The disorder, in about 20% of children, can affect the glomerulus. Renal involvement is more likely in older children and adults and is more likely to be associated with more severe renal disease. Glomerular

blood vessel damage and inflammation occur due to the deposition of immune complexes (usually IgA), resulting in nephritic syndrome (e.g., hematuria with minimal to no proteinuria). Nephrotic syndrome is not as common. With limited renal involvement (e.g., mild hematuria and proteinuria), therapy may not be required, and close monitoring may be all that is necessary. Those individuals with more renal involvement may need corticosteroids and other therapies such as those discussed with other nephropathies. The disorder is usually self-limiting, and complete remission occurs usually within 1 month but may take longer in those individuals who have more significant renal involvement.

Rapidly progressive glomerulonephritis (i.e., rapidly progressive crescentic glomerulonephritis) is a rare clinical syndrome with serious consequences if not diagnosed early. The disorder is a manifestation of severe glomerular injury. The disorder can manifest quickly over a period of days to months and is more common in adults over the age of 50. The disorder is characterized by extensive crescent formation (which is the shape of the Bowman capsule). There are three types or mechanisms of injury:

- **Type 1:** This type is an anti-glomerular basement membrane antibody disease (Goodpasture syndrome) with IgG antibodies forming against pulmonary and alveolar capillary membrane.
- **Type 2:** Immune complexes are deposited in the glomeruli due to multiple disorders that cause immune complex development such as lupus nephritis, IgA nephropathy, and postinfectious glomerulonephritis.
- **Type 3:** This type is a form of necrotizing glomerulonephritis called *Pauci-immune glomerulonephritis*, where there are few, if any, immune complexes. Rather, serum ANCA attack small blood vessels. This type of glomerulonephritis will develop with systemic diseases such as granulomatous disease (e.g., Wegener granulomatosis) or microscopic polyangiitis.

Fibrin, macrophages, and T cells cause inflammation with proliferation of these substances into the Bowman space regardless the mechanism of injury. Collagen and fibrous deposits develop into crescents, which decreases glomerular blood flow and, in turn, glomerular filtration rate.

Onset may be rapid with signs similar to other nephritic syndromes (e.g., oliguria, hematuria, edema, and hypertension) or insidious with fatigue and edema. Renal insufficiency as manifested by a serum creatinine of > 3 mg/dL is often present at diagnosis. Other manifestations may be present if there are other systemic diseases such as in pauci-immune glomerulonephritis. Those individuals with anti-GBM may have hemoptysis since the alveolar membranes are also a target of the immune complexes.

Diagnostic tests are similar to other disorders and geared toward looking for the underlying causes. Tests may include serum ANCA, antinuclear antibodies, and anti-GBM antibodies. Renal biopsy may be necessary. The number of crescents that form play a part in the severity of the disease, and those patients with fewer crescents have a better prognosis and a slower disease progression. Treatment consists of immunosuppressive therapy with corticosteroids or cyclophosphamide. Plasmapheresis may be considered to remove circulating antibodies.

Diagnostic Link

Proteinuria vs. Albuminuria

While the GFR is a measure of renal function, the presence of protein/albumin in urine is a sign of kidney damage. The two major groups of serum proteins are albumin and globulins, and these can be measured in the urine. The total amount of protein (albumin and nonalbumin) excreted by adults is usually 150 mg/day. Glomerular disorders are usually associated with the passage of large molecules such as albumin into the urine (i.e., albuminuria). Tubular disorders are usually associated with the passage of lower molecular weight proteins such as immunoglobulins into the urine . The urine dipstick primarily detects albumin and only when the levels are above 300 mg/day (formerly known as *macroalbuminuria*). However, diluted urine may reveal a false negative. Low levels of albumin in the urine are associated with kidney disease, an albumin-to-creatinine (ACR) ratio on a random (spot) urine sample or a 24-hour collection should be done. The ACR will detect albumin levels in the range of 30–300 mg/day (formerly called *microalbuminuria*). Detection of other proteins (including albumin) such as immunoglobulin light chains that are present in multiple myeloma can be accomplished with a screening tool known as the sulfosalicylic acid test.

Nephrotic Syndrome

Glomerular disorders resulting in nephrotic syndrome are a result of the immune injury affecting mainly podocytes (i.e., visceral epithelial cells) (Figure 7-18). Podocytes are an important barrier to proteins passing to the filtrate. Proteins also pass due to the loss of the negative charge on the endothelial and basement membrane that repelled proteins.

Injury, therefore, causes massive quantities of proteins to pass into the urine. The proteinuria for nephrotic syndrome is defined as 3.5 g/day or greater in adults and 50 mg/kg of body weight in children. The protein lost is mainly albumin, but other plasma proteins may be present in the urine (e.g., transferrin, clotting inhibitors). Glomerular inflammation is usually minimal, so hematuria is absent or minor. No red blood cell casts are present in the urine. Due to the massive protein loss, hypoalbuminemia occurs (serum < 3 g/dL). The colloid oncotic pressure decreases, causing water to go into the interstitial spaces, and generalized edema develops. Sodium and water are retained, worsening the edema. The decreased oncotic pressure causes the liver to produce more albumin, but it is insufficient to maintain levels in comparison to the decline. Additionally, the decreased oncotic pressure stimulates the liver to increase the production of lipids, so nephrotic syndrome causes hypercholesteremia (cholesterol > 300 mg/dL) and hypertriglyceridemia. The lipids can be present in the urine (lipiduria) and can be seen as fatty casts or oval fat bodies. Additionally, immunoglobulins are excreted in the urine; this loss of immune cells, in turn, increases the individual's risk for infection.

Nephrotic syndrome can be due to primary kidney disease such as minimal change disease, which is a common cause in children. Adults develop nephrotic syndrome usually due to systemic disorders such as diabetes, systemic lupus erythematosus, or amyloidosis. Membranous nephropathy is a common cause of primary kidney disease in adults that causes nephrotic syndrome.

Most cases of primary nephrotic syndrome in children are idiopathic. Among the idiopathic cases, many children histologically have podocyte loss and minimal changes on renal biopsy. Immunoglobulin deposition is absent. These minimal changes are termed **minimal change disease**, which is also known as lipoid nephrosis. Affected children are usually between the ages of 2 and 6 years old. Children with minimal change disease do not usually have hypertension and hematuria. Renal function may be normal or impaired due to intravascular volume depletion, and complement levels are normal. Due to the volume loss, there may be hemoconcentration and increased platelets with risk for hypercoagulation and thrombosis. Minimal change disease is usually treated with steroids.

A common cause of primary nephrotic syndrome in adults is **membranous nephropathy** (i.e., membranous glomerulonephritis). The disease, however, can also be associated with systemic disorders such as hepatitis B, autoimmune disorders and certain drugs (e.g., nonsteroidal anti-inflammatory drugs). The disorder is more common in White men but can occur in women and other ethnicities (e.g., there is higher incidence in China). The diagnosis reflects that the histologic changes occur in the basement membrane, which becomes thickened, but there is no cell proliferation as seen with other glomerular disorders. The membrane becomes thickened due to immune complex deposits formed from antibodies (e.g., IgG) and various antigens such as M-type phospholipase A2 receptors expressed on podocytes. Clinical manifestations are those of nephrotic syndrome (e.g., marked proteinuria and hypoalbuminemia), and diagnosis is made based on its presentation. Diagnostic tests can include a renal biopsy; however, serologic testing can detect antigens and antibodies associated with membranous nephropathy. Treatment includes immunosuppressive therapy (e.g., steroids), alkylating agents (e.g., cyclophosphamide), and calcineurin inhibitors (e.g., cyclosporine). Hypertension and kidney protection are accomplished with the use of angiotensin-converting enzyme inhibitors and/or angiotensin-2 receptor blockers. Some patients have complete remission while others progress to renal failure.

Focal segmental glomerulosclerosis is a histologic description for sclerotic lesions that occur in parts of the glomeruli (segmental) and some of the glomeruli (focal). The sclerosis is often present in adults and children with nephrotic syndrome. These lesions are more common in Blacks as compared to Whites. The disorder is often idiopathic. Patients can also have mild proteinuria with renal insufficiency that occurs due to glomerular injury from drugs (e.g., heroin and interferon) or viral infections such as human immunodeficiency virus. Genetic mutations can cause podocyte structural lesions and alter filtration barriers in the glomerulus (e.g., basement membrane). The genetic mutations will usually manifest as nephrotic syndrome in infancy and childhood.

IgA nephropathy (i.e., Berger disease) is a common cause of primary glomerulonephritis in adolescents and young adults (i.e., ages 15–30 years). The highest incidence is in Asians and Whites. IgA immune complexes are deposited in the mesangium. The inciting factors leading to the development of IgA nephropathy are unclear; however, there may be dysregulation in the synthesis and metabolism of IgA with mesangial cell affinity and reaction to the antibodies. The deposits cause cell proliferation, an inflammatory response with subsequent crescent formation, interstitial fibrosis, and segmental sclerosis.

BOX 7-4 Application to Practice

A 20-year-old Black woman is complaining of increasing fatigue, swelling in her legs, and darker urine. She denies any fever or other symptoms. She was diagnosed with systemic lupus erythematosus 1 year ago. She has been taking chloroquine, and she takes ibuprofen for joint pain about one or two times a month.

Physical examination: pulse 98 per minute; blood pressure 150/100 mmHg; remainder of exam is unremarkable except for 2+ pitting edema in her lower extremities.

Laboratory results: urinalysis with hematuria (10 RBCs per HPF) with no casts; proteinuria of 8 g/24 hr; low complement level; serum creatinine of 1.31 mg/dL.

A diagnosis of lupus nephritis is made pending renal biopsy results.

Answer the following questions:

1. What is the incidence and epidemiology of lupus nephritis?
2. Which clinical manifestations and laboratory findings are consistent with lupus nephritis? Explain why the clinical manifestations develop.
3. Describe how lupus nephritis develops.

BOX 7-5 Application to Practice

A 13-year-old boy presented to the clinic complaining of a sore throat that persisted for 2 days. After those 2 days, he developed fever, nausea, and malaise. A throat culture revealed the presence of group A beta-hemolytic streptococci, and the child was started on antibiotic therapy. The child's symptoms gradually improved, but approximately 2 weeks later, he returned to the clinic because the fever, nausea, and malaise returned. He became tachypneic and short of breath. The mother noted that his eyes were puffy, his ankles were swollen, and his urine was dark and cloudy.

On examination, the child's blood pressure was 148/100 mmHg, his pulse was 122 beats/minute, and his respirations were 35/minute. Orbital and ankle edema were present. Crackles were auscultated bilaterally. No heart murmurs were found. Slight tenderness to percussion over the flank areas was noted.

A chest X-ray showed evidence of congestion and edema in the lungs. The patient's hematocrit was 37%, and his WBC count was 11,200/mm^3. Blood urea nitrogen was 48 mg/dL (normal is less than 20 mg/dL). Urinalysis results showed that the patient's protein was 2+ (24-hour excretion was 0.8 g),

specific gravity was 1.012, and there were moderate amounts of RBCs and WBCs in the urine. Serum albumin was 4.1 g/dL (normal is 3.5–4.5).

1. Which evidence supports the conclusion that this patient has a kidney disease?
2. Which clinical pattern of kidney disease does this patient have? Explain the symptoms.
3. Which morphologic changes would you expect in the kidney?
4. What is the prognosis? What are the possible short- and long-term complications of this disease? Is it necessary to hospitalize the patient?

Clinical presentation may be asymptomatic and the disorder is found with incidental screening. The urine may reveal mild proteinuria or microscopic hematuria. Other patients may have episodes of gross hematuria with an upper respiratory infection. Patients can also complain of flank pain as the renal capsules stretch. Episodes of hematuria and proteinuria can recur for several years, and progression is gradual. Diagnosis is usually accomplished with a renal biopsy. Treatment is aimed at preventing chronic kidney disease through managing hypertension and kidney protection with the use of angiotensin-converting enzyme inhibitors and/or angiotensin-2 receptor blockers. Lipid levels should be low to reduce the cardiovascular risks associated with chronic kidney disease. Anti-inflammatory and immunosuppressive therapy benefits are not clear in IgA nephropathy and such therapy is usually reserved for renal disease that is progressing (e.g., increased serum creatinine or persistent proteinuria).

Chronic glomerulonephritis is a result of progressive types of glomerulonephritis that usually lead to chronic kidney disease. The underlying disorder may be difficult to determine as multiple glomerular changes may be present. Hyperlipidemia, hypertension, systemic lupus erythematosus, and diabetes mellitus are all associated with the development of chronic glomerulonephritis.

Kidney Injury and Disease

The pivotal role that the kidneys play in maintaining homeostasis becomes clear when these organs stop performing that role. *Renal failure* refers to the kidneys' inability to function adequately; it is classified as either acute or chronic. See chapter 6 for a discussion of fluid, electrolyte, and acid–base homeostasis.

Acute Kidney Injury

Acute kidney injury (AKI), formerly known as acute renal failure, refers to a sudden loss of renal function. The loss of renal function, which is generally reversible, most commonly occurs in critically ill, hospitalized patients. Causes include disorders such as sepsis, volume deficits (e.g., heart failure, cirrhosis), and nephrotoxic drugs (e.g., vancomycin). Prerenal disorders along with acute tubular necrosis are the most common cause of AKI in hospitalized patients. AKI has a mortality rate of 10–60% depending on the underlying etiology. Its causes are divided into three categories:

1. Prerenal conditions, which disrupt blood flow on its way to the kidneys:
   - Extremely low blood pressure or blood volume (e.g., hemorrhage, sepsis, dehydration, shock, and traumatic injury)
   - Heart dysfunction (e.g., myocardial infarction and heart failure)
   - Liver disease with portal hypertension

2. Intrarenal conditions, which directly damage the structures of the kidneys and can be further divided into vascular disease, glomerular disease, or tubular and interstitial disease:

- Reduced blood supply within the kidneys (e.g., atherosclerosis; renal vein thrombosis, renal aneurysm, and aortic dissection)
- Hemolytic uremic syndrome (associated with infection with certain strains of *E. coli*, in which bacterium toxins damage small blood vessels; it is the leading cause of acute kidney failure in children)
- Glomerular disorders (e.g., glomerulonephritis and acute interstitial nephritis [usually associated with an allergic reaction to certain nephrotoxic medications])
- Tubular disorders (e.g., obstructions from myoglobinuria, multiple myeloma light chains, uric acid casts)
- Toxic injury (usually from alcohol, cocaine, heavy metals, solvents, fuels, chemotherapy drugs, bowel preparations containing phosphate, and contrast dyes)

3. Postrenal conditions, which interfere with the urine excretion:

- Bilateral ureter obstruction (e.g., nephrolithiasis and tumors)
- Bladder obstruction and dysfunction (e.g., BPH, tumors, and nerve innervation disruption)

Acute tubular necrosis (ATN) or **acute tubular injury** is a common cause of intrarenal AKI. The most common cause of ATN is ischemia due to decreased renal perfusion. The exposure to nephrotoxic drugs and substances is another common cause. Many nephrons drain into a single collecting duct (Figure 7-2). A reduction in blood flow to the kidneys sets the stage for the development of ATN. The endothelial cells in the microcirculation of the kidneys become injured. The blood vessels become more permeable, and the inflammatory response is triggered. Leukocytes, macrophages, and complement are activated with release of chemical mediators (e.g., chemokines or tumor necrosis factor). These microcirculatory changes further contribute to the reduction in renal blood flow, further worsening tubular injury. Sodium, water, and transport of other substances is impaired, and the tubular border sheds. This shedding can result in tubular casts in the urine. The tubules can become obstructed from the cellular debris.

The intraluminal obstruction causes the pressure to rise in the lumen, and fluid backs up. The fluid moves from the lumen to the interstitium. Necrosis develops along multiple areas of the tubule. ATN is generally reversible.

Clinical Manifestations

AKI has an abrupt onset (usually over a period of 48 hours) and progresses through four phases. The progression through these phases is particularly characteristic of acute tubular necrosis. The individual is usually asymptomatic in the initial phase. Although renal damage is occurring, the nephrons that are still functioning compensate for those that are not. During the second (oliguric) phase, impaired glomerular filtration leads to solute and water reabsorption. This reabsorption decreases daily urine output to approximately 400 mL or less, such that waste products begin to accumulate (uremia). The second phase can last a few days to a few weeks. In the third (diuretic) phase, renal function gradually returns as healing and cellular regeneration occur. Diuresis occurs due to tubular damage that impairs the kidneys' ability to concentrate the urine. Daily urine output in this phase can be as much as 5 L. The excessive urine output can lead to dehydration and electrolyte imbalances. The third phase can last days to weeks. In the recovery stage, glomerular function gradually returns to normal. This final stage can persist for 3–12 months. Depending on the age and overall health of the individual, full renal function may be regained.

As previously mentioned, the initial phase of AKI is asymptomatic. As renal function is lost, symptoms appear. Clinical manifestations vary depending on the AKI phase. In the oliguric phase, manifestations include:

- Decreased urine output
- Electrolyte disturbances (usually increased levels)
- Fluid volume excess
- Azotemia
- Metabolic acidosis

In the diuretic phase, manifestations include:

- Increased urine output
- Electrolyte disturbances (usually decreased levels)
- Dehydration
- Hypotension

In the recovery phase, symptoms begin resolving.

Diagnosis and Treatment

The diagnostic criteria for AKI in adults and children are those defined by the Kidney Disease: Improving Global Outcomes guidelines and are as follows: 1) increase in serum creatinine by $\geq$ 0.3 mg/dL within a 48-hour period; or 2) increase in serum creatinine to > 1.5 times baseline, which has occurred in the prior 7 days; or 3) urine volume < 0.5 mL/kg/hour for 6 hours. Diagnostic procedures for AKI include those to identify both the renal injury and its underlying cause. These procedures consist of a history and physical examination. Often in the hospital, a cause can be identified (e.g., hypotension, sepsis, or drug administration). Evaluation of serum creatinine trends may reveal when an injury occurred particularly if the serum creatinine was normal and then suddenly increased. Diagnostic tests will include a BUN, blood chemistry, arterial blood gases, and complete blood count. Urine evaluation includes a urinalysis, urine osmolality, urine sodium, and fractional excretion of sodium. Distinguishing ATN from prerenal AKI can be determined by evaluating the concentration of the urine. With ATN, concentration is impaired, while in prerenal AKI the resorptive function is maintained. Urinalysis may reveal myoglobin or various casts (e.g., brown granular, tubular epithelial cells). Treatment strategies for AKI vary depending on the phase and the cause. As an example, volume replacement is indicated in hypovolemia. Different fluid and electrolyte disturbances occur in the second and third phases, requiring different strategies for these phases. Some patients (e.g., those with fluid overload, hyperkalemia, acidosis, and uremia) with AKI may require temporary dialysis (e.g., hemodialysis or peritoneal dialysis) until renal recovery occurs. Continuous renal replacement therapy (CRRT) is an alternative to hemodialysis. CRRT is preferred for patients who are hemodynamically unstable. Patients may have less hypotension than with hemodialysis as CRRT is continuous and slower. Solute removal with CRRT is also higher than with hemodialysis. Other supportive strategies include the following measures:

- A diet that is high in calories and carbohydrates but restricted in protein, sodium, potassium, and phosphates
- Hypertension management
- Anemia treatment with synthetic erythropoietin
- Infection prevention strategies (e.g., hand washing, limiting visitors, and aseptic technique)

Chronic Kidney Disease

Chronic kidney disease (CKD) consists of the gradual, irreversible loss of renal function. An estimated 23 million adults are living with CKD in the United States (NIH, 2013). Several conditions can initiate the slow, progressive destruction of the nephrons with diabetes mellitus and hypertension as the two most common causes. Renal diseases such as polycystic kidney disease, pyelonephritis, and glomerulonephritis damage nephrons in a variety of ways. Systemic illnesses such as lupus erythematosus and sickle cell anemia can cause CKD. Aging confers a risk for CKD as the kidneys generally become less efficient and are exposed to more conditions that can cause damage.

Regardless of which disorder has caused CKD, nephrons are progressively damaged. This damage results in the inability of the kidneys to perform critical filtration, resorptive, and endocrine functions. Inability of the kidney to perform results in water (e.g., increased volume) and electrolyte imbalances (e.g., hyperkalemia), accumulation of nitrogenous wastes (e.g., azotemia), acid–base imbalances (e.g., metabolic acidosis) as well as altered vitamin D, calcium, and phosphate balance (e.g., osteodystrophy). These alterations are usually slow to develop and often do not manifest until there is advanced renal disease as the kidneys have a remarkable capacity to compensate for failing nephrons. The compensatory mechanisms ultimately lead to further damage to surviving nephrons.

Two key factors are postulated to contribute to the progression of CKD—intraglomerular hypertension and glomerular hypertrophy. When nephrons are damaged and lost, surviving nephrons take over filtration function in an attempt to maintain GFR, a process known as hyperfiltration. There is adaptive renal vasodilation, reduction in glomerular permeability, and an adaptive rise in intraglomerular pressure in response to a reduced GFR. As a result, the glomeruli hypertrophy, which causes glomeruli injury. Further cellular mechanisms that are not completely understood include endothelial cell damage. Glomerular epithelial cells detach from the capillary wall, allowing water and solutes to pass more freely, but large molecules (e.g., IgM, fibrinogen) get trapped, producing hyaline casts and lumen narrowing. The mesangial cells produce cytokines and begin to expand, further crowding the capillary area. The structural and functional changes all lead to glomerulosclerosis (i.e., scarring).

Tubulointerstitial injury in CKD in the form of dilation and fibrosis is present even if the primary area of injury is the glomerulus. The tubulointerstitial injury is thought to occur due to vessel changes and accumulation of inflammatory substance in the tubules.

In 2002, the National Kidney Foundation Kidney Disease Outcomes Quality Initiative guidelines defined and classified CKD based on five stages (**TABLE 7-5**). In 2012, the guidelines were updated to include albuminuria as increased levels have been associated with increased mortality, cardiovascular events, and end-stage renal diseases. The definition and diagnosis of CKD is based on the following criteria:

1. Kidney damage for $\geq$ 3 months, as defined by structural or functional abnormalities of the kidney, with or without decreased GFR
2. GFR < 60 mL/min/1.73 m^2 for $\geq$ 3 months, with or without kidney damage

Kidney damage is defined as albuminuria (albumin excretion rate > 30 mg/24 hours; ACR > 30 mg/g), urine sediment abnormalities, electrolytes disorders due to tubular disorders, kidney disorders based on histology or structural abnormalities, and history of kidney transplant.

TABLE 7-5	CKD Stages Based on GFR and Albuminuria Levels
GFR stages	**GFR (mL/min/1.73 m^2)/term**
G1	$\geq$ 90 normal or high
G2	60–89 mildly decreased
G3a	45–59 mildly to moderately decreased
G3b	30–44 moderately to severely decreased
G4	15–29 severely decreased
G5	< 15 kidney failure or dialysis
Albuminuria stages	**AER mg/day**
A1	< 30 normal to mildly increased
A2	30–300 moderately increased
A3	> 300 severely increased

GFR = glomerular filtration rate; AER = albumin excretion ratio.

Clinical Manifestations

Clinical manifestations are complex and dependent on the degree of renal function lost. These manifestations also reflect the complications associated with CKD (**TABLE 7-6**). Initially, CKD is often asymptomatic because the remaining nephrons compensate for those lost to the disease. Clinical manifestations develop insidiously as 50% of the nephrons are destroyed. Multiple systems are affected as CKD progresses. These complications worsen as the renal function declines.

These manifestations include the following signs and symptoms:

- Hypertension (see chapter 4)
- Polyuria with pale urine (early)
- Oliguria or anuria (absent urine output) with dark-colored urine (late)
- Anemia
- Bruising and bleeding tendencies
- Electrolyte imbalances, specifically hyperkalemia, hypocalcemia, hypomagnesemia, and hyperphosphatemia
- Muscle twitches and cramps (related to hypocalcemia and hyperphosphatemia; see chapter 6)
- Pericarditis, pericardial effusion, pleuritis, and pleural effusion (secondary to uremia)
- Heart failure (see chapter 4)
- Respiratory distress and abnormal breath sounds (due to pulmonary edema associated with congestive heart failure; see chapter 4)
- Sudden weight change (usually increased because of fluid retention)
- Edema of the feet and ankles (due to fluid retention)
- Azotemia
- Peripheral neuropathy, restless legs syndrome, and seizures
- Nausea and vomiting
- Anorexia
- Malaise
- Fatigue and weakness
- Headaches that seem unrelated to any other cause
- Sleep disturbances
- Decreased mental alertness
- Flank pain
- Jaundice
- Persistent pruritus
- Recurrent infections (due to an impaired immune response because of uremia)

TABLE 7-6	Complications of Chronic Kidney Disease	
System	**Manifestations and etiology**	**Treatment**
General appearance	Tired, weak, sallow (yellow or pale) skin color due to anemia and toxins	Dialysis and epoetin alfa
Integumentary	Itching due to phosphate crystals and urea crystals (uremic frost) Dry, decreased sweating due to decreased oil and sweat gland activity	Dialysis and palliative care
Sensory	Metallic taste in mouth and fishy breath odor (uremic fetor) due to toxins	Dialysis
Cardiopulmonary	**Hypertension** Related to salt and water retention, erythropoietin (20% of patients on this therapy develop CKD), or increased renin production Accelerated renal damage if not controlled development of **heart failure**	Limiting salt and fluids Angiotensin-converting enzyme (ACE) inhibitors, angiotensin-2 receptor blockers and other agents
	Pericarditis Result of metabolic toxins Chest pain, fever, friction rub, and decreased cardiac output	Hemodialysis
	Heart disease Heart failure (in 75% of patients needing dialysis), **ischemic heart disease**, **cardiomyopathy** Result of increased workload of the heart (left ventricular hypertrophy) secondary to anemia, dialysis (shunting of blood), fluid overload, hypertension, hyperlipidemia, and atherosclerosis	Salt and fluid restriction Diuretics (loop) ACE inhibitors and angiotensin-2 receptor blockers
Hematologic	**Coagulopathy** Platelet dysfunction due to abnormal aggregation and adhesion Increased bleeding time Platelet count slightly decreased May have petechiae or purpura Increased risk of thrombosis	Desmopressin (causes release of factor VIII from endothelial cells)—used before surgery
	Anemia Related to decreased erythropoietin production (occurs when glomerular filtration rate falls below 20–25 mL/min), iron deficiency (e.g., anorexia, dietary restrictions, hemodialysis blood loss), uremia causes bone marrow suppression Red blood cell destruction due to hemodialysis	Epoetin alfa if hematocrit is below 33% (hemoglobin levels should increase no more than 1 g/dL every 3–4 weeks so hypertension does not develop) Intravenous iron for patients on dialysis (oral absorption of iron is poor)
Gastrointestinal	Anorexia, nausea, vomiting, hiccups, ulceration—related to metabolic toxins (e.g., ammonia) PTH	Dietary protein restriction Dialysis

(continues)

TABLE 7-6	Complications of Chronic Kidney Disease (*Continued*)	
System	**Manifestations and etiology**	**Treatment**
Endocrine	**Sexual dysfunction**	
	Decreased libido, impotence, and infertility	Dialysis and a healthy diet to restore fertility
	Decreased estrogen levels in women—no ovulation; menorrhagia; amenorrhea	
	Decreased testosterone levels in men	
	Glucose impairment	
	Glucose intolerance	Lower doses of hypoglycemic agents for some patients with diabetes
	Peripheral insulin resistance	
	Serum insulin high	
	Kidneys cannot clear insulin from the bloodstream	
Mineral metabolism	Renal osteodystrophy (disorder of calcium, phosphorus, and bone) leading to bone pain, fractures, muscle weakness, and calcium deposits in the blood vessels, soft tissue, heart, and lungs	
	Low glomerular filtration rate, slower phosphorus excretion, increased calcium excretion	Restriction of dietary phosphorus
	Increase in parathyroid hormone secretion, leading to a high bone turnover rate	Phosphorus-binding drugs such as calcium carbonate
	In stage V, buffering of excess hydrogen ions by leaching of large stores of calcium phosphate and calcium carbonate from the bones (bone demineralization)	Vitamin D (suppresses parathyroid hormone)
Neurologic	**Uremic encephalopathy**	
	Appears when glomerular filtration rate falls below 10–15 mL/min or because of hyperparathyroidism	Dialysis
	Symptoms: poor concentration (first sign) that progresses to confusion, asterixis, weakness, nystagmus, and hyperreflexia	
	Peripheral nervous system	
	Peripheral neuropathy (restless leg syndrome, distal pain and burning, and loss of deep tendon reflexes), usually symmetrical, lower limbs more commonly affected	
	Impotence and autonomic dysfunction	
Metabolic	**Hyperkalemia**	
	Glomerular filtration rate below 10–20 mL/min	Monitoring of cardiac status
	Hemolysis, trauma, and acidosis	Calcium chlorides, insulin, glucose (insulin moves potassium into cells), bicarbonate, or an exchange resin
	Diet high in citrus fruits/juices	
	Medications such as ACE inhibitors and nonsteroidal anti-inflammatory drugs	Dietary potassium restriction
Acid–base disorders	**Damaged kidneys**	
	Cannot produce enough ammonia or buffer hydrogen ions	Maintenance of serum bicarbonate above 21 mEq/L by giving alkali supplements such as sodium bicarbonate, calcium bicarbonate, or sodium citrate
	Arterial pH generally between 7.33 and 7.37	
	Buffering of excess hydrogen ions by large stores of calcium phosphate and calcium carbonate from the bones	

Modified from Story, L. (2017). *Pathophysiology: A Practical Approach* (3rd ed.). Burlington, MA: Jones & Bartlett Learning.

Diagnosis and Treatment

Diagnosis of CKD is based on the criteria previously discussed (e.g., GFR and ACR). Diagnostic procedures then focus on identifying the underlying cause and any complications that have developed as a result of the development of CKD.

The main goal of CKD treatment is to stop or slow disease progression, usually by controlling the underlying cause. Additionally, strategies to treat and prevent complications will be necessary (Table 7-6). Doses of any medications will likely need adjustments; with limited excretion capability, medication toxicity is probable when the usual doses are given. Without treatment, CKD has a mortality rate of 100%. Conservative management strategies are employed early but evolve into more aggressive measures as renal function declines and include renal replacement therapy with dialysis or kidney transplant. In children with CKD, transplant is the best option to allow for optimal growth and development and better outcomes.

CHAPTER SUMMARY

The urinary system maintains homeostasis through a complex filter (kidney) that can regulate pH, fluid, electrolytes, and endocrine functions (e.g., blood glucose). Additionally, the urinary system is the main site for excreting waste products and other harmful substances obtained from the food and water ingested orally. A functioning urinary system is crucial to maintaining health, and disease in this system can have detrimental effects on other systems and the body as a whole.

Prevention and early treatment of these diseases are paramount to avoiding these consequences. Maintaining a healthy lifestyle (e.g., drinking plenty of fluids, avoiding harmful chemicals, preventing sexually transmitted infection, exercising, and smoking cessation) can help preserve urinary health. Many chronic diseases, such as hypertension and diabetes mellitus, can lead to kidney disease, so controlling blood pressure and blood glucose is crucial.

REFERENCES AND RESOURCES

AAOS. (2004). *Paramedic: Anatomy and physiology*. Sudbury, MA: Jones and Bartlett Publishers.

American Cancer Society. (2016). Cancers that develop in children. Retrieved from https://www.cancer.org/cancer/cancer-in-children/types-of-childhood-cancers.html

American Urological Society. (2014). Diagnosis and treatment of interstitial cystitis/bladder pain syndrome. Retrieved from https://www.auanet.org/guidelines/interstitial-cystitis-(ic/bps)-guideline

Baumberger-Henry, M. (2008). *Fluid and electrolytes* (2nd ed.). Sudbury, MA: Jones and Bartlett Publishers.

Bonnegio, R. G. B., & Salant, D. J. (2018). Mechanisms of immune injury of the glomerulus. In T. W. Post (Ed.), *Uptodate*. Waltham, MA: UpToDate, Inc. Retrieved from https://uptodate.com

Chintagumpala, M., & Muscal, J. A. (2018). Treatment and prognosis for Wilms tumor. In T. W. Post (Ed.), *Uptodate*. Waltham, MA; UpToDate, Inc. Retrieved from https://uptodate.com

Chiras, D. (2015). *Human biology* (8th ed.). Burlington, MA: Jones & Bartlett Learning.

Crowley, L. V. (2017). *An introduction to human disease* (10th ed.). Burlington, MA: Jones & Bartlett Learning.

Curahn, G. C., Aronson, M. D., & Preminger, G. M. (2018). Diagnosis and acute management of suspected nephrolithiasis in adults. In T. W. Post (Ed.), *Uptodate*. Waltham, MA: UpToDate, Inc. Retrieved from https://uptodate.com

de Jong, Y., Pinckaers, J., Brinck, R., Nijeholt, A., & Dekkers, O. (2014). Urinating standing versus sitting: Position is of influence in men with prostate enlargement. A systematic review and meta-analysis. *PLOS ONE, 9*(7), e101329.

Elling, B., Elling, K., & Rothenberg, M. (2004). *Anatomy and physiology*. Sudbury, MA: Jones and Bartlett Publishers.

Gould, B. (2015). *Pathophysiology for the health professions* (5th ed.). Philadelphia, PA: Elsevier.

Hanno, P. M., Burks, D. A., Clemens, J. Q., Dmochowski, R. R., Erickson, D., Fitzgerald, M. P...Faraday, M. M. (2011). AUA guideline for the diagnosis and treatment of interstitial cystitis/bladder pain syndrome. *Journal of Urology, 185*, 2162–2170.

Hanno, P. M., Erickson, D., Moldwin, R., & Faraday, M. M. (2015). Diagnosis and treatment of interstitial cystitis/bladder pain syndrome: AUA guideline amendment. *Journal of Urology, 193*, 1545–1553.

Inker, L. A., Astor, B. C., Isakova, T., Lash, J. P., Peraltal, C. A., Tamura, M., & Feldman, H. I. (2014). KDOQI US commentary on the 2012 KDIGO clinical practice guideline for the evaluation and management of CKD. *American Journal of Kidney Diseases, 63*(5), 713–735.

Khwaja, A. (2012). KDIGO clinical practice guidelines for acute kidney injury. *Nephron Clinical Practice, 120*, c179–c184. doi: 10.1159/000339789

Madara, B., & Pomarico-Denino, V. (2008). *Quick look nursing: Pathophysiology* (2nd ed.). Sudbury, MA: Jones and Bartlett Publishers.

National Cancer Institute. (2016). Wilms tumor and other childhood kidney tumors treatment (PDQ): Health professional version. Retrieved from http://www.cancer.gov/types/kidney/hp/wilms-treatment-pdq#section/all

National Cancer Institute. (2018a). Bladder cancer treatment (PDQ). Retrieved from http://www.ncbi.nlm.nih.gov/pubmedhealth/PMH0032608/

National Cancer Institute. (2018b). Renal cell cancer treatment (PDQ): Health professional version. Retrieved from http://www.cancer.gov/types/kidney/hp/kidney-treatment-pdq#link/_228_toc

National Institutes of Health (NIH). (2013). Chronic kidney disease and kidney failure. Retrieved from http://report.nih.gov/NIHfactsheets/ViewFactSheet.aspx?csid=34&key=C

National Institutes of Health (NIH). (2015). Polycystic kidney disease. Retrieved from https://www.niddk.nih.gov/health-information/health-topics/kidney-disease/polycystic-kidney-disease-pkd/Pages/facts.aspx

National Kidney Foundation. (2002). Kidney disease outcome quality initiative clinical practice guidelines for chronic kidney disease: Evaluation, classification, and stratification. *American Journal of Kidney Diseases, 39*, S1.

Professional guide to pathophysiology (3rd ed.). (2010). Philadelphia, PA: Lippincott Williams & Wilkins.

Resnick, N., & Yalla, S. (1998). Geriatric incontinence and voiding dysfunction. In P. C. Walsh, A. B. Retik, E. D. Vaughan, & A. J. Wein (Eds.), *Campbell's urology* (7th ed.). Philadelphia, PA: W.B. Saunders.

Sevcenco, S., Spick, C., Helbich, T. H., Heinz, G., Shariat, S. F., Klingler, H. C., … Baltzer, P. A. (2016). Malignancy rates and diagnostic performance of the Bosniak classification for the diagnosis of cystic renal lesions in computed tomography—a systematic review and meta-analysis. *European Radiology, 27*(6), 2239–2247.

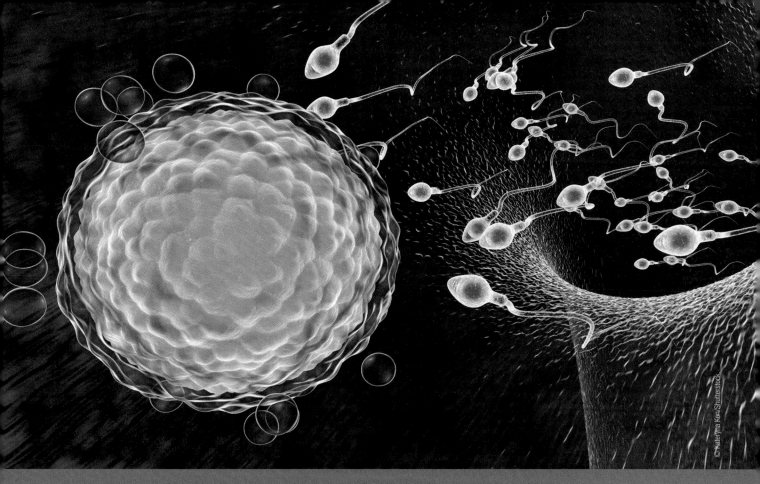

CHAPTER 8
Reproductive Function

LEARNING OBJECTIVES

- Discuss normal reproductive anatomy and physiology.
- Differentiate congenital reproductive disorders.
- Summarize issues with fertility.
- Differentiate penile, testicular, and scrotal disorders.
- Differentiate disorders that affect menstruation.
- Summarize disorders of pelvic support.
- Differentiate uterine and ovarian disorders.
- Differentiate breast disorders.

- Differentiate infectious disorders of the reproductive system.
- Summarize cancers of the reproductive system.
- Apply understanding of reproductive system alterations in describing various common disorders such as leiomyomas, erectile dysfunction, and sexually transmitted infections.
- Develop diagnostic and treatment considerations for various reproductive disorders.

The reproductive system is composed of the structures responsible for procreation; therefore, a healthy reproduction system is necessary for the survival of the species. This system is responsible for transmitting genetic material to offspring. The male reproductive system generates sperm and transports it to the female reproductive system. The female reproductive system produces ova. When a sperm fertilizes an ovum, the female reproductive system nurtures and safeguards the embryo as it develops into a fetus, with this process lasting until birth. The primary difference between the two systems is the varying hormone levels, which cause the reproductive system to develop differently.

Anatomy and Physiology

Normal Male Reproductive System

The male reproductive system includes organs involved in the generation (spermatogenesis) and transportation of sperm. These organs include the penis, scrotum, testes, duct system, and accessory glands (FIGURE 8-1; TABLE 8-1).

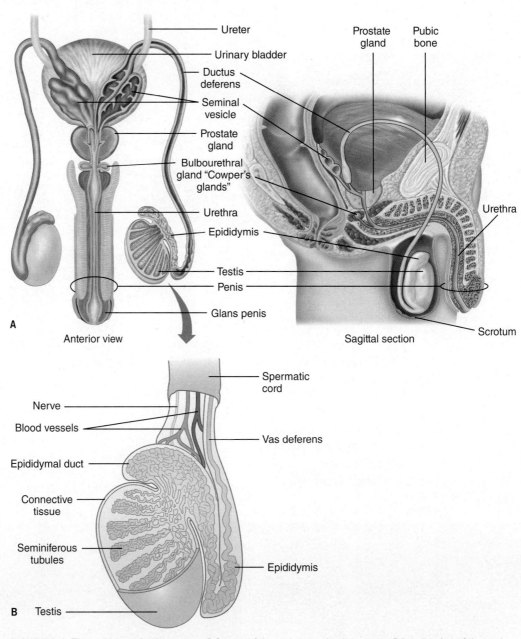

FIGURE 8-1 The male reproductive system. **A** Organs of the male reproductive system. **B** Interior view of the testis.

In addition to producing sperm, the male reproduction system produces sex hormones (mostly testosterone) that give males their distinct characteristics (e.g., facial hair, increased muscle mass, and low voice pitch). Parts of the male reproductive system work with the urinary system to aid in urinary elimination (e.g., penis and urethra). Because the male reproductive and urinary systems are integrated, disorders in one system generally affect the other system (see chapter 7 for more discussion of urinary function).

Penis

The penis is part of the male external genitalia; it contains erectile tissue that fills with blood during sexual arousal. The penis deposits sperm in the female reproductive system during sexual intercourse. The penis consists of three cylinders—the corpus spongiosum (which contains the urethra) and two corpora cavernosa (**FIGURE 8-2**). The penis structure includes the root, shaft, and glans (enlarged tip). Penis length can vary considerably, but the average length is 2–5 inches when flaccid and 4–7 inches when erect. Penis appearance can also vary from person to person.

A sheath of loose skin, called the *foreskin*, covers the glans penis at birth. The foreskin is often surgically removed (circumcision) shortly after birth for hygienic, cultural, or religious reasons. If the foreskin is not removed, it usually becomes fully retractable usually by the age of 3 due to frequent erections breaking up adhesions (i.e., foreskin to glans). The

TABLE 8-1	The Male Reproductive System
Component	**Function**
Testes	Produce sperm and male sex steroids
Epididymis	Store sperm; provide nourishment for sperm maturation
Vas deferens	Conduct sperm to urethra
Sex accessory glands	Produce seminal fluid that nourishes sperm
Urethra	Conduct sperm to the outside of the male body
Penis	Organ of copulation
Scrotum	Provide proper temperature for testes and protection due to several sensory receptors

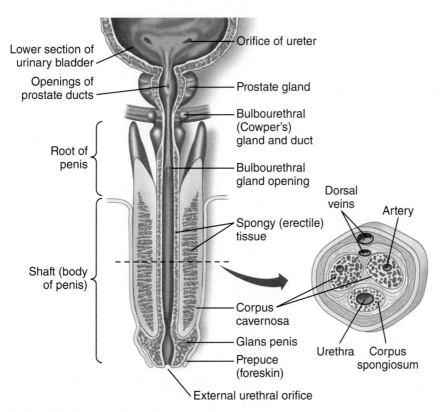

FIGURE 8-2 Anatomy of the penis.

glans produces an oily secretion that can combine with dead skin to form a cheesy substance called *smegma*. If the smegma is not regularly removed from under the foreskin, the penis can become irritated and infected. The glans also has an opening, or meatus, that allows for ejaculation (propulsion of sperm-containing fluid) and urination.

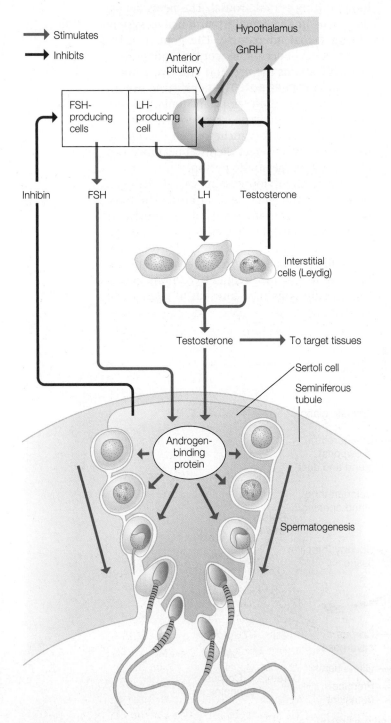

FIGURE 8-3 Hormonal control of testicular function: testosterone, FSH, and LH participate in a negative feedback loop.

Scrotum

The scrotum is a fibromuscular sac of skin just below the penis that contains the testes, epididymis, and lower spermatic cords. The scrotum maintains the proper testicular temperature for spermatogenesis by contracting to draw the testes closer to the body to warm them and relaxing to drop the testes farther from the body to cool them. Various sensory receptors to pain, pressure, touch, and temperature are on the scrotum to serve as a protective mechanism for the underlying testes.

Testes

The testes, or gonads, produce sperm (i.e., gametes) and the sex hormones testosterone and androgens. Spermatogenesis develops in most males by 16 years of age. Spermatogenesis, in contrast to ova production, occurs throughout life. The testes form in the abdominal cavity in utero and descend through the inguinal canal into the scrotum in approximately the seventh month of gestation when stimulated by rising testosterone levels. Occasionally, they will descend shortly after birth (usually by 3 months of age). Seminiferous tubules produce sperm, and the tubules are the bulk of testicular volume. The seminiferous tubules have specialized cells known as Sertoli cells that are necessary to provide nourishment to developing sperm (i.e., spermatids). Development takes about 70–80 days. The sperm then travel to a fingerlike projection on the posterior portion (in most men) of the testes known as the epididymis. The sperm mature during storage in the epididymis, making them capable of movement. The testes can produce approximately 50,000 sperm per minute.

The testes produce hormones (especially testosterone) in their Leydig cells. Other sources of testosterone and androgen are the adrenal glands (See chapter 10 on endocrine function).

The male sex and reproductive hormones are controlled by the hypothalamus, pituitary, and other feedback mechanisms (FIGURE 8-3). Neurotransmitters such as *norepinephrine* stimulate gonadotropin-releasing hormone (GnRH) from the hypothalamus, and the neurotransmitters, *serotonin* and *dopamine*, inhibit GnRH from the hypothalamus. GnRH stimulation occurs in a pulsatile fashion, which causes the production of luteinizing hormone (LH) and follicle-stimulating hormone (FSH) in the anterior pituitary. Prolactin release affects hormone production. These hormones cause stimulation of the testes. Subsequently, the various effects of these hormones are as follows:

- **LH:** Stimulates Leydig cells to produce and secrete testosterone (about 5–7 mg a day)
- **FSH:** Stimulates Sertoli cells (seminiferous tubules) promoting spermatogenesis
- **Inhibin:** Secreted by Sertoli cells; causes inhibition of FSH, which leads to reduction in spermatogonia (germ cells that eventually become sperm)

Testosterone is one of the main male sex hormones. Other hormones include 5-alpha-dihydrotestosterone (DHT) and estradiol. Testosterone, DHT, and estradiol hormones regulate LH secretion. Testosterone and DHT directly inhibit LH secretion from the pituitary gland while estradiol inhibits LH but does so by inhibiting GnRH from the hypothalamus. Inhibin is an important inhibitor of FSH with some effects from estradiol and minor regulation from testosterone.

The process of testosterone synthesis in the Leydig cells occurs in multiple steps (**FIGURE 8-4**). Testosterone, under LH stimulation, is produced initially by the conversion of cholesterol to pregnenolone then to dehydroepiandrosterone (DHEA) to androstenediol, and then to testosterone. In the testes, a small amount of testosterone is aromatized to estradiol or DHT. The enzyme, 5-alpha-reductase mediates the reduction of testosterone to DHT. Inhibition of this enzyme with 5-alpha-reductase inhibitors (e.g., finasteride [Proscar]) are used to treat benign prostatic hyperplasia. While some

estradiol is synthesized in the testes, most of the estradiol (estrone also) is produced in adipose tissue and other tissue such as the brain, skin, and bone. Estradiol effects include sexual function, bone growth, and body fat. While some DHT is produced in the testes, the majority is produced in the skin and liver. DHT is a potent androgen and is important in prostatic growth and male balding. Propecia, is another 5-alpha-reductase, that can be used for balding in men. See chapter 7 for a discussion of benign prostatic hyperplasia.

Testosterone in plasma is mostly bound to sex hormone–binding globulin (SHBG) and albumin. About 0.5–3% of testosterone is free (i.e., unbound). SHBG has a stronger bind to testosterone in comparison to albumin, so this testosterone is considered inactive. Serum SHBG increases with age; therefore; less testosterone is available as a man ages.

Testosterone and the metabolites (DHT and estradiol) give males their classic secondary sex characteristics (e.g., facial hair and deep voice) and sexual function (e.g., libido, erection, and satisfaction). Testosterone also regulates metabolism and protein anabolism (encourages skeletal growth and muscle development and lowers fat mass), and promotes potassium excretion and renal sodium reabsorption. Additionally, testosterone contributes to male pattern baldness and acne in some men. Testosterone increases erythropoiesis.

Duct System

The male reproductive system contains a complex tube structure to deliver sperm from the testes to the female reproductive system. This duct system includes the epididymis, vas deferens, spermatic cord, ejaculatory duct, and urethra. Once they are mature, sperm leave the epididymis and travel to the vas deferens. The testicular artery and venous plexus, lymph vessels, nerves, connective tissue, and cremaster muscle (which contracts or relaxes the scrotum) surround the vas deferens; together, these structures make up the spermatic cord. The spermatic cord essentially suspends the testes and is the testicular supply line. The vas deferens widens at the prostate, forming a pouch called the *ampulla*. The ampulla joins the seminal vesicles (a pair of pouches that secrete an alkaline ejaculatory fluid containing sugar, protein, and prostaglandins to nurture and protect the sperm) to form the ejaculatory duct. The sperm and the ejaculatory fluid join in the vesicles to form semen (i.e., ejaculate).

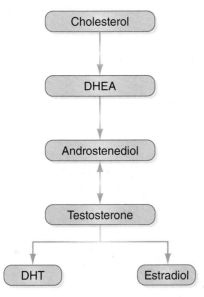

FIGURE 8-4 Testosterone synthesis and metabolism.

The semen flows from the ejaculatory duct to the urethra, where it is propelled from the penis during sexual intercourse.

Accessory Glands

The primary function of the accessory reproductive glands is to facilitate ejaculation. Sexual stimulation initiates the ejaculatory process. When a male is sexually stimulated, his sperm travel from the epididymis to the vas deferens to the seminal vesicles and ejaculatory duct. Fluid from the prostate gland (a chestnut-shaped gland located at the base of the urethra) mixes with the sperm and secretions of the seminal vesicles. This prostate fluid further decreases the ejaculatory fluid's acidity, increases sperm motility, and prolongs sperm life. The alkaline medium counteracts the acidity of vaginal secretions that would otherwise kill the sperm. The Cowper glands (two pea-sized glands found adjacent to the urethra) secrete another alkaline fluid into the urethra to neutralize acidity caused by urine transportation. The Cowper gland secretions can sometimes be seen at the meatus before ejaculation. This secretion aids in lubrication of the penis during sexual intercourse and may contain some sperm left over from a previous ejaculation; therefore, these secretions can cause pregnancy even if the penis is withdrawn prior to ejaculation.

Erection and Ejaculation

Erections start occurring in utero and continue throughout the life of a man. Penetration of the penis during sexual intercourse is accomplished due to the ability of the penis to become erect. An erection can occur with stimulation, which results in parasympathetic nerve impulses in the spinal cord (sacral area) to release nitric oxide; simultaneously sympathetic nerve fibers, which cause constriction, are inhibited.

The release of nitric oxide leads to arteriolar dilation, and blood fills in the corpora cavernosa and, to a lesser degree, the spongiosum of the penile shaft. The spongiosum does not fully expand so that semen can travel through the urethra. The filling of this tissue with blood causes expansion of the erectile tissue, and the penis enlarges and elongates (i.e., erection or tumescence). The erection is maintained due to the compression and constriction of the veins which prevents outward blood flow. Collagen fibers that surround the penis prevent curvature when the penis is erect.

The actual expulsion of semen from the penis (i.e., ejaculation) is the result of motor neurons stimulating muscular contractions of the glands and ducts of the reproductive system—particularly the ampulla, seminal vesicles, and bulbocavernosus muscle (the muscle surrounding the corpus spongiosum). During ejaculation, a valve at the bladder closes to prevent urine from entering the urethra and killing the sperm. An orgasm, the climax of pleasurable sensations, usually accompanies the ejaculation. Ejaculated semen contains sperm (about the volume of a pinhead) and secretions (about 2–6 mL [a tablespoon]) from the seminal vesicles, prostate, and Cowper glands. One ejaculation contains approximately 300 million sperm. While erections occur throughout life, ejaculation occurs with the commencement of spermatogenesis. After ejaculation or if there is cessation of stimulation of the penis, the reverse occurs in the vasculature; the veins dilate and blood flows outward from the arterioles causing detumescence (flaccidity).

Normal Female Reproductive System

The female reproductive tract is a complex system that includes organs to manage the generation of eggs (oogenesis), transportation of eggs (ovulation) for fertilization (impregnation), support of fetal development (gestation), birth of the fetus (parturition), and feeding of the offspring through lactation. To accomplish all these functions, the female reproductive system requires a delicate hormone balance and operational organs. These organs include the ovaries, fallopian tubes, uterus, vagina, external genitalia, and mammary glands (**FIGURE 8-5**, **FIGURE 8-6**, **FIGURE 8-7**, and **FIGURE 8-8**). In addition to facilitating the system's function, the hormones (specifically estrogen and progesterone) produced by the female reproductive system give females their distinct characteristics (e.g., enlarged breasts, wide hips, and high-pitched voice).

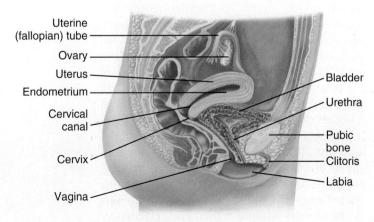

Uterine (fallopian) tube — Ovary — Uterus — Endometrium — Cervical canal — Cervix — Vagina — Bladder — Urethra — Pubic bone — Clitoris — Labia

FIGURE 8-5 Side view of the female reproductive system.

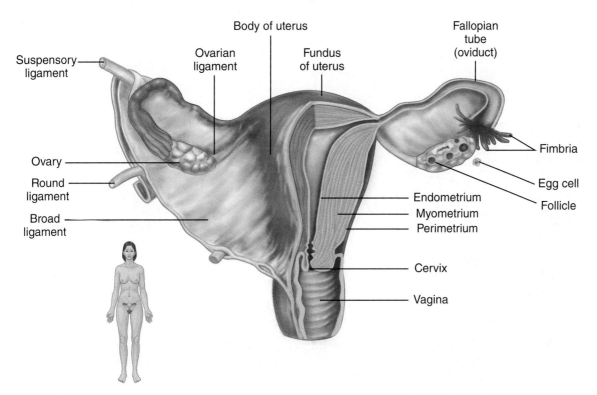

FIGURE 8-6 Front view of the female reproductive system.

The female reproductive system is intimately intertwined with the physiologic functions of nearby structures in the female pelvis. The female pelvis contains organs of the urinary and gastrointestinal systems along with organs for the reproductive system; thus, the female pelvis is the site for urination, defecation, menstruation, ovulation, copulation (sexual intercourse), impregnation, pregnancy, and parturition. Because of the close proximity of these three systems, problems in one system can lead to problems in the others.

Ovaries

The ovaries are paired, almond-shaped organs located on each side of the uterus (Figure 8-6; **FIGURE 8-9**). The suspensory and ovarian ligaments and the mesovarium (fold in the peritoneum) hold the ovaries in place. The ovaries produce hormones (primarily estrogen, progesterone, and inhibin) that regulate reproductive function and secondary sex characteristics (e.g., enlarged breasts, wide hips, and high-pitched voice). Estrogen is also produced in smaller amounts by breast and adipose tissue and during pregnancy by the placenta. The ovaries also produce testosterone and other androgens, but the levels are lower in women (e.g., up to 70 ng/dL) in comparison to men (e.g., up to 1,000 ng/dL). Men, likewise, have

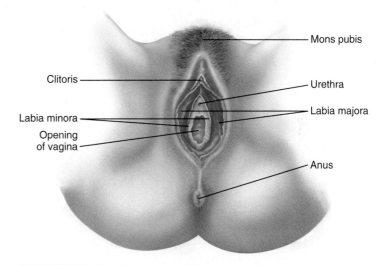

FIGURE 8-7 The female external genitalia.

lower levels of estrogen in comparison to women. The adrenal cortex production of androgens can be significant in women, while in men adrenal androgens are not as influential.

There are three types of estrogen—estradiol, estrone, and estriol. Estradiol is the most potent and prevalent, particularly up to menopause, at which time estrone becomes the predominant estrogen. Estradiol is produced in the ovarian follicles (theca cells and granulosa cells) under FSH stimulation, while the corpus luteum produces progesterone, estrogen, and inhibin

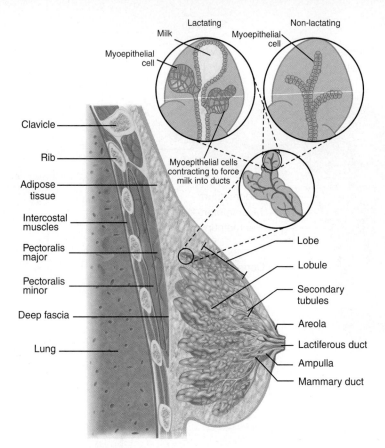

FIGURE 8-8 The female mammary glands.

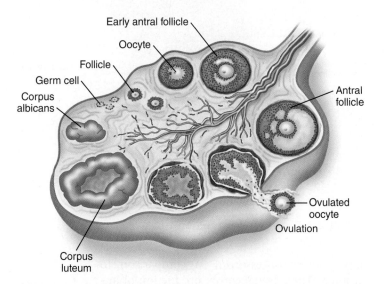

FIGURE 8-9 Structure of the ovary.

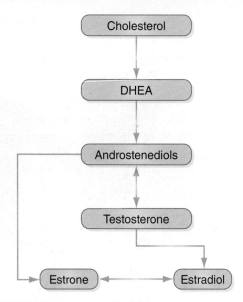

FIGURE 8-10 Estrogen synthesis.

under LH stimulation. In the ovaries, androgens are converted to estradiol and estrone. Estriol is a metabolite of estradiol and estrone. All estrogens are derived from androgens (**FIGURE 8-10**). Estrogen effects, like testosterone, are systemic. In the reproductive tract, estrogen is important in reproductive growth and maturation of the breast, uterus, fallopian tubes, and external genitalia. Nonreproductive effects include alteration of lipids, reduction of osteoclastic activity, inhibition of platelet adhesiveness, increases in collagen, maintenance of skin, and neuroprotection of memory and cognition. The lipid effects include increases in high-density lipoprotein and decreases in low-density lipoprotein; changes in osteoclastic activity includes reduction in bone breakdown; and skin maintenance refers to elasticity and healing.

Progesterone is mainly secreted by the corpus luteum and in small amounts by the follicles. During pregnancy, the placenta secretes progesterone. Progesterone principally targets the uterus, breasts, and brain. Progesterone can have antiestrogenic effects when progesterone levels are high (LH is inhibited) and estrogen is inhibited. Progesterone is used as a contraceptive because the estrogen inhibition prevents ovulation. Progesterone is a key hormone required in the maintenance of pregnancy because it allows the uterus to thicken (hypertrophy), prevents uterine contractions, prepares the breast for lactation, and protects the fetus from maternal antibodies.

The ovaries also contain the precursors to mature eggs (oocytes). During oogenesis, the oocytes mature into ova (mature eggs). By the 30th week of gestation, the female fetus has approximately 7 million follicles (biologic units, each containing a single oocyte). These 7 million follicles degenerate to approximately 2 million follicles by birth. By puberty approximately 400,000 follicles remain. Ova are not continually produced throughout a woman's lifetime, which is a key difference from spermatogenesis. All the ova in the ovaries remain in a state of prophase for as long as 45 years. During the reproductive years, the follicles mature as they are exposed to pituitary hormones—specifically, FSH and LH. During the ovulation phase of the menstrual cycle, the mature follicle ruptures, releasing the mature ovum into the fallopian tubes (FIGURE 8-11). The ovum travels to the uterus for fertilization by the sperm. Meiosis completion in egg cells occurs during fertilization. Fewer than 500 of each woman's ova mature and become fertile. Although approximately a dozen follicles begin developing during each cycle, usually only one makes it to ovulation. Multiple births (e.g., twins or triplets) may occur when more than one ovum is produced, released, and fertilized.

Once the mature follicle releases the ovum, the empty follicle (called the *corpus luteum*) secretes progesterone to signal the endometrium to prepare for fertilization. The release of an older woman's ova can result in abnormal meiosis and a higher risk for chromosomal abnormalities and congenital diseases. See chapter 1 for an explanation of prophase and meiosis.

Fallopian Tubes

The fallopian tubes are two cylindrical structures that extend from the fundus of the uterus to near the ovaries. The ends of the tubes near the ovaries are fimbriated (fringelike) to capture the ovum after ovulation. The tubes use a

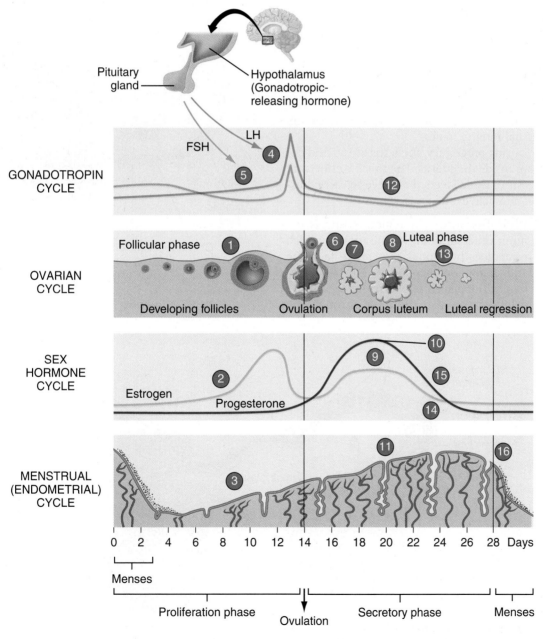

FIGURE 8-11 The menstrual cycle.

ciliary and muscular action to move the ovum toward the uterus as well as to assist sperm in moving from the uterus toward the ovum that is likely still in one of the tubes. If fertilization occurs, the same ciliary and muscular action moves the fertilized egg (zygote) from the tube to the uterus for implantation (**FIGURE 8-12**). Occasionally, the zygote does not reach the uterus but rather becomes implanted outside the uterus; this event is called an *ectopic pregnancy*. The most common site for ectopic pregnancies is the fallopian tubes. Ectopic pregnancies cannot develop normally and can be life threatening.

Uterus

The uterus is a hollow, pear-shaped organ held in place by the broad, round, and uterosacral ligaments. Usually, the uterus is tilted forward (anteverted) over the bladder, but it is tilted backward (retroverted) in approximately 20% of women. A woman with a retroverted uterus is more likely to experience menstrual discomfort or pain with intercourse (i.e., dyspareunia), but she should not experience any unusual fertility issues.

During pregnancy, the fetus grows and develops inside the uterus. The thick uterine wall consists of three layers that serve to carry, nurture, and deliver the fetus.

- **Endometrium:** The endometrium is the inner mucosal lining of the uterus, which undergoes hormonal changes to facilitate and maintain pregnancy. During pregnancy, the placenta (a vascular organ) develops to nourish the fetus through the

umbilical cord (which contains two arteries and one vein). The placenta attaches to the endometrium on one side and surrounds the fetus on the other (**FIGURE 8-13**). The uterus expels the placenta within a few minutes after birth. The endometrium is the lining that sheds during menses.

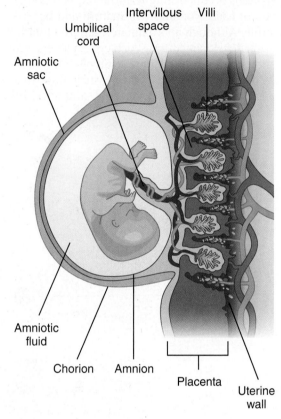

FIGURE 8-13 The developing placenta and embryo.

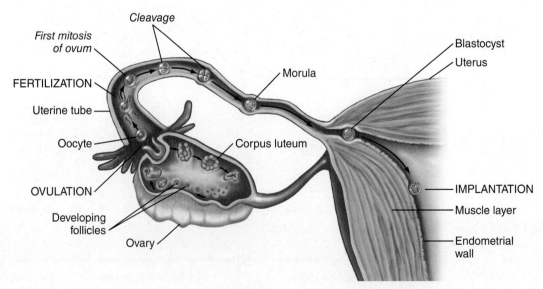

FIGURE 8-12 Fertilization and implantation of the embryo.

- **Myometrium:** The myometrium is the middle layer of the uterus; it consists of smooth muscle and a vascular system. During pregnancy, the vascular system radically increases to support the fetus. During childbirth, the myometrium contracts to push the fetus out through the vaginal canal. After childbirth or abortion (spontaneous or induced pregnancy termination), this layer contracts to constrict blood vessels and control bleeding.
- **Perimetrium:** The perimetrium is the outer, serous layer that covers all of the fundus and part of the corpus, but none of the cervix (the narrow opening from the uterus to the vagina). The incomplete coverage of this layer allows for surgical access into the uterus without requiring an incision into the peritoneum (the membrane that lines the abdominal cavity). The cervical glands secrete a mucus that covers the cervical os (opening) to provide protection against organisms traveling to the upper reproductive structures (e.g., the uterus). The mucus changes with the menstrual cycle and around ovulation becomes clear, slippery, and can be stretched between the fingers. The mucus protects the sperm from the acidic vaginal environment and helps sperm to move through the cervix.

The menstrual cycle (Figure 8-11) is a series of monthly changes that begin at puberty and continue through the reproductive years. The average age of onset of menstruation (menarche) is approximately 13 years. Hypothalamus maturation and subsequent hormone increases trigger the menstrual cycle. Initiation of this cycle is marked by the onset of menstruation (shedding of the endometrium). The menstrual cycle is usually a 28-day cycle (ranges from 25 to 28 days) that consists of two phases—the proliferative/follicular (estrogen-dominated) and secretory/luteal (progesterone-dominated) phases. The follicular phase lasts approximately 14–21 days and starts with menses and ends before the surge of LH. The luteal phase lasts approximately 14 days and begins with the LH surge and ends with onset of the next menstrual cycle.

At the beginning of the follicular phase, estrogen and progesterone levels are low, causing GnRH stimulation and FSH and LH secretion from the anterior pituitary gland. FSH release leads to estrogen production, and the follicles develop with both hormones. The LH also starts to rise. The small, select group of follicles then secretes inhibin, which starts suppression of FSH. Increasing estrogen also suppresses FSH and LH. While the follicle is developing, estrogen starts prepping the uterus by causing proliferation and leading to an increase in stringy cervical mucus (i.e., spinnbarkeit).

Estradiol levels peak around one day before ovulation. Normally, high estradiol and progesterone levels would cause FSH and LH suppression due to negative feedback mechanisms, but for poorly understood reasons, the reverse happens. The high hormone levels cause a positive feedback mechanism with increases in FSH and an LH surge. This surge marks the beginning of the luteal phase. About 36 hours after the LH surge, the oocyte is released from the follicle (i.e., ovulation occurs); it travels to the fallopian tubes, and the follicle becomes the corpus luteum. The remaining follicles are reabsorbed by the body. The corpus luteum secretes predominantly progesterone (referred to as the *secretory phase*) which causes several endometrial effects (e.g., maintaining thickened endometrium and glandular secretions).

At the end of the luteal (secretory) phase, the uterus is ready to receive and nourish a zygote. If fertilization does not occur, the LH and FSH start to decline, resulting in the corpus luteum producing less estrogen and progesterone. The corpus luteum atrophies (becomes corpus albicans). The thickened uterine lining sloughs off, signaling the beginning of menstruation. Menstruation expels the unfertilized ovum and maintains a healthy uterine lining that is prepared for fertilization.

If fertilization and pregnancy occur, the endometrium thickens, and vascularization develops. After implantation of the zygote (5–6 days after fertilization), the placenta secretes human chorionic gonadotropin to stimulate the corpus luteum to continue estrogen and progesterone production. The continued estrogen and progesterone production will suppress FSH and LH production, preventing further ovulation and menstruation. Human chorionic gonadotropin secretion continues until the placenta fully develops and begins making its own estrogen and progesterone, a phase that usually begins by the end of the first trimester.

The menstrual cycle continues to be repeated throughout a woman's reproductive years until estrogen levels begin to decline with age. As a result of the decreased estrogen levels, ovulation and menstruation become less frequent and more erratic. This change in the menstrual cycle usually begins between 45 and 55 years of age. Menopause refers to the complete cessation of the menstrual cycle. In addition to changes in the menstrual cycle, the declining estrogen levels associated with menopause can cause the following manifestations:

- Atrophy of the breasts and internal reproductive organs
- Decreased vaginal secretions (which can make sexual intercourse painful)
- Behavioral changes (e.g., irritability, anxiety, and depression)
- Headaches
- Insomnia (may be due to hot flashes, anxiety, or depression)
- Hot flashes (one of the hallmarks and most common symptom of perimenopause and menopause; usually worsens at night and causes sweating)
- Collagen decreases (results in increased wrinkling of skin)
- Decreased bone density
- Increased cardiovascular risks

These manifestations can vary in severity, but in most cases, they are mild and improve with time. Hormone replacement therapy can decrease severity of the symptoms (particularly hot flashes), but careful consideration should be given prior to initiating such therapy because it is associated with an increased risk of breast cancer, thrombus (blood clot), and stroke.

Vagina

The vagina is a hollow, tunnellike structure located between the bladder and the rectum and extends from the cervix to the external genitalia. This muscular canal is usually 2–4 inches in length, and it can expand in width (e.g., during parturition). The vagina serves as a passageway for sperm to travel to the fallopian tubes, for the body to discharge menstrual fluid, and to birth the fetus. Sperm enter the vagina when the male partner inserts his penis during sexual intercourse. Ejaculation propels the semen into this canal, where the sperm begin their journey to the fallopian tubes. In the mucosal lining of the vagina, Skene glands secrete a protective, lubricating fluid during sexual intercourse. Stimulation of the vagina can produce orgasm, but often clitoral stimulation is necessary, whether directly or indirectly, through vaginal intercourse. The vaginal wall is lubricated by the cervical mucous glands and transudate from the walls (the vagina has no mucous glands). The vagina is acidic due to normal bacterial flora production of lactic acid. This acidic environment serves a protective function against infections but is harmful to sperm. Adolescents have a more alkaline vaginal environment, placing them at greater risk for infections.

The vagina may contain a thin connective tissue that covers the external vaginal opening to some degree, called the *hymen* (FIGURE 8-14). All hymens have openings large enough to permit menstrual flow passage or tampon insertion, but the openings are generally too small to permit an erect penis to enter without tearing. Tearing of the hymen does not usually cause significant discomfort, but it may cause a few drops of blood to be noticed. In addition to sexual intercourse, physical activity can partially or completely tear the hymen; therefore, the absence or presence of the hymen is not a reliable indicator of virginity.

External Genitalia

The external female genitalia contain several structures that are collectively referred to as the *vulva*. These structures include the mons pubis, labia majora, labia minora, clitoris, and vestibule. The size, color, and shape of these structures as well as hair distribution and skin texture can vary significantly from person to person. The mons pubis is the pad of fat over the pubic bone (symphysis pubis) that becomes covered with hair after puberty. The labia majora are the two large, fatty skin folds that protect the perineum and aid in lubrication; they become prominent and darkened after puberty. The labia minora are two small, firm skin folds just inside the labia majora; they have a rich blood and nerve supply. The two labia minora connect at their upper portion to form the clitoris. The clitoris is very sensitive to stimulation and becomes filled with blood during sexual arousal, and stimulation of the clitoris is often required for orgasm. It

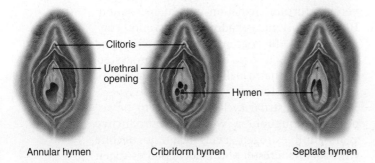

Clitoris

Urethral opening

Hymen

Annular hymen   Cribriform hymen   Septate hymen

FIGURE 8-14 The various types of hymens.

contains two corpora cavernosa, similar to the penis. Bartholin glands lie just within the labia minora and provide lubrication during sexual intercourse. The vestibule refers to the area that contains the urethral and vaginal opening.

Mammary Glands

The mammary glands are in the breasts. Although both males and females have mammary glands, they are functioning structures only in females. The mammary glands are not a reproductive organ per se, but they can have a role in sexual arousal and provide nourishment to the newborn. Each breast contains 15–20 clusters of milk-secreting mammary glands that open into the nipple. The mammary glands do not make milk unless stimulated to do so. Prolactin, a hormone released by the anterior pituitary gland, prompts milk production. During pregnancy, increased estrogen levels trigger prolactin secretion, which matures the mammary glands and prepares them for milk production. After childbirth, prolactin secretion initially decreases as the estrogen levels return to non-pregnancy levels, but the newborn's suckling then stimulates increased prolactin production.

Each breast in both sexes contains a nipple surrounded by an areola (area of pigmentation). The areolar glands (i.e., Montgomery glands) are sebaceous glands that produce secretions that protect and lubricate the nipple and areola during breastfeeding.

Congenital Disorders

Abnormalities of the urinary and reproductive systems are the most common congenital defects. Because of these systems' close relationship, an abnormality in one system will often lead to an abnormality in the other. Additionally, fetal development of both systems is intertwined. The reproductive system continues its development until birth; however, even though the system is formed at birth, it is incapable of reproduction until it matures during puberty. Numerous congenital disorders of the reproductive system are possible, most of which are structural problems. Sexual organs arise from the same fetal tissue, meaning the tissue that produces a penis in males will produce a clitoris in females. Therefore, the controlling factor are hormones, specifically androgens. The presence of male hormones leads to development of male reproductive organs while the absence leads to development of female reproductive organs. But if a fetus is genetically programmed to be male (XY) or female (XX) and

the androgens are deficient (usually causes male development issues) or excessive (usually causes female development issues) disorders can result. Some disorders cause mild symptoms (e.g., epispadias and hypospadias), whereas others may cause infertility and gender ambiguity (e.g., testicular or ovarian agenesis).

Epispadias

Epispadias refers to the condition in which the urethral meatus inner lining is exposed and occurs on the dorsal surface of the penis instead of the end (FIGURE 8-15). The urethral

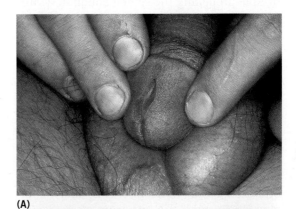

(A)

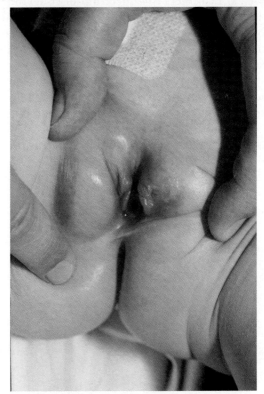

(B)

FIGURE 8-15 Epispadias. **(A)** Male. **(B)** Female.

opening may extend the entire length of the penis. Additionally, the penis may be shorter, be wider, or have an abnormal curve. Epispadias is rare (1 in 117,000 newborn boys) and usually develops during the first month of gestation (Jayachandran, Bythell, Platt, & Rankin, 2011). This malformation can also affect females (1 in 484,000 newborn girls), with the meatus often being placed in the clitoris. Epispadias is more likely to cause urination problems in men and sexual dissatisfaction in women. Men with epispadias are not necessarily infertile, but they may have trouble propelling the semen adequately during ejaculation. Both males and females with epispadias are at increased risk for urinary tract infections.

Urinary defects, such as bladder exstrophy (in which part or all of the bladder is present outside the body) (FIGURE 8-16), often occur with this type of congenital condition. Classic bladder exstrophy occurs in 3.3 per 100,000 births. Along with exstrophy, other organ systems such as the reproductive tract, digestive system, pelvic bone, and muscles are often exposed. Exstrophy–epispadias complex (EEC) refers to a spectrum of congenital abnormalities that includes epispadias, classic bladder exstrophy, cloaca exstrophy (the bladder and intestines are exposed at birth), and several variations. EEC occurs due to a rupture of fetal tissue (the cloacal membrane), leading to an embryologic defect in abdominal wall development (the lower abdominal contents herniate). This defect occurs during the first trimester. The prevalence of this condition ranges from 1 per 10,000 births (EEC involving classic exstrophy) to 1 per 200,000 births (EEC involving cloaca exstrophy).

The exact cause of epispadias and EEC is unknown, but these defects are thought to result from an event occurring early in pregnancy. Risk factors include parental history of epispadias or exstrophy (which carries a 500 times greater risk than the general population) and maternal factors including young age, high parity, and smoking.

Diagnosis of epispadias is typically made through a physical examination. Other procedures may be used to identify associated conditions and determine the severity of this congenital defect, including intravenous pyelogram (X-ray of the kidneys, bladder, and ureters using radioactive isotopes), pelvic X-ray, computed tomography (CT), magnetic resonance imaging (MRI), and ultrasound of the urinary system and genital structures. The diagnosis can be made prenatally with an ultrasound. In males, surgical procedures may use the foreskin to repair the defect, but urinary incontinence is common in postoperative patients. In patients with EEC, the goal is to protect the external structures (e.g., prevent injury, cover with plastic wrap, and use mist tents) until repair can be done. Surgical repair of EEC may also include closure of the abdominal wall and urinary or intestinal diversions. Multiple procedures may be required to achieve the desired cosmetic outcome, urine flow control, and sexual function.

Hypospadias

Hypospadias refers to the condition in which the urethral meatus is on the ventral surface of the penis instead of the end (FIGURE 8-17). According to the Centers for Disease Control and Prevention (CDC, 2016a), hypospadias is a commonly occurring congenital defect, affecting 5 out of 1,000 newborn boys. Like

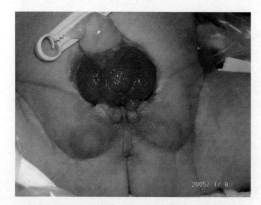

FIGURE 8-16 Bladder exstrophy.

Photo from Ebert, A. K., Reutter, H., Ludwig, M., & Rösch, W. H. (2009). The exstrophy-epispadias complex. Orphanet Journal of Rare Diseases, 4(1), 23.

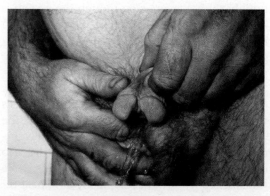

FIGURE 8-17 Hypospadias.

Courtesy of K. Mae Lennon, Tulane Medical School; Clement Benjamin/CDC.

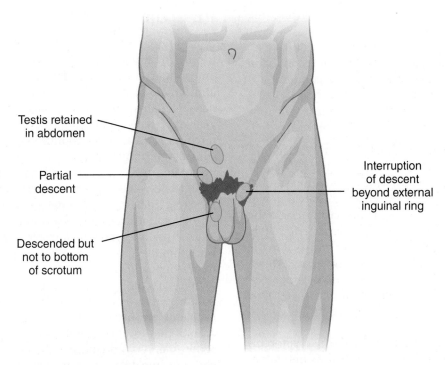

Testis retained
in abdomen

Partial
descent

Descended but
not to bottom
of scrotum

Interruption
of descent
beyond external
inguinal ring

FIGURE 8-18 Potential sites for cryptorchidism.

epispadias, hypospadias can vary in severity, and the opening can extend along the length of the penis or be located on the scrotum or perineum. Males with this condition may also have a downward curvature of the penis, called *chordee*, that becomes apparent with an erection. Hypospadias does not usually affect females. Hypospadias can occur with other congenital reproductive anomalies such as a bifid scrotum (lack of separation of labioscrotal fold) or cryptorchidism which can be the cause of gender ambiguity. This ambiguity may lead to inappropriate surgical gender assignment. Genetic studies prior to any gender assignment procedures can minimize this risk.

The exact cause of hypospadias is unknown, but it is thought to result from a disruption in androgen stimulation during development of the male external genitalia. The androgenic disruption is due to a combination of environmental exposure (e.g., medication exposure in utero) and genetic vulnerability. Risk increases with maternal factors such as age greater than 35 years, obesity, use of fertility treatments, and hormone therapy just before or during pregnancy.

Diagnosis of hypospadias is made through a physical examination. Imaging tests (e.g., MRI, CT, X-rays, and ultrasound) may be performed to identify other congenital defects. Surgical repair (often in stages) can improve the penis's appearance as well as the patient's urinary and sexual function. Surgery can be done as early as 4 months of age but should be undertaken before 18 months of age.

Cryptorchidism

Cryptorchidism is a common congenital genitourinary tract condition in which one or both testes do not descend from the abdomen to the scrotum prior to birth (**FIGURE 8-18**). Cryptorchidism means *hidden testis* and can also include an absent testis or testes. The absence occurs because the testes never developed or they atrophied. A case of bilateral absent testes is termed *anorchia*. Usually the undescended testes remain along the path of descent, but they can also deviate from that path, which is called *ectopic testes*. Approximately 2–5% of full-term males are born with one or two undescended testicles. Rarely, both testes are undescended. Risk factors for cryptorchidism include:

- Prematurity (birth before 37 weeks' gestation)
- Low birth weight
- Small size for gestational age
- Multiple fetuses (e.g., twins)
- Family history of cryptorchidism or other problems of genital development

- Maternal estrogen exposure during the first trimester
- Maternal alcohol use during pregnancy
- Maternal cigarette smoking or secondhand smoke exposure during pregnancy
- Maternal diabetes (type 1 diabetes, type 2 diabetes, or gestational diabetes)
- Parental exposure to some pesticides

Occasionally, a testicle that descended normally by birth may disappear later in childhood, often due to muscular reflexes that develop in puberty. A retractile testicle moves back and forth between the scrotum and the lower abdomen due to the cremasteric reflex. In this case, the testicle is easily returned to the scrotum through gentle manipulation. An ascending testicle, or acquired undescended testicle, refers to a testicle that has returned to the lower abdomen and cannot easily be guided back into the scrotum.

Diagnostic procedures for cryptorchidism include a history, physical examination, self-testicular examinations (the condition places the individual at increased risk for testicular cancer later in life), abdominal ultrasound, MRI, laparoscopy (visualization using a small camera through a small abdominal incision), and open abdominal exploratory surgery. Additionally, hormone levels and genetic studies can distinguish potential causes and complications.

In most cases, the testes descend by 9 months of age without treatment; however, cryptorchidism treatment should be done by 6 months of age because the testes are unlikely to descend after this time. Early treatment prevents permanent damage to the testicles and improves fertility during later life. Testes that do not naturally descend into the scrotum before birth are considered abnormal, and the individual is at increased risk for cancer and infertility even with repair. Treatment strategies include the following measures:

- Manual manipulation
- Hormonal therapy (specifically human chorionic gonadotropin and GnRH to induce descent)
- Surgical repair (either laparoscopic or open) such as orchidopexy (wherein a testicle is brought down in a pouch and stitched into place)
- Orchiectomy (testicle removal)
- Testicle implants
- Hormone replacement (specifically testosterone if the testicle is removed or damaged)

Infertility Issues

Infertility describes a biologic inability to contribute to reproduction. The ability to conceive and support a fetus requires functioning male and female reproductive systems. If a couple has been unsuccessful in conceiving after 1 year of actively trying (unprotected sexual intercourse at least once monthly), they should consult a fertility expert.

Male problems that can lead to infertility include decreased sperm or sperm abnormalities (e.g., defects in spermatogenesis and abnormal sperm transport), hormone deviations (e.g., usually hypogonadotropic hypogonadism), and physical impediments. Hypogonadotropic hypogonadism is due to hypothalamus or pituitary disorders that cause GnRH or gonadotropin deficiencies. Spermatogenesis problems are usually idiopathic. Multiple disorders that are congenital (e.g., Klinefelter syndrome, cryptorchidism), genetic (e.g., Y chromosome defects), or acquired (e.g., varicocele, antisperm antibodies) can affect testicular spermatogenesis. Sperm transport issues can be caused by any disorder affecting structures that are involved and deliver sperm, such as the epididymis, vas deferens, and ejaculatory ducts.

Diagnostic procedures for infertility in males include a history, physical examination, sperm analysis, cultures of penal drainage if infection is suspected, hormone analysis (e.g., FSH, LH, thyroid-stimulating hormone, testosterone, and prolactin), and imaging studies (e.g., ultrasound and vasography). Genetic testing may also be indicated (e.g., Y and X chromosome defects and *CFTR* gene mutations).

The most common female infertility problem is ovulation dysfunction. Other female infertility problems include hormone deviations (e.g., hyperprolactinemia), transport disorders (e.g., stenosis or tumors of the fallopian tubes or cervix), uterine defects (e.g., endometriosis, positioning, and placenta development), and pelvic adhesions (fibrotic tissue that binds organs together). Normally, women who ovulate have monthly menses and molimina (i.e., bloating, breast tenderness, and dysmenorrhea). An ovulatory cause of infertility is indicated if menses and molimina are absent or irregular. Many conditions can cause ovulation dysfunction (e.g., extreme exercise, eating disorders, and hyperprolactinemia), and they can be categorized as hypothalamic-pituitary in origin or as being due to other systemic origins (e.g., polycystic ovarian syndrome, thyroid disorders, and Cushing disease). Disorders that affect transport of the oocyte and sperm can be caused by tubal disease and pelvic adhesions. Tubal disease is usually due to pelvic inflammatory disease caused by sexually transmitted infections. Uterine fibroids (leiomyomata) and endometriosis, which also cause ovarian tissue damage and impair ovulation, are some uterine disorders that cause infertility.

Diagnostic procedures for infertility in females include a history, physical examination, ovulation testing, hysterosalpingography, ovarian reserve testing to determines the quality and quantity of eggs available, hormone analysis, imaging studies, and genetic testing. Hysterosalpingography is an X-ray of the uterus with radioactive isotopes; hormones analyzed can include FSH, LH, thyroid-stimulating hormone, prolactin, estrogen, and progesterone; and imaging studies can include ultrasound and hysterosonography.

Treatment for infertility includes the following measures:

- Lifestyle modifications (e.g., weight loss, stress reduction, and smoking cessation)
- Endocrinopathies
  - Human chorionic gonadotropin, GnRH, testosterone, and estrogen supplements, estrogen modulator
  - Estrogen receptor blockers (increase GnRH secretion)
  - Dopamine agonists (inhibit prolactin release)
  - Gonadotropins (stimulate gonadal steroid hormones)
- Immunotherapy for males with antisperm antibodies
- Alpha-sympathomimetic agents for males with retrograde ejaculation (closes the bladder neck)
- Collagen injections to the bladder neck
- Sperm treatment to wash and concentrate sperm
- Antimicrobial therapy if infection is present
- Coenzyme Q (may increase sperm quantity and quality)
- Metformin (decreases insulin resistance, making ovulation more likely to occur)
- Intrauterine insemination
- Tubal and uterine tumors/adhesions (removal of the tumor, breaking up adhesions)
- In vitro fertilization

Disorders of the Penis

Disorders of the penis can result in erectile issues as a result of vascular, neurogenic, or psychological issues. Penile disorders can impair urinary functioning such as those due to foreskin issues and sexual functioning. These disorders can be a manifestation of an underlying systemic disorder or due to local trauma or infection. Most can be managed with medications and surgery. Some penile disorders can potentially lead to penile necrosis and emergent care is necessary.

Erectile Dysfunction

Erectile dysfunction (ED), or impotence, refers to the recurring or consistent inability to attain or maintain a penile erection sufficient to complete sexual intercourse. Other sexual dysfunction disorders include diminished libido and abnormal ejaculation (e.g., premature). A decreased libido usually coexists with other sexual dysfunction, and most causes are the same as ED. The most common sexual disorder is ED. Although ED can occur at any age, it commonly starts around the age of 40 and becomes more of a problem in older men. Risk factors associated with ED development include obesity, smoking, sedentary lifestyle, and obstructive sleep apnea. Infrequent sexual intercourse (e.g., less than once per week) may be associated with or a consequence of higher ED risks. ED can be transient or permanent, depending on the etiology.

An erection results from psychological, neurologic, and vascular processes, as well as hormonal influences. ED can result from dysfunctions in any of these areas. Psychological causes include anxiety, depression, guilt, stress, and relationship issues. Normally, the brain receives perceived sensual input (e.g., visual erotic images and auditory stimuli) and signals are sent to an erection center in the spinal cord (T11–L2); there is also a sacral erection center (S2 to S4). The spinal cord then sends signals to divert blood to the corpora cavernosa. Neurologic disorders stroke, multiple sclerosis, or dementia can result in ED. Disruption in testosterone will cause decreased libido and ED. Testosterone maintains nitric oxide levels, which are a requisite for acquiring and maintaining an erection. Nitric oxide causes cavernosal relaxation so that blood flow is maximized, and the penis can engorge. Nitric oxide promotes the nucleotide cyclic guanosine monophosphate. This nucleotide causes smooth muscle relaxation with vasodilation and increased blood flow. The phosphodiesterase 5 enzyme inhibitors (e.g., sildenafil [Viagra]) prevent the breakdown of cyclic guanosine monophosphate. Cigarette smokers and patients with diabetes mellitus have low nitric oxide levels. Thyroid disorders such as hypothyroidism can alter testosterone production and prolactin disorders such as hyperprolactinemia can suppress gonadotropin secretion and thereby suppress testicular function both resulting in ED.

In addition to nitric oxide, a requisite for acquiring and maintaining an erection is adequate arterial blood flow. Cardiovascular disorders (e.g., arteriosclerosis and hypertension) are often associated and a common cause of ED. Cardiovascular disorders and ED have similar risk factors, and ED may even be an early warning sign of cardiovascular disease. Hyperlipidemia, diabetes mellitus, and smoking cause vascular dysfunction and, therefore, can lead to ED. In these disorders, endothelial dysfunction is the mechanism causing ED.

Pelvic trauma and prostate surgery can cause vascular and neurologic interruption and lead to ED. Pharmacotherapeutic agents can cause ED. Some common categories include antihypertensives, antidepressants, antipsychotics, and antiandrogens. Use of alcohol and other recreational substances such as cocaine can cause ED. Penile anatomic issues can cause ED such as those caused by Peyronie disease. In Peyronie disease a fibrotic plaque forms on the tunica albuginea (i.e., connective, fibrous tissue that surrounds the corpora cavernosa). The cause is unknown, but genetic predisposition, trauma, and local ischemia can lead to plaque formation. The plaque that develops leads to a curved or bent penis, a mass, pain, and ED. Peyronie disease can resolve without treatment or remain stable. Treatment can include oral pentoxifylline (nonspecific phosphodiesterase inhibitor) or intralesional injections with collagenase (breaks up collagen deposits). Penile traction therapy can be used in conjunction with medications.

Diagnostic procedures for ED consist of a history and physical examination. If the ED began suddenly and abruptly, the cause is usually psychogenic unless there is trauma or surgery associated with potential ED. If a man has ED but has nocturnal erections, a vascular and neurologic cause are more likely in comparison to a psychogenic cause. Detumescence after penetration is also usually psychological (e.g., anxiety). Laboratory evaluation usually begins with identifying common causes (e.g., cardiovascular disorders, diabetes mellitus) with glucose testing, a lipid profile, and testing thyroid hormone and testosterone levels. Comprehensive metabolic testing should also include an evaluation of the liver and kidney. Additional hormone analysis (e.g., sex hormone binding globulin, prolactin, and LH) may be necessary depending on clinical findings (e.g., gynecomastia and visual field defects). Nocturnal penile tumescence testing can be done to evaluate for psychogenic versus physiologic ED. This test can even be done with a monitoring device in a patient's own home during sleep. Ultrasound (e.g., of the penis and testicles, as well as transrectal ultrasound) and dynamic infusion cavernosometry and cavernosography may be necessary and can determine areas of vascular disorder, such as arterial obstruction or venous leakage. Cavernosography involves an X-ray of the penis after injecting contrast dye into penile blood vessels. A variety of treatment options are available, some of which are costly and are not covered by most insurance plans. When ED has a physiologic origin, identifying and resolving the cause is the priority. Treatment strategies include the following measures:

- Psychological counseling
- Testosterone replacement
- Phosphodiesterase 5 inhibitors (e.g., sildenafil, tadalafil [Cialis], and vardenafil [Levitra])
- Other medications (e.g., adrenergic antagonists)
- Herbal remedies (e.g., ginkgo, ginseng, and saw palmetto)
- Prostaglandin E injections directly into the corpus cavernosum or intraurethral insertion (similar to a suppository)
- Penis pumps or vacuum devices
- Surgical penile implants
- Vascular surgery

Just as with estrogen replacement in women, testosterone replacement must be carefully considered prior to initiating therapy because it is associated with an increased risk of myocardial infarction, stroke, and prostate cancer.

Phimosis and Paraphimosis

Phimosis occurs when the foreskin cannot be retracted from the glans penis. Physiologic phimosis—not being able to retract the foreskin—is common during the first 3 years of age, but the foreskin should become retractable as the child grows. Pathologic phimosis can result from poor hygiene, infections, and inflammation. Elderly men are at risk of this condition due to loss of skin elasticity and infrequent

Diagnostic Link

Laboratory Evaluation of Hypogonadism

Hypogonadism results in low testosterone levels and sperm production. Several laboratory tests can be done to determine whether the issue is due to primary disorder indicating disease of the testes or secondary disorder indicating disease of the pituitary or hypothalamus or a combination of both. Testosterone levels are normally highest in the early morning and slowly decline throughout the day. To be accurate, serum measurements should be done in the morning. Total testosterone is a measure of bound and free testosterone and is often the initial test to evaluate for testicular hypofunction. Free testosterone is a reflection of unbound active (i.e., bioavailable) testosterone. Low total and/or free testosterone is consistent with hypogonadism. Determination of whether the hypogonadism is primary or secondary often requires additional laboratory evaluation. Sex hormone binding globulin (SHBG) levels reflect the bound testosterone (some is also bound to albumin). Low levels of SBHG occur with common disorders such as obesity, insulin resistance, and type 2 diabetes mellitus. High levels of SHBG occur with aging and common disorders such as high estrogen levels and liver disease. High levels can result in less available free testosterone (i.e., more testosterone is bound to SHBG). Low levels mean there is more available unbound testosterone; however, testosterone levels can still be low, indicating possible hypogonadotropism. Gonadotropic hormone levels influencing testosterone levels include FSH, LH, and prolactin and are a reflection of pituitary response to changing testosterone levels. FSH and LH measurements can distinguish between primary and secondary hypogonadism. Low total and/or free testosterone with high FSH and LH is consistent with primary hypogonadism. Low testosterone and/or free testosterone with low FSH and LH (which may be inappropriately normal) is consistent with secondary hypogonadotropic hypogonadism. Elevated prolactin levels inhibit gonadotropin release and reflect secondary hypogonadotropic hypogonadism.

erections. Phimosis can lead to urinary obstruction and pain.

Paraphimosis refers to a condition in which the foreskin is retracted and cannot be returned over the glans penis. Paraphimosis may occur when the foreskin is forcibly retracted or when the patient or caregiver does not replace the foreskin during hygiene. In paraphimosis, the penis becomes constricted and the glans becomes edematous. If paraphimosis is not resolved, the lack of blood flow can lead to local skin necrosis and, rarely, infarction and gangrene, making it a medical emergency.

Treatment strategies for paraphimosis includes manual reduction, which requires pain control and swelling reduction or surgeries such as emergency circumcision and dorsal slit reduction, which involves cutting a constricting band of foreskin. Elective circumcision can be considered after the resolution of paraphimosis. Phimosis can be treated with circumcision, topical steroid cream, and foreskin stretching.

Priapism

Priapism is a prolonged (usually 4 hours or more), painful erection. The unwanted, unrelenting erection is not a result of sexual stimulation. Priapism usually results from too much blood shunting within the corpus cavernosum (referred to as *nonischemic* or *high-flow priapism*). Nonischemic priapism is usually caused by penile or perineal trauma. The more common type of priapism is due blood becoming trapped in the penis (referred to as *ischemic* or *low-flow priapism*). In ischemic priapism, the smooth muscles' relaxation is impaired, causing a compartment syndrome (i.e., increased pressure in a confined space). Nitric oxide dysfunction may be a mechanism for some priapism disorders. Priapism is most common in boys between 5 and 10 years old and in men 20 to 50 years of age. Priapism occurs in conjunction with a variety of blood, circulatory, and nervous dysfunctions, including:

- Sickle cell anemia (the most common cause in pediatric cases) *Blood becomes trapped*
- Leukemia and other hematologic disorders (e.g., multiple myeloma)
- Trauma (e.g., bicycling, urologic procedures)
- Tumors (e.g., prostate, bladder, and renal carcinomas; melanoma)
- Diabetes mellitus and other metabolic disorders (e.g., gout)
- Spinal cord injuries
- Neurologic diseases (e.g., multiple sclerosis and stroke)
- Medications (e.g., phosphodiesterase inhibitors, anticoagulants, and antianxiety agents)
- Alcohol and illicit drugs (e.g., cocaine, ecstasy, and marijuana)
- Poisonous venom (e.g., from a scorpion or black widow)

Diagnostic procedures can identify the type of priapism. They include a history, physical examination, penile arterial blood gases, complete blood count (CBC), and toxicology tests. With ischemic priapism, a Doppler ultrasound will show minimal or absent blood flow, so this test is useful in differentiating the two types of priapism. Other tests may be necessary to look for underlying disorders such as a CT or MRI for tumors. An erection lasting more than 4 hours is considered a urologic emergency warranting immediate medical attention. Without medical attention (urgent urologic consultation), priapism can lead to ischemia, necrosis, ED, and infertility, and the likelihood of complications is associated with the duration of the priapism. Nonischemic priapism does not usually lead to long-term issues.

Treatment focuses on managing the underlying cause and varies depending on the type of priapism. Strategies for ischemic (low-flow) priapism include the following:

- Needle aspiration of blood
- Injection of medications directly into the penis (e.g., alpha-adrenergic sympathomimetic agents)
- Surgical placement of a shunt

Strategies for nonischemic (high-flow) priapism include the following:

- Cold application
- Lower abdominal pressure
- Surgical repair of trauma

Additional interventions regardless of type include the following:

- Analgesics
- Sedation
- Hydration
- Urinary catheterization

Disorders of the Testes and Scrotum

Disorders of the testes and scrotum are usually structural in origin, and some can cause infertility (e.g., cryptorchidism). These disorders can be acquired or congenital, and most can be resolved with minimal residual effects. Infectious causes are discussed with sexually transmitted infections.

Hydrocele

A hydrocele is an accumulation of fluid between the layers of the tunica vaginalis (the membrane covering the testes) or along the spermatic cord (**FIGURE 8-19**). This condition can affect one or both testes. A hydrocele often occurs as a congenital defect, affecting approximately 10% of newborn males. In this case, the vas deferens does not close properly as the testes descend into the scrotum and peritoneal fluid drains from the abdomen. A congenital hydrocele usually disappears without treatment by 1 year of age. An inguinal hernia—a condition in which a section of the intestine passes through the abdominal wall—commonly occurs in infants with hydroceles. In adults, hydroceles

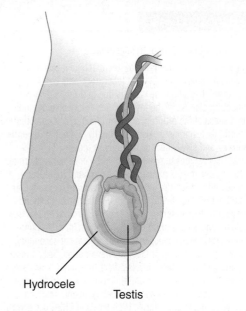

Hydrocele   Testis

FIGURE 8-19 Hydrocele.

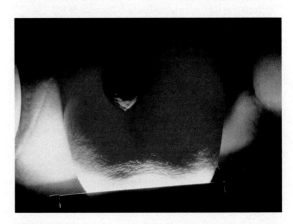

FIGURE 8-20 Transillumination of hydrocele.
© SPL/Science Source.

are commonly idiopathic. An acquired hydrocele occurs because of inflammation, infection, trauma, and tumors.

Hydroceles are usually painless, but the scrotum feels heavy. The fluid accumulation can be small or large, sometimes liters. The swelling generally worsens over the course of the day. This scrotum enlargement can be differentiated from other testicular disorders by transillumination (transmission of light through tissue). Hydroceles will transilluminate, whereas solid tumors will not (**FIGURE 8-20**).

Diagnostic procedures for hydroceles consist of a history, physical examination (including transillumination), and ultrasound. In most cases, the hydrocele resolves without any action other than treating the underlying cause. Strategies to encourage reabsorption of the fluid include scrotal elevation on a rolled towel, sitz baths (warm-water treatments for the perineum), and heat/cold application. Large amounts of fluid can compromise testicular blood flow, requiring aspiration, but surgical removal (hydrocelectomy) of the hydrocele sac is preferred due to recurrence with aspiration.

Spermatocele

A spermatocele is a benign, sperm-containing cyst that develops between the testis and the epididymis (FIGURE 8-21). If it is < 2 cm, it is called an *epididymal cyst*. Usually the cyst is painless, soft, and small, but it can grow quite large, leading to increased discomfort. Additionally,

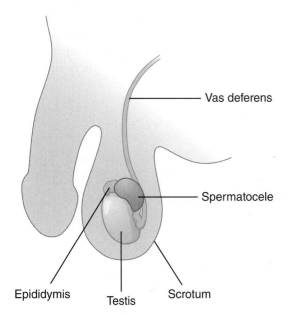

FIGURE 8-21 Spermatocele.

the cyst is moveable and may transilluminate light. The exact cause of this common condition is unknown, but it is thought to be caused by a blockage of the duct system, infection, inflammation, or trauma. Diagnostic procedures are similar to those for hydroceles. The cyst usually does not cause problems but may require surgical removal (spermatocelectomy) if it is large.

Varicocele

A varicocele is a dilated vein in the spermatic cord (FIGURE 8-22). Much like varicose veins in the leg, this condition results from valve issues that allow blood to pool in the veins. These valve issues can be caused by congenital defects (e.g., incompetent or absent valves) or obstructions (e.g., tumors and thrombi). Varicoceles are more common in men ages 15–25 (typically appear around puberty) and are often seen on the left side of the scrotum. For unknown reasons, they occur more frequently in infertile men (approximately 40% greater risk). Additionally, varicoceles are the most common cause of low sperm counts and decreased sperm quality because of testicular ischemia. Varicoceles that appear suddenly in an older man may be caused by a renal tumor that has blocked blood flow.

Varicoceles are much more common (approximately 80–90%) in the left testicle than in the right testicle because of several anatomic factors. These factors include the angle at which the left testicular vein enters the left renal vein, a lack of effective antireflux valves at the left testicular and renal vein juncture, and increased renal vein pressure. Unilateral

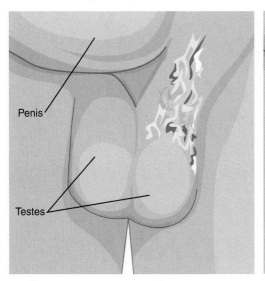
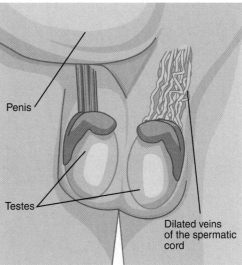

FIGURE 8-22 Varicocele.

right varicoceles are rare and are more likely to be due to obstruction (e.g., renal vein thrombosis and inferior vena cava obstruction) as the right gonadal vein empties into the inferior vena cava. Some varicoceles may be asymptomatic while some may cause mild pain that is described as dull and aching. Extensive varicoceles can be tender and painful. The dilated veins give the scrotum a bag-of-worms feeling upon palpation, and the blood pooling may give a sense of heaviness in the scrotum. The testicular heaviness and pain are usually present when standing, and lying down relieves the symptoms. To palpate or visualize smaller varicoceles, a Valsalva maneuver (i.e., bearing down) may be necessary, and varicoceles can disappear in a lying position. The testicle can atrophy due to an increased scrotal temperature. Additionally, men with varicoceles may experience fertility issues.

Diagnostic procedures for varicoceles are similar to those for hydroceles. In suspected underlying pathology (e.g., thrombosis), a CT of the abdomen with contrast is usually done. Treatment is often unnecessary unless the varicocele causes discomfort, impairs semen, or if testicular atrophy occurs, particularly in men who want to continue to have children. Treatment strategies include scrotal support (e.g., wearing briefs or a jock strap), surgical repair (open or laparoscopic), embolectomy, and sclerotherapy (injection of an irritant into the vein that causes the vessel to harden and fade).

Testicular Torsion

Testicular torsion refers to an abnormal rotation of the testes on the spermatic cord (FIGURE 8-23). Sudden scrotal edema and pain develop as the twisting compresses the blood vessels (reduces arterial flow and obstructs venous outflow),

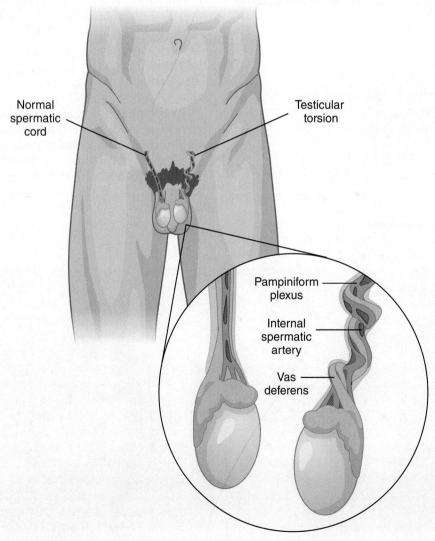

Normal spermatic cord

Testicular torsion

Pampiniform plexus

Internal spermatic artery

Vas deferens

FIGURE 8-23 Testicular torsion.

leading to ischemia and necrosis. Immediate treatment is required to restore blood flow and minimize testicular damage. After approximately 12 hours, irreversible ischemic damage can occur. Scrotal pain can also be due to torsion of the appendix testis or appendix epididymis (each a small tissue appendage left from embryonic development). These appendages are pedunculated and can also twist resulting in torsion. Torsion of the appendix testis or appendix epididymis is more likely in boys between 7 and 12 years of age.

Testicular torsion is more common during the first year of life with another peak incidence at puberty and up until the age of 18. It is most frequently caused by trauma, but it can also occur after strenuous exercise or spontaneously, especially in males whose testicles are not secured in the scrotum due to congenital differences. The primary manifestation is sudden, severe testicular pain (usually unilateral) with or without a predisposing event. Other manifestations may include scrotal swelling, nausea, vomiting, dizziness, and hematospermia (bloody semen). In children, nighttime testicular pain can be a sign of testicular torsion, possibly due to nocturnal sexual stimulation and cremasteric contractions. Physical exam findings may reveal a negative cremasteric reflex (normally when the inner thigh is stroked the testicle contracts up) and a testicular mass. The testicle can be high up (due to spermatic cord shortening), and instead of being longitudinal, the testicle may be in a transverse position (i.e., bell clapper deformity).

Diagnostic procedures include a history, physical examination, testicular Doppler ultrasound to determine blood flow, and scrotal ultrasound, which will reveal absent blood flow to the affected testicle. With appendage torsion, blood flow will be normal or even increased due to the inflammation. Surgery will be required to treat testicular torsion and should be performed within 6 hours to prevent testicular necrosis. Manual manipulation by rotating the testicle gently away from the midline may be used to untwist the testes, but surgery will be required to secure the testicle (orchiopexy) and prevent recurrence. Appendage torsion usually resolves within 10 days without surgery.

Disorders of Pelvic Support

Muscles, ligaments, and fascia normally support the bladder, uterus, and rectum in the female pelvis (Figure 8-5; Figure 8-6). These supportive structures weaken with age, excessive stretching (e.g., due to childbirth and chronic constipation), obesity, and trauma (e.g., large baby, forceps delivery, and hysterectomy). Decreasing hormone levels at the onset of menopause can further atrophy these structures. With weakened support, the organs can shift out of normal position, causing pelvic organ prolapse (i.e., herniation) into the vaginal walls.

Traditionally, pelvic organ prolapse has been categorized based on physical examination findings and presumptive organ prolapse (e.g., cystocele refers to bladder prolapse). Physical examination findings can be misleading, and a posterior collapse, which is usually associated with a rectal prolapse, may be due to another organ. Therefore, pelvic organ prolapse is preferably described based on the site that the prolapse is visualized rather than the suspected organ prolapse. These categories include:

- **Anterior compartment prolapse:** Usually associated with cystocele (i.e., bladder prolapse)
- **Posterior compartment prolapse:** Usually associated with rectocele (i.e., rectal prolapse)
- **Apical compartment prolapse:** Usually associated with uterine and cervical prolapse or the vaginal vault after hysterectomy

Other organs than can prolapse include the intestines (i.e., enterocele, sigmoidocele) and the urethra (i.e., urethrocele). In many women, more than one organ is affected.

Clinical Manifestations

Women can be asymptomatic or have symptoms related to the prolapsed organs. Pelvic organ prolapse often causes vaginal, urinary, defecatory, and sexual dysfunction. Most women will complain of vaginal or pelvic pressure (e.g., rectal pressure) and report a sensation of something coming out of their vagina. If the prolapse is beyond the vaginal opening (i.e., introitus), a woman may even see the organ (e.g., cervix). The urinary symptoms are the result of the organ (usually anterior or apical prolapse) kinking the urethra. This partial blockage results in variable symptoms of obstructions such as incomplete emptying, urine coming out slowly, or weak stream. Due to the variable obstruction symptoms, changing position or splinting may improve urine flow. Stress incontinence and overactive bladder symptoms (e.g., urgency and frequency) also occur. These urinary symptoms predispose women to cystitis (i.e., bladder infections). During sexual intercourse, urine can leak, and enuresis can also occur. Problems with defecation can occur with any type of prolapse because any of the organs cause pressure as they prolapse. Chronic constipation can even cause prolapse. However, bowel dysfunction is more common with posterior and apical prolapse (e.g., rectocele and uterine prolapse). The bowel symptoms include incomplete emptying and constipation. Due to difficulties with fecal emptying, applying pressure with a finger in the vagina or perineum can facilitate evacuation. Fecal incontinence, while not common, can occur with or without sexual intercourse. Pelvic organ prolapse may cause pain with sexual intercourse (i.e., dyspareunia) and women may avoid sexual activity due to concerns about incontinence or embarrassment regarding their body image.

When conducting a physical examination for pelvic organ prolapse, a woman is usually in a dorsal lithotomy position. The prolapse may be evident immediately upon visualization of the introitus or may be seen while the woman performs a Valsalva maneuver. The prolapse may be evident in a supine position. A bulge seen in the anterior wall (superior) of the vagina is classified as anterior compartment prolapse (FIGURE 8-24); a bulge of the posterior wall (inferior) of the vagina is classified as a posterior compartment prolapse; and visualization of the cervix descending into the vaginal vault (canal) is classified as an apical compartment prolapse. The simplified Pelvic Organ Prolapse Quantification can be used by general clinicians to grade the severity of the organ prolapse. This system involves measurements along anatomic points in the vagina.

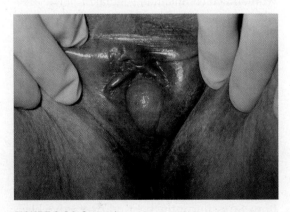

FIGURE 8-24 Cystocele.
© Dr. P. Marazzi/Science Source.

Diagnosis and Treatment

Diagnosis is usually made on findings of the history and physical examination. Diagnostic procedures are generally used to evaluate for bladder or bowel dysfunction. In asymptomatic women, treatment is not necessary. Treatment strategies include Kegel exercises (isometric exercises to strengthen the pelvic muscles) and avoidance of straining. A vaginal pessary device (a vaginally inserted ring that supports the bladder) is a nonsurgical option. A pessary must be removed and cleaned routinely. The effectiveness of estrogen therapy (if the woman is postmenopausal) is controversial. Incontinence interventions can include bladder training and protective garments. Various surgical options, such as vaginal mesh, are available.

Menstrual Disorders

The menstrual cycle can vary from woman to woman. The duration and the amount of menstrual bleeding fluctuate to some degree, but a standard pattern can be expected. The usual duration of menstruation is 4–8 days, and the usual amount of bleeding for the entire menstruation is usually ≤ 80 mL. The frequency ranges from 24 to 38 days. The normal menstrual cycle can be associated with pain and cramping (i.e., dysmenorrhea). The normal menstrual cycle can also be associated with various physical and emotional symptoms (i.e., premenstrual syndrome). A comparison can be made to a patient's baseline menstrual cycle if there is a complaint of a menstrual abnormality.

Menstrual disorders can encompass abnormalities in menstrual bleeding, dysmenorrhea, or premenstrual syndrome. Some menstrual disorders may be a manifestation of a minor, easily treatable problem, while other menstrual disorders are an indication of a serious problem.

Abnormal Uterine Bleeding

Abnormal uterine bleeding (AUB) is defined as a menstrual bleeding abnormality in the frequency of a cycle, volume of blood loss, or duration of flow. AUB also includes precocious puberty—menstrual bleeding prior to the usual start of menses. AUB is generally a manifestation of an underlying disorder. AUB generally presents as vaginal bleeding and refers to the uterus as the source of the bleeding. However, other genital tract sources can cause vaginal bleeding, including the cervix, the vaginal vault, the vulva. Urinary (e.g., hematuria) and gastrointestinal (e.g., rectal bleeding) disorders can be mistaken for uterine bleeding.

In 2011, the Menstrual Disorders working group of the International Federation of Gynecology and Obstetrics revised AUB terminology (Munro, Critchley, Broder, & Fraser 2011). The new terms replaced commonly used terms such as menorrhagia, metrorrhagia, polymenorrhea, and hypermenorrhea, which lacked a clear definition and led to confusion pertaining to diagnosis and treatments. As an example, menorrhagia was used in several ways to describe heavy menstrual bleeding regardless of timing (e.g., regular, irregular, or random). Dysfunctional uterine bleeding, often used to describe AUB, is also considered an outdated term. The new terminology has been an attempt to create a common language and definitions for describing AUB internationally. The new terminology has been adopted in the United States. Amenorrhea is a term that continues to be used. Menstrual bleeding key classifications are as follows:

- **Chronic AUB:** Uterine bleeding that has been abnormal in frequency, regularity, duration, and/or volume for at least the majority of the past 6 months.
- **Acute AUB:** A single episode of uterine bleeding (in a woman of reproductive age and nonpregnant) that is of sufficient quantity to require immediate intervention to prevent further blood loss.
- **Heavy menstrual bleeding (HMB):** Increased menstrual volume (daily or total monthly) as perceived by the woman and that interferes with various aspects of her life (e.g., physical or social).
- **Intermenstrual bleeding (IMB):** Menstrual bleeding that occurs between regular, well-defined cyclical menses. IMB can be random or predictable.
- **Amenorrhea:** Absence of menses.

Abnormal uterine bleeding causes can often be differentiated by age or reproductive transitions. The ages are divided as premenarche, early menarche, reproductive age, menopausal transition (i.e., perimenopause), and menopause. These categories exclude pregnancy-related AUB. The mechanism and causes of AUB are extensive and can include hormonal disorders, anatomic alterations, iatrogenic effect, systemic disorders, or a combination of several mechanisms.

Amenorrhea

Amenorrhea refers to the absence of menstruation. With this condition, menstruation may have never occurred or may have ceased. Amenorrhea is considered primary if menstruation has not occurred by 16 years of age. However, an evaluation for disorders should be carried out earlier than 16 if growth and sexual development (e.g., breast development and pubic and axillary hair) are absent. Genetic or anatomic abnormalities are the usual causes of **primary amenorrhea**, and the mechanism involves the hypothalamus, pituitary gland, ovaries, or other parts of the genital tract. Hypothalamic and pituitary tumors result in abnormal GnRH levels. Stress, sudden weight loss, and extreme reduction in body fat (such as caused by eating disorders or incurred by athletes) is termed *functional hypothalamic amenorrhea* as there is no underlying pathologic disease. Ovarian disorders can cause primary amenorrhea as a result of abnormal ovarian development (i.e., dysgenesis) due to disorders such as Turner syndrome. Congenital abnormalities can cause vaginal disorders such as transverse vaginal septum and vaginal agenesis, or they can cause uterine developmental disorders such as uterine agenesis. A simple defect that can occur without other disorders and causes amenorrhea is an imperforate hymen. A minor surgical procedure to perforate the hymen can be performed to allow normal menstrual flow.

Secondary amenorrhea is defined as absence of menses for more than 3 months in a female who had regular menstrual cycles or absence of menses for 6 months in a female who had irregular menses. Oligomenorrhea (i.e., infrequent menstrual bleeding) is defined as fewer than nine menstrual cycles per year or a cycle length that is longer than 35 days. The causes of oligomenorrhea are the same as for secondary amenorrhea. Oligomenorrhea is usually an anovulatory bleeding pattern. The most common cause of secondary amenorrhea is pregnancy during reproductive age and menopause (average onset age 51)—both normal physiologic conditions. Lactation will also cause amenorrhea. Pathologic causes of secondary amenorrhea, as with primary amenorrhea, include hypothalamus, pituitary, ovarian, or other genital tract disorders. Hypothalamic and pituitary disorders could be due to tumors (e.g., prolactinoma) and infiltrative diseases (e.g., sarcoidosis). Systemic diseases (e.g., histiocytosis and hemochromatosis) can lead to altered GnRH levels and subsequent secondary amenorrhea. Functional hypothalamic amenorrhea due to the same causes as in primary amenorrhea (e.g., stress and weight loss) can cause secondary amenorrhea. Ovarian disorders include ovarian tumors or, more often, primary ovarian failure or insufficiency at an early age (< 40 years). The causes of primary ovarian failure can include ovarian autoimmune destruction, dysgenesis, medication effects (e.g., from chemotherapy), or environmental toxins. Often the cause of primary ovarian insufficiency is unknown. Polycystic ovarian syndrome is a complex disorder with multiple hormonal alterations and can be a cause of secondary amenorrhea. A uterine cause of secondary amenorrhea is known as Asherman syndrome (i.e., intrauterine adhesions). The adhesions and scarring in the endometrial lining are usually the result of instrumentation (e.g., during dilatation and curettage or ablation).

Heavy and Intermenstrual Bleeding

HMB is one the most common types of AUB, and the terms are often used interchangeably even though amenorrhea is included in the AUB definition. The most common causes of HMB and IMB vary depending on whether the woman is pregnant, of reproductive age, or experiencing perimenopause or menopause. The causes of HMB and IMB in nonpregnant females can be categorized by the PALM-COEIN system. PALM refers to structural disorders, and COEIN refers to nonstructural disorders. The acronym refers to the following disorders:

P polyps (endometrial or cervical tumors that are usually benign)

A adenomyosis (endometrial type glands within the endometrium)

L leiomyoma (benign tumors of the uterine smooth muscle)

M malignancy (e.g., leiomyosarcoma [cancerous uterine tumor]) and hyperplasia (abnormal thickening of the endometrial lining, which may lead to uterine cancer)

C coagulopathy (bleeding disorders such as von Willebrand disease)

O ovulatory dysfunction (lack of ovulation due to several disorders or unknown reasons [e.g., stress, weight change, and thyroid disorders])

E endometrial disorder (primary disorder of the endometrium that usually causes regular, cyclic menses that are most likely ovulatory)

I iatrogenic disorder (result of medications [e.g., estrogen, progestin, and androgens] or intrauterine devices)

N not yet classified

During perimenopause, the menstrual cycle changes due to a normal physiologic reduction in ovarian hormone secretion that occurs with aging. However, AUB can also occur due to underlying pathology, and the most likely causes include structural disorders such as polyps, fibroids, and adenomyosis. Malignant disorders such as uterine cancer or leiomyosarcoma are more prevalent with aging.

Any bleeding after menopause (i.e., 1 year without a menstrual cycle) is considered abnormal. The causes often include endometrial polyps and malignant disorders. Hormone replacement therapy can also cause postmenopausal bleeding.

Learning Points

Menstruation in Early Menarche

AUB can be seen the initial 1–2 years after menarche. During this time, missed menses and infrequent menses, and even episodes of heavy menstrual bleeding can occur and are not necessarily a reflection of an abnormality. Commonly this abnormal pattern is due to an immature hypothalamic-pituitary-ovarian axis. These patterns are generally anovulatory; however, the transition to ovulatory, regular menses is not known and pregnancy can occur.

Dysmenorrhea

Dysmenorrhea is painful menstruation. Most women experience some mild lower abdominal cramping during menstruation, but with dysmenorrhea, the cramping pain impairs usual daily activities. The pain begins at the conclusion of ovulation and continues through menstruation. Primary dysmenorrhea may appear in early menarche and often has no known etiology. Dysmenorrhea may also appear later in life secondary to a number of conditions (e.g., endometriosis or reproductive cancers). In many cases of dysmenorrhea (especially the primary type), the condition resolves following childbirth and decreases with aging. The pathogenesis of dysmenorrhea, particularly primary, is excessive prostaglandin secretion which produces strong uterine muscle contractions and blood vessel constriction, intensifying the normal uterine ischemia associated with menstruation. These contractions and ischemia generate strong, intermittent abdominal pain that can radiate to the back, legs, and perineum. Excessive prostaglandins can also cause nausea, vomiting, diarrhea, headaches, and dizziness. Diagnostic procedures may be performed to identify the dysmenorrhea and underlying cause—specifically, a history, physical examination, pelvic ultrasound, laparoscopy, and hysteroscopy. Treatment strategies focus on relieving the discomfort and resolving the underlying etiology. These strategies include analgesics (especially nonsteroidal anti-inflammatory drugs [NSAIDs] because they inhibit prostaglandin secretion), oral contraceptives (which prohibit ovulation), and heat application or warm baths.

Premenstrual Syndrome

Premenstrual syndrome (PMS) refers to a group of physical and emotional symptoms that affect women during the menstrual cycle. Most women experience symptoms similar to PMS. The criteria for diagnosis of PMS, however, is the presence of at least one symptom that causes dysfunction (economic or social) 5 days before menstruation and is present for three consecutive menstrual cycles. PMS occurs more often in women between their late 20s and late 40s who have at least one child, a personal or family history of major depression, and a history of postpartum depression or affective mood disorder. The pathogenesis of PMS is poorly understood. During the luteal phase of the menstrual cycle (Figure 8-11), estrogen and progesterone are thought to normally cause neurotransmitter changes, particularly serotonin. PMS occurs during the luteal phase, so estrogen and progesterone levels are normal; however, there is possibly an abnormal response to the neurotransmitters.

Clinical manifestations of PMS include irritability, depression, mood swings, fatigue, headache, abdominal bloating, changes in bowel pattern, joint pain, breast tenderness, weight gain, and sleep disturbances. *Premenstrual dysphoric syndrome* is a severe form of PMS that is characterized by severe depression, tension, and irritability. Diagnostic procedures for PMS center on a thorough history (focusing on gynecologic complaints) and physical examination. Treatment strategies are individualized and often include hormone therapy such as oral contraceptives, diuretics, antidepressants (especially selective serotonin reuptake inhibitors), analgesics (specifically NSAIDs), and lifestyle measures (e.g., stress reduction regular exercise). Additional measures such as dietary changes (e.g., small frequent meals, decreasing sodium and sugar, or reduction in soda and caffeine) have yielded inconsistent results. Likewise, supplementation with vitamin B_6, calcium, magnesium, or primrose oil lack data regarding efficacy.

Disorders of the Uterus

The uterus is a crucial organ for reproduction in females. Conditions that affect the uterus include benign or malignant tumors, congenital disorders, infections, and hormonal imbalances that may affect menstruation and fertility. Benign and malignant tumors can include leiomyomas and leiomyosarcomas; congenital disorders can include abnormal uterine positioning and uterine agenesis; and infections can include endometritis and pelvic inflammatory disease.

Endometriosis

With endometriosis, the endometrium tissue begins growing and forming lesions in areas outside the uterus. Although such ectopic endometrial tissue most commonly occurs in the fallopian tubes, ovaries, and peritoneum, it can be found anywhere in the body. The endometrial lesions can be superficial or deep and are made of stromal and endometrial glands (like normal endometrial tissue). The abnormal endometrial tissue continues to act like normal endometrial tissue would during menstruation—thickening, breaking down, and bleeding—even though it is outside the uterus. The endometrial lesions, however, are estrogen dependent and resist the effects of progesterone. Without an outlet, the blood becomes trapped and irritates the surrounding tissue. Pain, cysts, scarring, and adhesions develop because of the inflammation, with the scarring and adhesions resulting in altered ovarian function, impaired fertilization, and implantation.

The exact cause of endometriosis is unclear, but numerous theories have been proposed. One theory holds that menstrual blood containing endometrial cells flows back through the fallopian tubes (called *retrograde menstruation*), takes root, and grows. Another theory proposes that the bloodstream carries endometrial cells to other sites in the body. Other theories speculate that a predisposition toward endometriosis may be carried in the genes of certain families or an inappropriate immune response may contribute to endometriosis development. Still other theories suggest that certain cells that are responsible for embryonic reproductive development are present within the abdomens of some women and these cells retain their ability to become endometrial cells under genetic or environmental influences later in life.

Risk factors for endometriosis include early onset of menstruation, late onset of menopause, nulliparity, short menses cycles ($\leq$ 27 days), heavy menstrual bleeding, low body mass index, being tall ($>$ 68 inches), severe physical or sexual abuse during childhood or adolescence, and disorders that obstruct menstrual flow.

Clinical Manifestations

Clinical manifestations depend on the severity of the endometriosis but often worsen as the endometriosis progresses (**FIGURE 8-25**). Most cases are diagnosed in patients between 25 and 35 years of age. Clinical manifestations are due to the inflammatory response and anatomic abnormalities. The types of manifestations are dependent on the lesion locations. The manifestations of endometriosis include the following:

- Dysmenorrhea—dull or crampy pelvic pain or pressure that begins before menses, lasts throughout menses, and can persist for a few days after the end of menses
- Low back pain
- Bowel dysfunction (e.g., dyschezia [pain with bowel movements], diarrhea, and constipation)
- Urinary dysfunction (e.g., frequency, urgency, and dysuria)
- Pain during or after sexual intercourse
- Infertility
- Adnexal (ovarian, fallopian tubes, or supporting ligaments) mass
- Pain during vaginal examination
- Uterus or cervix immobility or displacement upon pelvic examination

Diagnosis and Treatment

Diagnosis is usually made with a history, physical examination, and pelvic ultrasound. A laparoscopy confirms the diagnosis. Treatment strategies focus on minimizing discomfort and maximizing childbearing potential (if desired) and includes:

- Analgesics (particularly NSAIDs)
- Hormone therapy (e.g., estrogen and progestin together, progestin monotherapy, GnRH agonists and antagonists, and danazol)
- Surgical repair (laparoscopy or hysterectomy)

Mild

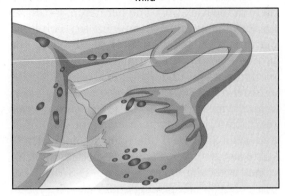

Moderate

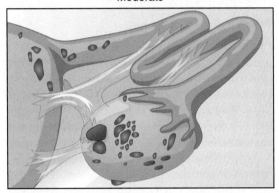

Severe

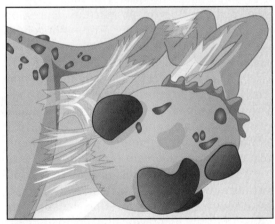

FIGURE 8-25 Stages of endometriosis.

Leiomyomas

A leiomyoma, or uterine fibroid, is a firm, rubbery growth of the smooth muscle of the myometrium (**FIGURE 8-26**). Leiomyomas are the most common benign pelvic tumors in women, and they are classified according to their location (**FIGURE 8-27**). At least 25% of women have symptomatic leiomyomas, but as many as 70% of all women have fibroids by

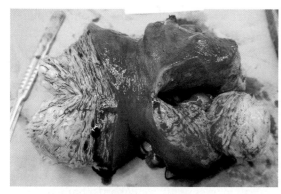

FIGURE 8-26 Leiomyomas.
© ChaiwatUD/Shutterstock.

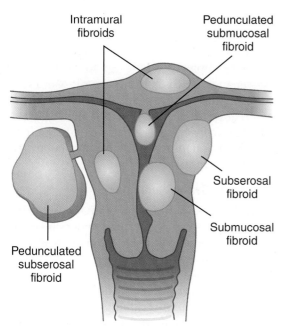

FIGURE 8-27 Leiomyoma classification.

the age of 50 (Zimmerman, Bernuit, Gerlinger, Schaefers, & Geppert, 2012). Leiomyomas are more frequent in Blacks, and the reason for this higher incidence is unknown. Other risk factors include obesity, advancing age, hypertension, and nulliparity. Other factors such as high consumption of red meat, low vitamin D levels, and alcohol are possibly associated. The cause of leiomyomas is unknown, but tumor growth is monoclonal—involving the expansion of a single cell. Most tumors seem to grow during the menstruation years in the presence of estrogen and shrink after menopause. Tumor growth was thought to increase during pregnancy, but recent research suggests that growth actually levels off during

pregnancy. Leiomyomas usually occur as multiple, well-defined, unencapsulated masses.

Clinical Manifestations

Most leiomyomas are asymptomatic and go undetected. Clinical manifestations depend on the leiomyoma size, which can range from microscopic to weighing several pounds, and location. The growing fibroid can cause pressure on adjacent structures. Pressure from the fibroid can result in symptoms such as pelvic pain, bladder dysfunction, dyspareunia, and constipation.

Heavy menstrual bleeding (volume and/ or duration) and the passage of clots can cause dysmenorrhea. Risk for heavy menstrual bleeding usually occurs with submucosal and intramural fibroids, but the risk is low with subserosal fibroids. Degenerating fibroids can cause pelvic pain. Although they do not usually interfere with fertility, leiomyomas do increase the risk of spontaneous abortion and preterm labor slightly. The risk for fertility and pregnancy problems increases as the tumor size increases. Physical examination findings consistent with a leiomyoma include an enlarged, mobile, and irregularly shaped uterus. Leiomyomas that have prolapsed or are on the cervix can be infrequently seen during a vaginal speculum exam. A large, fixed, immobile uterus or one that is rapidly enlarging may be due to a malignant tumor such as leiomyosarcoma instead of a benign leiomyoma

Diagnosis and Treatment

Diagnosis is made with a history, physical examination, and pelvic and transvaginal ultrasound. A CBC is done to evaluate for anemia. Other diagnostic procedures can include hysteroscopy (uterine endoscopy), biopsy (to rule out malignancy), laparoscopy, and MRI. Most leiomyomas are harmless and do not require treatment. Symptom severity and childbearing intentions should be considered when choosing treatment options. Treatment strategies include simple monitoring. Hormone therapy (e.g., GnRH agonists/antagonists and progestin) can be used to shrink the fibroid and reduce symptoms. Oral contraceptives with estrogen-progestin (i.e., combined) can be used to reduce risk of fibroid development and menstrual bleeding, but the combined hormones may cause fibroid growth. Other treatment strategies include analgesics such as NSAIDs; surgery such as myomectomy or hysterectomy; myolysis (laparoscopic laser treatment); endometrial ablation, which uses heat to destroy the uterine lining; and uterine artery embolization, which obstructs uterine blood supply. Additionally, anemia treatment may be necessary.

Disorders of the Ovaries

A variety of benign and malignant conditions can affect the ovaries. Ovarian disorders can be congenital, such as hypogonadism and Turner syndrome, or acquired, such as ovarian cancer, but many have a genetic basis. While some disorders, such as functional cysts, are simple, others, such as polycystic ovarian syndrome, are complex and cause systemic issues. Ovarian disorders can affect the woman's hormonal balance and fertility status.

Ovarian Cysts

Ovarian cysts are benign, fluid-filled sacs on the ovary. Often the cyst forms during the ovulation process when a follicle or follicles are stimulated. Instead of the dominant follicle releasing the egg, the fluid stays in the follicle or the nondominant follicles do not get reabsorbed or regress, creating a follicular cyst. Inadequate development of the corpus luteum can cause a corpus luteum cyst. Because these cysts form during normal physiologic events, they are termed *functional cysts*. Follicular cysts are more common, but corpus luteum cysts can cause more symptoms. Other ovarian cysts include dermoid cysts (i.e., ovarian teratoma), which develop from ovarian germ cells. While the functional and dermoid cysts are benign, a small number (< 3%) of dermoid cysts can become malignant. In most cases, they disappear without treatment. On occasion, however, they rupture, causing discomfort. This common condition most frequently occurs during the childbearing years. Complications are rare, but ovarian cysts can lead to hemorrhage, peritonitis, infertility, and amenorrhea.

When present, abdominal pain or discomfort is the most prevalent clinical manifestation. Pain occurs when the cyst bleeds, ruptures, twists, or exerts pressure on nearby structures. Pain may also be associated with bowel movements and sexual intercourse. Other clinical manifestations include abnormal menstrual bleeding and abdominal distention. A mass on the ovaries may be felt if the cyst has not completely collapsed. Although rare, ovarian cysts can cause an ovarian torsion (similar to testicular torsion), cutting off blood flow and leading to potential for ovarian necrosis. Prompt recognition of ovarian torsion (the patient has acute, severe unilateral pelvic pain) and emergency surgery are necessary.

Diagnosis is accomplished with a history and physical examination. Human chorionic gonadotropin should be performed to assess for pregnancy, particularly ectopic pregnancy. A pelvic and transvaginal ultrasound or an MRI may be necessary. If the imaging studies reveal masses with malignant characteristics, then a biopsy is necessary. A CBC can evaluate for anemia due to bleeding. A CA-125 serum biomarker can evaluate for ovarian cancer. Evaluation for different tumors in the ovary, such as germ cell tumor, may be accomplished by measuring various serum markers (e.g., alpha fetoprotein or inhibin).

Treatment strategies for benign cysts can include simply following up to evaluate for cyst changes such as enlargement. Most cysts resolve without treatment. Oral contraceptives can reduce the incidence of cyst development. An ovarian cystectomy (removal of a cyst from an ovary) or oophorectomy (removal of ovary) may be necessary.

Polycystic Ovary Syndrome

Polycystic ovary syndrome (PCOS) is considered one of the most common endocrine disorders, affecting approximately 5 million women of reproductive age (CDC, 2019). The syndrome is characterized by functional ovarian hyperandrogenism (present in 90% of women with PCOS) and insulin-resistant hyperinsulinemia (present in 50% of women with PCOS) leading to menstrual and ovulatory dysfunction (FIGURE 8-28). The pathogenesis is complex, and the etiology is mostly unknown and theoretical. The syndrome is thought, however, to begin in utero with a resulting congenital dysfunction that causes a predisposition to subsequent development of PCOS. The congenital factors can be hereditary or acquired. The congenital dysfunction predominantly affects the ovaries. In congenitally predisposed individuals, epigenetic and environmental factors (e.g., obesity and insulin resistance) result in PCOS.

The syndrome manifestations become evident during puberty and adolescence. During puberty, GnRH release normally occurs, triggering LH release and FSH release. The LH release stimulates the ovarian theca cells to produce androgens (e.g., androstenedione). The

FSH release stimulates ovarian granulosa cells to produce estrogen. Ovarian theca androgens are important as they are precursors for estrogen production and fertility (follicle growth and development). The balance between the theca cell androgen production and granulosa cell estrogen production, despite triggering by LH and FSH, is regulated within the ovaries. Theca cell and granulosa cell factors respond to androgen and estrogen levels and basically ignore or respond to LH and other mediators (e.g., inhibin). Small contributions of androgens also come from the adrenal glands.

In PCOS, the dysfunctional ovarian theca cells are overly sensitive to LH and oversecrete androgens. The excessive androgens also affect the granulosa cells as they normally rely on the theca cell coordination to start progesterone and continue preovulatory follicle development. The excess androgens cause the growth of a lot of small follicles. Increased LH causes premature luteinization of the follicle (the one that would have been dominant) and the follicle does not mature. This results in oligo-anovulation. While ovarian dysfunction is primary in PCOS, the excess androgen production also causes an impairment in the GnRH negative feedback mechanism, causing more GnRH secretion. As a result, LH secretion increases, and the ovaries respond by producing more androgens. It is theorized that most likely androgen excess leads to LH excess rather than LH excesses causing androgen excesses. LH causes increased abnormal secretion of estradiol, which in turn suppresses FSH. Therefore, FSH levels are usually low. In a small number of women with PCOS (8%) androgen excesses are due to isolated primary functional adrenal hyperandrogenism. Some women have a combination of both ovarian and adrenal dysfunction causing hyperandrogenism.

Insulin-resistant hyperinsulinemia is the second most common characteristic of PCOS and is present in approximately 50% of patients. The insulin resistance causes a compensatory excess insulin secretion (hyperinsulinemia). In PCOS, the muscle is resistant to the metabolic effects of insulin but the ovaries, fat tissue, and adrenal glands remain responsive to insulin; in other words, they are not resistant. The insulin perpetuates theca and granulosa cells to produce more androgens and more small follicles. Hyperinsulinemia contributes to obesity. The reason for obesity in PCOS is not well understood.

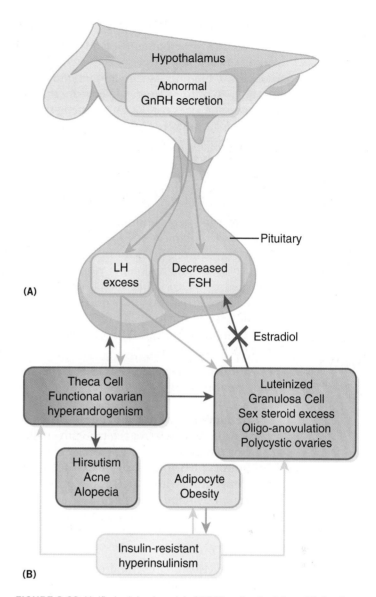

FIGURE 8-28 Unified minimal model of PCOS pathophysiology. (A) Ovarian hyperandrogenism is nearly universal in PCOS and can account for all the cardinal clinical features of the syndrome: hyperandrogenemia, oligo-anovulation, and polycystic ovaries (1). Pituitary LH secretion is necessary to sustain the ovarian androgen excess but is not sufficient to cause it. (B) About half of patients with functional ovarian hyperandrogenism have insulin-resistant hyperinsulinism (2). Insulin-resistant hyperinsulinism acts on theca cells to aggravate hyperandrogenism, synergizes with androgen to prematurely luteinize granulosa cells, and stimulates adipogenesis. The increased hyperandrogenemia provokes LH excess (3), which then acts on both theca and luteinized granulosa cells to worsen hyperandrogenism. LH also stimulates luteinized granulosa cells to secrete estradiol (4), which suppresses FSH secretion. These hyperinsulinism-initiated changes in granulosa cell function further exacerbate PCOM and further hinder ovulation. Obesity increases insulin resistance, and the resultant increased hyperinsulinism further aggravates hyperandrogenism. Heaviness of lines and fonts represents severity. Both functional ovarian hyperandrogenism and insulin resistance typically have an intrinsic basis. This model does not exclude the possibility that the unknown intrinsic ovarian defects that underpin the ovarian steroidogenic dysfunction also involve granulosa cell folliculogenesis as well. The figure also does not depict other associated defects, such as the functional adrenal hyperandrogenism that often accompanies the ovarian hyperandrogenism and the contribution of excess adiposity to peripheral androgen production and gonadotropin suppression.

Inherited traits and disorders that increase risk for PCOS development include abnormal ovarian morphology (form), elevated testosterone, sex-binding hormone globulin, and metabolic syndrome (e.g., defects in insulin resistance and obesity). Various genetic markers are being evaluated (e.g., *DENND1A [DENN domain-containing protein 1A]*, which encodes a protein that is overexpressed and leads to increased steroid hormone production). A maternal history of PCOS is also a risk for PCOS development.

There have been multiple definitions and criteria for describing PCOS since the syndrome was first recognized in 1935. In 2012, an NIH evidence-based methodology workshop was conducted on PCOS (Johnson, Kaplan, Ouyang, & Rizza, 2012). At the workshop criteria were developed for four different phenotypes (observable characteristics from the genotype) for PCOS in adults:

- **Phenotype (classic PCOS):** Hyperandrogenism, oligo-anovulation, and polycystic ovary
- **Phenotype 2 (hyperandrogenic anovulation):** Hyperandrogenism with oligo-anovulation
- **Phenotype 3 (ovulatory PCOS):** Hyperandrogenism with a polycystic ovary but without ovulatory dysfunction
- **Phenotype 4 (nonhyperandrogenic PCOS):** Oligo-anovulation and a polycystic ovary

The severity of hyperandrogenism, menstrual disorders, and symptoms decreases from phenotype 1 to phenotype 4. Criteria for adolescents with PCOS varies somewhat from adult criteria as menstrual disorders and other hyperandrogenic symptoms (e.g., acne) are common and can be normal during adolescence. The criteria for PCOS in adolescence is as follows:

- Abnormal uterine bleeding pattern that is not explained by other disorders and is abnormal for gynecologic developmental age. Symptoms persistent (e.g., > 1 year).
- Evidence of hyperandrogenism—persistent testosterone elevation, moderate to severe hirsutism, and moderate to severe inflammatory acne.

Clinical Manifestations

There are multiple potential causes, and the various phenotypes result in different clinical manifestations. Functional ovarian hyperandrogenism is the cause of most clinical features in PCOS. The clinical manifestations as a result of excess androgens include:

- Skin manifestations—hirsutism (abnormal facial and body hair), acne, and male pattern baldness
- Menstrual disorders—infrequent menses (oligomenorrhea) and anovulation; episodes of heavy menstrual bleeding can occur
- Obesity
- Ovarian cysts—usually multiple and small

Polycystic ovary syndrome increases the risk for developing obesity, insulin resistance, diabetes mellitus, dyslipidemia, and cancer (especially endometrial and breast cancers). Women may also have a higher incidence of sleep apnea, depression, or nonalcoholic fatty liver disease.

Diagnosis and Treatment

Diagnosis of PCOS is accomplished with a history, physical examination, and hormone levels (e.g., testosterone, LH, FSH, and estradiol). A transvaginal ultrasound may reveal cysts. The absence of cysts does not rule out PCOS, and the presence of cysts does not confirm diagnosis. Additional tests can evaluate for glucose and lipid abnormalities (e.g., hemoglobin A1c, lipid panel, etc.).

Weight loss with diet and exercise may improve symptoms and ovulation. Hormonal therapy (e.g., combined oral contraceptives and progestin-only treatment) will improve symptoms of hyperandrogenism, regulate menses, and protect the endometrium from hyperplasia. Spironolactone can be added to the oral contraceptives to further lower androgen levels. Metformin can be used to improve insulin sensitivity and can restore ovulation. Fertility issues need to be addressed, and ovulation can be induced (e.g., with clomiphene). Any other complications (e.g., depression) or manifestations of the disorder should also be treated.

Disorders of the Breasts

Breast disorders can be benign (e.g., fibrocystic breast disease) or malignant (e.g., breast cancer). Most breast disorders are not life threatening; however, malignancies should always be ruled out when breast symptoms are noted. These conditions can affect lactation, breastfeeding, and self-image.

Benign Breast Masses

Benign breast masses are often detected by palpation and/or on imaging studies such as a mammogram. Breast masses can occur anywhere

BOX 8-1 Application to Practice

Abnormal uterine bleeding is a common gynecologic complaint. Review the following scenarios and determine a likely cause and describe the mechanism that leads to the abnormal bleeding pattern.

Scenario 1: A 13-year-old girl is having episodes of amenorrhea and infrequent menses. Her menarche was at the age of 12, she denies being sexually active, and a urine pregnancy test is negative.

Scenario 2: A 60-year-old woman who has been in menopause for 5 years is having episodes of menstrual bleeding for the past 2 months. She said sometimes it is just spotting but at times she has worn a small sanitary pad. She is overweight and says despite her efforts she struggles to lose weight.

Scenario 3: A 21-year-old woman is having episodes of amenorrhea and infrequent menses. Her menarche was at the age of 14 and her menses have sometimes been regular. She is overweight and says despite her efforts to lose weight, she does not do so. She is generally very healthy otherwise and the only medication she is taking is doxycycline for acne, which she feels is getting worse. She said her mother's menstrual pattern was the same and that her mother told her she had trouble getting pregnant (the patient is an only child). She is sexually active, her partner uses condoms consistently, and her urine pregnancy is negative.

---

in breast tissue such as the ducts, lobules, and connective tissue. While many masses are benign, some are associated with an increased risk of breast cancer. Breast masses are categorized based on their tissue type, which includes nonproliferative lesions, proliferative lesions without atypia, and lesions with atypical hyperplasia. The types of common masses included in these categorization and risk of breast cancer are as follows:

- **Nonproliferative:** The most common type of masses are breast cysts, which are usually fluid-filled masses that can be solitary, multiple, or in clusters. Cysts are classified as simple, complex, and complicated. The cancer risk for each type of cyst is as follows: simple cyst not associated with cancer; complex rarely associated with cancer ($< 1\%$); and complicated with slightly higher association with cancer than others ($1–23\%$). *Fibrocystic changes* or *fibrocystic disease* are terms that are commonly used by clinicians in reference to nonproliferative disease, but this description encompasses many types of breast masses and therefore is nonspecific.
- **Proliferative without atypia:** The most common type of breast mass overall is a fibroadenoma, which is a solid mass containing glandular and fibrous tissue that can be solitary or multiple. Simple fibroadenoma are not associated with an increased cancer risk, while complex fibroadenomas confer a slightly increased risk.

- **Atypical hyperplasia:** These masses can be ductal or lobular and are associated with ductal carcinoma in situ or lobular carcinoma in situ, respectively.

There are many other breast masses that are considered benign, such as lipomas, fat necrosis (mass that occurs after trauma), galactoceles (masses caused by obstructed milk ducts), and adenomas. There are also many benign breast masses usually associated with low or varying risks for breast cancer, such as ductal papillomas (solitary or multiple) and sclerosing adenosis (lobular mass). Masses can become more prominent and painful during menstruation because of hormone fluctuations. During perimenopause and menopause, hormonal changes and lobular decreases can result in increased breast masses. Although the exact cause is unknown, the condition is thought to be a result of hormones. Breast cysts are more frequent during the childbearing years than in the postmenopausal years.

Clinical Manifestations

Clinical manifestations of breast masses can include changes such as increases in size or pain before or during menstruation. The breast mass can be solitary (most common) or multiple or occur in clusters. Some masses are large while others are small. The mass can feel smooth or firm and is often discrete (distinct or separate). The consistency can be rubbery, squishy, grapelike, and even hard. Physical examination findings alone are insufficient to determine whether a mass is benign or malignant. Nipple discharge is not common with benign breast masses, and any discharge that is spontaneous, persistent, or bloody is consistent with breast cancer.

Diagnosis and Treatment

Diagnostic procedures for breast masses consist of a history with a focus on breast cancer risk and a physical examination. Masses are evaluated with an ultrasound, which by itself is often sufficient for women < 30 years of age. Further testing, however, regardless of age, is dependent on the ultrasound findings. A biopsy to rule out breast cancer can be done with fine needle aspiration, core biopsy (a piece of mass removed), or excisional biopsy (whole mass is removed). Mammograms are often done, particularly for older women with masses. Usually no treatment is required for masses that have no risks for cancer. When necessary, treatment strategies are largely symptomatic and include needle aspiration of fluid, surgical removal of cysts, analgesics (e.g., NSAIDs or acetaminophen), a supportive bra, heat/cold application, limitation of dietary fat, and avoidance of caffeine and chocolate (although research is inconclusive about this strategy). Vitamin E, vitamin B_6, magnesium, and evening primrose oil may improve symptoms, but the use of these supplements remains controversial. Additionally, oral contraceptives can minimize symptoms. Danazol is an androgen that can reduce breast nodules and pain but is associated with significant side effects (e.g., weight gain, irregular menses). Due to these androgenic side effects, danazol is usually reserved for women who have severe pain not responsive to other treatments. Benign breast masses that are associated with a risk of breast cancer need to be monitored more often. Chemoprevention with use of drugs such as selective estrogen modulators (e.g., tamoxifen) can be considered; however, risks and benefits should be thoroughly evaluated.

Mastitis

Mastitis refers to an inflammation of the breast tissue that can be associated with infection and lactation. This condition usually develops within 6 weeks of childbirth. In most cases, a staphylococcal or streptococcal bacterium is introduced to the nipple through the breastfeeding process, but mastitis can also occur in the absence of lactation or breastfeeding. Impaired nipple or skin integrity increases the likelihood of mastitis developing. The infection

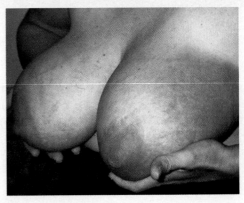

FIGURE 8-29 Mastitis.
Courtesy of Sarah Coulter-Danner.

usually invades the breast's fatty tissue, triggering an inflammatory response (e.g., edema, redness, warmth). The edema puts pressure on the milk ducts, causing pain and palpable lumps. Despite popular belief to the contrary, breastfeeding can occur in the presence of mastitis, but it may be uncomfortable. In some cases, however, flow of milk may become blocked and abscesses can develop.

Clinical manifestations usually appear suddenly and include the following signs and symptoms:

- Breast tenderness, swelling, redness, and warmth (**FIGURE 8-29**)
- Breast lumps
- Pain or a burning sensation continuously or while breastfeeding
- Flulike symptoms (e.g., fever, malaise, chills, nausea, and vomiting)
- Nipple discharge (usually purulent)
- Enlarged nearby axillary lymph nodes

Diagnostic procedures for mastitis include a history, physical examination, and cultures of drainage and/or breastmilk. Treatment strategies consist of antibiotic therapy, adequate hydration, rest, analgesics (e.g., acetaminophen and NSAIDs), supportive bra, heat/cold application, adequate milk expression, and needle aspiration. During treatment, breastfeeding is safe and should be encouraged (except if the mother is human immunodeficiency virus [HIV] positive).

Reproductive Tract Infections

Infections can occur anywhere along the reproductive tract or organs. There are various modes of transmission. Infections can arise from the urinary system or be sexually transmitted.

Some infections are due to alterations in the host such as an alteration in vaginal flora seen in candidiasis. Many of the infections are easily resolved with treatment, however some infections are lifelong and periodic exacerbations can occur. Infections that are untreated can have detrimental effects such as infertility.

Prostatitis

Prostatitis refers to inflammation of the prostate, which can be either acute or chronic. Prostatitis may be caused by a variety of conditions (e.g., bacteria, sperm, trauma, stress, and urinary catheter) that trigger the inflammatory process. Normally, the prostate has protective mechanisms to prevent ascending infection such as the flushing action of urination and ejaculation. Additionally, it contains secretions that have an antimicrobial action (possibly attributable to their zinc content). However, owing to its close proximity to the urinary system, urethra, or bladder, bacteria can migrate through the prostate ducts, and there is intraprostatic reflux of urine. The most common pathogen causing prostatitis is gram-negative *Escherichia coli*. Prostatitis is more common in young and middle-aged men and those in immunocompromised states. Prostatitis with epididymitis and urethritis leads to sexually transmitted infections (especially chlamydia and gonorrhea).

Prostatitis is classified into four categories.

- **Category 1:** Acute bacterial prostatitis
  - Usually seen in younger men
  - Usually results from a urinary tract infection (often *E. coli*) or sexually transmitted (often *N. gonorrhoeae* and *C. trachomatis*)
  - Least common
  - Easiest to diagnose and treat, but can be life threatening
- **Category 2:** Chronic bacterial prostatitis
  - Usually results from recurrent urinary tract infection
  - Relatively uncommon
  - Persists longer than 3 months
  - Indolent (causes little to no pain)
- **Category 3:** Chronic prostatitis/chronic pelvic pain
  - No clear etiology and may be inflammatory or noninflammatory
  - No bacteria are present, but immune cells can be found
  - Most common and least understood
  - Manifestations last longer than 3 months; can disappear and reappear without warning

- **Category 4:** Asymptomatic inflammatory prostatitis
  - No clear etiology
  - No bacteria are present, but immune cells can be found
  - May be associated with infertility

Clinical Manifestations

Clinical manifestations of prostatitis vary depending on the type. These manifestations include the following signs and symptoms:

- Dysuria
- Difficulty urinating, such as dribbling or hesitancy
- Urinary frequency and urgency
- Nocturia
- Pain in the abdomen, groin, lower back, perineum, or genitals
- Painful ejaculation
- Indications of infection such as fever, chills, and myalgia (with acute bacterial prostatitis)
- Recurrent urinary tract infections (with chronic bacterial prostatitis)

Diagnosis and Treatment

Diagnostic procedures for prostatitis consist of a history, physical examination (including a digital rectal examination), and urine gram stain and culture. Men with acute bacterial prostatitis are acutely ill (e.g., fever and malaise), and symptoms are not subtle as in chronic forms of prostatitis. The digital exam with acute prostatitis should be performed gently as a vigorous exam can result in bacteremia. The exam is also very painful. The prostate will also be edematous. With acute prostatitis, the urine will be positive for pyuria (white blood cells) and bacteriuria. Treatment strategies include long-term antibiotics. Hospitalization may be necessary for those with presumptive bacteremia or urinary retention. A urinary catheter should not be inserted with acute prostatitis due to the risk of septicemia and rupture of a prostatic abscess, if present. Abscesses should be suspected when treatment has been delayed or when symptoms do not improve with antibiotic therapy. Diagnosis of an abscess can be confirmed with a transrectal ultrasound of the prostate or a CT scan.

Diagnostic tests for chronic prostatitis include urine and prostatic fluid samples. The prostate fluid sample culture will be positive for pathogens in chronic bacterial prostatitis. The urine sample may be negative or positive for pathogens. Other diagnostic procedures may include cystoscopy, urodynamic studies, CT scan, or transrectal ultrasound, which may reveal prostatic calculi.

Treatment strategies for chronic bacterial prostatitis, as with acute, include long-term organism-specific antibiotic therapy, analgesics (e.g., NSAIDs and acetaminophen), antipyretics, adequate hydration, and sitz bath. Other strategies can include treatment for urinary symptoms (e.g., alpha blockers and anticholinergics), and acupuncture and extracorporeal therapy may be beneficial for chronic pelvic pain.

Epididymitis

Epididymitis describes an inflammation of the epididymis, the duct connecting the testes to the vas deferens. It is a common cause of scrotal pain in adults. Ascending bacterial infections or sexually transmitted infections usually initiate this inflammatory process. Bacteria, most commonly *E. coli* and *Pseudomonas aeruginosa*, frequently spread to the epididymis from the urinary system. Urinary tract infections, particularly from obstructions due to benign prostatic hypertrophy or other urethral strictures, are the most frequent etiology in men > 35 years of age. Gonorrhea and chlamydia are the typical sexually transmitted culprits (**TABLE 8-2**). Sexually transmitted infections are more frequent in men < 35 years of age. In boys (prior to puberty) or adolescents who are not sexually active, the causative organisms are usually viruses (e.g., adenoviruses) or atypical bacteria such as *Mycoplasma pneumoniae*. Men who engage in insertive anal sex, regardless of age, are at risk of epididymitis due to enteric bacteria (e.g., *E. coli*). The urethral or bladder bacteria ascend from the vas deferens to the epididymis. Some other causes of epididymitis include *Mycobacterium tuberculosis* and the antidysrhythmic medication amiodarone (Cordarone). *Mycobacterium* results in chronic epididymitis with symptoms of pain in the scrotum, testicle, or epididymis lasting longer than 6 weeks and should be suspected in those with a history of tuberculosis or recent exposure. Risk factors for developing epididymitis include the following conditions:

- Being uncircumcised
- Recent surgery or a history of structural problems in the urinary tract
- Urinary catheterization
- Sexual intercourse with more than one partner and failure to use condoms

TABLE 8-2	Sexually Transmitted Infections
Disease characterization	**Common STI pathogens**
Urethritis, cervicitis	*Neisseria gonorrhoeae*, *Chlamydia trachomatis*, *Mycoplasma genitalium*
Epididymitis	*N. gonorrhoeae*, *C. trachomatis* Men engaging in insertive anal intercourse: *Escherichia coli*
Pelvic inflammatory disease*	*N. gonorrhoeae*, *C. trachomatis*, *M. genitalium*
Prostatitis	*N. gonorrhoeae*, *C. trachomatis*
Vaginal discharge	*Trichomonas vaginalis*
Ulcers	*Treponema pallidum* (syphilis) Herpes simplex virus 1 and 2 (genital herpes)
Condyloma (warts)	Human papillomavirus type 6 and type 11 (*Condyloma acuminata*) *T. pallidum* (condyloma lata)

*Often polymicrobial

The inflammatory and infectious process can lead to abscesses, fistulas (the cutaneous scrotal type), infertility, testicular necrosis, and chronic epididymitis.

Clinical Manifestations

Clinical manifestations of epididymitis reflect the inflammatory and infectious processes:

- Indicators of infection (e.g., fever, chills, and myalgia)
- Testicular tenderness (acute onset) and edema; can develop scrotal wall erythema (epididymo-orchitis) and fluid accumulation (like a hydrocele)
- Prehn sign (elevating the scrotum relieves pain)
- Penile discharge
- Bloody semen (i.e., hematospermia)
- Painful ejaculation
- Dysuria
- Groin pain

Diagnosis and Treatment

Diagnostic procedures for epididymitis focus on identifying the causative agent and consist of a history, physical examination, urinalysis, cultures (urine and penile discharge), and sexually transmitted infection testing particularly for gonorrhea and chlamydia. Treatment

BOX 8-2 Application to Practice

Epididymitis and testicular torsion are both causes of scrotal pain. Testicular torsion requires prompt recognition and surgical intervention to avoid testicular damage. Epididymitis is easily managed with antibiotics. Differentiation between the two disorders is important. Review the case and answer the questions.

Case: A 15-year-old presents to the emergency department complaining of sudden onset of right-sided scrotal and groin pain. He states the pain is constant and extreme. He said it started about 2 hours ago during basketball practice at school, but he denies any trauma to the scrotum. He is worried that he has a sexually transmitted infection as he just started having sexual intercourse with his girlfriend and he did not use condoms. He says he feels nauseated and thinks he is going to vomit. He said he noticed this same pain once before, but it went away within a few seconds and he did not tell anyone.

Vital signs: Temperature 98.9° F; pulse 100 beats per minute; respirations 20 breaths per minute; blood pressure 120/70 mmHg.

Physical examination reveals a healthy-appearing adolescent who is anxious and grimacing. The patient has edema and erythema of his right scrotum. His scrotum is tender, and the patient only tolerated superficial palpation.

1. The most likely diagnosis based on his history is:
   a. Epididymitis
   b. Testicular torsion
2. Erythema and edema of the scrotum are only present with epididymitis.
   a. True
   b. False
3. Which of the following clinical manifestations are consistent with epididymitis, and which are consistent with testicular torsion?
   a. Positive Prehn sign
   b. Negative cremasteric reflex
   c. Testis elevated on affected side
   d. Fever
      1. Testicular torsion
      2. Epididymitis
4. Which diagnostic test is most appropriate to confirm the suspected diagnosis?
   a. A complete blood count with differential
   b. An MRI of the scrotum
   c. A Doppler ultrasound of the scrotum
   d. A urine culture and sensitivity
5. Discuss the treatment plans for testicular torsion and epididymitis.

---

strategies center on eliminating the infection and decreasing discomfort. These interventions include the following measures:

- Antibiotic therapy
- Analgesics (especially NSAIDs)
- Bed rest
- Scrotal support (wearing briefs instead of boxers) and elevation (on a rolled towel)
- Cold application
- Screening and treatment of sexual partners

Within 3 days of starting antibiotics, the symptoms should improve. Lack of symptom improvement may indicate other causes of testicular pain or complications of epididymitis (e.g., abscess). Further diagnostic testing may include a scrotal ultrasound.

Candidiasis

Candidiasis is a yeast infection caused by the common fungus *Candida albicans*. This condition usually occurs as an opportunistic infection that can arise anywhere in the body (especially the skin and the gastrointestinal tract), but the focus of the discussion here is the infection's effects on the reproductive system.

In the reproductive system, candidiasis most frequently occurs in the vulva and vagina (i.e., vulvovaginal candidiasis) and is a common cause of vaginitis (inflammation of the vagina). *Candida* and many other microorganisms are part of the normal flora present in the vagina, which usually exist in a balanced state. Imbalance may occur in the presence of vaginal pH changes; normally, the vagina is slightly acidic. This acidic state is mainly maintained by lactobacillus that break glycogen down into lactic acid. Antibiotic therapy can increase vaginal pH (making it more alkaline), leading to yeast overgrowth. Other factors contributing to such imbalance include decreased immune response (e.g., due to corticosteroid medications or HIV). Candidiasis is more common in those with increased estrogen level and increased glucose in the vaginal secretions which can occur with pregnancy, oral contraceptive use, diabetes mellitus, and obesity. Bubble baths and feminine products can also alter the delicate pH balance. Synthetic and tight-fitting clothes will also increase the risk of *Candida* infection. Candidiasis is not sexually transmitted, but men may develop balanitis (inflammation of the glans penis) after having sexual intercourse with an infected partner (especially if a partner has recurrent vaginal candidiasis). If the foreskin is also affected, then the condition is termed *balanoposthitis*. Balanitis is more common in men with diabetes mellitus and those who are uncircumcised.

Clinical Manifestations

Clinical manifestations of candidiasis include the following signs and symptoms:

- A thick, white vaginal discharge that is curdlike (resembles cottage cheese) and nonodorous
- Vulvar erythema and edema
- Vaginal and labial pruritus (can be intense) and burning
- White patches on the vaginal wall
- Dysuria (burning occurs when urine touches the vulva rather than while it is exiting)
- Painful sexual intercourse

At times, the vaginal discharge can be thin, loose, and watery as opposed to the typical thick, white discharge. Men have similar symptoms such as white curdlike exudate, pruritis, and erythematous small papules or white patches on the penis and foreskin.

Diagnosis and Treatment

Vulvovaginal candidiasis diagnosis is often made clinically but is best evaluated with in-office vaginal microscopy. The vaginal discharge is placed on a slide and 10% potassium hydroxide (KOH) is added onto the slide. The KOH destroys cellular elements so that yeast buds, hyphae, and pseudohyphae can be visualized in the presence of a *Candida* infection (FIGURE 8-30). The vaginal pH with candidiasis is usually normal (4.0–4.5). A culture of the discharge can be performed, particularly if manifestations are consistent with candidiasis yet microscopy was negative. *Candida glabrata* is responsible for approximately 10% of vulvovaginal candidiasis, and the organism is usually not seen with microscopy. Balanitis or balanoposthitis diagnosis can also be made with a history, physical examination, and an in-office microscopic evaluation of the exudate.

Treatment focuses on reestablishing normal flora balance, minimizing tissue irritation,

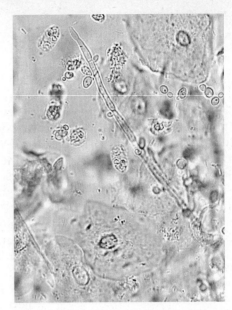

FIGURE 8-30 Polymorphonuclear granulocyte leukocytes PMNs and yeast pseudohyphae.
Courtesy of University of Washington STD Prevention Training Center.

and increasing comfort. Treatment strategies can also be used for prevention of candidiasis:

- Antifungal agents (available in oral or topical forms; some are available without a prescription)
- Perineum care (including cleaning from front to back, keeping the perineum area clean and dry, avoiding soap and rinsing with water only, and taking warm—not hot—baths)
- Avoidance of douching
- Resisting the urge to scratch
- Practicing safe sex (tissue irritation increases the risk for contracting a sexually transmitted infection)
- Avoidance of feminine hygiene sprays, fragrances, or powders in the genital area
- Avoidance of extremely tight-fitting clothing (which may cause irritation)
- Wearing cotton underwear or cotton-crotch panty hose and avoiding underwear made of silk or nylon (these materials are not very absorbent and restrict airflow, increasing sweating in the genital area and irritation)
- Controlling blood glucose (if diabetic)
- Eating yogurt with live cultures or taking *Lactobacillus acidophilus* or probiotic tablets (a practice for which effectiveness, however, is questionable and controversial)

Most cases of uncomplicated candidiasis (e.g., ≤ 3 episodes a year, mild to moderate symptoms, or in healthy, nonpregnant females) can be treated at home and without medical supervision. Self-management is not recommended in situations that may be due to a more complicated infection such as:

- Symptoms are severe
- Fever or pelvic pain is present
- The patient has a negative history for candidiasis
- Pregnancy
- Immunosuppression or uncontrolled diabetes mellitus
- Other vaginal infections are present or possibly present
- The patient has recurrent infections (≥ 4 episodes a year)

If self-management strategies are not successful, a healthcare provider should be consulted.

Sexually Transmitted Infections

Sexually transmitted infections (STIs), sometimes referred to as *sexually transmitted diseases*, encompass a broad range of infections that can be contracted through sexual contact (including oral–genital contact, anal contact, and vaginal intercourse). More than 30 different sexually transmissible bacteria, viruses, and parasites have been identified; some of these pathogens can also be transmitted from mother to child during pregnancy and childbirth as well as through blood contact (e.g., HIV and syphilis). Some STIs result from ectoparasites such as pediculosis pubis caused by *Phthirus pubis* (i.e., crab louse) and scabies caused by *Sarcoptes scabiei*. Some STIs (e.g., chlamydia and gonorrhea) are easily eradicated with appropriate treatment, whereas others (e.g., genital herpes and condylomata acuminata) persist for a lifetime. See chapter 2 for a discussion of HIV. See chapter 13 for a discussion of *Sarcoptes scabiei*.

The CDC reported that 2,295,739 cases of STIs were reported in 2017 alone (CDC, 2017). Many STIs go undiagnosed and not all STIs are reportable therefore making the incidence much higher. Laws mandate that three STIs be reported to the CDC: chlamydia, gonorrhea, and syphilis. In 2017, increases were seen in the prevalence of all three of these nationally reported STIs. Other STIs are not required to be reported (e.g., genital herpes and condylomata acuminata); therefore, their actual prevalence may be much higher than the CDC's estimates.

STI prevalence rates vary depending on the geographic region within and outside the United States. STI rates have been increasing in the United States despite education efforts directed toward their prevention. Since 2013, chlamydia rates have increased 22%, gonorrhea rates have increased 67%, and syphilis rates have increased 76% (CDC, 2018). Some of this increase may be attributed to changes in societal attitudes toward sex and pregnancy (e.g., less fear, less sexual education, and more media inundation) as well as changes in screening practices (e.g., less funding for local and state screening programs).

Bacterial STIs

Bacterial STIs are common and are usually treated with minimal residual effects. Screening generally focuses on identifying the causative organism through cultures of exudate, rapid assay tests, and fluorescent antibody tests. Bacterial STIs, particularly gonorrhea and chlamydia, can cause a spectrum of disorders but are often characterized by urethritis, cervicitis, epididymitis, and pelvic inflammatory disease (Table 8-2). The bacteria causing syphilis is categorized as one of several STIs that can cause a genital ulcer. Treatment of bacterial STIs usually requires a simple course of antibiotics. If taken properly, the antibiotics will resolve the infection. Reinfection is common, but it can be minimized by refraining from sexual activity until bacteria are eradicated, by practicing safe sex (e.g., using condoms and dental dams), and by sexual partners receiving treatment.

Chlamydia

Chlamydia is caused by *Chlamydia trachomatis*, an intracellular parasitic bacterium that requires a host cell to reproduce. Chlamydia is the most commonly reported STI in the United States; more than 1.7 million cases were reported to the CDC in 2017. According to the CDC (2018), chlamydia rates have increased by 22% since 2013. Chlamydia rates are high across all groups and regions in the United States, but the burden of chlamydia is the highest in women, American Indians/Alaska Natives, Blacks, and persons living in the District of Columbia (CDC, 2017).

Chlamydia can be transmitted through sexual contact and infects the mucosal epithelium along the urogenital tract. There are 11 serotypes labeled from A through K. Genotypes D–K cause urogenital, rectal, pharyngeal, and conjunctival infections. Mother-to-child transmission during childbirth, many times, occurs in the form of neonatal conjunctivitis (an eye infection that can lead to blindness). Chlamydia can cause pharyngitis. Another chlamydia species, *Chlamydia pneumoniae*, causes pneumonia, and this organism is not sexually transmitted. Chlamydia genotypes A–C can cause trachoma, a non–sexually transmitted conjunctivitis and are the leading causes of infectious blindness worldwide. The incubation period for sexually transmitted chlamydia is 7–14 days after infection; however, the period of infectivity is not clear in asymptomatic cases. See chapter 14 for a discussion of trachoma. See chapter 5 for a discussion of pharyngitis.

Clinical Manifestations

Often called the *silent STI*, chlamydia is usually asymptomatic in both males and females. Chlamydia most commonly infects the cervix, causing cervicitis. In men, the urethra is the most commonly infected site, and infection results in urethritis. In men, chlamydia is a common cause of sexually transmitted causes of epididymitis and prostatitis, and it is associated with pelvic inflammatory disease in women. Chlamydia can cause proctitis (inflammation of the distal rectal mucosa) particularly in men who engage in receptive anal intercourse. Chlamydia can be isolated in the throat but it is generally asymptomatic. When present, clinical manifestations include the following signs and symptoms:

- Mucopurulent endocervical discharge from the cervix and cervical friability (bleeds easily when endocervix touched)
- Vaginal discharge that is purulent or mucopurulent (usually comes from the cervix, not the vagina)
- Mucoid, mucopurulent, or watery penile discharge
- Menstrual disorders such as intermenstrual or postcoital bleeding
- Dysuria
- Painful sexual intercourse (dyspareunia)
- Rectal pain and mucopurulent discharge

Complications of untreated chlamydia include pelvic inflammatory disease, which can then lead to infertility and chronic pelvic pain. Chlamydia during pregnancy can cause complications such as premature membrane rupture and preterm delivery. Reactive arthritis (i.e., Reiter syndrome) is an uncommon chlamydia-associated disorder in men. Reactive arthritis manifestations include a triad of symptoms—urethritis, arthritis (e.g., acute onset, knee pain), and uveitis (iris redness and swelling).

Diagnosis and Treatment

Because of this STI's high prevalence and potential to cause neonatal complications, it is recommended that all pregnant women be screened for chlamydia and receive treatment if they are found to be infected. The U.S. Preventive Services Task Force (2014) also recommends annually screening all sexually active women who are < 25 years old (LeFevre, 2014). Guidelines have not been established for screening in men or older women; however, screening should be offered to those engaging in riskier behaviors such as having multiple partners or unprotected sexual intercourse.

Diagnosis is made with a history and physical examination. Diagnostic testing can be accomplished in several manners. The source of the specimen can be a urine sample or swabs of the genitourinary tract—vaginal, endocervical, or urethral (men). The diagnostic technique that is most accurate and considered the gold standard is nucleic acid amplification testing (NAAT). With this method, detection is made by amplification of the DNA or RNA of a pathogen (e.g., *C. trachomatis*). NAAT can be done on urine or vaginal or endocervical specimens. Some NAAT (e.g., Xpert CT/NG) can provide results within 90 minutes. Chlamydia antibodies may take several weeks to appear in the serum, so antibody testing is not often used. Due to the availability of better tests, culture tests are rarely used. Antigen testing and DNA genetic probe methods can be used but require a swab from the urethra or cervix.

Learning Points

Chlamydia and Genital Ulcers

Lymphogranuloma venereum (LGV) is caused by *C. trachomatis* serovars L 1-3. LGV causes a lymphoproliferative reaction as the infection spreads from the primary site to draining lymph nodes. This reaction is in contrast to mucosal chlamydial infection which is usually confined to the site of infection. The incidence is highest in tropical and subtropical areas of the world, however, LGV has been increasingly reported in men who have sex with men particularly in temperate climates (e.g. Western Europe, parts of North America [large outbreak in New York]). HIV is a risk factor. The initial infection is a genital ulcer with an incubation period of 3-12 days. The ulcer heals and is often missed as it is usually small and there are no other symptoms. Subsequently 2-6 weeks after the initial infection severe inflammation and invasive infection appear in the inguinal and/or femoral lymph nodes. Buboes (large, painful, lymph nodes) that are unilateral can develop. In those who are exposed rectally proctocolitis may occur with or without a urogenital ulcer and manifest as rectal bleeding, mucoid discharge, anal pain, constipation, fever, and tensemus. Clinical presentation can vary and diagnostic testing is not standardized making diagnosis difficult. Antibiotics are the treatment of choice and the buboes may need to be drained.

Treatment usually consists of antibiotics such as azithromycin (Zithromax) (usually one dose) or doxycycline (usually one week of therapy). Erythromycin or quinolones (e.g., levofloxacin) are alternative choices. Gonorrhea often occurs as a coinfection, and treatment may be necessary. Sexual partners, usually those within 60 days prior to infection, should also be screened and treated. If the last sexual exposure was > 60 days ago, then the most recent sexual partner should be screened and treated. Subsequent testing for cure is not necessary, and a repeat NAAT within 3 weeks may be positive due to the presence of nonviable organisms. Medication resistance is uncommon. There is, however, a high rate of reinfection, and appropriate follow-up (usually within 3 months) and testing for new infection may be necessary. Pregnant women are usually retested. Additionally, avoiding vaginal childbirth by electing to have a cesarean section delivery may decrease the chances of mother-to-child transmission. Patients should avoid sexual intercourse until 7 days after completion of therapy.

Gonorrhea

Gonorrhea (referred to colloquially as the *clap*) is caused by *N. gonorrhoeae*, an aerobic bacterium that has developed many drug-resistant strains. The incidence of gonorrhea was declining, but the CDC (2018) reported a 67% increase since 2013; gonorrhea remains a very commonly reported disease to the CDC. According to the CDC (2017), gonorrhea rates are highest in men, Blacks and American Indians/ Alaska Natives, and for persons living in the District of Columbia.

The *N. gonorrhoeae* bacterium attaches to the epithelial mucosa of the urethra, cervix, mouth or anus, causing irritation and inflammation. The *N. gonorrhoeae* bacterium can adapt to the genital tracts, change its surface structure (like a chameleon changes color), multiply in various forms, and avoid the immune system. Gonorrhea is transmissible through sexual contact and from mother to infant during childbirth. Mother-to-child transmission usually results in neonatal conjunctivitis. Gonorrhea can also cause pharyngitis and transmission is more common with fellatio in comparison to cunnilingus. Outside the body, the bacterium dies within a few seconds.

Clinical Manifestations

Gonorrhea is often asymptomatic. Clinical manifestations, if they occur, usually do not appear until 2–10 days after infection exposure, but the incubation period is usually 2–5 days for men. Gonorrhea most commonly infects the cervix, causing cervicitis, but the urethra is also often coinfected in women as opposed to chlamydia. In men, the urethra is the most common infected site and results in urethritis. In men, gonorrhea can be a cause of sexually transmitted epididymitis, although more often it is chlamydia alone or as a coinfection. In women, gonorrhea is associated with pelvic inflammatory disease. Gonorrhea can cause proctitis (inflammation of the distal rectal mucosa), particularly in men who engage in receptive anal intercourse. Men are more likely than women to experience symptoms. When present, clinical manifestations are similar to those of chlamydia and include the following signs and symptoms:

- Mucopurulent endocervical discharge (can be more copious than with chlamydia) and cervical friability (bleeds easily when endocervix touched)
- Vaginal discharge that is purulent or mucopurulent (usually from the cervix, not the vagina) (**FIGURE 8-31**)
- Mucoid, mucopurulent or watery penile discharge (spontaneous, more copious than with chlamydia)
- Menstrual disorders, including intermenstrual or postcoital bleeding or heavy menstrual bleeding
- Dysuria
- Painful sexual intercourse (dyspareunia)

Complications of untreated gonorrhea include pelvic inflammatory disease, which can then lead to infertility and chronic pain. Gonorrhea during pregnancy can cause complications

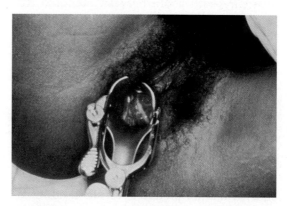

FIGURE 8-31 Gonococcal infection.
Courtesy of CDC.

such as premature membrane rupture, preterm delivery, and spontaneous abortion. Additionally, gonorrhea can spread to other locations in the body (disseminated gonococcal infection); in such a case, complications may include purulent arthritis (usually of the hands, wrists, ankles, knees, and elbows), tenosynovitis (tendon inflammation usually in the wrists/hands and ankles/feet), dermatitis (usually of the hands and lower extremities), and endocarditis.

Diagnosis and Treatment

Because of this STI's high prevalence and potential to cause neonatal complications, it is recommended that all pregnant women be screened for gonorrhea and receive treatment if they are infected. The U.S. Preventive Services Task Force (2014) also recommends annually screening all sexually active women who are < 25 years old (LeFevre, 2014). Guidelines have not been established for screening in men or older women; however, screening should be offered in those engaging in riskier behaviors such as having multiple partners or unprotected sexual intercourse.

Diagnosis is made with a history, physical examination, and several testing options. The source of the specimen can be a urine sample or swabs of the genitourinary tract—vaginal, endocervical, or urethral (men). As with chlamydia, the diagnostic technique that is most accurate and considered the gold standard is NAAT. With this method, detection is made by amplification of the DNA or RNA of a pathogen (e.g., *N. gonorrhoeae*). NAAT can be done on urine or vaginal or endocervical specimens. Some NAAT (e.g., Xpert CT/NG) can provide results within 90 minutes. Gonorrhea antibodies may take several weeks to appear in the serum, so this test is not often used. Antibiotic resistance with gonorrhea can occur, so culture of the discharge can be sent to evaluate for antibiotic susceptibilities. Antigen testing and DNA genetic probe methods can be used but require a swab from the urethra or cervix.

Treatment usually consists of antibiotics with ceftriaxone (cephalosporin) in one dose and azithromycin in one dose. Gonorrhea resistance to multiple classifications of antibiotics is becoming a worldwide problem, and there is an increased prevalence in men having sex with men. Other antibiotics such as doxycycline, while not preferred, can be used. Chlamydia often occurs as a coinfection, but it is already covered with the usual treatment of

azithromycin for gonorrhea. Sexual partners, usually those within 60 days prior to infection, should also be screened and treated. If the last sexual exposure was > 60 days ago, then the most recent sexual partner should be screened and treated. Subsequent testing for cure is usually not necessary, but treatment failure due to antibiotic resistance can occur. A repeat NAAT should not be done within 2 weeks after infection as there may be a false positive due to the presence of nonviable organisms. A culture to test for cure can be done 7 days after therapy is completed. If symptoms recur soon after completion of therapy (e.g., within 5 days), treatment failure or reinfection are possibilities. Appropriate follow-up (usually within 3 months) is recommended. Pregnant women, however, are usually retested. Additionally, avoiding vaginal childbirth by electing to have a cesarean section delivery may decrease the chance of mother-to-child transmission. Patients should avoid sexual intercourse until 7 days after completion of therapy.

Bacterial Vaginosis

Bacterial vaginosis (BV) is a common cause of vaginal discharge. BV occurs as result of a reduction in vaginal flora, *Lactobacillus*, with an increase in a variety of bacterial species and anaerobes (e.g., *Gardnerella vaginalis*). The prevalence is highest in women of reproductive age. BV is not classified as an STI. However, BV only occurs in sexually active women, and BV risk is associated with increased number of sexual partners, whether they are male or female.

Lactobacillus produces hydrogen peroxide, which maintains a low pH and is a natural microbicide that prevents the overgrowth of normal anaerobic bacteria in the vagina. A decrease in *Lactobacillus* results in a pH rise, and bacterial anaerobes multiply. The bacterial overgrowth produces enzymes causing the breakdown of proteins in the vagina, resulting in volatile amine production. These amines cause the symptoms that occur in BV, such as a foul-smelling vaginal discharge. *G. vaginalis* has long been recognized as one of the key pathogens in BV. It is theorized that this organism forms a film on the wall of the vaginal epithelium, and other bacteria adhere to this film and accumulate.

Clinical Manifestations

Most women with BV are asymptomatic. Manifestations, if present, include increased vaginal discharge that is off-white/gray, thin with an unpleasant fishy odor that worsens after sexual intercourse or menses. Other symptoms, such as dysuria and dyspareunia, occur with coinfection rather than BV alone. BV is often described when discussing vaginitis; however, BV does not cause vaginal inflammation like vulvovaginal candidiasis and trichomoniasis (two other common causes of vaginal discharge). BV is a risk factor for development of several STIs (e.g., herpes simplex 2 virus, gonorrhea, and chlamydia).

Diagnosis and Treatment

Diagnosis is made based on a history, physical examination, and the presence of at least three of the Amsel criteria: 1) characteristic vaginal discharge, 2) elevated pH, 3) clue cells (FIGURE 8-32), and 4) fishy odor. Vaginal microscopy is recommended to evaluate for the presence of clue cells on a saline wet mount slide (discharge is placed on a slide and normal saline is placed on top). Clue cells are vaginal epithelial cells that are full of adherent coccobacilli giving the cell a roughened, stippled appearance. Additionally, a strong, fishy odor is produced when a drop of KOH is placed on a swab with vaginal discharge if BV is present—termed a *positive whiff test* or *positive amine test*. A culture is not useful in BV due to the complex vaginal flora changes and because many organisms that would cause a positive culture are in women without BV.

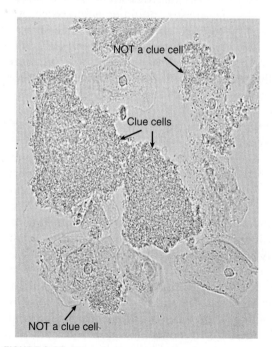

FIGURE 8-32 Clue cells.

Courtesy of University of Washington STD Prevention Training Center.

BV can resolve spontaneously without treatment; however, treatment is usually initiated to relieve symptoms and prevent the risk of getting other STIs. Treatment consists of antibiotics such as metronidazole or clindamycin. These medications can be administered intravaginally or taken orally. If oral doses are given, they should be administered over time as opposed to the one-dose regimen used for trichomoniasis (discussed later in this chapter). Treatment of asymptomatic sexual partners is not necessary as transmission is not from the male partner. Incidence of BV in women who have sex with women is higher, and these sexual partners should be evaluated and treated if symptomatic. Recurrence of BV within 1 year is high and may be due to reinfection or treatment failure.

Pelvic Inflammatory Disease

Pelvic inflammatory disease (PID) is a general term that refers to an acute infection of the female reproductive system (e.g., endometritis [uterus], oophoritis [ovaries], and salpingitis [fallopian tubes]). PID is usually a result of a sexually transmitted infection that ascends to the upper genital tract and is not usually used in reference to pelvic infections due to other causes (e.g., cervical surgery). Pelvic infections from another source of infection, however, can cause similar manifestations as PID due to STIs. The focus of this section will be on PID due to STIs. According to the CDC (2016b), PID diagnoses have declined in recent years, but an average of 5% of all U.S. women will have PID in their lifetime.

In this infection, bacteria (often gonorrhea or chlamydia) usually ascend through the reproductive tract. *Mycoplasma genitalium* is another common organism. PID, however, is often polymicrobial, and often the exact microbe is unknown. Risk factors for PID are the same as for acquiring other STIs (e.g., multiple sexual partners, sexual intercourse with an infected partner, or history of prior STIs or PID). PID most commonly occurs in women 15 to 25 years of age.

In PID, organisms enter the upper genital tract through the endocervical canal as a result of cervical disruption (e.g., cervicitis). The normally protective endocervical canal is breached, and the normal vaginal flora is altered, allowing ascension of pathogens into the upper genital tract. The infection triggers the inflammatory response, resulting in mucosal irritation, edema, and purulent exudate. The edema and exudate can obstruct the reproductive structures, and the exudate can migrate to the peritoneal cavity through the uterus and fallopian tube openings, increasing the risk of peritonitis. Abscesses (tubo-ovarian) and septicemia (bacterial blood infection) can develop and become life threatening. The liver and peritoneal surfaces can become inflamed and result in a syndrome known as Fitz-Hugh–Curtis or perihepatitis. This complication occurs in up to 14% of women with PID (NORD, 2009). Perihepatitis is thought to occur as a result of bacteria traveling through the blood or lymphatics to the right upper quadrant or possibly due to an autoimmune reaction to *C. trachomatis* or *N. gonorrhoeae*. Manifestation includes severe right upper quadrant pain. Adhesions and strictures frequently result from PID, leading to chronic pelvic pain, ectopic pregnancies, infertility, and problems with surrounding structures.

Clinical Manifestations

Clinical manifestations of PID vary slightly depending on the severity of the infection. Manifestations can be subtle or severe and include the following:

- Indications of infection such as fever, chills, myalgia, and leukocytosis (with acute forms and more likely to indicate peritonitis or pelvic abscess)
- Pain or tenderness in the pelvis, lower abdomen, or lower back (sudden and severe with acute forms and more likely to indicate peritonitis or pelvic abscess)
- Dysmenorrhea—a bacterial invasion is more likely during or shortly after menses
- Abnormal vaginal and cervical discharge (usually purulent)
- Postcoital bleeding; intermenstrual bleeding, or heavy menses
- Dyspareunia
- Urinary frequency and dysuria

Bimanual pelvic examination findings include cervical motion tenderness (pain when the examiner moves the cervix) and uterine and adnexal tenderness, as well as purulent endocervical and/or vaginal discharge.

Diagnosis and Treatment

Diagnosing PID consists of a history and physical examination. A presumptive clinical diagnosis is made in young, sexually active women (especially if they are engaging in risky sexual behaviors) with lower abdominal or pelvic pain and pelvic exam findings of cervical motion or uterine and adnexal tenderness. Because PID

can result in serious reproductive disorders, treatment should be given with just the presence of clinical findings. Additional manifestations can further support the diagnosis (e.g., mucopurulent discharge). Diagnostic tests include evaluation for chlamydia and gonorrhea (e.g., NAAT testing of discharge) and other pathogens. Ultrasound, CT, or MRI of the pelvis may reveal various findings such as thickened, fluid-filled fallopian tubes). A CBC may reveal and infection with increased leukocytes. Laparoscopy can also be done.

Treatment strategies include broad-spectrum antibiotic coverage due to the polymicrobial pathogens that are commonly present with PID. A majority of women with uncomplicated PID can be treated on an outpatient basis. Hospitalization may be necessary for patients with severe systemic manifestations (e.g., fever and severe abdominal pain), complicated PID (e.g., tubo-ovarian abscess), inability to tolerate oral medications, pregnancy, or possible nonadherence to therapy. Follow-up to evaluate for improvement should be done within 3 days. Screening and treatment of sexual partners (usually those within the last 60 days prior to the onset of symptoms) is important to prevent spreading and reinfection. If the last sexual exposure was > 60 days prior, then the most recent sexual partner should be screened and treated. Sexual activity should be delayed until after completion of therapy, resolution of symptoms, and treatment of partner(s). Practicing safe sex should be emphasized. Abscesses may need treatment with needle aspiration or surgical removal. As with gonorrhea and chlamydia, follow-up should be conducted at 3 months due to higher reinfection rates.

Syphilis

Syphilis is an ulcerative infection caused by *Treponema pallidum*, a spiral-shaped (spirochete) bacterium that requires a warm, moist environment to survive (FIGURE 8-33). According to the CDC (2018), syphilis rates have increased by 76% since 2013, including a significant increase in congenital syphilis. Syphilis is transmitted through skin or mucous membrane contact with infected, ulcerative lesions (chancres). Additionally, the bacterium can cross from the mother through the placental barrier to the fetus after the fourth month of gestation (congenital syphilis). *T. pallidum* causes infection wherever the pathogen is introduced such as in the mouth or on the genitals or breasts. Syphilitic lesions also provide an

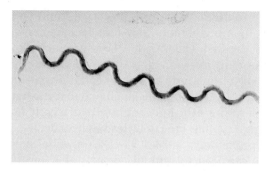

FIGURE 8-33 *T. pallidum*, the spirochete that causes syphilis.

Courtesy of Bill Schwartz/CDC.

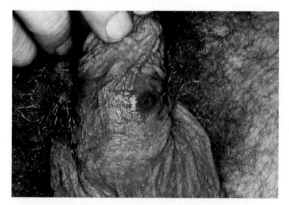

FIGURE 8-34 Chancre characteristic of primary syphilis.

Courtesy of Dr. Gavin Hart and Dr. N.J. Fiumara/CDC.

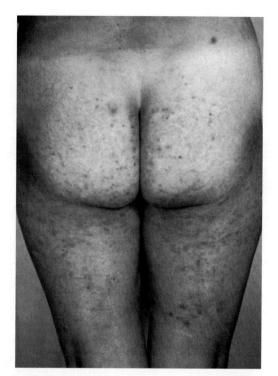

FIGURE 8-35 Skin rash characteristic of secondary syphilis.

Courtesy of J. Pledger, BSS/VD/CDC.

opportunity for the transmission and acquiring other STIs.

When a person becomes infected with syphilis, *T. pallidum* begins to replicate and forms the characteristic ulcerative lesion (i.e., chancre). Some organisms go to the lymph nodes and then start spreading throughout the body. Syphilitic infection causes activation of the innate and adaptive cellular immune response. The humoral immune response begins (antibodies start developing). The chancre may heal due to this immune response. The body's immune response alone, however, is insufficient to keep the spirochetes from spreading, so antibiotic treatment is necessary to avoid disease progression.

Syphilis occurs in stages, each with its own clinical manifestations:

- **Primary syphilis:** Primary syphilis (also known as early syphilis) is the first stage. Painless chancres (usually one) form at the site of infection about 2–3 weeks after the initial infection is acquired (FIGURE 8-34), along with local lymphadenopathy (enlarged lymph nodes). The chancres can appear up to 90 days after initial infection. The chancres often go unnoticed and disappear about 4–6 weeks later, even without treatment. The chancres begin as a papule then ulcerate, and the lesions are hard, have raised edges, and are usually about 2 cm in size. The ulcers can have different appearances, so syphilis should be considered in any painless genital ulcer. The bacteria become dormant, and no other symptoms are present. Because the individual may not test positive during this stage, the test should be repeated later. Even if he or she tests negative, the infected individual is contagious during this stage.

- **Secondary syphilis:** Secondary syphilis (also part of early syphilis) occurs about 2–8 weeks after the first chancres form. Approximately 33% of those individuals with infection who do not receive treatment for primary syphilis will develop this second stage, which is characterized by a generalized, nonpruritic, brown-red rash (FIGURE 8-35). Most commonly the rash is on the trunk, extremities, and palms and soles (FIGURE 8-36). The rash tends to be symmetric and is macular (flat) or papular (raised) and scaly. The rash, however, can take on different appearances (e.g., smooth or nodular). Condyloma lata are wartlike skin lesions that usually occur on the mouth, perineum, anus, vulva, and inner thighs. Mucous patches can develop in

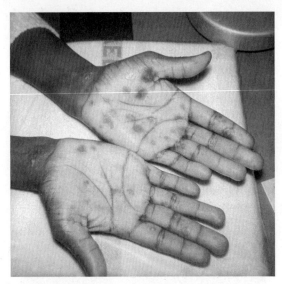

FIGURE 8-36 Syphilis affecting the hands.
Courtesy of CDC.

the mouth. Other symptoms include malaise, fever, patchy hair loss, malaise, headache, myalgia (muscle ache), arthralgia, sore throat, poor appetite, and weight loss. Lymph nodes in the neck, axilla, groin, and epitrochlea are usually enlarged. Other findings can include hepatitis, gastric lining inflammation and ulceration, and renal abnormalities (e.g., acute nephritis). These symptoms will often go away without treatment, and again, the bacteria become dormant. The individual will test positive (if untreated) and is contagious during this stage, especially with direct contact with the rash. Condyloma lata lesions are highly contagious.

- **Latent or tertiary syphilis:** Latent or tertiary syphilis is the final stage of syphilis. The early latency stage begins when the secondary symptoms disappear and usually occurs within the first year of infection. The late latency stage starts after 1 year and can last for years. During latency periods, there are no symptoms. Tertiary syphilis is a symptomatic stage, and manifestations occur in the cardiovascular system (e.g., aortic dilation and aortic valve regurgitation) or granulomatous, nodular lesions (i.e., gummas) can develop in different organs throughout the body, usually the skin and bones. Multiple central nervous system manifestations can occur with late syphilis, such as progressive dementia and ataxia. Tertiary syphilis manifestations can occur as late as 30 years after infection. The individual will test positive (if untreated).

In utero, the fetus is protected from syphilis by a membrane known as Langhans layer for the first 4 months of the pregnancy. Consequently, screening and treating the mother prior to the fourth month of gestation can significantly decrease the likelihood that the fetus will contract the infection. Untreated early maternal syphilis infections lead to fetal demise in approximately 40% of cases. Congenital syphilis can lead to multiple defects affecting the bones, teeth, liver, lungs, and nervous system.

Diagnosis and Treatment

Diagnostic procedures include a history and physical examination. Diagnostic tests include nontreponemal and treponemal serologic tests. Nontreponemal tests (e.g., venereal disease research laboratory test or rapid plasma reagin) are measures of biomarkers released from the spirochete and IgG and IgM antibodies are reported as a titer. As an example, a nontreponemal test titer may be reported as 1:32, which reflects the dilution ratio. The nontreponemal tests are nonspecific and there can be false positive rates, and require evaluation with a treponemal test. Nontreponemal test titers are used to evaluate treatment success (e.g., the titers should decrease by fourfold, that is, 1:32 to 1:8). Nontreponemal tests will eventually become negative after treatment. Treponemal tests (e.g., fluorescent treponemal antibody absorption) measure antibodies directed against specific treponemal antigens, so it is more specific than nontreponemal tests. The tests are reported as reactive or nonreactive. The test results will remain positive for life in a patient with syphilis, even if treated, so only a nontreponemal test can be used to evaluate for reinfection. Nontreponemal tests have usually been used initially because they were easier and cheaper; however, newer versions of treponemal tests are easier and are being used for initial testing. Treatment usually consists of antibiotics such as penicillin (preferred), a penicillin derivative, doxycycline, or tetracycline.

Viral STIs

Many STIs are caused by viruses. In terms of their severity, these infections can range from minor (e.g., condylomata acuminata) to life threatening (e.g., HIV). Viral STIs can also lead to several reproductive cancers (e.g., human papillomavirus). *Molluscum contagiosum*, caused by a poxvirus, is sexually transmitted in adults. Viral infections are the most difficult STIs to treat because viruses are highly adaptive and elusive. Treatment options for the various infections depend on the causative virus.

Genital Herpes

Genital herpes is an infection that causes blisters (vesicles) on the genitals and in the reproductive tract. Genital herpes is caused by the herpes simplex virus (HSV), which belongs to a family containing more than 70 herpes viruses. Some other common viruses in this family include cytomegalovirus (which can cause mental retardation and fetal demise with maternal infections), varicella-zoster virus (which causes chickenpox and shingles), and Epstein-Barr virus (which can cause infectious mononucleosis and lymphoma).

HSV occurs in two forms—HSV type 1 and HSV type 2. Generally, HSV type 1 infections occur above the waist, whereas HSV type 2 infections occur below the waist. HSV type 1 infection most frequently manifests as a cold sore (a small blister on the mouth or nose). Most cases of genital herpes (70%) are caused by HSV type 2. HSV type 2 infections can also spread above the waist, and HSV type 1 infections can spread below the waist through oral–genital sexual contact. HSV type 2 is also transmissible through direct skin-to-skin contact. Although the risk of transmission is greatest when lesions are present, HSV can be spread when lesions are not apparent or when lesions are not present (i.e., they are asymptomatic or subclinical viral shedding has occurred). HSV type 2 is also transmissible from mother to child.

Contracting genital herpes during pregnancy creates the greatest risk to the fetus—spontaneous abortion. HSV can also be transmitted to the infant during childbirth if an active genital herpes infection is present at the time of delivery. Transmission of this infection during childbirth can result in encephalitis and brain damage. If lesions are present at the time of birth, a cesarean section should be performed to minimize these risks. Rarely, HSV can be transmitted to the fetus through the placenta, causing an infection prior to birth. Pregnant women should be monitored for genital herpes throughout their pregnancy.

Genital herpes is not a reportable disease to the CDC; however, data from healthcare clinics indicate that the prevalence of genital herpes has been increasing for the last 50 years, albeit with declining numbers of cases (incidence) occurring in the most recent years. According

to the CDC (2017), rates of genital herpes are highest in Blacks.

Both types of HSV infections are characterized by recurrent episodes of the lesions. Most people with HSV type 2 will experience recurrence of the lesions; however, recurrence is much less frequent with HSV type 1. The virus causes an initial infection at the entry site, but then it travels along the dermatome to the nerve root, where it remains protected and dormant until the next outbreak (recurrence), which will occur at the same site. In either case, the lesions appear and progress similarly. Recurrent episodes begin with a tingling or burning sensation at the site just before the lesion appears (prodrome). The lesions first appear as vesicles (< 0.5 cm clear fluid filled lesions [blister]) surrounded by erythema. These vesicles rupture, leaving behind a painful ulcerative lesion with watery exudate (**FIGURE 8-37**). Ultimately, a crust forms over the ulcer, and it heals

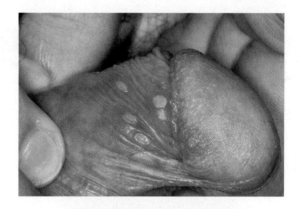

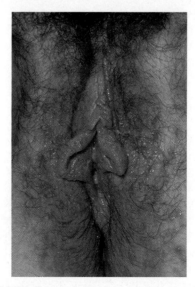

FIGURE 8-37 Genital herpes blisters on the external genitalia.
© Mediscan/Visuals Unlimited, Inc; © Dr P. Marazzi/Science Source.

spontaneously in 3–4 weeks. Because genital herpes creates an opening in the skin, the individual is at risk for contracting other STIs.

Clinical Manifestations

Genital herpes manifestations are dependent on whether the lesions occur shortly after being infected for the first time (i.e., primary infection), whether the lesions occur for the first time after antibodies have developed, or whether the lesions are due to recurrent infection.

Primary herpes genitalis begins at the actual time of infection and antibody development. The time from exposure to this primary infection can range from 2 to 12 days. This first occurrence of the infection can be either very painful, mildly painful, or completely asymptomatic (75% of cases). When present, clinical manifestations associated with this stage include multiple painful 1–2 mm vesicular lesions that can be pruritic and accompanied by malaise, low-grade fever, and groin lymph node enlargement. The lesions can be in the vulvar area or on the cervix, penis, buttocks, or thighs. The lesions usually heal in about 10–20 days. Viral shedding is high during this first stage, making transmission more likely.

There is a period when herpes genitalis antibodies are formed. Antibodies do not protect an individual against reinfection, but they do tend to make the recurrent episodes less severe. The virus travels up the nerve root and becomes dormant (FIGURE 8-38). The individual is asymptomatic while the virus is dormant. The lesions can appear for the first time after antibodies are already formed. This first episode is considered nonprimary as the actual time of infection occurred in the past. A first presentation with antibodies already formed will cause a presentation

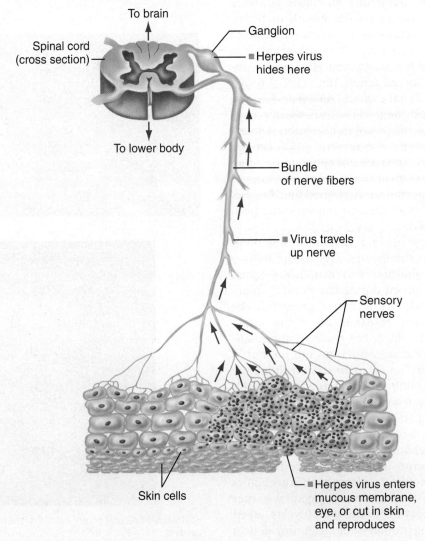

FIGURE 8-38 Herpes simplex virus movement in the nervous system.

with fewer lesions and fewer systemic symptoms in comparison to primary infection.

Recurrent herpes genitalis is characterized by the reactivation of the virus and clinical manifestations. During this stage, the virus travels back down the nerve root to the skin and causes a vesicle at the same site as with the first stage. The duration of lesions is usually shorter (< 10 days), and viral shedding usually occurs for up to 5 days. The number of recurrences varies from none to many in a lifetime. Factors that can trigger a recurrence include stress, menstruation, and illness.

Diagnosis and Treatment

Diagnosis for genital herpes is based on a history, physical examination, and confirmation with laboratory testing. Diagnostic testing is dependent on whether lesions are present or not. If lesions are present, vesicular fluid should be sent for viral culture. The blister might need to be unroofed to acquire the fluid. Viral cultures are best performed early in the disease course. Polymerase chain reaction viral DNA or RNA of the lesion or serum can also be done. Both tests can differentiate between HSV 1 and HSV 2. Serologic testing can detect antibodies to HSV 1 or HSV 2. Genital herpes is a significant public concern because the lesions and symptoms are not always apparent, transmission can occur with or without symptoms, and no cure exists. Genital herpes can cause a great deal of psychological stress for patients because of the ongoing fear of outbreaks and the need to disclose the information about their infection status to partners.

Treatment options include antiviral medications that can suppress the number of outbreaks as well as minimize the severity and duration of the first infection and recurrences. Avoiding recurrence triggers, especially stress, can also prevent outbreaks. Implementing stress reduction strategies (e.g., yoga, meditation, journaling, and distraction) is advised. Secondary bacterial infections can develop from the lesions, so proper hygiene (e.g., washing the area with soap and water several times a day, keeping the area dry, and wearing loose-fitting clothing and cotton underwear) is advised during outbreaks. Because the risk of transmission is highest when lesions are present, sexual activity should be avoided during outbreaks. Due to the lifelong implications of genital herpes, prevention is the best treatment strategy. Prevention strategies center on safe sex practices such as using condoms and limiting sexual partners.

Learning Points

Uncommon Causes of Genital Ulcers

Syphilis and herpes are the most common causes of genital ulcers. LGV is another STI that presents as an ulcer along with two other uncommon organisms: chancroid (organism: *Haemophilus ducreyi*) and granuloma inguinale (organism: *Klebsiella granulomatis*). Chancroid is rare in the United States; however, because few laboratories are able to test for the organism, the actual incidence is unknown. Chancroid starts with a genital papule that erupts into multiple ulcers with pus draining from lymph nodes. The ulcers are painful and are 1-2 cm in diameter. Buboes may develop. Granuloma inguinale (i.e., donovanosis) is rare in the United States. Manifestations include slowly progressive painless ulcers that have raised rolled edges and usually without lymphadenopathy.

Condylomata Acuminata

Condylomata acuminata, or anogenital warts, are benign growths caused by human papillomavirus (HPV). More than 200 different types of HPV exist, several of which can cause condylomata acuminata. HPV can only infect humans and can cause mucosal or cutaneous disorders. Condylomata acuminata can occur on the external genitals, vaginal wall, cervix, anus, thighs, lips, mouth, and throat. The genotypes causing most genital warts (90%) are types 6 and 11. In addition to condylomata acuminata, HPV infection can lead to the development of reproductive tract cancer in women (cervical, vulvar, and vaginal) and penile cancer in men. HPV can also cause oropharyngeal and anal cancers. There are various genotypes that cause cancer such as 16 and 18. HPV can have an incubation period that lasts up to 6 months. The immune system clears most HPV within 2 years (about 90%), though some infections persist. Most sexually active men and women will contract HPV at some point in their lives as HPV can be contracted with just skin-to-skin contact. Transmission can occur from mother to fetus.

Clinical Manifestations

Condylomata acuminata may be asymptomatic, depending on their location. Transmission, as with other viruses, can occur without the presence of a lesion. The time from infection to the development of lesions can be 3 weeks to 8 months. The lesions vary in appearance, texture, and size (**FIGURE 8-39**; **FIGURE 8-40**). Growths can be raised, flat, rough, smooth, flesh-colored, white, gray, pink, cauliflower-like, large, or barely visible. Additional symptoms may include abnormal bleeding, discharge, or itching.

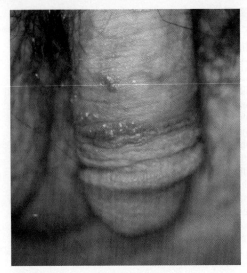

FIGURE 8-39 Genital warts on the penis.
Courtesy of Dr. M.F. Rein/CDC.

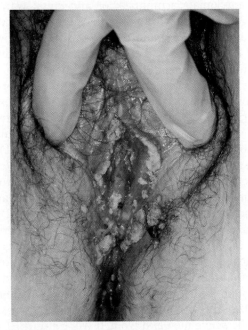

FIGURE 8-40 Genital warts on the vagina.
Courtesy of Joe Millar/CDC.

Diagnosis and Treatment

Diagnosis of condylomata acuminata is based on a history and clinical findings. While there are no treatments for HPV itself, treatments exist for the serious conditions that HPV can cause (e.g., cervical cancer). A vaccine is available to prevent HPV infections. Various HPV vaccines can provide protection anywhere from two to nine of the most common types of HPV that cause cancer and genital warts. Vaccination is recommended for both males and females (ideally to be administered around 11 or 12 years of age, before sexual activity is

initiated). Using condoms and dental dams can also reduce the risk of HPV transmission.

Most condylomata acuminata are harmless, but they can be removed for aesthetic purposes. Removal of the growths will not cure the underlying condition, so the growths may reappear. Condylomata acuminata can be removed using chemicals (e.g., podophyllin), cryosurgery (freezing the tissue with liquid nitrogen), electrocauterization (heating the tissue with electricity), laser therapy (burning the tissue with a light), or surgical excision.

As with other STIs, sexual partners of individuals with HPV infection should also be screened and treated. Condylomata acuminata can be fatal if transmitted to infants at birth, so cesarean section deliveries are advised for pregnant women with this STI.

Learning Points

Adult Male Circumcision and STIs

Adult male circumcision can reduce the rate of transmission of sexually transmitted infections, particularly HIV and genital ulcers, warts, and herpes simplex virus and possibly other STIs such as gonorrhea and chlamydia. Removal of the foreskin allows the skin on the glans penis to keratinize (create a protective thickening), which provides a protection against organisms. Additionally, the prepuce has Langerhans cells that HIV targets. In addition to circumcision reducing risk in men, women who have sexual partners who are circumcised also have a reduced risk of an STI.

Protozoan STIs

Like candidiasis infections, protozoan infections often arise when the body's natural defenses are altered; unlike candidiasis, however, some of these infections can be transmitted through sexual contact. Protozoan STIs are usually easily treated and resolve with minimal issues.

Trichomoniasis

Trichomoniasis (colloquially referred to as the *trich*) is caused by *Trichomonas vaginalis*, a one-celled anaerobic organism. This extracellular parasite can burrow under the mucosal lining. In men, the organism primarily resides in the urethra and, in most cases, causes no symptoms. In women, the organism resides in the vagina, and the infection becomes symptomatic when vaginal microbial imbalance occurs. The *T. vaginalis* organism cannot survive in the mouth or the rectum. The incidence, in contrast to other STIs, is higher in men and women > 40 years of age, but another peak is seen in women around the age of 20. Coinfection with bacterial vaginosis and STIs is common. Trichomonas can cause complications in women (e.g., PID in HIV-infected women, and infertility), and trichomonas can be associated with disorders such as prostatitis and epididymitis in men.

Myth Busters

A common misconception is that condoms protect users against all STIs. While condoms are highly effective against most STIs, some of these infections have been known to spread despite condom use. Some STIs can be transferred through sexual contact that does not involve insertion intercourse (e.g., skin to skin contact of genitalia and oral sex).

Another common misconception is that condoms can break off or slip off easily. Some are concerned that a condom may not fit; however, there are many different shapes and sizes. When used properly this is unlikely. Proper use includes: 1) using throughout the whole sexual act; 2) using only latex condoms with no oil-based lubricants; 3) checking expiration dates on condoms; 4) keeping condoms away from extreme heat; 5) removing the condom while the penis is erect and holding the rim of the condom prior to withdrawal; 6) not reusing condoms; and 7) checking for tears or breakage after withdrawal. Some may think two condoms are better than one but simultaneous use increases friction leading to a higher likelihood of tears or breaks. STIs that can spread through skin-to-skin contact even with a condom in place include HPV, HSV, and syphilis. Additional strategies, such as receiving the HPV vaccination, receiving genital herpes suppression therapy, and treating syphilis early, can decrease the likelihood of contracting and spreading these infections.

BOX 8-3 Application to Practice

Most women at some point in their life will get a vaginal infection. Vaginal infection can be characterized by complaints of vaginal discharge. Three common causes of vaginal discharge are bacterial vaginosis, trichomoniasis, and vulvovaginal candidiasis. Review the following case and answer the questions.

Case: A 40-year-old woman comes in complaining of an increased thin whitish vaginal discharge that started about 5 days ago. She said it is so much that she needs to wear a small sanitary pad. She also noted that she had a funny odor after having sexual intercourse, and she says the odor continues despite her attempts to control it with douching. Physical examination reveals a thin white discharge around the vaginal wall with no erythema. Examination of the discharge includes a positive KOH whiff test and a vaginal pH > 4.5. Vaginal microscopy reveals clue cells.

1. What is a likely cause of the vaginal discharge?
   a. Trichomoniasis
   b. Bacterial vaginosis
   c. Vulvovaginal candidiasis
2. Which of the clinical manifestations confirms the diagnosis?
   a. The thin white discharge
   b. Malodorous discharge
   c. Presence of clue cells on a saline wet mount slide

3. The cause of this vaginal discharge disorder is due to:
   a. An alteration in the vaginal flora
   b. Overgrowth of yeast due to antibiotic use
   c. A sexually transmitted organism, *T. pallidum*
4. Which is the primary treatment of this vaginal discharge disorder?
   a. Fluconazole
   b. Metronidazole
   c. Clindamycin
5. Describe the mode of transmission, common organism, clinical manifestations, and treatment of the other two diagnoses not chosen in question 1.

Clinical Manifestations

Up to 75% of men and women with trichomoniasis are asymptomatic. In men, the infection is often transient and resolves in a few weeks without treatment. If symptoms are present, they are similar to infections causing urethritis (e.g., clear or mucopurulent penile discharge and dysuria). In women, the primary clinical manifestation is copious amounts of odorous, frothy, thin, white or yellow-green vaginal discharge. This discharge can irritate the vagina and vulva. The cervix can develop petechiae, which can appear like the surface of a strawberry (termed a *strawberry cervix*), but this appearance occurs in < 2% of cases. Additional symptoms may include itching, painful intercourse, and dysuria. *Trichomonas* can infect the paraurethral glands. Women can remain asymptomatic carriers for several months. Trichomoniasis during pregnancy can cause complications such as premature rupture of membranes or preterm delivery. Newborns who contract the infection during delivery can have a fever, respiratory problems, urinary tract infections, and vaginal discharge.

Diagnosis and Treatment

Diagnostic procedures for trichomoniasis include a history and physical examination. As with vulvovaginal candidiasis and bacterial vaginosis (two other common causes of vaginal discharge), vaginal microscopy is important in evaluating the vaginal discharge. On a wet mount slide, mobile trichomonads can be seen (**FIGURE 8-41**). The vaginal pH is usually > 4.5. Other diagnostic tests can include NAAT for *Trichomonas* RNA. Rapid tests (e.g., results can be provided in 45 minutes) can evaluate for antigen or DNA. Cultures can be used, but it can take a week to obtain results. Trichomonads can sometimes be seen in a liquid Pap smear, but a liquid Pap smear should not be used for diagnosis because of many false positives. In men, microscopy is not accurate and a NAAT or culture is the preferred test. Trichomoniasis is easily treated with metronidazole (Flagyl), an antibiotic that treats bacteria and parasite infections usually as a one-time dose (e.g., 2 grams). Intravaginal metronidazole therapy is not as effective for trichomoniasis treatment. Sexual partners should also be treated to prevent reinfection. Follow-up testing is often done due to the high risk of reinfection. Repeat testing can be done as soon as 2 weeks and up to 3 months after treatment completion. Untreated or prolonged infections can increase the risk of

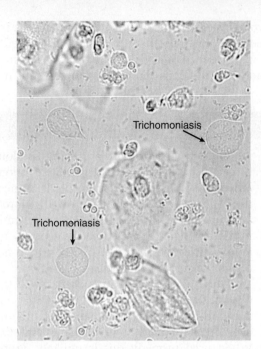

FIGURE 8-41 Wet prep: Trichomoniasis.
University of Washington STD Prevention Training Center.

cervical cancer and HIV. Patients should avoid sexual intercourse until 7 days after completion of therapy.

Cancers

Malignancies of the reproductive system may either originate in the reproductive tract or spread there from other sites. Some of these cancers have high rates of successful treatment (e.g., testicular cancer), whereas others have high mortality rates (e.g., ovarian cancer). Typical cancer diagnosis, staging, and treatments are generally utilized with these tumors (see chapter 1 for more on cellular function).

Penile Cancer

Penile cancer is a rare malignancy. The most common type is squamous cell carcinoma. Its exact cause is unknown, but risk is thought to be increased by various penile disorders or conditions such as the presence of smegma, being uncircumcised, poor hygiene, phimosis, and HPV infections. Penile cancer usually occurs in older men. Penile cancer appears as a thick, gray-white lesion (Bowen lesion) or a red, shiny lesion (erythroplasia of Queyrat) (**FIGURE 8-42**) or a painless lump. Inguinal lymphadenopathy may also be present. Prognosis is good with early diagnosis and treatment, but a penectomy (removal of the penis) may be required if the cancer is extensive or does not respond to the

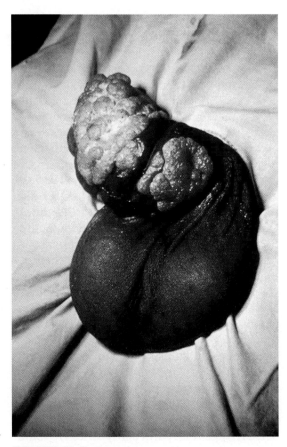

FIGURE 8-42 Penile cancer.

Courtesy of William R. Smart/Susan Lindsley/CDC.

usual cancer treatments (e.g., chemotherapy, radiation, and surgical excision).

Prostate Cancer

Prostate cancer is the most common cancer among men, particularly Blacks (American Cancer Society, 2019). The most common type is adenocarcinoma. The tumors are slow growing, and 80% of cases are diagnosed while the cancer is still confined to the prostate, improving the prognosis. Prostate cancer is the second leading cause of cancer deaths in the United States, but the 5- and 10-year survival rates for this disease are improving. Prognosis improves with early diagnosis and treatment and worsens with advancing age. Increased screening with prostate-specific antigen (PSA) and prostate biopsy for those with elevated PSA have contributed to these newly improved survival rates. The exact cause of prostate cancer remains unknown, but men's risk is thought to increase with age (the peak is between 65 and 75 years of age). However, prostate cancer in Black men usually occurs at a younger age. A family history (first-degree relatives) or a family history of other cancers such as breast, ovarian, or pancreatic cancer increases prostate cancer risk. Breast cancer variants may contribute to the development of prostate cancer, particularly aggressive forms, and other common genetic factors are being explored. Consumption of high-fat diet, and androgen hormone replacement (some tumors are androgen dependent) and other risk factors (e.g., STIs) may contribute to prostate cancer development.

As the tumor grows, the prostate enlarges and impedes the urethra; therefore, prostate cancer presents with similar clinical manifestations as benign prostatic hyperplasia (e.g., urinary difficulties and erectile dysfunction). Additional manifestations may include bloody semen and hematuria. Digital rectal exam may reveal prostate nodules, induration, or asymmetry, however a rectal exam can only detect tumors on the posterior and lateral aspects of the gland (areas palpable via the rectum). Men, however, are often asymptomatic when diagnosed. If prostate cancer metastasizes, the bones are usually affected, and bone pain is a likely complaint. See chapter 7 for a discussion of benign prostatic hypertrophy.

Diagnostic procedures to evaluate the prostate include measurements of PSA level, which is elevated in any prostate enlargement. Free PSA, which measures unbound PSA, can differentiate between benign prostatic hypertrophy and prostate cancer. The free PSA measurement is used to calculate the ratio of free to total PSA and a low ratio (< 15%) is suspicious for prostate cancer. Prostatic acid phosphatase (which is high in prostate cancer) testing may be used. Biopsy, however, is necessary to make the diagnosis. Prostate cancer treatment follows the path of the usual cancer treatments and can vary depending on the cancer stage. If the cancer is diagnosed in an early stage, careful observation (called *active surveillance*) instead of immediate treatment is appropriate for many patients. Treatment includes a combination of a radical prostatectomy (complete prostate removal), radiation, and orchiectomy (removal of the testes) or antitestosterone drug therapy. These treatments often impact the patient's quality of life due to their side effects or complications (e.g., urinary and erectile dysfunction), which may be short or long term. Researchers are exploring new biologic markers in an effort to improve the differential diagnosis between indolent and aggressive prostate cancer so as to minimize unnecessary treatment of the indolent variant (American Cancer Society, 2019).

Testicular Cancer

Testicular cancer is an uncommon cancer. Men ages 15–35 years old and White men are at higher risk of developing this type of cancer than other groups. Most cases of testicular cancer occur due to germ cell tumors, which can be a slow-growing (seminoma) tumor or, less commonly, a fast-growing (nonseminoma) tumor. Risk for developing testicular cancer is thought to be increased by family history, infection, trauma, tobacco use, testicular abnormalities (e.g., atrophy or dysgenesis), and cryptorchidism. Testicular cancer usually affects one testicle, but it can affect both. Metastasis, when it happens, usually occurs to the nearby lymph nodes, lungs, liver, bone, and brain.

Testicular cancer is often asymptomatic. When present, clinical manifestations usually include a hard, painless, palpable mass that does not transilluminate; testicular discomfort or pain; testicle enlargement; and gynecomastia (femalelike breasts).

Testicular cancer is highly curable even when it has metastasized to other sites. Early diagnosis and treatment enhance prognosis. Monthly testicular self-examinations are the cornerstone of early detection. The evaluation of a testicular mass begins with a bilateral scrotal ultrasound. A CT scan of the abdomen and pelvis and a chest X-ray or CT of the chest are done to evaluate for metastasis. Other diagnostic procedures include measurement of tumor markers such as alpha fetoprotein, beta human chorionic gonadotropin, and lactate dehydrogenase. In most cases, an orchiectomy is advised to evaluate the tissue histology and control the tumor but chemotherapy and radiation may also be used to treat this disease. Prior to orchiectomy, semen can be preserved in case of a desire to preserve fertility. Testicular cancer can reoccur in the remaining testicle, so testicular self-examinations and follow-up are crucial.

Breast Cancer

Breast cancer is the most common malignancy in women and the second leading cause of cancer death in women (American Cancer Society, 2019). While breast cancer can occur in men, its rates are highest in White women, although Black women are more likely to die from it. The risk of breast cancer increases with advancing age (most occur in women > 50 years of age). Hormonal alterations throughout life increase chances of cell mutations and breast cancer risk. Risk factors for breast cancer include early menarche, late menopause, nulliparity or pregnancy after 30, and no history of breastfeeding. Other risk factors include a history of benign atypical hyperplasia and chest-wall radiation.

A family history (up to 10% of breast cancers) and inherited genetic predisposition—usually due to defects on the *BRCA1* and *BRCA2* genes—increase breast cancer risk. Obesity and excessive alcohol consumption (more than one to two drinks per day) can also increase breast cancer risk. Exogenous estrogen exposure (e.g., oral contraceptives, hormone replacement therapy) may increase the risk for breast cancer, although current formulations have minimized this risk. In many circumstances of breast cancer, there are no identifiable risks. See chapter 1 for discussion of BRCA1 and BRCA2 mutations.

As with many cancers, breast cancer is a clonal disease. Cells reproduce due to a combination of an inherited germline cell variant that causes susceptibility to breast cancer development and somatic cell mutations (noninherited) (e.g., *p53* mutation), along with environmental factors, which can then also cause cancer cells to reproduce. Breast cancer is a hormonally dependent disorder. Inherited defective genes, particularly *BRCA1* mutations can cause breast cancer in up to 80% of women and ovarian cancer in 33% of women. Breast cancers due to *BRCA1* are almost always negative for receptors to estrogen (ER), progesterone, and human epidermal receptor 2 (HER2)—these are termed *triple negative cancers*. These cancers tend to be very aggressive. *BRCA1* tumors can also be associated with ER-positive breast cancer.

There are many types of breast cancer, and each type can have different pathology, genetic basis, and clinical manifestations. Breast cancers are mainly adenocarcinomas (i.e., glandular tissue cancer). Most breast cancers originate in the epithelial lining of the duct system (structures that carry milk from the lobules), but such a malignancy may also arise in the lobules (structures that produce milk). Breast cancers are categorized by histologic type, and the most common type of invasive breast cancer is infiltrating ductal carcinoma (i.e., invasive ductal carcinoma) that is nonspecific, which accounts for approximately 75–80% of all breast cancers. There are several other rare subtypes of invasive ductal carcinoma such as tubular carcinoma, medullary carcinoma, and mucinous carcinoma. The second most common histologic type is infiltrating lobular carcinoma (i.e., invasive lobular carcinoma). Other uncommon types of breast cancers include Paget disease (starts in ducts and spreads to nipple and areola), sarcomas, and lymphomas. Noninvasive breast cancer includes ductal carcinoma in situ (DCIS) which consists of malignant epithelial cells that have not invaded the stroma (i.e., cells have remained in situ) but rather are confined in the breast ducts. Lobular carcinoma in situ (LCIS) malignant cells are confined in the lobules. Both DCIS and LCIS are considered cancer precursors, although cancer may never develop. The risk for progression depends on several factors such as the grade of the lesion (e.g., low or high risk), the hormone receptor status (e.g., positive for the human epidermal receptor 2), and the age and race of the woman (young, Black women have a higher risk for invasiveness). DCIS is more common than LCIS, and the risk for future invasive cancer is somewhat higher than with LCIS.

Breast cancers can be described by molecular subtypes that are based on the genes a cancer expresses, creating a genomic profile. The various subtypes have different rates of progression, prognosis, and response to therapy. There are several molecular subtypes such as luminal A, luminal B, triple negative, basal-like, HER2 enriched, and normal-like. These subtypes are described based on whether the cancer is hormone receptor positive or negative for estrogen and/or progesterone, or HER2 negative or positive. The Ki-67 protein level can be used to determine the degree of tumor proliferation along with several other prognostic profiling tools (e.g., Oncotype Dx). As an example the normal-like molecular subtype is described as a hormone-receptor positive (estrogen-receptor and/or progesterone-receptor), HER2-negative breast cancer with low levels of the protein Ki-67. While advances have been made, intensive research efforts are ongoing to determine and refine the use of genomic profiling.

Clinical Manifestations

Breast cancer manifestations can vary. The tumor can infiltrate the surrounding tissue and adhere to the skin, causing dimpling. In its early stages, the tumor moves freely, but it becomes fixed as the cancer progresses. Most classic breast masses will be one dominant, hard, immovable mass with irregular borders (uneven edges). The upper quadrant of the breast is where a majority of breast cancers occur. Small masses (< 1 cm) are often not palpable. As the disease advances, nearby axillary lymph nodes may become enlarged and palpable. Skin changes can include erythema, dimpling, or puckering that looks like the peel of an orange (FIGURE 8-43). The nipple can be laterally displaced or retracted, with spontaneous discharge (e.g., bloody). Metastasis can occur early depending on the type of breast cancer, and in most cases, several nodes are affected at the time of diagnosis. Widespread metastasis quickly follows and usually involves the lungs, bone, and liver, which manifests as cough, bone pain, and nausea and jaundice, respectively. Further indications that the cancer has metastasized include skin ulcers, edema in the arm next to the affected breast, and weight loss.

Early diagnosis and treatment are crucial to positive outcomes. Regular breast self-examinations allow women to become familiar with their breasts and is particularly important for women at increased risk. Another

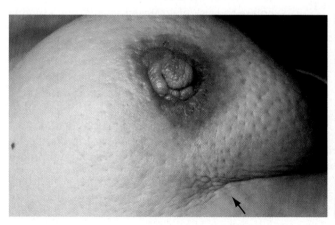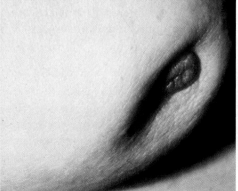

FIGURE 8-43 Changes in the breast caused by advanced breast cancer.

Courtesy of Leonard V. Crowley, MD, Century College.

diagnostic procedure specific to breast cancer is the mammogram (which can detect masses as small as 1 mm), but like other screening tools, it is not perfect. Most (95%) of the 10% of women who have abnormal mammograms do not have cancer (American Cancer Society, 2019).

Currently, screening guidelines vary depending on the recommending organization. Screening should generally begin around the age of 40–45 in women with an average risk. The screening can be annual or biennial. As women get older (between 50 and 55) screening frequency recommendations vary from annual to biennial (American Cancer Society, 2018; U.S. Preventive Services Task Force, 2018). After age 75 mammogram benefits are inconclusive but can be continued if life expectancy is longer than 10 years. (American Cancer Society, 2018). Women in high-risk groups should start annual mammograms sooner (typically age 30) in addition to receiving an annual MRI. Men at high risk for breast cancer should have a clinical exam yearly and learn how to do breast self-examination starting at age 35.

Diagnosis and Treatment

Recent advances in breast cancer treatments (especially in chemotherapies) have significantly increased survival rates for this disease. Treatment strategies vary depending on the stage, but usually breast cancer requires an aggressive, multimethod treatment (e.g., chemotherapy, radiation, surgery, and hormone therapy) to improve outcomes. The life-threatening nature of breast cancer, along with the changes in body image that result from treatment, can increase the need for coping and support interventions (e.g., support groups and counseling). Those patients with evidence of breast cancer (e.g., *BRCA1* or high DCIS) may be offered prophylactic therapies such as hormone therapy or surgery.

Cervical Cancer

Cervical cancer rates have been declining in recent years with advancements in screening. Cervical cytology screening (i.e., Pap smear)—the long-standing cervical screening method—can now detect precancerous changes (dysplasia). Procedures can be performed to remove these precancerous cells, limiting the likelihood of these changes progressing to permanent malignant changes (**FIGURE 8-44**). The precancerous cells are 100%

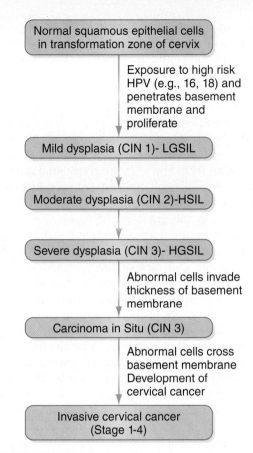

FIGURE 8-44 Development of cervical cancer.

treatable; however, malignant changes can return if carcinogen exposure continues. Almost all cervical cancers (99.7%) are caused by HPV infection with subtypes 16 and 18 accounting for 70% of cancers. The latency period from exposure to HPV to development of cervical cancer is 10–15 years, making it a slow-developing cancer. Most risk factors for cervical cancer are the same as those that increase the risk of contracting HPV (e.g., having multiple sex partners and not practicing safe sex). According to the National Cancer Institute (2016), Hispanic women have the highest incidence of cervical cancer, while Black women have the highest mortality rates from this disease.

Early-stage cervical cancer is usually asymptomatic. When present, clinical manifestations include the following signs and symptoms:

- Continuous vaginal discharge, which may be pale, watery, pink, brown, bloody, or foul smelling
- Abnormal uterine bleeding (intermenstrual or postcoital bleeding)

Indications of advanced cervical cancer include the following conditions:

- Anorexia
- Weight loss
- Fatigue
- Pelvic, back, or leg pain
- Unilateral lower extremity edema
- Heavy menstrual bleeding
- Leaking of urine or feces from the vagina
- Bone fractures

The Pap smear remains the cornerstone of early cervical cancer detection. An abnormal cervical cytology indicates the need for a cervical biopsy and removal of a portion of the cervix (i.e., cervical conization). Administration of the HPV vaccine, however, may prevent the cancer. Precancerous and early malignant changes can be treated using a loop electrosurgical excision procedure, cryotherapy, and laser therapy. Advanced cancer will require chemotherapy, radiation, and surgery (usually a hysterectomy). The survival rate is usually 100% when cervical cancer is treated early, but the rate decreases as the disease advances.

Endometrial Cancer and Uterine Sarcoma

Endometrial cancer, or cancer of the uterus, is a common malignancy in women. According to the American Cancer Society (2019), endometrial cancer is the fourth most frequent cancer in women and the sixth leading cause of cancer death in women, with a 5-year survival rate of approximately 82%. White women have the highest prevalence rates, but Black women have the highest mortality rates. Most endometrial cancers (80%) are endometrioid (a type of adenocarcinoma). The exact cause of this disease is unknown, but unopposed estrogen (i.e., estrogen without opposing progesterone) may be a major factor in its development. Unopposed estrogen is more likely in women with prolonged episodes of amenorrhea and anovulation (e.g., PCOS) or obesity. Additional risk factors for developing endometrial cancer include diabetes mellitus and hypertension.

The most significant finding indicating the possible presence of endometrial cancer is abnormal painless vaginal bleeding (the cancer erodes the endometrium), especially after menopause. After the age 45, any menstrual disorders such as intermenstrual or heavy menstrual bleeding may be due to endometrial cancer. Additional clinical manifestations that are usually late signs include nonbloody vaginal discharge, pelvic pain, weight loss, palpable pelvic mass, and pain during sexual intercourse.

The Pap smear does not detect cancers above the cervix, but some Pap smear findings can be due to malignant cells including adenocarcinoma, atypical glandular cells, and the presence of endometrial cells in women ≥ 40 years of age. Endometrial biopsy is the diagnostic procedure of choice when this malignancy is suspected. Transvaginal ultrasound with the finding of a thickened endometrium in a postmenopausal woman is suspicious for endometrial cancer. If diagnosed early, endometrial cancer can be successfully treated with chemotherapy, radiation, hysterectomy, and hormone therapy.

Uterine sarcoma is a malignant uterine tumor and is not as common as endometrial carcinoma. These tumors are rare, accounting for only 3% of uterine cancers, and the incidence increases with aging. These tumors arise from the myometrium or connective tissue. The types of sarcoma include endometrial stromal sarcomas, leiomyosarcoma, and adenosarcoma. These tumors can be aggressive but can be found at an early stage. The most common manifestations are postmenopausal bleeding, AUB in premenopausal women, abdominal or pelvic pain, and pressure and abdominal distention. Physical examination findings reveal an enlarged uterus. Diagnosis is often made during a myomectomy or hysterectomy, as imaging studies such as an ultrasound do not differentiate benign from malignant tumors. Endometrial biopsy is not reliable. Treatment can include hormone therapy, chemotherapy, radiation, and surgery.

Ovarian Cancer

Ovarian cancer is a relatively common cancer in women. According to the American Cancer Society (2019), ovarian cancer incidence rates have declined, but this disease remains the fifth leading cause of cancer death in women. Prevalence and mortality rates are the highest in White women. Ovarian cancer causes concern because there is no reliable screening test for this disease, it is difficult to treat, and it has often metastasized at the time of diagnosis. However, advances in treatment are improving the survival rates (5-year survival rates are approximately 46%).

Most ovarian cancers (95%) form in epithelial cells, and the remainder are from other cells (e.g., germ cell tumors). Risk factors for developing ovarian cancer include genetic predisposition (defects on the *BRCA1* and *BRCA2* genes), advancing age, infertility or

Myth Busters

Several misconceptions around breast cancer warrant discussion.

Myth 1: Breast implants, use of antiperspirant, and wearing underwire bras increase breast cancer risk.

Facts: There is *no* evidence that links these factors to breast cancer. Breast implants can make it more difficult to detect tumors with a breast self-examination depending on the surgical technique used to insert the implants. Placing the implants behind the muscle wall can improve the ability to detect any tumors. Nevertheless, breast implants, antiperspirant, and underwire bras do *not* increase breast cancer risk.

Myth 2: Only older women need to worry about breast cancer.

Facts: Breast cancer risk does increase with age, but women of *all* ages can develop breast cancer.

Myth 3: Breast cancer always runs in families.

Facts: Family history does increase the likelihood of developing breast cancer, but *most* women who develop breast cancer *do not* have a family history of breast cancer.

Myth 4: There is no need to worry about breast cancer if no *BRCA1* and *BRCA2* mutation is present.

Facts: *BRCA1* and *BRCA2* mutations do increase breast cancer risk, but 90–95% of women who are diagnosed with breast cancer *do not* have either a family history or this genetic mutation.

Data from American Cancer Society (2019). What are the risk factors for breast cancer? Retrieved from http://www.cancer.org/cancer/breast cancer/detailedguide/breast-cancer-risk-factors

nulligravida (never pregnant), excessive estrogen exposure, obesity, and androgen hormone therapy.

Early clinical manifestations of ovarian cancer can be vague, and the more common symptoms include abdominal distention (bloating), pelvic or abdominal pain, eating disturbances (e.g., feeling full quickly), and urinary frequency or urgency. Additional symptoms are not as specific and can include bowel pattern changes, gastrointestinal discomfort (e.g., gas, indigestion, and nausea), pain during sexual intercourse, malaise, and menstruation changes.

CA-125, a protein that is produced in response to several conditions, including ovarian cancer, is often examined as a part of the diagnostic and treatment process. Because it is not specific to ovarian cancer, imaging studies (e.g., pelvic and transvaginal ultrasound) and a biopsy are still required for definitive diagnosis. During treatment, a declining CA-125 level is considered a favorable response to interventions. Surgery and chemotherapy are the preferred treatment strategies. Surgery may include a bilateral salpingo-oophorectomy (removal of both ovaries and fallopian tubes) and a hysterectomy.

CHAPTER SUMMARY

The reproductive systems in males and females are responsible for procreation and hormone balance. Disorders of the reproductive system range from harmless to life threatening. These disorders are most often infections or tumors (benign and malignant). Reproductive function is closely connected with the endocrine, cardiovascular, and nervous systems and, therefore, can affect those systems. Maintaining reproductive health can decrease the likelihood of issues within this system. Strategies to promote reproductive health include practicing safe sex; abstaining from alcohol, smoking, and illicit drug use; maintaining a healthy weight; and limiting exposure to radiation and chemicals.

REFERENCES AND RESOURCES

AAOS. (2004). *Paramedic: Anatomy and physiology*. Sudbury, MA: Jones and Bartlett Publishers.

American Cancer Society. (2018). American cancer society breast cancer screening guideline (2015). Retrieved from https://www.cancer.org/healthy/find-cancer-early/cancer-screening-guidelines/american-cancer-society-guidelines-for-the-early-detection-of-cancer.html

American Cancer Society. (2019). Cancer facts & figures 2019. Retrieved from https://www.cancer.org/content/dam/cancer-org/research/cancer-facts-and-statistics/annual-cancer-facts-and-figures/2019/cancer-facts-and-figures-2019.pdf

Centers for Disease Control and Prevention (CDC). (2015a). Chlamydia statistics. Retrieved from https://www.cdc.gov/std/chlamydia/stats.htm

Centers for Disease Control and Prevention (CDC). (2015b). Sexually transmitted treatment guidelines. Retrieved from https://www.cdc.gov/std/tg2015/default.htm

Centers for Disease Control and Prevention (CDC). (2016a). Facts about hypospadias. Retrieved from http://www.cdc.gov/ncbddd/birthdefects/Hypospadias.html#ref

Centers for Disease Control and Prevention (CDC). (2016b). Pelvic inflammatory disease. Retrieved from https://www.cdc.gov/std/pid/stdfact-pid-detailed.htm

Centers for Disease Control and Prevention (CDC) (2017). Sexually transmitted surveillance 2017. Retrieved from https://www.cdc.gov/std/stats17/default.htm

Centers for Disease Control and Prevention (CDC). (2018). Sexually transmitted disease surveillance. Retrieved from https://www.cdc.gov/std/stats17/default.htm

Centers for Disease Control and Prevention (CDC). (2019). Polycystic ovary syndrome (PCOS) and diabetes. Retrieved from https://www.cdc.gov/diabetes/basics/pcos.html

Chiras, D. (2015). *Human biology* (8th ed.). Burlington, MA: Jones & Bartlett Learning.

Cunningham, G. R. (2018). Overview of male sexual dysfunction. In K. A. Martin (Ed.), *Uptodate*.

Elling, B., Elling, K., & Rothenberg, M. (2004). *Anatomy and physiology*. Sudbury, MA: Jones and Bartlett Publishers.

Fraser, I. S., Critchley, H. O. D., Broder, M., & Munro, M. G. (2011). The FIGO recommendations on terminologies and definitions for normal and abnormal uterine bleeding. *Seminars in Reproductive Medicine, 29*(5), 383–390.

Gould, B. (2015). *Pathophysiology for the health professions* (5th ed.). Philadelphia, PA: Elsevier.

Greenger, J., Bruess, C., & Conklin, S. (2014). *Exploring the dimensions of human sexuality* (5th ed.). Sudbury, MA: Jones & Bartlett Learning.

Hayes, D. F., & Lippman, M. E. Breast cancer. In J. Jameson, A. S. Fauci, D. L. Kasper, S. L. Hauser, D. L. Longo, & J. Loscalzo (Eds.). *Harrison's principles of internal medicine* (20th ed.). New York, NY: McGraw-Hill. Retrieved from http://accessmedicine.mhmedical.com.ezproxy.fiu.edu/content.aspx?bookid=2129&sectionid=192015612

Jayachandran, D., Bythell, M., Platt, M., & Rankin, J. (2011). Register based study of bladder exstrophy-epispadias complex: Prevalence, associated anomalies, prenatal diagnosis and survival. *Journal of Urology, 186*(5), 2056–2060.

Johnson, T. R. B., Kaplan, L. K., Ouyang, P., & Rizza, R. A. (2012, December). Executive summary. *Evidence-based methodology workshop on polycystic ovarian syndrome*. National Institute of Health, Bethesda, Maryland. Retrieved from https://prevention.nih.gov/sites/default/files/2018-06/FinalReport.pdf

LeFevre, M. L., & U. S. Preventive Services Task Force. (2014). Screening for chlamydia and gonorrhea: U.S. Preventive Task Force recommendation statement. *Annals of Internal Medicine, 161*(12), 902.

Meyer, T. (2016). Diagnostic procedures to detect *Chlamydia trachomatis* infections. *Microorganisms, 4*(3), 25. doi:10.3390/microorganisms4030025

Moini, J. (2016). *Anatomy and physiology for health professionals* (2nd ed.). Burlington, MA: Jones & Bartlett Learning.

Munro, M. G., Critchley, H. O., Broder, M. S., & Fraser, I. S. (2011). FIGO classification system (PALM-COEIN) for causes of abnormal uterine bleeding in nongravid women of reproductive age. *International Journal of Gynecology and Obstetrics, 113*, 3–13. Retrieved from https://www.figo.org/sites/default/files/uploads/IJGO/papers/AUB%20Classification.pdf

National Cancer Institute. (2016). Cervical cancer. Retrieved from http://seer.cancer.gov/statfacts/html/cervix.html

National Institutes of Health (NIH). (2013). Premenstrual syndrome. Retrieved from http://www.ncbi.nlm.nih.gov/pubmedhealth/PMH0072449/

National Organization of Rare Disorders (NORD). (2009). Fitz Hugh Curtis syndrome. Retrieved from https://rarediseases.org/rare-diseases/fitz-hugh-curtis-syndrome/

Professional guide to pathophysiology (3rd ed.). (2010). Philadelphia, PA: Lippincott Williams & Wilkins.

Rosenfield, R. L., & Ehrmann, D. A. (2016). The pathogenesis of polycystic ovary syndrome (PCOS): The hypothesis of PCOS as functional ovarian hyperandrogenism revisited. *Endocrine Reviews, 37*(5), 467–520. doi:10.1210/er.2015-1104

U.S. Preventive Services Task Force (2018). Final update summary: Breast cancer: Screening. Retrieved from https://www.uspreventiveservicestaskforce.org/Page/Document/UpdateSummaryFinal/breast-cancer-screening1

World Health Organization. (2019). Sexually transmitted infections. Retrieved from https://www.who.int/news-room/fact-sheets/detail/sexually-transmitted-infections-(stis)

Zimmerman, A., Bernuit, D., Gerlinger, C., Schaefers, M., & Geppert, K. (2012). Prevalence, symptoms and management of uterine fibroids: An international internet-based survey of 21,746 women. *British Medical Journal Women's Health, 12*(6). Retrieved from https://www.ncbi.nlm.nih.gov/pmc/articles/PMC3342149/

The gastrointestinal (GI) system, or digestive system, consists of structures responsible for consumption, digestion, and elimination of food (FIGURE 9-1). These processes provide the essential nutrients, water, and electrolytes required for the body's physiologic activities. Structures of the GI system include an alimentary canal through which food is passed and accessory organs that aid digestion (FIGURE 9-2). The alimentary canal includes the oral cavity, pharynx, esophagus, stomach, small intestine, large intestine, and anus. The accessory organs include the salivary glands, liver, gallbladder, bile ducts, and pancreas.

Disorders of the GI system can result in nutritional deficits and metabolic imbalances. These conditions vary from mild (e.g., constipation) to life threatening (e.g., pancreatitis) in severity and often present as vague, nonspecific manifestations that reflect a disruption in the system's normal functioning.

Anatomy and Physiology

The GI tract is divided into upper and lower divisions, which will be further discussed in upcoming sections. Additionally, the liver, gallbladder, and pancreas are collectively referred to as the *hepatobiliary system* because of their close location to each other and their complementary functions. The walls of the GI tract have four layers (FIGURE 9-3). The mucosa is the innermost layer that produces mucus. Mucus facilitates movement of the GI contents and protects the GI tissue from the extreme pH conditions of the GI tract (the stomach's pH is in the range of 1–2) necessary for digestion. The epithelial mucosa cells have a high turnover rate because of erosion associated with food passage and the highly acidic environment. The submucosa layer consists of connective tissue that includes blood vessels,

nerves, lymphatics, and secretory glands. The muscle layer includes circular and longitudinal smooth muscle layers. This layer contracts in a wavelike motion to propel food through the GI tract, an action called *peristalsis*. The serosa is the outer layer of the wall; however, the outer layer of the esophagus is adventitia. Within the layers of the GI tract are three neuronal plexuses that make up the enteric nervous system. These plexuses include the submucosal plexus (Meissner plexus), myenteric plexus (Auerbach plexus), and the subserosal plexus.

The peritoneum is the large serous membrane that lines the abdominal cavity. The outer parietal peritoneum layer covers the abdominal wall as well as the top of the bladder and uterus. The inner visceral peritoneum layer encases the abdominal organs. This double-walled membrane is similar to the pericardial sac and the pleural membrane. The peritoneal cavity is the space between these two layers; it contains serous fluid to decrease friction and facilitate movement. The mesentery is a double-layer peritoneum that is a serous membrane. The mesentery is continuous with the serosa that contains blood vessels and nerves that supply the intestinal wall. It supports and connects the organs and intestines while allowing flexibility to accommodate peristalsis and varying content volumes.

Upper Gastrointestinal Tract

The upper GI tract includes the oral cavity, pharynx, esophagus, and stomach (Figure 9-2). Food usually enters the GI tract through the mouth (consumption), where chemical and mechanical digestion begins. Issues with the mouth or swallowing can create a need to bypass the mouth and esophagus and introduce the food or a food supplement directly into the stomach or small intestine. Chewing, or mastication, pulverizes the food into small

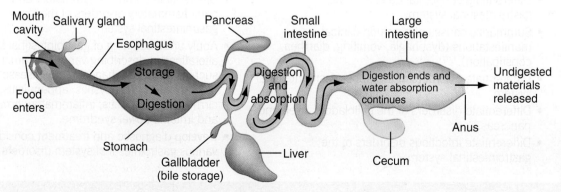

FIGURE 9-1 Functions of the gastrointestinal system.

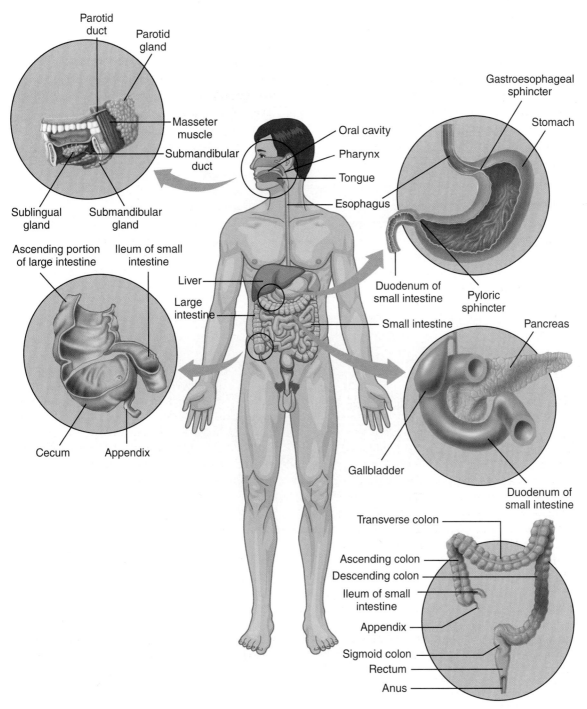

FIGURE 9-2 The structures of the gastrointestinal system.

pieces, and saliva from the salivary glands moistens and further breaks down the food (**TABLE 9-1**). Saliva contains enzymes (e.g., salivary α-amylase), which start the process of carbohydrate digestion and antibodies (e.g., IgA) that can kill or neutralize bacteria. Saliva also consists of water, mucus, and electrolytes (e.g., potassium and sodium). The smell, taste, feel, and thought of food triggers the olfactory nerve (cranial nerve II) to initiate saliva and gastric acid secretion. Various receptors located throughout the mouth can distinguish tastes (e.g., salty and bitter), and their stimulation adds to the satisfaction of eating. Saliva secretion is controlled by the autonomic nervous system. Parasympathetic cholinergic fiber stimulation inhibits salivation, and sympathetic adrenergic stimulation leads to salivation. Healthy teeth and gums play a key role in maintaining adequate nutrition.

The tongue pushes the semisolid food mass (bolus) to the back of the throat, where it is

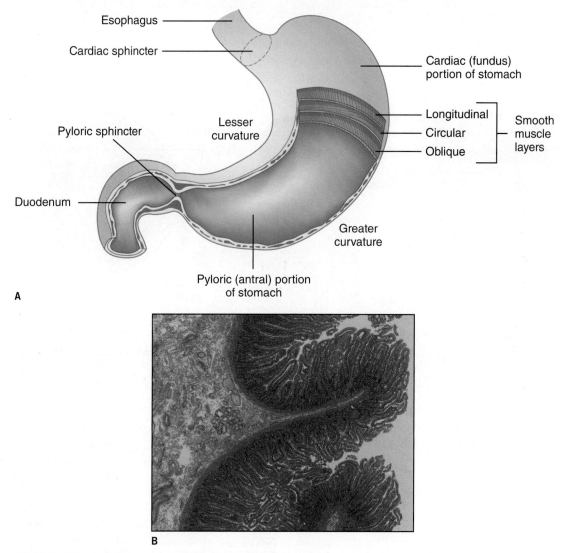

FIGURE 9-3 The layers of the gastrointestinal tract.

B: © Donna Beer Stolz, PhD, Center for Biologic Imaging, University of Pittsburgh Medical School.

TABLE 9-1	Digestive Juices and Hormones and Actions*	
Source	**Type**	**Action**
Salivary glands	Bicarbonate	Moistens food
	Salivary lipase	Digests fat
Stomach	Hydrochloric acid	Digests protein
		Kills bacteria
	Pepsin	Digests protein
	Gastric lipase	Digests fat
	Intrinsic factor	Aids in absorption of vitamin B_{12} in the small intestine
	Mucus	Protects stomach lining
	Gastrin	Stimulates gastric acid secretion, histamine, and pepsinogen
	Histamine	Stimulates gastric acid secretion
	Ghrelin	Stimulates hunger (hypothalamus)
	Somatostatin	Inhibits gastrin, gastric acid secretion, histamine, and pepsinogen

Source	Type	Action
Liver	Bile acids	Dissolve fats
	Cholesterol	Excreted in bile
	Phospholipids	Aid in absorption of fats
	Immunoglobulins	Act as antibodies
Small intestine	Motilin	Increases motility in GI tract
	Secretin	Inhibits gastric acid secretion; stimulates production of bicarbonate
	Cholecystokinin	Stimulates gallbladder to release bile and pancreas to release pancreatic juice; decreases rate of gastric emptying
	Serotonin	Activates GI immune response; stimulates intestines (e.g., secretion, motility)
Pancreas	Bicarbonate	Protects digestive enzymes
		Neutralizes acid
	Water	Carries enzymes
	Amylase	Digests starch and glycogen
	Lipases	Digest fats
	Proteases	Digest protein

*Partial list of types and actions

swallowed (**FIGURE 9-4**). All activities up to the creation of a bolus are under voluntary control. Food passing the trigeminal (cranial nerve V) glossopharyngeal nerve (cranial nerve IX), and vagus (cranial nerve X) initiates the swallowing reflex, which is an involuntary action. These nerves relay information to the swallowing center in the medulla and pons; the swallowing center then coordinates the movement of the food from the mouth through the pharynx and into the esophagus with use of the trigeminal, glossopharyngeal, vagus, and hypoglossal (cranial nerve XII). This orchestrated movement prevents food from entering the nearby trachea and lungs (a phenomenon called *aspiration*). The esophagus has muscular rings to move the food toward the stomach (**FIGURE 9-5**). As the food nears the stomach, the normally closed lower esophageal sphincter (LES) relaxes to allow the food to enter the stomach. The LES also prevents the stomach contents from refluxing into the esophagus. Relaxation of the LES occurs as a result of vagal impulses and the hormones progesterone, secretin, and glucagon. However, vagal stimulation through cholinergic fibers will increase LES sphincter tone along with the hormone gastrin.

The stomach is an expandable food and liquid reservoir. When it is empty, the stomach wall shrinks, forming wrinkles called *rugae* (**FIGURE 9-6**). Prior to the arrival of food into the stomach, gastric acid secretion begins in preparation for the arrival of food. As the stomach fills, the rugae unfold and the wall stretches to accommodate a volume up to 4 liters. Rugae inside the gastric glands have different cells that secrete various substances. These cells include parietal cells that secrete hydrochloric acid, intrinsic factor, and gastroferrin; mucous cells that secrete an alkaline mucus; chief cells that secrete pepsinogen (a precursor to pepsin); G cells that release gastrin; D cells that secrete somatostatin; and enterochromaffin cells that secrete histamine. Parietal cells (i.e., oxyntic cells) are found mainly in the fundus while G cells are in the pyloric glands of the antrum. Some gastric secretions are released directly into the stomach, while others are secreted into the blood and then travel to the stomach or intended tissue. Inside the stomach, hydrochloric acid and enzymes (Table 9-1) further chemically digest the food, and peristaltic churning further mechanically digests the food. This new food mixture is referred to as *chyme*. The highly acidic nature of chyme aids in digestion and destroys bacteria. The epithelial cells of the stomach's inner lining are densely packed together to prevent damage to the tissues through contact with the acidic stomach contents. For additional protection, bicarbonate is secreted to neutralize the acid, and numerous glands are in the stomach. These glands coat the inner lining of the stomach with a thick layer of mucus. Nutrients are not absorbed in the stomach; instead, the food is simply prepared for absorption. However, alcohol, nonsteroidal anti-inflammatory drugs (NSAIDs), and aspirin are absorbed in the stomach. Chyme leaves the stomach through

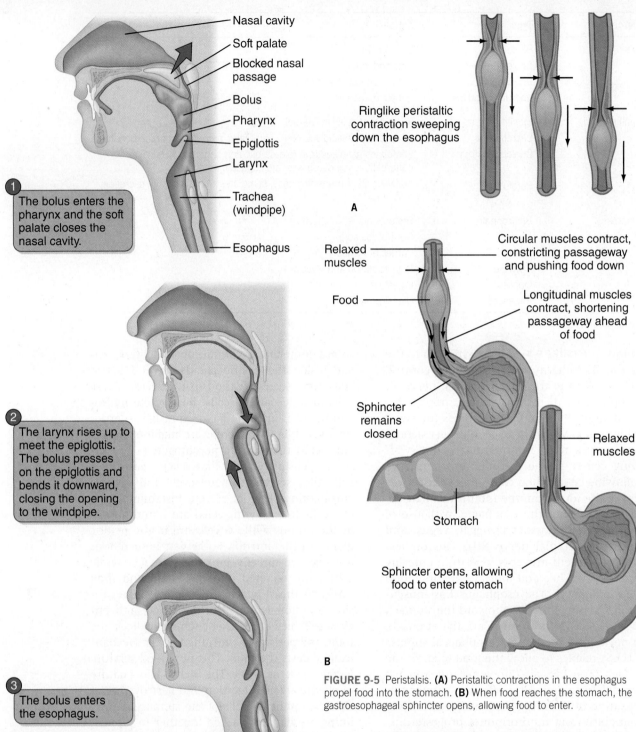

FIGURE 9-4 Swallowing.

1 The bolus enters the pharynx and the soft palate closes the nasal cavity.

2 The larynx rises up to meet the epiglottis. The bolus presses on the epiglottis and bends it downward, closing the opening to the windpipe.

3 The bolus enters the esophagus.

Ringlike peristaltic contraction sweeping down the esophagus

A

Relaxed muscles

Food

Circular muscles contract, constricting passageway and pushing food down

Longitudinal muscles contract, shortening passageway ahead of food

Sphincter remains closed

Stomach

Relaxed muscles

Sphincter opens, allowing food to enter stomach

B

FIGURE 9-5 Peristalsis. **(A)** Peristaltic contractions in the esophagus propel food into the stomach. **(B)** When food reaches the stomach, the gastroesophageal sphincter opens, allowing food to enter.

the pyloric sphincter in small (1–3 mL), intermittent amounts. As it passes through the pyloric sphincter into the duodenum, liver and pancreatic secretions (Table 9-1) are added to continue the digestion process. Much like the

LES, the pyloric sphincter prevents reflux of bile from the small intestines into the stomach. In addition to extrinsic sympathetic and parasympathetic innervation, the stomach is controlled by the intrinsic plexuses of the enteric nervous system.

Lower Gastrointestinal Tract

The lower GI tract comprises the small intestine (duodenum, jejunum, and ileum), large intestine (cecum, colon, and rectum), and anus

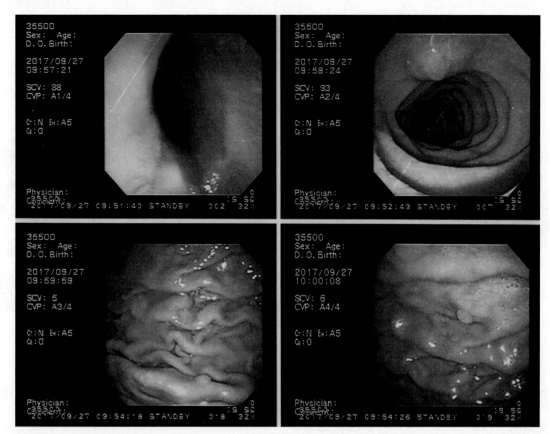

FIGURE 9-6 Rugae of the stomach.
© Captain Hook/Shutterstock.

(Figure 9-2). The small intestine is the longest section of the GI tract (approximately 20 feet long in adults). This length allows for adequate nutrient absorption as the small intestine continues the digestion process. The duodenum, which is located retroperitoneally, in conjunction with digestive juices from the liver and pancreas, are important sites for mixing of food. Carbohydrate, protein, fat, bile, vitamins, and minerals are digested and absorbed in different locations of the small intestines. In the small intestine, the enzymes that have been secreted into the GI tract break the large food molecules into smaller molecules, which are then absorbed. These smaller molecules are transported to the circulatory and lymphatic system. Muscular rings slowly move the food mixture through the small intestine using a peristaltic wave motion. The wall of the small intestine contains numerous circular folds (plicae circulars) covered with villi and microvilli, particularly in the jejunum and ileum (**FIGURE 9-7**). These projections increase the surface area available for absorption of nutrients. Each villus contains capillaries, nerves, and lymphatic vessels that play key roles in this absorption. In between the villi are the intestinal

glands (i.e., crypts of Lieberkühn) that are the sites where stem cells differentiate into multiple types of cells (e.g., goblet cells and enterocytes). The small intestine also contains cells that secrete fluid to neutralize pH and enzymes to facilitate digestion. Much like the stomach, the small intestine produces a large amount of protective mucus. Immune cells such as lymphocytes, plasma cells, and macrophages are located beneath the villus in lymph nodules in areas known as **Peyer patches**. These cells act as a defense against microorganisms. Antimicrobial peptides, immunoglobulins, and enzymes are produced as part the defensive role of the GI tract. As with other parts of the GI tract, intestinal motility is under the control of the vagus nerve, the enteric nervous system, and various hormones.

After making its long journey through the small intestine, the chyme ultimately reaches the large intestine (in approximately 3–5 hours). The large intestine is approximately 5 feet long and about twice the diameter of the small intestine. The large intestine does not contain villi. The large intestine has few enzyme-secreting cells but has a large number of goblet cells and enterocytes

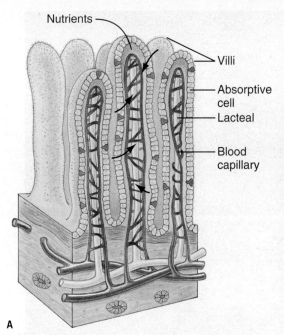

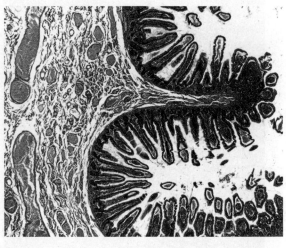

A

B

FIGURE 9-7 Villi of the small intestines.

B: © Donna Beer Stolz, PhD, Center for Biologic Imaging, University of Pittsburgh Medical School.

(absorptive cells). The cecum and colon muscle layers are structured into a succession of pouches called *haustra* with a band of muscle (teniae coli) that runs through the haustra (Figure 9-2). This structure gives the intestine a gathered look. The small intestine ends in a pouch called the *cecum*. The appendix is also attached to the cecum. This small, wormlike structure seemingly has no function, but it does have plenty of potential to cause harm. The ileocecal valve is a sphincter that controls flow of digested material from the ileum to the cecum and prevents substances from refluxing into the small intestine. The ileocecal valve is normally closed, and peristalsis from the ileum will stimulate intrinsic fibers and cause the valve to open. The colon makes up most of the large intestine. Unlike the coiled small intestine, the colon has three relatively straight sections—termed the *ascending*, *transverse*, and *descending* colons. The descending colon becomes the sigmoid colon.

The mixture entering the colon from the small intestine includes water, unabsorbed food molecules, indigestible food remnants (e.g., cellulose), and electrolytes (sodium and potassium). The colon absorbs 90% of the water and electrolytes, and *Escherichia coli* feed off the undigested or unabsorbed food remnants. *E. coli* organisms constitute a large population of bacteria normally found in the GI tract. These bacteria synthesize several key vitamins (e.g., vitamins B_{12}, B_1, B_2, and K) that are later

absorbed by the large intestine. As the chyme moves through the colon, it changes into a fecal mass. The fecal mass is moved through the colon by way of segmental movements passing the mass from the haustra. Peristaltic movements further promote colonic emptying. Feces contain the remaining undigested or unabsorbed remnants along with bacteria (one-third of the feces). Feces also introduce mucus (approximately 300 mL daily) to aid in bowel movements, even in times of decreased dietary intake. Because the feces are denser than the contents in the small intestines, the colon's muscular rings must be thicker to propel the feces until they reach the rectum (this usually takes approximately 18 hours). The movement of feces from the sigmoid colon to the rectum is controlled by the rectosigmoid sphincter. The rectum serves as a reservoir to store the feces.

Much like the bladder, the rectum expands when feces enter this area, stimulating the stretch receptors in the sigmoid colon and rectal wall. These receptors send an impulse through the enteric nervous system and spinal cord (which controls the external sphincter) to elicit the defecation reflex. During defecation, the internal and external anal sphincters relax, and the rectum contracts to expel the feces. Stool passage is best accomplished in a squatting or sitting type position as the puborectal muscles relax and the anorectal angle straightens. Gravitational forces also assist with stool passage. Defecation is consciously controlled (except in infants and young children) and may require assistance from abdominal muscles. The Valsalva maneuver, which involves taking a breath and then pushing, causes an increase in intrathoracic and intra-abdominal pressure and facilitates the passage of stool. Defecation control requires both appropriate muscular and nervous function. The urge to defecate can be delayed up to a point through voluntary contraction of the external sphincter, but the longer the feces remain in the large intestine, the more water from them will be absorbed, making the feces more difficult to expel.

In addition to the nerves that control defecation, the enteric nervous system and the sympathetic and parasympathetic nervous systems innervate the GI tract. Activation of the sympathetic nervous system slows digestive activity, whereas activation of the parasympathetic nervous system increases digestive activity.

Liver

The liver is an organ that is a hub of activity. This large organ performs as many as 500 different functions. Some of the liver's primary roles are vital for homeostasis and include the following:

- Metabolize carbohydrates, protein, and fats.
- Synthesize glucose, protein (albumin, globulins—alpha and beta), amino acids, enzymes, cholesterol, triglycerides, and clotting factors.
- Store glucose (glycogen), fats (lipids), and micronutrients (e.g., iron, copper, and vitamin B_{12}) and release them when needed.
- Detoxify the blood of potentially harmful chemicals (e.g., alcohol, nicotine, and medications).
- Maintain intravascular fluid volume through the production of circulating proteins (see chapter 6).
- Metabolize medications to prepare them for excretion.
- Produce bile (necessary for emulsification of fat and fat-soluble vitamins).
- Inactivate and prepare hormones for excretion.
- Remove damaged or old erythrocytes from blood to recycle iron and protein (see chapter 3).
- Serve as a blood reservoir (stores approximately 450 mL of blood that can be used when needed).
- Convert fatty acids to ketones.

A tough membrane (Glisson capsule) protects this crucial organ. The liver has a dual blood supply. The liver is a small part of the body weight (approximately 2.5%) but receives 25% of cardiac output. The hepatic artery carries oxygenated blood from the general circulation to the liver at a rate of approximately 300 mL per minute to nourish the liver. The portal vein carries partially deoxygenated blood from the stomach, pancreas, spleen, and gallbladder as well as from the small and large intestines, to the liver at a rate of approximately 1,000 mL per minute so that the liver can process nutrients and digestion by-products.

The liver is one of the few body organs that can regenerate. As much as 75% of the liver tissue can be lost or removed, yet the remaining liver tissue can slowly regenerate into a whole liver again. This regeneration occurs primarily due to certain liver cells (hepatocytes) that act as stem cells. A single hepatocyte can divide into two daughter cells. During regeneration, steps should be taken to protect the liver from damage (e.g., avoiding hepatotoxic medications and substances).

In addition to providing regeneration capabilities, the hepatocytes produce bile and perform most of the liver's other activities. The hepatocytes constantly produce bile at a rate of approximately 600–1,200 mL per day. Bile is a green or yellowish liquid that contains water, bile salts (formed from cholesterol), conjugated bilirubin, cholesterol, and electrolytes (including bicarbonate). Bile salts are necessary to emulsify fats and fat-soluble vitamins (A, D, E, and K) so that they can be absorbed in the small intestine. The distal ileum reabsorbs most of the bile and returns it to the liver through the portal vein for recycling. The bicarbonate ions in the bile neutralize the acidic gastric contents so that the intestinal and pancreatic enzymes can perform their functions. The bile flows from the liver through a duct system to either the gallbladder for storage or on to the duodenum (see FIGURE 9-8). The gallbladder is a small (usually no larger than a golf ball), saclike organ located on the undersurface of the liver that serves as a reservoir for bile. In addition to storing the bile, the gallbladder concentrates it by removing water and electrolytes, leaving bile salts, bile pigments, and cholesterol. The presence of chyme in the small intestine triggers the gallbladder to contract, releasing bile into yet another duct system, where it travels to the small intestine. The hormone cholecystokinin, which is produced by the small intestine

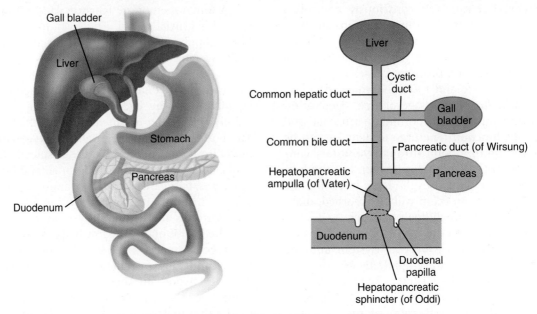

FIGURE 9-8 Gross anatomy of the human liver and gallbladder. The liver, gallbladder, stomach, pancreas, and duodenum, with a detail of the related ducts. Hepatopancreatic sphincter of Oddi, hepatopancreatic ampulla of Vater, duodenum, duodenal papilla, pancreatic duct of Wirsung, cystic duct, common bile duct, common hepatic duct, pancreas, stomach, liver, gallbladder.

when there is fat, also controls gallbladder contraction. If the gallbladder requires surgical removal, the bile constantly flows directly from the liver to the small intestine.

Pancreas

The pancreas is an organ that is nestled underneath the stomach and liver (with the head tucked under the duodenum and the tail touching the spleen). It has exocrine and endocrine functions. The exocrine functions include producing enzymes, electrolytes (e.g., bicarbonate ions), and water necessary for digestion (Table 9-1). A duct system (see Figure 9-8) carries these substances to the duodenum to join the chyme. The endocrine functions include producing hormones (insulin, glycogen, somatostatin, and pancreatic polypeptide) to help regulate blood glucose, thereby maintaining homeostasis. See chapter 10 for more on endocrine function.

Gastrointestinal Changes Associated With Aging

The GI system undergoes a few changes with aging. The stomach lining may shrink and become inflamed, leading to atrophic gastritis. Stomach acid production occasionally can decrease (a condition called achlorhydria) because of atrophic gastritis. Achlorhydria can cause decreased intrinsic factor production, resulting in vitamin B_{12} deficiency and slow digestion. Changes in the liver associated with age include reduced

blood flow, delayed drug clearance, and a diminished capacity to regenerate damaged liver cells. Additionally, changes in the metabolism and absorption of lactose, calcium, and iron can occur. In particular, the small intestine absorbs less calcium with advancing age, so increased calcium intake is needed to prevent bone mineral loss and osteoporosis. The production of some enzymes, such as lactase (which aids in the digestion of lactose, a sugar found in dairy products), declines with age. Peristalsis also decreases with age, increasing the risk of constipation. Intestinal microflora changes can result in increased susceptibility to disease.

Understanding Conditions That Affect the Gastrointestinal System

When considering alterations in the GI system, organizing them based on their basic underlying pathophysiology can increase understanding. These concepts are based on the two major underlying pathologic issues—altered nutrition and impaired bowel elimination that result in alterations in movement of intestinal content and disruption in secretory and absorptive functions. Conditions that alter nutritional status include issues with consuming, digesting, and absorbing food. Examples of these conditions include cleft lip, pancreatitis, and celiac disease, respectively. Regardless of the cause

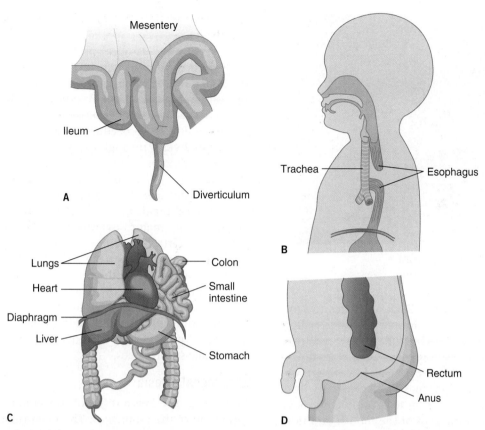

FIGURE 9-9 Diagram of gastrointestinal malformations. **A**. Meckel's diverticulum, **B**. Esophageal atresia with distal tracheoesophageal fistula (type C), **C**. Congenital diaphragmatic hernia, **D**. Imperforate anus

of the altered nutrition, the result is similar—inadequate nutritional states in which individuals may be underweight, malnourished, and vitamin deficient. Conditions impairing bowel elimination generally manifest as constipation and diarrhea. These issues may be either the primary condition or a symptom of another condition. Additionally, conditions that cause altered nutrition may cause issues with elimination.

Disorders of the Upper Gastrointestinal Tract and Accessory Organs

Disorders of the upper GI tract generally cause issues with nutrition and range in severity from mild to life threatening. These disorders can be congenital or acquired (e.g., peptic ulcers). Upper gastrointestinal tract disorders can result in manifestations such as dysphagia or vomiting. Depending on their severity, most of these disorders can be resolved or managed with minimal residual effects.

Congenital Defects

Congenital defects of the digestive system can affect the upper and the lower GI tract (to be

discussed later in chapter) (**FIGURE 9-9**). These congenital disorders, including cleft lip, cleft palate, and pyloric stenosis, are common and not usually life threatening, but they may cause nutritional and self-image issues.

Cleft Lip and Cleft Palate

Cleft lip and cleft palate are the most common types of congenital craniofacial malformations that are apparent at birth. The Centers for Disease Control and Prevention (CDC, 2017a) estimates that cleft palate without cleft lip occurs in 1 of every 2,650 births in the United States, and cleft lip with or without cleft palate occurs in 1 of every 4,440 births. Some infants with cleft lip or palate have other anomalies, and there are over 100 syndromes associated with clefts. These conditions usually develop between the fourth and ninth weeks of gestation and are multifactorial in origin. Such defects have been associated with genetic mutations, maternal diabetes, drugs (e.g., anticonvulsants), toxins, viruses, vitamin deficiencies, alcohol consumption, and cigarette smoking. Clefts are most frequent in children of Native American, Hispanic, and Asian descent, whereas Black children are the least likely to have a cleft. Males are twice as likely as females to have a cleft lip. Females,

Risk factors

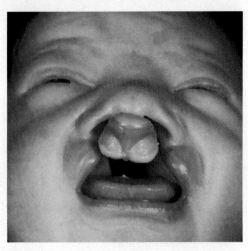

FIGURE 9-10 Cleft lip and palate.
Courtesy of Leonard V. Crowley, MD, Century College.

Complications

however, are twice as likely as males to have a cleft palate. A cleft lip and palate can affect the appearance of an individual's face and may lead to feeding issues, speech problems, ear infections (e.g., otitis media), and hearing problems. The conditions may vary in severity from a small notch in the lip to a complete groove that runs into the roof of the mouth and nose (**FIGURE 9-10**). These defects may occur either separately or together.

Clinical Manifestations

Cleft lip may appear unilaterally or bilaterally (on either side of the midline of the upper lip). This defect results from failure of the maxillary processes and nasal elevations or upper lip to fuse during development. Cleft palate results from failure of the hard and soft palates to fuse in development, creating an opening between the oral and nasal cavities. At times, a cleft palate may just involve the muscles, and the cleft palate may be covered by the mouth lining (i.e., submucous cleft palate) often making these types of defects difficult to see. In addition to lip and palate deformities, teeth and nose malformations may be present. Feeding problems result from these deficits due to an insufficient ability to suck. An infant with a cleft lip and/or palate is also at high risk for aspiration when the nasal cavity is open. The inability to make sounds using the lips and tongue impairs speech development.

Diagnosis and Treatment

Diagnostic procedures for cleft lip/palate consist of a history, physical examination, and prenatal ultrasound. Orofacial clefts can often be detected after 12 weeks' gestation. Treatment

strategies for cleft lip/palate include temporary measures (e.g., special nipples or dental appliances) until surgical procedures are recommended. Surgical repair of the defect is necessary to close the gap. Cleft lip repair is recommended before age 3 months, and cleft palate repair is recommended by 18 months of age. Follow-up procedures are often necessary from 2 years through the adolescent years and depending on the type of cleft. Treatment can span over 20 years. Cosmetic plastic surgery can improve the appearance of the defect. Surgical repair in utero is currently being explored. The major advantage of surgical repair before birth is little or no scarring. Speech therapy, including language and eating interventions, as well as orthodontist consultation can promote normal growth and development. Additionally, a multidisciplinary team (including an audiologist, speech and language therapist, and a pediatrician) is frequently required to manage severe cases.

Esophageal Atresia

Esophageal atresia is a result of congenital malformation of the esophagus. The malformation leads to two separate esophageal sections—an upper and a lower section that are not connected (Figure 9-9). There are four types (type A, B, C, and D) with two separate sections, and most cases (88%) are associated with a tracheoesophageal fistula (TEF) (type C). The CDC (2017b) estimates that esophageal atresia occurs in 1 of every 4,300 pregnancies. Most of the cases of esophageal atresia with TEF involve the lower half of the esophagus connecting with the trachea. A tracheoesophageal fistula can also occur without esophageal atresia and this is termed type E. Many cases of esophageal atresia are associated with other congenital anomalies such as anal atresia, cardiac defects, and renal defects. The risk of esophageal atresia is higher in infants as their father's age increases and if their mothers used assistive reproductive technology to become pregnant.

Clinical Manifestations

Prenatally, esophageal atresia should be suspected when there is polyhydramnios (excess amniotic fluid), however many cases are not detected prenatally. Clinical manifestations of esophageal atresia are dependent on whether a TEF is present or absent. Manifestations in the infant occur immediately after birth. Saliva and secretions are unable to descend the esophagus because the upper esophagus is closed off. The infant will start drooling, choking, and have difficulty breathing. The infant may choke with feeding, as he or she is unable to swallow during feedings. If there is no TEF, the infant may have a scaphoid-shaped abdomen with no gas because food and liquids are not going through from the esophagus to the stomach. If there is a TEF with the distal esophagus section, the abdomen can become distended, causing breathing difficulties. The gastric contents can also reflux through the fistula, leading to an aspiration pneumonia, which is associated with a higher incidence of death. Complications of esophageal atresia with or without TEF include recurrent aspiration, pneumonia, and atelectasis.

Diagnosis and Treatment

Diagnosis is usually made at birth. The atresia is evaluated by attempting to pass a catheter into the stomach and an inability to do so is suspicious for atresia. The catheter location is assessed with an X-ray, and the catheter will be curled up in the upper esophageal pouch with an atresia. The TEF may be evident on chest X-ray, and the GI tract will be filled with gas. Diagnostic tests for the evaluation of other associated abnormalities may include an echocardiogram, renal sonogram, and X-ray of the spine and limbs. Once a diagnosis is made, initial treatment will include continuous suction of the esophagus to prevent complications (e.g.,

---

Diagnostic Link

Liver Injury

Measurement of liver enzymes is a common serologic test. These enzymes are markers of liver injury and include ALT, AST, ALP, and bilirubin. ALT is mainly in the liver, and elevated serum levels are a marker of liver injury while AST is present in the liver and other organs (e.g., cardiac and skeletal muscle, kidney, and brain) and therefore elevated levels can be indicative of an injury to the liver and/or other organs. ALT, therefore, is a better marker of liver injury in comparison to AST. The magnitude of the aminotransferase elevations can vary depending on the type of liver injury. As an example, acute viral hepatitis and ischemic hepatitis can cause levels to go up 25 and 50 times the upper limits of normal, respectively. Fatty liver disease not due to alcohol, on the other hand, can cause milder elevations (e.g., < 4 times the upper limit of normal). Alkaline phosphatase is derived from the bone and liver, and elevated serum levels can indicate injury in either organ. The γ-glutamyl transpeptidase (GGT) can confirm that the elevated ALP is due to liver injury as the γ-glutamyl transpeptidase rises with liver injury but not with bone disorders. Lactic dehydrogenase is found in the liver and in tissue throughout the body. While it is elevated with liver injury, elevations can also occur with many other disorders, so it is not as specific as other markers for liver injury.

---

choking and pneumonia). Surgical repair of the esophageal defects and TEF is the mainstay of treatment. Surgery may need to be performed in stages, such as when the gap between the upper and lower pouch of the esophagus is too large. With a large gap, surgery may have to be postponed until the esophagus grows longer, usually in a few months.

Pyloric Stenosis

Pyloric stenosis, also known as infantile hypertrophic pyloric stenosis, is a narrowing and obstruction of the pyloric sphincter. The pyloric sphincter muscle fibers become thick and stiff, making it difficult for the stomach to empty food into the small intestine. This condition can be present at birth, or it may develop later in life (rarely in children older than 6 months). Most cases present at approximately 3 weeks of life. The exact cause of pyloric stenosis is unknown, but it is thought to be multifactorial—that is, a combination of environmental and hereditary factors. Use of macrolides such as azithromycin and erythromycin in early infancy has demonstrated a strong association with increased pyloric stenosis risk. Evidence also suggests that exposure in utero with breastfeeding due to maternal use or increases this risk. Although it is the most common cause of intestinal obstructions in infancy, pyloric stenosis is relatively uncommon (occurring in 2–4 infants per 1,000 births) (Singh & Sinert, 2015). Pyloric stenosis is most common in Whites and in males.

Clinical Manifestations

Clinical manifestations of pyloric stenosis usually appear within several weeks (3–6) after birth. In the congenital form, the hypertrophied pyloric muscle can be palpated as a hard, olive-shaped mass in the abdomen (right upper quadrant), and vomiting (usually after every feeding, often projectile, and sometimes with hematemesis being noted) is usually the first symptom. Additional manifestations include the following signs and symptoms: persistent hunger (the infant often wants to eat soon after vomiting), regurgitation, belching, abdominal pain, failure to gain weight, and wavelike stomach contractions that result from the increased peristaltic effort to pass food through the narrowed areas. Dehydration, electrolyte imbalances, and pH disturbances (usually metabolic alkalosis) may occur; however, advances in diagnostic imaging have led to earlier diagnosis and a decreased incidence of dehydration. Hyperbilirubinemia can be associated with pyloric stenosis, known as the icteropyloric syndrome. The hyperbilirubinemia can be conjugated or unconjugated (more common).

Diagnosis and Treatment

Diagnostic procedures for pyloric stenosis include a history, physical examination, abdominal ultrasound, blood chemistry (to identify and monitor fluid and electrolyte imbalances), and a complete blood count (to rule out other causes such as infection). A test of bilirubin and liver enzymes, aspartate aminotransferase (AST), alanine aminotransferase (ALT), and alkaline phosphatase (ALP) is performed when an infant has jaundice. Surgical repair called *pyloromyotomy* is recommended to open the sphincter, but balloon dilation may be used in high-surgical-risk infants. Additionally, fluid, electrolyte, and pH imbalances may need correction. Signs and symptoms usually resolve within 24 hours of surgical repair. In most cases, feedings are restarted within 8 hours of surgery.

Diagnostic Link

Bilirubin Measurement

Bilirubin is another marker of liver injury or function, but it is not as good of a marker as other measures such as ALT. Bilirubin is a by-product of heme metabolism (mainly hemoglobin breakdown), and the breakdown results in unconjugated bilirubin (not water soluble). The unconjugated bilirubin is sent to the liver for conjugation (it is water soluble) where most is readily cleared from the body through bile and out into the small intestines and in feces. Measurements can be direct, reflecting conjugated bilirubin, or indirect, reflecting unconjugated bilirubin. Bilirubin levels reflect the balance between production and clearance, so high levels can occur with increased production, decreased use, and too little excretion. High unconjugated levels reflect too much bilirubin that has not been conjugated by the liver so there is either too much heme being metabolized (as in sickle cell anemia) at a rate that is higher than the liver can handle or there is a problem with the liver's conjugating capacity (e.g., Gilbert syndrome). High conjugated bilirubin, which has already been processed by the liver, can indicate there is a problem with the secretion of the bilirubin into the bile, preventing it from exiting (e.g., biliary obstruction, hepatitis) and causing it to back up into the blood.

Dysphagia

Dysphagia, or difficulty swallowing, usually develops secondary to a condition that causes mechanical obstruction of the esophagus or impaired esophageal motility (FIGURE 9-11). Dysphagia may be due to a disorder in the pharynx (i.e., oropharyngeal dysphagia), which is characterized by difficulty initiating swallowing, or or esophagus (i.e., esophageal dysphagia), which is characterized by difficulty swallowing after initiating a swallow. Dysphagia can occur as a result of intrinsic (originating with the esophagus lumen) or extrinsic (originating outside the esophagus lumen) mechanical obstruction. Numerous conditions can lead to dysphagia:

- Mechanical obstructions, including those caused by the following:
  - Congenital atresia (congenital separation of the upper and lower esophagus)
  - Esophageal stenosis or stricture (may be developmental or acquired)
  - Esophageal diverticula (outpouching of the esophageal wall)
  - Esophagitis (e.g., infectious, eosinophilic)
  - Tumors (esophageal or of nearby structures)
- Neurologic disorders, including those caused by the following:
  - Stroke
  - Cerebral damage (e.g., traumatic brain injury)
  - Achalasia (failure of the LES to relax because of loss of innervations)
  - Parkinson disease
  - Alzheimer disease
  - Huntington disease
  - Cerebral palsy
  - Multiple sclerosis
  - Amyotrophic lateral sclerosis
  - Guillain-Barré syndrome
- Muscular disorders, including those caused by muscular dystrophy

Functional dysphagia is a sense of solid and/or liquid food lodging, sticking, or passing abnormally through the esophagus. With functional dysphagia, there is no evidence of esophageal, mucosal, or structural abnormality, and the dysphagia is not attributable to other disorders such as achalasia or gastroesophageal reflux disease. Dysphagia can also have iatrogenic causes, resulting from many head and neck surgeries and procedures such as laryngectomy, tracheostomy, endotracheal intubation, esophageal dilatation, or radiation. Dysphagia can also occur as a result of medication side effects. Medications that relax the muscles, suppress the nervous system, or damage the mucosa, such as sedatives, narcotics, antipsychotics, NSAIDs, or potassium chloride tablets, may cause dysphagia. Dysphagia has likewise been associated with several psychiatric conditions, including anxiety, depression, somatoform disorders, hypochondriasis, conversion disorders, and eating disorders. Dysphagia can have an acute and

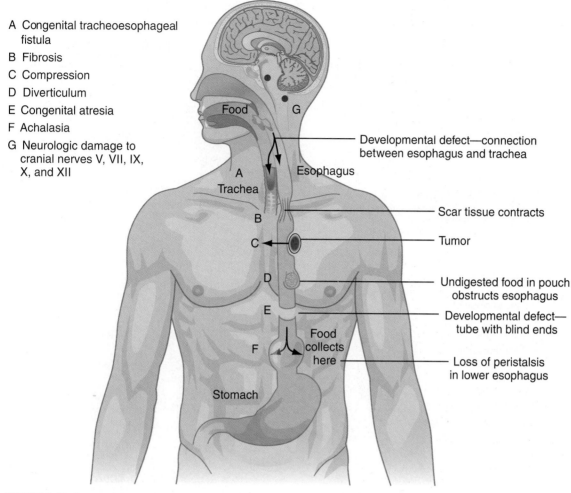

A Congenital tracheoesophageal fistula
B Fibrosis
C Compression
D Diverticulum
E Congenital atresia
F Achalasia
G Neurologic damage to cranial nerves V, VII, IX, X, and XII

Food
G
Developmental defect—connection between esophagus and trachea
Esophagus
A
Trachea
B
Scar tissue contracts
C
Tumor
D
Undigested food in pouch obstructs esophagus
E
Developmental defect—tube with blind ends
F
Food collects here
Loss of peristalsis in lower esophagus
Stomach

FIGURE 9-11 Causes of dysphagia.

sudden onset, and generally, this onset is due to food that is impacted in the esophagus (usually beef or chicken) that completely blocks off the esophagus. In these circumstances, the food is extracted or pushed into the stomach with a grasping device during an upper endoscopy.

Clinical manifestations include a sensation of food being stuck in the throat, choking, coughing, pocketing food in the cheeks, difficulty forming a food bolus, delayed swallowing, and painful swallowing (odynophagia). Dysphagia may occur with solids, liquids, or with both, and the distinction is important to determine the probable underlying disorder. As an example, difficulty only with swallowing solid foods may indicate that the esophageal lumen has a stricture. Dysphagia can be intermittent (e.g., esophageal spasms) or progressive (e.g., due to peptic stricture or achalasia). Dysphagia not only causes alterations in nutrition, but also poses an aspiration risk.

Diagnostic procedures focus on identifying the underlying cause and consist of a history, physical examination, barium swallow, chest and neck X-rays, esophageal pH measurement, esophageal manometry, upper endoscopy, flexible endoscopic evaluation of swallowing with sensory testing, videofluoroscopic swallow study, and esophagogastroduodenoscopy (EGD). Manometry measures the movement and pressure in the esophagus and stomach through a small nasogastric tube. Flexible endoscopic evaluation of swallowing with sensory testing uses a small, lighted camera to view the mouth and throat while examining how the swallowing mechanism responds to such stimuli as a puff of air, food, or liquids. A videofluoroscopic swallow study is a videotaped X-ray of the entire swallowing process in which foods or liquids along with the mineral barium are consumed. EGD is a visualization of the esophagus, stomach, and duodenum using a small, lighted camera. Treatment strategies are specific for the causative condition and can include surgery (e.g., myotomy [cutting of the muscle] and endoscopic balloon dilation) or botulinum toxin injection to allow the muscle to relax to facilitate swallowing.

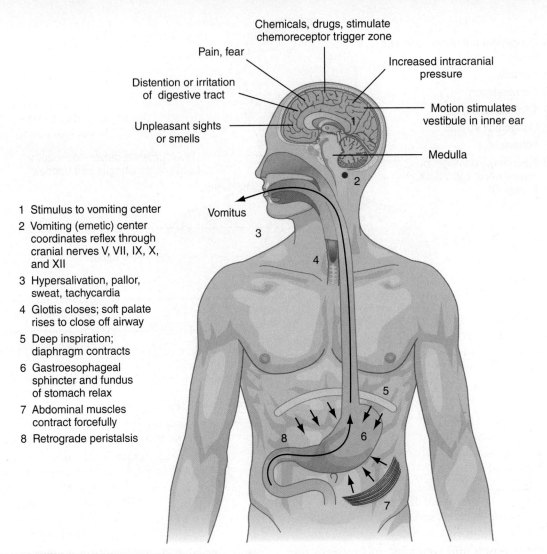

Pain, fear

Chemicals, drugs, stimulate chemoreceptor trigger zone

Distention or irritation of digestive tract

Increased intracranial pressure

Unpleasant sights or smells

Motion stimulates vestibule in inner ear

Medulla

Vomitus

1 Stimulus to vomiting center
2 Vomiting (emetic) center coordinates reflex through cranial nerves V, VII, IX, X, and XII
3 Hypersalivation, pallor, sweat, tachycardia
4 Glottis closes; soft palate rises to close off airway
5 Deep inspiration; diaphragm contracts
6 Gastroesophageal sphincter and fundus of stomach relax
7 Abdominal muscles contract forcefully
8 Retrograde peristalsis

FIGURE 9-12 Vomiting reflex.

Additionally, interventions are employed to maintain the patient's nutritional status and prevent aspiration (e.g., soft or pureed foods, thickened liquids, small bites, and no use of straws).

Vomiting

Vomiting, or emesis, is the involuntary or voluntary forceful ejection of chyme from the stomach up through the esophagus and out the mouth. Vomiting is a common event that results from a wide range of conditions. It may be protective (e.g., with drug overdose or infections) or result from reverse peristalsis (e.g., with intestinal obstructions). Increased intracranial pressure can cause sudden projectile vomiting. Additionally, vomiting may be associated with other symptoms such as severe pain (e.g., migraines or renal calculi). The medulla coordinates vomiting, and drugs, toxins, and chemicals can stimulate this vomiting center. See chapter 11 for details on neural function.

Regardless of the cause, vomiting requires the collaboration of several structures (**FIGURE 9-12**). Involuntary vomiting occurs through the following sequence:

1. A deep breath is taken.
2. The glottis closes and the soft palate rises.
3. Respirations cease to minimize the risk of aspiration.
4. The gastroesophageal sphincter relaxes.
5. The abdominal muscles contract, squeezing the stomach against the diaphragm and forcing the chyme upward into the esophagus.
6. Reverse peristaltic waves eject chyme out of the mouth.

Vomiting may be preceded by nausea (a subjective urge to vomit) or retching (a strong unproductive effort to vomit). Recurrent vomiting can be exhausting because of the strong muscular contractions. Additionally, recurrent vomiting can lead to fluid, electrolyte, and pH imbalances. Aspiration of chyme into the lungs can cause serious damage and inflammation. This event can occur if the individual is supine or unconscious when vomiting occurs. Aspiration can also occur when the vomiting or cough reflex is suppressed from drugs (e.g., anesthesia or narcotics) or disease (e.g., stroke).

The characteristics of the contents vomited (called *vomitus*) are significant and can illuminate the underlying cause of the vomiting event. Hematemesis describes the condition in which blood is present in the vomitus. Blood in vomitus has a characteristic brown, granular appearance similar to coffee grounds. This appearance results from protein in the blood being partially digested in the stomach. Blood in the stomach is irritating to the gastric mucosa, so the stomach attempts to expel it. Hematemesis can occur from several conditions that can cause upper GI bleeding (e.g., gastric ulcers and esophageal varices). Yellow- or green-colored vomitus usually indicates the presence of bile. This type of vomitus can occur as a result of a GI tract obstruction. A deep brown color of vomitus may indicate content from the lower intestine, possibly fecal. This type of vomitus frequently results from intestinal obstruction. Conditions that impair gastric emptying (e.g., pyloric stenosis) can cause recurrent vomiting of undigested food.

The force with which the vomiting occurs is important. Projectile vomiting occurs when the vomitus exits the mouth with such force that it is propelled over a short but significant distance. It is often sudden, with excessive vomitus with each attack, and not preceded with nausea.

Projectile vomiting is associated with intestinal obstructions, delayed gastric emptying, increased intracranial pressure, poisoning, and overeating.

Diagnostic procedures for vomiting focus on identifying causative agents as well as fluid, electrolyte, and pH imbalances (usually metabolic alkalosis). These procedures vary and may include a history, physical examination, and blood chemistry, among others. Treatment strategies center on the cessation of vomiting, maintaining hydration, restoring acid–base balance, and correcting electrolyte alterations. These strategies may vary depending on the severity of the vomiting:

- Antiemetic medications (e.g., dimenhydrinate [Dramamine], ondansetron [Zofran], and promethazine [Phenergan])
- Oral or intravenous fluid replacement
- Correcting any electrolyte imbalances (see chapter 6)
- Restoring acid–base balance (see chapter 6)

Hiatal Hernia

A hiatal hernia occurs when a section of the stomach protrudes upward through an opening (hiatus) in the diaphragm into the thoracic cavity. There are two categories of hiatal hernia—sliding hernia (type I) and paraesophageal hernia (types II, III, and IV). A sliding hiatal hernia is the most common type, accounting for approximately 95% of cases. With a sliding hernia, the gastroesophageal (GE) junction is displaced above the diaphragm. The stomach remains aligned, and the stomach fundus remains below the GE junction (FIGURE 9-13). With paraesophageal hernias,

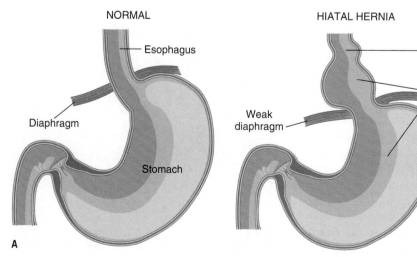
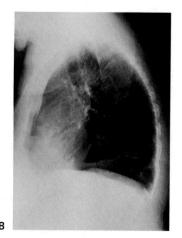

FIGURE 9-13 Sliding hiatal hernia.

the GE junction remains below the diaphragm, and the stomach fundus herniates through the hiatus (type II). Paraesophageal hernias, however, can result in both the GE junction and the fundus herniating (type III—a combination of type I and type II). The combination type is the most common of the paraesophageal hiatal herniations. When there is a large opening, the stomach and other organs (e.g., colon, pancreas) can also herniate (type IV). Sliding hiatal hernias develop from GE junction disruption that is progressive, while paraesophageal hernias usually occur as a result of laxity of the ligaments that hold the stomach in place. The cause of the hernias is not clear; however, they are more likely to occur with congenital malformation (e.g., short esophagus, large hiatal opening), iatrogenic factors (e.g., the patient is postgastrectomy or has had lower esophageal surgeries), or trauma. Factors exacerbating sliding hiatal hernias include activities that increase intrathoracic pressure (e.g., coughing, vomiting, or straining to defecate) or increased intra-abdominal pressure (e.g., pregnancy and obesity). Risk factors associated with hiatal hernias include advancing age and smoking. Small hiatal hernias may go undetected and rarely cause problems. Large hiatal hernias can cause chyme to reflux into the esophagus, irritating the mucosa. When the stomach protrudes through the diaphragm (paraesophageal), it creates a pouch (hernia sac). This sac can alter blood flow. There is also an increased risk for ulcer development and strangulation of the sac that can lead to ischemia, perforation, bleeding, and obstruction.

Risk factors [handwritten annotation]

Clinical Manifestations

A hiatal hernia by itself rarely causes symptoms. Clinical manifestations in a sliding hiatal hernia reflect the inflammation of the esophagus and stomach due to reflux of gastric acid, air, or bile. These manifestations include indigestion, heartburn (pyrosis), frequent belching, nausea, chest pain, strictures, and dysphagia. Manifestations worsen with recumbent positioning, eating (especially after large meals), bending over, and coughing. Conversely, these symptoms often improve when standing as the organ returns to its usual position. Additionally, a soft upper abdominal mass (protruding stomach pouch) may be visualized especially when intra-abdominal pressure is increased such as by coughing, laughing, or straining. With paraesophageal hernias, reflux symptoms are not as common, but the patient may experience fullness after eating, epigastric or substernal pain, nausea, and retching due to the herniation.

Diagnosis and Treatment

Diagnostic procedures for hiatal hernia consist of a history, physical examination, barium swallow, upper GI tract X-rays, manometry, and EGD. Treatment strategies focus on relieving inflammation by decreasing regurgitation of chyme and healing the mucosa. Such strategies include eating small, frequent meals (six small meals per day), avoiding alcohol, assuming a high Fowler position after meals, sleeping with the head of the bed elevated 6 inches, smoking cessation, losing weight (if overweight), as well as taking antacids, acid-reducing agents (e.g., histamine$_2$ blockers and proton pump inhibitors), and mucosal barrier agents. Surgical repair (e.g., fundoplication) may be necessary for hiatal hernias, particularly for paraesophageal hernias, not relieved by these strategies.

Gastroesophageal Reflux Disease

Gastroesophageal reflux disease (GERD) is a condition where chyme (acid, pepsin) periodically backs up from the stomach into the esophagus. Occasionally, bile can back up into the esophagus. The presence of these gastric secretions irritates the esophageal mucosa (**FIGURE 9-14**). Mechanisms for development of GERD are a result of abnormalities in the LES (e.g., relaxation, decreased pressure, or GE disruption). Reflux can also occur due to issues with acid clearance. Normally, the esophagus clears the acid via peristalsis, and bicarbonate in saliva neutralizes acid. Impairment of these protective mechanisms as a result of

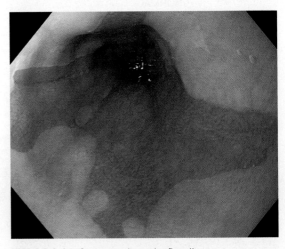

FIGURE 9-14 Gastroesophageal reflux disease.
© Gastrolab/Science Source.

impaired esophageal peristalsis and problems with saliva bicarbonate neutralizing the acid (e.g., decreased saliva production) can result in GERD. Gastric motility issues such as pyloric stricture or gastroparesis can result in a higher likelihood of reflux because chyme sitting in the stomach for prolonged periods can become more acidic, increasing the risk for chyme to reflux. Various factors can cause or contribute to LES abnormalities and development of GERD. Pressure changes may originate from many sources such as obesity, pregnancy, or other circumstances (e.g. coughing or bending) that increase intra-abdominal pressure. Smoking, drinking alcohol, certain foods, and certain medications can alter LES pressure. Foods that alter LES pressure include chocolate, caffeine, carbonated beverages, citrus fruit, tomatoes, spicy or fatty foods, and peppermint. Medications with LES-altering effects include nitrates, sedatives, beta blockers, calcium channel blockers, and anticholinergic agents. GERD can cause esophagitis (esophageal inflammation), usually through activation of the immune system (e.g., cytokine release). Esophagitis is typically diagnosed based on endoscopy findings (termed *erosive* or *reflux* esophagitis) because not all patients affected by GERD have esophageal injury (termed *nonerosive reflux disease*). Conversely, those patients with esophagitis may have minimal GERD symptoms. Reflux esophagitis is not so much a consequence of increased acid secretion but rather occurs due to the amount of time the reflux is in contact with the esophageal mucosa. Another key determinant to the amount of injury caused by reflux is the acidity of that reflux (the more acidic the higher chance of injury). Physiologic reflux is a normal reflux that occurs after eating, and this type of reflux does not cause symptoms and is short lived.

Clinical Manifestations

GERD varies in severity depending on the degree of LES weakness. Clinical manifestations include heartburn (early), which is described as epigastric or retrosternal pain (usually after a meal or when recumbent), and regurgitation of food, which is described as a gastric content coming back up into the throat or mouth. This reflux can lead to a "sour taste." Other symptoms can include nausea (usually after eating), dry cough, laryngitis, pharyngitis, and sensation of a lump in the throat. Some patients with GERD may hypersalivate (i.e., they have water brash). Symptoms such

as dysphagia and odynophagia may occur with GERD. These symptoms are usually indicative of long-standing heartburn and mucosal injury or ulceration and not a simple, uncomplicated GERD. The pain associated with GERD is often confused with angina and may warrant steps to rule out cardiac disease. See chapter 4 for further discussion of cardiovascular function.

GERD can result in esophageal and nonesophageal complications such esophagitis, Barrett esophagus (normal esophageal squamous epithelium becomes metaplastic columnar epithelium), strictures, ulcerations, esophageal cancer, asthma exacerbation, and chronic laryngitis. GERD is one of the top three reasons for a chronic cough (the other two are asthma and postnasal drip) in the absence of smoking and use of angiotensin-converting enzymes. Risk for Barrett esophagus, considered a precursor to adenocarcinoma of the esophagus, is higher in those with long-standing GERD (at least 5 years) and the presence of other criteria (e.g., obesity, smoking).

GERD complications or other possible diagnosis, such as gastrointestinal malignancy, should be suspected in individuals with symptoms other than heartburn and regurgitation (e.g., dysphagia and odynophagia). Other concerning features include GI bleeding (e.g., melena and hematochezia), persistent vomiting, new onset dyspepsia after age 60, anorexia, unexplained weight loss, anemia, or a first-degree relative with GI cancer.

Diagnosis and Treatment

Diagnosis of GERD is generally made clinically based on a history and physical examination in those with heartburn and/or regurgitation. Diagnostic testing is usually not necessary; however, testing is indicated in the presence of symptoms other than heartburn and regurgitation or if there is concern for the presence of GERD complications, such as Barrett esophagus, or other disorders like GI malignancy. Diagnostic testing with concerning presentations will include an EGD. Esophageal pH monitoring and esophagus manometry may also be done. Treatment strategies focus on balancing pressures and reducing acid, including the following:

- Eating small, frequent meals and avoiding eating 2–3 hours before bedtime
- Assuming a high Fowler position for 2–3 hours after meals
- Elevating the head of the bed approximately 6 inches

- Losing weight
- Avoiding triggers (e.g., trigger foods, alcohol, medications, and nicotine)
- Avoiding medications that cause gastric irritation (e.g., aspirin and other NSAIDs)
- Avoiding clothing that is restrictive around the waist
- Taking certain drugs and herbal remedies, including:
  - Acid-reducing agents (e.g., proton pump inhibitors and histamine$_2$ blockers)
  - Mucosal barrier agents (e.g., sucralfate, sodium alginate)
  - Antacids (e.g., Maalox and Tums) for symptom relief, not preventive
  - Herbal therapies (e.g., licorice, slippery elm, and chamomile)
- Having surgery (e.g., Nissen fundoplication or implantation of a reflux management device)

Gastritis

Gastritis refers to an inflammation of the stomach's mucosal lining. The inflammation can involve the entire stomach or a region. Acute mucosal injury can also occur with minimal or no inflammation (i.e., gastropathy). Gastritis can be either acute or chronic; each type has its own presentation, although this can vary.

Acute gastritis is commonly caused by infections or autoimmune conditions. Infections are often due to *Helicobacter pylori*, which is a gram-negative spiral bacterium transmitted through the fecal–oral route. Most *H. pylori* exposure occurs during childhood, and most infections are asymptomatic. Acute infection with *H. pylori*, however, can cause acute gastritis. Other organisms (e.g., *E. coli*, streptococci, staphylococci) can also cause acute gastritis. Neutrophilic infiltration characterizes acute gastritis. Gastritis can be caused by internal and external irritants. These irritants can include bile reflux, alcohol, cocaine, and medications (e.g., NSAIDs, chemotherapy agents, and alendronate). Severe stress due to major surgery, traumatic injury, burns, or severe infections can cause acute gastritis because of tissue ischemia and decreased gastric motility resulting from the stress response. Acute gastritis can be a mild, transient irritation, or it can be a severe ulceration with hemorrhage. It usually develops suddenly and is likely to be accompanied by nausea and epigastric pain.

Chronic gastritis is associated with the presence of lymphocytes, plasma cells, and macrophages, as opposed to acute gastritis where there is neutrophil infiltration. Chronic gastritis generally proceeds through phases. Initially, the gastritis is superficial, then the inflammation extends deeper in the mucosa and the gastric glands are affected. The final phase is **gastric atrophy**, during which glandular structures are lost. Chronic gastritis can be characterized as type A or type B based on the location of the injury, or both types can coexist (type AB). Type A is less common than type B and generally affects the fundus and the body of the stomach while sparing the antrum. Type A is associated with autoimmune processes (e.g., pernicious anemia and Hashimoto disease) that results in autoantibody development against parietal cells or intrinsic factor. The H$^+$-K+ATPase is the specific antigen targeted by the autoantibodies. Because the parietal cells are the target with type A (i.e., autoimmune gastritis), achlorhydria (reduced or absent hydrochloric acid) occurs and results in increased gastrin production by G cells found in the antrum. Hypergastrinemia occurs as a result of the increased gastrin and causes hyperplasia of the cells. The cellular changes can increase the risk for gastric tumors and gastric cancer development. The resulting lack of intrinsic factor can cause vitamin B$_{12}$ deficiency (see chapter 3 for more on hematopoietic function.).

Type B is usually the result of a *H. pylori* infection. In contrast to type A, the stomach antrum is affected, but the fundus and body can also become infected. *H. pylori* embeds itself in the mucous layer, activating toxins and enzymes that cause inflammation. *H. pylori* is equipped with flagella that help it move, molecules that help it adhere, and enzymes that neutralize the gastric acid in its immediate vicinity (see **FIGURE 9-15**).

Why some people experience complications from *H. pylori* infections and others do not is not clear; however, genetic vulnerability, lifestyle behaviors such as smoking, and different strains of *H. pylori* may increase susceptibility to the bacterium's effects. Long-term use of NSAIDs (e.g., ibuprofen or naproxen) can contribute to chronic gastritis by reducing cyclooxygenase, a key substance that helps preserve the mucosal lining. Alcohol and smoking can also contribute to chronic gastritis development.

Clinical Manifestations

The clinical manifestations of gastritis reflect injury of the mucosal lining. These symptoms include indigestion, heartburn, epigastric pain, nausea, vomiting, anorexia, and malaise. The

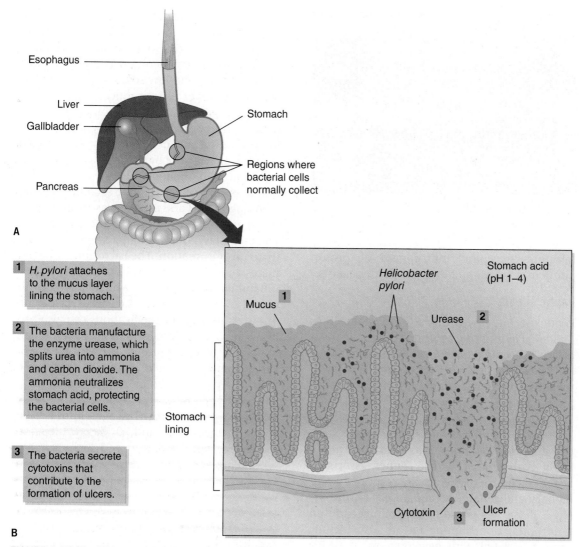

FIGURE 9-15 The **(A)** location and **(B)** progression of peptic ulcers associated with *Helicobacter pylori* infection. *H. pylori* produce toxic virulence factors such as urease and cytotoxins that act at different levels of infection. Urease neutralizes stomach acidity by degrading urea present on epithelial cells, whereas cytotoxins are involved in the development of ulcers.

presence of hematemesis and dark, tarry stools can indicate ulceration and bleeding. Chronic gastritis develops gradually and can last for months to years. It is likely to be accompanied by a dull epigastric pain and a sensation of fullness after minimal intake. Nausea and vomiting may occur. In some cases, chronic gastritis can be asymptomatic. As with acute gastritis, GI bleeding may occur.

Chronic gastritis increases the risk for peptic ulcers, gastric cancer, anemia, and hemorrhage.

Diagnosis and Treatment

Diagnosis of gastritis consists of a history and a physical examination along with diagnostic tests to evaluate for the cause. Imaging tests can include an EGD to evaluate the mucosal lining and *H. pylori* testing. Active

H. pylori infection is evaluated with the urea (produced by *H. pylori*) breath test or *H. pylori* stool antigen. Serum *H. pylori* antibodies will not distinguish between acute or prior infection. Additional tests often include a complete blood count (CBC; to identify anemia) and stool analysis for occult blood). Acute gastritis is often self-limiting and resolves within a few days. Irritants should be identified and discontinued or avoided. Treatment strategies vary depending on the underlying etiology. For instance, bacterial infections, such as those caused by *H. pylori*, require antibiotic therapy. Chronic disease management is important to limit any complications associated with this inflammation. In addition to etiology-specific interventions, pharmacologic management may include antacids, acid-reducing agents (e.g.,

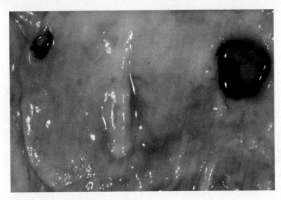

FIGURE 9-16 Peptic ulcer.

© Jose Luis Calvo/Shutterstock.

histamine₂-receptor antagonists or proton pump inhibitors), and mucosal barrier agents.

Peptic Ulcers

Peptic ulcer disease (PUD) refers to stomach or duodenal lesions that extend through the muscularis mucosae (**FIGURE 9-16**). The incidence of PUD has been declining in recent years, but it remains a common condition that affects approximately 4.5 million people in the United States each year (Anand, 2015). The two common risk factors for developing PUD are NSAID use and *H. pylori* infections—both are more likely with advancing age. Other associated factors include chronic disease (especially pulmonary and renal) and certain gastric tumors (e.g., those associated with Zollinger-Ellison syndrome). Contributing factors also include those associated with development of GERD (e.g., stress, smoking, and alcohol use). Family history of ulcer disease, particularly duodenal ulcer, confers a risk.

Ulcers vary in severity from superficial erosions to complete penetration through muscle, damaging blood vessels and even eroding through the GI tract wall. Regardless of its etiology, PUD develops because of an imbalance between destructive forces (e.g., excess acid production) and protective mechanisms (e.g., decreased mucus production). The imbalance generally occurs as a result of a superimposed process (e.g., *H. pylori* infection or NSAID use) as opposed to a primary defect in normal secretory, protective, and repair mechanisms.

Duodenal ulcers account for 80% of cases as opposed to gastric ulcers. Duodenal ulcer onset is typically between the age of 20 and 50 years. Duodenal ulcers are most commonly associated with excessive gastric acid with or without *H. pylori* infections. *H. pylori*, however, is associated in a majority (95%) of cases. The proposed mechanism by which *H. pylori* results in duodenal ulcer formation is not well understood (Figure 9-15). Some theories include increased gastric acid secretion as a result of more gastrin release and low somatostatin. The bacterium, however also produces gastric urease which cleaves urea into ammonia and carbon dioxide. This reaction ultimately leads to acid neutralization and allows the organism to colonize and survive the harsh acidic environment. Infection with duodenal ulcers causes a reduction in duodenal bicarbonate secretion, further lowering the pH and causing gastric metaplasia (i.e., gastric epithelial cells in the duodenum). The metaplasia causes an increased susceptibility to ulcer formation. The bacterium also stimulates an immune response with the release of inflammatory cytokines, which may contribute to ulcer formation. Increased NSAID use or other ulcerogenic medications can also promote duodenal ulcer formation. Patients with duodenal ulcers typically present with epigastric pain that is relieved in the presence of food. The pain may be more common at night.

Gastric ulcers, by comparison, are less frequent but more deadly. The age of onset is between the ages of 50 and 70. Gastric ulcers are associated with NSAID use, which increases with aging (e.g., to treat arthritis). *H. pylori* infection is also associated with gastric ulcer formation, but the incidence is somewhat lower (e.g., 60–80%) in comparison to the incidence in duodenal ulcer. Depending on the ulcer's location in the stomach (e.g., antrum versus the body), acid level secretion may be normal, low, or high. As an example, ulceration in the distal antrum may have decreased antral somatostatin from D cells (inhibit gastrin G cells) and resulting increase in gastric acid secretion. An ulcer closer to the body (midportion of the stomach) is a reflection of atrophy of glands that contain parietal cells (oxyntic glands0 resulting in lower acid secretion. Gastric cancer risk is higher in those patients with gastric ulcers but not for those with duodenal ulcers. In contrast to duodenal ulcers, the pain experienced with gastric ulcers typically worsens with eating.

Stress ulcers describe PUD that develops because of a major physiologic stressor on the body (e.g., large burns, trauma, sepsis, surgery, or head injury). Stress ulcers associated with burns are generally called *Curling ulcers*, whereas stress ulcers associated with head injuries are generally called *Cushing ulcers*. Stress ulcers develop due to local tissue ischemia, tissue acidosis, entry of bile salts into the stomach, and decreased GI motility. Such ulcers most frequently develop in the stomach, and multiple ulcers can form within hours of the precipitating event. Often hemorrhage is the first indicator of a stress ulcer because the ulcer develops rapidly and tends to be masked by the primary problem.

Zollinger-Ellison syndrome is caused by duodenal or pancreatic neuroendocrine tumors, referred to as *gastrinomas*, that secrete gastrin. The tumors are sometimes cancerous. The incidence is rare (approximately 0.5 to 2 per million). The average age of diagnosis is between 20 and 50 years of age, and men have a higher incidence in comparison to women. The excessive gastrin causes parietal cells and enterochromaffin-like cells (histamine secreting) to produce an excessive quantity of gastric acid. The clinical manifestations are the same as those with other ulcers, but chronic diarrhea is present in many cases. The diarrhea is a result of the high acid content affecting reabsorption, the inactivation of digestive enzymes, and the inhibition of sodium and water absorption by gastrin. Treatment will be similar to that for other ulcers, and tumor resection can reduce metastasis.

Clinical Manifestations

Complications of PUD may involve GI hemorrhage, obstruction, perforation, bowel penetration, and peritonitis. Clinical manifestations of PUD resemble those associated with other conditions of GI inflammation (e.g., gastritis and GERD) and include:

- Epigastric or abdominal pain
- Abdominal cramping
- Heartburn
- Indigestion
- Chest pain
- Nausea and vomiting (may include hematemesis—bright red blood or coffee ground appearance)
- Melena (dark, tarry stools)
- Fatigue
- Weight loss

Diagnosis and Treatment

Diagnosis of PUD consists of a history and physical examination, but the diagnosis is confirmed with an EGD. A CT of the abdomen can also identify ulcers (nonperforated ulcers). Evaluation for the cause will include testing for *H. pylori*, a CBC to identify anemia, and a stool analysis (occult blood). Serum gastrin levels may be measured to evaluate for a gastrinoma.

Treatment strategies include those discussed for gastritis. Additionally, surgical repair may be necessary for perforated or bleeding ulcers.

Prevention is crucial with stress ulcers to improve patient outcomes. Prophylactic medications (e.g., acid-reducing agents) are administered to persons at risk for developing stress ulcers.

Cholelithiasis

Cholelithiasis, or gallstones, is a common condition (affecting 10–20% of all people in the United States) in which stones (calculi) of varying sizes and shapes form inside the gallbladder (Heuman, Allan, & Mihas, 2016) (**FIGURE 9-17**).

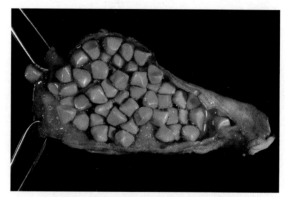

A

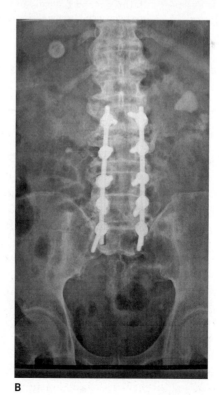

B

FIGURE 9-17 Cholelithiasis.
Courtesy of Leonard V. Crowley, MD, Century College; © Casa nayafana/Shutterstock.

Risk factors

Cholelithiasis is more common in fair-skinned women. Other risk factors include advancing age, obesity, diet (high fat, high cholesterol, and low fiber), rapid weight loss (like that associated with bariatric surgery), pregnancy, hormone replacement, certain chronic diseases (e.g., diabetes mellitus, hyperlipidemia, and liver disease), and long-term parenteral nutrition. Three types of calculi can develop in the gallbladder or nearby ducts (**TABLE 9-2**; FIGURE 9-18), and the presence of calculi can cause inflammation or infection in the biliary system (cholecystitis).

TABLE 9-2	Types of Cholelithiasis
Type	**Characteristics**
Cholesterol	Most common
	Can be small or large, single or multiple
	Can cause obstruction, pain (biliary colic), and jaundice
	Strong association with female hormones
	Increased incidence with obesity, extreme dieting, and hypercholesterolemia
Bilirubin (pigmented)	Usually multiple, small, black stones
	More common in Asians and in persons with chronic diseases that cause hemolysis (e.g., sickle cell anemia)
Mixed	Usually found in large numbers
	Bilirubin center surrounded by cholesterol and calcium

Small calculi are often asymptomatic and excreted with the bile. Larger calculi are likely to obstruct bile flow and cause clinical manifestations. Biliary colic is caused by the contraction of the gallbladder while it is trying to move a stone (or biliary sludge) through the gallbladder outlet or cystic duct. Pressure in the gallbladder builds, leading to visceral pain.

Clinical Manifestations

Most individuals with gallstones are asymptomatic, and the stones are found incidentally during abdominal imaging for other reasons. Of those who are asymptomatic, up to 25% can develop symptomatic disease (it can occur as late as 10 years after), and complication risk is low. In those patients with symptomatic gallstones, biliary colic is the typical manifestation. Biliary colic is a pain located in the right upper quadrant or epigastric area that can radiate to the back or right shoulder. The pain lasts from 30 minutes to 6 hours and usually peaks within 1 hour. The pain is described as intense and dull. Nausea, vomiting, and diaphoresis can accompany the pain. The pain usually occurs after eating a fatty meal, but the pain may be nocturnal for some patients. Physical examination may reveal no findings, particularly if no pain is present. The pain can recur, and the frequency can be variable (from hours to years). Those patients with biliary colic are at increased risk for complications.

Prior to complications, affected individuals will usually have had episodes of biliary colic, and symptoms of complications as an initial presentation are unusual. The most

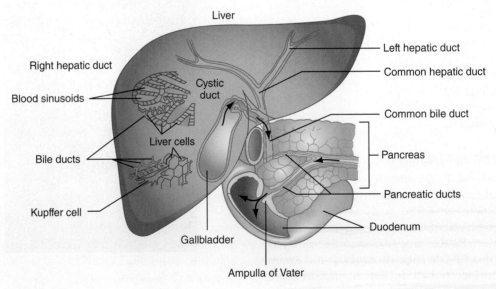

FIGURE 9-18 Location of cholelithiasis.

Cholelithiasis → Cholecystitis / → Choledocolithiasis → Cholangitis

common complication of gallstones is **acute cholecystitis**, which is gallbladder inflammation as a result of cystic duct obstruction. The manifestations are the same as those of biliary colic. However, the pain is steady, severe, and typically prolonged (> 4 hours) and is accompanied by fever and leukocytosis. The Murphy sign is positive (pain is elicited when the patient takes a deep breath and upon palpation of the right upper quadrant). While most episodes of acute cholecystitis are due to gallstones, a few cases (< 10%) are acalculous. The cause of acalculous cholecystitis is gallbladder ischemia and stasis, and many risk factors are associated with development of this disorder (e.g., leukemia, AIDS, burns, diabetes mellitus, and renal disease). Gallstones can also be present in the common bile duct (i.e., **choledocholithiasis**) and results in **acute cholangitis** (stasis and infection in the biliary tract). The manifestations of choledocholithiasis include biliary colic symptoms and abnormal liver tests (i.e., elevated bilirubin and ALP). Acute cholangitis will cause fever, jaundice, and abdominal pain (Charcot triad). Gallstones can obstruct the pancreatic duct or the ampulla of Vater (leading to bile reflux into the duct); both obstructions can lead to acute pancreatitis. Other less common complications of gallstones include gallbladder gangrene, gallbladder cancer, and common hepatic duct obstruction. Additionally, inflammation can lead to gallbladder rupture. Gallstone disease is responsible for approximately 10,000 deaths annually in the United States—7,000 are attributed to acute complications and 3,000 are attributed to gallbladder cancer (Heuman, Allen, & Mihas, 2016).

Diagnosis and Treatment

Diagnostic procedures for cholelithiasis consist of a history, physical examination, and an abdominal ultrasound, which is very sensitive in detecting gallstones. An endoscopic ultrasound can be performed to detect even very small stones. Other tests that may detect gallstones include an abdominal X-ray, but only a small percentage of stones are radio-opaque, allowing them to be visible on X-ray. An abdominal computed tomography (CT) may identify gallstones. Other tests can include endoscopic retrograde cholangiopancreatography, magnetic resonance cholangiopancreatography, and percutaneous transhepatic cholangiogram. Serum laboratory tests can include bilirubin levels, liver function tests, pancreatic enzymes (e.g.,

amylase and lipase), and a CBC. Treatment strategies for an acute attack will include pain management, usually with NSAIDs. Opioids can be used, but all (e.g., meperidine, morphine) have the potential to increase sphincter of Oddi pressure, which could worsen pain. Treatment strategies focus on removing the calculi, restoring bile flow, preventing reoccurrence, and include the following:

- Low-fat diet
- Medications to dissolve the calculi (e.g., bile acids)
- Antibiotic therapy (if infection is present)
- Lithotripsy (e.g., extracorporeal shock wave)
- Surgically creating an opening for drainage (choledochostomy)
- Laparoscopic removal of calculi (through cholecystostomy tube) or gallbladder (cholecystectomy)

Disorders of the Liver

Disorders of the liver are usually serious and often life threatening. The liver's involvement in so many of the body's activities results in a situation that can be complex to manage when this organ's functions become disrupted. Liver disorders are often acquired through ingestion of hepatotoxic substances (e.g., medications or alcohol) or infections.

Hepatitis

Hepatitis is an inflammation of the liver that can be caused by infections (usually viral), alcohol, medications such as acetaminophen (Tylenol), antiseizure agents, and antibiotics; or autoimmune disease such as systemic lupus erythematosus, rheumatoid arthritis, and scleroderma. Hepatitis can be acute, chronic, or fulminant, such as in liver failure. Additionally, this disease can be active or nonactive. People with nonviral hepatitis usually recover, but some people develop liver failure, liver cancer, or cirrhosis. Nonviral hepatitis is not contagious, whereas viral hepatitis is contagious. Like individuals with nonviral hepatitis, people with viral hepatitis usually recover in time with no residual damage. Advancing age and comorbidity increase the likelihood of liver failure, liver cancer, or cirrhosis in patients with hepatitis. Both viral and nonviral hepatitis can result in hepatic cell destruction, necrosis, autolysis, hyperplasia, and scarring.

Viral hepatitis accounts for approximately 50% of all cases of acute hepatitis in the United

States (Buggs & Dronen, 2014). There are five types of viral hepatitis, each with its own general characteristics (**TABLE 9-3**). In the United States, viral hepatitis is most commonly caused by hepatitis A (HAV), hepatitis B (HBV), and hepatitis C (HCV). According to the CDC (2015b), rates of hepatitis A and B declined from 2000 to 2014, whereas hepatitis C cases

TABLE 9-3	Types of Viral Hepatitis				
Characteristic	**Type A**	**Type B**	**Type C**	**Type D**	**Type E**
Mode of transmission	Waterborne Fecal–oral/blood Venereal	Perinatal Blood/skin Venereal	Venereal Blood/skin	Venereal Blood	Waterborne Fecal–oral/blood Perinatal
Incubation period (range in days)	15–42	42–160	14–160	28–49	14–56
Onset	Abrupt	Insidious	Insidious	Insidious	Abrupt
Symptoms					
Fever	Common	Uncommon	Uncommon	Common	Common
Nausea/vomiting	Common	Common	Common	Common	Common
Jaundice	More common in adults than children	Occasionally	Uncommon	Common	Common
Outcome					
Severity	Mild	Moderate	Mild	Mild to severe	Mild
Fulminating hepatitis	< 1%	< 1%	Rare	3–4% with coinfection with hepatitis B	0.3–3% 20% in pregnant women
Mortality rate	Low (< 1%)	Low (1–3%)	Low (2%)	High (5%)	Moderate; high with pregnancy
Chronic hepatitis	No	Yes (5–10%)	Yes (80%)	< 5% with coinfection 80% with superinfection	Rare (immuno-compromised)
Carrier state	No	Yes (1 million in United States)	Yes	Yes	No
Relapse	Yes	Yes	Persistent	Unknown	Unknown
Carcinoma	No	Yes (25–40%)	Yes (25–30%)	No increase above that for hepatitis B	Unknown but not likely
Develop cirrhosis	No	40%	30%	Yes, with superinfection	Rare since chronic rare
Source of virus	Feces	Blood/blood-derived body fluids	Blood/blood-derived body fluids	Blood/blood-derived body fluids	Feces
Route of transmission	Fecal–oral	Percutaneous permucosal	Percutaneous permucosal	Percutaneous permucosal	Fecal–oral
Chronic infection	No	Yes	Yes	Yes	Yes
Prevention	Preexposure/ postexposure immunization	Preexposure/ postexposure immunization	Blood donor screening; all born between 1945 and 1965 should be screened; risk behavior modification	Preexposure/ postexposure HBV immunization; risk behavior modification	Ensure safe drinking water

have increased since 2000. Additionally, several genotypes for hepatitis B and C are possible. Hepatitis D can replicate independently, but HBV is necessary for the HDV virion (virus particle) to assemble and be secreted. Therefore, those patients with HDV are always dually infected with HBV.

Clinical Manifestations

Acute hepatitis proceeds through four distinct phases—an asymptomatic incubation phase and three symptomatic phases. Clinical manifestations for each symptomatic phase include the following signs and symptoms:

- **Prodromal phase**: Starts 2 weeks after exposure to the virus; includes viral symptoms such as abdominal pain, nausea, vomiting, malaise, anorexia, low-grade fever, and headache
- **Icteric phase**: Begins 1–2 weeks after the prodromal phase and lasts up to 6 weeks; includes jaundice, pruritus, dark tea-colored urine (bilirubinuria) or clay-colored stools (lack bilirubin), hepatomegaly, and right upper quadrant pain

- **Recovery phase**: Resolution of jaundice approximately 6–8 weeks after exposure; enlarged liver for as long as 3 months

Chronic hepatitis, usually as a result of hepatitis B and C, is characterized by continued hepatic disease lasting longer than 6 months. Its symptom severity and disease progression vary depending on the degree of liver damage. An individual can live with chronic hepatitis for years (i.e., carrier state) but his or her health can quickly deteriorate with declining liver integrity. Chronic hepatitis can lead to cirrhosis and liver cancer. Fulminant hepatitis is an uncommon, rapidly progressing form that can quickly lead to liver failure, hepatic encephalopathy, or death within 3 weeks. Extrahepatic manifestations can occur with acute or chronic hepatitis and include rash and arthralgias.

Diagnosis and Treatment

Diagnostic procedures for hepatitis include a history and physical examination, but diagnosis is confirmed with a serum hepatitis profile (**TABLE 9-4**). Additional tests may include liver function tests, clotting studies, liver biopsy, and

TABLE 9-4 **Viral Hepatitis Profile**

Virus	Hepatitis B surface antigen (HBsAG)	Hepatitis B surface antibody (anti-HBs)	Hepatitis B core-total antibody (anti-HBc)	Hepatitis B core-IgM antibody (anti-HBc) IgM	Interpretation
Hepatitis B vaccine	-	Positive	-	-	Indicates immunity—core is negative with vaccine
Hepatitis B infection	Positive	Negative	Positive	Positive	Acute active infection
	Positive	Negative	Positive	Negative	Chronic infection*
	Negative	Positive	Positive	Negative	Previous infection and immunity

Virus	Hepatitis C (anti-HCV)			Interpretation	
Hepatitis C	Positive			Previous or present infection	

Virus	Hepatitis A (anti-HAV) IgM antibody	Hepatitis A (anti-HAV) total		Interpretations	
Hepatitis A	Positive	Negative		Acute infection	
	Negative	Positive		Immunity	

* HBeAg—if positive, indicates active replication virus; anti-HBe—if positive, indicates antibody has developed; virus nonreplicating.
HBsAG—protein on surface of virus indicates acute or chronic infection.
anti-HBs—indicates recovery and immunity.
anti-HBc—indicates previous or ongoing infection; remains for life.
anti-HBc—IgM; indicates acute infection (≤ 6 months).

abdominal ultrasound. Treatment strategies concentrate on prevention, and vaccinations are the cornerstone of hepatitis prevention. Vaccinations are available for HAV and HBV. HAV vaccination is recommended for all children starting at age 1 year, travelers to certain countries, men who have sex with men, intravenous drug users, persons with long-term liver disease, persons requiring repeated blood transfusions (e.g., those with hemophilia), and others at risk for exposure (e.g., living with someone who is hepatitis A positive). HBV vaccination is recommended for all infants beginning at birth, older children and adolescents who were not vaccinated previously, and adults at risk of developing this form of hepatitis (e.g., healthcare workers, men who have sex with men, and intravenous drug users). HBV vaccination is also recommended to prevent HDV infection as HDV requires HBV infection for development. Prevention also includes limiting exposure to the virus (e.g., by limiting exposure to blood, body fluids, and feces).

Once viral hepatitis is contracted, there is no method of destroying the virus. Most cases of HAV and hepatitis E will resolve with no treatment, and care is supportive. The treatment of other types of viral hepatitis is dependent on the degree of liver damage or other circumstances such as pregnancy. Hepatitis can be treated with interferon injections to improve the immune response and antiviral (e.g., nucleotide or nucleoside analogs) medications to decrease viral replication (see chapter 2 for further discussion of immunity).

Additional strategies include rest, adequate nutrition (a diet high in carbohydrates, protein, and vitamins), increased hydration, and avoidance of alcohol. Affected individuals should be counseled on methods to avoid transmission, which can include not sharing toothbrushes or shaving equipment and covering wounds to prevent potential blood exposure. Hygienic practices are important and include hand washing as well as avoiding water and raw foods (foods should be cooked at a high temperature) in areas with poor sanitation. Liver transplant may be necessary in those patients with advanced liver diseases. The most common indication for liver transplantation in the United States is chronic HCV infection.

Cirrhosis

Cirrhosis refers to chronic, progressive, irreversible, diffuse damage to the liver resulting in decreased liver function (**FIGURE 9-19**). The causes of cirrhosis are hepatitis, alcoholic liver disease, nonalcoholic fatty liver disease, and hemochromatosis. Other conditions that can lead to cirrhosis can include autoimmune conditions (e.g., primary biliary cirrhosis),

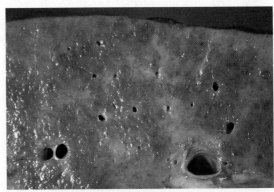

A

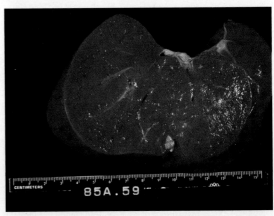

B

FIGURE 9-19 (A) Cirrhosis. **(B)** A normal liver.

A: Courtesy of Dr. Edwin P. Ewing, Jr./CDC; B: © Clark Overton/Medical Images.

Learning Points

Acute Liver Failure

Acetaminophen in nontherapeutic ranges (> 4 grams/day) is the most common cause of acute liver failure (50%) in the United States. While most cases are due to intentional overingestion during a suicide attempt, some individuals inadvertently take high doses when not taking medications as directed or when taking multiple medications that contain acetaminophen. Inadvertent, inappropriate dosing is a more common cause in young children. Liver toxicity is dose dependent, and toxicity is likely with doses of greater than 250 mg/kg or 12 grams over 24 hours. Toxicity threshold in children is usually 150 mg/kg. Clinical manifestations can be mild in the first 24 hours and are poor predictors of who will develop toxicity. Jaundice, hepatic encephalopathy, bleeding, lactic acidosis, hypoglycemia, and multiorgan failure may occur within 4 days if the person survives. Liver enzymes are exceedingly high (often > 10,000 IU/L) and prothrombin time are prolonged. Early identification and management increases chance of survival. Activated charcoal can be effective within 4 hours of acetaminophen ingestion. Acetylcysteine (Mucomyst) is an antidote and is best administered within 8 hours of ingestion.

hepatotoxic medications, hepatic venous obstruction (e.g., right-sided heart failure), and hereditary metabolic disorders (e.g., glycogen storage disease). Hepatitis C infection and chronic alcohol abuse are the most frequent causes of cirrhosis in the United States (Wolf, 2015). Nonalcoholic fatty liver disease, also known as nonalcoholic steatohepatitis, is becoming a more common cause of cirrhosis, reflecting the rising rates of obesity.

Liver fibrosis development in cirrhosis occurs at different rates depending on the underlying cause of the cirrhosis and the general health of the patient. The extracellular matrix of the liver includes various molecules (e.g., collagen, growth factors, glycosaminoglycans). With fibrosis, the extracellular matrix becomes degraded by proteases, which in turn affects the normal functioning of cells. The degradation occurs as a result of the activation of cells, particularly stellate cells, which release chemokines and other mediators. Production of collagens is increased along with other extracellular matrix components, and destructive liver enzyme production is increased. Regenerative nodules eventually develop, giving the liver a cobbly appearance; the liver blood flow is impaired; and bile flow is obstructed—all of which contribute to liver failure. Cirrhosis develops due to ongoing injury and progressive fibrosis. Cirrhosis may take as long as 40 years to develop. While cirrhosis is generally considered irreversible, early stages of fibrosis may be reversible. As an example, hepatitis C treatment can lead to reversal of fibrosis. The time frame from reversible to irreversible damage is unclear. Several advancements have been made in understanding the process of fibrogenesis and regression of fibrosis, leading to new antifibrotic therapies.

Clinical Manifestations

Clinical manifestations of cirrhosis are similar regardless of the underlying cause. These manifestations can range from nonspecific symptoms such as anorexia, fatigue, and weight loss seen in compensated cirrhosis to manifestations that reflect decompensation and failure of the liver to accomplish its many functions (FIGURE 9-20). As cirrhosis progresses, pressures rise in the hepatic artery and the portal vein (portal hypertension) as a result of the resistance created by abnormal liver changes (e.g., fibrosis, nodules) as well as due to the increased release of vasoconstrictors (e.g., norepinephrine) and reduction in release of vasodilators. Cirrhosis is an intrahepatic cause

of portal hypertension and is one of the most common causes of portal hypertension in the United States. Portal hypertension is present in almost 60% of patients with cirrhosis. Prehepatic (e.g., portal vein thrombosis or stenosis) and posthepatic (e.g., right-sided heart failure) disorders can also lead to portal hypertension. Many consequences can result from portal hypertension because the portal vein receives blood from most of the GI tract. As the pressure rises in the portal system vessels, the veins become engorged, and varicosities (FIGURE 9-21) commonly develop in the esophagus, stomach, abdominal wall (caput medusa), spleen, and rectum (hemorrhoids). Bleeding, either slow or severe, can occur along these overstretched vessels—particularly in the esophagus. Varices will cause hematemesis (reflects acute bleeding) and/or melena (reflects chronic bleeding). Esophageal bleeding has a high mortality and reoccurrence rate. Nearby organs utilizing the same circulation (e.g., the spleen, pancreas, and stomach) enlarge as pressures rise. Platelets become sequestered in the congested spleen (i.e., hypersplenism), causing thrombocytopenia that contributes to bleeding. Hypersplenism can cause neutropenia. See chapter 4 for more on cardiovascular function.

Fluid accumulates in the peritoneal cavity (a condition referred to as *ascites*) as the portal hypertension pushes fluid back into the abdominal cavity and the damaged liver can no longer produce sufficient amounts of albumin (a protein responsible for maintaining colloidal pressure and fluid balance in the vessels; see chapter 6 for discussion of fluid homeostasis).

Ascites also develops as a result of vasodilation (due to substances such as increased nitric oxide) of splanchnic arteries in response to increased portal pressure, which causes increased portal venous inflow. The ascites then worsens the portal hypertension and contributes to systemic hypotension. Patients can accumulate up to 2 L of fluid in the peritoneal cavity. Ascites causes weight gain, dyspnea, and early satiety due to the increasing abdominal pressure. An abdomen with ascites appears distended and is dull to percussion (normal is tympanic). The vasodilation in the splanchnic arterial system causes poor circulation and activation of the renin–angiotensin–aldosterone system and sodium retention. Sodium retention leads to extracellular fluid volume and contributes to ascites as well as the development of peripheral edema. Changes in protein metabolism result in decreased protein clotting factors, muscle wasting, and hyperlipidemia.

Effects of Hepatic Failure and Portal Hypertension

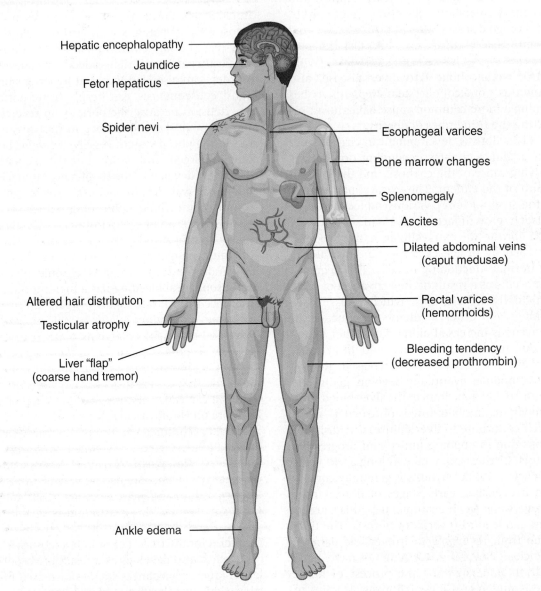

Hepatic encephalopathy

Jaundice

Fetor hepaticus

Spider nevi

Esophageal varices

Bone marrow changes

Splenomegaly

Ascites

Dilated abdominal veins
(caput medusae)

Altered hair distribution

Testicular atrophy

Rectal varices
(hemorrhoids)

Liver "flap"
(coarse hand tremor)

Bleeding tendency
(decreased prothrombin)

Ankle edema

FIGURE 9-20 Effects of cirrhosis.

Poor nutritional absorption in the intestines and poor dietary intake also contribute to malnutrition. Changes in glucose metabolism can lead to hyperglycemia or hypoglycemia. Malabsorption of vitamin D and calcium increases the risk for bone loss, resulting osteopenia and osteoporosis (see chapter 12 for more on musculoskeletal function).

Bile accumulation in the liver causes inflammation and necrosis. Because it cannot flow through the duct system to the intestine, bile enters the bloodstream and causes jaundice. Fats cannot be digested, and fat-soluble vitamins cannot be absorbed without the presence

of bile. Additionally, the stools become clay colored without the presence of bile. The kidneys attempt to compensate for the excessive bile in the blood by increasing excretion, causing the urine to become dark. The kidneys can start to decline in function (i.e., they develop **hepatorenal syndrome**) as a result of the splanchnic artery vasodilation and other poorly understood changes in renal arterial circulation. The kidney decline will manifest as an increase in serum creatinine. The excessive bile is also excreted in the sweat, causing bile salts to accumulate on the skin. These bile salts cause intense itching. Estrogen builds up in both sexes, as the

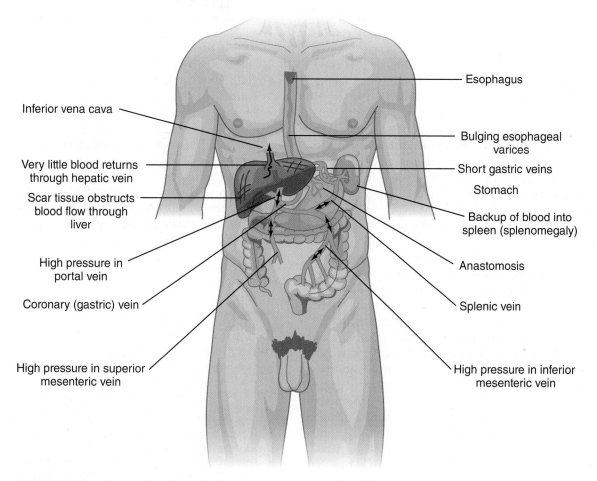

Inferior vena cava

Very little blood returns
through hepatic vein

Scar tissue obstructs
blood flow through
liver

High pressure in
portal vein

Coronary (gastric) vein

High pressure in superior
mesenteric vein

Esophagus

Bulging esophageal
varices

Short gastric veins

Stomach

Backup of blood into
spleen (splenomegaly)

Anastomosis

Splenic vein

High pressure in inferior
mesenteric vein

FIGURE 9-21 Development of esophageal varices.

liver can no longer inactivate the hormone. Excessive estrogen produces female characteristics in men and irregular menstruation (anovulation) in women. Men develop hypogonadism with impotence, infertility, and testicular atrophy. Numerous toxins and waste products also accumulate as the liver fails to detoxify the blood. In particular, the buildup of ammonia produces neurologic impairment (i.e., **hepatic encephalopathy**) that presents as cognitive and mental status changes (e.g., confusion, disorientation, disordered sleep, and lethargy) as well as hand tremors (asterixis). Ulcers and GI bleeding occur as the excessive bile and inflammation impair the mucosa. GI bleeding, in combination with a high-protein diet, renal failure, and infection, can cause protein levels to increase. Excessive protein levels lead to the rapid onset of encephalopathy. Spontaneous bacterial peritonitis, usually as a result of *E. coli*, may also occur because of compromised host defenses and bacterial overgrowth common in persons with cirrhosis. The bacteria translocate from the

intestines to the mesenteric lymph and then spread into the ascitic fluid, leading to potential bacteremia. Spontaneous bacterial peritonitis may cause fever, abdominal pain, altered mental status, and acute kidney injury. Liver damage can alter the pulmonary vasculature, resulting in hypoxemia (i.e., **hepatopulmonary syndrome**), and the increased portal pressures can also cause pulmonary artery vasoconstriction and pulmonary hypertension (i.e., **portopulmonary hypertension**).

Diagnosis and Treatment

Diagnostic procedures for cirrhosis include a history and physical examination. An abdominal ultrasound can be used to detect cirrhosis and manifestations such as ascites and splenomegaly. A liver biopsy is confirmatory but not always necessary particularly if the cause is known (e.g., alcoholism). Other tests can include an abdominal CT and abdominal magnetic resonance imaging (MRI). Laboratory tests will include a CBC, liver enzyme panel, clotting studies, platelet count, and stool examination for occult blood. Endoscopy can be performed to identify esophageal varices. Since there are more therapies aimed at reversing fibrosis, new noninvasive markers are being evaluated to measure and categorize the stages of fibrosis. Some of these markers include FibroSpect (evaluate markers associated with matrix breakdown such as hyaluronic acid and inhibitors of metalloproteinases) or calculation of the aspartate-to-AST to platelet ratio, and elastography (use of ultrasound and MRI to estimate liver stiffness).

Treatment strategies for cirrhosis are complex and vary depending on the underlying cause. The general treatment goals are aimed at slowing or reversing liver disease, preventing and treating complications, and managing clinical manifestations. Hepatitis-related cirrhosis is treated with antiviral agents and interferon. Alcohol and drugs should be completely avoided. Hepatotoxic medication doses may need to be adjusted if discontinuation is not possible. Vaccinations for hepatitis A and B should be administered to avoid further liver injury. Nutritional imbalances (usually treated with total parenteral nutrition [TPN]) and metabolic dysfunction are corrected to manage complications and promote optimal health. Bile acid–binding agents can aid bile excretion. Portal hypertension is treated with a surgically implanted shunt. Antacids and acid-reducing agents can minimize GI inflammation.

Specific complication management for the various aspects of cirrhosis includes:

- Varices
  - Nonselective beta blocker and endoscopic variceal ligation to prevent bleeding
  - During acute bleeding, vasoconstrictive agents such as somatostatin, octreotide, or terlipressin and temporary balloon tamponade (e.g., use of Sengstaken-Blakemore tube) until variceal ligation, or esophageal sclerotherapy (injection of a sclerosing agent such as sodium morrhuate into varices)
  - As a last resort, transjugular intrahepatic portosystemic shunt and other surgeries (e.g., portacaval shunts); highly effective but high mortality rate
- Ascites—diuretics (e.g., spironolactone, furosemide), sodium restriction, therapeutic paracentesis (removal of fluid), or transjugular intrahepatic portosystemic shunt
- Spontaneous bacterial peritonitis—administration of antibiotics

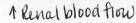 ↑ Renal blood flow

- Hepatorenal syndrome—administration of albumin, alpha agonists (e.g., midodrine), and agents like those for varices (e.g., terlipressin, octreotide); liver transplantation
- Pulmonary complications—liver transplantation
- Hepatic encephalopathy—correct underlying cause (e.g., GI bleeding), hydration, correction of electrolyte imbalances, lactulose (type of laxative that can promote ammonia excretion in stools), nonabsorbable antibiotics (e.g., rifaximin) that can suppress intestinal flora and decrease endogenous ammonia production

A liver transplant usually offers the best outcome for individuals with cirrhosis, but not all patients are candidates for this therapy.

Learning Points

Fatty Liver Disease

Hepatic steatosis, also known as fatty liver disease, can occur as a result of chronic alcohol ingestion (alcoholic steatosis) or nonalcoholic causes (e.g., obesity, metabolic syndrome, type 2 diabetes mellitus). Nonalcoholic steatosis is termed *nonalcoholic fatty liver disease*, or it is termed *nonalcoholic steatohepatitis* if hepatitis is present. The primary disorder in development of fatty liver disease is insulin resistance, which leads to lipolysis (lipid triglycerides broken down into glycerol and free fatty acids), increased synthesis of triglycerides, and uptake of free fatty acids. Fat, primarily triglycerides, infiltrate the hepatocytes. Fatty liver disease, regardless of type, can cause cirrhosis. Treatment strategies are aimed at managing the underlying causes such as weight loss, alcohol cessation, dyslipidemia control, and type 2 diabetes mellitus control.

Diagnostic Link

Liver Function

While various serum tests (e.g., ALT, AST, and ALP) are commonly termed *liver function tests*, these markers reflect injury more than they do function (e.g., they can be normal with advanced liver disease or be abnormal due to other nonhepatic disorders). Some of the common serum markers that reflect function are albumin and prothrombin time, which reflect the liver's synthesizing capacity. The liver is the site of albumin production, and low levels can indicate abnormal liver function. The liver is also the site of the synthesis of 11 blood coagulation proteins (e.g., fibrinogen, factor VII), and prothrombin is a commonly measured coagulation protein. High prothrombin levels can indicate abnormal liver function. Bilirubin is conjugated in the liver, and abnormalities can indicate abnormal liver function (see *Diagnostic Link—Bilirubin Measurement* box pertaining to bilirubin). Each of these tests has limitations regarding the accuracy of liver function, and several other markers indicate function (e.g., indocyanine green clearance); however, they are usually not used in clinical practice.

BOX 9-1 Application to Practice

A 55-year-old woman is complaining of right upper quadrant pain for the past 5 hours. She said she has had two or three similar episodes in the past; however, they only lasted 1 hour, and the pain was not as severe as with this episode. She thought the prior episodes were due to heartburn, and she has taken over-the-counter antacids with some relief but this time she has not had relief. This episode is rated as an 8 of 10 scale (0 no pain, 10 severe pain). The pain is constant and does not radiate. She says the pain started a few hours after she had lunch (states she ate a fast-food burger). She feels nauseous but has not vomited. She has been getting chills but also feels sweaty. She feels warm but does not know if she has a fever as she has not checked her temperature.

Past medical history: type 2 diabetes mellitus and dyslipidemia.

Medications: metformin 1,000-mg 1 tablet twice a day; atorvastatin 10-mg 1 tablet a day; and estrogen/progestin hormone replacement therapy 0.3-mg/1.5-mg 1 tablet a day.

Social history: does not smoke or drink alcohol; works as a cashier in a grocery store, is married, and has no children.

Vital signs: temperature 101.0° F, heart rate 110 beats per minute, respiratory rate 20 breaths per minute, blood pressure 140/80 mmHg, body mass index 31 kg/m². Answer the following questions pertaining to this case.

1. What is the most likely diagnosis based on this history, vital signs, and body mass index?
2. What are the data to support the diagnosis chosen in 1?
3. What are expected physical examination findings?
4. What are the expected findings on a complete blood count and abdominal ultrasound that would support the most likely diagnosis?

Alcoholics must refrain from all alcohol consumption for a minimum of 6 months to be considered for transplant. Some hepatitis infections (hepatitis B more than C) can return after transplant, so patients with such infections may not be considered as good candidates for this treatment. Additionally, patients with any evidence of cancer are not considered transplant candidates.

Disorders of the Pancreas

Disorders of the pancreas are frequently grave. The pancreas has a significant role in maintaining homeostasis by regulating electrolytes, water, and glucose. Consequently, conditions affecting the pancreas can have a global impact on the individual's health. Most often, the gallbladder is affected by pancreatic disorders because of the intricate relationship between these two organs.

Pancreatitis

Pancreatitis is an inflammation of the pancreas that can be either acute or chronic. Causes of pancreatitis include cholelithiasis (the most common acute cause), alcohol abuse (the most common chronic cause), biliary dysfunction, hepatotoxic drugs, metabolic disorders (e.g., hypertriglyceridemia, hyperglycemia), trauma, renal failure, endocrine disorders (e.g., hyperthyroidism), pancreatic tumors, and penetrating peptic ulcer. When the pancreas is injured or its function is disrupted, the pancreatic acinar cells are activated and release pancreatic enzymes (phospholipase A, lipase, and elastase) that leak into the pancreatic tissue and initiate autodigestion. Trypsin and elastase are activated proteases that, along with lipase, break down tissue and cell membranes, resulting in edema, vascular damage, hemorrhage, and necrosis. Pancreatic tissue is replaced by fibrosis and dysfunction of the islets of Langerhans and acinar cells resulting in exocrine and endocrine changes

Acute pancreatitis is considered a medical emergency (FIGURE 9-22). The mortality rate from this condition is approximately 15%, but the rate increases with advancing age and comorbidity. Serious complications can develop with acute pancreatitis, including acute respiratory distress syndrome, renal failure, disseminated intravascular coagulation, systemic inflammatory response, and sepsis. Pseudocyst or abscess can form and cause pancreatic fluids and necrotic debris to collect in cystlike pockets. Large pseudocysts or abscesses that rupture can cause complications such as internal bleeding and infection (e.g., peritonitis). Recurrent acute pancreatitis episodes can lead

ACUTE PANCREATITIS

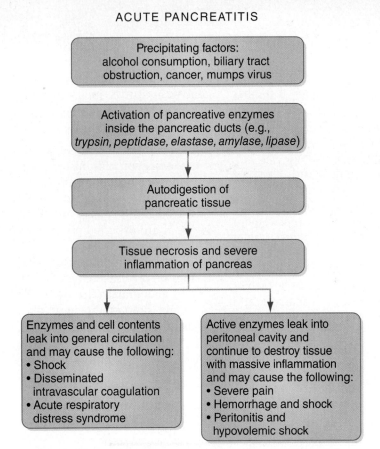

Precipitating factors: alcohol consumption, biliary tract obstruction, cancer, mumps virus

↓

Activation of pancreative enzymes inside the pancreatic ducts (e.g., *trypsin, peptidase, elastase, amylase, lipase*)

↓

Autodigestion of pancreatic tissue

↓

Tissue necrosis and severe inflammation of pancreas

Enzymes and cell contents leak into general circulation and may cause the following:
• Shock
• Disseminated intravascular coagulation
• Acute respiratory distress syndrome

Active enzymes leak into peritoneal cavity and continue to destroy tissue with massive inflammation and may cause the following:
• Severe pain
• Hemorrhage and shock
• Peritonitis and hypovolemic shock

FIGURE 9-22 Effects of acute pancreatitis.

to progressive and permanent damage and chronic pancreatitis.

Chronic pancreatitis can damage insulin-producing cells in the pancreas, leading to the development of diabetes mellitus. Both acute and chronic pancreatitis can decrease pancreatic enzyme production, and these enzymes are necessary for digestion and absorption. Malnutrition and weight loss may occur, even when food intake remains stable. Long-standing inflammation caused by chronic pancreatitis can initiate cellular mutations and lead to pancreatic cancer. See chapter 10 for discussion of diabetes.

Clinical Manifestations

Clinical manifestations vary depending on whether the pancreatitis is acute or chronic. Manifestations of acute pancreatitis are usually sudden and severe; in contrast, manifestations of chronic pancreatitis tend to be insidious. Monitoring for the development of complications is crucial to achieve positive patient outcomes. Clinical manifestations of acute pancreatitis are dependent on the severity (mild, moderate, or severe) and include the following symptoms:

• Epigastric or midabdominal pain that radiates to the back, worsens after eating, and is somewhat relieved by leaning forward or pulling the knees toward the chest
• Nausea and vomiting
• Mild jaundice
• Fever
• Blood pressure and pulse changes (may be increased or decreased), tachypnea
• Retroperitoneal bleeding (severe cases) resulting in periumbilical ecchymosis (Cullen sign) or flank ecchymosis (Grey-Turner sign)

Clinical manifestations of chronic pancreatitis include these symptoms:

• Epigastric or midabdominal pain that radiates to the back, worsens after eating, and is somewhat relieved by leaning forward or pulling the knees toward the chest
• Pancreatic insufficiency—fat malabsorption causing steatorrhea (loose, oily, fatty, odorous stools)
• Malnutrition—unintentional weight loss

Diagnosis and Treatment

Diagnostic procedures for pancreatitis include those to verify the pancreatitis and those to identify complications. These procedures will consist of a history and physical examination. Serum amylase and lipase levels will be elevated during episodes of acute pancreatitis, usually up to three times their normal limits. Amylase levels rise within 12 hours after onset of acute pancreatitis and returns to normal within 5 days. Lipase levels rise within 8 hours and return to normal within 14 days. Since lipase levels remain elevated longer, they are a more reliable marker of acute pancreatitis. Immune markers, such as C-reactive protein, will be elevated and can be used as a marker of severity. A CBC may reveal leukocytosis and an increased hematocrit due to hemoconcentration. A chemistry profile may reveal an elevated blood urea nitrogen, hypocalcemia, and glucose abnormalities (high or low). Other laboratory testing that can be performed includes a liver enzymes panel, measurement of serum bilirubin level, arterial blood gases, and stool analysis (lipid and trypsin levels). Imaging studies will include either an abdominal CT with contrast, abdominal MRI, or abdominal ultrasound. Additional testing may include an

BOX 9-2 Application to Practice

K.S. is a 35-year-old man who has been homeless for the past 5 years. He presents to the health department complaining of flulike symptoms and abdominal pain. K.S. has multiple tattoos and piercings. He admits to intravenous drug use and unprotected sexual behavior with multiple female partners. Blood tests reveal that K.S.'s liver enzymes are elevated. The healthcare provider suspects some type of hepatitis.

1. Considering K.S.'s lifestyle, which type or types of hepatitis has he most likely contracted? Explain your choice or choices.
   a. Hepatitis A
   b. Hepatitis B
   c. Hepatitis C

2. How would you expect a differential diagnosis of hepatitis to be confirmed?
   a. Presence of viral particles in stool
   b. Elevated bilirubin and prothrombin time and low albumin
   c. Presence of the specific hepatitis antibodies in the blood
   d. Inflammation of the liver on ultrasound

3. Choose all of the following results that are consistent with an acute episode of hepatitis B infection. Discuss what each test measures.
   a. Anti-HBs positive
   b. Anti-HBc (IgM) positive
   c. HBsAg positive
   d. HBsAG negative

4. K.S.'s girlfriend is also developing similar symptoms. Which of the following factors likely explains the onset of the girlfriend's symptoms?
   a. They probably ate the same food.
   b. They likely obtained the virus from contaminated water.
   c. They probably infected each other through sexual contact or drug activity.
   d. They likely became infected because of poor living conditions.

---

endoscopic retrograde cholangiopancreatography or a magnetic resonance imaging cholangiopancreatography. These imaging studies are also used in the evaluation of chronic pancreatitis. Laboratory evaluations may be normal in chronic pancreatitis.

Management of pancreatitis requires early treatment and aggressive strategies to prevent complications. Patients with severe pancreatitis as well as altered vital signs (e.g., pulse < 40 or > 150 beats/minute) or other parameters (e.g., abnormal electrolytes) will likely need to be closely monitored in an intensive care unit. Treatment strategies will be dependent on the severity of the pancreatitis and will include the following measures:

- Resting the pancreas by fasting, administering intravenous nutrition (e.g., TPN), and gradually advancing the diet from clear liquids as tolerated to a low-fat, low-residue diet; if oral nutrition not tolerated, feedings can be administered enterally (e.g., nasojejunal tube)
- Pancreatic enzyme supplements when the diet is resumed
- Maintaining hydration status with intravenous fluids

- Inserting a nasogastric tube with intermittent suction for persistent nausea and vomiting
- Antiemetic agents (if vomiting is present)
- Pain management (usually includes intravenous narcotic agents and analgesics)
- Antacids and acid-reducing agents
- Anticholinergic agents (which reduce vagal stimulation, decrease GI motility, and inhibit pancreatic enzyme secretion)
- Antibiotic therapy (if infection is present)
- Insulin (which treats hyperglycemia secondary to temporary or permanent pancreatic damage and TPN)
- Identifying and treating complications early (e.g., blood transfusions for hemorrhage, dialysis for renal failure, airway management for acute respiratory distress syndrome, surgical drain for abscesses, pancreatic debridement, and laparotomy for biliary obstruction)

Prevention of disease progression becomes the focus after an episode of acute pancreatitis and for chronic pancreatitis. Lifestyle modifications (e.g., cessation of alcohol and smoking) can prevent progression. Long-term pain management may be necessary (e.g., analgesics, nerve blocks).

Disorders of the Lower Gastrointestinal Tract

Disorders of the lower GI tract can alter nutrition or impair elimination. These conditions range in severity from mild (e.g., diarrhea and constipation) to life threatening (e.g., appendicitis and peritonitis) and can be either congenital (e.g., celiac disease) or acquired (e.g., intestinal obstruction). Depending on their severity, most of these disorders can be resolved or managed with minimal residual effects.

Diarrhea

Diarrhea refers to a change in bowel pattern characterized by an increased frequency, amount, and water content of the stool. This condition can result from an increase in fluid secretion (it is secretory), a decrease in fluid absorption (it is osmotic), or an alteration in GI peristalsis (motility is affected). Diarrhea can be acute (three or more loose stools per day and lasting < 14 days) or chronic (lasting longer than 4 weeks) and may be attributed to many conditions. Acute diarrhea is often caused by viral (more common) or bacterial infections (more common in severe cases).

Gastroenteritis is an intestinal disease manifested by acute onset of diarrhea, nausea, and vomiting due to an infection. Diarrhea can also be triggered by certain medications (e.g., antibiotics, antacids, and laxatives). Depending on the cause, acute diarrhea is usually self-limiting. Causes of chronic diarrhea are usually noninfectious and include inflammatory bowel diseases (e.g., Crohn disease and ulcerative colitis), malabsorption syndromes (e.g., celiac disease), endocrine disorders (e.g., thyroid disorders), chemotherapy, and radiation. In developing countries, chronic diarrhea is more commonly due to chronic infection of the GI tract (e.g., bacterial, parasitic).

Clinical manifestations of diarrhea vary depending on the underlying etiology. When this condition originates in the small intestine, stools are large, loose, and provoked by eating. Diarrhea originating in the small intestine is usually accompanied by pain in the right lower quadrant of the abdomen along with bloating and gas. Additionally, fever and occult blood in the stool are uncommon. Many organisms have been implicated in small bowel diarrhea, including *E. coli*, *Salmonella*, *Vibrio cholerae*, and *Giardia lamblia*. When diarrhea originates in the large intestine, stools are small and frequent. Diarrhea originating in the large

intestine is frequently accompanied by pain and cramping in the left lower quadrant of the abdomen along with painful defecation. Fever and bloody or mucoid type stool is more common in large intestine diarrhea than with small intestine diarrhea. Many organisms have been implicated in large intestine diarrhea, including *Clostridioides difficile*, *Shigella*, and *Campylobacter*. Nausea and vomiting may also be present.

Blood in the stool may present as frank blood (bright red blood on the surface of the stool), occult blood (small amounts of blood hidden in the stool indicative of lower GI tract disorders as the cause), or melena (dark, tarry stool from a significant amount of bleeding higher up in the GI tract). Additionally, bowel sounds may be hyperactive. Fluid, electrolyte, and pH (usually metabolic acidosis) imbalances can develop regardless of whether the diarrhea is acute or chronic (see chapter 6 for further details on fluid, electrolyte, and acid–base homeostasis).

Diagnostic procedures for diarrhea focus on identifying the underlying cause and any complications. These procedures may include a history (including usual bowel pattern and completion of the Bristol stool chart [FIGURE 9-23]) and physical examination. Additional testing is not generally indicated in acute diarrhea as most cases are self-limiting. Certain geographic regions in the world may have a higher prevalence of pathogenic intestinal organisms, so a travel history may provide clues to the source of the diarrhea. As an example, epidemics are often caused by *S. dysenteriae* and *V. cholerae* and are likely to occur in resource-limited countries such as parts of Central America, Africa, and South Asia. The CDC maintains information pertaining to outbreaks, recommended vaccines, and other travel-related health advice, and this information can be accessed at https://wwwnc.cdc.gov/travel. While diagnostic testing is usually not indicated, there are circumstances (e.g., severe presentations, immunocompromised patients, elderly patients, and public health concerns such as diarrhea in food handlers) that warrant stool analysis (e.g., ova and parasites, cultures, and occult blood). A CBC, blood chemistry, and other laboratory testing may also be indicated. Imaging studies may be necessary for those patients with complications such as peritonitis and bowel perforation, including an abdominal CT.

Treatment strategies vary depending on the underlying etiology. Maintaining hydration status and correcting electrolyte and pH imbalances is crucial to managing acute or chronic diarrhea (see chapter 6 for further details on fluid, electrolyte, and acid–base homeostasis).

Acute diarrhea with infectious origins usually improves with short-term fasting. Generally, food consumption slows GI motility, allowing bacterial and viral toxins to increase. As toxin levels rise, diarrhea can become more severe. Antidiarrheal agents may be withheld for the same reason. Antibiotics may be necessary depending on the infectious agent. In non-infectious diarrhea, antidiarrheal agents slow GI motility and increase fluid absorption. Some additional medications that may be administered include anticholinergic and antispasmodic agents. Probiotics can maintain normal flora and reduce the duration of diarrhea. When oral intake is recommended, a clear liquid diet is usually ordered until the diarrhea subsides. At that time, the diet is advanced to a regular diet as tolerated. Dairy products and fatty foods are probably best avoided as both may aggravate diarrhea. Dietary fiber can be used to manage chronic diarrhea; the fiber acts like a sponge to absorb the excess water and increase bulk in the stool. Management of chronic diarrhea involves treating the underlying cause. Meticulous skin care can maintain skin integrity, especially in cases of bowel incontinence.

Constipation

Constipation refers to a change in bowel pattern characterized by infrequent passage of stool. Bowel patterns vary from person to person, so the decrease in frequency is in reference to the individual's typical bowel pattern. With constipation, the stool remains in the large intestine longer than usual. The longer the stool remains in the large intestine, the more water is removed from the stool. Consequently, the stool becomes hard and difficult to pass. Constipation is often caused by a low-fiber diet, inadequate physical activity, insufficient fluid intake, delaying the urge to defecate, or laxative abuse (which smooths intestinal rugae). Stress (sympathetic nervous system stimulation slows GI motility) and travel can also contribute to constipation or other changes in bowel habits. Diseases of the bowel such as irritable bowel syndrome, pregnancy, and medications such as narcotics, anticholinergic agents, and iron supplements can cause constipation. Other causes include mental health problems such as depression, neurologic diseases (e.g., stroke, Parkinson disease, and spinal cord injuries), and colon cancer. In addition, constipation is common in children

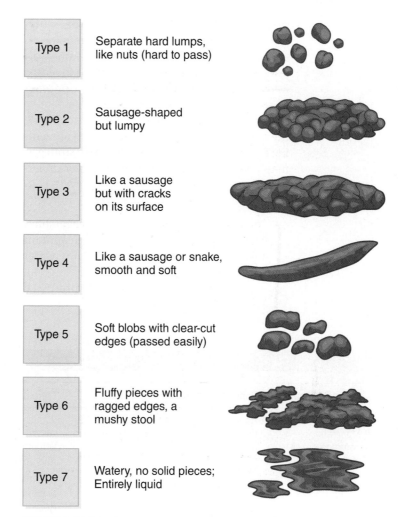

Type 1	Separate hard lumps, like nuts (hard to pass)	
Type 2	Sausage-shaped but lumpy	
Type 3	Like a sausage but with cracks on its surface	
Type 4	Like a sausage or snake, smooth and soft	
Type 5	Soft blobs with clear-cut edges (passed easily)	
Type 6	Fluffy pieces with ragged edges, a mushy stool	
Type 7	Watery, no solid pieces; Entirely liquid	

FIGURE 9-23 Bristol stool chart.

Data from: Lewis, S., & Heaton, K. (1997). Stool form scale as a useful guide to intestinal transit time. *Scandinavian Journal of Gastroenterology*, 32(9), 920–924.

who are toilet training, especially if they are not ready for training or are scared of toileting.

Constipation may involve pain during the passage of a bowel movement, inability to pass stool after straining or pushing for more than 10 minutes, or no bowel movements for more than 3 days. Additionally, bowel sounds may be hypoactive. The passage of large, wide stools may tear the mucosal membrane of the anus, especially in children. This tearing can cause bleeding and cause an anal fissure to develop. Chronic constipation can lead to pH disturbances (usually metabolic alkalosis), hemorrhoids (swollen, inflamed veins in the rectum or anus), diverticulitis, impaction, intestinal obstruction, and fistulas. See chapter 6 for discussion of metabolic alkalosis.

Diagnostic procedures for constipation focus on identifying the underlying cause. These procedures consist of a history (including usual bowel pattern and completion of the Bristol stool chart [Figure 9-23]), physical examination (may include a digital rectal examination), abdominal X-ray, upper GI series, barium swallow, colonoscopy (for visualization of the large intestine), and proctosigmoidoscopy (for visualization of the lower bowel).

Treatment strategies focus on reestablishing the individual's usual bowel pattern and preventing future constipation episodes. These strategies may involve managing or removing any underlying causes. Strategies to treat and prevent constipation may include the following measures:

- Increasing dietary fiber (e.g., vegetables, fruit, and whole grains) with concomitant increase in hydration (specifically water and juices)
- Avoid constipating foods (e.g., processed sugar, white flour, and red meat)
- Increasing physical activity
- Defecating when the initial urge is sensed
- Taking stool softeners (incorporates lipids and water into the stool)
- Limiting use of laxatives and enemas
- Digitally removing an impaction if present

Intestinal Obstruction

An intestinal obstruction refers to blockage of intestinal contents in the small intestine (where it is most common) or the large intestine. Intestinal obstructions have two types of causes—mechanical and functional. Mechanical obstructions consist of physical barriers, whereas functional obstructions result from GI tract physiologic dysfunction. Mechanical obstructions can occur due to foreign bodies, tumors, adhesions, hernias, intussusception (telescoping of a portion of the intestine into another portion) (TABLE 9-5), volvulus

TABLE 9-5	Causes of Intestinal Obstruction in Children		
Cause/incidence	Pathophysiology	Typical manifestations	Treatment
Intestinal Malrotation—common cause of congenital abnormality of the small intestine	Abnormal rotation of the small intestine during embryonic development—results in cecum and colon up in right upper quadrant and fixated with peritoneal bands across duodenum Complications include: peritoneal bands that cross the duodenum can compress the duodenum and cause obstruction; loose loops of bowel can twists upon themselves (volvulus) around the mesenteric artery leading to ischemia and necrosis	Vomiting usually bilious (green or bright yellow) and is intermittent or persistent. Vomiting occurs after feeding Abdominal distension Abdominal tenderness Malabsorption Diarrhea Peritonitis (indicates volvulus and perforation) Hematochezia (indicates bowel ischemia) Hypovolemia and septic shock	Surgery (endoscopic or open) includes a Ladd procedure—moving of the duodenum which is then held in place through creation of adhesions to prevent volvulus
Hirschsprung Disease (congenital aganglionic megacolon)	Pre-ganglionic intestinal cells do not migrate completely during intestinal fetal development. This results in an inability of the colon to relax (due to lack of motor stimulation) and feces movement is impaired, the colon distends (i.e., megacolon) leading to colon obstruction Complications include enterocolitis which can lead to sepsis	Failure to pass meconium within 48 hours of life Bilious emesis Abdominal distension Watery stool around the impacted feces Constipation	Surgery involves resection of the aganglionic bowel and anastomosis of normal bowel proximal to the anus
Intussusception—most common cause of intestinal obstruction in children under 2 years old	Invagination (telescoping) of a part of the intestine into a more distal part. The mesentery is also in invaginated causing impeded venous and lymphatic flow resulting in edema. Most cases are idiopathic. Complications include: Bowel ischemia, perforation and peritonitis	Sudden onset of intermittent, severe, crampy/colicky and progressive abdominal pain. The pain causes inconsolable crying and drawing up of the legs toward the abdomen. Vomiting that is initially nonbilious then becomes bilious (worsening obstruction). Bloody stool or stool mixed with blood and mucus (looks like currant jelly) Sausage shaped mass on the right side of the abdomen	With no evidence of bowel perforation a nonoperative reduction using hydrostatic or air pressure with an enema. If the child is unstable and if nonoperative reduction not successful then surgery is necessary- either reduction or resection

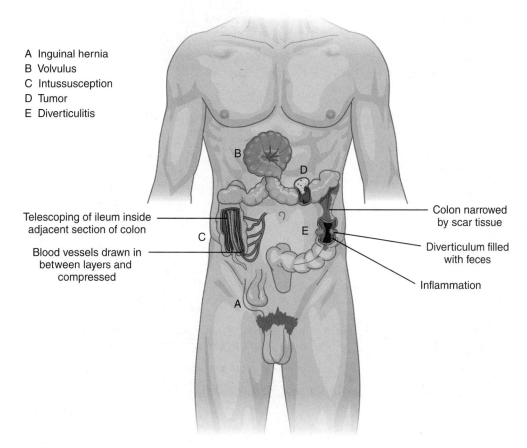

A Inguinal hernia
B Volvulus
C Intussusception
D Tumor
E Diverticulitis

Telescoping of ileum inside adjacent section of colon

Blood vessels drawn in between layers and compressed

Colon narrowed by scar tissue

Diverticulum filled with feces

Inflammation

FIGURE 9-24 Causes of intestinal obstruction.

(twisting of the intestine), strictures, Crohn disease, diverticulitis, Hirschsprung disease (also known as congenital megacolon), and fecal impaction (**FIGURE 9-24**). Postoperative adhesions and hernias account for approximately 90% of all mechanical small intestine obstructions. Tumors, diverticulitis, and volvulus are the most common causes of mechanical large intestine obstructions. Functional obstructions, also called *paralytic ileuses*, usually result from neurologic impairment such as spinal cord injury; intra-abdominal surgery complications; chemical, electrolyte, and mineral disturbances; intra-abdominal infections such as peritonitis and pancreatitis; abdominal blood supply impairment; renal and lung disease; and use of certain medications such as narcotics.

Depending on the cause and location, intestinal obstructions can develop either suddenly or gradually. Additionally, the obstruction can be either partial or complete. Tumors are also likely to be associated with gradual and partial obstruction. Chyme and gas initially accumulate at the site of the blockage. Over time, saliva, gastric juices, bile, and pancreatic secretions begin to collect as the blockage lingers.

This GI fluid buildup increases serum electrolytes and protein and causes abdominal distention and pain. Intestinal blood flow can become impaired, leading to strangulation and necrosis. Intestinal contents will begin to seep into the peritoneal cavity as the pressure at the blockage increases. These complications are more likely to develop with a complete obstruction. If a complete obstruction goes untreated, death can occur within hours due to shock and cardiovascular collapse. Additional complications include perforation, pH imbalances, and fluid disturbances.

Clinical Manifestations

The following manifestations are a result of the GI tract blockage (**FIGURE 9-25**):

- Abdominal distention
- Abdominal cramping and colicky pain
- Nausea and vomiting (usually gastric or bile contents)
- Constipation and inability to pass flatus
- Diarrhea (some of the intestinal liquid passes around the obstruction)
- Borborygmi (audible bowel sounds; associated with mechanical obstruction)

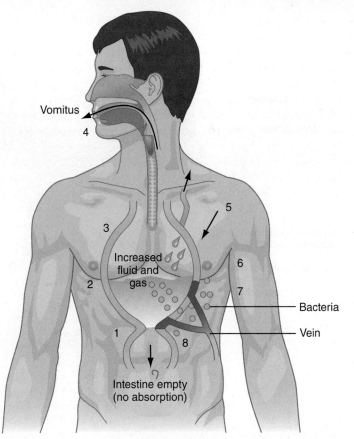

1 Site of obstruction
2 Increased fluid and gas lead to distention
3 Distention causes increased peristalsis to force contents past obstruction, leading to colicky pain
4 Severe vomiting from distention and pain leads to dehydration and electrolyte imbalance
5 Increased pressure on wall causes more fluid to enter intestine
6 Decreased blood pressure and hypovolemic shock as fluid shift into intestine continues (third spacing)
7 Continued pressure on intestinal wall causes edema and ischemia of wall and decreased peristalsis
8 Prolonged ischemia causes increased permeability and necrosis of wall; intestinal bacteria and toxins leak into blood and peritoneal cavity (peritonitis)

Vomitus

Increased fluid and gas

Bacteria

Vein

Intestine empty (no absorption)

FIGURE 9-25 Effects of intestinal obstruction.

- Intestinal rushes (forcible intestinal contractions; associated with mechanical obstruction)
- Decreased or absent bowel sounds
- Anorexia
- Restlessness, diaphoresis, tachycardia progressing to weakness, confusion, and shock

Diagnosis and Treatment

Diagnostic procedures for intestinal obstruction are directed at identifying the obstruction, the underlying etiology, and complications. These manifestations consist of a history (including the usual bowel pattern), physical examination, blood chemistry, and CBC. Arterial blood gases, serum lactate, and blood cultures are performed for those patients who present with systemic signs such as fever, tachycardia, and hypotension. Imaging is necessary to confirm the diagnosis and usually includes an abdominal CT and abdominal X-ray. Other studies can include an abdominal ultrasound and contrast studies.

Treatment strategies depend on the underlying cause. Such strategies generally focus on correcting fluid, electrolyte, and pH imbalances; decompressing the bowel; and reestablishing

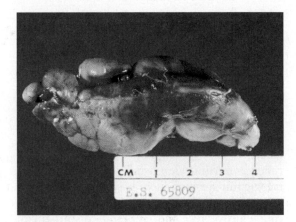

FIGURE 9-26 Appendicitis.
Courtesy of Leonard V. Crowley, MD, Century College.

bowel movements. A nasogastric tube with intermittent suctioning is inserted to decompress the bowel and relieve vomiting. Ambulation can help restore peristalsis. Laxatives should not be used in most cases until the obstruction is resolved. Surgery is frequently necessary to relieve mechanical obstruction.

Appendicitis

Appendicitis refers to an inflammation of the vermiform appendix (**FIGURE 9-26**). The incidence of appendicitis is highest between the ages of 10 and 19 years old. Appendicitis occurs as a result of obstruction, possibly caused by hard stool (fecaliths), calculi, tumors, and infections. The inflammation process triggers local tissue edema, which obstructs the small structure. As fluid builds inside the appendix, microorganisms proliferate. The appendix fills with purulent exudate, and the stretched, edematous wall compresses area blood vessels. With blood flow compromised, ischemia and necrosis develop. The pressure inside the appendix escalates, forcing bacteria and toxins out to surrounding structures. Abscesses and peritonitis can develop as bacteria escape, and gangrene can result from the worsening necrosis. The pressure inside the appendix will continue to intensify until the appendix ruptures or perforates, releasing its contents. This release can accelerate peritonitis, which can be life threatening.

Clinical Manifestations

Clinical manifestations reflect the pathogenesis characteristic of appendicitis. These manifestations vary significantly in severity, from asymptomatic to sudden and severe. The first symptom is often pain near the umbilicus. As swelling increases, the pain tends to move to the lower right quadrant of the abdomen (McBurney point). The pain gradually intensifies (over approximately 12–24 hours). It is often aggravated by movement, so patients tend to guard their abdomen. Due to normal anatomic variations, this pain may occur anywhere in the abdomen. The pain will temporarily subside if the appendix ruptures, but then will return and escalate as peritonitis develops. Anorexia, nausea, and vomiting are other classic manifestations of appendicitis in addition to pain. Abdominal distention and bowel pattern changes can also be associated with appendicitis. Other manifestations reflect the inflammation and infectious process (e.g., fever, chills, and leukocytosis). Various clinical maneuvers each with varying accuracy can be used to evaluate for physical signs of appendicitis, such as the psoas sign. This sign involves passively extending the right hip, which will elicit right lower quadrant pain if the appendix is inflamed. Additionally, the patient should be monitored for signs and symptoms of peritonitis (e.g., abdominal rigidity, tachycardia, and hypotension).

Diagnosis and Treatment

Urgent diagnosis and treatment are crucial for positive patient outcomes. Diagnostic procedures include a history and physical examination. A CBC with differential will reveal leukocytosis with increased bands (immature neutrophils) and mature neutrophils. An abdominal CT with or without contrast is preferred; however, an MRI or abdominal ultrasound can be performed and is the recommended imaging for pregnant women and children. Because of the life-threatening nature of appendicitis, surgery remains the cornerstone of treatment. In fact, appendicitis is one of the most common indications for emergency surgery in the United States. Performing the surgery prior to rupture of the appendix is paramount. Laparoscopic or open surgical procedure can be performed for nonperforated and perforated appendices, and the decision is based on surgeon preference, patient age, and condition. If the appendix ruptures, all of the appendix fragments and infectious materials are removed, and extensive irrigation of the abdominal cavity is performed to flush out any remaining bacteria. The wound may be left open to heal by secondary intention to decrease the risk of infection. Peritoneal drains may be inserted for abscesses. Long-term antibiotic therapy may be necessary to prevent and resolve any infections. Analgesics will be necessary to manage pain before and after surgery. Additionally, the patient should avoid activities that increase intra-abdominal pressure (e.g., straining and coughing).

Peritonitis

Peritonitis is an inflammation of the peritoneum, the membrane that lines the abdominal wall and abdominal organs. Peritonitis usually presents as an acute condition and has an inpatient hospital mortality rate of up to 20%. Treatment centers on resolving the underlying cause. The inflammation may result from chemical irritation (e.g., ruptured gallbladder or spleen) or direct organism invasion (e.g., appendicitis and peritoneal dialysis) (FIGURE 9-27). Chemical irritation will lead to a bacterial invasion if not quickly treated. Peritonitis is also categorized as primary or secondary. Primary peritonitis occurs as a result of infection spreading from the blood or lymph. Secondary peritonitis occurs as a result of pathology of a visceral organ (e.g., perforation, trauma). Most cases of primary (spontaneous) peritonitis are due to advanced cirrhosis. The inflammatory response triggered by the chemical increases intestinal wall permeability. In turn, the increased permeability allows for passage of enteric bacteria. Necrosis or perforation of

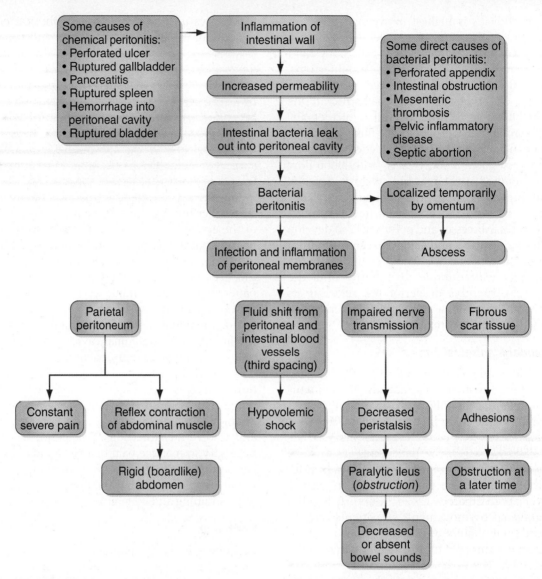

FIGURE 9-27 Development of peritonitis.

the intestinal wall also creates an opportunity for an enteric bacteria invasion. The most common organisms in spontaneous bacterial peritonitis are gram-negative *E. coli* and *Klebsiella* species. Secondary peritonitis due to perforation in comparison to spontaneous peritonitis is usually polymicrobial, and the organisms involved are also often *E. coli* and other gram-negative rods.

Several protective mechanisms are activated along with the inflammatory response in an attempt to localize the problem. These mechanisms include producing a thick, sticky exudate that bonds nearby structures and temporarily seals them off. Abscesses may form as the body attempts to wall off the infections. Peristalsis may slow down as a response to the inflammation, decreasing the spread of toxins and bacteria. These mechanisms merely slow the progression, however. If the underlying cause is not treated,

the condition can become critical as septic shock and multisystem organ failure develop.

Clinical Manifestations

Clinical manifestations reflect the inflammatory and infectious processes. These manifestations tend to be sudden and severe. The classic manifestation of peritonitis is abdominal rigidity. A rigid, boardlike abdomen develops because of a reflexive abdominal muscle spasm that occurs in response to the peritoneal inflammation. Inflamed tissue creates abdominal tenderness and pain. Rebound tenderness, pain that is worse upon removal of pressure, indicates parietal peritoneal inflammation. Large volumes of fluid can leak into the peritoneal cavity (a phenomenon called *third spacing*), leading to hypovolemic shock. This fluid contains protein and electrolytes, making it an optimal medium for bacterial growth. Nausea and vomiting are common responses to the intestinal irritation. Persistent inflammation impairs nerve conduction, which decreases peristalsis. This decreased peristalsis can, in turn, lead to intestinal obstruction. Sepsis develops as the bacteria and toxins migrate to the circulatory system through the inflamed membranes. Fever, malaise, and leukocytosis occur because of the infectious process. Additionally, the patient should be monitored for signs of septic shock and multisystem organ failure(e.g., tachycardia, hypotension, restlessness, and diaphoresis). See chapter 4 for details on cardiovascular function.

Diagnosis and Treatment

Diagnostic procedures for peritonitis consist of a history, physical examination, CBC, abdominal X-ray (flat and upright), abdominal ultrasound, and abdominal CT. Paracentesis is performed to obtain peritoneal fluid for analysis (e.g., gram stain, culture, cell count with differential, and albumin). Other laboratory tests will include chemistry panel, liver enzymes, and other tests based on suspected underlying cause and patient status. Treatment strategies vary based on the underlying cause. The patient's prognosis depends on the underlying cause along with the implementation of early and aggressive treatment. Management often includes surgical repair of the chemical leak and draining of the infected fluid. Long-term antibiotic therapy specific to the causative organism will be required. In addition, correction of any fluid and electrolyte imbalance may be required. Insertion of a nasogastric tube with intermittent suction can relieve abdominal distention and treat intestinal obstructions. TPN will be necessary to maintain nutritional status until the peritonitis is resolved.

Celiac Disease

Celiac disease (also known as celiac sprue or gluten-sensitive enteropathy) is an inherited, autoimmune, malabsorption disorder of the small intestine. Although it is considered primarily a childhood disease, this condition can develop at any age. Celiac disease results from a combination of the immune response to environmental factors (dietary gluten and related proteins) and genetic predisposition. It affects approximately 1% of the general population worldwide. Celiac disease is most common in Whites and in females.

The most common gene locus with celiac is the HLA-DQ2 and HLA-DQ8. This genotype is essential to confer the disease, but their presence alone is insufficient to develop the disease. Other genes and environmental factors must also be

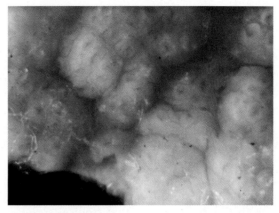

FIGURE 9-28 Effects of celiac disease on intestinal villi.
© Biophoto Associates/Science Source.

present. Celiac disease results from a defect in the intestinal enzymes that prevent further digestion of gliadin—a product of gluten digestion. The triggering gluten proteins are ingredients in grains, wheat, barley, and rye. The combination of digestive dysfunction and immune activities creates a toxic environment for the intestinal villi. The villi atrophy and flatten. The fingerlike grooves between the villi (i.e., crypts) develop hyperplasia and elongate, resulting in decreased enzyme production and making less surface area available for nutrient absorption (**FIGURE 9-28**). Eventually, the malnutrition associated with celiac disease can cause vitamin deficiencies that deprive the brain, peripheral nervous system, bones, liver, and other organs of vital nourishment. These nutritional deficits, in turn, can lead to other illnesses. Celiac disease is associated with many conditions, including:

- Anemia (e.g., iron deficiency anemia)
- Arthralgia (bone and joint pain)
- Myalgia (muscle pain)
- Bone disease (e.g., osteoporosis, kyphoscoliosis, and fractures)
- Dental enamel defects and discoloration
- Growth and development delays in children
- Hair loss
- Hypoglycemia
- Mouth ulcers
- Increased bleeding tendencies (e.g., bruising and nose bleeds)
- Neurobehavioral or psychiatric disorders (e.g., depression, anxiety, and sleep problems)
- Neurologic disorders (e.g., seizures and peripheral neuropathy)
- Risk of malignancy (e.g., intestinal cancers and non-Hodgkin lymphoma)
- Skin disorders (e.g., dermatitis herpetiformis and eczema)

- Vitamin or mineral deficiency, either single or multiple nutrient (e.g., iron, folate, vitamin B_{12}, and vitamin K)
- Endocrine disorders (e.g., menstrual dysfunction, thyroid disease, type 1 diabetes, and adrenal insufficiency)

Tropical sprue is a small intestine disease characterized by malabsorption of nutrients, and a differential diagnosis is celiac disease. The disorder also causes endoscopic findings like those of celiac disease, such as villi atrophy and elongated crypts. The distinctions between the disorders are that tropical sprue is probably infectious in origin (bacterial, viral, parasitic, or amoebic) and occurs in tropical regions, especially India, Southeast Asia, Central America, South America, and the Caribbean. Tropical sprue should be suspected in anyone who has chronic diarrhea ($>$ 1 month) and who has traveled to prevalent regions. Tropical sprue can be resolved with antibiotic therapy, unlike celiac disease, which becomes a lifelong condition.

Clinical Manifestations

Clinical manifestations of celiac disease vary significantly from person to person—a factor that often delays diagnosis. In infants, clinical manifestations generally appear as gluten (e.g., in cereals) is added to their diet (usually around 4–6 months of age). Most of the clinical manifestations are GI in nature, but occasionally there are no GI symptoms. Other manifestations include arthritis and skin disorders. Some patients have silent/subclinical celiac disease—they have no symptoms but are seropositive for the disorder. The GI manifestations in infants and younger children are generally more intense than in older children and adults. The GI clinical manifestations may include the following symptoms:

- Abdominal pain
- Abdominal distention, bloating, gas, and indigestion
- Anorexia
- Diarrhea (chronic or occasional)—bulky, foul smelling, and possibly floating
- Constipation (not as common)
- Changes in appetite (usually decreased)
- Lactose intolerance (common upon diagnosis; usually goes away following treatment)
- Nausea and vomiting
- Steatorrhea

- Unexplained weight loss (although people can be overweight or of normal weight upon diagnosis)
- Signs of vitamin deficiencies (e.g., bruising, fatigue, hair loss, paresthesia, and mouth ulcers)

Manifestations that are not GI in nature may include irritability, lethargy, malaise, and behavioral changes. Additionally, the individual with celiac disease should be monitored for development of complications.

Diagnosis and Treatment

Diagnostic procedures for celiac disease consist of a history, physical examination, celiac blood panel, and EGD with duodenal biopsy. The celiac blood panel includes serum antibody assays that can be divided into two groups:

1. **Autoantibody testing**: Immunoglobulin A antibody-endomysium antibodies (EMA-IgA) and immunoglobulin A anti-tissue transglutaminase (tTG-IgA)
2. **Antibodies targeting gliadin**: Immunoglobulin A antigliadin antibodies (AGA-IgA, AGA-IgG) and deamidated gliadin peptide antibody (DGP-IGA, DGP-IgG)

Other tests that can be considered include stool tests to evaluate for fat malabsorption, a lactose tolerance test, and a d-xylose test.

Dietary management is the cornerstone of treatment. Most people (approximately 90%) with celiac disease are effectively managed by eliminating gluten from their diet. Dietary changes may also be used as a part of the diagnosis. The individual is given a gluten-free diet to assess whether the symptoms improve. A gluten-free diet involves avoiding wheat and wheat products—rice and corn can be substituted. Once gluten is removed from the diet, the intestinal mucosa will return to normal after a few weeks. Even when symptoms are controlled with diet, the individual with celiac disease remains at risk for intestinal cancers; consequently, he or she should be periodically monitored for cancer development. Additionally, long-term support may be necessary for children and parents of children with celiac disease. If gluten is reintroduced into the diet, relapses can occur.

Inflammatory Bowel Disease

Inflammatory bowel disease (IBD) describes chronic inflammation of the GI tract, usually the intestines. IBD is chiefly seen in women, Whites, persons of Jewish descent (Ashkenazi Jews), and smokers. It encompasses two disorders—Crohn disease and ulcerative colitis. Both conditions are characterized by periods of exacerbations and remissions that can vary in severity.

The exact cause of IBD is unknown, and the pathogenesis is poorly understood. This disease is thought to be caused by a genetically associated autoimmune state that occurs as a result of a dysregulated response by the mucosal immune system to the intestinal microbiota (**TABLE 9-6**). The GI immune system either reacts excessively or inadequately to intestinal microbiota, resulting in an imbalance in the immune response and development of IBD. The immune dysregulation causes alterations in the epithelial barrier, immune cells (e.g., T cells), and abnormal secretion of immune-related mediators. Immune cells located in the intestinal mucosa are stimulated to release inflammatory mediators (e.g., histamine, prostaglandins, leukotrienes, and cytokines). These mediators alter the function and neural activity of the secretory and smooth muscle cells in the GI tract. The immune response may also be directed at other intraintestinal antigens (e.g., dietary products or tobacco smoke). Fluid, electrolyte, and pH imbalances develop. IBD can be painful, debilitating, and life threatening. Additionally, children have a more extensive intestinal involvement, and the disorder progresses rapidly in comparison to the progression in adults.

Crohn Disease

Crohn disease is an insidious, slow-developing, progressive condition that often emerges in adolescence. Its exact cause is unknown, but T-cell activation leading to tissue damage has been implicated. This condition usually affects the intestines, particularly the distal ileum (most common), ileum and cecum, or the ileum and entire colon (it usually spares the rectum); however, it may occur anywhere along the GI tract from the mouth to the anus. When the disorder involves the colon only, it may be difficult to distinguish from ulcerative colitis. Crohn disease is characterized by patchy areas of inflammation involving the full thickness (transmural) of the intestinal wall and ulcerations. These patchy areas and ulcerations, often called *skip lesions*, are separated by areas of normal tissue. The ulcers combine to form fissures divided by nodules (thickened

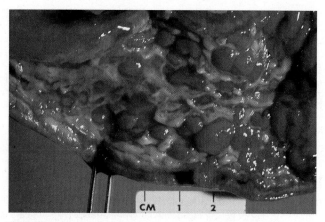

FIGURE 9-29 Crohn disease.
Courtesy of Leonard V. Crowley, MD, Century College.

elevations), giving the intestinal wall a cobblestone appearance (**FIGURE 9-29**). Eventually, the entire wall becomes thick and rigid, and the intestinal lumen becomes narrowed and potentially obstructed. Granulomas—that is, nodules consisting of epithelial and immune cells—develop on the intestinal wall and nearby lymph nodes because of the chronic inflammation. Over time, the damaged intestinal wall loses the ability to process and absorb food. The inflammation also stimulates intestinal motility, decreasing digestion and absorption.

Complications of Crohn disease can include malnutrition; anemia (e.g., iron deficiency); micronutrient deficiencies (e.g., vitamin D); and fluid, electrolyte, and pH imbalances. Intestinal complications can include the development of obstructions (e.g., small bowel), adhesions, abscesses, fistulas (e.g., bowel to bowel, bowel to bladder, bowel to vagina), and perforations.

Clinical Manifestations

Clinical manifestations of Crohn disease reflect the inflammatory process and the digestive dysfunction (Table 9-6). These manifestations, which intensify during exacerbations, include the following symptoms:

Intestinal Manifestations
- Abdominal cramping and pain (typically in the right lower quadrant and may occur with defecation)
- Diarrhea (usually watery)
- Steatorrhea
- Constipation (as the intestinal lumen narrows)
- Palpable abdominal mass (thickened intestinal wall)

| TABLE 9-6 | Comparison of Inflammatory Bowel Disease and Irritable Bowel Syndrome |

	Inflammatory bowel disease		Irritable bowel syndrome
	Ulcerative colitis	**Crohn disease**	
Epidemiology	Gradual, progressive onset	Insidious onset	Late teens/early adulthood
	Peak ages 15 to 30	Ages 15 to 40	
	Whites ≫ Blacks	Female ≫ male	Female ≫ male
	Female ≫ male		
Pathology	Possible autoimmune infection triggers in those with familial tendency	Possible autoimmune infection triggers in those with a genetic predisposition	Cause unknown
	Continuous, irregular superficial inflammation of mucosal layer of colon and rectum	Skipping ulcerations involving mucosal and submucosal layers along the entire GI tract; 80% with small intestine involvement	Increased bowel response to stimuli and visceral hypersensitivity
		Strictures/fistulas common	Altered perception of central nervous system
Signs and Symptoms			
Abdominal pain	Intermittent, mild crampy tenderness	Crampy or steady	Sharp, burning; may be diffuse or left lower quadrant
		Periumbilical or right lower quadrant	
Mass present	No	Common	No
Bleeding	Common	Occasionally	No
Diarrhea	Frequent watery stools with blood and mucus	Chronic, recurrent, may have some blood particularly if colon involved	Intermittent, predominant
			Variation of symptoms with individuals
Perianal lesions	No	One-third develop perianal abscesses or fistulas	No
Weight loss	With severe diarrhea	Common	No
Fever/malaise	During severe exacerbation	With exacerbation and abscess formation	No
Psychological	As a result of long-standing disease	As a result of long-standing disease	Exacerbation with stressful situations
Course/prognosis	75–80% relapse after first attack	Recurrent, progressive	Chronic, intermittent
	Most have mild to moderate disease	Typically need surgery after 7 years to treat/repair fistulas or abscesses	Rare functional limitations
	Routine colonoscopy with biopsy after having the disease for 7–8 years because of increased colon cancer risk	Shortened life span	

- Hematochezia (if ulcers begin bleeding)
- Anorexia
- Perianal fissures/fistulas
- Weight loss
- Delayed growth and development (e.g., poor weight gain)
- Delayed puberty

Extraintestinal Manifestations
- Mouth ulcers
- Arthralgia
- Skin disorders (e.g., erythema nodosum)
- Kidney stones
- Eye inflammation (e.g., uveitis and iritis)

Diagnosis and Treatment

Diagnostic procedures for Crohn disease consist of a history, physical examination, stool analysis (including cultures and occult blood), CBC, blood chemistry with liver enzyme evaluation, C-reactive protein levels, and erythrocyte sedimentation rate. Colonoscopy will be done to evaluate the lower GI tract, while abdominal CT, abdominal MRI, barium studies (swallow and enema), or a capsule endoscopy (use of pill with a camera) may be used to evaluate the small bowel. Biopsies are also performed. Serologic markers (e.g., antineutrophil cytoplasmic antibodies) and stool markers (e.g., calprotectin) are usually done, however the accuracy of these tests is unclear. Treatment strategies focus on nutritional support, symptom relief, and complication minimization. Dietary management usually includes 1) a low-residue, high-calorie, high-protein diet; 2) oral nutritional supplements (e.g., Ensure and Sustacal); 3) multivitamin supplements; and 4) TPN as the disease progresses. Pharmacologic management usually includes 1) antidiarrheal agents; 2) aminosalicylates (5-ASAs; to treat mild to moderate inflammation); 3) glucocorticoids (to treat moderate to severe inflammation); 4) immune modulators (e.g., thiopurines and tumor necrosis factor-α blocking agents) to suppress inflammatory response); 5) biologic agents (e.g., infliximab or adalimumab; to treat severe unresponsive Crohn disease); 6) analgesics; and 7) antibiotics if infection is present. Surgical intestine resection may be necessary as the disease progresses and complications develop. Additional strategies involve stress management (e.g., exercise, meditation, deep breathing, biofeedback, and acupuncture) and support (e.g., group involvement and counseling). There may be an increased risk for certain cancers (e.g., colon cancer), so appropriate screenings should be conducted.

Ulcerative Colitis

Ulcerative colitis is a progressive condition of the rectum and colon mucosa that usually develops in the second or third decade of life. Inflammation triggered by T-cell accumulation in the colon mucosa causes epithelium loss, surface erosion, and ulceration. The ulceration begins in the rectum and extends in a continuous segment to involve the entire colon. Ulcerative colitis rarely affects the small intestine. The mucosa becomes inflamed, edematous, and frail. Necrosis of the epithelial tissue (specifically at the base of the crypts of Lieberkühn) can result in abscesses, known as crypt abscesses. As the body attempts to heal, granulation tissue forms, but the tissue remains fragile and bleeds easily. The ulcers merge together, creating large areas of stripped mucosa. Nutritional, fluid, electrolyte, and pH imbalances develop due to the lack of an

adequate surface area for absorption. Complications of ulcerative colitis include the following conditions: malnutrition; anemia (e.g., iron deficiency); micronutrient deficiencies (e.g., vitamin D); and fluid, electrolyte, and pH imbalances. Intestinal complications can include the development of strictures and fistulas (e.g., bowel to bowel, bowel to bladder, bowel to vagina), pseudopolyps, perforations, and hemorrhage. Toxic megacolon is a life-threatening condition caused by rapid dilation of the large intestine and systemic toxicity (e.g., fever, tachycardia, leukocytosis). Liver disease can occur as a result of inflammation and scarring of the bile ducts.

Clinical Manifestations

Clinical manifestations of ulcerative colitis reflect the inflammatory process and digestive dysfunction, and symptoms can range from mild to severe (Table 9-6). As is the case with Crohn disease, these manifestations intensify during exacerbations. Manifestations usually include the following symptoms:

Intestinal Manifestations

- Diarrhea (usually frequent [as many as 20 daily], watery stools containing blood and mucus)
- Tenesmus (persistent rectal spasms associated with the need to defecate) and urgency
- Proctitis (inflammation of the rectum)
- Abdominal cramping
- Nausea and vomiting
- Weight loss

Extraintestinal Manifestations

- Arthralgia
- Skin disorders (e.g., erythema nodosum)
- Eye inflammation (e.g., uveitis, iritis)

Diagnosis and Treatment

Diagnostic procedures for ulcerative colitis are the same as those for Crohn disease. Treatment strategies are also similar to those used for Crohn disease and focus on nutritional support, symptom relief, and complication minimization. Dietary management usually includes 1) a high-fiber, high-calorie, high-protein diet; 2) oral nutritional supplements (e.g., Ensure or Sustacal); 3) multivitamin supplements; and 4) TPN as the disease progresses. Pharmacologic management usually includes 1) antidiarrheal agents; 2) antispasmodics;

3) anticholinergics; 4) aminosalicylates to treat mild to moderate inflammation; 5) glucocorticoids to treat moderate to severe inflammation; 6) immune modulators to suppress inflammatory response; 7) biologic agents; 8) analgesics; and 9) antibiotics if infection is present. Surgical intervention (e.g., ileostomy or colostomy) may be necessary as the disease progresses and complications develop. Additional strategies involve stress management (e.g., exercise, meditation, deep breathing, biofeedback, and acupuncture) and support (e.g., group involvement and counseling). There may be an increased risk for certain cancers (e.g., colon cancer), so appropriate screenings should be conducted.

Irritable Bowel Syndrome

Irritable bowel syndrome (IBS) refers to a chronic functional GI condition characterized by exacerbations often associated with stress. IBS includes alterations in bowel pattern and abdominal pain not explained by structural or biochemical abnormalities. IBS is similar to IBD, but in contrast to IBD, IBS is less serious, is noninflammatory, and does not cause permanent intestinal damage (Table 9-6). IBS is more common in women than in men. Its exact cause is unknown, but three theories of its etiology include altered GI motility, visceral hyperalgesia, and psychopathology. IBS is thought to be an intensified response to stimuli that is characterized by increased intestinal motility and contractions. People with IBS may have a low tolerance for stretching and pain in the intestinal smooth muscle, causing them to respond to stimuli to which people without IBS do not respond. Evolving theories of the pathogenesis include a possible role of inflammation, an alteration in the intestinal microbiota, food sensitivity, and possible genetic predisposition. IBS is associated with other conditions such as fibromyalgia, GERD, depression, and anxiety. Complications of IBS include hemorrhoids, nutritional deficits, social issues, and sexual discomfort.

Clinical Manifestations

Clinical manifestations vary from person to person. Stress, mood disorders (e.g., anxiety and depression), food, and hormone changes (e.g., menstruation) often worsen symptoms. These manifestations usually include the following symptoms:

- Abdominal distention, fullness, flatus, and bloating

- Intermittent, abdominal, crampy pain exacerbated by eating and relieved by defecation
- Chronic and frequent constipation, usually accompanied by pain (i.e., Bristol stool chart type 1 and 2)
- Chronic and frequent diarrhea, usually accompanied by pain (i.e., Bristol stool chart type 6 and 7)
- Alternating diarrhea and constipation with or without interspersed normal bowel habits
- Nonbloody stool that may contain mucus
- Bowel urgency and tenesmus
- Sensation of incomplete emptying after a bowel movement
- Intolerance to certain foods (usually gas-forming foods and those containing sorbitol, lactose, and gluten)
- Emotional distress
- Anorexia

Diagnosis and Treatment

Diagnosis is based on clinical presentation (**TABLE 9-7**) and is often made by excluding other GI disorders. Diagnostic procedures consist of a history and physical examination which is generally normal. The diagnosis of IBS is made using the Rome IV criteria. Diagnostic testing is not necessary for the diagnosis of IBS, but tests are performed to exclude other diagnoses. These tests can include stool analysis (including cultures and occult blood), celiac blood panel, C-reactive protein, abdominal X-ray, abdominal CT, abdominal MRI, barium studies (swallow and enema),

TABLE 9-7	**Rome IV Criteria**

Recurrent abdominal pain on average at least 1 day/week in the last 3 months, associated with two or more of the following criteria:

1. Relieved by defecation
2. Associated with changes in stool frequency
3. Associated with changes in stool form (appearance)

Symptoms That Support Diagnosis of IBS

Abnormal stool frequency (> 3/day or > 3/week)

Abnormal stool form (lumpy and hard or watery and loose)

Abnormal stool passage (straining, urgency, feeling of incomplete evacuation)

Passage of mucus

Bloating or feeling of abdominal distention

sigmoidoscopy, colonoscopy, and biopsy. Diagnostic testing should be performed for those patients with concerning symptoms usually not associated with IBS such as unexplained weight loss, rectal bleeding, age of onset after age 50, nocturnal diarrhea, progressive abdominal pain, laboratory abnormalities (e.g., iron deficiency anemia), or family history of IBD or GI cancer.

Treatment focuses on management of symptoms and may vary depending on those symptoms. Initial therapies involve dietary modification with avoidance of gas-producing foods (e.g., beans, bananas, carrots, celery). The FODMAP diet (fermentable oligo-, di-, monosaccharides, and polyols) involves reduction or exclusion of short-chain carbohydrates that are poorly absorbed or that increase osmosis. In some cases, lactose and gluten avoidance may improve symptoms. Maintaining a regular eating pattern and avoiding large meals is recommended. Other strategies involve avoiding triggers, stress management (through techniques such as exercise, meditation, deep breathing, biofeedback, and acupuncture), and support (e.g., group involvement, counseling, and psychotherapy). Pharmacologic strategies for abdominal pain can include antispasmodics and antidepressants. Pharmacologic agents for constipation may include laxatives (e.g., psyllium), chloride channel activators (e.g., lubiprostone [Amitiza]), which works by increasing intestinal fluid and intestinal motility, or guanylate cyclase agonists (e.g., linaclotide [Linzess]) which work by increasing intestinal fluid and intestinal transit. Pharmacologic strategies for diarrhea may include antidiarrheal agents (e.g., loperamide) and bile acid sequestrants. Eluxadoline (Viberzi) is a mu-opioid receptor agonist and delta-opioid receptor antagonist that can be used for IBS related diarrhea. Probiotics can be used, however, their efficacy is uncertain.

Diverticular Disease

Diverticular disease refers to conditions related to the development of diverticula. Diverticula (singular, *diverticulum*) are outwardly bulging pouches of the intestinal wall that develop when mucosa sections or large intestine submucosa layers herniate through a weak point in the muscular layer (e.g., where arteries penetrate the muscle layer) (**FIGURE 9-30**). Diverticula may be congenital or acquired. The causes of diverticula development are unknown, but they are thought to be caused by abnormal motility of the colon. In those patients with diverticula, the colon exhibits exaggerated segmental contractions and increased intraluminal pressure. The reasons for the abnormal motility are unclear, but the increased pressure may occur as a result of structural changes in the intestinal wall (e.g., thickened circular muscle layer and luminal narrowing). The incidence increases after age 60. Risk factors for the development of symptoms include a diet low in fiber and high in red meat and fat, obesity, physical inactivity, smoking, and medications (e.g., steroids, opiates, and NSAIDs). Diverticular disease is rare in developing countries where high-fiber diets are typical but is more common in developed countries where processed foods and low-fiber diets are widely consumed. In addition to diet, poor bowel habits (e.g., straining and delaying defecation) can contribute to developing diverticula.

Meckel diverticulum is a common congenital malformation of the GI tract that results in herniation of all layers of the small bowel wall, not just the mucosa as in diverticular disease. Meckel diverticulum can be described using the rule of 2s—the incidence occurs in approximately 2% of the population; the male-to-female ratio is 2:1; the diverticulum is found 2 feet from the ileocecal valve and is 2 inches long; and approximately 2% develop a complication over their lifetime, typically before the age of 2. Meckel diverticulum usually causes no symptoms. If symptoms occur, they usually consist of GI bleeding, abdominal pain, or perforation signs. Surgery (e.g., small bowel resection and simple diverticulectomy) is performed for those patients with symptoms.

Most cases of diverticular disease are asymptomatic and are discovered incidentally. Diverticulosis describes asymptomatic diverticular disease, usually with multiple diverticula present. Diverticulitis refers to a state in which diverticula have become inflamed. The wall of the diverticula erodes due to the increased pressure and food particles that are thick or hardened. Focal necrosis and perforation, usually microperforations, occur in addition to inflammation. Diverticulitis can be acute or chronic. While some cases of diverticulitis are uncomplicated, several serious complications can occur, such as obstructions, infection, abscess (usually due to a walled-off perforation), fistula, large perforation, peritonitis (e.g., fecal peritonitis), hemorrhage, and shock.

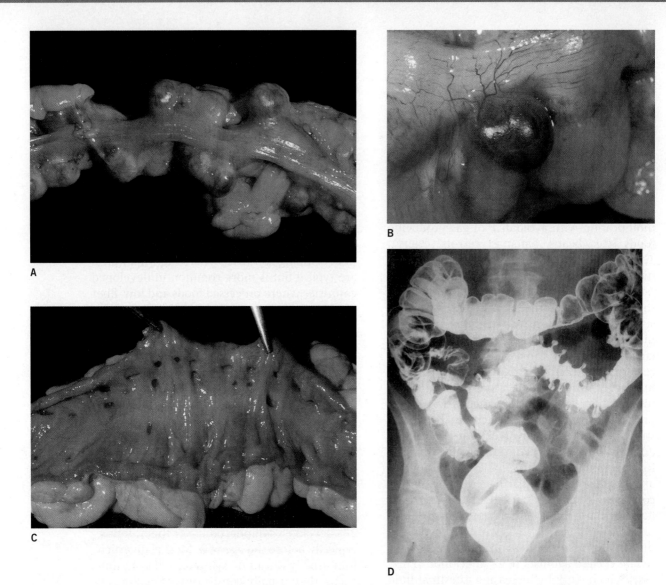

FIGURE 9-30 Diverticula. **(A)** Exterior of the colon illustrating several diverticula projecting through the wall of the colon. **(B)** A closer view of the diverticulum. **(C)** Interior of the colon, illustrating openings of multiple diverticula. **(D)** Diverticula of the colon demonstrated by injection of barium contrast material into the colon.

Courtesy of Leonard V. Crowley, MD, Century College.

Clinical Manifestations

Diverticulitis usually manifests with abdominal tenderness (often in the left lower quadrant). However, cecal diverticulitis is more common in Asian populations and will present with right lower quadrant pain. The pain is constant and may be present for days before the patient seeks care. Other clinical manifestations that may be present include a low-grade fever, abdominal distention, constipation, diarrhea, nausea, vomiting, a palpable abdominal mass, and leukocytosis. While diverticulosis is generally asymptomatic, painless bleeding (hematochezia) that is usually mild and self-limiting can occur, but it can be more severe. Diverticular disease may also present with

persistent abdominal pain without inflammation (i.e., smoldering diverticulitis).

Diagnosis and Treatment

Diverticula are often noted on diagnostic imaging performed for other purposes such as colonoscopy for colorectal cancer screening. During an episode of acute diverticulitis, diagnostic procedures consist of a history, physical examination, and an abdominal CT with contrast (preferred) or abdominal ultrasound. Laboratory studies will include a CBC, and a finding of leukocytosis is consistent with acute disease. Complicated acute diverticulitis requires inpatient treatment with management of complications (e.g., obstruction). Other

[handwritten notes:] ! Hx: ~~Ree~~ Constipation ↑ Risk / Ask about frequency of diverticulitis - each time bowel thins ↑ RC: perf.

inpatient management will include administration of intravenous antibiotics, pain medications, and intravenous fluids. Bowel rest may be necessary, or oral nutrition should start with clear liquid diet, advancing to a regular diet. Outpatient care will consist of oral antibiotics and modified diet if necessary. With outpatient care, short-term follow-up is important (e.g., repeat evaluation in 2–3 days).

Long-term treatment strategies include consumption of a high-fiber diet, adequate hydration, proper bowel habits (e.g., defecating when urge is sensed and not straining). A low-residue diet (i.e., avoiding foods with seeds, nuts, and corn) is thought to help, but no evidence supports this notion. Consuming nuts, seeds, and corn also do not *cause* diverticular disease. A colon resection may be necessary for some patients whose symptoms do not resolve.

Cancers

Malignancies of the GI system may originate in the GI tract or spread there from other sites. These cancers can lead to altered nutrition as well as impaired elimination depending on their location. Some GI cancers have moderate treatment success rates (e.g., colorectal cancer), whereas others have high mortality rates (e.g., oral and pancreatic cancer). Typical cancer diagnosis, staging, and treatments are usually employed with cancers involving the GI system (see chapter 1 for details on cellular function).

Oral Cancer

Oral cancer can occur anywhere in the mouth, but most cases involve squamous cell carcinomas of the tongue and mouth floor (FIGURE 9-31). Approximately 75% of cases can be attributed to use of smoked and smokeless tobacco. Alcohol consumption also significantly increases the risk of developing oral cancer. Combined alcohol and tobacco use can increase this risk by as much as 100 times. Chewing areca nuts (from an areca palm) also increases the of oral cancer. Additional risk factors include viral infections (especially with human papillomavirus), immunodeficiencies, inadequate nutrition, poor dental hygiene, chronic irritation (e.g., from dentures), and exposure to ultraviolet light (as in cancer of the lips).

Incidence rates of oral cancer have slightly decreased since 1980. Men are twice as likely as women to develop oral cancer. According to the American Cancer Society (2016), oral cancer is the eighth most frequent cancer in men.

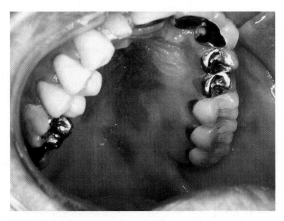

FIGURE 9-31 Oral cancer.
Courtesy of Sol Silverman, Jr., DDS, University of California, San Francisco/CDC.

Prevalence and mortality rates are the highest in Black men; however, overall mortality rates have decreased since 1980.

In its early stages, oral cancer is very treatable. Unfortunately, most cases are advanced by the time the diagnosis is made because the cancer tends to be hidden. Oral cancer has a 5-year survival rate of 63%—a rate that has significantly improved since 1990.

Oral cancer is often preceded by premalignant lesions that appear as a white patch (leukoplakia) or a red patch (erythroplakia) that is usually persistent (e.g., > 3 weeks) and asymptomatic. These lesions then develop into a nodule or an ulcerative lesion. Multiple lesions may be present. These lesions persist, do not heal, and bleed easily. Additional manifestations include a lump, thickening, or soreness in the mouth, throat, or tongue as well as difficulty chewing or swallowing food. Oral cancer often metastasizes to the neck lymph nodes and the esophagus.

Treatment primarily consists of surgery and radiation, but surgery may be difficult depending on the location. Chemotherapy may be added for patients with advanced disease. Speech therapy is often necessary after treatment to improve chewing, swallowing, and speech.

Esophageal Cancer

Much like oral cancer, esophageal cancer is usually a squamous cell carcinoma or adenocarcinoma, and it most often affects men. Incidence rates of esophageal cancer have remained steady, but the mortality rates have increased since 1980. According to the American Cancer Society (2016), esophageal cancer is the seventh leading cause of cancer death in men, even though it did not make the list of top 10 cancers in men. Rates are fairly equal across racial and ethnic groups.

The distal esophagus is the most common site at which this adenocarcinoma develops, and the middle esophagus is a more common location for squamous cell carcinoma. Esophageal cancer is associated with chronic irritation (e.g., GERD, achalasia, hiatal hernia, alcohol abuse, and use of smoked and smokeless tobacco), obesity, and Barrett esophagus. Smoking and alcohol abuse are major risk factors for squamous cell carcinoma, but Barrett esophagus is the most common risk factor for adenocarcinoma. These tumors can grow to match the circumference of the esophagus, creating a stricture, or they can grow out into the lumen of the esophagus, creating an obstruction. Complications include esophageal obstruction, respiratory compromise, and esophageal bleeding.

Esophageal cancer is usually asymptomatic in its early stages, delaying its diagnosis and treatment. Because of the usually late diagnosis, the prognosis is poor for patients with esophageal cancer. Clinical manifestations, when present, typically include dysphagia and weight loss. Other signs can include odynophagia, chest pain (not related to eating), hematemesis, hoarseness/cough due to laryngeal nerve compression, and halitosis. Chronic blood loss may cause iron deficiency anemia. Endoscopy with a biopsy is necessary to confirm the diagnosis. Surgery is the treatment of choice, but chemotherapy and radiation are also frequently included in management. Speech therapy will likely be necessary following treatment.

Gastric Cancer

Gastric cancer occurs in several forms, but adenocarcinoma (an ulcerative lesion) is the most frequently encountered type. Incidence and mortality rates of gastric cancer in the United States have declined since 1980. Nevertheless, gastric cancer remains extremely prevalent worldwide (it is the fifth most common type of cancer) and is the third most deadly cancer worldwide (WHO, 2015). Japan has particularly high rates of gastric cancer. Gastric cancer is prevalent in men and Asians and Pacific Islanders, but mortality rates are highest among Black men. Gastric cancer has a 5-year survival rate of approximately 29%.

Gastric cancer is strongly associated with increased intake of salted, cured, pickled, preserved (containing nitrates and nitrites), and smoked foods. A low-fiber diet and constipation can increase the risk of developing this cancer because they prolong the time over which the intestinal wall is exposed to these substances. Additional risk factors include family history, *H. pylori* infections, smoking, alcohol consumption, obesity, pernicious anemia, Epstein-Barr virus (in some populations), chronic atrophic gastritis, gastric ulcers, and gastric polyps. A small percentage (1–3%) of gastric cancers are familial.

Gastric cancer is asymptomatic, or symptoms may be nonspecific in its early stages, which often delays its diagnosis and treatment. Nonspecific symptoms can include dyspepsia, nausea, decreased appetite, and mild epigastric pain. When present, clinical manifestations include the following symptoms:

- Abdominal pain and fullness
- Epigastric discomfort
- Palpable abdominal mass
- Dark stools, possibly melena
- Dysphagia that worsens over time
- Excessive belching
- Anorexia
- Nausea and vomiting
- Hematemesis
- Premature abdominal fullness after meals
- Unintentional weight loss
- Weakness and fatigue

Endoscopy with biopsy confirms the diagnosis. Additionally, barium studies may be necessary. Surgical removal of the stomach (gastrectomy) is the only curative treatment. Endoscopic resection may be done in certain cases (e.g., early stages, no lymph node involvement). Chemotherapy and radiation are also used as curative and palliative measures. *H. pylori* infection should be treated. Nutritional support (e.g., TPN) and supplements (e.g., vitamin B_{12} and iron) will be needed before, during, and after treatment. Screening for gastric cancer with contrast radiography and upper endoscopy is being performed in some countries with a high incidence (e.g., Japan and Korea).

Liver Cancer

Liver cancer most commonly occurs as a secondary tumor that has metastasized from the breast, lung, or other GI structures (FIGURE 9-32). Incidence and mortality rates of liver cancer in the United States have tripled since 1980. According to the American Cancer Society (2016), liver cancer is the 10th most common cancer in men and the 5th deadliest cancer in men. Worldwide, liver cancer is the 2nd most common cancer (WHO, 2015). Most primary tumors (termed *hepatocellular carcinomas*) are caused by chronic cirrhosis or

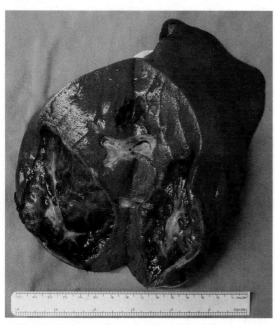

FIGURE 9-32 Liver cancer.
© Medicine-R/Shutterstock.

hepatitis infection (HBV and HCV). Liver cancer is most prevalent among men as well as Asians and Pacific Islanders. It has a 5-year survival rate of approximately 17%.

Liver cancer may either be asymptomatic or produce mild symptoms initially. Clinical manifestations are similar to those of other liver diseases:

- Anorexia
- Fever
- Jaundice
- Nausea and vomiting
- Abdominal pain (usually in the upper right quadrant)
- Hepatomegaly
- Splenomegaly
- Portal hypertension
- Edema, third spacing (accumulation of fluid in tissue or body cavities), and ascites
- Paraneoplastic syndrome (manifestations and diseases that result from cancer such as hypoglycemia, hypercalcemia, and severe diarrhea)
- Diaphoresis
- Weight loss

Treatment strategies vary depending on the primary site and progression of the cancer. Chemotherapy is used systemically when metastasis is evident or may be injected directly into localized tumors. Common sites of metastasis are the heart and the lung. Other areas are the brain, kidney, and spleen. If the tumor is small, a section of the liver may be surgically removed (a procedure called a *hepatectomy*). If the cancer has spread throughout the liver or has caused significant damage, a liver transplant will be the best option if metastasis has not occurred. Several nontraditional cancer treatment procedures are also available to treat liver cancer. Cryoablation is a procedure that uses extreme cold to destroy cancer cells by injecting liquid nitrogen into the tumor. Radiofrequency ablation uses electric current to heat and destroy cancer cells. Pure alcohol can also be injected into the tumor to dry and eventually kill the cancer cells.

Pancreatic Cancer

Pancreatic cancer is an aggressive malignancy—most commonly a ductal adenocarcinoma that arises from exocrine cells. Endocrine tumors (in the islets of Langerhans) are rare. Pancreatic cancer can quickly spread to nearby structures (e.g., stomach, intestines, spleen, liver, and lungs). Its incidence and mortality rates have remained steady since 1980. According to the American Cancer Society (2016), pancreatic cancer is the ninth most common cancer in women, and it is the fourth leading cause of cancer deaths in men and women.

Pancreatic cancer occurs most frequently in men and Blacks. Other risk factors include family history, obesity, chronic pancreatitis, long-standing diabetes mellitus, cirrhosis, alcohol abuse, and tobacco use. Inherited susceptibility may occur in those individuals with non-O blood groups (e.g., type A, AB, or B).

The overall 5-year survival rate for this disease is a mere 7%. This dismal prognosis is due largely to the asymptomatic nature of pancreatic cancer and the lack of a reliable early detection method. Clinical manifestations do not generally develop until the cancer is well advanced and has metastasized, delaying diagnosis and treatment. These manifestations may include the following signs and symptoms:

- Upper abdominal (usually epigastric) pain that may radiate to the back (pain worsens as cancer progresses), has insidious onset, is intermittent, and worse with eating or lying supine
- Jaundice, often with pruritus, dark urine, and clay-colored stools
- Steatorrhea
- Indigestion
- Anorexia
- Weight loss

- Depression
- Malnutrition
- Hyperglycemia or recent onset of diabetes mellitus
- Increased clotting tendencies

No effective treatment has been developed for pancreatic cancer. Pancreaticoduodenectomy (Whipple procedure) is recommended for decompression of obstructed ducts. Surgical resection of tumors or total pancreatectomy may be performed, but tumor recurrence rate can be high. Chemotherapy and radiation are often used as palliative treatment or in combination with surgery. Biliary blockages that develop may require repair through surgery or endoscopy. Pain management and nutritional support are often necessary. As with other life-limiting diseases, palliative care is important.

Colorectal Cancer

Colorectal cancer (CRC) most often develops from an adenomatous polyp. The large bowel is the most common site for cancer development, with a smaller proportion affecting the rectum. A majority of the tumors are adenocarcinomas. According to WHO (2015), CRC is the fourth most common cancer worldwide. According to the American Cancer Society (2016), CRC is the third most common and most fatal cancer in men and women in the United States, although its rates have been declining since 1980. Incidence and mortality rates are the highest among men and Blacks. The 5-year survival rate for CRC is a robust 65%.

Dietary factors that have been associated with CRC include excessive intake of fat, calories, red meat, processed meat, and alcohol as well as deficient intake of fiber. Other risk factors involve genetics, family history (e.g., familial adenomatous polyposis has a 100% risk of CRC as well as hereditary nonpolyposis CRC), advancing age, obesity, tobacco use, physical inactivity, IBD, and history of abdominal irradiation.

Like many other GI cancers, CRC remains asymptomatic until it is well advanced. Manifestations are also dependent on the location of the tumor (the right side includes the cecum and ascending colon, and the left side includes the descending colon). When present, clinical manifestations may include the following symptoms:

- Lower abdominal pain and tenderness
- Blood in the stool (occult or frank)
- Diarrhea, constipation, or other change in bowel habits

- Intestinal obstruction
- Narrow stools
- Unexplained anemia (usually iron-deficiency anemia)
- Unintentional weight loss

Routine screening can dramatically improve prognosis. The 5-year survival rate for colorectal cancer if detected when it is localized to the large intestine is approximately 90%. The U.S. Preventive Services Task Force (2016) recommends regular colorectal screening beginning at 50 years of age for both sexes (earlier if risk factors are present). The American Cancer Society lowered the recommended age for screening to 45 for people at average risks in 2018 (Wolf et. al, 2018). The screening tests and recommended intervals depending on test performed are identified here:

- A high-sensitivity fecal occult blood test (which checks for hidden blood in three consecutive stool samples) should be administered every year.
- A fecal immunochemical test (which is more accurate than the fecal occult blood test) should be administered every year.
- A fecal immunochemical test for DNA should be administered every 1–3 years.
- Flexible sigmoidoscopy should be administered every 5 years.
- CT colonography (i.e., virtual colonoscopy) should be administered every 5 years
- Colonoscopy (preferred screening test) should be administered every 10 years.

During colonoscopy, adenomatous polyps can be removed (polypectomy). Progression from a polyp to cancer can occur over 10-15 years, but hereditary nonpolyposis can progress over a shorter time (e.g., 3 years). Colonoscopy is also used as a diagnostic test when symptoms are present, and it can be used as a follow-up test when the results of another colorectal cancer screening test are unclear or abnormal. Additionally, early (stage 0) cancer cells can be removed during the colonoscopy.

Cancers stage I through III require extensive surgery (colon resection). Chemotherapy and radiation use vary depending on the cancer stage. The patient may require a temporary or permanent colostomy (usually with lower rectal tumors) because of the colon resection. Because colorectal cancer often reoccurs, lifestyle changes (e.g., diet and physical activity) and follow-up screenings are crucial to long-term survival.

BOX 9-3 Application to Practice

In which of the following cases would gastrointestinal cancer be a risk and what would be the likely type of cancer?

1. A 40-year-old man who smokes and has a duodenal ulcer.
2. A 50-year-old woman with long-standing GERD and recent evidence of Barrett esophagus on upper endoscopy.
3. A 60-year-old obese woman with a history of alcohol abuse and chronic pancreatitis.
4. A 25-year-old man who contracted hepatitis A on an international trip.
5. A 60-year-old woman with type 2 diabetes mellitus and a history of long-standing constipation and consuming one or two alcoholic drinks every other day.
6. A 25-year-old with a history of Hashimoto thyroiditis and Crohn disease.

BOX 9-4 Application to Practice

Now that we have discussed conditions of the GI system, let us put that knowledge into practice. While working in the clinic, you encounter the following patients. Which patient would be at greatest risk for developing an intestinal obstruction?

- An adult diagnosed with cirrhosis of the liver
- An individual eating a low-fiber, high-fat diet
- A Jewish patient who smokes and consumes large amounts of caffeine
- An elderly patient who is on bed rest because of postoperative abdominal surgery

When determining who is at greatest risk, just start counting risk factors—the patient with the most risk factors "wins." Here, we start with the adult with cirrhosis. This patient has no risk factors for developing an intestinal obstruction. The patient with a low-fiber, high-fat diet may be at risk because consuming low-fiber diet can put individuals at risk for constipation. Keep this patient on the short list. Next, consider the Jewish patient. This patient does not have any risk factors, so eliminate this individual. Finally, the elderly patient has three risk factors—advancing age, immobility, and abdominal surgery. With three risk factors, the elderly patient is at the most risk for developing an intestinal obstruction.

CHAPTER SUMMARY

The GI system is responsible for ingestion, absorption, and removal of food. These functions obtain the essential nutrients, water, and electrolytes the body needs to maintain many physiologic activities and homeostasis. Disorders of the GI tract range in severity from harmless to life threatening. These disorders can be congenital, infectious, structural, or cancerous in nature. Regardless of the pathogenesis, GI disorders often create short- or long-term nutritional deficits or elimination issues that can affect the individual's overall health. Promoting GI health focuses primarily on dietary strategies that include following a well-balanced diet, reducing alcohol consumption, and maintaining a healthy weight. Other lifestyle factors to promote GI health includes avoiding smoking and engaging in regular physical activity. CRC screening is highly effective and should commence at the age of 50.

REFERENCES AND RESOURCES

American Cancer Society. (2016). Cancer facts and figures 2016. Retrieved from http://www.cancer.org/acs/groups/content/@research/documents/document/acspc-047079.pdf

Anand, B. (2015). Peptic ulcer disease. *Medscape.* Retrieved from http://emedicine.medscape.com/article/181753-overview#a3

Buggs, A., & Dronen, S. (2014). Viral hepatitis. *Medscape.* Retrieved from http://emedicine.medscape.com/article/775507-overview

Centers for Disease Control and Prevention (CDC). (2017a). Facts about cleft lip and cleft palate. Retrieved from http://www.cdc.gov/ncbddd/birthdefects/CleftLip.html

Centers for Disease Control and Prevention (CDC). (2017b). Facts about esophageal atresia. Retrieved from https://www.cdc.gov/ncbddd/birthdefects/esophagealatresia.html

Centers for Disease Control and Prevention (CDC). (2015b). Viral hepatitis surveillance, United States 2014. Retrieved from https://www.cdc.gov/hepatitis/statistics/2014surveillance/pdfs/2014hepsurveillancerpt.pdf

Chiras, D. (2015). *Human biology* (8th ed.). Burlington, MA: Jones & Bartlett Learning.

Crowley, L. V. (2017). *An introduction to human disease* (10th ed.). Burlington, MA: Jones & Bartlett Learning.

Elling, B., Elling, K., & Rothenberg, M. (2004). *Anatomy and physiology.* Sudbury, MA: Jones and Bartlett Publishers.

Gould, B. (2015). *Pathophysiology for the health professions* (5th ed.). Philadelphia, PA: Elsevier.

Heuman, D., Allen, J., & Mihas, A. (2016). Gallstones (cholelithiasis). *Medscape.* Retrieved from http://emedicine.medscape.com/article/175667-overview#a1

Hoffenberg, E. J., Furuta, G. T., Kobak, G., Walker, T., Soden, J., Kramer, R. E., & Brumbaugh, D. Gastrointestinal tract. In W. W. Hay, Jr., M. J. Levin, R. R. Deterding,

M. J. Abzug (Eds.), *Current diagnosis & treatment: Pediatrics* (24th ed.). New York, NY: McGraw-Hill. Retrieved from http://accessmedicine.mhmedical.com.ezproxy.fiu.edu/content.aspx?bookid=2390&sectionid=189079593

Madara, B., & Pomarico-Denino, V. (2008). *Quick look nursing: Pathophysiology* (2nd ed.). Sudbury, MA: Jones and Bartlett Publishers.

Professional guide to pathophysiology (3rd ed.). (2010). Philadelphia, PA: Lippincott Williams & Wilkins.

Singh, J., & Sinert, R. (2015). Pediatric pyloric stenosis. *Medscape.* Retrieved from http://emedicine.medscape.com/article/803489-overview#a6

U.S. Preventive Services Task Force. (2016). Colorectal cancer: Screening recommendations. Retrieved from http://www.uspreventiveservicestaskforce.org/Page/Document/UpdateSummaryFinal/colorectal-cancer-screening2?ds=1&s=colorectal

Valle, J. (2018). Peptic ulcer disease and related disorders. In J. Jameson, A. S. Fauci, D. L. Kasper, S. L. Hauser, D. L. Longo, & J. Loscalzo (Eds.), *Harrison's principles of internal medicine* (20th ed.). New York, NY: McGraw-Hill.

Wolf, D. (2015). Cirrhosis. *Medscape.* Retrieved from http://emedicine.medscape.com/article/185856-overview#a1

Wolf, A. M., Fontham, E. T., Church, T. R., Flowers, C. R., Guerra, C. E., LaMonte, S. J., Etzioni, R., McKenna, M. T., Oeffinger, K. C., Shih, Y. T., Walter, L. C., Andrews, K. S., Brawley, O. W., Brooks, D., Fedewa, S. A., Manassaram-Baptiste, D., Siegel, R. L., Wender, R. C. and Smith, R. A. (2018), Colorectal cancer screening for average-risk adults: 2018 guideline update from the American Cancer Society. CA: A Cancer Journal for Clinicians, 68: 250-281. doi:10.3322/caac.21457

World Health Organization (WHO). (2015). Cancer fact sheet. Retrieved from http://www.who.int/mediacentre/factsheets/fs297/en/

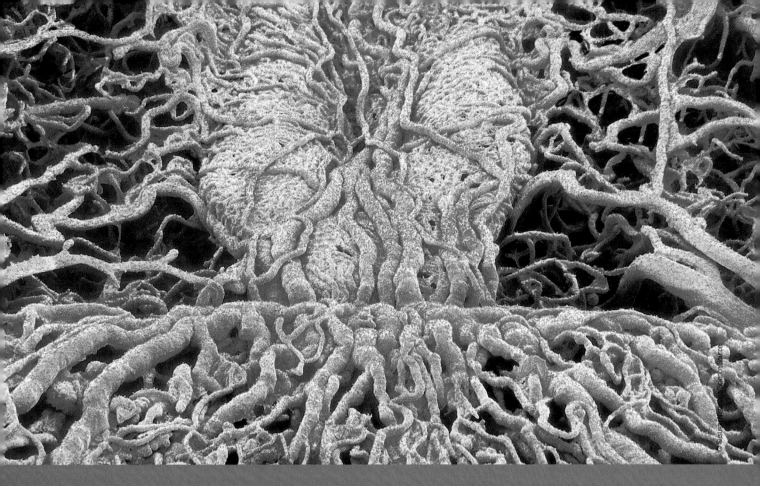

CHAPTER 10
Endocrine Function

LEARNING OBJECTIVES

- Discuss normal endocrine anatomy and physiology.
- Differentiate disorders of the hypothalamus and pituitary gland.
- Explain the pathogenesis, consequences, and complications of diabetes mellitus.
- Differentiate the types of diabetes mellitus.
- Differentiate disorders of the thyroid gland.

- Differentiate disorders of the parathyroid gland.
- Differentiate disorders of the adrenal glands.
- Apply understanding of endocrine system alterations in describing various common disorders such as diabetes mellitus, hypothyroidism, hyperthyroidism.
- Develop diagnostic and treatment considerations for various endocrine disorders.

The endocrine system consists of glands located throughout the body (FIGURE 10-1) that are responsible for producing and secreting a wide range of hormones and chemical transmitters. These hormones serve as chemical messengers, traveling to various sites to regulate several processes, including 1) growth and development, 2) metabolism, 3) sexual function, 4) reproduction, and 5) mood stability. Hormones influence these processes by binding to receptors on the surface or within their target cells. Only small amounts of these potent substances are required to make a significant impact at the cellular and organism levels. Consequently, subtle fluctuations in hormone levels can disrupt the body's delicate balance. Disorders of the endocrine system can result from insufficient or excessive amounts of these hormones that alter their specific function. Causes of these disorders vary but include genetic alterations, lifestyle behaviors, and tumors. The severity of these endocrine disorders can range from mild conditions that are easily managed to life-shortening or life-threatening conditions.

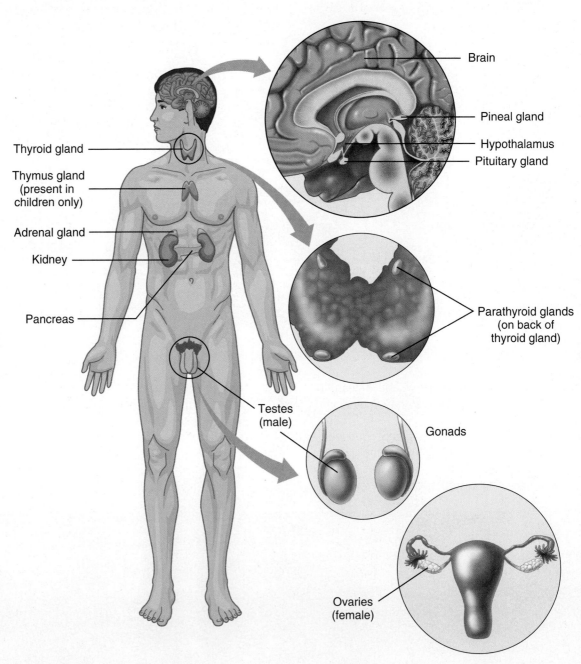

FIGURE 10-1 The human endocrine system.

Anatomy and Physiology

Hormonal Regulation

The endocrine system is a complex messaging and control system that interacts with several body functions. It uses hormones to orchestrate these multifaceted communication and control operations. Endocrine glands located throughout the body produce and secrete these hormones. The term *endocrine* refers to the act of secreting substances directly into the bloodstream (**FIGURE 10-2**) rather than in a duct (like the exocrine glands of the gastrointestinal tract). In addition to these structures, reproductive glands (e.g., testes and ovaries) produce hormones (see chapter 8 for more on reproductive function).

Hormones can be classified or described in regard to their action (e.g., altering serum and glucose levels), source (e.g., anterior pituitary gland), or chemical structure. They can also be divided into four categories based on chemical composition: 1) steroids (e.g., androgens,

glucocorticoids, and thyroid hormones), which are lipid soluble; 2) proteins or polypeptides (e.g., insulin and growth hormone), which are water soluble; 3) amines and amino acids (e.g., epinephrine), which are water soluble; and 4) fatty acid derivatives (e.g., prostaglandins).

Hormone release is influenced by the nervous system (e.g., autonomic control of beta cells), other chemical substances (e.g., glucose and sodium), and one endocrine gland influencing another (e.g., the adrenal cortex influences pancreatic secretions). Hormone secretion can also occur in various patterns (e.g., circadian or pulsatile). Release of hormones from their respective glands is primarily controlled by a negative feedback system but may occasionally be controlled by a positive feedback system. In a negative feedback loop, the product (in this case, hormones) of a biochemical process inhibits its own production—the hormone is released only when its levels decline, and production stops when its levels rise (e.g., insulin is released

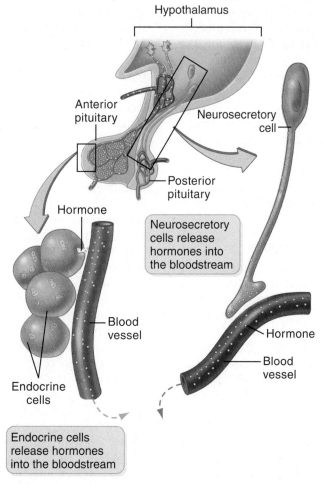

FIGURE 10-2 Endocrine release of hormones.

in response to serum glucose levels). In the endocrine system, a positive feedback loop is rare and occurs when the hormone is released when levels are high, and production stops when its levels are low (e.g., the release of oxytocin during childbirth). Tropic hormones regulate endocrine glands to produce other hormones (e.g., thyroid-stimulating hormone). Nontropic hormones (e.g., cortisol) directly stimulate cellular metabolism and other activities.

Once released from the gland, hormones travel through the circulatory system to their target cells in other glands and tissues. Multiple hormone signals continuously interact with these target cells, but these cells respond only to their specific hormone. This selective response is due to protein receptors located in the cell membrane or the cytoplasm. The number of receptors on the target cells and the sensitivity of the receptors to the hormones (i.e., affinity) can change depending on hormone concentration. Upregulation is the process where low hormone levels cause an increase in the number of cell receptors. Conversely, downregulation is the process where high levels of hormone decrease the number of receptors or decrease the cell's affinity to the hormone. For hormones to cause a reaction, they must be in a free (i.e., unbound) form. Water-soluble hormones (e.g., insulin) are already circulating in free forms while lipid-soluble hormones (e.g., glucocorticoids) are bound to a carrier protein. A lipid-soluble hormone reaches its target cell, dissociates from its carrier protein, and then enters the cell. Once the hormone has acted on the target cells, the liver metabolizes the hormone and the kidneys excrete it to prevent a cumulative effect.

Pituitary Gland and Hypothalamus

Roughly the size of a pea, the pituitary gland (i.e., hypophysis) is located at the base of the brain. The gland is located in a depression in the sphenoid bone known as the sella turcica. This gland can be divided into two parts—the anterior (adenohypophysis) pituitary gland and the posterior (neurohypophysis) pituitary gland. The pituitary gland is often referred to as the *master gland* despite that it mainly functions as an intermediary, receiving input from the hypothalamus and peripheral endocrine glands. Despite its small size, this gland secretes several hormones that influence many different body functions (FIGURE 10-3; TABLE 10-1). The hypothalamus, which is the basal (bottom) portion of

the diencephalon, regulates the pituitary gland. The hypothalamus is connected to the pituitary gland through the pituitary stalk (i.e., infundibulum) and connects the nervous and endocrine systems. It contains receptors that monitor hormone, nutrient, and ion levels. When activated, these receptors stimulate neurosecretory neurons in the hypothalamus to synthesize and secrete various types of releasing and inhibiting hormones (Figure 10-2). These hypothalamus hormones, in turn, regulate the hormones produced by the anterior pituitary gland (a relationship known as the hypothalamic-pituitary axis). The hypothalamus hormones travel to the anterior pituitary, and then pituitary capillaries transport the pituitary hormones to the peripheral circulation via the internal jugular veins (i.e., portal circulation). The hypothalamus neurosecretory neurons also synthesize the posterior pituitary hormones—antidiuretic hormone (ADH) and oxytocin. The posterior pituitary hormones, in contrast to the anterior pituitary hormones, travel through a nerve tract and not a circulation portal (Figure 10-2). The posterior pituitary stores and releases ADH and oxytocin, and they are released directly into the systemic circulation. The key neurotransmitters of the nervous system, glutamate (excitatory) and gamma-aminobutyric acid (inhibitory), regulate the posterior pituitary hormones. The posterior pituitary hormones have a direct effect on peripheral tissue (i.e., they bypass target glands).

Pancreas

The pancreas is an organ with both exocrine digestive functions and endocrine functions. The pancreas lies underneath the liver and between the two kidneys in the retroperitoneum (the space behind the peritoneum) (FIGURE 10-4). Its endocrine functions are carried out by the islets of Langerhans, which are situated among the many small acini (cell clusters that produce digestive enzymes) in the pancreas. The human pancreas contains approximately 1 million islets of Langerhans, and each islet of Langerhans contains five types of cells: 1) alpha cells, which secrete glucagon; 2) beta cells, which secrete insulin and amylin; 3) delta cells, which secrete somatostatin and gastrin; 4) pancreatic polypeptide cells, which secrete a pancreatic polypeptide (stimulates gastric acid secretion and antagonizes cholecystokinin); and 5) epsilon cells, which secrete ghrelin. See chapter 9 for a discussion of the functions of the pancreas.

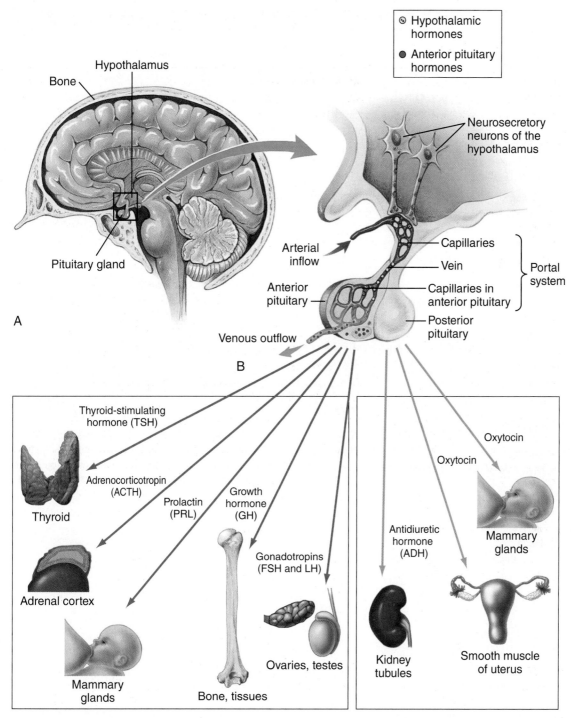

FIGURE 10-3 The pituitary gland. **(A)** A cross-section of the brain showing the location of the pituitary and the hypothalamus. **(B)** The structure of the pituitary gland. Releasing and inhibiting hormones travel via the portal system from the hypothalamus to the anterior pituitary, where they affect hormone secretion.

The regulation of glucose is reflected in the balance between energy intake and energy use with insulin as a key hormonal regulator. Glucagon is released when serum glucose levels fall, insulin levels drop, or glucose needs increase (e.g., with exercise) (**FIGURE 10-5**). Glucagon stimulates the breakdown of glycogen to glucose (i.e., glycogenolysis) in the liver, which raises serum glucose levels. Gluconeogenesis (synthesis of glucose) occurs when glucagon stimulates the liver and, to a small extent, the kidneys (renal medulla). Glucagon also decreases the uptake of glucose in skeletal muscle and fat

TABLE 10-1	Hormones Secreted by the Hypothalamus and Pituitary Gland	

Hormone		Function
Hypothalamus **Stimulation** Growth hormone–releasing hormone (GHRH): stimulates release Substance P: stimulates secretion **Inhibition** Somatostatin: inhibits release	*Anterior pituitary gland* Growth hormone (GH)	Stimulates cell growth and fat breakdown. Primary targets are muscle and bone, where GH stimulates amino acid uptake and protein synthesis.
Stimulation Thyrotropin-releasing hormone: stimulates release **Inhibition** Somatostatin: inhibits release	Thyroid-stimulating hormone (TSH)	Stimulates release of thyroxine and triiodothyronine.
Stimulation Corticotropin-releasing hormone (CRH): stimulates release **Inhibition** Substance P: inhibits synthesis and release	Adrenocorticotropic hormone (ACTH)	Stimulates secretion of hormones by the adrenal cortex, especially glucocorticoids.
Stimulation Gonadotropin-releasing hormone (GnRH): stimulates release Substance P: stimulates secretion	Gonadotropins: follicle-stimulating hormone (FSH) and luteinizing hormone (LH)	Stimulates gamete production and hormone production by the gonads.
Stimulation Prolactin-releasing hormone: stimulates secretion Thyrotropin-releasing hormone: stimulates release Substance P: stimulates secretion **Inhibition** Prolactin-inhibiting hormone: inhibits secretion Dopamine: inhibits synthesis and secretion	Prolactin	Stimulates breast development during pregnancy and milk production postpartum. Suppresses ovarian function during breastfeeding.
Posterior pituitary gland Antidiuretic hormone (ADH): **Stimulation**: glutamate **Inhibition**: gamma-aminobutyric acid	Melanocyte-stimulating hormone	Has a function in promoting secretion of melanin (darkens skin).
		Stimulates water reabsorption by nephrons of the kidney.
Stimulation: glutamate **Inhibition**: gamma-aminobutyric acid	Oxytocin	Stimulates breasts to release milk and uterine contractions during birth.

(insulin-sensitive tissue) and promotes the release of amino acids and fatty acids (lipolysis). Sympathetic stimulation causes glucagon release. Conversely, high blood glucose inhibits glucagon release. Insulin is released when serum glucose levels increase. Insulin stimulates cellular uptake of glucose, which in turn decreases serum glucose levels. Amylin is

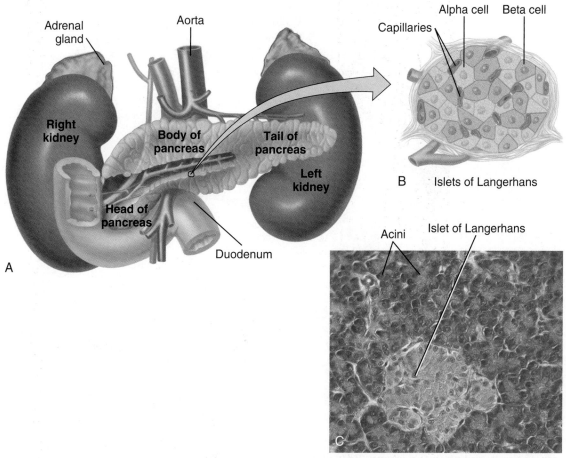

FIGURE 10-4 The pancreas. **(A)** The pancreas produces two hormones, insulin and glucagon, as well as digestive enzymes. **(B)** Hormones are produced by specialized cells within the islets of Langerhans. **(C)** The islets of Langerhans are located among the acini, very small groups of digestive enzyme–producing cells of the pancreas.

C: © Jubal Harshaw/Shutterstock.

released from the beta cells along with insulin. Insulin also promotes the storage of carbohydrates, fats, and proteins. Amylin has a synergistic relationship with insulin in controlling glucose. Amylin stimulation results in glucose control by suppressing glucagon, delaying gastric emptying, and increasing satiety (feeling of fullness). Somatostatin in the pancreas regulates insulin, glucagon, and pancreatic peptide by inhibiting their secretion. Pancreatic polypeptide is thought to regulate some of the other pancreatic activities (e.g., inhibiting cholecystokinin).

Several hormones are secreted in the gastrointestinal tract that affect pancreatic hormones and in turn glucose regulation. These hormones include incretins from the small intestine and ghrelin from the stomach. The key types of incretin hormones are glucagon-like peptide-1 and glucose-dependent insulinotropic polypeptide. After a meal, the incretins cause insulin release and inhibit glucagon release. Incretins also delay gastric emptying and decrease appetite. Dipeptidyl peptidase 4 is the enzyme causing the breakdown of the incretins. There are medication categories used in the treatment of type 2 diabetes mellitus that target incretin and dipeptidyl peptidase 4. Finally, ghrelin stimulates hunger.

Learning Points

Glucose Concepts

Several concepts pertain to synthesis of glucose. Understanding the differences is important. Glycogenesis is the formation of glycogen from glucose, and, conversely, glycogenolysis is the breakdown of glycogen to glucose. Glycogenolysis occurs in the muscle and liver. Gluconeogenesis is the formation of glucose from various chemicals such as pyruvate, and conversely glycolysis is the breakdown of glucose to pyruvate.

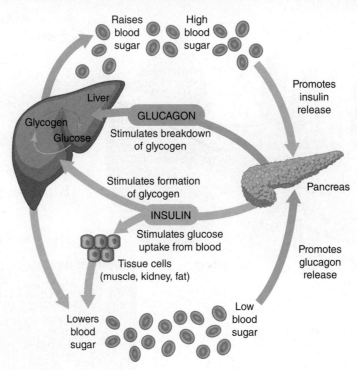

FIGURE 10-5 Glucose metabolism.

Thyroid Gland

The thyroid gland (**FIGURE 10-6**) is located at the base of the neck below the larynx. This gland consists of two lobes, one on either side of the trachea, which are connected by a thin band of tissue (isthmus) that extends across the anterior aspect of the trachea. The thyroid is a highly vascular gland that contains several functional units called *follicles*. These follicles produce three hormones: 1) thyroxine, or T_4; 2) triiodothyronine, or T_3; and 3) thyrocalcitonin, or calcitonin.

Together, T_3 and T_4 account for 95% of circulating thyroid hormones; they regulate cellular metabolism as well as growth and development. The hypothalamus, through the release of thyrotropin-releasing hormone, stimulates the pituitary gland to produce thyroid-stimulating hormone (TSH) using a negative feedback system. TSH, in turn, drives the thyroid to produce T_3 and T_4 (i.e., thyroxine). Most of the T_4 is produced by the thyroid gland (approximately 90%) while only a small amount (approximately 10%) of T_3 is produced by the gland. The remainder of T_3 is produced when T_4 is converted to T_3 in body tissues. The thyroid requires iodine to synthesize these hormones. The thyroid hormones remain attached to a protein known as thyroglobulin until they are released. As with other hormones, the bound thyroid hormones are not active while the unbound (free) form is active. Somatostatin from the hypothalamus inhibits the releases of TSH. With aging, thyroid hormone secretion declines, but the rate of thyroid hormone removal from the bloodstream slows down; therefore, a balance is usually maintained. TSH secretion is thought to increase with aging; however, determining if this is a normal part of aging or hypothyroidism can be difficult.

Calcitonin, along with parathyroid hormone, regulates serum calcium levels. Calcitonin alters serum calcium levels by inhibiting osteoclast activity (which decreases calcium release from the bone) and stimulating osteoblast activity (which increases calcium deposits in the bone). Calcitonin lowers serum phosphate levels. Calcitonin regulates calcium and phosphate by decreasing renal tubular reabsorption and possibly decreasing gastrointestinal absorption. Calcitonin is also regulated with a negative feedback system and is secreted when serum calcium levels are high.

Parathyroid Glands

The parathyroid glands, usually four in number, are located on the posterior surface of the thyroid. Each parathyroid gland secretes parathyroid hormone (PTH). PTH works in the

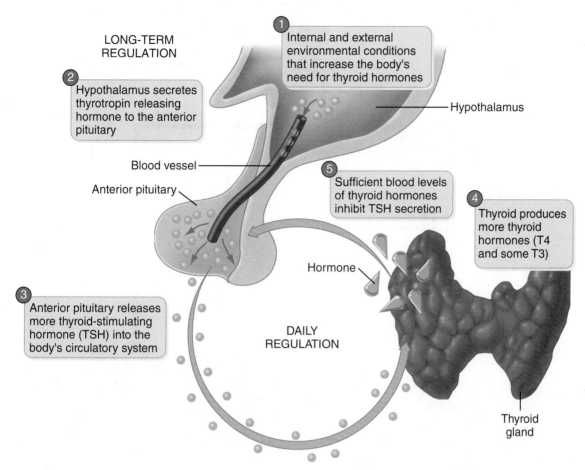

FIGURE 10-6 The thyroid gland.

opposite way to calcitonin to regulate serum calcium levels, and PTH is more important than calcitonin in calcium regulation. Specifically, PTH is secreted when serum calcium levels drop. This hormone increases serum calcium levels by increasing osteoclast activity (which increases calcium release from the bone) as well as by increasing absorption of calcium in the gastrointestinal tract and kidneys. PTH conversely decreases serum phosphate levels. Calcium levels are also regulated through the action of PTH on the kidney, PTH stimulates vitamin D, and, together, they increase calcium and phosphate absorption in the intestines. See chapter 6 for a discussion of calcium regulation.

Adrenal Glands

The adrenal glands are located on each kidney. Each adrenal gland has an inner portion, or medulla, and an outer portion, or cortex. The hypothalamus influences both portions of the adrenal glands, albeit by different mechanisms.

The adrenal cortex is regulated by negative feedback involving the hypothalamus and adrenocorticotropic hormones; the medulla is regulated by nerve impulses from the hypothalamus. The medulla produces epinephrine (about 30%) and norepinephrine (minor amounts) during times of stress. The majority of epinephrine is released from nerve endings. Epinephrine and norepinephrine mediate the fight-or-flight response of the sympathetic nervous system (**FIGURE 10-7**). The adrenal catecholamines (e.g., epinephrine and norepinephrine) are also regulated by glucocorticoids and ACTH (increases in both of these cause release of catecholamines).

The cortex has three separate regions that produce different steroids. The outermost region of the adrenal cortex secretes mineralocorticoids. The principal mineralocorticoid is aldosterone, which acts to conserve sodium and, in turn, water in the body. Aldosterone is primarily regulated by the renin–angiotensin–aldosterone system. The middle region of the adrenal cortex secretes glucocorticoids. The principal glucocorticoid is cortisol, which increases serum glucose levels. Other glucocorticoids secreted include cortisone and

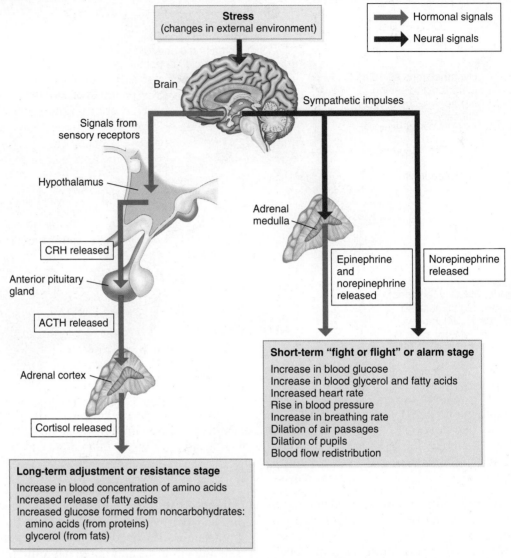

FIGURE 10-7 Stress response.

corticosterone. Glucocorticoids have effects on multiple systems such as the metabolic, neurologic, immune, and musculoskeletal systems. The glucocorticoids are released during stress (Figure 10-7). In addition, cortisol is released in a diurnal (i.e., circadian) pattern. Just before a person awakens, cortisol levels rise, and throughout the day, the levels slowly decline (this pattern is assuming regular sleep–wake patterns). Lastly, the innermost region of the cortex secretes gonadocorticoids, or sex hormones. Male hormones (e.g., androgen) and female hormones (e.g., estrogen) are secreted in minimal amounts in both sexes by the adrenal cortex, but the hormones from the testes and ovaries usually mask their effect. In females, the masculinization effect of androgen

secretion may become evident after menopause, when estrogen levels from the ovaries decrease. The innermost layer also secretes mineralocorticoids, aldosterone, and glucocorticoids. See chapters 4 and 6 for more information on aldosterone.

Understanding Conditions That Affect the Endocrine System

When considering alterations in the endocrine system, organizing them based on their basic underlying pathophysiology can increase understanding. These concepts focus on inadequate or excessive functioning of the glands. Hormone alterations can be due to 1) inadequate hormones (e.g., decreased production due to missing precursor, inadequate free active hormone, hormone destruction), 2) abnormal delivery (e.g., impaired blood supply), 3) abnormal regulation (e.g., feedback mechanism impaired), and 4) abnormal amount (e.g., ectopic hormone production from a tumor). Production may be adequate, and the regulatory and delivery system may be intact; however, the target gland response may be inappropriate. Inappropriate target gland response is usually a result of problems on the cell surface where receptors are located or problems within the cell. Examples of target gland receptor dysfunction include an inadequate number of receptors and antibodies attacking receptors. Endocrine system disorders can also be categorized by the primary location of the disorder such as hypothalamic or pituitary (e.g., anterior versus posterior) and the target gland affected (e.g., thyroid or adrenal). Once you understand the normal function of the glands and the hormones they produce, it becomes clear that those functions can be either insufficient or exaggerated. In most cases of hypofunctioning, something has destroyed the gland (e.g., tumors or autoimmune conditions). Treatment for hypofunctioning usually centers on hormone replacement. In most cases of hyperfunctioning, something is overstimulating the gland or secreting hormonelike substances (e.g., tumors). Treatment for hyperfunctioning usually centers on giving medications to block hormone production, removing the cause (e.g., a tumor), or removing part or all of the gland.

Disorders of the Pituitary Gland

Disorders of the pituitary gland can have significant consequences because of the many hormones and processes this gland influences. Pituitary gland disorders can stem from dysfunction of the hypothalamus or from just the pituitary gland (anterior, posterior, or both). Hypothalamic hormones cause inhibition or release of anterior pituitary hormones. Hypothalamic disorders will, therefore, lead to clinical manifestations that reflect the pituitary hormone altered. Like most endocrine disorders, pituitary gland disorders result in either increased or decreased levels of hormones associated with the gland (Table 10-1). These conditions can be caused by multiple disorders such as tumors (most common), infection, trauma, and necrosis.

Hyperpituitarism

Hyperpituitarism is a condition in which the pituitary gland secretes excessive amounts of one or all of the anterior pituitary hormones (Table 10-1). The most common causes are benign pituitary adenomas (primary pituitary carcinoma is rare). The adenomas (i.e., glandular tumors) are usually a result of genetic mutations such as those in multiple endocrine neoplasia type 1 or aryl hydrocarbon receptor-interacting protein. The adenomas usually develop from a cell of origin that secretes hormones (e.g., lactotroph adenoma that is formed from cells that secrete prolactin). Adenomas can form from any cell in the anterior pituitary. The adenomas secrete an excessive amount of hormone of the same type from the cell from which they originated (e.g., an adenoma from somatotroph cells will secrete excessive growth hormone). While the adenoma causes excesses, deficiencies in hormone production can occur. These deficiencies are the result of the destruction or compression of the pituitary gland by the growing adenoma. The tumor can cause pituitary gland infarction, and hemorrhaging can occur into the tumor and gland (apoplexy). While some adenomas can secrete excessive hormones, many are nonfunctional or silent and do not hypersecrete hormones.

Clinical Manifestations

Hyperpituitarism is a progressive disorder that can occur suddenly but usually develops slowly. Clinical manifestations vary greatly depending on the hormones affected and the severity of those alterations. The manifestations are usually a result of the expanding adenoma in the small enclosed space where the pituitary is located. Hormonal manifestations can be minimal to absent as many adenomas are nonfunctional. In nonfunctional adenomas, the manifestations are due to the mass and a failing pituitary (i.e., hormone deficiency). Some tumors cause hypersecretion of certain hormones (i.e., the cell origin of the tumor), and manifestations will be a result of the hypersecretion of a specific hormone (e.g., hyperprolactinemia from a lactotroph adenoma). In summary, manifestations are due to the expanding adenoma and possible hormone excesses or deficiencies.

The size of the adenoma can also influence the presence of manifestations. Microadenoma

(< 1 cm) manifestations are more likely to be due to hormone excesses, and macroadenoma (> 1 cm) manifestations are likely to be due to the mass. The mass manifestations usually include headache and visual disturbances (the pituitary gland is located near the optic chiasm). The visual disturbances can include loss of vision, visual field loss, or double vision. The expanding mass can impinge upon cranial nerves that traverse the gland (i.e., cranial nerve III, IV, and parts of V and VI; see chapter 11 on neural function).

Hormonal manifestations will be dependent on whether the tumor secretes excess hormones and the type it is secreting. The types of primary adenomas and the associated hormone excess include:

- **Lactotroph (i.e., prolactinoma):** This causes increased prolactin, further causing hypogonadism in women (e.g., in premenopausal infertility, oligomenorrhea, and galactorrhea) and men (e.g., decreased libido, impotence, infertility, gynecomastia, and galactorrhea). Lactotrophs are among the most common types of adenomas.

- **Somatotroph:** This causes increased growth hormone leading to acromegaly (adults) and gigantism (children) (**FIGURE 10-8**). Somatotrophs are common types of adenomas.
- **Corticotroph:** This causes increased ACTH, in turn causing central Cushing disease.
- **Gonadotroph:** This causes increased LH and FSH, resulting in precocious puberty and ovarian hyperstimulation. These tumors are rare.
- **Thyrotroph:** This type of tumor is usually nonfunctioning, and of the tumors that are functioning, which are extremely rare, can cause hyperthyroidism.

Lactotrophic and somatotrophic adenomas can also occur in combination and cause manifestations of prolactin and growth hormone excesses.

Diagnosis and Treatment

Diagnosis of hyperpituitarism is often delayed because of its varying presentation. Diagnostic procedures usually include a history and physical examination with vision testing. Diagnostic

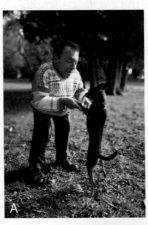
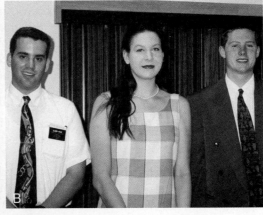
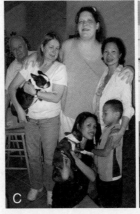
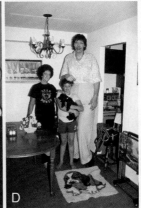

FIGURE 10-8 A person with acromegaly **A** as a child, **B** as a teenager, **C** as an adult, and **D** gigantism.

testing will include magnetic resonance imaging (MRI), which is the best imaging technique for adenomas. A brain computed tomography (CT), usually that is contrast enhanced, can be also be done. Serum prolactin, insulin-like growth factor-1 (IGF-1), and cortisol levels are usually measured. All levels will be high depending on the type of adenoma (e.g., high cortisol with a corticotroph adenoma). Other hormone levels such as TSH, FSH, and LH may be evaluated if there are suspicions for imbalances in these hormones.

Treatment strategies depend on the underlying etiology and the hormone affected. Tumors will likely require medications for tumor suppression, surgery, radiation, and chemotherapy, but they often reoccur. Additionally, analogues that inhibit hormone production may be given.

Diagnostic Link

Serum Hormone Levels

Evaluating the pituitary gland and target gland hormones can be useful in determining whether the problem is in the hypothalamus/pituitary or the target gland (e.g., serum ACTH and cortisol). Serum hormone levels (e.g., cortisol) are usually obtained in the morning (e.g., between 8 a.m. and 10 a.m.). Some serum hormones may require pharmacologic agents to evaluate a response to the stimulation (e.g., metyrapone test reduces cortisol, and ACTH should increase if secretion is intact). Growth hormone effects are dependent on insulin-like growth factors (IGFs) produced in the liver. Therefore, IGFs and GH should be measured. IGF-1 levels are usually constant as they are dependent on GH while circulating GH varies throughout the day. Therefore, IGF-1 measures may be a better reflection of GH abnormalities.

Hypopituitarism

Hypopituitarism is a rare, complex condition in which the pituitary gland does not produce sufficient amounts of some or all (panhypopituitarism) of its hormones. Hypopituitarism usually affects the anterior pituitary hormones (e.g., TSH, growth hormone, ACTH, FSH, LH, prolactin, and melanocyte-stimulating hormone). As a result, the gland or process that the hormone controls is impaired. Hypopituitarism may result from disorders that affect the pituitary or the hypothalamus. Those causes can be divided into tumors within the hypothalamus or pituitary, extrapituitary tumors (i.e., tumors outside the pituitary), and nontumors.

Pituitary Causes
- Congenital defects (e.g., pituitary hypoplasia or aplasia) and genetic mutations

- Pituitary surgery or radiation
- Infections, such as meningitis and tuberculosis
- Pituitary tumors, such as pituitary adenomas, which are the most common type of tumor associated with hypopituitarism (see the *Hyperpituitarism* section)
- Infiltrative disorders, such as hemochromatosis (a condition resulting in excessive iron absorption) or lymphocytic hypophysitis (an abnormal infiltration of lymphocytes and enlargement of the pituitary)
- Pituitary infarction (Sheehan syndrome), which occurs due to postpartum hemorrhage

Hypothalamic Causes
- Tumors that originate in the hypothalamus (e.g., benign craniopharyngiomas) or tumors from metastasis (e.g., lung cancer)
- Infections (e.g., meningitis, tuberculosis)
- Infiltrative disorders, such as histiocytosis X (an abnormal immune condition that results in tissue damage) or sarcoidosis (an abnormal inflammatory condition that results in tissue damage)
- Traumatic brain injury
- Radiation-induced damage (e.g., brain tumor treatment)

Clinical Manifestations

Hypopituitarism can result in several manifestations depending on the hormones involved. The severity of these conditions reflects the degree of hormone deficit. Hypopituitarism is a progressive disorder that can occur suddenly (e.g., pituitary hemorrhage) but usually develops slowly (e.g., years after radiation therapy). Clinical manifestations vary greatly depending on the hormones affected and the severity of those alterations. In general, GH, LH, and FSH are more likely to be affected than ACTH or TSH. Manifestations may also be due to the underlying causes, such as a tumor causing compression (e.g., headaches or visual disturbance). Comprehensive discussions of manifestations are found in the individual target gland or hormone sections. General manifestations of hormone deficiency include:

- **GH deficiency:** Delayed growth and development (e.g., weight-to-height ratio increase, immature-appearing face such as undeveloped nasal bridge, frontal protrusion, infantile voice, diminished hair growth) (FIGURE 10-9)

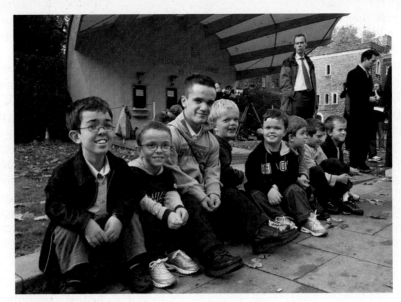

FIGURE 10-9 Dwarfism.
© Marion Bull / Alamy Stock Photo.

- **FSH/LH deficiency:** Impaired reproductive system (e.g., infertility, amenorrhea, irregular menses, hot flashes)
- **TSH deficiency:** Central hypothyroidism with decreased metabolic activity (e.g., fatigue, cold sensitivity, weight gain, constipation)
- **ACTH deficiency:** Secondary adrenal insufficiency usually due to cortisol deficiency (e.g., weakness, nausea, anorexia, hypotension). ACTH deficiency is a serious disorder than can be life threatening. ACTH deficiency from pituitary disorders (i.e., secondary adrenal insufficiency) does not cause alterations in aldosterone as seen in ACTH deficiency due to adrenal gland disorder (i.e., primary adrenal insufficiency).
- **ADH deficiency:** Excessive urination

Diagnosis and Treatment

Diagnosis of hypopituitarism is often delayed because of its variable presentation. Hypopituitarism, even severe deficiencies, may cause few or no clinical manifestations. Diagnostic procedures usually include a history and physical examination. Diagnostic testing includes measurement of serum hormone levels; findings consistent with hypopituitarism include low ACTH levels. Normally during times of stress, the levels of ACTH rise. To evaluate ACTH reserve, medications such as metyrapone can be administered to evoke a stress response. With pharmacologic provocation, a low ACTH level reflects a lack of a response (i.e., deficiency).

Serum GH and IGF levels can be evaluated. Medications can be administered to evaluate whether GH release can be stimulated. Low GH levels with an attempt at stimulation reflect a GH deficiency. Thyroid hormone measurement of TSH, T_3, and T_4 should be done. With hypopituitarism, TSH levels are suppressed, resulting in low T_4 and T_3 which is in contrast to thyroid gland where the TSH and thyroid hormones have an inverse relationship (one is up, the other is down). The hypothalamus produces thyrotropin-releasing hormone, which can be measured; however, these laboratory measurements are only available outside of the United States. Men will have LH and testosterone levels evaluated while women will have FSH, LH, and estradiol levels evaluated. With hypothalamic or pituitary disorders, the testosterone and estradiol will be low, and the gonadotropic hormones (i.e., FSH, LH) will be low or normal (reflecting deficiency). Primary disorders of the target glands (i.e., ovarian failure or testicular hypofunction), in contrast to hypothalamic or pituitary disorders, causes high FSH and LH with low estradiol levels (in women), and low testosterone levels with normal LH in men. Additional diagnostic tests for hypopituitarism include pituitary MRI or brain CT and X-rays (to identify any bone abnormalities). See chapter 8 for more on reproductive function.

Lifelong hormone replacement therapy is the cornerstone of treatment. Resolving and treating the underlying cause, such as cancer, is also important when possible. Life-threatening deficiencies, such as those potentially seen in

ACTH deficiency, require emergent care. Additional strategies, such as infertility treatments and counseling, depend on the specific hormones affected.

Prolactin Disorders: Prolactinemia

Prolactin disorders usually result in high prolactin levels. Deficient levels rarely occur in isolation but instead occur with other hormone deficiencies. Prolactinemia (high prolactin levels) is a result of disorders of the hypothalamus or anterior pituitary. Lactotroph adenomas (i.e., prolactinomas) cause prolactinemia, and they are some of the most common types of pituitary adenomas. Hyperprolactinemia can be caused by interference of the dopamine inhibitory effect on prolactin. Dopamine interference can be due to several medications that are dopamine receptor antagonists (they block dopamine), such as neuroleptics (e.g., antipsychotics including haloperidol and chlorpromazine). Many other medications can increase prolactin levels such as opioids, antihypertensive agents, and H_2 antihistamines, but not all the medications in these categories result in high prolactin levels (e.g., verapamil is the only calcium channel blocker associated with hyperprolactinemia). Genetic mutations can result in a familial hyperprolactinemia. Systemic disorders, such as chronic kidney disease, result in a decreased excretion of prolactin, resulting in high serum levels. The normal range of prolactin is approximately 20 ng/mL. In general, prolactinomas cause the highest elevations of prolactin (e.g., up to 50,000 ng/mL) while most other causes will have smaller elevations (usually not > 200 ng/mL). High prolactin levels can also be due to normal physiologic states, such as pregnancy or from nipple stimulation during breastfeeding.

Clinical manifestations of hyperprolactinemia will include hypogonadism due to inhibition of GnRH. The GnRH inhibition suppresses LH and possibly FSH and, in turn, this suppression usually results in gonadotropic suppression. This suppression in premenopausal women manifests as infertility, oligomenorrhea, and galactorrhea; in men, manifestations include decreased libido, impotence, infertility, gynecomastia, and galactorrhea. Evaluation and treatment are geared toward determining and treating the underlying cause.

Growth Hormone Disorders

Growth hormone excesses result in **acromegaly** in adults and **gigantism** in children. Growth hormone deficits result in **dwarfism** (Figure 10-9).

The most common causes of growth hormone excesses are adenomas. More than 300 conditions cause short stature. Growth hormone deficiency as one of the causes of dwarfism is generally due to GHRH deficiency as a result of tumors, GHRH receptor mutations, pituitary agenesis (failure of organ development), or panhypopituitarism.

Gigantism is a result of excess GH and IGF-1 causing excess skeletal growth before epiphyseal growth plate closure. The growth is rapid and usually affects stature, causing rapid height increase before weight gain or concurrent with weight gain. The condition is often caused by a tumor (e.g., adenoma), but the condition is rare.

Acromegaly is also a result of excess GH and IGF-1 in adults. The onset is usually around the age of 40–59 years of age. In contrast to gigantism, the progression is usually insidious and slow with most adults having manifestations 12 years prior to diagnosis. The excess growth effects of GH and IGF-1 do not occur in the long bones as the epiphyseal plates have closed. Rather the excessive GH and IGF-1 lead to soft tissue and connective tissue growth and proliferation. Excessive GH and IGF-1 results in the characteristic appearance of a person with acromegaly, which includes:

- **Soft tissue and skin changes:** Skin thickens; patients develop large hands and feet with paresthesias and carpal tunnel syndrome, an enlarged nose as well as a protruding forehead and jaw, teeth that are spread apart, tongue enlargement (i.e., macroglossia), deepening voice, excessive sweating (i.e., hyperhidrosis), malodor, and sleep apnea as a result of macroglossia.
- **Bones and joints:** Knees, ankles, hips, spine, and other joints become hypertrophic leading to back pain and other musculoskeletal disorders (e.g., kyphosis).
- **Organ enlargement:** Thyroid (goiter) function can be normal or abnormal; cardiovascular issues (primary cause of death) such as ventricular hypertrophy, hypertension, and cardiomyopathy can occur.
- **Metabolic changes:** Fat and carbohydrate metabolism changes result in decrease glucose use, increased glucose production by the liver, and increased insulin production leading to hyperinsulinemia, insulin resistance, and impaired glucose tolerance or diabetes mellitus.

Children with growth hormone deficiency due to congenital disorders usually have growth failure soon after birth, and in neonates, hypoglycemia and seizures can occur. As the child ages, facial features are immature, stature is short, and obesity may be present. Puberty may be delayed, and boys may have microcephalus (i.e., a small penis). Acquired GH deficiency in older children may be due to tumors. GH deficiency in adults is usually due to hypothalamic pituitary tumors.

Diagnosis and treatment of gigantism, acromegaly, and dwarfism is based on determining the underlying cause (e.g., MRI, serum hormone levels) and targeting treatment to the cause (e.g., surgery, medications to suppress hormone secretion).

Antidiuretic Hormone (Vasopressin) Disorders

Antidiuretic hormone (ADH) excesses (i.e., vasopressin, arginine, and vasopressin) lead to a disorder known as **syndrome of inappropriate antidiuretic hormone secretion** (SIADH). **Diabetes insipidus** (DI) is characterized by low levels of ADH. Both SIADH and DI are a result of posterior pituitary disorders.

In SIADH, water is retained, and total body water increases as a result of the increased levels of ADH. Dilutional hyponatremia and hypo-osmolality occurs as a result of excess total body water. Conversely, urine osmolality increases as a result of urine concentration (particularly with sodium). The excesses may be due to increased ADH secretion/release (pituitary or ectopic) or increased effect. Central nervous system disorders (e.g., stroke, trauma, and psychosis) can cause SIADH. Small cell lung carcinoma is the most common tumor causing ectopic ADH production. Several drug categories are associated with SIADH, such as antidepressants, anticonvulsants, antipsychotics, anticancer drugs, and antidiabetic drugs. Iatrogenic causes include surgery (usually pituitary), hormone administration (e.g., vasopressin for gastrointestinal bleeding), and infections (e.g., HIV and pneumonia).

SIADH should be suspected when hyponatremia (serum levels < 135 mEq/L), hypo-osmolality (serum osmolality < 280 mOsm/kg), and increased urine hyperosmolality (> 100 mOsm/kg) are present. The manifestations are due to hyponatremia and dependent on the rapidity and severity of the sodium decrease. Manifestations are usually the same as from other causes of hyponatremia (e.g., nausea, vomiting, confusion, weakness, and cramping). Treatment is based on the underlying cause and management of the hyponatremia (see chapter 6 for discussion of sodium imbalance.).

DI occurs as a result of insufficient ADH. This deficiency leads to polyuria and polydipsia. Causes can be either due to insufficient secretion of ADH due to hypothalamus or pituitary disorders (i.e., neurogenic or central DI) or as a result of inadequate renal tubule response to ADH (i.e., nephrogenic DI). Nephrogenic DI may be due to genetic or inherited disorders (e.g., vasopressin receptor gene mutation), which are uncommon. Acquired nephrogenic DI occurs when renal tubules are damaged due to drugs such as lithium, loop diuretics, or certain general anesthetics or due to disorders such as bilateral urinary tract obstruction and polycystic kidney disease.

In up to 50% of cases, neurogenic DI is due to idiopathic causes, and autoimmune processes may lead to the destruction of ADH-secreting cells in the hypothalamus. Other causes include hypothalamus or pituitary damage such as trauma, surgery, or hypoxic encephalopathy; benign or malignant tumors; metastatic cancer; infiltrative disorders; and uncommon familial and congenital diseases, such as Wolfram syndrome or congenital hypopituitarism, respectively.

Clinical manifestations of DI include polyuria (urine output 3 L/day in adults or 2 L/m^2 in children), nocturia, and polydipsia. The serum osmolality (> 295 mOsm/kg) and sodium (> 145 mEq/L) are high due to the water loss, and these high levels lead to polydipsia. Hypernatremia can worsen if a patient with DI has impaired thirst or inability to drink or if fluids are not replaced.

Treatment will be based on the underlying cause. DI (whether nephrogenic or neurogenic) treatment generally involves reduction of sodium intake (e.g., low-protein, low-sodium diet). Thiazide diuretics may be administered to improve water retention and thereby less water is delivered to ADH sites in the collecting tubules and this reduces urine output. Because of the polyuria, the bladder can easily become dilated, so adequate emptying using double-voiding techniques is recommended. Carbamazepine and chlorpropamide potentiate ADH action and can be considered. Nonsteroidal anti-inflammatory drugs may be beneficial as they inhibit prostaglandin synthesis and, therefore, essentially block the antagonistic action of prostaglandins on ADH. Neurogenic treatment of DI often includes administration of desmopressin (ADH analog).

Diabetes Mellitus

Diabetes mellitus (DM) refers to a group of conditions characterized by hyperglycemia (high serum glucose levels) resulting from defects in insulin production, insulin action, or both. Glucose is a vital energy source for the body, but insulin is required for glucose to travel into the cell, where it can be used. Insulin acts like a key that unlocks the cell membrane and allows the glucose to enter. Impaired insulin production or action results in abnormal carbohydrate, protein, and fat metabolism because of the glucose transportation issue. Some cells, such as those in the brain, digestive tract, and skeletal muscles, can use glucose without insulin to some degree. DM can occur in three main forms—type 1, type 2, and gestational diabetes—each with its own pathogenesis (**TABLE 10-2**).

An estimated 422 million people worldwide have DM (World Health Organization, 2016). DM is extremely common in the United States—approximately 30.3 million Americans have diabetes and another 84.1 million have prediabetes (more than 1 out of 3 adults) (Centers for Disease Control and Prevention [CDC], 2017). DM incidence is relatively equal across genders, and it is most common in people older than 65 years of age, with nearly 25% of this population having DM. DM is most frequent among Native Americans, Blacks (non-Hispanic), and Latinos (CDC, 2017). In 2017, DM accounted for $327 billion in medical costs in the United States. Although DM was only the seventh most common listed cause of death on U.S. death certificates in 2015, it likely played a role in many more deaths because this disease contributes to several complications (e.g., heart disease, stroke, and kidney disease).

Type 1 Diabetes

Type 1 diabetes was previously called *insulin-dependent DM* and *juvenile-onset DM* (Table 10-2). These terms are no longer used. Type 1 DM accounts for approximately 5% of all newly diagnosed cases of DM. Type 1 DM develops when the body's immune system destroys pancreatic beta cells, leading to progressive loss of insulin secretion. To survive, people with type 1 DM must obtain insulin delivered by injection or a pump. This form of DM usually strikes children and young adults (usually less than 20 years of age), although its onset can occur at any age. Type 1 DM accounts for 5–10% of all diagnosed cases in adults (after the age of 30). The exact cause of type 1 diabetes is unknown, but most likely a viral or environmental trigger in genetically susceptible people causes an autoimmune reaction. Initially in the course of the disease, there may be a short period (sometimes 1–2 years) termed the *honeymoon phase* where there are still residual beta cells producing insulin, but as more and more insulin is needed, as during an infection or puberty, the insulin reserve disappears and insulin becomes near absent to absent.

Type 1 DM is associated with multiple genes with one of the major susceptibility genes found on the human leukocyte antigen region of chromosome 6. This region of the chromosome has genes that encodes for class II major histocompatibility complex, which is involved in the immune response. See chapter 2 for details on immunity.

TABLE 10-2	Comparison of Type 1 and Type 2 Diabetes	
	Type 1	**Type 2**
Age	Usually in children or young adults	Usually after age 40, and incidence increases with age
Onset	Generally abrupt	More often insidious
	Often diagnosed after infection	Patients often obese
	Diabetic ketoacidosis	HHNK
Treatment	Insulin	Diet, exercise, medication (oral or noninsulin injectables)
		Insulin may be required in severe cases
Complications	Occur early, often severe	Full range of complications may be present at diagnosis
Insulin levels	Low or absent	Frequently normal or high

Data from: Sheila Grossman (2014). *Porth's Pathophysiology: Concepts of Altered Health States*, Wolters Kluwer Health Lippincott Williams & Wilkins.

Many other gene loci are being discovered and evaluated for association with type 1 DM development. While inheritance of certain human leukocyte antigen types increases risk of type 1 DM, up to 80% of patients with type 1 DM do not have an affected relative. With type 1 DM, beta cells are destroyed by the immune system (e.g., cytotoxic CD8 and T lymphocytes), and while there is sparing of other pancreatic cells (e.g., alpha and delta cells), hormonal patterns from these cells are altered. An example of this alteration is the impaired response of glucagon from alpha cells to hypoglycemia in type 1 DM. The reason beta cells are selected and targeted for destruction is unknown. Type 1 DM cannot be prevented.

Type 2 Diabetes

Type 2 diabetes was previously called *non–insulin-dependent DM* and *adult-onset DM*. These terms are no longer used as some individuals with type 2 DM require insulin, and type 2 DM can occur in any age group. In adults, type 2 DM accounts for approximately 90–95% of all newly diagnosed DM cases. This form of diabetes usually begins as insulin resistance, a disorder in which the body's cells do not use insulin properly. As the need for insulin rises, the pancreas gradually loses its ability to produce insulin. Type 2 DM is associated with advancing age, obesity, family history of DM, history of gestational DM, impaired glucose metabolism, and physical inactivity. Blacks, Latinos, Native Americans, Asians, Native Hawaiians, and other Pacific Islanders are at particularly high risk for type 2 DM and its complications. Type 2 DM in children and adolescents, although still rare, is being diagnosed more frequently among Native Americans, Blacks, Latinos, Asians, and Pacific Islanders.

The common phenotype in DM is hyperglycemia, but various ethnic groups may have different pathogenesis. As an example, some Asian populations develop type 2 DM while young and with a low body mass index, and some Latino populations have a greater incidence of insulin resistance. Development of type 2 DM is considered multifactorial and polygenic. Multiple genes and environmental influences such as obesity, poor nutrition, and inactivity contribute to the development. A significant risk for type 2 DM is heritable, which is in contrast to the lower familial incidence in type 1 DM risk. As with type 1 DM, several loci are being evaluated for association with DM development.

The pathogenesis of type 2 DM starts with insulin resistance, which refers to insulin's inability to act upon target tissues (fat, muscle, and liver, which are insulin sensitive tissue). The lack of glucose use causes the liver to produce more glucose in response. Both these processes, lack of use and increased production) lead to hyperglycemia. Hyperinsulinemia occurs as a compensatory response. Ultimately, the beta cells struggle with maintaining the hyperinsulinemic state, so insulin secretion decreases, hepatic glucose production increases, and beta cell failure occurs. Glucagon additionally increases hepatic glucose production due to the inadequate insulin suppression further compounding the hyperglycemia.

The genesis of insulin resistance is unclear, but a known risk factor for type 2 DM development is obesity. Obesity is present in approximately 80% of patients with type 2 DM, and when weight is lost, insulin responsiveness improves. Obesity, particularly when fat is in a central or visceral location, may be related to the development of insulin resistance through various mechanisms. Free fatty acids are extremely high in the plasma of obese individuals and may contribute to impaired glucose uptake and decreased insulin secretion. Adipocytes (cells that store fat) release adipokines such as leptin, adiponectin, resistin, and other chemicals such as tumor necrosis factor-alpha, which stimulate inflammatory activity. These various factors released from adipose tissue may be increased or decreased and contribute to the development of type 2 DM (e.g., leptin is increased while adiponectin is decreased). Adiponectin is one of the adipokines that has been extensively evaluated. Adiponectin is a protective adipokine that reduces free fatty acid and is associated with glycemic control, reduced inflammation, and improved lipid profiles. Low levels of adiponectin are found in obesity. The role of other adipokines, such as leptin and resistin, in diabetes development is still unclear. In type 2 DM, several inflammatory markers (e.g., C-reactive protein, interleukins) are increased. Low-grade systemic inflammation is a characteristic of type 2 DM. Medications, such as thiazolidinediones used for type 2 DM, have an anti-inflammatory property. Receptor alterations contribute to insulin resistance, specifically postreceptor defects.

The mechanism by which insulin secretion decreases is unclear. Amylin, which is stored in the beta cell and is cosecreted with insulin, may contribute to islet cell destruction through the depositions of amyloid deposits. With beta cell decline, amylin becomes deficient in type 2 DM (and type 1 DM). Pramlintide is an amylin analog that is used in DM treatment to reduce blood glucose. Pramlintide specifically targets postprandial blood glucose levels and slows gastric emptying, promotes satiety, and suppresses abnormal postprandial glucagon rise. Chronic hyperglycemia and inflammatory markers in the islet environment may contribute to impaired islet functioning and destruction. Altered functioning of glucagon-like peptide-1 may reduce insulin secretion.

Gestational Diabetes

Gestational DM is a form of glucose intolerance diagnosed during pregnancy (usually the second or third trimester). DM in the first trimester is considered preexisting and pregestational. Metabolic needs increase during pregnancy, and the normal pregnancy state is one of insulin resistance that occurs to ensure the fetus is adequately nourished. Various hormones are secreted by the placenta that are diabetogenic (cause diabetes), including GH, CRH, prolactin, progesterone, and placental lactogen. Gestational DM occurs in women whose pancreas are unable to function effectively to overcome the insulin-resistant state in pregnancy. Gestational DM occurs most frequently among Blacks, Hispanics, and Native Americans. Other risk factors include obesity and a family history of DM. During pregnancy, gestational DM requires treatment (usually lifestyle changes and insulin) to normalize maternal blood glucose levels to avoid fetal complications. Immediately after pregnancy, 5–10% of women with gestational DM are diagnosed with DM, usually type 2. Women who have had gestational DM have a 40–60% chance of developing DM within 10 years. Children who are born to mothers with gestational DM have an increased risk for development of DM.

Metabolic Syndrome

Metabolic syndrome (i.e., insulin resistance syndrome) is a cluster of risk factors that occur together—specifically, hyperglycemia, hypertension, hypercholesterolemia, and increased waist circumference. Metabolic syndrome is not a form of DM but is related to DM because metabolic syndrome increases the risk of cardiovascular disease, DM, and stroke. The diagnostic criteria for metabolic syndrome include the presence of three or more of those risk factors. Treatment strategies focus on lifestyle changes such as weight loss, dietary changes, and physical activity to prevent development of complications.

Clinical Manifestations and Complications

The clinical manifestations of DM can range from asymptomaticity to life-threatening diabetic ketoacidosis (DKA). The presentation of type 1 DM or type 2 DM can also vary. Most patients with type 2 DM are asymptomatic, and the diagnosis usually is made during a routine laboratory evaluation or during DM screening. In type 2 DM, symptoms of hyperglycemia are often recalled on retrospect (e.g., upon questioning, the patient may have noted polyuria or paresthesias). Patients with type 2 DM have often had impaired glucose tolerance for years prior to diagnosis. Some patients, upon initial diagnosis, present with complications of DM such as erectile dysfunction. In contrast, in type 1 DM, DKA may be the initial manifestation. Adults with type 1 DM tend to have a more gradual beta cell destruction and a longer period of hyperglycemia symptomaticity in comparison to children. Insulin therapy may not initially be necessary as autoimmune insulin deficiency occurs later. This type of DM is commonly termed *latent autoimmune diabetes of adults*.

The manifestations of DM, which are a direct result of hyperglycemia, include the following:

- Glucosuria (glucose is excreted in the urine to lower serum levels)
- Polyuria (increased urine output because of the osmotic effects of the glucosuria)
- Polydipsia (increased thirst because of the dehydration caused by the increased urine output)
- Polyphagia (increased appetite because of the energy loss as glucose is excreted)
- Weight loss (from increased fat catabolism)
- Blurred vision (excessive glucose changes the shape and flexibility of the lens of the eye, decreasing the ability to focus and causing blurred vision)
- Fatigue (because of a lack of an energy source)
- Nausea, vomiting, and abdominal pain (associated with sudden onset of type 1 diabetes)

DM can result in an array of acute and chronic complications. Acute complications are related to excessive alterations in blood glucose, either too high or too low, that can be life threatening. **Hypoglycemia** (low serum glucose level) may result from insufficient dietary intake, increased physical activity, and diabetic pharmacologic therapy (e.g., too intensive, side effect of medication, or excessive use) and is more common with insulin. **Hyperglycemia** may be a result of excessive dietary carbohydrate intake as well as insufficient or inappropriate diabetic pharmacologic therapy. Two serious complications of DM reflect extreme hyperglycemia—**diabetic ketoacidosis**

(DKA) and **hyperosmolar hyperglycemic nonketotic state** (HHNK). The major causes for the development of DKA and HHNK are insulin deficiency and/or resistance as well as glucagon excess. Often, patients manifest with varying degrees of clinical manifestations precipitated by hyperglycemia (**FIGURE 10-10**).

DKA development is usually associated with type 1 DM and is more likely to occur at a young age. HHNK development occurs in patients with type 2 DM and is more likely to occur in older patients. DKA has a higher prevalence in comparison to HHNK, but mortality is higher with HHNK. In DKA and HHNK, the various metabolic abnormalities and the pathogenesis are as follows:

- **Severe hyperglycemia:** HHNK serum glucose levels are usually much higher (e.g., > 1,000 mg/dL) than in DKA (e.g., < 800 mg/dL). The severe hyperglycemia is a result of impaired glucose use in tissues (muscle and fat) and insulin deficiency. Severe hyperglycemia leads to fatty acid (lipolysis) and protein breakdown (proteolysis). The oxidized fatty acids are

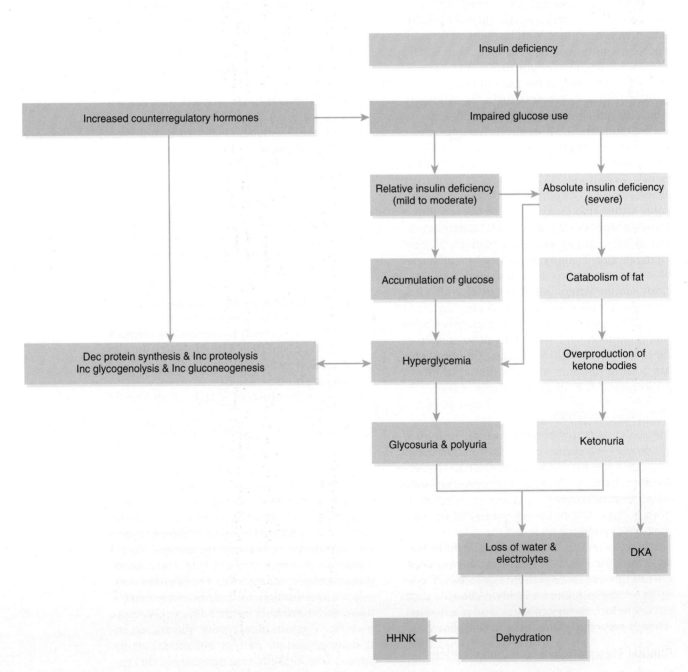

FIGURE 10-10 Major metabolic derangements in diabetes mellitus.

delivered to the liver, which results in gluconeogenesis. Insulin also suppresses the effects of glucagon contributing to the hyperglycemia. Counterregulatory hormone release such as catecholamines, which promote glycogenolysis; cortisol, which promotes gluconeogenesis; and GH, which decreases use of glucose in the periphery, oppose the action of insulin. The relatively lower glucose levels in DKA are due to the higher renal excretion of glucose because patients are younger and their glomerular filtration rates (GFRs) are high. Conversely, the osmotic diuresis eventually leads to dehydration and a reduced GFR. The severe hyperglycemia in older adults with HHNK can be a result of preexisting reduced GFR that is more prevalent in older patients.

- **Ketones:** The development of ketones is a result of the degradation of fatty acids. When glucose is not used as an energy source, the body begins using fat (where fuel is stored for energy. Initially, the liver uses the energy from fatty acids (small amount) and then releases the remainder into the circulation as ketones. An excessive number of ketones is a characteristic of DKA. The greater the insulin deficiency (e.g., type 1 DM), the greater the need to use fat as an energy source and, therefore, ketone development is higher. To convert carbohydrates to glucose as an energy source, insulin is a requirement. The relative absence of ketone development in HHNK is unclear. However, insulin is thought to be necessary to suppress lipolysis and gluconeogenesis. The amount of insulin needed to suppress lipolysis is much lower than the amount needed to suppress gluconeogenesis. In HHNK, the insulin deficiency is not as severe, leading to less lipolysis and a reduction in ketone formation.
- **Metabolic acidosis:** Excessive ketones cause ketoacidosis, an anion gap metabolic acidosis (see chapter 6 on *fluid, electrolyte, and acid–base homeostasis*).
- **Hyperosmolality and hyponatremia:** Hyperglycemia leads to an osmotic diuresis with a resulting elevated plasma osmolality and a dilutional hyponatremia. Most of the urine excreted does not have a higher number of electrolytes, thereby also contributing to a higher plasma osmolality. These alterations are more prevalent in HHNK in comparison to DKA.

- **Potassium:** In DKA and HHNK, potassium deficits and excesses are present. The deficits are a result of excess urinary excretion due to the osmotic diuresis. Glycogen and protein breakdown in the cells contribute to potassium loss. DKA and HHNK can also lead to serum hyperkalemia. Insulin deficiency leads to a decrease in the uptake of potassium by the cells. The hyperosmolality causes water to move out of the cell, and potassium levels are increased in the cell. The higher concentration causes potassium to shift out of the cell. The water also drags potassium out of the cell.
- **Inflammation:** Various inflammatory cytokines are generated during hyperglycemic crises.

Hypoglycemia

Hypoglycemia is defined as a low plasma blood glucose level with or without symptoms that may result in harm. A common alert value is usually < 70 mg/dL; however, the actual glycemic threshold that can induce symptoms (e.g., dizziness and sweating) and activate counterregulatory responses (e.g., glucagon secretion) can vary. If symptoms are present, they are caused by an autonomic response to a low glucose and include tremor, palpitations, anxiety, sweating, hunger, and paresthesias. Symptoms mediated by the actual low glucose (neuroglycopenia) include dizziness, weakness, drowsiness, confusion, and delirium, as well as seizure and coma with extremely low levels. The neuroglycopenic symptoms are more common in older adults or those with long-term diabetes.

Chronic complications are a direct result of long-term excessive glucose levels, especially when DM is not adequately managed. Over time, increased glucose levels contribute to thickening and hardening of vessel walls (much in the same way that the sugar in icing hardens on a cake), causing diffuse ischemia and necrosis. DM complications reflect these circulatory changes. Complications are also the result of the abnormal lipids such as increased triglycerides and reduced protective high-density lipoprotein (see chapter 4 for more on cardiovascular function). Adequate DM management is the best strategy to prevent chronic complications. Vascular complications can affect large vessels and small vessels. Macrovascular complications include atherosclerotic diseases such as coronary artery disease, peripheral artery disease, and cerebral vascular disease. Microvascular complications include retinopathy,

TABLE 10-3 | Types of Diabetic Neuropathies

Type	Characteristics	Clinical Manifestations
Polyneuropathy (diffuse)- involve multiple nerves	Distal Symmetrical Primarily sensory	Pain or loss of sensation (described as numbness and tingling) in extremities most commonly the feet/legs but can involve hands; worse at night; muscle weakness, if present, usually mild; lower extremities reflexes may be absent
	Autonomic*	Cardiovascular- postural hypotension, arrhythmias Eye- dry eyes, decreased pupillary reaction Mouth- dry mouth Gastrointestinal- gastroparesis, anorexia, early satiety, bloating, diarrhea or constipation Genitourinary- incontinence, urinary retention; in men impotence, ejaculatory and erectile disorder; in women vaginal dryness, impaired orgasm, and low libido Integument- impaired sweating (too much or too little) Hypoglycemia unawareness
Mononeuropathy (focal)- involve single	Asymmetric Commonly affects femoral, sciatic, and peroneal nerves and median and ulnar nerve	Lower extremity nerves affected: Pain in low back or hips and can radiate to thighs and knees; Pain described as deep aching with intermittent stabbing or piercing sensation weakness in legs; muscle atrophy; absent reflexes on affected side Upper extremity nerves affected: Wrist and elbow- arm/hand weakness and decreased sensation in fingers

*partial list of autonomic manifestations

nephropathy, and neuropathy. DM complications include:

- **Coronary artery disease:** Myocardial infarction is the most common type of heart disease and the most common cause of death in those with DM. Myocardial infarctions tend to be silent with DM due to diminished sensation from neuropathy. Heart failure is more prevalent in DM. Heart disease death rates are two to four times higher in people with DM.
- **Peripheral artery disease:** Diminished blood flow leads to ulcers and gangrene. Approximately 60% of nontraumatic amputations are due to DM.
- **Cerebral vascular disease:** Ischemic and lacunar infarcts are the most common types, and occurrence rates are two to four times higher in people with DM.
- **Hypertension:** Of the people with DM, 75% also have hypertension.
- **Hypercholesterolemia:** Diabetes decreases high density lipoprotein (i.e., good cholesterol) and increases low density lipoprotein (i.e., bad cholesterol) and triglycerides, increasing the risk of cardiovascular disease.
- **Diabetic retinopathy:** This is a leading cause of blindness.
- **Diabetic neuropathy:** Diabetic neuropathy (**TABLE 10-3**) occurs due to diminished nutrients to nerves resulting from decreased blood supply and nerve demyelination. Approximately 70% of people with DM have neuropathy (pain and numbness in the hands and feet). Neuropathy contributes to amputation rates due to unawareness of pain or foot ulcers.

Diagnosis and Treatment

Diagnosis is usually made with laboratory evaluation of glucose status. Evaluating glucose status is used for for assessing the effectiveness of DM management (**TABLE 10-4**). Diagnostic procedures include a history and physical examination. The various glucose tests include fasting blood glucose test, oral glucose tolerance test (most accurate for diagnosis in pregnancy), random blood glucose test, and hemoglobin A1c (HgbA1c; an average of glucose control for the previous 2–3 months).

Treatment strategies for DM vary depending on the type, but dietary changes (American Diabetic Association recommendations) and exercise are the first line of treatment. Management also includes glucose self-monitoring, weight loss (if the patient is overweight), oral or noninsulin injectable hyperglycemia medications (**TABLE 10-5**), insulin, and complication management. Insulin can be administered as a bolus. Insulin used for a bolus is rapid and

TABLE 10-4	Diagnostic Procedures and Treatment Goals for Diabetes Mellitus

Criteria for Diagnosis of Prediabetes

HgbA1c 5.7–6.4%

or

Impaired fasting glucose 100–125 mg/dL (fasting plasma glucose)

or

Impaired glucose tolerance 140–199 mg/dL (2-hour post 75 g glucose challenge)

Criteria for Diagnosis of Diabetes

HgbA1c $\geq$ 6.5%

or

Fasting plasma glucose $\geq$ 126 mg/dL*

or

2-hour plasma glucose $\geq$ 200 mg/dL* post 75 g glucose challenge

or

Random plasma glucose $\geq$ 200 mg/dL with symptoms (polyuria, polydipsia, and unexplained weight loss)

Treatment Goals for the ABCs of Diabetes

HgbA1c
Should be less than 7% for patients in general.

Preprandial capillary plasma glucose 70–130 mg/dL.

Peak postprandial capillary plasma glucose $\leq$ 180 mg/dL (usually 1–2 hours after the start of a meal). Be alert to the impact of hemoglobin variants on HgbA1c values.

*Blood Pressure***
Systolic $\leq$ 130 mmHg

Diastolic $\leq$ 80 mmHg

Cholesterol: Lipid Profile
LDL cholesterol $\leq$ 100 mg/dL

HDL cholesterol

- Men $\geq$ 40 mg/dL

- Women $\geq$ 50 mg/dL

Triglycerides $\leq$ 150 mg/dL

* Repeat to confirm on a subsequent day unless symptoms are present.
Data from American Diabetes Association. (2019). American Diabetes Association standards of medical care. *Diabetes Care, 42* (Suppl. 1), S1–S240.
** < 140/90 mmHg target acceptable for those with low cardiovascular risks.

short acting. Bolus administration is usually administered around mealtime and can be administered at a fixed dose or based on blood glucose values measured by the patient. Basal insulin is considered a background insulin and the effect is to keep glucose under control during fasting and to maintain a steady state. Basal insulin is intermediate and long acting, and it is usually administered once or twice a day. In addition, bariatric and metabolic surgeries have shown promise as potential cures for DM.

TABLE 10-5	Common Noninsulin Glucose-Lowering Drugs and Mechanism of Action
Medication class	**Main mechanism of action**
Biguanides	Decrease hepatic glucose output
Sulfonylureas	Stimulate sustained insulin release
Sodium/glucose cotransporter 2 inhibitors—glucoretics	Decrease glucose reabsorption in kidneys
Dipeptidyl peptidase-4 inhibitors—incretin enhancers	Prolong action of gut hormones Increase insulin secretion Delay gastric emptying
Glucagon-like peptide-1 receptor agonists—incretin mimetics	Increase insulin release with food Slow gastric emptying Promote satiety Suppress glucagon
Amylin mimetics	Slow gastric emptying Suppress glucagon Promote satiety

Obesity

Obesity is a chronic metabolic and endocrine disorder characterized by abnormal or excessive fat accumulation. Obesity is defined as a body mass index (BMI) of 30 kg/m^2 or greater. Overweight is defined as a BMI of 25 kg/m^2 or greater. The BMI is calculated using weight in kilograms divided by the square of height in meters. Obesity in children is defined as BMI at or above the 95th percentile for age and sex (based on CDC growth charts). The incidence of obesity worldwide has tripled since 1975; 650 million adults are obese, and 381 million persons under the age of 19 are either overweight or obese (WHO, 2019). Obesity is on the rise in the United States with 93.3 million (39.8%) adults affected and 13.7 million (18.5%) children and adolescents affected (CDC, 2018). The incidence is higher in Hispanics and Blacks in both adults and children. Obesity rates increase with aging; however, middle-aged adults (40–59 years) have a slightly higher incidence (approximately 1%) in comparison to adults over 60 years.

Obesity develops as a result of an imbalance between caloric intake (higher) and energy expenditure (lower). The reasons for the imbalance are multifactorial and complex. The various factors involved in obesity development include genetic, epigenetic, physiologic, environmental, behavioral, and sociocultural factors. Heritability of obesity has been demonstrated in twin studies and adoptee studies where the obese adoptees—even twins who were raised in separate environments—had BMIs closer to their biologic parents. While it is well known that obesity is heritable, identifying the genes has been challenging. Genetic loci have been found with BMI and waist-to-hip ratios. The *FTO* gene on chromosome 16 has demonstrated the strongest link with obesity, with the variant changing adipocytes from an energy-using fat (beige fat) to an energy-storing type of fat (white fat). There are also several single-gene defects causing various disorders associated with obesity such as abnormalities on chromosome 15 that cause Prader-Willi syndrome. This syndrome is associated with obesity, behavioral problems, and cognitive impairments.

Energy expenditure is determined by resting (basal) metabolic processes, which include energy needed for processes such as cellular membrane exchanges and heart, lung, and gastrointestinal function. Most energy expenditure (approximately 70%) is used for these basal metabolic processes even though this is the energy needed during a physically inactive state. The basal metabolic rate is also defined as the minimum number of calories needed to live. About 10% of energy is used to process food (called the *thermogenic response*), and the remaining 20% is used for activity. Low-energy expenditure such as what occurs in a sedentary lifestyle will cause weight gain. Interestingly, weight gain is associated with an increase in energy expenditure while weight loss results in lower energy expenditure, which can cause many frustrations in weight-loss attempts and in maintenance of weight loss. Energy expenditure is also influenced by types of food ingested, with some foods expending more energy than others. However, determining the optimum types of food that would increase energy expenditure in attempts to lose weight is complex and not simply measured by food thermogenesis.

Different types of fat in the body will influence energy expenditure. Fat or adipose tissue types include white adipose fat, brown adipose fat, and beige adipose fat. White adipose fat is the most abundant in the body and is responsible for the many functions of fat. Some key functions include the storage of excess calories as an energy reserve. Adipokines (hormones and cytokines) released by adipocytes (fat cells) also regulate metabolism and activate immune processes. Excesses of white fat cause dysregulation of these multiple adipokines. White adipose fat is found deep within the body (visceral fat) and in the periphery as subcutaneous fat. Increases in visceral fat predominantly around the intra-abdominal cavity (belly fat) are associated with increased complications such as cardiovascular and diabetes mellitus risk. With aging, gonadal and growth hormone naturally declines, resulting in an increase in visceral fat in men, while in women, decreases in estrogen (usually due to menopause) and growth hormone contribute to increases in visceral fat. This, in part, may be a reason why fat mass increases during middle age. White fat can become beige fat, which is an energy-expending type of fat. Investigations are underway to determine how to stimulate this conversion so that weight loss can be achieved. Brown fat is considered a good fat and primarily regulates energy usage, particularly maintenance of warmth in newborns, and usage peaks around puberty. Brown fat expends energy like beige fat. The amount of brown fat decreases with age but continues to remain metabolically active and is stimulated with exposure to cold weather. Brown fat is located mainly in the upper torso in the neck and clavicular area. The more active the brown fat, the lower the BMI and body fat percentage. Leaner individuals have more brown fat, and investigations are underway to determine how to increase and stimulate brown fat.

Body weight and fat stores are regulated by the central and peripheral nervous system. The central nervous system receives afferent signals from the periphery regarding food needs and fuel use. In the hypothalamus, there are orexigenic neurons (e.g., neuropeptide Y, melanin-concentrating hormone, and orexin A and B) that when stimulated lead to decreased metabolism and mechanisms to increase calories by promoting appetite and stimulation of eating. In contrast, anorexigenic neurons, when stimulated, increase metabolism and suppress appetite and eating. These opposing neuron activations are necessary for balancing food intake and energy use. The hypothalamus also connects with areas of the cortex that are associated with memory, pleasure, and reward, and these areas can be activated by food and the feeling of satiety. Activation of these areas can override physiologic intake and energy expenditure stimuli leading to overeating, or the desire for only certain foods. The signals that are received by the hypothalamus come from the periphery via the circulation and the autonomic nervous system. Some of the sensory signals originate in the fat and gastrointestinal tract. Leptin is a key hormone that is primarily secreted by white fat adipocytes; its role is to send signals to the brain regarding the adequacy of energy reserves. When a person overeats, leptin levels increase dramatically, and when the person fasts, levels decrease. Leptin levels are correlated with body fat mass, and the levels increase in proportion to the number of adipocytes. Leptin's key action is decreasing food intake, but the high levels in obese individuals are ineffective in suppressing appetite. This ineffective response is due to resistance or tolerance to the effects of leptin. The reason for the development of resistance is unclear. There is also a single gene defect that causes leptin deficiency and obesity.

Several gastrointestinal hormones are involved in regulation of food intake. These hormones are either associated with appetite stimulation and increases in food intake (i.e., they are orexins), or they are associated with appetite suppression and inhibit food intake (i.e., they are anorexins). Some of these hormones are listed next.

Increase Food Intake

- **Ghrelin**: Ghrelin is produced in the stomach and duodenum, and it stimulates growth hormone and food intake. Levels increase when a person is fasting and decrease after eating. Food types that suppress ghrelin the most are carbohydrates, followed by protein and lipids. Diet and exercise-related weight loss causes increases in ghrelin as a compensatory mechanism, thereby making maintenance of weight loss challenging.

Inhibit Food Intake

- **Glucagon-like-peptide-1**: This is an incretin hormone produced in the intestines. Stimulation causes insulin release, slows gastric emptying, and suppresses appetite. Levels may be low in obese individuals.
- **Cholecystokinin**: Cholecystokinin is secreted by the intestines. Stimulation causes gallbladder release of bile and release of pancreatic enzymes and insulin and slows gastric emptying. Levels may be low in obese individuals.
- **Pancreatic polypeptide and peptide YY 3-36**: These are produced by the pancreatic polypeptide cells; they inhibit gastric motility, cause satiation, and decrease appetite. Levels may be decreased in obesity.
- **Oxyntomodulin**: This is a peptide hormone found in the colon that causes appetite suppression.
- **Amylin**: Amylin is released from the beta cells and has a synergistic relationship with insulin. Stimulation results in glucose control by suppressing glucagon, delaying gastric emptying, and increasing satiety. Levels may be increased in obesity, but there is resistance to the effects.

Obesity is associated with many complications, particularly cardiometabolic disorders such as dyslipidemia, hypertension, diabetes mellitus type 2, polycystic ovary syndrome, and nonalcoholic fatty liver disease. Several of these disorders are partly the result of the chronic, low-grade inflammatory state created by adipocytes in white fat. Immune cells in the white fat release various inflammatory cytokines (e.g., interleukin-6 and tumor necrosis factor). The inflammatory state is further maintained by various adipokines such as adiponectin (anti-inflammatory), leptin, and resistin (promotes inflammation). Adiponectin levels are decreased, while leptin and resistin levels are increased in obesity. The excess fat of obesity is associated with various biomechanical disorders such as gastroesophageal reflux disease, osteoarthritis, sleep apnea, and urinary incontinence. Various cancers are associated with obesity such as colon, pancreatic, breast, and endometrial cancer. Approximately 40% of all cancers diagnosed are attributed to obesity and overweight (Steele et al., 2017). Reproductive effects include abnormal menses and infertility. Psychosocial problems arising from stigma and low self-esteem are associated with obesity and can cause depression.

Clinical Manifestations

Obesity manifestations will be related to the complications that they cause. Some individuals are obese but develop no complications; these individuals are considered metabolically healthy obese. However, not all components of metabolic health are measurable, and the impact may therefore be underestimated. Fat distribution may confer different degrees of risk for obesity-related complications. Those with a greater visceral fat distribution (such persons are commonly referred to as having an apple shape) are at risk for more complications in comparison to those whose fat distribution is in the subcutaneous or buttocks and thigh region (such persons are commonly referred to as having a pear shape).

Diagnosis and Treatment

Diagnosis is made based on anthropometric measurements of height and weight and calculation of BMI. BMI limitations include overestimation of body fat in athletes or those with a muscular build and underestimation of body fat in older persons and others who have lost muscle mass. Other diagnostic tools can include the measurement of the waist circumference—usually for those with a BMI less than 35 kg/m² (above this, waist measurement adds little prediction for risks). In a woman, a high waist circumference is > 88 cm (> 35 inches), and in a man a high waist circumference is > 102 cm (> 40 inches). The waist-to-hip ratio can be calculated to evaluate for body shape and fat distribution. Growth chart percentiles and BMI are used in the diagnosis of obesity in children. Other components of body composition analysis can be done with techniques such as bioelectrical impedance to evaluate fat mass (which measures the rate at which a low electrical current travels through the body—fat slows this rate), air/water displacement plethysmography, or dual-energy X-ray absorptiometry. A history and physical examination are important to evaluate for complications of obesity. Diagnostic testing is done based on risk and complications associated with obesity and will generally include a lipid profile and electrolyte, glucose, renal function, and liver enzyme analysis.

Treatment strategies center on weight and fat reduction. Lifestyle and behavioral therapies will include healthy eating and physical activity. There are various proposed diet modalities to achieve weight loss such as low-calorie, low-fat/low-calorie, moderate-fat/low-calorie, and low-carbohydrate diets. The most important component of weight loss, however, is not the type of diet but rather adherence to the diet. Adherence can be facilitated with dietary counseling or support groups and behavioral therapy (e.g., self-monitoring with food diaries, stimulus control). If weight loss is not achieved with comprehensive lifestyle strategies, then pharmacologic therapies can be added. The medications available include orlistat (alters fat digestion and increases fecal excretion), lorcaserin (a serotonin agonist that reduces food intake), phentermine/topiramate (which suppresses appetite and increases satiety), naltrexone/bupropion (which suppresses appetite and controls cravings and overeating behaviors), and liraglutide (which has glucagon-like peptide-1 effects). Bariatric surgery is another strategy that is indicated for those with a BMI of 40 kg/m^2 or higher and for those with a BMI of 30 to 39.9 kg/m^2 with obesity comorbidities or difficulties with controlling their diabetes. There are various techniques for bariatric surgery. The most commonly performed procedures are Roux-en-Y bypass and sleeve gastrectomy. Other techniques include intragastric balloon therapy, vagal blockage, and aspiration therapy.

Disorders of the Thyroid Gland

Because of the thyroid hormones' responsibilities, disorders of the thyroid have a significant impact on metabolic activities. These disorders usually result in either an increase or a decrease in the thyroid hormones. Several etiologies can give rise to these conditions, including tumors, congenital defects, damage (e.g., from surgery, radiation, or infections), and aging. These conditions are usually easily managed with medications and surgery.

Goiter and Thyroid Nodules

A goiter refers to an abnormal growth of the thyroid gland. Thyroid nodules are also abnormal growths on the thyroid gland, and they can occur with or without a goiter. A goiter is usually painless but can be painful. Goiters may affect the respiratory and gastrointestinal systems. The enlargement is not necessarily malignant. Goiters can occur in hyperthyroidism, hypothyroidism, and euthyroid thyroid states. Thyroid nodules are common and can be single or multiple. Most nodules are benign; however, up to 15% of nodules are malignant. Thyroid hormone levels are usually normal, but a nodule may produce excess hormone levels, leading to hyperthyroidism.

Iodine deficiency is the most common cause of goiters worldwide. Iodine deficiency leads to decreased T$_3$ and T$_4$ production, and TSH production increases in an attempt to compensate for the low levels of these thyroid hormones. Iodine deficiency in the United States is not common, and goiters in the United States are usually due to the presence of thyroid nodules and autoimmune thyroid disorders. Increased levels of TSH lead to thyroid hyperplasia and hypertrophy. A similar reaction occurs in both hyperthyroidism and hypothyroidism states. Many goiters grow slowly and are asymptomatic. Nodules are usually asymptomatic. Goiters, however, can cause obstructive-type symptoms due to compression of the trachea, and nodules, and, if large enough, may also compress the trachea or esophagus. These symptoms vary and depend on the goiter size and the tracheal diameter. Symptoms such as dyspnea, cough, or a choking sensation can be due to compression. A thyroid ultrasound is usually done to evaluate the thyroid gland and to determine whether a nodule is solid or cystic. With an ultrasound, the size of the nodules can be determined, and cancerous and noncancerous nodule characteristics can be evaluated. After an ultrasound, a fine-needle biopsy is normally done to evaluate if the nodule is benign or cancerous.

Hypothyroidism

Hypothyroidism refers to a condition in which the thyroid does not produce sufficient amounts of the thyroid hormones. This endocrine disorder is relatively common (affecting 1 out of 500 Americans) and is more common in women than men. Hypothyroidism can be congenital (e.g., absent thyroid gland) or acquired as a result of hypothalamus, pituitary, or thyroid (primary hypothyroidism; the most common) dysfunction. Several conditions can result in hypothyroidism. Hypothyroidism risk increases with age, especially in persons older than 50 years.

In many cases, a previous or current inflammation of the thyroid gland (thyroiditis) leaves a large percentage of thyroid cells damaged and incapable of producing sufficient hormone amounts. Causes of thyroiditis include infections, medications such as lithium or amiodarone, and trauma. Trauma that induces thyroiditis can involve vigorous manipulation during surgery or a seat belt injury in a car accident. However, the most common cause of thyroiditis, which can cause thyroid gland failure, is called *chronic autoimmune thyroiditis* (also called *Hashimoto thyroiditis*). Chronic autoimmune thyroiditis occurs due to genetic susceptibility and environmental triggers (e.g., pregnancy). In chronic autoimmune thyroiditis, antibodies and T cells destroy thyroid antigen cells. The types of thyroid antigens include thyroglobulin, thyroid peroxidase (TPO), and TSH receptor. Under normal circumstances, the thyroid follicle cells take up thyroglobulin when stimulated by TSH. TPO is the enzyme that oxidizes iodide to iodine, which is necessary for thyroglobulin to yield thyroxine (T_4) and triiodothyronine (T_3). T_4 is deiodinated in the peripheral tissues to form T_3. In chronic autoimmune thyroiditis, B cells in the thyroid gland produce IgG-type antibodies to thyroglobulin and TPO. The T cells secrete cytokines, regulate an immune response, and ultimately, destroy the thyroid cells. Thyrotropin receptor antibodies (i.e., thyroid-stimulating immunoglobulin) are present in Graves disease (hyperthyroidism) and chronic autoimmune thyroiditis (atrophic type).

A variant of chronic autoimmune thyroiditis is postpartum thyroiditis. As with chronic autoimmune thyroiditis, there is an autoimmune destruction of the gland. High levels of anti-TPO antibodies are often detected in pregnancy and persist after delivery. Risk factors for development of postpartum thyroiditis include women with type 1 DM, family history, and history of postpartum thyroiditis with prior pregnancies. Postpartum thyroiditis usually occurs within 1 year after childbirth and can also occur after an abortion (e.g., spontaneous or induced). In postpartum thyroiditis, the thyroid gland initially produces large amounts of T_3 and T_4 as follicular cells are being destroyed. The high levels of thyroid gland hormones result in hyperthyroidism. Eventually, the follicular cells can no longer produce the hormones, and hormone levels decrease. Hypothyroidism occurs and thyroid hormone levels are decreased in response to increased TSH levels. The inflammation of thyroiditis can subside, the gland can begin functioning normally again, and the woman can remain euthyroid. However, hypothyroidism or goiter can remain. Even if the hypothyroidism resolves, the woman is at risk for development of permanent hypothyroidism in the future. The second major cause of hypothyroidism, after chronic autoimmune thyroiditis, is iatrogenic (resulting from medical treatments). The treatment of many thyroid conditions, such as hyperthyroidism, warrants partial or complete surgical removal of the thyroid gland. If the total

remaining thyroid hormone–producing cells are not able to meet the needs of the body, hypothyroidism develops. This result is often the goal of surgery for thyroid cancer. Similarly, goiters and some other thyroid conditions can be treated with radioactive iodine therapy. The aim of the radioactive iodine therapy (for benign conditions) is to kill a portion of the thyroid to prevent goiters from growing larger or developing into hyperthyroidism. Occasionally, the radioactive iodine treatment can damage too many cells, but this consequence is usually preferred over the original problem.

Clinical Manifestations

The clinical manifestations of hypothyroidism vary widely, depending on the severity of the hormone deficiency. Generally, clinical manifestations tend to be insidious and develop slowly, often over a number of years. Abrupt manifestations can occur after thyroidectomy or sudden cessation of thyroid hormone replacement therapy. These clinical manifestations reflect the decreased thyroid activity (e.g., metabolism) and deposition of glycosaminoglycans (connective tissue compounds such as chondroitin sulfate) around tissues (**TABLE 10-6**).

Severe hypothyroidism, known as myxedema coma, is rare. Myxedema coma is more likely to occur in those individuals with long-standing hypothyroidism or poorly controlled hypothyroidism in combination with a precipitating event such as infection or opioid administration. Older women are more commonly affected. When it occurs, myxedema coma can be life threatening. Clinical manifestations include marked hypotension, respiratory depression, hypothermia, hyponatremia, hypoglycemia, lethargy, and coma.

Diagnosis and Treatment

Diagnostic procedures for hypothyroidism include a history, physical examination, serum thyroid hormone levels, and serum TSH. Diagnosis is made based on laboratory results of the thyroid levels and TSH. Primary hypothyroidism (thyroid gland disorder) results in a high serum TSH and low serum-free T_4, total T_4, and total T_3. Conversion of T_4 to T_3 increases in the early stages of hypothyroidism, so T_3 levels may be normal. If the TSH is high and the T_3 and T_4 are normal, the patient is diagnosed with subclinical hypothyroidism. Central hypothyroidism (pituitary or hypothalamus disorder) results in a low serum TSH and low thyroid hormones. Antithyroid antibodies,

TABLE 10-6 Hypothyroidism and Hyperthyroidism Clinical Manifestations

System	Hypothyroidism	Hyperthyroidism
General	Fatigue, sluggishness Cold intolerance Slow speech Peripheral edema (hands, feet)	Restlessness, nervousness, anxiousness, irritability, impaired concentration Heat intolerance Insomnia
Skin	Cool, pale, dry, rough Diminished perspiration Hair: coarse, loss/thinning Nails: brittle	Warm, smooth Diaphoresis Hair: fine, thinning Nails: onycholysis, softening Shins: raised, pigmented papules (pretibial myxedema)
Hematologic	Increased bleeding risk Anemia (pernicious—gastric atrophy, iron deficiency)	
Head	Puffy face, hoarseness Eyes: periorbital edema Nose: rhinitis Mouth: macroglossia Neck: goiter (painful or painless)	Eyes: exophthalmos (**FIGURE 10-11**) with staring Neck: goiter (painful or painless)
Cardiovascular	Decreased heart rate Hypercholesteremia	Increased heart rate Hypertension Atrial fibrillation
Respiratory	Dyspnea with exertion	Dyspnea with exertion
Gastrointestinal	Constipation Weight gain	Diarrhea Weight loss (usually sudden) Increased appetite
Reproductive	Abnormal menses (absent, irregular (frequent/infrequent), heavy (more common) Infertility Erectile dysfunction, decreased libido	Abnormal menses (oligomenorrhea, amenorrhea Infertility Erectile dysfunction, decreased libido
Neurologic	Depression Carpal tunnel syndrome Decreased deep tendon reflexes	Fine tremor (usually hands)
Musculoskeletal	Muscle weakness/cramps, myalgias, arthralgias	

particularly anti-TPO and antithyroglobulin, may also be evaluated. Elevated levels indicate chronic autoimmune thyroiditis.

Hypothyroidism is easily managed with thyroid hormone replacement with T_4 (e.g., levothyroxine [Synthroid]). The effectiveness of the dose is usually evaluated 6 weeks after initiation of therapy with a TSH measurement. Six weeks is when steady-state TSH levels are expected with replacement therapy. Lower doses are recommended when initiating thyroid-replacement therapy in the elderly to

avoid the risk of inducing cardiovascular syndromes. T_3 therapy (usually combined with T_4) may be attempted for some patients (e.g., those with persistent symptomaticity after thyroidectomy despite adequate T_4 replacement), but monotherapy with T_4 is almost always sufficient. Hormone replacement for subclinical hypothyroidism is usually recommended when TSH levels are ≥ 10 mU/L. Hormone replacement for patients with values between 4.5 and 10 mU/L is controversial; however, monitoring TSH levels is recommended to evaluate

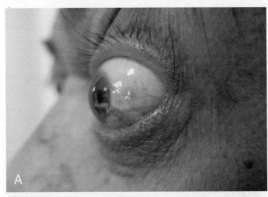

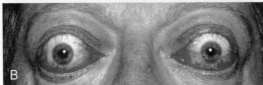

FIGURE 10-11 Exophthalmos.

A: © Casa nayafana/Shutterstock; **B:** © SPL/Science Source.

for potential progression to hypothyroidism. Central hypothyroidism is also treated with T$_4$ replacement therapy and other strategies to manage the cause (usually pituitary adenoma).

Hyperthyroidism

Hyperthyroidism refers to a condition of excessive levels of thyroid hormones. This overabundance of thyroid hormones results in a hypermetabolic state. The incidence is higher in women than in men. Older age and smoking are risk factors. Hyperthyroidism can result from a variety of conditions, and these disorders can be distinguished using a 24-hour radioiodine uptake scan. The scan is used to measure the amount of radioactive iodine that is taken up by the thyroid gland after oral administration. This test is only for nonpregnant patients. The presence of uptake usually indicates that there is new hormone synthesis. No uptake indicates a destroyed or inflamed thyroid gland, and the thyroid hormones are coming from preformed hormones or an ectopic source. Hyperthyroid disorders are outlined in the following lists.

Normal or High Radioiodine Uptake
- **Graves disease:** This disease is an autoimmune condition with TSH receptor antibodies, which stimulate thyroid hormone production; the condition may be precipitated by excessive iodine or medications (e.g., lithium).
- **Thyroid adenomas/toxic multinodular goiter:** This adenoma/goiter causes thyroid hyperplasia with cells that produce hormones independent from TSH regulation.

- **Excessive iodine:** The excess can occur after administration for scanning or due to iodine-rich medications such as amiodarone.

Near-Absent Radioiodine Uptake
- Thyroiditis from multiple causes (e.g., radiation, medications such as lithium, amiodarone).
- Excess thyroid hormone replacement.
- Ectopic production (e.g., thyroid cancer metastasis)

Clinical Manifestations

Hyperthyroidism can mimic other health problems, and its clinical manifestations may be overt, leading to a high suspicion of hyperthyroidism, or they can vary, making diagnosis difficult (Table 10-6).

Older patients tend to have predominant cardiovascular manifestations such as tachycardia or atrial fibrillation, dyspnea, and edema. The manifestations are a result of a hypermetabolic state.

Learning Points

Hyperthyroidism and Hypothyroidism Manifestations

Hypothyroidism and hyperthyroidism present differently. When considering the clinical manifestations of these disorders, think about what increasing or decreasing thyroid hormones would do in the body. With hypothyroidism, the hormone levels are decreased and so are all the clinical manifestations (e.g., bradycardia, hypotension, depression, and constipation), with the exception of weight gain. With hyperthyroidism, the hormone levels are increased and so are all the clinical manifestations (e.g., tachycardia, hypertension, anxiety, and diarrhea), with the exception of weight loss.

Thyroid crisis (storm) is a sudden worsening of hyperthyroidism symptoms that may occur with long-term, untreated hyperthyroidism and may be precipitated by such factors as infection, stress, or surgery. Thyroid crisis is rare and is a medical emergency. Thyroid crisis is characterized by high temperature (e.g., 104 to 106° F), tachycardia (> 140 beats per minute), decreased mental alertness, abdominal pain, and an exaggeration of any hyperthyroid manifestations (Table 10-6). Additional complications of hyperthyroidism include cardiomyopathy, heart failure, and osteoporosis.

Diagnosis and Treatment

Diagnostic procedures for hyperthyroidism include a history, physical examination, serum thyroid hormone levels, and serum TSH. With hyperthyroidism, the serum TSH will be low and the T$_4$ and T$_3$ will be high. The T$_3$ increases more than the T$_4$. Central hyperthyroidism will result in a low TSH and normal T$_3$ and T$_4$. This pattern may also be present in subclinical hyperthyroidism. Thyroid-stimulating immunoglobulin will be positive with Graves disease. The anti-TPO antibody may also be positive with Graves syndrome but not as often as in chronic autoimmune thyroiditis (Hashimoto's thyroiditis). A radioactive iodine uptake test is usually indicated when there is nodular thyroid disease, and results can aid in diagnosing the cause of hyperthyroidism. Hyperthyroidism can usually be easily managed with medication and surgery. Beta blockers can be used to manage symptoms such as tachycardia, anxiety, and heat intolerance. In circumstances where there is increased hormone synthesis (i.e., normal or increased radioiodine uptake disorders) treatments are geared during reducing synthesis. Pharmacologic treatment usually includes radioactive iodine (which shrinks the gland) as well as antithyroid agents, such as methimazole (the primary drug), to decrease hormone production or propylthiouracil which is safe during pregnancy. Surgical removal of the thyroid (thyroidectomy) with subsequent hormone replacement is warranted when the patient does not respond to or tolerate medications. Even with treatment, exophthalmos usually remains. Strategies to improve the discomfort associated with exophthalmos include cool compresses, wearing sunglasses, eye lubricants, and elevating the head of the bed. Increasing caloric and calcium intake is crucial to maintain weight and prevent bone loss. For hyperthyroidism with near-absent radioiodine uptake due to thyroiditis, hormone-synthesis-blocking agents will not be effective since new hormones are not being produced. The treatment, therefore, is symptom control (e.g., via a beta blocker) or anti-inflammatory medications such as nonsteroidal anti-inflammatory drugs.

Disorders of the Parathyroid Glands

Parathyroid disorders result in an increase or decrease in PTH. Because of PTH's effects, disorders of the parathyroid have a significant impact on calcium balance that has a domino effect on other electrolytes (phosphorus and magnesium). Several etiologies can result in

these conditions, including tumors, congenital defects, damage (e.g., from surgery, radiation, or infections), and renal failure. These conditions are usually easily managed with medications and surgery. See chapter 6 for a discussion of calcium regulation.

Hypoparathyroidism

Hypoparathyroidism refers to a condition in which the parathyroid gland does not produce sufficient amounts of PTH. Hypoparathyroidism, which is uncommon, can be caused by congenital or genetic defects—a lack of one or more of the four parathyroid glands, abnormal PTH synthesis, or mutations of calcium-sensing receptors. It can also be caused by damage following surgery, autoimmune conditions, or metabolic alkalosis. Rare causes of hypoparathyroidism include radiation and infiltrative disorders (e.g., metastasis or hemochromatosis). Hypomagnesemia from multiple causes such as chronic alcoholism or malabsorption suppresses PTH. Correction of the magnesium levels returns PTH levels to normal. PTH deficiency results in hypocalcemia and a subsequent increase in phosphorus levels.

Clinical Manifestations

Clinical manifestations reflect electrolyte and pH imbalances, particularly hypocalcemia (see Table 6-6). Hypocalcemia results in an excitatory nerve and muscle response from stimuli.

Acute manifestations will typically include neuromuscular irritability (i.e., tetany) with symptoms such as paresthesias (perioral, hands, and feet), muscle cramping, carpopedal spasms, and seizures along with other manifestations. Acute manifestations can occur after parathyroid or neck surgery (e.g., thyroid surgery). Chronic manifestations that are not present in acute causes include basal ganglia calcifications (cause movement disorders or dementia), cataract development, and skin changes (e.g., dry, coarse, sparse hair, and brittle nails).

Diagnosis and Treatment

Diagnostic procedures for hypoparathyroidism include a history, physical examination, and serum PTH with serum calcium evaluation. Serum calcium and PTH will be low and serum phosphate levels will be high. Acute manifestations will typically include neuromuscular irritability (i.e., tetany) with symptoms such as paresthesias (perioral, hands, and feet), muscle cramping, carpopedal spasms, and seizures along with other manifestations.

BOX 10-1 Application to Practice

Thyroid Function Panel Reference Range

(handwritten note in left margin): TSH will show abnml VS - may need to see sooner than 6 wks.

Test	Reference range*
TSH	0.450–4.500 mU/mL
Thyroxine (T_4), total	4.6–12.0 mcg/dL
Thyroxine (T_4), free (direct)	0.7–1.9 mcg/dL
Free thyroxine index (calculated)	4–11
Triiodothyronine (T_3), total	80–180 ng/dL

* Reference range may vary from one laboratory to another.

Review the following case and answer the questions.

Case 1: Ms. Jefferson is a 50-year-old woman who comes into the clinic to review her laboratory results from 2 weeks prior. She is in good health and has no complaints. Her laboratory values are normal except for the following:

TSH = 30 mU/L; T_4 = 3.0 mcg/dL; free T_4 = 0.5 mcg/dL; free thyroxine index = 3.0; T_3 = 90 ng/dL

1. Based on these lab findings Ms. Jefferson is diagnosed with which thyroid disorder?
   a. Hyperthyroidism
   b. Subclinical hyperthyroidism
   c. Hypothyroidism *(circled)*
   d. Subclinical hypothyroidism

2. The lack of symptoms in the type of thyroid disorder Ms. Jefferson has is uncommon. Answer True or False *(False circled)*

3. Ms. Jefferson's thyroid disorder is most likely caused by what?
   a. A pituitary adenoma (i.e., thyrotroph)
   b. Chronic autoimmune thyroiditis (i.e., Hashimoto thyroiditis) *(circled)*
   c. Autoimmune Graves disease
   d. Iodine deficiency

4. Treatment of Ms. Jefferson's thyroid disorder will include what?
   a. Thyroid hormone replacement with T_4 *(circled)*
   b. Thyroid hormone replacement with T_3
   c. Beta blocker
   d. No therapy indicated

5. Ms. Jefferson asks when she should return to evaluate her thyroid disorder. You should respond:
   a. An annual evaluation should be sufficient.
   b. Return to have a TSH level done 6 weeks after starting therapy. *(circled)*
   c. Six months from now.

6. Ms. Jefferson asks what are some possible symptoms of her thyroid disorder? Select all that apply.
   a. Weight gain *(circled)*
   b. Diarrhea
   c. Anxiety
   d. Palpitations
   e. Fatigue *(circled)*
   f. Cold intolerance *(circled)*

Acute manifestations can occur after parathyroid or neck surgery (e.g., thyroid surgery). Chronic manifestations that are not present in acute causes include basal ganglia calcifications (cause movement disorders or dementia), cataract development, and skin changes (e.g., dry, coarse, sparse hair, and brittle nails). Treatment regimens generally include calcium and vitamin D administration. The addition of PTH replacement is rarely necessary and is indicated when calcium levels are not maintained. Other strategies generally focus on correcting electrolyte and pH imbalances such as replacement of magnesium for hypomagnesemia (see chapter 6 for more on fluid, electrolyte, and acid–base homeostasis).

Hyperparathyroidism

Hyperparathyroidism refers to a condition of excessive PTH production by the parathyroid gland. Primary hyperparathyroidism is due to parathyroid gland disorders, which are usually caused by adenomas (most common cause), tumors (due to genetic mutations), hyperplasia, or radiation exposure. Secondary hyperparathyroidism is due to chronic hypocalcemia (e.g., kidney disease, decreased intestinal absorption, and chronic vitamin D deficiency). Hyperparathyroidism will result in hypercalcemia. The excessive calcium levels can lead to decreases in phosphorus levels, increases in magnesium levels, and metabolic acidosis. The clinical manifestations of hyperparathyroidism

BOX 10-2 Application to Practice

Differentiating the relationship between serum calcium and PTH levels can be a bit confusing. Understanding the underlying mechanisms for the alterations can assist in interpreting these laboratory values. The following are possible laboratory findings. Answer the following questions.

1. Explain the mechanism by which the serum calcium and serum PTH is high with primary hyperparathyroidism.
2. Explain the mechanism by which the serum calcium is high and the serum PTH is low with a nonparathyroid disorder such as breast malignancy.
3. Explain the mechanism by which the serum calcium is low and the serum PTH is high with secondary hyperparathyroidism.

reflect these electrolyte and pH imbalances (see Table 6-5). See chapter 6 for more on fluid, electrolyte, and acid–base homeostasis.

Diagnosis and Treatment

Diagnostic procedures for hyperparathyroidism include a history, physical examination, serum PTH, and serum calcium evaluation. Serum PTH and calcium will be high with hyperparathyroidism. If the calcium levels are high and the PTH is low, then the high calcium levels may be due to malignancy (usually breast, lung, or multiple myeloma), or excessive calcium or vitamin D intake. Low serum calcium with high PTH is consistent with secondary hyperparathyroidism. Treatment varies depending on the underlying etiology. Tumors will likely require surgery and radiation. Calcitonin may be administered to shift the calcium from the bloodstream to the bones. Calcimimetic agents may be administered to mimic calcium circulating in the blood and, in turn, may lead to decreased PTH production. Bisphosphonates can decrease the loss of calcium from the bone and lessen osteoporosis. Phosphates may be administered to correct phosphorus deficits, which will decrease calcium levels. Increasing fluid intake (either oral or intravenous) will increase renal excretion of calcium. Additionally, magnesium and pH imbalances may need correction (see chapter 6 for more on fluid, electrolyte, and acid–base homeostasis).

Disorders of the Adrenal Glands

Adrenal gland disorders may affect one or both areas of the adrenal gland. These disorders result in an increase or a decrease in one or more adrenal hormones. Depending on the hormone affected and the severity of the condition, adrenal gland disorders can have serious consequences. Several etiologies can result in these conditions, including tumors, congenital defects, medications (e.g., corticosteroids), and damage (e.g., from surgery, radiation, or infections). These disorders are usually easily managed with medications and surgery, but they can become life threatening if not managed promptly.

Pheochromocytoma

Pheochromocytoma is a rare tumor of the adrenal medulla. The tumor excretes epinephrine and norepinephrine and can be life threatening because of the effects of these hormones (e.g., increased blood pressure and tachycardia). Other tumors that are catecholamine secreting include paragangliomas (extra-adrenal pheochromocytomas), which are clinically similar and treated the same. Pheochromocytoma can occur as a single tumor or as multiple tumors in one or both adrenal glands and is only malignant in 10% of cases. The exact cause is unknown, and the tumors are often sporadic. Some tumors are associated with inherited mutations (e.g., neurofibromatosis type 1 gene). The tumors can occur at any age but are more common in early to middle adulthood for hereditary tumors and older people (40–50 years of age) for sporadic types.

Clinical Manifestations

Clinical manifestations reflect the fight-or-flight response and occur in unpredictable attacks that usually last 15 to 20 minutes, but some manifestations can be sustained. The classic triad is the episodic occurrence of headache, diaphoresis, and tachycardia, and while many patients have these symptoms individually, they do not necessarily have all three classic symptoms together. The manifestations include the following symptoms:

- Hypertension (sustained or paroxysmal is the most common sign)
- Tachycardia
- Profound diaphoresis
- Mild or severe headaches with variable duration
- Dysrhythmias
- Forceful palpitations
- Chest pain
- Hyperglycemia
- Abdominal pain
- Anxiety
- Feeling of extreme fright
- Pallor
- Weight loss
- Difficulty sleeping

Diagnosis and Treatment

Diagnostic procedures for pheochromocytoma include a history, physical examination, serum catecholamines (norepinephrine, epinephrine, and dopamine) and metanephrines, as well as urine catecholamines and metanephrines. Metanephrines are metabolites of epinephrine. Radiologic evaluation will include an abdominal and pelvic CT or abdominal and pelvic MRI. An *m*-iodobenzylguanidine scintiscan (a nuclear scan to confirm pheochromocytoma) can be used if the CT or MRI is negative, and there is continued suspicion or if there are multiple tumors. Genetic testing may be necessary for patients suspected of familial disease. If not promptly treated, pheochromocytoma can lead to hypertensive crisis, stroke, kidney disease, psychosis, and seizures. Surgical removal of the tumor or adrenal gland is the cornerstone of treatment. Administration of antihypertensive medications (e.g., alpha blockers and beta blockers) is often necessary until surgery can be performed. Metastatic pheochromocytoma may require additional treatment, such as radioactive iodine.

Cushing Syndrome

Cushing syndrome refers to a condition characterized by excessive amounts of glucocorticoids, specifically cortisol. The most common cause of this excess, called *hypercortisolism*, is iatrogenic, resulting from ingestion of glucocorticoid medications; however, the incidence is often underreported. When these medications are ingested, they mimic the body's own

hormones. Cushing syndrome can also be caused by excess ACTH production, usually from a pituitary adenoma (the second most common cause of Cushing syndrome), and this state is termed *Cushing disease*. Cushing disease is ACTH dependent, which refers to ACTH stimulating excess cortisol production while the negative feedback mechanism is impaired. Normal pulsatile cortisol secretion or increased cortisol response during stress is impaired. Cushing disease can occur at any age. An ectopic nonpituitary tumor such as from small cell lung cancer, which is more common in older adults, is another form of ACTH-dependent hypercortisolism. Benign or malignant adrenal gland tumors that secrete cortisol are a form of ACTH-independent hypercortisolism. This condition is the least common cause of Cushing syndrome. Adrenal carcinoma is the cause of 50% of childhood Cushing syndrome.

Glucocorticoids are essential for life but can produce serious effects when present in excessive amounts (FIGURE 10-12). Manifestations can also be the result of androgen deficit or excess. Some

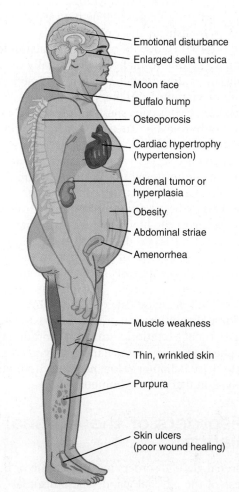

FIGURE 10-12 Signs and symptoms of Cushing syndrome.

- Emotional disturbance
- Enlarged sella turcica
- Moon face
- Buffalo hump
- Osteoporosis
- Cardiac hypertrophy (hypertension)
- Adrenal tumor or hyperplasia
- Obesity
- Abdominal striae
- Amenorrhea
- Muscle weakness
- Thin, wrinkled skin
- Purpura
- Skin ulcers (poor wound healing)

BOX 10-3 Application to Practice

A 50-year-old woman with an 8-year history of diabetes mellitus presents with difficulty controlling her blood sugars for the past 2 weeks. Her self-monitoring blood glucose readings have been in the 200s–300s for 2 weeks. She has managed her type 2 DM with diet, exercise, and metformin 1,000 mg twice a day. Her last glycosylated hemoglobin (HgbA1c) level, which was measured 2 months ago, was 6.8%. She has had asthma since age 18. She felt her asthma was getting worse for the past 6 months as she was having increased dyspnea and dry cough. She has managed her asthma with a daily combined long-acting beta-2 adrenergic agonist, an inhaled corticosteroid, and montelukast. She also uses her short-acting beta-2 adrenergic agonist, albuterol, about once a day. She went to her pulmonologist about 2 months ago and was diagnosed with severe asthma. A decision was made to start her on oral prednisone (corticosteroid). The

first month she took 5 mg a day with some relief, but the symptoms returned, so her prednisone dose was increased to 10 mg a day. She has been taking the 10 mg dose for 3 weeks. She says her breathing is better, but she feels increasingly tired and like she is gaining weight. See chapter 8 on respiratory function.

Physical examination reveals an anxious woman with blood pressure of 144/92 mmHg, pulse of 90, respiratory rate of 20, and weight of 190 pounds. She is talking in full sentences. Lung sounds are clear bilaterally. No accessory muscles are being used. No cyanosis is present.

1. Which of the following is the most likely cause of this patient's loss of glucose control?
   a. Inhaled corticosteroid
   b. Prednisone therapy
   c. Asthma exacerbation
   d. Albuterol
2. All of the following actions are important for this patient to

learn regarding glucocorticoid therapy, but which is the most important?
   a. Monitor cuts for healing
   b. Take the medication with food
   c. Do not stop taking the medication abruptly *adrenal crisis*
   d. Contact her healthcare provider if she has any manifestations of infection
3. Which of the following endocrine conditions is this patient at risk of developing?
   a. Hyperthyroidism
   b. Pheochromocytoma
   c. Addison disease
   d. Cushing syndrome
4. Given this patient's acute loss of glucose control, which of the following interventions would be ordered for this patient?
   a. Insulin as needed per routine sliding scale (dosing based on blood glucose levels)
   b. Increase exercise
   c. Decrease caloric intake
   d. Decrease prednisone dose

tumors secrete only glucocorticoids (e.g., adrenal adenomas) while others can cause excesses in both cortisol and androgens (e.g., adrenal cancer in women). Therefore, the clinical manifestations of Cushing syndrome are a direct result of the excessive amounts of glucocorticoids and possible androgen excess. The clinical manifestations of Cushing syndrome can be metabolic, dermatologic, infectious, cardiovascular, reproductive, musculoskeletal, or neuropsychiatric.

Metabolic
- Glucose intolerance—insulin resistance from obesity; cortisol stimulation of gluconeogenesis
- Delayed growth and development
- Obesity (especially around the trunk) (FIGURE 10-13)

- A fatty pad between the shoulders known as a buffalo hump; fat accumulation in the cheeks known as moon face

Dermatologic
- Hirsutism (abnormal hair growth); thin hair, oily facial skin, acne due to androgen excess in women (usually adrenal carcinoma); other virilizing signs (e.g., deep voice) if androgen is very high
- Broad purple striae (marks) on the abdomen, thighs, and breasts
- Thin skin that bruises easily—catabolic effects of glucocorticoids
- Skin atrophy—loss of subcutaneous fat
- Hyperpigmentation due to increased ACTH, which binds to melanocyte-stimulating hormone receptors

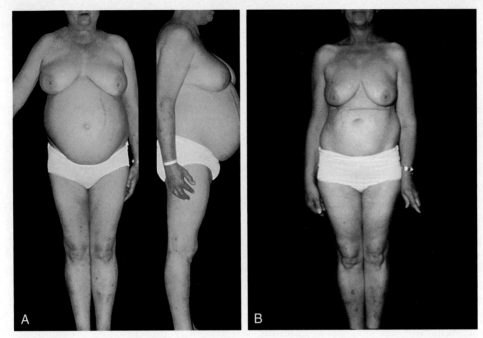

FIGURE 10-13 Cushing disease before and after treatment. **A** Before treatment, front and side views of subject, illustrating trunk obesity with relatively thin extremities. **B** After treatment, illustrating normal body configuration.

Courtesy of Leonard V. Crowley, MD, Century College.

Infectious

- Increased risk and frequency of infections due to glucocorticoid suppression of immune function
- Delayed wound healing

Cardiovascular

- Hypertension resulting from multifactorial causes such as increased liver production of angiotensinogen; increased sensitivity to adrenergic agonists
- Dyslipidemia
- Edema
- Hypokalemia

Reproductive

- Changes in menstruation due to GnRH suppression caused by hypercortisolism
- Decreased libido
- Erectile dysfunction

Musculoskeletal

- Osteoporosis—decreased intestinal calcium absorption, decreased renal calcium reabsorption, decreased bone formation with increased bone resorption
- Muscle weakness and wasting—catabolic effects of glucocorticoids

Neuropsychiatric

- Mood changes (e.g., depression, anxiety) and psychosis due to excess cortisol

Diagnostic procedures for Cushing syndrome include a history, physical examination, and serum hormone levels (e.g., cortisol and ACTH). Adrenal and pituitary CT and MRI may be necessary to evaluate for an underlying cause. Other tests are used to further evaluate manifestations or complications of hypercortisolism and can include serum glucose, complete blood count (CBC), blood chemistry, and bone density studies. Treatment varies depending on the underlying cause. Gradual tapering of any glucocorticoids being administered is crucial. If these glucocorticoids are suddenly discontinued, the adrenal gland does not have the opportunity to initiate its own production of hormones, leading to an adrenal crisis. Tumors will likely require surgical removal and radiation. Medications can be used to control cortisol production (e.g., ketoconazole [Nizoral], mitotane [Lysodren], and metyrapone [Metopirone]), control the effects of cortisol (e.g., mifepristone [Korlym]), and decrease ACTH production (e.g., pasireotide [Signifor]). Interventions may be necessary to manage specific complications as they develop (e.g., osteoporosis, DM, and hypertension).

Addison Disease

Addison disease refers to a deficiency of adrenal cortex hormones (glucocorticoids, mineralocorticoids, and androgens). It can be caused by damage resulting from autoimmune conditions (the most common cause), infections (e.g., tuberculosis, human immunodeficiency virus, fungal infections, and meningitis), hemorrhage, and tumors. Additionally, Addison disease may result from pituitary dysfunction that results in insufficient ACTH levels.

Clinical Manifestations

Clinical manifestations reflect the glucocorticoid and mineralocorticoid deficiency and usually develop slowly over weeks to months. Androgen deficiency may be apparent in women only because the testes, not adrenals, are the primary source of androgen in men. The manifestations include laboratory abnormalities and metabolic, dermatologic, cardiovascular, gastrointestinal, reproductive, musculoskeletal, and neuropsychiatric manifestations:

Laboratory Abnormalities
- Electrolyte disturbances (particularly hyperkalemia, hyponatremia, and hypochloremia)
- Hypoglycemia

Metabolic Manifestations
- Unintentional weight loss due to anorexia or dehydration

Dermatologic Manifestations
- Patchy hyperpigmentation of areas exposed to light (e.g., face and hands), lips, and oral mucosa
- Patchy depigmentation (vitiligo)
- Pallor

Cardiovascular Manifestations
- Postural hypotension due to mineralocorticoid deficiency

Gastrointestinal Manifestations
- Nausea and vomiting
- Abdominal pain
- Salt craving
- Diarrhea (can alternate with constipation)

Reproductive Manifestations
- Decreased axillary and pubic hair (women)
- Loss of libido (women)

Musculoskeletal Manifestations
- Myalgia and arthralgia
- Weakness

Neuropsychiatric Manifestations
- Mood changes (e.g., depression) and psychosis

Adrenal crisis (i.e., Addisonian crisis) will manifest as shock with hypotension, dehydration, fever, confusion, and other nonspecific manifestations seen in Addison disease (e.g., hyperpigmentation, vitiligo). Adrenal crisis can be precipitated by an acute stressor in someone with Addison disease, acute adrenal gland destruction (e.g., bilateral infarction of the gland), or abrupt withdrawal of glucocorticoid therapy. Adrenal crisis may be the initial presentation of Addison disease.

Treatment of this disease requires lifelong hormone replacement with glucocorticoid and mineralocorticoid therapy. Increases in hormone doses may be required during times of infections, stress, and trauma. The patient should wear a medical alert bracelet and carry extra medication at all times.

Learning Points

Glucocorticoid Adverse Effects

Glucocorticoids such as prednisone and prednisolone are medications that are commonly used for various disorders (e.g., asthma, rheumatic disease, lupus, and transplant rejection). The major adverse effects occur with oral and systemic use. The adverse effects are a result of the inhibition of the hypothalamic-pituitary-adrenal (HPA) function with resulting CRH and ACTH suppression. The suppression causes adrenal atrophy, and cortisol secretion diminishes. The only source of glucocorticoid then becomes the exogenous glucocorticoid. Withdrawal of the exogenous glucocorticoid can lead to adrenal crisis. The occurrence and degree of CRH and ACTH suppression are related to the potency, dose, and duration of glucocorticoid therapy. Minimizing adverse glucocorticoid effects and identifying patients with HPA suppression is important. Various principles of glucocorticoid therapy include 1) use glucocorticoids only if there is objective evidence of benefit; 2) use glucocorticoids only after other therapies have failed; 3) use glucocorticoids with a specific end point in mind and when response can be objectively measured; and 4) administer glucocorticoids in sufficient amounts and duration to get a desired response and for no longer than is necessary. The glucocorticoid should be discontinued if there is no response to glucocorticoid administration, complications arise, or the maximum benefit is achieved. Those patients likely to develop HPA suppression include glucocorticoid use for longer than 3 weeks particularly if greater than 10 mg of prednisone or equivalent daily or the presence of Cushing syndrome manifestations. To avoid HPA suppression, the glucocorticoids should be tapered slowly. Those patients receiving short-term therapy (even if high doses) are not likely to develop HPA suppression. Those patients with long-term low doses are not likely to develop HPA suppression; however, other long-term complications of glucocorticoid use such as osteoporosis can develop.

CHAPTER SUMMARY

The endocrine system is responsible for producing a wide range of hormones necessary for a variety of processes. Endocrine disorders are often caused by congenital defects, tumors, or gland damage. These conditions vary from harmless to life threatening, and most are managed easily with medications and surgery. Clinical manifestations of these conditions reflect the hormones affected and the degree of deviation. Regardless of the disorder and the severity, lifelong management is necessary to prevent significant complications or death.

REFERENCES AND RESOURCES

AAOS. (2004). *Paramedic: Anatomy and physiology*. Sudbury, MA: Jones and Bartlett Publishers.

American Diabetes Association. (2019). American Diabetes Association standards of medical care. *Diabetes Care, 42* (Suppl. 1), S1–S240.

Centers for Disease Control and Prevention (CDC). (2017). Diabetes basics. Retrieved from https://www.cdc.gov/diabetes/basics/diabetes.html

Centers for Disease Control and Preventions (CDC). (2018). Overweight and obesity. Retrieved from https://www.cdc.gov/obesity/data/index.html

Chiras, D. (2015). *Human biology* (8th ed.). Burlington, MA: Jones & Bartlett Learning.

Elling, B., Elling, K., & Rothenberg, M. (2004). *Anatomy and physiology*. Sudbury, MA: Jones and Bartlett Publishers.

Else, T., & Hammer, G. D. (2019). Disorders of the hypothalamus & pituitary gland. In G. D. Hammer & S. J. McPhee (Eds.), *Pathophysiology of disease: An introduction to clinical medicine* (8th ed.). New York, NY: McGraw-Hill.

Garvey, W. T., Mechanick, J. I., Brett, E. M., Garber, A. J., Hurley, D. L. Jastreboff, A. M, … Plodkowski, R. (2016). American Association of Clinical Endocrinologists and American College of Endocrinology comprehensive clinical practice guidelines for medical care for patients with obesity. *Endocrine Practice, 22*.

Gould, B. (2015). *Pathophysiology for the health professions* (5th ed.). Philadelphia, PA: Elsevier.

Hart, M., & Loeffler, A. (2015). *Introduction to human disease: Pathophysiology for health professionals* (6th ed.). Burlington, MA: Jones & Bartlett Learning.

Madara, B., & Pomarico-Denino, V. (2008). *Pathophysiology* (2nd ed.). Sudbury, MA: Jones and Bartlett Publishers.

Nieman, L. K. (2019). Pharmacologic use of glucocorticoids. In K. A. Martin (Ed.), *Uptodate*.

Powers, A. C., Niswender, K. D., & Evans-Molina, C. (2018). Diabetes mellitus: Diagnosis, classification, and pathophysiology. In J. Jameson, A. S. Fauci, D. L. Kasper, S. L. Hauser, D. L. Longo, & J. Loscalzo (Eds.), *Harrison's principles of internal medicine* (20th ed.). New York, NY: McGraw-Hill.

Perreault, L. (2019). Genetic contribution and pathophysiology of obesity. In L. Kunins (Ed.), *Uptodate*

Professional guide to pathophysiology (3rd ed.). (2010). Philadelphia, PA: Lippincott Williams & Wilkins.

Snyder, P. J. (2018). Diagnostic testing for hypopituitarism. In K. A. Martin (Ed.), *Uptodate*

Steele, C. B., Thomas, C. C., Henley, S. J., Massetti, G. M., Galuska, D. A., Agurs-Collins, T., Puckett, M., & Richardson, L. C. (2017). Vital signs: Trends in incidence of cancers associated with overweight and obesity—United States, 2005-2014. *Morbidity and Mortality Weekly Report, 66* (39), 1052.

Sterns, R. H. (2017). Pathophysiology and etiology of the syndrome of inappropriate antidiuretic hormone secretion (SIADH). In J. P. Forman (Ed.), *Uptodate*.

World Health Organization. (2016). Diabetes. Retrieved from http://www.who.int/mediacentre/factsheets/fs312/en/index.html

World Health Organization. (2019). Overweight and obesity. Retrieved from https://www.who.int/en/news-room/fact-sheets/detail/obesity-and-overweight

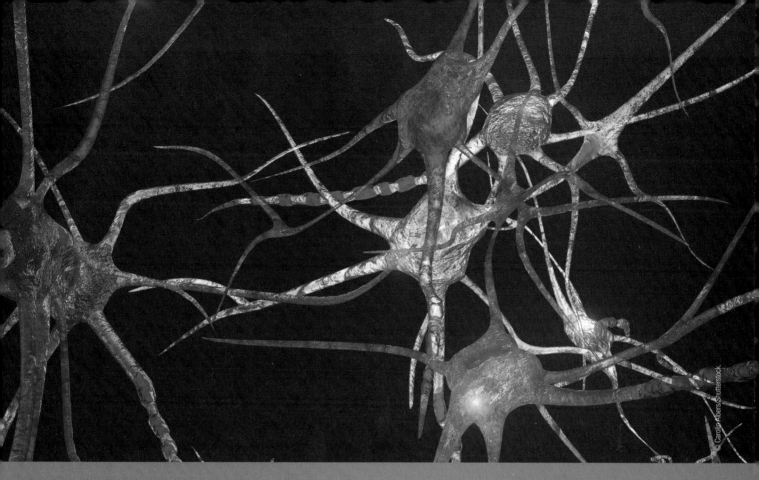

CHAPTER 11
Neural Function

LEARNING OBJECTIVES

- Discuss normal neural anatomy and physiology.
- Differentiate congenital neurologic disorders.
- Differentiate traumatic neurologic disorders.
- Summarize mechanisms and causes of increased intracranial pressure.
- Differentiate intracranial bleeding disorders.
- Differentiate infectious neurologic disorders.
- Differentiate vascular neurologic disorders.
- Differentiate types of headache disorders.
- Differentiate types of seizure disorders.
- Differentiate chronic degenerative neurologic disorders.
- Differentiate types of dementia.

- Differentiate cancers of the nervous system.
- Summarize structural and functional alterations associated with various mental health disorders.
- Summarize schizophrenia.
- Differentiate mood disorders.
- Differentiate anxiety disorders.
- Apply understanding of neural system alterations in describing various common disorders such as headaches, dementia, depression, anxiety, spinal cord injuries, and multiple sclerosis.
- Develop diagnostic and treatment considerations for various neural system disorders.

The nervous system consists of complex structures that control many body functions and cognition. The functions this system manages include: 1) structures such as muscles, glands, and organs; 2) heart rate; 3) blood flow; 4) breathing; 5) digestion; 6) urination; and 7) defecation. The nervous system is involved in a variety of cognitive functions such as perception, memory, and attention, as well as emotional and behavioral regulation. The nervous system works with other systems to maintain homeostasis by receiving and responding to input from the environment. Disorders of the nervous system include physical and psychological disorders that may be acute or chronic; regardless of their severity, these conditions often have grave or life-altering effects on the body. Causes of these disorders include congenital defects, trauma, infections, tumors, chemical imbalances, and vascular changes.

Anatomy and Physiology

The nervous system is an intricate network of specialized cells and tissue that receive and react to environmental stimuli on physiologic and cognitive levels. To communicate this input, these structures conduct electric impulses between the brain and the rest of the body. The nervous system consists of three main components: the brain, the spinal cord, and the nerves. The brain and spinal cord make up the central nervous system (CNS), and the cranial and spinal nerves make up the peripheral nervous system (PNS).

Central Nervous System

The skull and vertebral column house and protect the brain and spinal cord. Additionally, a set of three tough membranes, called the *meninges*, encase the CNS (FIGURE 11-1). The dura mater is the outer and toughest layer. The arachnoid layer is the middle layer, named for its spider web–like vascular system. The pia mater is the innermost layer that rests directly on the brain and spinal cord. Cerebrospinal fluid (CSF) is a plasmalike liquid that fills the space between the arachnoid and pia mater layers to provide additional cushioning and support to the CNS. The choroid plexus cells in the brain's ventricles continuously produce the CSF. Approximately 600 mL of CSF is produced per day in adults, and 50 mL is produced in newborns. The composition of CSF is similar to plasma and contains electrolytes (e.g., sodium and potassium), glucose, proteins (e.g., albumin and gamma globulin), and red and white blood cells. There are four ventricles that are interconnected, hollow areas (cavities) of the brain that the CSF fills and where it flows freely between them through openings known as foramens (e.g., foramen of Monro) and aqueducts (e.g., aqueduct of Sylvius) that act as canals. Up to 150 mL (25%) of CSF circulates

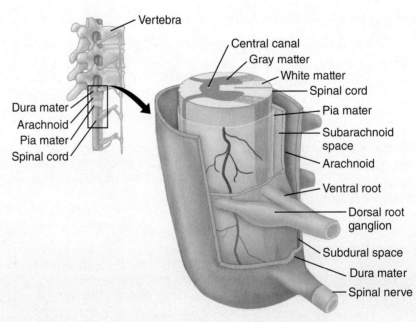

FIGURE 11-1 The meninges enclose the brain and the spinal cord.

within the ventricles, and excess CSF drains into the bloodstream.

The brain is located within the skull and contains billions of neurons. Neural tissue consists of two basic types of cells—neuroglia and neurons. Neuroglia cells play several important supportive roles in the nervous system. Neuroglial cells are more numerous than neurons. These cells scaffold neural tissue and isolate and protect neuron cell membranes. Additionally, neuroglia cells regulate interstitial fluid, defend the neurons against pathogens, and assist with neural repair.

Neuroglial cells consist of astrocytes, oligodendrocytes, Schwann cells, microglia, and ependymal cells. Each of these cell types has specific functions. Astrocytes form the framework of the brain and spinal cord (central nervous system) and form the blood–brain barrier. Ependymal cells form the epithelial lining of the central nervous system and produce cerebrospinal fluid. The oligodendrocytes are responsible for the development of myelin in the central nervous system. Schwann (neurilemma) cells produce myelin in the peripheral nervous system. Schwann cells also provide metabolic support. Schwann cell transplantation for therapeutic purposes is in a preclinical trial phase. Microglia have phagocytic activities.

Neurons are the fundamental unit of the nervous system; they generate bioelectrical impulses and transmit these signals from one area of the body to another. Neurons occur in several sizes and shapes, but all share similar characteristics. Neurons do not have the ability to divide (except for olfactory neurons, which can divide throughout life); thus, when these cells are lost due to aging or injury, they cannot be replaced. Not all cell death results in loss of functioning. For example, if neurons become damaged in one area of the brain, neurons in other areas can eventually assume responsibility for those functions. In the PNS, severed nerves can regenerate to a point to reestablish connections with the tissue they once supplied. In the brain or spinal cord, severed axons cannot be repaired. Severed spinal cord nerves result in paralysis and loss of sensation below the area of damage. In addition to being unable to divide, nerve cells require a constant supply of oxygen and glucose. This characteristic makes neurons vulnerable to the effects of hypoxia and hypoglycemia. Neurons can begin dying within minutes of these events.

Most neurons have a spherical cell body that houses the nucleus, most of the cytoplasm, and organelles. Neurons contain projections called *axons* and *dendrites* that make connections with nearby cells (FIGURE 11-2). Axons transmit impulses away from the cell body (i.e., the soma), whereas dendrites transmit impulses toward the cell body. Dendrites on a neuron are not to be confused with dendritic cells, which are antigen-presenting cells in the immune system. Groupings of soma in the central nervous system are called *nuclei* (e.g., subthalamic nuclei), while soma collections in the peripheral nervous system are called *ganglions* (e.g., posterior dorsal root ganglion). However, there is some crossover with terms as the basal ganglia is a group of CNS soma. When the axon reaches its destination, it often branches into several small fibers that terminate into miniscule bulges, called *terminal boutons*. These terminal boutons communicate with neurons, muscle fibers, or glands. Axons can communicate with several different neurons or influence one single neuron. Axons may be surrounded by a myelin sheath made of lipids, which increases the rate of impulse transmission to approximately 400 times faster than is possible in unmyelinated nerves (FIGURE 11-3). Schwann cells produce the myelin sheath in the PNS, and oligodendrocytes produce myelin in the CNS; these cells are separated by nodes of Ranvier. Nutrient exchange can occur at the nodes but not where there is myelin. Because of the myelin, impulses move at greater speeds down the axon, jumping from one node to the next, much like stones skipping across water. Bundles of these myelinated nerves are referred to as *white matter*. Impulses move in a slow, wavelike pattern in unmyelinated nerves. The larger the axon, the faster the impulse transmission. Gaps between the neurons are referred to as *synapses*. Each of these gaps includes a presynaptic terminal (e.g., a terminal bouton or some similar structure), a synaptic cleft (the space between neurons), and a postsynaptic cell membrane (FIGURE 11-4). The presynaptic and postsynaptic terminals are opposite ends of the nerve. Presynaptic neurons relay impulses toward the synapse, while postsynaptic neurons relay impulses away from the synapse. Throughout life, brain synapse numbers and strength can change, and the ability to do so is termed *neuroplasticity* or *synaptic plasticity*.

Electrical impulses of the nervous system are not like the electrical current that powers appliances, which is formed by the flow of electrons. Instead, small ionic changes such as potassium, sodium, and calcium moving

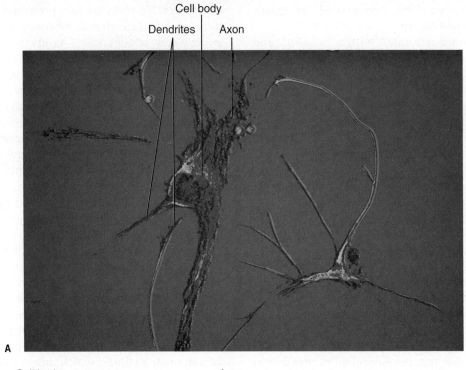

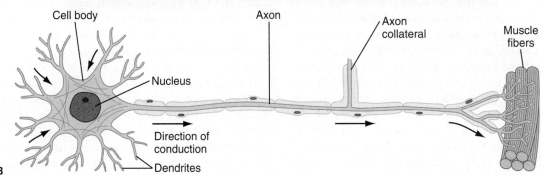

FIGURE 11-2 A neuron. **(A)** A scanning electron micrograph of the cell body and dendrites. **(B)** Collateral branches may occur along the length of the axon. In motor neurons, when the axon terminates, it branches many times, ending in individual muscle fibers.

A: © Geostock/Photodisc/Getty Images.

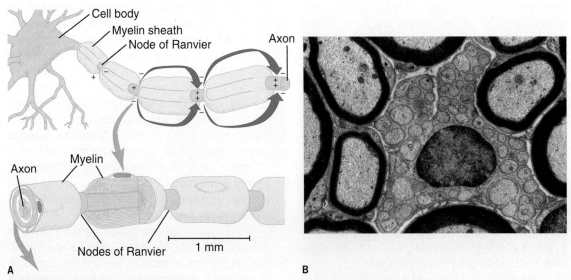

FIGURE 11-3 A myelinated nerve. **(A)** The myelin sheath allows impulses to "jump" from node to node, greatly accelerating the rate of transmission. **(B)** A transmission electron micrograph of an axon in the cross section, showing a myelin sheath.

B: © Jose Luis Calvo/Shutterstock.

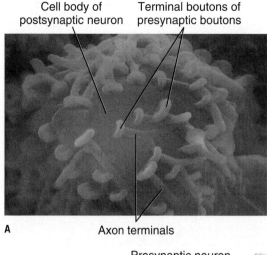

Cell body of postsynaptic neuron

Terminal boutons of presynaptic boutons

A   **Axon terminals**

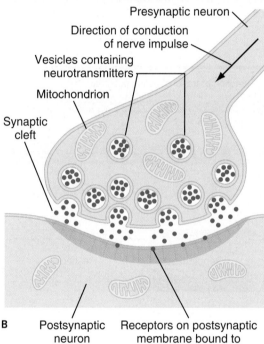

Presynaptic neuron

Direction of conduction of nerve impulse

Vesicles containing neurotransmitters

Mitochondrion

Synaptic cleft

B   Postsynaptic neuron   Receptors on postsynaptic membrane bound to neurotransmitter

Synaptic vesicles   Presynaptic neuron

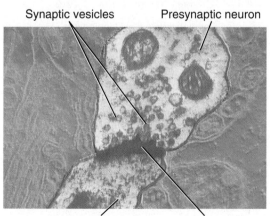

Postsynaptic neuron   Synaptic cleft

C

across cell membranes generate neural impulses (action potential) (**FIGURE 11-5**). Usually several potentials, whether excitatory or inhibitory, are necessary for impulse transmission; this concept is known as summation. The plasma side of the neuron membrane has a slight charge at rest, or resting potential, because of the sodium ions concentrated on the outside of the cell. When the neuron is stimulated, protein gates open and sodium flows into the cell. The rapid inflow of positively charged sodium ions increases the charge—a process called *depolarization*. This is the same process that occurs in the cardiac cells. Immediately following depolarization, the cell membrane returns to its resting state through the rapid outflow of the positively charged potassium ions. When generated, these impulses travel down the nerve to trigger the release of neurotransmitters from vesicles in the presynaptic terminal. The neurotransmitters cross the synaptic cleft, albeit only in one direction, to stimulate an electrical reaction in nearby neurons. The neurotransmitters bind to a receptor on the postsynaptic membrane. Synaptic transmission of the impulse takes a mere millisecond. This electrical reaction passes through those neurons to the next synapse, where the process is repeated. At each synaptic transmission, a small burst of neurotransmitters is released and then removed. Neurotransmitters are either destroyed by enzymes or reabsorbed by the postsynaptic membrane to be recycled for the next transmission. Whereas some neurotransmitters stimulate the action potentials of neurons, other neurotransmitters inhibit action potentials (see **TABLE 11-1**). Some common neurotransmitters include acetylcholine, norepinephrine, dopamine, and serotonin.

The brain is an organ with millions of neurons and an extensive circuitry that allows for

FIGURE 11-4 The function of neurotransmitters in the synaptic cleft. **(A)** A scanning electron micrograph showing the terminal boutons of an axon ending on the cell body of another neuron. **(B)** The arrival of the impulse stimulates the release of neurotransmitters held in synaptic vesicles in the axon terminals. The neurotransmitter diffuses across the synaptic cleft and binds to the postsynaptic membrane, where it elicits another action potential that travels down the dendrite to the cell body. **(C)** A transmission electron micrograph showing the details of the synapse.

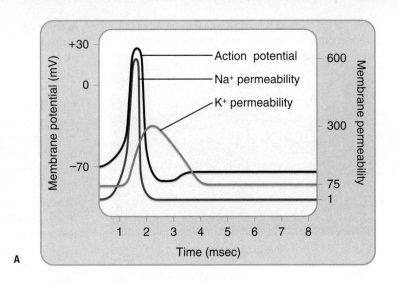

A

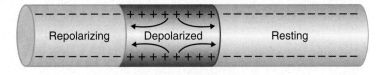

Direction of travel of action potential

The end of the axon away from the neuron's body becomes depolarized in response to a signal.

B

Depolarization extends through the axon as the initial part of the membrane repolarizes.

C

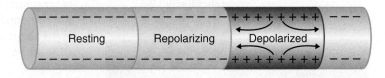

Action potential spreads across the axon.

D

FIGURE 11-5 Action potential. **(A)** Stimulating the neuron creates a bioelectric impulse, which is recorded as an action potential. The resulting potential shifts from 270 millivolts to 130 millivolts. The membrane is said to be depolarized. This graph shows the shift in potential and the change in the permeability of sodium (Na^+) and potassium (K^+) ions, which is largely responsible for the action potential. **(B)** The influx of sodium ions and the depolarization that occur at the point of stimulation. **(C)** The impulse travels along the membrane as a wave of depolarization. **(D)** The efflux of potassium ions restores the resting potential, allowing the neuron to transmit additional impulses almost immediately.

| TABLE 11-1 | Substances That Are Neurotransmitters or Neuromodulators |

Substance	Location	Effect	Clinical example
Acetylcholine	Many parts of the brain, spinal cord, neuromuscular junction of skeletal muscle, and many ANS synapses	Excitatory or inhibitory	Alzheimer disease (a type of dementia) is associated with a decrease in the number of acetylcholine-secreting neurons. Muscle weakness caused by myasthenia gravis result from an autoimmune response to acetylcholine receptors on the postsynaptic terminal.
Monoamines			
Norepinephrine	Many areas of the brain and spinal cord; also in some ANS synapses	Excitatory or inhibitory	CNS: Sleep-wake cycles and mood. Cocaine and amphetamines* result in overstimulation of postsynaptic neurons. PNS: Sympathetic nerve transmission.
Serotonin	Many areas of the brain and spinal cord	Generally inhibitory	Is involved with mood, anxiety, and sleep induction. Levels of serotonin are elevated in schizophrenia (delusions, hallucinations, withdrawal).
Dopamine	Some areas of the brain and ANS synapses	Generally excitatory	Parkinson disease (depression of voluntary motor control) results from destruction of dopamine-secreting neurons. Drugs used to increase dopamine can induce vomiting and hallucinations.
Histamine	Posterior hypothalamus	Excitatory (H1 and H2 receptors) and inhibitory (H3 receptors)	There is no clear indication of histamine-associated pathologic conditions. Histamine is involved with arousal and attention and links to other brain transmitter systems.
Amino acids			
Gamma-aminobutyric acid (GABA)	Most neurons of the CNS have GABA receptors	Majority of postsynaptic inhibition in the brain	Drugs that increase GABA function have been used to treat epilepsy by inhibiting excessive discharge of neurons.
Glycine	Spinal cord	Most postsynaptic inhibition in the spinal cord	Glycine receptors are inhibited by strychnine.
Glutamate and aspartate	Widespread in brain and spinal cord	Excitatory	Drugs that block glutamate or aspartate, such as riluzole, are used to treat amyotrophic lateral sclerosis. These drugs might prevent overexcitation from seizures and neural degeneration.
Neuropeptides			
Endorphins and enkephalins	Widely distributed in the CNS and PNS	Generally inhibitory	Morphine and heroin bind to endorphin and encephalin receptors on presynaptic neurons and reduce pain by blocking the release of neurotransmitter.
Substance P	Spinal cord, brain, and sensory neurons associated with pain, GI tract	Generally excitatory	Substance P is neurotransmitter involved in pain transmission pathways. Blocking release of substance P by morphine reduces pain.
Vasoactive intestinal peptide	Gastrointestinal tract	Generally excitatory	Stimulates secretion, vasodilation, and smooth muscle relaxation (vasodilation, sphincter relaxation).

*Increase the release and block the reuptake of norepinephrine.

ANS, autonomic nervous system; *CNS*, central nervous system; *GI*, gastrointestinal; *PNS*, peripheral nervous system.

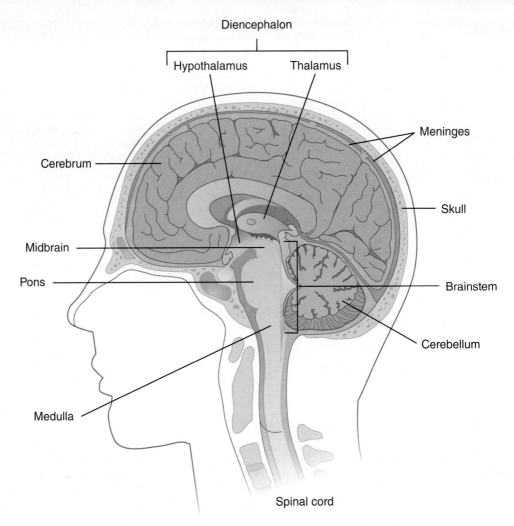

FIGURE 11-6 The major regions of the brain.

thought, emotion, intellect, and receiving and relaying signals from the environment in response to stimuli. The major regions of the brain include the cerebrum (including the cerebral cortex), diencephalon (thalamus and hypothalamus), brainstem (midbrain, pons, and medulla), and cerebellum (**FIGURE 11-6**). The cerebrum and diencephalon are also part of the structural region known as the **forebrain**, and the **hindbrain** encompasses the cerebellum and pons. The **midbrain** is composed of several nerve tracts and is the portion of the brainstem that connects the forebrain and hindbrain. The cerebrum is the largest of the regions (accounting for 80% of the brain's total mass) and controls the higher thought processes. A thin layer of gray matter, referred to as the *cerebral cortex*, surrounds the cerebrum. The gray matter is the area where information is received, integrated, stored, and transmitted. A thick central core of white matter lies beneath the gray matter. This white matter contains bundles of myelinated axons that transmit impulses from the cerebral cortex to the spinal cord, enhancing communication and coordination of activities. The cerebrum is divided into right and left hemispheres by a longitudinal fissure (deep grooves). Although minor shifts of one hemisphere into the other may occur, impinging of one hemisphere on the other can have significant—even life-threatening—effects. Numerous folds, or gyri, increase the surface area of the cerebrum. The grooves in between the gyri are called *sulci*. At birth, only a minimal set of gyri is present, but these folds increase as the brain develops into adulthood. The right side of the cerebral cortex controls the left side of the body, and the left side of the cerebral cortex controls the right side of the body (term for opposite side of the body is contralateral). As an example, a stroke in the left hemisphere will cause right-sided body symptoms such as hemiparesis.

Within each hemisphere of the brain are subdivisions called *lobes*; each lobe is named for the bone of the skull that covers it (FIGURE 11-7). The frontal lobe facilitates voluntary motor activity and plays a role in personality traits. The parietal lobe receives and interprets sensory input, with the exception of smell, hearing, and vision stimuli. The occipital lobe processes visual information. The temporal lobe plays an essential role in hearing, smell, and memory. Areas within and across these lobes can be classified as three types—motor, sensory, and association. These areas stimulate muscle activity, receive sensory information, and integrate information and initiate coordinated responses, respectively.

The diencephalon includes the thalamus and hypothalamus (FIGURE 11-8). The thalamus receives and relays most of the sensory input, affects mood, and initiates body movements, especially those associated with fear or anger. The subthalamus participates in motor activities, but the functions of the epithalamus—especially the pineal body—are unclear. The hypothalamus is

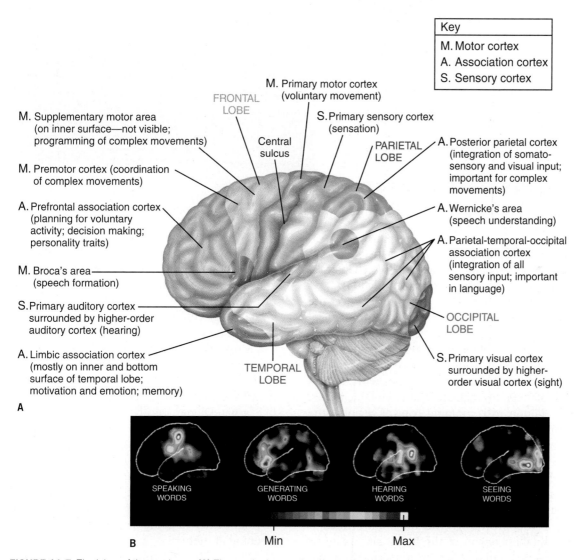

Key
M. Motor cortex
A. Association cortex
S. Sensory cortex

M. Primary motor cortex (voluntary movement)
FRONTAL LOBE
S. Primary sensory cortex (sensation)
Central sulcus
PARIETAL LOBE

M. Supplementary motor area (on inner surface—not visible; programming of complex movements)

M. Premotor cortex (coordination of complex movements)

A. Prefrontal association cortex (planning for voluntary activity; decision making; personality traits)

M. Broca's area (speech formation)

S. Primary auditory cortex surrounded by higher-order auditory cortex (hearing)

A. Limbic association cortex (mostly on inner and bottom surface of temporal lobe; motivation and emotion; memory)

TEMPORAL LOBE

A. Posterior parietal cortex (integration of somato-sensory and visual input; important for complex movements)

A. Wernicke's area (speech understanding)

A. Parietal-temporal-occipital association cortex (integration of all sensory input; important in language)

OCCIPITAL LOBE

S. Primary visual cortex surrounded by higher-order visual cortex (sight)

A

SPEAKING WORDS   GENERATING WORDS   HEARING WORDS   SEEING WORDS

B   Min   Max

FIGURE 11-7 The lobes of the cerebrum. **(A)** The cerebral cortex has three principal functions: receiving sensory input, integrating sensory information, and generating motor responses. Special sensory areas handle vision, smell, taste, and hearing. **(B)** A positron emission tomography (PET) scan reveals the locations of increased blood flow in the brain during performance of certain tasks.

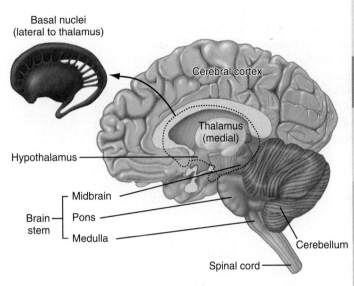

Cerebral cortex
- Receives sensory information from skin, muscles, glands, and organs
- Sends messages to move skeletal muscles
- Integrates incoming and outgoing nerve impulses
- Performs associative activities such as thinking, learning, and remembering

Basal nuclei
- Plays a role in the coordination of slow, sustained movements
- Suppresses useless patterns of movement

Thalamus
- Relays most sensory information from the spinal cord and certain parts of the brain to the cerebral cortex
- Interprets certain sensory messages such as those of pain, temperature, and pressure

Hypothalamus
- Controls various homeostatic functions such as body temperature, respiration, and heart rate
- Directs hormone secretions of the pituitary

Cerebellum
- Coordinates subconscious movements of skeletal muscles
- Contributes to muscle tone, posture, balance, and equilibrium

Brainstem
- Origin of many cranial nerves
- Reflex center for movements of eyeballs, head, and trunk
- Regulates heart rate and breathing
- Plays a role in consciousness
- Transmits impulses between brain and spinal cord

FIGURE 11-8 The regions of the brain and their functions, including the thalamus and hypothalamus.

the most inferior portion of the diencephalon; it regulates many bodily functions (see chapter 10 for more details about endocrine function).

The brainstem and cerebellum connect the brain to the spinal cord. This structure is crucial for many basic body functions (e.g., maintaining heart rate, blood pressure, and respiration), and injury to the brainstem can easily result in death. The brainstem collaborates with the hypothalamus to regulate these vital activities. In addition to containing control regions, the brainstem serves as the main thoroughfare for information traveling to and from the brain. Of the 12 cranial nerves, 10 exit from the brainstem. The pons (means *bridge* in Latin) serves as a relay station between the cerebellum and brainstem and contains nerves that regulate sleep and breathing. The midbrain, which is the smallest region of the brain, acts as a sort of relay station for auditory and visual information. It controls the visual and auditory systems and eye movement. The substantia nigra is gray matter located in the midbrain containing a tract that produces dopamine, an important excitatory neurotransmitter involved in motivation

and motor control. The medulla (medulla oblongata) is a conduction pathway for ascending and descending nerve tracts. It coordinates heart rate, peripheral vascular resistance, breathing, swallowing, vomiting, coughing, and sneezing (Figure 11-6).

Most of the many nerve fibers passing through the brainstem have branches that terminate in a region of the brainstem called the *reticular formation*. The reticular formation acts like a gatekeeper, receiving all incoming and outgoing information. It sends impulses to the cerebral cortex through specialized nerve fibers. These fibers, in turn, make up the reticular activation system (**FIGURE 11-9**). The reticular formation and the reticular activation system are responsible for alertness during the day, and their ongoing activation can prevent sleeping at night.

The cerebellum communicates with other regions of the brain to coordinate the synergistic motion of muscle movement (reflexive, involuntary) and balance as well as cognition. The cerebellum, in contrast to the cerebral cortex, has same side body control, meaning

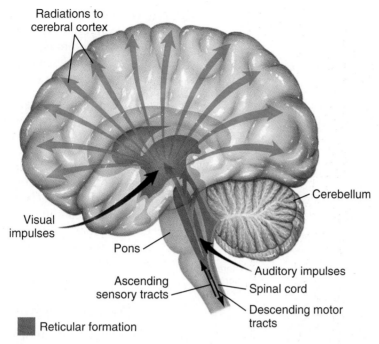

FIGURE 11-9 The reticular activation system.

Labels: Radiations to cerebral cortex; Cerebellum; Visual impulses; Pons; Auditory impulses; Ascending sensory tracts; Spinal cord; Descending motor tracts; Reticular formation

the left cerebellum controls the left side of the body (term for same side of the body is ipsilateral). Deep within the cerebrum, diencephalon, and midbrain is a set of key structures called the *basal ganglia*. The basal ganglia or basal nuclei play a pivotal role in coordination, voluntary motor movement, and posture, along with cognitive and emotional functions. The basal ganglia includes the substantia nigra along with several other nuclei (e.g., lentiform nuclei and the striatum). Portions of the cerebrum and diencephalon constitute the limbic system (**FIGURE 11-10**). The limbic system is a set of structures that includes the hypothalamus, **amygdala**, **hippocampus**, and thalamus; each structure works to influence instinctive behavior, emotions, motivation, mood, pain, and pleasure. The amygdala is often referred to as the *aggression center* as stimulation can lead to anger, violence, fear, and anxiety. Benzodiazepines and alcohol affect the amygdala by inhibiting amygdala response and resulting in a mellowing effect and disinhibited behavior. The hippocampus helps in the formation of new memories and is involved in short-term memories becoming long-term memory. Damage to the hippocampus can lead to difficulties forming new memories; however, old memories may remain intact.

Limbic System

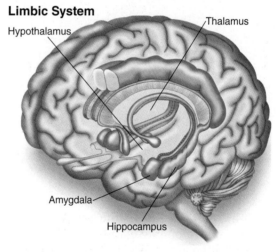

Labels: Hypothalamus; Thalamus; Amygdala; Hippocampus

FIGURE 11-10 The limbic system. The odd assortment of structures shown in blue is the limbic system. The limbic system is the seat of emotions, such as joy, and instincts; it is home to other functions as well.

The spinal cord, which starts from the medulla oblongata, exits the skull through the opening in the skull, called the *foramen magnum*. The spinal cord extends through the vertebral canal to the second lumbar vertebra. At this point, the spinal cord transitions into individual nerve roots referred to as the *cauda equina*. The spinal cord consists of 31 pairs of spinal nerves (part of the PNS) that branch off at regular intervals (**FIGURE 11-11**).

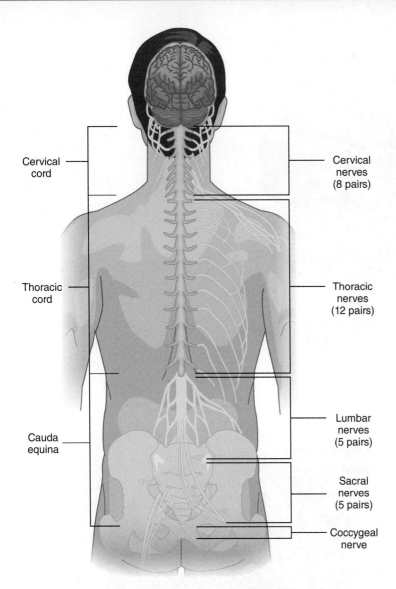

Cervical cord

Thoracic cord

Cauda equina

Cervical nerves (8 pairs)

Thoracic nerves (12 pairs)

Lumbar nerves (5 pairs)

Sacral nerves (5 pairs)

Coccygeal nerve

FIGURE 11-11 The spinal cord.

The central portion of the spinal cord is an *H*-shaped area of gray matter, which contains nerve cell bodies. White matter consisting of nerve fiber tracts, or pathways, surrounds the gray matter). Ascending fibers, also known as afferent tracts, carry sensory information in the form of action potentials from the periphery back to the brain. Descending fibers, also known as efferent tracts, carry motor impulses in the form of action potentials from the brain to the PNS. The white matter has a variety of tracts that communicate specific ascending or descending input. The tracts are named according to where they start and end. As an example, the corticospinal tract carries impulses from the cortex to the spinal cord, so it is a descending (efferent) pathway. Tracts are

grouped into columns based on their locations such as the anterior (ventral), lateral, and posterior (dorsal) columns. Ascending tracts are in all columns while descending tracts are only in the lateral and anterior columns. The following are the various tracts:

- Anterior spinothalamic tracts permit sensations of light touch, pressure, tickling, and itching.
- Lateral spinothalamic tracts allow the sensations of pain and temperature.
- Spinocerebellar tracts establish the body's position in relation to the cerebellum.
- Corticospinal tracts coordinate movements, especially in the hands.
- Vestibulospinal tracts are responsible for involuntary movements.
- Reticulospinal tracts are also responsible for involuntary movements.

The spinal reflex arcs refer to the process that creates an unconscious, involuntary response to stimuli (**FIGURE 11-12**). Most sensory neurons involved in the reflex arc do not pass directly to the brain but rather synapse in the spinal cord. By bypassing the brain the motor neurons can be activated quickly for a response. The brain, however, may receive sensory signals that "something" has occurred and there are times when the brain can prevent a reflex action. An example of this arc can be seen when the patella is gently tapped with a reflex hammer. The tendon stretch reflex is elicited when the patella is tapped, causing quadriceps contraction that results in the lower leg sharply moving forward (called *extension*) and then backward (called *flexion*). The flexor reflex is a withdrawal reflex that occurs in response to touching an unpleasant stimulus (e.g., extreme heat) (**FIGURE 11-13**). This reflex causes the muscles of a limb to withdraw the limb from the source of the stimulus without any conscious action. The tracts of the spinal cord and brain regulate these impulses. Chapter 14 contains detailed information pertaining to the various steps in sensory and motor pathways as they apply in particular to pain transmission.

Motor neurons are described as upper motor neurons and lower motor neurons. Upper motor neurons are those pathways located in the CNS (e.g., corticospinal tract neurons). Lower motor neurons describe peripheral neurons that directly influence muscle activity. Upper motor neurons form synapses with interneurons that synapse with lower

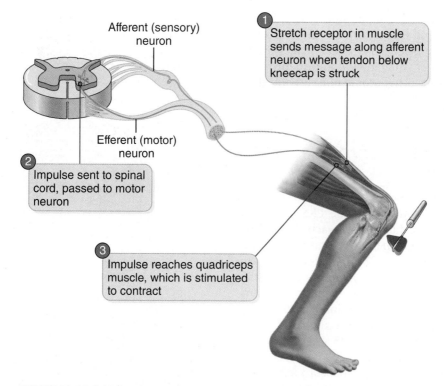

1. Stretch receptor in muscle sends message along afferent neuron when tendon below kneecap is struck

2. Impulse sent to spinal cord, passed to motor neuron

3. Impulse reaches quadriceps muscle, which is stimulated to contract

Afferent (sensory) neuron

Efferent (motor) neuron

FIGURE 11-12 Spinal cord nerve tracts.

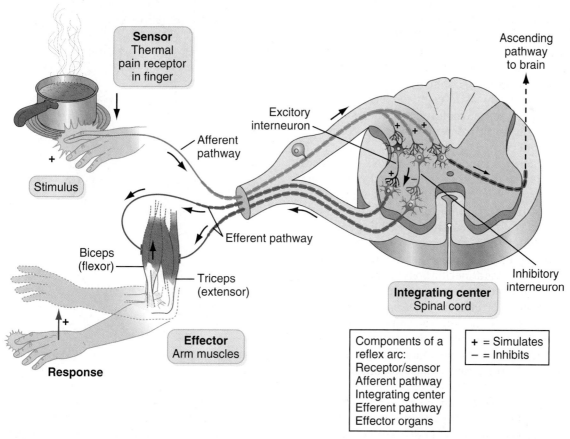

Sensor
Thermal pain receptor in finger

Stimulus

Afferent pathway

Ascending pathway to brain

Excitory interneuron

Inhibitory interneuron

Biceps (flexor)

Triceps (extensor)

Efferent pathway

Integrating center
Spinal cord

Effector
Arm muscles

Response

Components of a reflex arc:
Receptor/sensor
Afferent pathway
Integrating center
Efferent pathway
Effector organs

+ = Simulates
− = Inhibits

FIGURE 11-13 The spinal reflex arc. When you accidentally touch a hot pan on the stove, you withdraw your hand before your brain even knows what is happening. This reaction occurs because of a reflex arc. Sensory fibers send impulses to the spinal cord. The sensory impulses stimulate motor neurons in the spinal cord. This stimulation 1) causes muscle contraction in the flexor muscles and 2) inhibits muscle contraction in the extensor muscles, allowing you to withdraw your hand. Nerve impulses also ascend to the brain to let it know what is happening.

motor neurons. In general, upper motor neuron damage will lead to contracture and spastic type paralysis (e.g., a stroke damages upper motor neurons) while lower motor neuron injury will result in hypotonic muscles and flaccid type paralysis (e.g., amyotrophic lateral sclerosis).

Peripheral Nervous System

The PNS comprises the spinal nerves and cranial nerves. The nerves of the PNS consist of bundles of nerve fibers, with each fiber being part of the neuron. These nerves transport messages to and from the CNS. The nerves end on receptors that respond to a variety of internal and external stimuli. The 31 spinal nerve pairs (8 cervical, 12 thoracic, 5 lumbar, 5 sacral, and 1 coccygeal) branch directly off the spinal cord to make up the PNS (Figure 11-11). Each spinal nerve pair is named for the vertebral level at which it exits the spinal cord (e.g., C3 is the 3rd cervical nerve and T12 is the 12th thoracic nerve) except that C1 exits below its corresponding vertebrae. Each spinal nerve pair innervates specific areas of the body (**FIGURE 11-14**). Ganglia comprise collections of nerve cell bodies outside the CNS. Spinal nerves arise from several small nerves called *rootlets* along the dorsal and ventral surfaces of the spinal cord (**FIGURE 11-15**). Approximately six to eight rootlets combine to form each dorsal root and ventral root. These roots, in turn, come together to form the spinal nerve.

Each spinal nerve of the PNS comprises two types of nerves—sensory and motor. The sensory nerves, or afferent nerves, carry impulses (regarding information) from the body to the brain. A dermatome is the area of the skin innervated by a given pair of spinal sensory nerves. Each spinal nerve, with the exception of C1, has a specific body surface area from which it obtains sensory information. The motor nerves, or efferent nerves, carry impulses regarding action from the brain to the corresponding muscle receptor, resulting in muscle contraction and movement. Interneurons connect the sensory and motor neurons in the spinal cord.

Sometimes several nerves intersect to form an organized collaboration, or plexus. Four plexuses occur in the body—cervical (located at C1 to C4), brachial (located at C5 to T1),

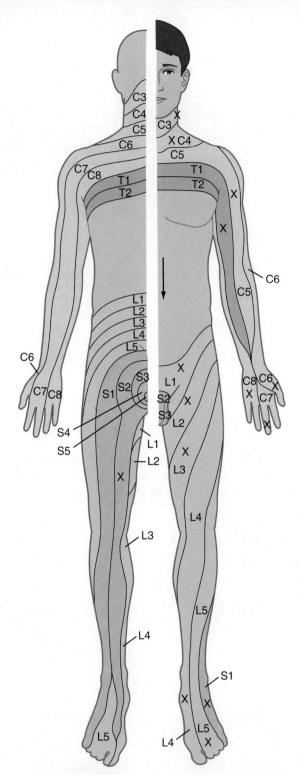

FIGURE 11-14 Spinal nerve innervation.

lumbar (located at L1 to L4), and sacral (located at L4 to S4). These plexuses branch into the peripheral nerves that supply sensory and motor functions to many areas of the body. The thoracic nerves are an exception and do not

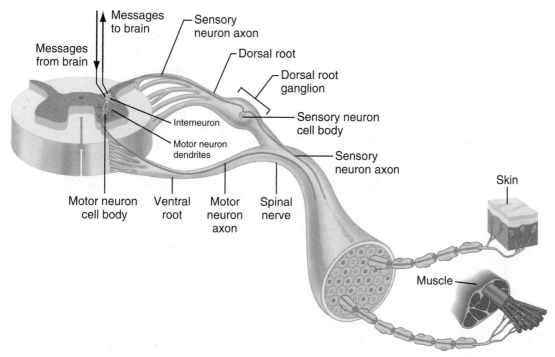

FIGURE 11-15 The dorsal root ganglion.

form a plexus; rather, the nerves pass through the intercostal spaces to innervate the thorax.

The brain is responsible for a variety of physiologically vital functions and cognitive activities. It accomplishes these functions in part through the set of cranial nerves. Twelve pairs of cranial nerves branch directly from the base of the brain (**FIGURE 11-16**). Some of the cranial nerves carry only sensory fibers (I, II, and VIII), others carry only motor fibers (III, IV, VI, XI, and XII), and a few carry both types of fibers (V, VII, IX, and X). Each nerve travels from the brain through the foramen to its destination.

Autonomic Nervous System

The autonomic nervous system (ANS) controls smooth muscles and is responsible for the fight-or-flight response. The autonomic nervous system is often considered to be part of the PNS; however, components are also located in the CNS (e.g., in the hypothalamus). The autonomic nervous system, which is not under conscious control, affects such activities as heart rate, blood pressure, and intestinal motility. This system has two subdivisions—sympathetic and parasympathetic. The two divisions have an antagonistic effect on each other that aids in maintaining homeostasis

(**FIGURE 11-17**). The sympathetic innervations run from the first thoracic spinal region to the second lumbar spinal region and are responsible for the fight-or-flight response; this response is initiated when a person is startled or faced with danger and is augmented by secretions of the adrenal medulla (**FIGURE 11-18**). In contrast, the parasympathetic innervations are in the cranial nerve nuclei and the sacral spinal region, and they are responsible for the rest-and-digest response. Neurotransmitters and receptors are important in the autonomic nervous system because sympathetic and parasympathetic innervations will stimulate or inhibit these sites, leading to the physiologic response (**TABLE 11-2**). The motor portion of the ANS consists of preganglionic, myelinated neurons and postganglionic, unmyelinated neurons. The preganglionic neurons, whether sympathetic or parasympathetic, release acetylcholine, resulting in cholinergic transmission.

The parasympathetic postganglionic neurons (like preganglion neurons) release acetylcholine, and effects are centered on a particular function. The sympathetic postganglionic neurons release norepinephrine, resulting in adrenergic transmission and can result in a generalized, widespread system effect. Some sympathetic postganglionic neurons (e.g., sweat gland innervation) release acetylcholine.

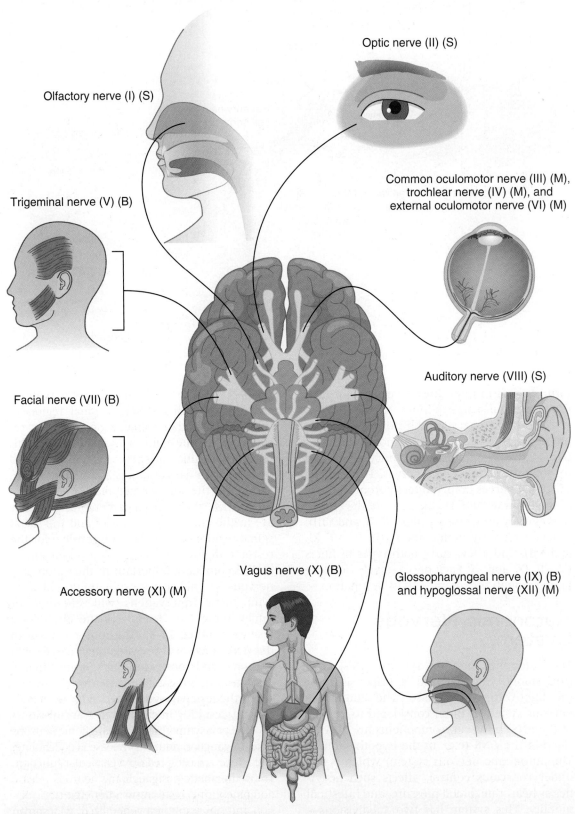

FIGURE 11-16 The cranial nerves.

(S)- sensory
(M)- Motor
(B)- both motor and sensory

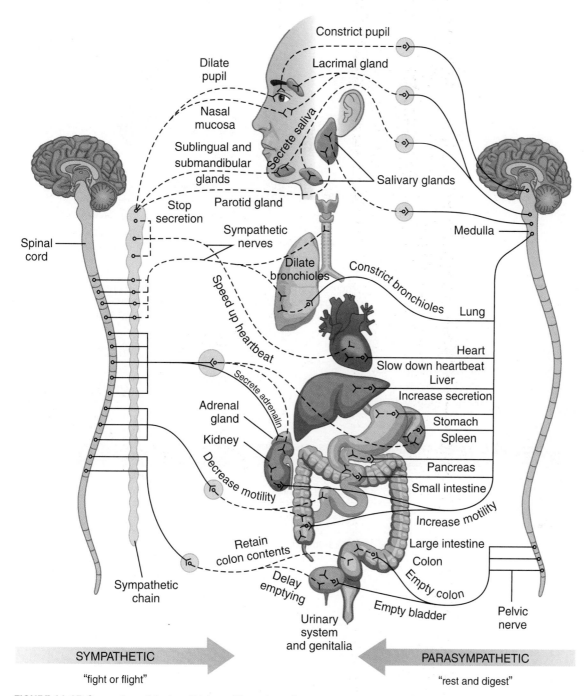

FIGURE 11-17 Comparison of the two divisions of the autonomic nervous system.

There are different types of cholinergic or adrenergic receptors on effector organs. Cholinergic receptors are nicotinic and muscarinic. At the synapse, acetylcholine is degraded by the enzyme acetylcholinesterase. Adrenergic receptors are beta (β) and alpha (α). At the synapse, norepinephrine is degraded by the enzyme catechol-o-methyl transferase (COMT).

Drugs that inhibit this COMT are used to treat Parkinson disease. Acetylcholine and norepinephrine can also be reabsorbed the by the preganglionic neurons. The effects of the neurotransmitter will be dependent on the receptors present on the target organ (may be one or multiple) and the receptor stimulated. As an example, sympathetic stimulation of

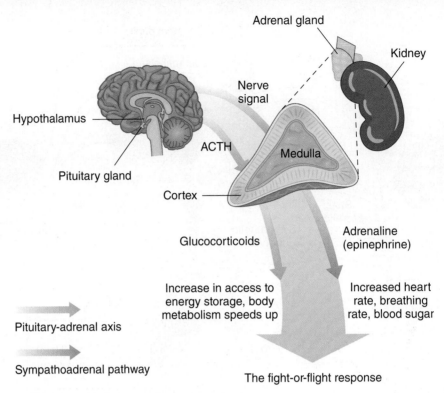

FIGURE 11-18 Physiologic response to stress.

TABLE 11-2	Types of Autonomic Receptors		
Neurotransmitter	**Receptor**	**Primary locations**	**Responses**
Acetylcholine (cholinergic)	Nicotinic	Postganglionic neurons	Stimulation of smooth muscle and gland secretions
	Muscarinic	Parasympathetic target: organs other than the heart	Stimulation of smooth muscle and gland secretions
		Heart	Decreased heart rate and force of contraction
Norepinephrine (adrenergic)	α_1	All sympathetic target organs except the heart	Constriction of blood vessels, dilation of pupils
	α_2	Presynaptic adrenergic nerve terminals	Inhibition of release of norepinephrine
	β_1	Heart and kidneys	Increased heart rate and force of contraction; release of renin
	β_2	All sympathetic target organs (in heart B1 predominates)	

α-receptors results in vasoconstriction, while stimulation of β-receptors results in vasodilation. Some medications can also stimulate or inhibit these receptors. See chapter 4 for discussion of cardiovascular ANS receptors.

Blood Supply to the CNS

The brain receives most of its blood supply from the internal carotid arteries, which form the anterior circulation (**FIGURE 11-19**). The spinal cord is supplied by vertebral arteries and arteries that branch off the descending aorta. The brain is also supplied by the vertebral arteries, which form the posterior circulation. These various branches interconnect in various ways. The internal carotid artery branches into several arteries; a main one is the anterior cerebral artery that continues as the middle cerebral artery. The vertebral arteries branch into

BOX 11-1 Application to Practice

Answer the following questions as they pertain to autonomic receptor activation and expected responses.

Case 1: A patient with chronic obstructive lung disease is prescribed a long-acting antimuscarinic agent. The expected therapeutic effect of this medication is:

1. Blocks muscarinic receptors in the airway, leading to smooth muscle constriction
2. Blocks muscarinic receptors in the airway, leading to smooth muscle relaxation

Case 2: A patient with chronic obstructive lung disease is prescribed a long-acting beta agonist. The expected therapeutic effect of this medication is:

1. Stimulates beta-2 adrenergic receptors, resulting in increased heart rate leading to increased oxygenation
2. Stimulates beta-2 adrenergic receptors, resulting in airway smooth muscle relaxation

Case 3: A 60-year-old woman is taking the following medications: lisinopril and metoprolol for hypertension and oxybutynin for an overactive bladder. She is complaining of increased constipation and dry mouth. The symptoms are deemed to be due to medication side effects.

Which of the medications is the likely cause of these symptoms, and why does this medication causes these symptoms?

Case 4: A 55-year-old man is in the intensive care unit in cardiogenic shock after coronary artery bypass surgery. He is unstable as his blood pressure has been very low (e.g., average 80/40 mmHg, average mean arterial pressure of 53) and his heart rate is high (e.g., average between 100 and 120 beats per minute). He is receiving a continuous infusion of Levophed (norepinephrine) and epinephrine as well as metoprolol every 6 hours intravenous push as needed.

Describe the intended therapeutic effects of the three intravenous medications he is receiving on his cardiovascular system.

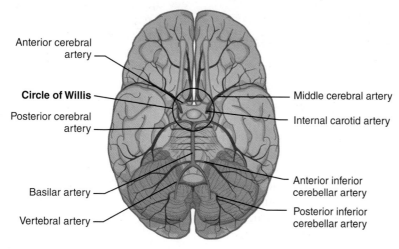

FIGURE 11-19 Blood supply of the brain.

several arteries (e.g., meningeal anterior and posterior inferior cerebellar artery) and then form the basilar artery. The terminal branches of the vertebral and carotid arteries also connect to form the circle of Willis at the base of the brain. The veins of the brain eventually drain into the internal jugular veins. Spinal cord veins are parallel to the arteries and drain via various sinuses.

The blood–brain barrier is an important vascular component of the brain that keeps the neurons from being exposed to potentially harmful substances (e.g., infectious agents and neurotoxins) (**FIGURE 11-20**). The lipid membrane of the blood–brain barrier is so tightly packed with endothelial cells that penetrating it is like trying to get through a brick wall. Some substances, such as water, carbon dioxide, and oxygen, can easily cross the membrane, while plasma proteins and large lipid molecules are incapable of permeation. Determining how to penetrate the blood–brain barrier for therapeutic purposes to treat CNS disorders, such as Alzheimer disease or depression, is an area

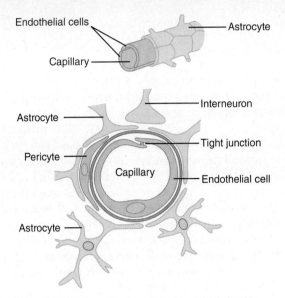

Endothelial cells

Astrocyte

Capillary

Astrocyte

Interneuron

Pericyte

Tight junction

Capillary

Endothelial cell

Astrocyte

FIGURE 11-20 The structure of the blood–brain barrier.

of continued research. As an example, drugs can be encapsulated in nanoparticles to protect them from degradation, allowing the drugs to attach to epithelial cells and giving them more time to cross the barrier. The nanoparticles can deliver hydrophobic and protein-based drugs.

Understanding Conditions That Affect the Nervous System

When considering alterations in the nervous system, organizing them based on their basic underlying pathophysiology and common anatomic origin can increase understanding. Conditions of the nervous system are usually complex, affecting many areas of function. For example, these disorders may lead to impaired physical mobility, chronic pain, impairments in thought processes and social interaction, incontinence, risk for injury, and self-care deficit, just to name a few possibilities. Patients experiencing these neurologic conditions often require vigilance to manage the complexity of the situation.

Congenital Neurologic Disorders

Congenital defects of the nervous system are often serious, with lifelong consequences. These disorders often have limited treatment options and require long-term management of complications.

Hydrocephalus

Hydrocephalus is a condition in which excess CSF accumulates within the ventricles and subarachnoid spaces in the brain. This accumulation leads to dilation of the ventricles and compresses the brain and blood vessels (**FIGURE 11-21**). The pressure from the excess CSF thins the cortex, causing severe brain damage. The CSF accumulates when the flow of this fluid is disrupted (referred to as *noncommunicating* or an *obstructive hydrocephalus*) or when too much CSF is made or not properly absorbed by the bloodstream (referred to as *communicating hydrocephalus*). Obstructive hydrocephalus is the most common type, while hydrocephalus due to excess production is rare. The obstructions can occur at the aqueduct of Sylvius, the ventricles, or the foramen of Monro. Overlaps can happen, so obstruction and absorption issues can occur together. Hydrocephalus is a common condition that may be present at birth (in an estimated 1 out of 500 births) or develop later in life (another 6,000 children younger than 2 years of age develop it each year) (National Hydrocephalus Foundation, 2014). Risk factors for hydrocephalus at any age include prematurity, pregnancy complications, nervous system tumors, CNS infections, cerebral hemorrhage, and severe head injuries. More than 50% of hydrocephalus cases are due to congenital defects with myelomeningocele being one of the most common causes of congenital hydrocephalus. If left untreated, hydrocephalus is often fatal (60% mortality rate). Adults can also be diagnosed with hydrocephalus, commonly due to enlarged ventricles without increased cerebral pressure, so it is termed *normal pressure hydrocephalus*. This type of hydrocephalus can be idiopathic or be due to other disorders (secondary). Idiopathic cases in adults are rare and usually occur after the age of 60. The prognosis depends on early treatment and comorbidity.

Clinical Manifestations

Clinical manifestations of hydrocephalus reflect the increased intracranial pressure (ICP). These manifestations vary by age group, underlying etiology, and disease progression. In infants, clinical manifestations are dependent on whether the cranial sutures have fused. If they have not fused, the signs of increased intracranial pressure (ICP) may be absent to mild. The rate of ICP rise (acute) and duration (longer period) will affect clinical manifestations.

Myth Busters

Some myths surrounding the brain warrant discussion.

Myth 1: The brain is gray.

The living, pulsing brain currently residing in your skull is not just a dull, bland, gray organ like the image often depicted in movies; instead, the brain is also white, black, and red. Like many myths, this one has a grain of truth, because much of the brain is gray. Sometimes the entire brain is referred to as *gray matter*. However, the brain also contains white matter, which comprises nerve fibers that connect the gray matter. The black component is called *substantia nigra*, which is Latin for *black substance*. The substantia nigra has a black color because of neuromelanin, a specialized type of pigment. Finally, the brain is red in some areas because of the many blood vessels it contains.

Myth 2: Listening to classical music, especially by Mozart, increases intelligence.

How did this myth get started? In the 1950s, a physician named Albert Tomatis claimed he had successfully used Mozart's music to help people with speech and auditory disorders. In the 1990s, 36 students in a study at the University of California at Irvine listened to 10 minutes of a Mozart sonata before taking an IQ test. The study reported that the students' IQ scores went up by about 8 points—and thus the Mozart effect was born. Multiple products have been sold based on this assumption. However, the original University of California at Irvine study remains controversial within the scientific community. Other scientists have been unable to replicate the original results, and current scientific evidence does not support the contention that listening to Mozart—or any other classical music, for that matter—increases intelligence. However, some evidence indicates that learning an instrument improves concentration, self-confidence, and coordination. Mozart's music certainly cannot hurt you, and you might even enjoy it if you try listening to this music; however, you will not get any smarter because of this activity.

Myth 3: You use only 10% of your brain.

This myth is probably one of the most well-known legends about the brain. This assumption seems puzzling at first glance. We have the biggest brain in proportion to our bodies of any animal, so why would we not use all of it? Many people have jumped on this idea, writing books and selling products that claim to tap into the other 90%. Believers in psychic abilities use this claim as proof, suggesting that people with these abilities have tapped into the rest of their brains.

In fact, this myth is false. In addition to 100 billion neurons, the brain is full of other types of cells that are continually in use. Significant neurologic deficits can occur from even minor damage depending on the location, so it is highly unlikely that we could function with only 10% of our brain in use. Brain scans have shown that no matter what we are doing, our brains are always active. Some areas are more active at any one time than others, but unless we have brain damage, no one part of the brain is completely turned off. Thus there is no hidden, extra potential you can tap into, in terms of actual brain space.

Myth 4: Games like sudoku and Brain Age keep your brain young.

There is some truth to this myth! Continued mental engagement has benefits, and puzzles can help you get good at a specific skill, such as memorizing grocery lists or hand–eye coordination. Most evidence, however, suggests practicing a task helps you get better only at that particular task. Far better for mental function is physical exercise. Regular physical fitness exercise is especially effective in the elderly, who may suffer from gradual problems with cognitive function such as planning ahead and abstract thinking.

Those with rapid progression will have earlier manifestations. The clinical manifestations often include the following:

- An unusually large head (**FIGURE 11-22**)
- A rapid increase in the head size
- A bulging fontanelle, or soft spot, on the top of the head
- Vomiting (often projectile)
- Dilated scalp veins
- Prominence of forehead (frontal bossing)

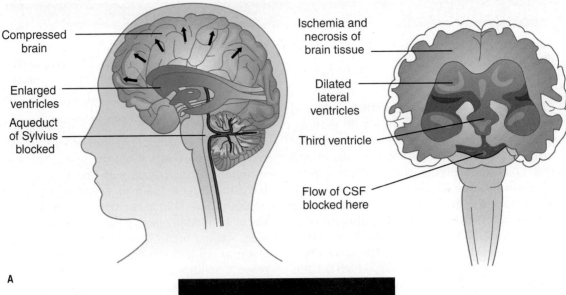

A

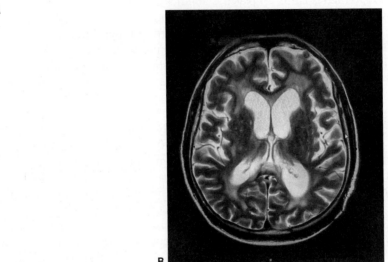

B

FIGURE 11-21 Hydrocephalus development.
B: © O_Akira/Shutterstock.

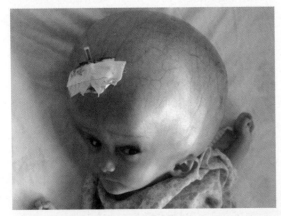

FIGURE 11-22 Hydrocephalus.
© Angela kay Agnew/Shutterstock.

- Spasticity of the extremities
- Lethargy
- Irritability
- High-pitched cry

- Feeding difficulties
- Seizures
- Eyes that gaze downward (setting-sun appearance)
- Developmental delays

In older children and adults, the head cannot enlarge because the sutures have closed. Clinical manifestations in these groups may include the following signs and symptoms:

- Headache, usually early in the morning when the pressure is highest while the patient is lying down; followed by vomiting
- Nausea
- Blurred vision or diplopia (double vision)
- Sluggish pupil response to light; eyes that gaze downward (setting-sun appearance)
- Problems with balance, coordination, or gait
- Extreme fatigue
- Slowing or regression of development

- Memory loss
- Confusion
- Urinary incontinence
- Irritability
- Personality, memory, or cognition changes
- Impaired performance in school or work

Normal pressure hydrocephalus is a slow-developing disorder, and many of the usual manifestations, such as headache or visual changes, are not typically present. Adults who have normal pressure hydrocephalus will usually have three key manifestations—one must be gait dysfunction, and the other two are cognitive impairment and urinary incontinence. The gait dysfunction is generally characterized as slow, with small steps, and a wide base. The cognitive impairment can include impaired executive functioning (conceptualization and ability to determine effective behavior), apathy, decreased attention and concentration, and psychomotor slowing. The urinary manifestations may start as urgency and then evolve into incontinence. Because of its symptoms, this disorder can easily be confused with dementia (e.g., Alzheimer disease).

Diagnosis and Treatment

Diagnostic procedures for hydrocephalus may be performed during pregnancy or after birth. These procedures consist of a history and physical examination (including head circumference measurement and a comprehensive neurologic assessment). Neuroimaging of various types can include head computed tomography (CT), head magnetic resonance imaging (MRI), skull X-ray, cranial ultrasound, and prenatal ultrasound.

The goal of treatment is to minimize brain damage and reduce or eliminate symptoms by reducing CSF. Blockages are surgically removed, if possible. If the blockage cannot be removed, a shunt may be placed within the brain to allow CSF to flow around the blocked area. The shunt tubing travels to another part of the body, such as the peritoneal cavity (ventriculoperitoneal) or right atrium (ventriculoatrial), where the extra CSF can be drained and absorbed. Shunt replacement may be needed periodically if it becomes blocked or infected or as a child grows. Antibiotic therapy will treat hydrocephalus caused by an infection or if a shunt infection develops. A temporary external ventricular drain can be used to relieve acute pressure. An endoscopic third ventriculostomy can also be performed to relieve pressure without replacing the shunt. Additionally,

the area producing too much CSF may be cauterized. Diuretics, such as furosemide and acetazolamide, can be used temporarily if a patient cannot go to surgery. Follow-up examinations generally continue throughout a child's life to monitor developmental progress and to manage any intellectual, neurologic, or physical problems. Adults with normal pressure hydrocephalus often have symptom improvement after shunting. An interprofessional team can provide emotional support and assistance with the care of those patients who have significant brain damage. The team would be made up of nurses, occupational therapists, educational specialists, social services personnel, and support groups.

Spina Bifida

Although rates have been declining over the last 15 years, spina bifida remains the second most common birth defect in the United States, affecting approximately 1 child in every 1,500 births each year (CDC, 2015c). Spina bifida is a neural tube defect that can vary in severity from mild to debilitating. Neural tube development begins early in pregnancy, starting at the cervical area and progressing toward the lumbar area, and the neural tube usually closes by the 4th week of gestation. In spina bifida, the posterior spinous processes on the vertebrae fail to fuse. This opening permits the meninges and spinal cord to herniate, resulting in neurologic impairment. The lumbar area of the vertebrae is most commonly the site of the defect. Spinal dysraphism is an umbrella term used to describe congenital defects of the spine. In addition to spina bifida, other types of spinal dysraphism include several defects such as a split cord malformation in which the spinal cord develops into two distinct cords; lipomas, which are fatty tumors; or other types of spinal cord tumors, such as dermoid tumors.

The exact cause of spina bifida is unknown, but it is thought to result from genetic and environmental influences. Spina bifida is most common in Hispanic and White populations, with females being more affected than males. Maternal risk factors for development of this defect in a child include family history of neural defects, folate deficiency (thought to be a key factor), certain medications (e.g., antiseizure agents), diabetes mellitus, prepregnancy obesity, and increased body temperature such as that caused by fever, hot tubs, saunas, and tanning beds. Most of these risk factors are likely to cause open spina bifida, while risk factors for the closed types of spina bifida are unclear.

Complications of spina bifida include physical and neurologic impairments as well as hydrocephalus and meningitis. Children with spina bifida are usually of normal intelligence, but they may have learning problems because of the chronic nature of the condition.

Spina bifida occurs in three forms, each varying in severity (**FIGURE 11-23**):

1. **Spina bifida occulta:** Spina bifida occulta is the mildest and most common form. It results in a small gap in one or more of the vertebrae. The spinal nerves and meninges do not usually protrude through the opening, so most children with this form have no clinical manifestations and experience no neurologic deficits. However, other associated anomalies, such as split spinal cord malformation, may be present. The defect may not be evident other than sacrococcygeal skin lesions such as a dimple, birthmark, or tuft of hair over the site. However, those children with other anomalies will have neurologic symptoms, and with some defects, manifestations can be present as the child ages or even become apparent in adulthood, although this is not common.

2. **Meningocele:** Meningocele is a rare form that involves the same bony defect as in spina bifida occulta, but the meninges protrude through the vertebral opening. The meninges and CSF form a sac on the surface of the infant's back. Transillumination (shining a light through the tissue) can confirm the absence of nerve tissue in the

sac. Because the spinal cord develops normally, neurologic impairment is usually not present, and these membranes can be removed by surgery with little or no damage to nerve pathways. However, infection or rupture of the sac can lead to neurologic impairment.

3. **Myelomeningocele:** This form, also known as open spina bifida, is the most severe form. In this variant, the spinal canal remains open along several vertebrae in the lower or middle back. The meninges, spinal cord, spinal nerves, and CSF protrude through this large opening at birth and form a sac on the infant's back (**FIGURE 11-24**). Skin covers the sac in some cases. However, tissues and nerves are exposed in most cases, making the infant vulnerable to life-threatening infections. Neurologic impairment (often including paralysis), bowel and bladder problems (e.g., incontinence, urinary tract infections, and constipation), seizures, and other medical complications (e.g., skin conditions and latex allergies) are common.

Clinical manifestations depend on the type and severity of spina bifida. Diagnostic procedures may be performed during pregnancy or after birth. These procedures may include a history, physical examination, check of maternal serum and amniotic fluid alpha fetoprotein levels (high levels indicate a possible neural tube or other congenital defect), prenatal ultrasound, spinal X-ray, spinal CT, and spinal MRI.

Treatment strategies vary depending on the type and severity. For instance, spina bifida occulta often requires no treatment.

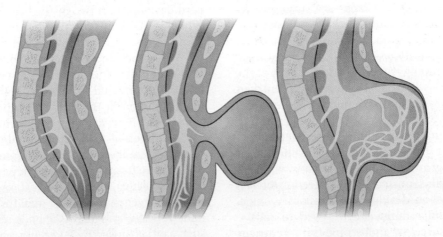

Spina bifida occulta   Meningocele   Myelomeningocele

FIGURE 11-23 Most common types of spina bifida.

BOX 11-2 Application to Practice

M.S. is a 26-year-old woman who is pregnant with her first child. Her husband accompanied her to all her prenatal visits. An ultrasound during a routine visit at 34 weeks' gestation revealed that the baby had hydrocephalus and a myelomeningocele. The parents were initially devastated but remained very excited about the birth of their first child. M.S. was scheduled for a cesarean section at 38 weeks' gestation, and the couple was anxious

about their child's condition and care following birth.

M.S. delivered a baby boy by cesarean section; he was transferred to the pediatric intensive care unit. On admission to the nursery, the baby's vital signs and weight were within normal limits, but his head circumference was large. He had bulging fontanelles and a high-pitched cry. The nurse noted a saclike projection in the lumbar region of his spine.

1. Discuss the rationale for delivering the infant by cesarean section.
2. Discuss the significance of the infant's clinical manifestations.
3. Discuss the acute and long-term treatment strategies for the infant.
4. Discuss the complications associated with myelomeningocele.

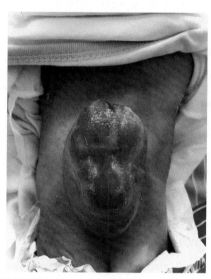

FIGURE 11-24 Myelomeningocele.
© Hugely/Shutterstock.

Surgery is the mainstay of treatment for the other two types; however, the appropriate timing of the surgery (in utero, immediately after birth, or delayed) remains a topic of debate. Surgery usually includes replacing the meninges and closing the vertebral opening. A shunt may be placed during surgery to control hydrocephalus. Performing the surgical repair in utero may enhance outcomes but will not restore lost neurologic functioning. Additional risk may be incurred with this procedure, including premature delivery and death. If spina bifida is diagnosed before birth, cesarean delivery is preferred to prevent rupture of the sac or damage to any exposed nerves. Long-term support from an interprofessional team (e.g., a nurse, physical therapist, social worker, and an education specialist) will be

necessary to limit complications and promote positive outcomes.

Cerebral Palsy

Cerebral palsy (CP) refers to a group of non-progressive disorders that appear in infancy or early childhood and permanently affect motor movement and muscle coordination. In addition to motor dysfunction, other cerebral functioning may be affected (e.g., cognition and communication). CP usually results from damage to the cerebellum during the prenatal period (often during childbirth), but it can also occur at any time during the first 3 years of life, when the brain is developing. In addition, this disorder can occur because of brain abnormalities. In the United States, CP is the leading cause of childhood disability, affecting approximately 3–4 out of 1,000 births (CDC, 2016a). CP is more common in males, in Blacks, and in persons of lower socioeconomic status.

Although CP is not curable, the right treatment can make a significant impact on the child's prognosis; however, these therapies are costly. According to the CDC (2016a), the average lifetime costs (direct and indirect) for one person with CP are estimated to be $921,000 (in 2003 dollars). The estimated lifetime costs (direct and indirect) for all people with CP who were born in 2000 will total $11.5 billion (in 2003 dollars).

CP is a multifactorial disorder, and many risk factors coexist in CP development. Direct causal relationships in the development of CP have not been established. The following factors contribute to the development of CP:

- Prematurity—the lower the gestational age, the higher the incidence

- Low birth weight—the lower the birth weight, the higher the incidence
- Breech births
- Multiple fetuses
- Hypoxia
- Hypoglycemia (in either the mother or the child)
- Cerebral hemorrhage
- Neurologic infections (e.g., meningitis and encephalitis)
- Head injury
- Maternal infections during pregnancy (e.g., rubella and varicella)
- Maternal exposure to toxins during pregnancy (e.g., mercury)
- Maternal smoking and heavy alcohol use
- Abnormal placenta
- Antepartum hemorrhage
- Severe jaundice

Clinical Manifestations

CP is classified according to the movement disorder involved, which reflects the area of the brain affected: spasticity (stiff muscles), dyskinesia (uncontrolled movements), or ataxia (poor balance and coordination). Spasticity is present in 80% of cases. In most patients, one or more movement disorders are present.

Clinical manifestations of CP may or may not be evident at birth, and the average age at diagnosis is 18–24 months. These manifestations vary from mild to severe in their effects. CP may affect the entire body (resulting in quadriplegia) or just one area (resulting in diplegia); it may affect one side or both sides of the body. Clinical manifestations can change over time as the brain matures. Manifestations may include the following signs and symptoms:

Neurobehavioral Signs
- Irritability, poor sleep, frequent vomiting, difficult to console and handle, and inadequate visual attention

Developmental Reflexes
- Persistence or exaggeration of early reflexes (e.g., Moro reflex)

Motor Tone and Posture
- Tone may be normal, increased (stiff), or decreased (flaccid)
- Poor head control
- Mouth—tongue retraction and thrust, grimacing, and abnormal jaw movement
- Motor milestones delay and varying abnormalities by age (normal developmental milestones up until age 5 can be accessed at www.cdc.gov/ncbddd/actearly/milestones/index.html)
- By 6 months, inability to roll over or bring hands together or to mouth
- By 8 months, not sitting, or by 10 months, crawling lopsided or in unusual manner (e.g., hopping on knees)
- By 18 months, not walking

Spastic Subtype
- Spastic movements
- Abnormal reflexes—hyperreflexia and clonus
- Impaired fine-motor function, difficulty with individual movement, and slow voluntary movements that take a lot of effort
- Atrophy below the waist
- Sensory disturbances (e.g., difficulty identifying an object simply by touch)
- Spastic quadriplegia with associated impairment such as severe intellectual disability, vision issues, and feeding and pulmonary disorders

Dyskinetic Subtype
- Choreoathetosis, which refers to rapid, irregular, and unpredictable contractions of muscles (individual or groups)
- Dystonia, which refers to involuntary, sustained muscle contraction leading to twisting and repetitive postures or movements

Ataxic Subtype
- Ataxic movement, which refers to abnormal, uncoordinated, voluntary movements
- Slow, jerky, and explosive speech

Complications of CP result because of these clinical manifestations:

- Balance and coordination issues
- Contractures (shortening of a muscle causing severe limitation in movement)
- Scoliosis
- Malnutrition
- Communication issues and speech delays
- Learning or cognition difficulties
- Seizures (occur in approximately 50% of patients)
- Vision and hearing issues
- Urinary incontinence
- Constipation
- Osteoporosis
- Chronic pain
- Injury

Diagnosis and Treatment

Diagnostic procedures for CP include a history, physical examination (including serial monitoring for developmental milestones), head CT, head MRI, and electroencephalogram (EEG) as well as hearing and vision screening. Treatment strategies focus on maximizing functioning and minimizing complications. Management is long term in nature and requires an interprofessional team (e.g., the primary care provider, nurses, a social worker, a physical therapist, an occupational therapist, a speech therapist, a dietitian, and education specialists). Therapeutic strategies often include the following measures:

- Muscle relaxants
- Botulinum toxin type A (Botox) injections directly into spastic muscles
- Antiseizure medications
- Pain management (e.g., massage therapy and analgesics)
- Physical therapy
- Occupational therapy
- Speech therapy
- Nutritional support
- Home safety (e.g., remove rugs)
- Braces and orthopedic devices (e.g., splints)
- Ambulation devices (e.g., walker and wheelchair)
- Constipation prevention (e.g., high-fiber diet, adequate water intake, and stool softeners)
- Glasses and hearing aids
- Surgical procedures to relieve contractures or to sever nerves of spastic muscles
- Support groups (especially for caregivers)
- Individualized education program

Infectious Neurologic Disorders

Nervous system infections can have serious effects by triggering the infectious and inflammatory response. These infections can be caused by a number of bacterial, viral, and fungal pathogens. Regardless of the causative agent, neurologic compromise (either temporary or permanent) can result. Early diagnosis and treatment is imperative for positive outcomes.

Meningitis

Meningitis refers to an inflammation of the meninges (membranes surrounding the brain and spinal cord), usually resulting from an infection. The CSF may also become affected. Bacteria, commonly *Neisseria meningitides* (meningococcus) and *Streptococcus pneumoniae* (pneumococcus), are causative organisms, as are other bacteria, such as *Haemophilus influenzae* and drug-resistant *S. pneumoniae*. Viruses (e.g., enterovirus, West Nile virus, influenza, human immunodeficiency virus [HIV], and herpes) are also a common cause of this infection. Viral meningitis is also known as aseptic meningitis (negative bacterial cultures with meningeal inflammation). The mode of transmission and mechanism by which the organism enters the CNS are dependent on the type of organism and host factors (e.g., if the patient is immunocompromised or has comorbid illnesses). The mode of transmission is generally through respiratory secretions and saliva. Other modes include the oral–fecal route (e.g., enteroviruses) and bites by mosquitoes, ticks, or rabid animals. These infectious agents invade the meninges through the blood or nearby structures (e.g., infective endocarditis) or by direct access (e.g., wounds and iatrogenic devices such as shunts). Additional causes of meningitis include chemical irritants, tumors, fungi, parasites, amoebas, and allergens. The infection or irritant triggers the inflammatory process, leading to swelling of the meninges, increased ICP, localized areas of brain ischemia, and neuronal apoptosis.

Risk factors for developing meningitis include age younger than 25 years, living in a community setting (e.g., a college dormitory), pregnancy, working with animals, and immunodeficiency. Depending on the cause of the infection, meningitis can be self-limiting (as with viral meningitis) or life-threatening (as with acute bacterial meningitis). Complications of meningitis may include permanent neurologic damage, seizures, hearing loss, blindness, speech difficulties, learning disabilities, behavior problems, paralysis, acute renal failure, adrenal gland failure, cerebral edema, septicemia, shock, and death.

Clinical Manifestations

Clinical manifestations of meningitis result from the inflammation of the meninges. Initially, these manifestations mimic those associated with an influenza infection (e.g., fever, chills, and malaise). Viral meningitis manifestations are similar to those of bacterial meningitis; however, they are typically not as severe. The clinical manifestations, which usually arise suddenly, include the following signs and symptoms:

- Fever (usually > 100.4° F [38° C]) and chills
- Mental status changes (e.g., confusion and lethargy)

- Stiff neck (meningismus or nuchal rigidity)
- Nausea and vomiting
- Photophobia
- Severe headache
- Agitation
- Bulging fontanelle
- Decreased consciousness
- Opisthotonos (abnormal positioning that involves rigidity and severe arching of the back with the head thrown backward)
- Myalgias
- Poor feeding or irritability in children
- Tachypnea
- Tachycardia
- Rash (e.g., petechiae and palpable purpura)

Diagnosis and Treatment

Diagnostic procedures for meningitis include a history, physical examination, throat cultures, lumbar puncture with CSF analysis, polymerase chain reaction test, and head CT. Treatment varies depending on the underlying etiology. Strategies may include antibiotics (if the infection is bacterial in origin), antivirals (usually reserved for those cases caused by a herpes virus), hydration, and fever management. Empiric antibiotics can be administered until a determination of a viral or bacterial process can be made. Additional strategies are geared toward managing complications as they develop (e.g., seizures, cerebral edema, and shock). Vaccinations, including those for *H. influenzae*, pneumococcal, and meningococcal infections, are the cornerstone of meningitis prevention. Meningococcal conjugate vaccines are recommended by the CDC (2019b) for preteens 11–12 years old with a booster given at the age of 16, and it is recommended for other age groups if there are risks (e.g., HIV-positive patients and those actively serving in the military). Serogroup B meningococcal vaccine is recommended for ages 10 and older who are at risk (e.g., outbreak of serogroup B meningococcus and sickle cell disease).

Encephalitis

Encephalitis refers to an inflammation of the brain, and when the spinal cord is involved, it is termed *encephalomyelitis*. The disorder usually results from an infection. A virus (e.g., coxsackievirus, echovirus, poliovirus, adenovirus, herpes virus, cytomegalovirus, Eastern equine encephalitis virus, West Nile virus, St. Louis virus, measles, or mumps) most frequently causes this infection. Viral exposure occurs through respiratory inhalation of droplets, ingestion of contaminated food or beverages, insect bites (especially mosquitoes and parasites), and skin contact. Encephalitis can also result from bacterial infections such as Lyme disease, tuberculosis, and syphilis. Noninfectious causes of encephalitis include allergic reactions (especially to vaccinations) and autoimmune conditions. The infection or other etiologic process triggers the inflammatory response, which causes vasodilation, increased capillary permeability, and leukocyte infiltration. This inflammatory process can cause nerve cell degeneration and diffuse brain destruction. Encephalitis is classified as either primary or secondary. Primary encephalitis involves a direct infection of the brain and spinal cord. In secondary encephalitis, an infection first occurs elsewhere in the body and then travels to the brain.

Most cases of encephalitis are mild and self-limiting, but in rare cases this condition can be severe and life threatening. Those individuals who are particularly vulnerable to more severe progression of encephalitis include immunocompromised persons (e.g., those with acquired immune deficiency syndrome [AIDS]), young children, older adults, persons living in high-incidence areas, and persons who are frequently outdoors. Complications of encephalitis include cerebral edema, cerebral hemorrhage, and brain damage.

Clinical Manifestations

Clinical manifestations of encephalitis result from the meningeal irritation and neurologic damage associated with the inflammatory response. These manifestations are similar to those noted in meningitis but have a more gradual onset. In most cases, clinical manifestations are mild and go undetected. When present, manifestations of encephalitis may include the following signs and symptoms:

- Flulike symptoms (e.g., fever, lethargy, and joint pain)
- Headache
- Neck rigidity
- Confusion and hallucinations
- Personality changes (e.g., flat affect, impaired judgment, and withdrawal from social interactions)
- Diplopia and photophobia
- Seizures
- Muscle weakness
- Ataxia
- Paresthesia or paralysis

- Loss of consciousness
- Tremors
- Abnormal deep tendon reflexes
- Rash
- Bulging fontanelle (in infants)

Diagnosis and Treatment

Diagnostic procedures for encephalitis include a history, physical examination, head CT, head MRI, EEG, lumbar puncture with CSF analysis, polymerase chain reaction test, and serum viral antibodies. Encephalitis is usually self-limiting, so treatment is largely supportive. Treatment strategies often include the following measures:

- Rest
- Adequate nutrition, including plenty of fluids
- Respiratory support (e.g., oxygen therapy or endotracheal intubation with mechanical ventilation) for severe cases
- Reorientation and emotional support
- Analgesics and antipyretics to relieve headaches and fever
- Antiviral agents if viral
- Antibiotic therapy if bacterial
- Corticosteroids to reduce cerebral edema
- Antiseizure agents
- Sedatives to treat irritability and restlessness
- Physical, speech, and occupational therapy as necessary for any residual neurologic dysfunction

Infection by many of the encephalitis-causative organisms can be prevented. Prevention strategies include vaccinations, wearing protective clothing when outside (e.g., long-sleeve shirts), using mosquito repellant, and eliminating water sources around the home (e.g., standing water in containers).

Zika Virus Disease

Infections caused by the Zika virus are a growing worldwide health concern. Zika virus is a flavivirus (in the same family as dengue, yellow fever, and West Nile virus) that is transmitted primarily by mosquitos (Navalkele, Chandrasekar, & Levine, 2016). In 1952, this virus was first discovered in Uganda and the United Republic of Tanzania (WHO, 2016). Since then, several outbreaks—usually involving a mild illness—have been recorded in Africa, the Americas, Asia, and the Pacific. In 2015, Brazil reported a large outbreak causing more severe neurologic complications. Within a short period of time, cases of Zika virus disease were noted in Florida (tracked to foreign travel to Zika-affected regions), and then the virus spread across the southeast United States. As of September 2016, nearly 3,000 cases of Zika had been diagnosed in the United States. Transmission of the infection in these cases has been attributed to foreign travel (most common), local mosquito spread, sexual transmission, and laboratory exposure (CDC, 2016c). In addition to being carried by mosquitos, the Zika virus can be transmitted from mother to fetus, through sexual contact, via blood transfusion, and organ transplantation.

Clinical Manifestations

In most cases, Zika virus infection causes a mild, self-limiting illness. In fact, more than 80% of the cases go unnoticed. The incubation period is thought to be 3–12 days. Most individuals will not experience any manifestations, but even when they do, manifestations are usually mild. Manifestations may include the following signs and symptoms:

- Flulike symptoms (e.g., fever, lethargy, and joint pain)
- Rash—erythematous macules and papules over face, trunk, extremities, palms, and soles
- Nonpurulent conjunctivitis
- Muscle and joint pain
- Weakness and lack of energy
- Headache
- Dysesthesia (unpleasant abnormal sense of touch manifested as burning or itching) due to nerve involvement

In rare cases, complications of Zika infection can be severe. The most severe complications occur with maternal–fetal transmission and may include miscarriage and microcephaly (**FIGURE 11-25**). Additionally, the Zika virus can

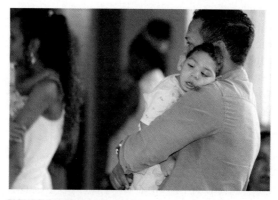

FIGURE 11-25 Microcephaly.
© Joa Souza/Shutterstock.

cause Guillain-Barré syndrome, myelitis, and meningoencephalitis.

Diagnosis and Treatment

Diagnostic procedures for Zika virus disease include a history, physical examination, and body fluid examination (e.g., blood, urine, saliva, and semen). The body fluids can be examined with real-time reverse-transcription polymerase chain reaction, which will detect Zika virus RNA and is recommended if the patient experiences symptoms for more than 14 days. While a positive Zika virus RNA confirms the diagnosis, a negative test does not exclude the disease, and an antibody should be conducted. High titers of Zika virus antibodies for IgM just indicate a flavivirus infection (also positive in dengue infection) and is not specific to the type. Treatment is primarily supportive and includes rest, hydration, analgesics, and antipyretics. Aspirin and nonsteroidal anti-inflammatory drugs should not be given until the patient is confirmed as not having a dengue infection as these drugs can cause hemorrhage in dengue. Men and women, whether symptomatic or not, need to refrain from engaging in unprotected sex for a few months after infection (the time frame varies from 8 weeks to 6 months). Prevention is paramount. It includes wearing protective covering, minimizing outdoor exposure, using an insect repellant containing DEET (N,N-diethyl-meta-toluamide), using condoms, and abstaining from unprotected sex while pregnant if there is risk of exposure (e.g., travel to mosquito transmission areas or if the partner is infected).

Traumatic Neurologic Disorders

Traumatic neurologic disorders vary significantly in severity and presentation depending on the location and extent of damage. Even minor injuries to the nervous system can have substantial effects on neurologic functioning. Traumatic injuries to the nervous system can result from a number of events that cause physical damage (e.g., motor vehicle accidents, gunshot wounds, and falls). Commonly, a number of these traumatic conditions overlap and occur concurrently (e.g., subdural hematoma and increased intracranial pressure).

Brain Injuries

A traumatic brain injury (TBI) is usually caused by a sudden and violent blow or jolt to the head (called a *closed injury*) or a penetrating head wound (known as an *open injury*) that disrupts the normal brain function. However, not all blows or jolts to the head result in a TBI. With such injuries, the brain collides with the skull and any penetrating objects (**FIGURE 11-26**). These events can bruise the brain, damage nerve fibers, and cause hemorrhaging.

According to the CDC (2019a), the main causes of TBI are falls (52%), motor vehicle accidents (20%), struck or hit against an object (28%). Intentional self harm has become the most common cause of death from TBI, surpassing motor vehicle accidents. TBIs range from mild to severe (e.g., from a brief change in mental status or consciousness to an extended period of unconsciousness or amnesia after the injury). Such injuries contribute to a substantial number of deaths and cases of permanent disability annually. According to the CDC (2019a), 2.87 million American sustained a TBI in 2014 and 556,800 died from this injury. The leading cause of TBI leading to emergency room and hospitalizations varied by age and include:

- Falls highest in 0-17 year old and over age 55
- Being struck by or against an object highest in 5 - 14 year olds
- Motor vehicle crashes high in adolescents and 15 to 44 year olds

Many TBIs result in a wide range of long-term and potentially life-altering complications such as changes in thinking, sensation, language, or emotions. These injuries can increase the risk for seizures, migraine headaches, chronic traumatic encephalopathy, Alzheimer disease, and Parkinson disease. Multiple mild TBIs can have a cumulative effect and result in neurologic dysfunction, cognitive deficits, and death. This damage can be seen in professional football players and the continuing research related to long-term effects of TBIs experienced by members of this group. These athletes, especially those who encounter routine impacts (e.g., linemen), have higher rates of cognitive deficits (e.g., memory impairment), depression, and possible neurologic diseases (e.g., Alzheimer disease and Parkinson disease).

TBIs are categorized as mild (i.e., concussion), moderate, or severe and can be either closed or open. Closed TBIs often result in a variety of conditions. Concussion describes a momentary interruption of brain function. Concussions usually result from a mild blow to the head that causes sudden movement of the brain, disrupting neurologic functioning. They may or may not lead to a loss of consciousness. Amnesia, confusion, sleep disturbances, dizziness, vertigo, and headaches may follow a

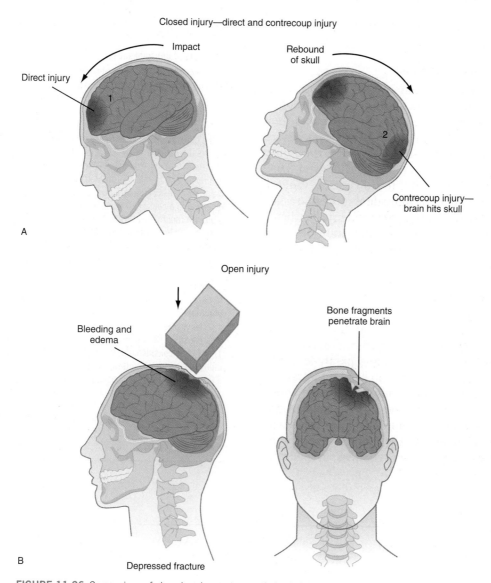

Closed injury—direct and contrecoup injury

Impact

Direct injury

Rebound
of skull

Contrecoup injury—
brain hits skull

A

Open injury

Bleeding and
edema

Bone fragments
penetrate brain

B

Depressed fracture

FIGURE 11-26 Comparison of closed and open traumatic brain injury.

concussion (i.e., postconcussive syndrome) for weeks or months; however, most are improved or resolved after one month. Cerebral contusion refers to a bruising of the brain accompanied by rupture of small blood vessels and edema. Most contusions result from a blunt blow to the head that causes the brain to make sudden impact with the skull. The initial area where the brain impacts the skull is referred to as the *coup*. The brain then rebounds and impacts the opposite side of the skull, causing another area of damage referred to as the contrecoup (Figure 11-26). Contusions vary in severity depending on the extent of damage (e.g., focal or diffuse axonal injury; cerebral infarction and necrosis), presence of cerebral edema, and increased ICP. Bleeding can occur as a result of vessel injury. The types of bleeding can include epidural, subdural, subarachnoid, and intracerebral hematomas. The presence and severity of residual effects depend on these factors.

Open TBIs can result in serious issues. In addition to the tissue damage from the impact of the brain with the skull, such injuries can cause damage owing to the penetrating object and skull fragments. The skull fractures as the object breaches it. Much like when an egg is broken, the skull usually ends up in multiple pieces when it is struck by an external force. The resulting fracture may take the form of a linear skull fracture (a simple crack), a comminuted skull fracture (several fracture lines), a compound skull fracture (a fracture where the brain tissue is exposed), a depressed skull fracture (displacement of the bone fragments into the brain), or a basilar skull fracture (located at the base of the skull and usually accompanied by CSF leakage). In addition to the brain damage from impact and penetrating objects, open TBIs carry a higher risk for developing infections because they permit direct access to the brain by infectious organisms. As discussed in previous sections, infections of the nervous system can have serious consequences.

Clinical Manifestations

Clinical manifestations of TBIs may be vague and develop slowly, or they may be sudden and severe. Symptoms may improve and then suddenly worsen. The outward appearance of the head is not an indication of the injury severity—serious injuries can occur even while the skin and the skull remain intact. When a TBI is suspected, the individual should be asked to give an account of the accident. Not being able to recall details is an indication of a TBI. The Glasgow Coma Scale (FIGURE 11-27) is the most commonly used clinical scale to grade the severity of the TBI. Mild TBI are classified as having a score of 13–15, while 9–12 is a moderate injury, and 8 or less is considered a severe injury. Limitations of the Glasgow Coma Scale include the use of medications that alter cognition (e.g., sedatives and paralytics), substance abuse (e.g., alcohol), and endotracheal intubation. Mild TBI findings were previously discussed. Manifestations of neurologic and cardiopulmonary compromise are likely with moderate to severe TBI. Some of the manifestations may include changes in behavior

Learning Points

Disorders of Consciousness

Consciousness is a state of wakefulness and awareness, and both must be present for the patient to be deemed conscious. Wakefulness is mediated by the reticular activating system in the brainstem and is evaluated with eye opening to command or to stimuli such as pain. Opening eyes is the clinical sign of wakefulness; however, just opening eyes is insufficient for the clinician to determine awareness. The ability to think and perceive indicates awareness and is a result of multiple coordinated activities throughout the brain. Awareness is determined by evaluating a purposeful response to a command, such as squeezing a hand or appropriate (nonreflexive) response to painful stimuli. Disorders of consciousness proceed into three levels—coma, vegetative state, and minimally conscious state. A coma is defined as a lack of awareness and lack of wakefulness. A coma generally lasts up to 3 weeks, after which a person goes into a vegetative state. The vegetative state can be a transition from coma to recovery, but it can also become permanent until death.

The vegetative state is defined as wakefulness without awareness. In TBI, the vegetative state must last more than 1 year to be considered permanent. In nontraumatic brain injury due to anoxic causes, the vegetative state must last 3 months in order to be considered permanent. A person can also transition from a coma to a minimally conscious state or from a vegetative state to a minimally conscious state. In a minimally conscious state, there is wakefulness and intermittent limited purposeful activities (e.g., following simple commands).

Parameter	Score	Response
Eye opening	Spontaneous	4
	To voice	3
	To pain	2
	No response	1
Best verbal response	Oriented, converses	5
	Disoriented, converses	4
	Inappropriate words	3
	Incomprehensible sounds	2
	No response or intubated	1
Best motor response	Follows commands	6
	Localizes response (pushes away stimulus)	5
	Withdraws	4
	Abnormal flexion (decorticate)	3
	Abnormal extension (decerebrate)	2
	No response	1

FIGURE 11-27 Glasgow Coma Scale.

Reproduced from Teasdale, G. & Jennett, B. (1974). Assessment of coma and impaired consciousness: A practical solution. *The Lancet*, 2, 81–84. Copyright (1974), with permission from Elsevier.

(e.g., irritability or unusual behavior), restlessness, or lethargy. There may be a loss of consciousness that can be prolonged (e.g., days to weeks), and retrograde amnesia may be present upon awakening. Brainstem injury and increased ICP signs include pupil asymmetry, unilateral or bilateral fixed and dilated pupils, posturing (decorticate or decerebrate; FIGURE 11-28), respiratory depression, irregular breathing pattern, hypertension, and bradycardia. TBI is a common cause of death and disability. For those who survive, neurologic deficits can include impairments such as altered motor movements (e.g., lack of coordination), changes in behavior, altered reasoning, and difficulty with written or verbal communication. The disabilities may be permanent. Some patients may remain in a vegetative or minimally conscious state.

Diagnosis and Treatment

Diagnostic procedures for TBI consist of a history, physical examination (including using the Glasgow Coma Scale) (Figure 11-27), head CT, head MRI, and ICP monitoring. Treatment strategies vary depending on the severity and the time since injury. Immediate emergency care for TBI focuses on limiting brain damage. Mild injuries usually require no treatment other than rest, analgesics (specifically acetaminophen [Tylenol]) if headache is present, and 24-hour observation in the hospital or at home if there is a reliable caregiver. Nonsteroidal anti-inflammatory drugs (NSAIDs), such as aspirin and ibuprofen (Motrin), should be avoided because they can increase bleeding risk. Cold compresses can be applied to any outward edema. Moderate to severe brain injuries usually require hospitalization, and patients with such damage often need intensive care. Blood pressure control and cerebral perfusion pressure must be maintained to prevent further injury. Ventilatory management and avoidance of hypoxia and abnormal carbon dioxide levels (high or low) are often necessary as these alterations can aggravate cerebral ischemia. Glucose levels (high or low) can worsen outcomes, so levels need to be maintained within a normal range. Patients with TBIs can display episodes of sympathetic hyperactivity such as tachycardia, hyperthermia, and diaphoresis. These episodes are managed with sedation (e.g., propofol, fentanyl, or midazolam) and cardiovascular agents (e.g., propranolol or clonidine). Hyperthermia or fever will worsen outcomes, so antipyretics and external cooling

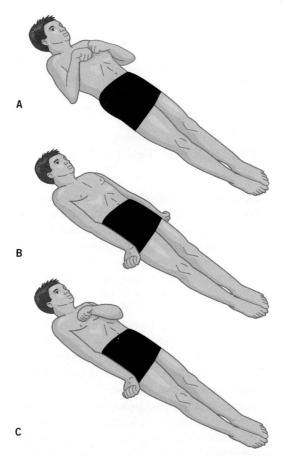

FIGURE 11-28 Decorticate and decerebrate posturing. (A) Decorticate response: flexion of the arms, wrists, and fingers with adduction in the upper extremities; extension, internal rotation, and plantar flexion in the lower extremities. (B) Decerebrate response: all four extremities in rigid extension with hyperpronation of the forearms and plantar extension of the feet. (C) Decorticate response on the left side of the body and decerebrate response on the right side of the body.

devices may be necessary. Intracranial pressure can be managed by elevating the head of the bed to a minimum of 30° and maintaining the head in a neutral position. Osmotic diuretics (e.g., mannitol) or hypertonic saline may be given to reduce cerebral edema. Antiseizure medications may be necessary for prevention and treatment. A barbiturate coma with pentobarbital and thiopental may be necessary if ICP is refractory to other strategies. Therapeutic hypothermia can reduce ICP, but whether outcomes are improved is unclear. Surgery can be performed to remove blood or repair fractures. The rehabilitative phase is usually long and requires physical, speech, and occupational therapy to minimize and/or improve residual neurologic dysfunction.

Prevention strategies for TBIs include wearing a seat belt when driving or riding in a motor vehicle, using appropriate child safety seats, wearing a helmet when appropriate (e.g., when playing sports, riding a bicycle, or skating), making the home safe (e.g., removing tripping hazards, having adequate lighting, and using safety gates), storing firearms in locked cabinets, never driving impaired, and supervising children when playing.

Increased Intracranial Pressure

Increased intracranial pressure describes increased volume (fluid or tissue) in the limited space of the cranial cavity. Increased ICP may occur because of a TBI and other conditions that would increase the volume in the skull (e.g., tumor, hydrocephalus, cerebral edema, and hemorrhage). The delicate pressure–volume relationship among ICP; volume of CSF (contributes 10%), blood (contributes 10%), and brain tissue (contributes 80%); and cerebral perfusion is explained by the Monro-Kellie hypothesis (FIGURE 11-29). The Monro-Kellie hypothesis states that the cranial cavity is incompressible, and the volume inside the cavity is fixed (normal ICP is 60–200 mm H_2O or 4–15 mmHg) as ICP is a function of the volume and the compliance of each component. The skull and its components (blood, CSF, and brain tissue) create a state of volume equilibrium, such that any increase in the volume of one component must be compensated by a decrease in the volume of another component. This compensation is primarily accomplished by shifts in the CSF and, to a lesser extent, blood volume as brain tissue volume remains relatively constant. These fluids respond to increases in the volume of the remaining components. For example, an area of bleeding into the brain tissue (e.g., epidural hematoma) will be compensated for by the downward displacement of CSF and venous blood. Transient increases in ICP routinely occur with position changes, coughing, or sneezing. These compensatory mechanisms are able to maintain a normal ICP for changes in volume up to a point (approximately 100–120 mL of volume increases).

In addition to shifting volumes, the brain has two other compensatory mechanisms to maintain tissue perfusion—autoregulation and Cushing reflex. With autoregulation, the blood vessels dilate to increase blood flow and constrict if the ICP is increased. Cushing reflex is a complex cascade of events that results in increased blood pressure. When the mean arterial pressure (average blood pressure) drops below the ICP, the hypothalamus increases sympathetic stimulation. This stimulation causes vasoconstriction, increased cardiac contractility, and increased cardiac output. If unresolved, the increased ICP eventually leads to a trio of effects known as Cushing triad—increased blood pressure, bradycardia, and changes in respiratory pattern (FIGURE 11-30). Baroreceptors in the carotid arteries detect the increase in blood pressure, triggering a parasympathetic response through vagal

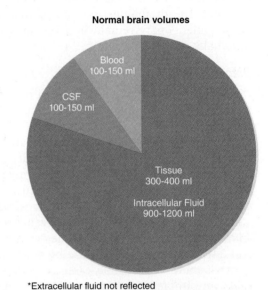

*Extracellular fluid not reflected

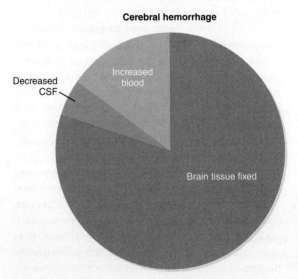

FIGURE 11-29 Monro-Kellie hypothesis.

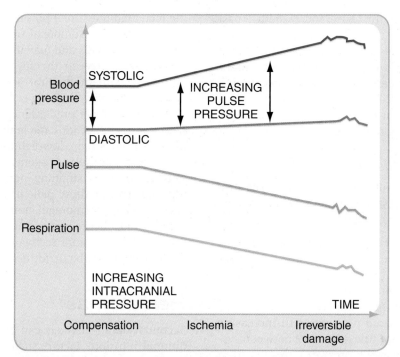

FIGURE 11-30 Vital sign changes with increased intracranial pressure.

stimulation that induces bradycardia. Bradycardia may also be stimulated by the increased ICP impinging on the vagal nerve, causing a parasympathetic response. As pressure increases inside the skull, space becomes limited and the brain tissue shifts downward. An irregular respiratory pattern, called *Cheyne-Stokes respiration* (deeper, faster breathing followed by slower breathing and apneic episodes), and bradypnea typically result from increased pressure on the brainstem due to swelling or from brainstem herniation.

Herniation—a feared complication of increased ICP—involves the displacement of brain tissue from a place of high pressure to a place of lower pressure. Several types of herniation are possible (**FIGURE 11-31**). In transtentorial (central) herniation, the cerebral hemispheres, diencephalon, and midbrain are displaced downward. The pressure created by this type of herniation impairs the cerebral blood flow, CSF, reticular activation system, and respirations. Uncal (uncinate) herniation occurs when the uncus (the hooklike anterior end of the hippocampal gyrus) of the temporal lobe shifts downward past the tentorium cerebelli (the extension of the dura mater that separates the cerebellum from the inferior portion of the occipital lobes). This type of herniation

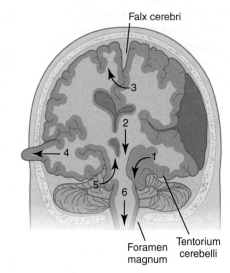

FIGURE 11-31 Types of herniation.

creates pressure on cranial nerve III, the posterior cerebral artery, and the reticular activation system. Cerebellar, or tonsillar (infratentorial), herniation occurs when the cerebellar tonsils (the rounded lobules on the undersurface of each cerebellar hemisphere) are pushed downward through the foramen magnum. This type of herniation compresses the brainstem and vital centers, causing death. Cerebellar herniations can also go upwards due to pressure.

Regardless of the cause, increased ICP past the point of compensation compresses cerebral blood vessels and other structures as it shifts the brain's contents. Eventually, brain tissue dies. Increased ICP is a life-threatening situation that requires prompt treatment. If left unresolved, it causes declining neurologic function, leading to death.

Clinical Manifestations

The clinical manifestations of increased ICP vary depending on the patient's age and reflect the effects of the rising pressures:

- Decreasing level of consciousness (results from pressure on the brainstem and cerebral cortex)
- Vomiting, often projectile (results from pressure on the medulla)
- Increasing blood pressure with increasing pulse pressure (the difference between systolic and diastolic pressure) (results from Cushing reflex)
- Bradycardia (response to the increasing blood pressure)
- Papilledema (results from increased pressure exerted by CSF, which causes swelling around the optic disk)
- Fixed and dilated pupils (results from pressure on cranial nerve III)
- Posturing (Figure 11-28)

Two manifestations of increased ICP are unique to infants:

1. Separated sutures
2. Bulging fontanelle

Manifestations in older children and adults include the following symptoms:

- Behavior changes
- Severe headache (results from stretching of the dura and walls of the large blood vessels)
- Lethargy
- Neurologic deficits
- Seizures

Diagnosis and Treatment

Diagnostic procedures for increased ICP consist of a history, physical examination (including completing the Glasgow Coma Scale), head CT, head MRI, and ICP monitoring. Increased ICP requires prompt diagnosis and treatment for optimal patient outcomes. Treatment strategies vary depending on the underlying etiology, and attempts should be made to resolve the source of the increased pressure if possible (e.g., remove a tumor or blood). Additional strategies are similar to those for TBIs and may include respiratory support (e.g., oxygen therapy or endotracheal intubation with mechanical ventilation), semi-Fowler positioning, draining excess CSF, osmotic diuretics or hypertonic saline, corticosteroids (used for CNS infections and brain tumors), seizure precautions (e.g., low lighting and minimal stimulation), antiseizure agents, sedatives, stool softeners (because straining increases ICP), antiulcer agents (for those patients at high risk for stress ulcers), thermoregulation, blood pressure control, and glucose management. Rarely, surgical removal of a skull segment (decompressive craniectomy) may be performed.

Hematomas

Secondary brain damage can be caused by additional injurious factors such as hemorrhaging. A hematoma is a collection of blood in the tissue that develops from ruptured blood vessels. Hematomas, which can develop immediately or slowly because of a TBI or surgery, are classified by their location (**FIGURE 11-32**).

- Epidural hematomas result from bleeding between the dura and skull, usually caused by an arterial tear (e.g., the middle meningeal artery at the skull base is a common location). Because of the location, epidural hematomas do not cross sutural margins. These bleeds are more common in adolescents and young adults as a result of trauma (e.g., accidents and assaults). Skull fractures are present in most patients with an epidural hematoma. Clinical manifestations of epidural hematomas include marked neurologic dysfunction that usually develops within a few hours of injury. The typical symptom pattern of an epidural hematoma is a brief loss of consciousness, followed by a short period of alertness, then deterioration over a period of hours manifested as headache, vomiting, confusion, aphasia, seizures, and hemiparesis, and loss of consciousness again. This pattern may not appear in all people.
- Subdural hematomas develop between the dura and the arachnoid, and are frequently caused by a small venous tear and, in fewer cases, an arterial rupture (**FIGURE 11-33**). In contrast to epidural hematomas, these bleeds can cross sutural margins but not dural attachments. Because they are usually

TYPES OF INTRACRANIAL HEMATOMAS

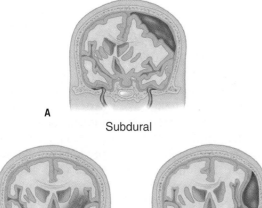

A

Subdural

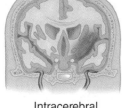

Intracerebral

B

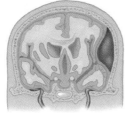

Epidural

C

FIGURE 11-32 Types of hematomas. **(A)** Beneath the dura but outside the brain (subdural hematoma). **(B)** Within the substance of the brain tissue (intracerebral hematoma). **(C)** Outside the dura and under the skull (epidural hematoma).

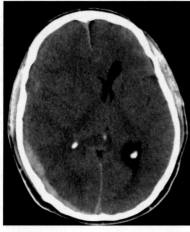

FIGURE 11-33 Midline shift associated with right-sided subdural hematoma.
Courtesy of Dr. Jason W. Schroeder, MD.

the result of a venous tear, these types of hematomas generally develop slowly. Subdural hematomas follow several patterns. With acute subdural hematomas, manifestations of neurologic deficits present within 24 hours of an injury. Manifestations are similar to other those of other head injuries (e.g., headache and vomiting) and a lucid interval may also appear followed by deterioration and coma. This type of hematoma progresses rapidly and has a high mortality. With subacute subdural hematomas, ICP increases over a period of about a week after the injury. With chronic subdural hematomas, manifestations develop several weeks (usually 2 weeks or longer) after the injury because of a slow leak. The manifestations with chronic subdural hematoma appear insidiously, can be transient, and fluctuate. The manifestations include headache, light-headedness, sleepiness, and personality changes (e.g., apathy). Chronic subdural hematomas are more common in elderly adults because of the brain atrophy that occurs with age, which gives the hematoma more space to develop. Atrophy is also prevalent with chronic alcohol abuse or in those with prior TBIs.

- Intracerebral hematomas result from bleeding in the brain tissue itself. These types of hematomas are caused by contusion or shearing injuries but, more commonly, result from hypertension or vascular abnormalities (a common cause in children). Intracerebral hematomas are a common cause of hemorrhagic stroke.

- A subarachnoid hemorrhage results from bleeding in the space between the arachnoid and the pia. This type of hemorrhage is often due to the rupture of an intracranial aneurysm or vascular malformations while trauma is a less common cause. The primary clinical presentation is a severe headache that has a sudden onset and is worse near the back of the head or wherever the aneurysm is located. The headache is often described as the worst headache of the patient's life and is often the only symptom.

In all types of hematomas, the bleeding leads to localized pressure on nearby tissue and increases ICP. Blood may coagulate and form a solid mass. The hematoma becomes encapsulated by fibroblasts, and blood cells within the capsule lyse. The fluid from the hemolysis exerts osmotic pressure, drawing more fluid into the capsule. This edema increases the size of the mass, applying pressure on the surrounding tissue and increasing ICP. Bleeding can trigger vasospasms, worsening ischemia. Additionally, increasing ICP can result in herniation. Chronic subdural hematomas can also expand and cause a recurrent bleed referred to as an *acute-on-chronic bleed*.

Diagnosis and Treatment

Diagnostic procedures for all types of hematomas and hemorrhaging consist of a history, physical examination (including completing the Glasgow Coma Scale), head CT, head MRI, cerebral angiogram, and intracranial pressure monitor. Treatment strategies depend on the location and bleeding severity. No treatment may be required in mild cases in which the volume is small and the bleeding has ceased. For many patients, surgical removal of the blood through a burr hole or a craniotomy is required. In some cases, however, removal of the blood may not be possible. In these situations, patients may experience significant residual neurologic deficits that require physical, speech, and occupational therapy. Strategies similar to those used for TBIs and increased ICP (e.g., respiratory management, seizure precautions, and thermoregulation) may be required.

Learning Points

Head Injury

Immediately following a head injury, some key actions should be avoided:

- Do *not* apply direct pressure to a bleeding site; cover the wound with sterile gauze.
- Do *not* wash a head wound that is deep or bleeding profusely.
- Do *not* remove any object sticking out of a wound.
- Do *not* move the person unless it is absolutely necessary.
- Do *not* shake the person if he or she seems dazed.
- Do *not* remove a helmet if you suspect a serious head injury.
- Do *not* pick up a fallen child with any sign of a head injury.
- Do *not* drink alcohol within 48 hours of a serious head injury.

Spinal Cord Injuries

Spinal cord injuries (SCIs) result from direct injury to the spinal cord or indirectly from damage to surrounding bones, tissues, or blood vessels. SCIs are most common in Whites and in males (National Spinal Cord Injury Statistical Center, 2016). The average age for experiencing an SCI has increased from 29 years in the 1970s to 42 years today. SCIs are often caused by motor vehicle accidents, falls, violence, and sports injuries. Minor injuries to the spinal cord can occur because of weakening vertebral structures (e.g., rheumatoid arthritis or osteoporosis). Direct damage can occur if the spinal cord is pulled, pressed sideways, or compressed (FIGURE 11-34). Such damage may occur, for example, if the head, neck, or

back twists abnormally during an accident or injury. A fracture, dislocation, ligament tear, or intervertebral disc disruption or herniation may accompany the SCI. The cord can also be partially or completely transected as a result of penetrating injuries (e.g., gunshot or knife wounds).

The primary injury occurs when there is direct impact to the cord. After the injury, a cascade of secondary events ensues, leading to further injury. The proposed mechanisms for these secondary insults are predominantly theoretic. The impact to the spinal cord disrupts the microvasculature, and the gray matter is highly metabolic and the most vulnerable to vascular disruption. Autoregulatory mechanisms designed to maintain adequate perfusion may fail. Ischemia and hypoxia result from the vascular disruption. The ischemia produces free radicals (e.g., superoxide), which cause cell membrane damage. The free radicals damage mitochondrial DNA and cellular enzymes, leading to the buildup of toxic metabolites and cell death. Ischemia in cells triggers glutamate (excitatory neurotransmitter) accumulation, and the glutamate acts on N-methyl-D aspartate (NMDA) receptors, which opens ion channels resulting in the influx of calcium and the activation of more destructive enzymes. Adenosine triphosphate is lost in the cell, and sodium and water enter the cell body. Inflammatory cells also secrete destructive enzymes and inflammatory cytokines (e.g., interleukins and interferon), resulting in further cell damage. The secondary injuries ultimately lead to SCI inflammation, edema, imbalance in neural connections, capillary permeability alterations with ion abnormalities, and cell death.

Hemorrhage, fluid accumulation, and edema can occur inside or outside the spinal cord (but within the spinal canal) and can occur immediately or within hours of the injury. The accumulation of blood or fluid can compress the spinal cord and damage it. The edema peaks around the sixth day after injury and begins to decrease after the ninth day. Eventually, the edema is replaced with a hemorrhagic necrosis. Spinal shock is different than neurogenic shock and refers to a temporary altered physiologic state with suppression of neurologic function because of spinal cord compression. In other words, the spinal cord is shocked by injury. The cause of the shock is thought to be due to accumulation of potassium that is released from injured cells. The potassium alterations lead to reduced axon impulse

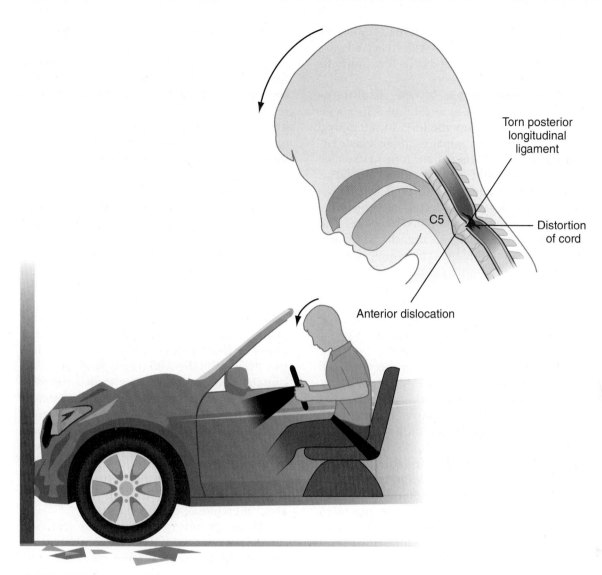

Torn posterior
longitudinal
ligament

C5

Distortion
of cord

Anterior dislocation

FIGURE 11-34 Spinal cord injuries.

transmission. In spinal shock, neurologic function gradually returns (see chapter 4 for discussion of types of shock.).

Clinical Manifestations

SCIs result in a significant loss of neurologic functioning, often requiring extensive, long-term management. SCIs can also result in death, either immediately due to the injury or because of complications (e.g., pneumonia, embolism, or septicemia). The degree of dysfunction depends on the severity of the injury and its location (Figure 11-14). The injury may result in a partial or complete disruption of the neurons and neural tracts anywhere along the spinal cord. SCIs are classified based on the location of damage (e.g., C4, T12) and the degree of function lost.

Immediately after an SCI, spinal shock can develop and consists of the following manifestations below the level of injury: flaccid paralysis, lack of sensation (anesthesia), and loss of reflex activity. Bowel and bladder control are lost. The sympathetic system is also disrupted above the level of injury resulting in vasodilation and decreased blood pressure. Temperature control is impaired, and the patient's body temperature assumes the ambient temperature (poikilothermia). The poor temperature control is a result of the inability of the hypothalamus to regulate temperature through normal mechanisms (e.g., vasoconstriction and increased metabolic rate). Resolving spinal shock usually becomes evident with the return of reflexes such as the perianal reflex (the reflex contraction of the external anal sphincter).

Manifestations of spinal shock may resolve or spastic paresis may develop with hyperreflexia. Spinal shock duration can be a few hours to several months.

Neurogenic shock, a type of distributive shock, can occur as a result of SCIs above thoracic level 6. Below the level of the injury, sympathetic tone is impaired or blocked, resulting in a loss of sympathetic tone in vascular smooth muscle and massive vasodilation. The vasodilation causes blood to pool in the venous system, leading to decreased venous return, cardiac output, and blood pressure. The compensatory mechanisms of tachycardia and vasoconstriction from the sympathetic nervous system are not present in response to hypotension. However, the parasympathetic response remains intact and is unopposed, so the patient will have bradycardia. In neurogenic shock, the patient will have a triad of bradycardia, vasodilation, and hypotension. Neurogenic shock can also occur with spinal shock. Neurogenic shock can last for several weeks after the injury.

Autonomic dysreflexia can also occur as a result of SCIs above thoracic level 6. Autonomic dysreflexia occurs within a few weeks (e.g., after spinal shock) or within 1 year of the injury. The manifestations of autonomic dysreflexia are the loss of coordinated heart rate and vascular response to various stimuli. Essentially, there is an exaggerated sympathetic response of generalized vasoconstriction and hypertension to a noxious stimuli below the level of injury. Above the injury, the parasympathetic system is stimulated. As a compensatory mechanism to reduce blood pressure, the parasympathetic response includes vasodilation and bradycardia. The compensatory parasympathetic response is insufficient to overcome the hypertension as motor signals are unable to travel through the injured cord. The types of noxious stimuli that can trigger this response commonly include a distended bladder or constipation. Other stimuli can include pressure injuries, fractures, or sexual activity. In addition, hypertension manifestations can include headache, diaphoresis, anxiety, nausea, bradycardia, or tachycardia.

SCI dysfunction will depend on the level of the injury (e.g., cervical, thoracic, or lumbar; FIGURE 11-35), the location of the injury (e.g., anterior), and the severity of the injury (e.g., incomplete). An injury to one of the eight cervical segments of the spinal cord causes quadriplegia (tetraplegia)—loss of all or most function in all four limbs. Patients with cervical injuries are likely to have difficulty breathing as a result of paralysis of respiratory muscles, often requiring intubation with mechanical ventilation. Injury to the thoracic, lumbar, or sacral regions causes paraplegia—loss of lower extremity function. The severity of SCI is often described based on the American Spinal Injury Association classification. The classes (from A to D) are based on the sensory and motor impairments after an injury. Class A is a complete spinal cord injury with complete paralysis, while classes B–D are types of incomplete injuries. The individual may experience complete cord injury with no sensation and complete paralysis below the level of injury. Incomplete cord injuries result in varying degrees of sensory and motor function below the level of injury. With incomplete injuries, sensation may remain more intact than motor function because sensory tracts are farther away from the cord (more peripheral). Incomplete quadriplegia is the most frequently occurring injury, occurring in approximately 30% of SCIs. The spinal cord does not extend beyond the first to second lumbar vertebra, so injuries at and below this level do not cause SCIs. However, they may cause cauda equina syndrome (injury to the nerve roots in the area of the cauda equina) (see chapter 12 for details about musculoskeletal function).

There are several incomplete spinal cord syndromes, such as central cord syndrome, anterior cord syndrome, posterior cord syndrome, and Brown-Sequard syndrome (FIGURE 11-36). These syndromes can occur as a result traumatic SCI, but other neurologic disorders (e.g., tumors and multiple sclerosis) can cause these syndromes. The different syndromes produce various motor and sensory deficits.

Diagnosis and Treatment

Diagnostic procedures for SCIs consist of a history and physical examination. Assessment priorities should be evaluated using the ABCDE assessment format. This format includes:

A Airway management with attention to spinal immobilization

B Breathing and ventilation

C Circulation and cardiac status

D Disability, neurologic deficit, and gross deformity

E Exposure (completely disrobe the patient, examine for associated injuries, and maintain a warm environment)

After this initial assessment, a thorough neurologic evaluation of the SCI should be conducted. Initial imaging studies include X-rays, CT scans, or MRI of the spine. Other imaging studies can include somatosensory-evoked potential testing or magnetic stimulation and spinal myelogram (X-ray using contrast dye). These injuries are always medical emergencies requiring immediate treatment. Therapeutic strategies include both immediate interventions starting in the field and interventions continuing in the emergency department to minimize residual effects and long-term interventions to limit complications. SCI patients will require intensive medical care. Immediate strategies may include the following measures:

- Immobilization of the spine
- Neurogenic shock management with intravenous fluids, blood transfusions, and pharmacologic vasopressors to maintain an adequate blood pressure (a mean arterial pressure of at least 85 mmHg), including atropine or external pacing for bradycardia
- Corticosteroid agents to reduce swelling (efficacy controversial)
- Spinal traction to reduce fractures and immobilize the spine
- Surgical repair of vertebral fractures or surgical removal of the fluid compressing the spinal cord (decompression laminectomy)
- Respiratory management (e.g., oxygen therapy, endotracheal intubation with mechanical ventilation, and chest physical therapy)
- Venous and pulmonary thromboembolism prophylactic treatment (e.g., low molecular weight heparin, intermittent pneumatic compression, and graduated compression stockings)
- Skin care and pressure injury prevention
- Pain management
- Urinary catheterization to avoid bladder distention
- Gastrointestinal ulcer prevention (e.g., use of proton pump inhibitors)
- Temperature maintenance
- Nutritional support (e.g., enteral or parenteral feeding)
- Bed rest

Chronic complications of SCIs are multisystem. The highest rates of mortality with an SCI occur within the first year. Life expectancy improves past 1 year; however, the neurologic level (e.g., cervical injuries reduce life expectancy) and severity as well as age at time of

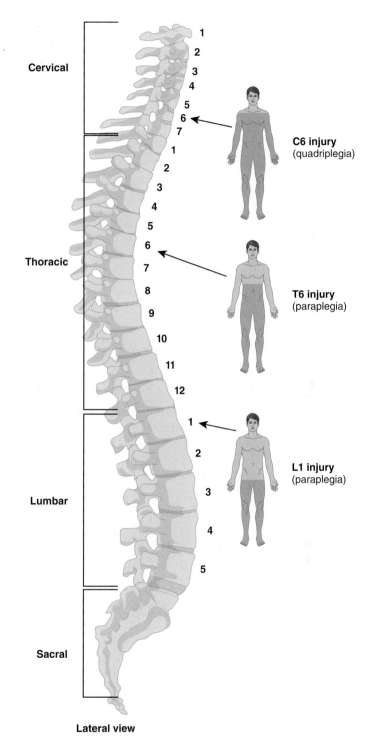

FIGURE 11-35 Spinal cord injury.

injury will impact life expectancy. The various complications include autonomic dysreflexia, coronary artery disease, pulmonary infections, neurogenic bladder, urinary infections, vesicoureteral reflux, renal calculi, renal failure, sexual dysfunction, impotence, impaired fertility (high incidence in men), constipation, osteoporosis, heterotopic ossification (bone

Central Cord Syndrome

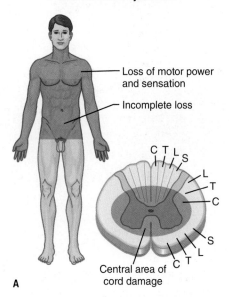

Loss of motor power and sensation

Incomplete loss

Central area of cord damage

A

Brown-Sèquard syndrome

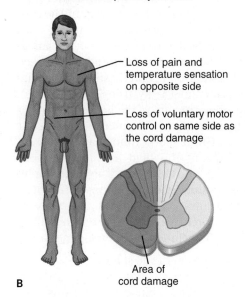

Loss of pain and temperature sensation on opposite side

Loss of voluntary motor control on same side as the cord damage

Area of cord damage

B

Anterior Cord Syndrome

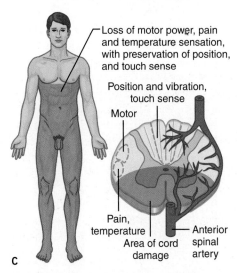

Loss of motor power, pain and temperature sensation, with preservation of position, and touch sense

Position and vibration, touch sense

Motor

Pain, temperature

Area of cord damage

Anterior spinal artery

C

Posterior Cord Syndrome

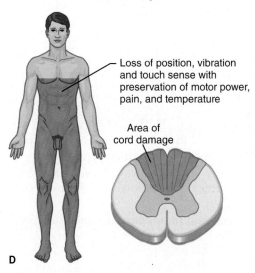

Loss of position, vibration and touch sense with preservation of motor power, pain, and temperature

Area of cord damage

D

FIGURE 11-36 Incomplete cord symptoms.

deposition within the soft tissue around the joints), muscle contracture, pressure injuries, muscle spasticity, chronic pain syndrome, psychiatric comorbidities (e.g., depression, substance abuse), and temperature imbalance.

Long-term strategies are aimed at addressing the complications and may include the following interventions:

- Physical, occupational, and speech therapy
- Psychological counseling and support groups
- Mobility assistive devices (e.g., a wheelchair and walking assistance system)
- Electronic devices (e.g., brain–computer interface, functional electronic stimulation systems, and electronic aids for daily living)

- Long-term respiratory management (e.g., mechanical ventilation)
- Meticulous skin care
- Bowel and bladder training or management (e.g., catheterization, stool softeners, anticholinergics, and alpha blockers)
- Antispasmodic agents and botulinum toxin type A (Botox) injections to treat muscle spasms or other agents such as baclofen
- Pain management including antiseizure medications (e.g., pregabalin), antidepressants, medical marijuana
- Nutritional support
- Prompt treatment of infections (pneumonia is the leading cause of death)
- Infertility treatment (e.g., artificial insemination) and high-risk pregnancy management

- Autonomic dysreflexia management (e.g., remove tight-fitting garments, sit upright to reduce blood pressure, correct noxious stimuli [e.g., catheterize]) and prophylactic treatment (e.g., nifedipine)

Vascular Neurologic Disorders

Vascular neurologic disorders generally involve ischemic injuries to the brain resulting from occlusion of blood flow or hemorrhage. These disorders vary significantly in their severity and presentation depending on the location and extent of damage. Often they result in some degree of neurologic dysfunction. These conditions may occur due to congenital abnormalities or chronic diseases such as hypertension, hypercholesterolemia, and atherosclerosis.

Cerebrovascular Accident

A cerebrovascular accident (CVA), or stroke, refers to an interruption of cerebral blood supply (**FIGURE 11-37**). A CVA is an infarction of the brain, so it is often referred to as a *brain attack*. This kind of interruption in the brain's blood flow may result from a brain ischemia (e.g., thrombus, embolus, or plaque) or brain hemorrhage (e.g., cerebral aneurysm, arteriovenous malformation, or hypertension). Thus, there are two major types of stroke—ischemic and hemorrhagic. Ischemic strokes are the most common (87%), but hemorrhagic strokes are the most deadly. Even 5 minutes (sometimes less) of altered tissue perfusion can lead to irreversible cell damage from the lack of oxygen and glucose. Stroke can result in significant neurologic dysfunction and death; in fact, someone has a stroke every 40 seconds, someone dies of a stroke every 3.70 minutes, and 389 deaths are due to strokes daily (AHA, 2019). Stroke is the chief cause of long-term disability and fifth leading cause of death in the United States (AHA, 2019).

CVA incidence and mortality rates are highest in the southeastern United States, often referred to as the *Stroke Belt*. The costs associated with this widespread problem and its extensive consequences are estimated at $34 billion annually in the United States (CDC, 2015d). In the United States, CVA prevalence and mortality are highest among Blacks. Additional risk factors include sedentary lifestyle, obesity, hypertension, smoking, hyperlipidemia, diabetes mellitus, unhealthy diet, renal dysfunction, and atherosclerosis. Pharmacologic agents (e.g., oral contraceptives,

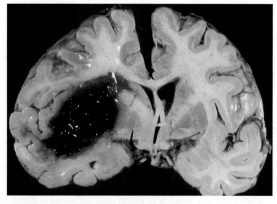

FIGURE 11-37 Cerebrovascular accident (CVA), or stroke.
Courtesy of Leonard V. Crowley, MD, Century College.

cocaine, amphetamines, and heroin) can increase stroke risk.

Ischemic and hemorrhagic stroke are divided into subtypes each with varying causes, clinical manifestations, outcomes, and treatment strategies. Hemorrhagic stroke subtypes include intracerebral hemorrhage and subarachnoid hemorrhage, which were previously discussed. Ischemic strokes are caused by thrombosis, and embolism with atherosclerosis is a common underlying pathology. Ischemic strokes are less common in children and younger adults, and the vasculature abnormalities are not usually due to atherosclerosis but rather noninflammatory (e.g., arterial dissection and sickle cell disease) and inflammatory (e.g., vasculitis) disorders. The obstruction caused by an embolus can be partial or complete and result in injury to a specific part of the brain that is supplied by the obstructed vessel. Ischemic stroke subtype characteristics include:

- **Thrombotic strokes** are a result of localized arterial occlusion. The occlusion can occur in large or small vessels, and the process can occur gradually (e.g., over several years as occurs in atherosclerosis) or acutely (e.g., platelets form a thrombus on plaque). Large-vessel diseases involve extracranial arteries (e.g., internal carotids and vertebral arteries) and intracranial arteries (e.g., circle of Willis and branches). The most common cause of large-vessel disease is atherosclerosis. Large-vessel disease causes local blood flow issues and reduces blood flow beyond the area of obstruction. Small-vessel disease affects small arteries and arterioles that supply deep brain structures, and ischemic lesions usually affect the basal ganglia, internal capsule, thalamus, and the pons. Small-vessel disease leads to what is termed **lacunar strokes**. These small-vessel strokes are a cause of 25% of ischemic strokes.

- **Embolic strokes** are also a result of arterial occlusion, but the source of the thrombus is from particles of debris that have originated outside the brain. The obstruction can be due to clots but also other debris (e.g., fat, air, or foreign body). Treating the source of the thrombus, if not local (i.e., formed in the brain) is important to prevent further strokes. The source of the thrombus that has embolized is often coming from the heart (e.g., atrial fibrillation or recent myocardial infarction). Other areas include the aorta or common carotid artery. In some circumstances, an embolic source cannot be identified. Atrial fibrillation is implicated in up to 25% of embolic strokes. Embolic strokes tend to affect cortical areas of the brain as opposed to lacunar strokes, which tend to affect the subcortical areas.

Regardless of the type of ischemic stroke, the consequences of a reduction in blood flow are the same. The brain has minimal energy stores of its own, so it relies on blood to deliver all its nutrients. While the brain receives 20% of the body's cardiac output, even brief interruptions in blood flow can lead to ischemia and infarction (cell death).

In an ischemic stroke, there is an area (the one supplied by a vessel) that necroses if ischemia is prolonged, and this damage is irreversible. This infarcted core, or destined-to-die core, is surrounded by possible tissue that can be saved known as the **penumbra**. The focus of treatment strategies are centered on protecting the penumbra, and this treatment usually needs to be accomplished within 3 hours.

As with spinal cord ischemia, a similar cascade of events occurs with brain ischemia that results in cell death. Cerebral autoregulatory mechanisms fail. Reduced cerebral blood flow causes decreased protein synthesis, and energy is sought from glucose; however, glucose use drops and anaerobic glycolysis leads to lactic acid buildup as blood flow worsens. Neurons then start to fail, and the neuronal membrane stability is disrupted. The excitatory neurotransmitter glutamate is released with ischemia. The glutamate release acts on NMDA receptors, which open ion channels, resulting in intracellular calcium and sodium (along with water) influx and potassium efflux. Sodium and water influx leads to edema, and the ion abnormalities

contribute to recurring glutamate stimulation and a phenomenon known as excitotoxicity. Nitric oxide, a free radical that normally causes beneficial vasodilation, is produced in large quantities, further compounding neuronal injury. Nitric oxide can react with other free radicals (e.g., superoxide) and damage mitochondrial DNA leading to the buildup of toxic metabolites and cell death. Excessive amounts of reactive oxygen species (normal by-products of oxidative metabolism) further damage the cells. Inflammatory cells also secrete destructive enzymes and inflammatory cytokines (e.g., interleukins, interferon), resulting in additional cell damage. Ultimately, infarction ensues.

Ischemia and infarction effects on the brain tissue and vascular integrity can be profound and result in cerebral edema. Brain tissue membrane alterations that cause water accumulation cause a **cytotoxic edema**, while blood–brain barrier vascular alterations allow large molecules (e.g., proteins) to go into the extracellular volume leading to **vasogenic edema**. Cerebral edema is a secondary complication of stroke. The edema can be severe enough, in up to 10% of ischemic strokes, to cause an increase in brain volume with increased ICP and brain herniation.

Transient ischemic attacks (TIAs) are defined as transient episodes of neurologic dysfunction caused by focal brain, spinal cord, or retinal ischemia without infarction. Prior definitions incorporated duration of symptoms (e.g., < 24 hours); however, brief episodes of ischemia can cause infarct. Additionally, short duration of symptom (e.g., < 1 hour) can be associated with permanent injury. In other words, duration of symptoms is not reliable in distinguishing what ischemic events will lead to infarction. Emphasizing tissue injury as the end point rather than time more accurately reflects whether infarct is absent or present and encourages earlier testing to identify the brain injury. TIAs serve as warning signs that a stroke may be impending; approximately one in three people who experience a TIA will eventually have a stroke, with about half of these strokes occurring within 1 year of the TIA. However, not all strokes are preceded by a TIA.

Clinical Manifestations

Clinical manifestations of ischemic stroke and TIA are similar and are dependent on the affected arterial flow. TIA neurologic deficits, however, tend to resolve quickly (usually within minutes to an hour). Some strokes are minor and nondisabling while other stroke manifestations improve with time and therapy, but they may also persist, creating complications. Hemorrhagic strokes can be somewhat distinguished from ischemic strokes by the course and symptoms. Subarachnoid hemorrhage symptoms are instant and not focal (i.e., they usually involve regions supplied by more than one artery). Strokes from intracerebral hemorrhage will not display an early period of improvement as in thrombotic strokes and decline is progressive. Thrombotic strokes may manifest with progression of symptoms with periods of improvement (this occurs in steps rather than all at once). The symptoms may evolve over hours or days. Embolic strokes tend to have a sudden onset, and usually the maximal deficit is at presentation and does not progress. Embolic stroke manifestations can improve quickly.

A key feature of ischemic stroke is a sudden loss of focal brain function. The manifestations of ischemic stroke are dependent on the brain area supplied by the obstructed artery. While there can be minor variations based on which vessel is involved, stroke manifestations in general can be described based on whether the anterior circulation or the posterior circulation is affected FIGURE 11-38 and FIGURE 11-39. The anterior circulation includes the middle cerebral artery, which

supplies the lateral anterior and central portions of the cerebral hemispheres, and the anterior cerebral artery, which supplies the portions of the frontal lobe. The posterior circulation includes the vertebral arteries, the basilar arteries, and the posterior cerebral arteries, which supply vertebrobasilar structures (e.g., the back of the cerebral hemispheres, thalamus, midbrain, and brainstem). Manifestations will include deficits of the motor (common), language, sensory, and cognitive systems (TABLE 11-3).

Diagnosis and Treatment

The diagnosis of a stroke is based on a history and physical examination with attention initially in evaluating airway, breathing, and circulatory status, as other medical conditions often coexist with stroke. Determining whether the CVA is ischemic or hemorrhagic in origin prior to treatment is crucial because the interventions vary depending on the type. Additionally, some interventions for ischemic strokes can worsen hemorrhagic strokes (e.g., thrombolytic agents). A noncontrast CT of the head is often the first test to accomplish this goal. Several modalities (CT perfusion imaging and CT angiography) can enhance a noncontrast CT to better visualize site of

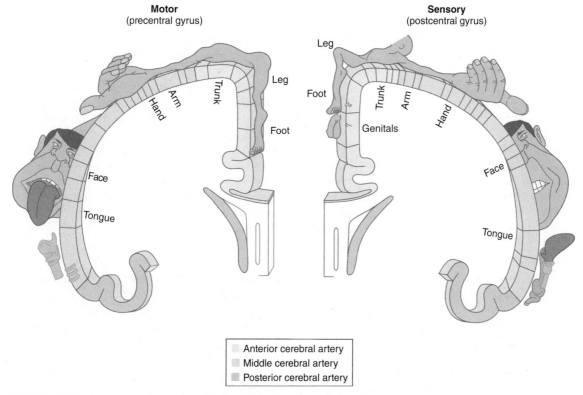

FIGURE 11-38 Homunculus of sensory and motor cortex with arterial blood supply.

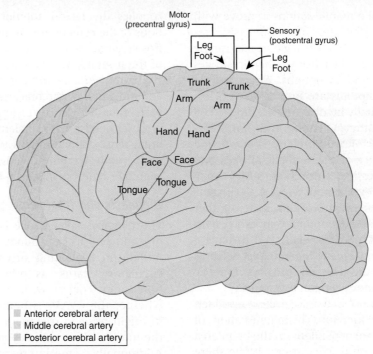

FIGURE 11-39 Location of motor and sensory gyrus and relation to lobes and arterial blood supply (lateral view).

TABLE 11-3 | **Major Cerebral Vessels and Manifestations of Stroke**

Major Cerebral Arteries	Arteries Included*	Brain Area Supplied	Clinical Manifestations***
Anterior Circulation	Anterior cerebral artery Middle cerebral artery**	Cerebral cortex Subcortical white matter Basal ganglia Internal capsule	Headache Apraxia- difficulty with motor planning to perform tasks or movement Aphasia- loss of ability to understand or express speech Agnosia- inability to interpret sensation – unable to identify (e.g., things, persons, smells) Hemiparesis Hemisensory deficits Visual field defects
Posterior (Vertebrobasilar) Circulation	Vertebral artery Basilar artery Posterior cerebral artery Cerebellar arteries	Brainstem Cerebellum Thalamus Portions of occipital and temporal lobe	Altered consciousness/Coma Drop attacks (sudden collapse without loss of consciousness) Nausea Vomiting Vertigo Ataxia Crossed sensorimotor symptoms (face on one side affected with opposite side limbs affected) Cranial nerve palsies- (e.g., diplopia, dysarthria) Visual field defects

*Partial list of arteries

**Most commonly occluded in stroke

***Manifestations can overlap between anterior and posterior circulation ischemia

BOX 11-3 Application to Practice

Anna Bryant, a 65-year-old White female, is brought to the emergency department by her daughter, Pat. Ms. Bryant complains of right-sided weakness and a headache that started about 2 hours ago. Her daughter states she found her in bed early this morning and noticed she was having trouble speaking. Ms. Bryant has a history of type 2 diabetes mellitus, for which she takes metformin and rheumatoid arthritis, which she manages with naproxen. She used to smoke but quit 5 years ago. She does not drink alcohol or use illicit drugs.

Her vital signs are as follows: Temperature 99.0° F; heart rate 94 beats per minute and irregular; respirations 20 breaths per minute; blood pressure 150/90 mmHg; and oxygen saturation 95%. Upon assessment, Ms. Bryant is alert, but has trouble answering questions. Her speech is slurred, and she appears frightened.

1. Based on her manifestations which cerebral artery is likely affected?
   a. Vertebral artery
   b. Basilar artery
   c. Posterior cerebral artery
   d. Middle cerebral artery
2. Which type of stroke is Ms. Bryant likely having?
   a. Ischemic embolic stroke
   b. Ischemic thrombotic stroke
   c. Subarachnoid hemorrhage
   d. Intracerebral hemorrhage
3. Where in the brain is the lesion?
   a. Right hemisphere
   b. Left hemisphere
4. Based on her history and physical examination findings, what is a possible etiology for a stroke in Ms. Bryant?
   a. Endocarditis
   b. Rheumatoid arthritis
   c. Atrial fibrillation
   d. Illicit drug use

5. What diagnostic tests should be ordered in the acute phase? Select all that apply
   a. 12-lead electrocardiogram
   b. Hemoglobin A_{1C}
   c. Noncontrast CT
   d. Lipid profile
6. What are treatment strategies for this acute stroke? Select all that apply.
   a. Intravenous thrombolytic therapy administration
   b. Systemic cooling to decrease risk of cerebral edema
   c. Antihypertensive agents to reduce mean arterial pressure to 80 (e.g., 100/70 mmHg)
   d. Statin administration

occlusion, infarct core, penumbra, and collateral circulation. A head MRI can also be used and can detect ischemia earlier than the CT. Ultrasounds are used to evaluate the extracranial (e.g., carotid arteries) and intracranial (e.g., circle of Willis) blood vessels. Cerebral angiography (i.e., arteriogram) is an invasive technique used to evaluate the cerebral vessels (e.g., degree of stenosis, evidence of dissection, vascular malformations, and vasculitis). Other diagnostic tests will include an electrocardiogram (many stroke patients also have coronary artery disease), an echocardiogram (determining the emboli source). Lab tests will include serum clotting studies, blood chemistry, and a complete blood count.

Early treatment will improve stroke outcomes. Optimally, treatment should be delivered within 3 hours of symptom onset, so persons or family members of persons who seem to be experiencing a stroke should make note of when the symptoms began. Ischemic strokes are treated with thrombolytic agents such as alteplase (to dissolve any clots) and

aspirin (to limit platelet activity). This treatment is contraindicated in persons with a recent history of bleeding issues. Additionally, procedures such as angioplasty or carotid endarterectomy may be necessary in patients with ischemic strokes. Surgical repair of aneurysms or arteriovenous malformations and blood removal may be required in patients with hemorrhagic strokes. Corticosteroids may also be administered with either type of CVA to reduce cerebral edema, and antihypertensive agents may be used to slowly (e.g., no more than 15% decrease in first 24 hours) and cautiously to reduce blood pressure. Prophylaxis for venous thromboembolism should be initiated (e.g., pneumatic compression stockings). All patients with an ischemic stroke should be started on a statin agent to reduce the risk of recurrent stroke and cardiovascular events. Statin therapy is used, independent of cholesterol levels. Statins, in addition to lipid-lowering effects, are thought to have antiatherothrombotic properties and may stabilize plaque, reduce inflammation, slow carotid disease progression, improve endothelial function, and reduce embolic stroke. Electrolyte and serum glucose alterations need to be corrected to prevent further injury. Elevating the head of the bed and maintaining proper body position in the same manner as those with other types of brain injury is important due to possible aspiration, increases in intracranial pressure, and cardiopulmonary decompensation. An interprofessional approach (using a team consisting of a nurse, physical therapist, speech therapist, occupational therapist, dietitian, and social worker) should be initiated as soon as the patient is stable and may be required on a long-term basis to minimize or prevent complications. Depending on the degree of dysfunction, strategies may be necessary to prevent complications of immobility (e.g., constipation, impaired skin integrity, contractures, and infections).

TIA diagnostic testing will be the same as those for stroke and should be performed expeditiously (e.g., within 2 days) as immediate evaluation and treatment reduces the risk of recurrent stroke. Stroke risk after a TIA is highest within 90 days.

Treatment strategies for TIAs focus on preventing the occurrence of a CVA. These strategies typically include managing any underlying conditions such as hypertension, atherosclerosis, and diabetes mellitus. Medications, such as antiplatelet aggregation agents (e.g., aspirin and clopidogrel [Plavix]) or anticoagulants (e.g., warfarin [Coumadin]), may be used to prevent clotting. Statin therapy is implemented to reduce stroke risk. Angioplasty (balloon dilation) can be undertaken to open narrowed arteries, or a carotid endarterectomy (surgical removal of plaque) may be performed to increase cerebral blood flow. Lifestyle management includes smoking cessation, minimizing dietary cholesterol and fat, increasing dietary fruits and vegetables, exercising regularly, limiting alcohol consumption, and eliminating illicit drug use.

Learning Points

Hypoxic-Ischemic Brain Injury

Brain ischemia can be due to systemic hypoperfusion causing diffuse areas of the brain to be injured, which is in contrast to thrombosis or emboli where regions are affected. Neurologic signs, in contrast to other causes of stroke, are usually bilateral and nonfocal (i.e., not confined to one region). The causes of the hypoperfusion include any disorders that affect cardiac output (e.g., acute myocardial infarctions or pulmonary embolism).

Cerebral Aneurysm

A cerebral aneurysm is a localized outpouching (ballooning out) of a cerebral artery. This weakening of the artery may occur as a congenital defect, or it may develop later in life because of conditions such as hypertension, cigarette smoking, connective tissue disease (e.g., Marfan syndrome), TBI, and arterial wall infection (FIGURE 11-40; FIGURE 11-41). Risk factors include hereditary syndromes (e.g., polycystic kidney disease) and familial factors even without a hereditary syndrome. Women are at higher risk after menopause, alluding to a possible link to estrogen deficiency, which results in reduction

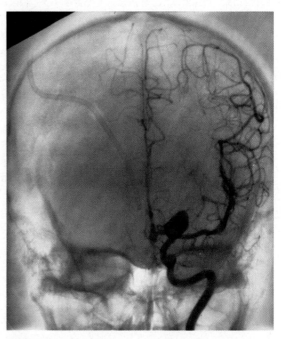

FIGURE 11-40 Cerebral aneurysm.
Courtesy of Michael Hart.

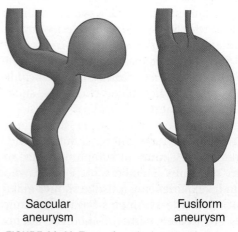

Saccular aneurysm   Fusiform aneurysm

FIGURE 11-41 Types of cerebral aneurysms.

of collagen in tissues. The bulging artery segment in an aneurysm can put pressure on surrounding tissue. Additionally, the aneurysm may leak or rupture, causing a CVA or death. Several types of aneurysms are possible, but most cerebral aneurysms are saccular (berry) forms. Cerebral aneurysms most frequently occur in the anterior circulation (85%), usually as multiple aneurysms on the circle of Willis.

Many cerebral aneurysms remain asymptomatic until they grow large enough to compress surrounding structures or they rupture. The most common cause of subarachnoid hemorrhage is a ruptured intracranial saccular aneurysm. Clinical manifestations that may appear as the aneurysm compresses nearby structures include cranial nerve III dysfunction (e.g., diplopia, ptosis, pupillary dilation, and loss of vision), headache, facial pain eye pain, neck pain, and pyramidal tract dysfunction (e.g., hyperreflexia and decreased fine motor coordination). A sudden, severe headache is an indication that the aneurysm has ruptured. The risk of an aneurysm rupture increases with the size of the aneurysm. However, it is proposed that small aneurysms can also rupture, usually soon after formation because they have not had time to stabilize and harden. While all aneurysms regardless of location can rupture, incidence is higher in posterior circulation aneurysms. Manifestations resemble those associated with increased ICP and CVA once a rupture has occurred.

Often diagnosis occurs inadvertently with a head CT or MRI. Additional diagnostic procedures include a history, physical examination, cerebral arteriography, and EEG. If discovered prior to rupture, treatment strategies include possible surgical repair and managing contributing factors (e.g., hypertension). Unruptured aneurysms may require routine monitoring (e.g., every year for 3 years) with a magnetic resonance angiography or CT angiography. Rupture is a medical emergency that requires immediate surgical repair. Additional strategies are similar to those for a CVA and subarachnoid hemorrhage.

Arteriovenous Malformations

An arteriovenous malformation (AVM) is a rare disorder of the cerebrovascular system where arteries and veins are connected together in a tangled mass. There is an absence of a capillary network in this mass. Single or multiple vessels may be involved. This rare disorder (incidence is 0.1% of the population) occurs as a result of sporadic congenital developmental vascular lesions or may be associated with hereditary syndromes. AVMs can also just develop without any prior anomaly, as a de novo brain lesion. AVMs are more common in males than females. In addition to AVM, there are three other types of cerebral vascular malformations: developmental venous anomalies (most common of the total four types), capillary telangiectasia, and cavernous malformation. Venous anomalies and capillary telangiectasia, are usually benign while cavernous malformation and AVM are likely to cause neurologic injury. AVM is considered the most lethal of the four types of cerebral vascular malformations. The high pressure of arterial blood flowing into the veins in an AVM can cause development of aneurysms. AVMs and associated aneurysms can rupture and lead to hemorrhage (e.g., intracerebral, subarachnoid hemorrhage) and stroke.

The most common age for the presentation of an AVM is between the ages of 10 and 40 years, and manifestations will depend on the location and the age of the affected individual. An AVM may cause no symptoms. Intracranial hemorrhage may be the first presentation in up to 50% of patients, and symptoms will be similar to other brain hemorrhages depending on location. Up to 25% of those with AVMs can present with a seizure. Headaches can occur with AVM and tend to be vague and not fall into any specific headache pattern (see the *Headache Disorders* section). Other manifestations are not as common and can include speech, vision, and movement difficulties.

An AVM can be found incidentally during brain imaging done for other reasons. In those with clinical manifestations, the diagnosis is made with brain imaging with a CT or MRI, and an angiography can be done with both modalities. The goal of treatment is to reduce complications of an AVM. Treatment options can include excision, focused radiation therapy, or endovascular embolization. If intracranial hemorrhages or seizures occur, they are treated similarly to hemorrhage and seizures due to other causes.

Headache Disorders

Headaches are a common form of pain within the United States and globally. As with low back pain, most individuals at some point in their life will experience a headache. Headaches are categorized as primary or secondary. Primary headaches are common and often are benign; however, they can be recurrent and significantly impact quality of life. Secondary headaches can be due to several underlying disorders. Some headaches can cause permanent disability and are life threatening (e.g., those due to intracerebral bleed or ruptured cerebral aneurysm). Of the primary headaches, 90% fall under three categories—migraine, tension-type, and cluster headache.

Migraine Headaches

Migraine headaches are severe headaches generally associated with systemic complaints. Migraine headaches are the most common type headache for which affected individuals seek medical care. The incidence of migraine is higher in women in comparison to men and tends to run in families. There are several migraine subtypes that fall under two categories—migraine with aura or migraine without aura (most common).

Migraines were once thought to be caused by vascular changes, predominantly vasodilation, but this theory has changed. Migraine is a result of a wave of self-propagating neuronal and glial depolarization that spreads across the cerebral cortex. This wave is termed *cortical spreading depression* of Leão. Cortical spreading depression causes the aura of migraine, activates the afferent trigeminal nerves, and activates and upregulates matrix metalloproteinases (protein enzymes that degrade tissue). The proteases alter the blood–brain barrier. The trigeminal nerve innervates several cerebral vessels and activation leads to inflammation around the meninges and the resulting headache. Trigeminal nerve stimulation also causes the release of several vasoactive peptides such as substance P, calcitonin gene-related peptide, and neurokinin A, which leads to vasodilation (mainly from calcitonin gene-related peptide release). Eventually, the neurogenic inflammation leads to neuronal sensitization. The neurons begin to become responsive to all types of stimuli—nociceptive and nonnociceptive. Serotonin receptors are activated; however, the role of serotonin in migraine pathogenesis is unclear. While it is well known that migraines are inherited, the genetic basis is probably attributable to multiple genetic variations, but genetic links to migraine development are largely unknown.

Clinical Manifestations

Most individuals affected with migraines (i.e., migraineurs) experience a prodrome (early symptom of an illness). Prodromal manifestations are often related to affective changes and can include irritability, euphoria, depression yawning, food cravings, and constipation. The prodrome can occur 1–2 days prior to the onset of the headache. After the prodrome, some migraineurs have an aura characterized by one or more focal neurologic symptoms. Generally, auras precede the migraine, but some auras occur with the migraine. The auras last about an hour and can be visual (e.g., small area of vision loss), sensory (e.g., tingling in a limb or side of the face), or language (e.g., wording struggles, dysphagia). Motor auras (e.g., weakness in a limb) are not common. Migraineurs can also have a migraine without an aura.

The sensitization that occurs with migraines is thought to account for the typical characterizations of migraine, which include a throbbing or pulsatile pain quality often accompanied by nausea and vomiting. Photophobia (sensitivity to light) and phonophobia (sensitivity to sounds) can occur. Some migraineurs develop skin sensitivity, and innocuous stimuli like hair brushing can trigger pain pathways. Typically, migraine headaches are unilateral and can spread throughout the head; however, they usually begin as bilateral in children with migraines. Untreated migraines can last for hours or days. Migraines have multiple triggers that can include emotional stress, hormonal changes in women (e.g., menstruation), sleep disturbances, odors, alcohol, and weather changes.

Diagnosis and Treatment

The diagnosis of a migraine is made based on a history and physical examination. Criteria for the diagnosis of migraine and other headaches have been developed and are updated by the International Headache Society. Diagnostic tests such as neuroimaging studies are not necessary for diagnosis but should be performed in the presence of certain findings (e.g., first or worse headache or abnormal neurologic physical examination). If necessary, neuroimaging studies can include a head CT or MRI.

Treatment strategies include two categories of pharmacotherapeutics, those for acute episodes and those to prevent episodes. Abortive (acute episodes) medications are used to manage acute symptoms and include NSAIDSs and acetaminophen; however, overuse of these medications can cause rebound headaches. Triptans (serotonin agonists) (e.g., sumatriptan, zolmitriptan) can be used alone or in combination

BOX 11-4 Application to Practice

A 45-year-old Hispanic female, Ms. Rodriguez, presents to the clinic complaining of sudden onset headache. She states this headache is different from her previous migraine headaches. The headache pain is described as a 10 on a scale of 0–10 with 10 being the worst pain. The pain is nonradiating, and she has mild photophobia. She did not get relief with sumatriptan (Imitrex), which previously provided relief for her migraines. She feels nauseous and states she vomited twice.

Physical examination findings are as follows:

Vital signs: Temperature 98.8° F; heart rate 88 beats per minute; respirations 20 breaths per minute; blood pressure 150/95 mmHg; oxygen saturation 100% on room air

General appearance: Alert, in mild discomfort due to pain

Head, eyes, ears, nose, and throat: normocephalic, atraumatic; pupils equal, round, reactive to light and accommodation; sclera nonicteric; extraocular movements intact; no nystagmus; optic disc margins are sharp with no evidence of papilledema or hemorrhaging noted.

Lungs: clear to auscultation bilaterally

Cardiac: Regular rate and rhythm; S1, S2 with no murmur

Abdomen: Soft, depressible, nontender, no organomegaly

Neuro: Cranial nerves II–XII intact; muscle strength 5/5; deep tendon reflexes 2+ and symmetrical throughout; no pronator drift; negative Romberg sign; coordination intact; gait steady

Questions

1. What is your differential diagnosis?
2. What are your risk factors for meningitis? Subarachnoid hemorrhage (SAH)?
3. What imaging would you like to do?
4. Discuss the difference between a headache that presents gradually as compared to a headache that presents suddenly?
5. What other history to you want to obtain from this patient?
6. What clinical findings would you anticipate with meningitis?
7. What clinical findings would you anticipate with SAH?

Contributor: Dana Sherman, DNP, ANP-BC, FNP-BC

---

with NSAIDs. Ergots can be used, but the side effects (e.g., nausea and vomiting), and risks (e.g., hypertension, ischemia complications) are higher than with other agents. Parenteral dexamethasone can prevent headache recurrence. Opioids and barbiturates are not as effective as other drugs and have addictive potential, so they should be used only when other therapies have failed. Preventive pharmacotherapeutic therapy can be used when headaches are frequent, long-lasting, or affect quality of life. Various preventive agents include beta blockers (e.g., metoprolol), antidepressants (particularly tricyclics such as amitriptyline), serotonin-norepinephrine reuptake inhibitors (e.g., venlafaxine), and anticonvulsants (e.g., topiramate, valproate, or gabapentin). The latest medication category for prevention is the calcitonin gene-related peptide antagonists that are monoclonal antibodies, and trials are in progress to evaluate their efficacy as abortive agents. Calcitonin gene-related peptide antagonists are thought to mediate trigeminal pain transmission and vascular inflammation. Various other preventive agents include herbal medications such as extract of butterbur root, which is a shrub. Other agents such as feverfew (herbal medication), magnesium, riboflavin (oral vitamin B_{12}),

Learning Points

Red Flags of Headaches

The following clinical situations indicate that a headache may be an ominous manifestation of an underlying disorder. These clinical situations include:

- Headaches described as the first or worst headache of the patient's life
- Changes in usual headache characteristics such as new or unexplained neurologic manifestations and change in the pattern, frequency, or severity
- Headaches that tend to remain on the same side
- Headaches that are nonresponsive to treatment
- Headaches that are new onset after the age of 50 or associated with meningeal signs (e.g., fever, stiff neck)
- Headache in those with cancer or HIV
- Physical neurologic findings (e.g., papilledema, abnormal reflexes, or motor dysfunction) or personality and cognitive changes

subcutaneous histamine, botulinum toxin, co-enzyme Q10, and melatonin may be effective; however, data is insufficient in confirming their efficacy in migraine prevention. Adequate sleep, regular aerobic exercise, biofeedback, relaxation techniques, transcutaneous electrical nerve stimulation, and acupuncture are treatment strategies that may be beneficial.

Tension-Type Headaches

Tension-type headaches (TTH) (i.e., stress headache), like migraines, are common and occur as a result of hypersensitivity of nerve fibers. TTHs may be episodic (infrequent and frequent), and chronic tension headaches can arise from the episodic headaches. TTHs are usually infrequent (headache less frequently than 1 day a month) episodic headaches. Migraines can occur with TTH and cause or aggravate a TTH. This type of headache is equally prevalent in men and women.

While stress and tension can trigger a TTH, the underlying mechanism in TTHs, particularly chronic type, is a result of central nervous hypersensitivity with the development of central sensitization. An episodic TTH is probably also the result of peripheral nervous system hypersensitivity and the development of peripheral sensitization. A TTH, particularly the episodic type, can result due to deficient inhibition of descending pain pathways. Muscle hypersensitivity may also play a role in TTHs, particularly in episodic TTHs. Genetic factors and vascular issues are not prevalent in TTHs as in migraines. See chapter 14 for details about sensory function.

Clinical Manifestations

TTH manifestations are generally mild to moderate, so most affected individuals do not seek medical care, but rather they self-treat (e.g., by taking acetaminophen). TTH pain is described as nonthrobbing. Affected individuals will describe their head as feeling dull, full, or like it has a tight cap or band around it. The headache is bilateral, and no symptoms are associated with a TTH like those with migraines (e.g., nausea or photophobia). Muscle tenderness in the head, neck, or shoulders often accompanies the headache. The neurologic examination is normal with a TTH. Triggers can include stress, tension, and migraines.

Diagnosis and Treatment

Diagnosis is made clinically based on the history and physical examination. Diagnostic testing is not necessary. Diagnostic criteria have been developed by the International Headache Society. Treatment strategies focus on symptom relief. Pharmacotherapeutic agents typically include NSAIDs, acetaminophen, or aspirin, and these agents can be combined with caffeine. Other pharmacotherapeutic agents can include intramuscular ketorolac, diphenhydramine, chlorpromazine, or metoclopramide. Ice packs may provide relief. Opioids and barbiturates should be avoided. Overuse of pharmacotherapeutic agents (e.g., NSAIDs) may cause headaches. Preventive measures include similar strategies as with migraines (e.g., adequate sleep, relaxation techniques). The benefit of preventive pharmacotherapeutic agents is not established; however, tricyclic antidepressants may be helpful.

Cluster Headaches

Cluster headaches are characterized by short bursts of unilateral orbital pain that can occur several times per day. The incidence is higher in men by four to one in comparison to women, and the headaches can start at any age. The overall prevalence is <1%. Smoking may be a risk factor for the development of a cluster headache.

The cause of the headaches is not well understood, but a leading theory is that the headaches are thought to occur due to activation of the hypothalamus and triggering of the trigeminal nerve (ophthalmic V1 division) autonomic reflex. For these reasons, cluster headaches are categorized as trigeminal autonomic cephalgias. Another theory is that there is inflammation of the walls of the cavernous sinus (the cavity near the sphenoid and the temporal bone), which injures sympathetic fibers that traverse in the sinus.

Clinical Manifestations

The two key features of cluster headaches are the trigeminal distribution of the pain and the unilateral and same-side autonomic features. The headaches are described as having a throbbing or stabbing quality that is severe. Along with the headache, lacrimation, rhinorrhea, nasal congestion, conjunctival redness, and eyelid edema can occur due to activation of the parasympathetic outflow portion of the facial nerve (cranial nerve VII). Ptosis (drooping of an upper eyelid) and miosis (pupillary constriction) occur due to a temporary blockage of the sympathetic outflow portion of the facial nerve. Sweating and increased blood flow to the headache side are other manifestations. While those with migraines prefer to stay still, those with cluster headaches tend to be very agitated and restless and will move around. During a single cluster attack, the headache and symptoms are all on one side, but during subsequent attacks the symptoms can switch to the other side. The headache can last for a few minutes to hours and the cluster attack can consist of up to eight headaches during one episode. These cluster attacks can occur daily for a few weeks (e.g., 6–12 weeks). Remissions can last longer than a year. The headaches are relapsing and remitting in nature, and the single attacks (i.e., clustering) are regular. This cyclical and regular pattern may be due to hypothalamic activation and possibly alteration in circadian patterns; however these associations are poorly understood. Chronic cluster headaches, which occur in 10–20% of patients, are defined as cluster headaches without significant periods of remission (i.e., 1 year without remission or remissions that last < 3 months).

Diagnosis and Treatment

The diagnosis of cluster headaches is made clinically based on a history and physical examination. Criteria for the diagnosis of cluster headaches as with other headache disorders have been developed and are updated by the International Headache Society. Diagnostic tests such as neuroimaging studies are not necessary for diagnosis but can be performed at initial diagnosis and should be performed in the presence of certain findings (e.g., first or worse headache or abnormal neurologic physical examination). If necessary, neuroimaging studies can include a CT or MRI of the brain.

Treatment strategies include those to abort the acute headache and those to prevent recurrent attacks. Oxygen and subcutaneous or intranasal triptans (intranasal agents are administered opposite the side of the headache) are used to abort the acute attack. Additional pharmacotherapeutic agents for an acute attack can include intranasal lidocaine (administered on the same side of the headache), oral ergotamine, or intravenous dihydroergotamine. Newer medications such as octreotide (mimic of somatostatin) are under investigation. Preventive therapy is initiated immediately during the commencement of a cluster as acute therapies will abort a single attack but not recurring ones. Preventive therapy consists of verapamil (a calcium channel blocker), glucocorticoids, and ergotamine. Chronic or refractory cluster headache management is complex, and additional medications may include topiramate, lithium, and other medications whose efficacy is limited (e.g., valproate). Nerve blocks (e.g., greater occipital) and neurostimulation techniques (e.g., vagus nerve stimulation) may be helpful.

Seizure Disorders

A seizure is a transient physical or behavioral alteration that results from abnormal electrical activity in the brain. Mechanisms that may be responsible for this abnormal electrical activity include altered membrane ion channels, altered extracellular electrolytes, and imbalances in excitatory and inhibitory neurotransmitters. Some neurons are hypersensitive or remain in a partial state of depolarization, increasing excitability. Seizures can be provoked or unprovoked. Any insult to the brain can provoke a seizure. Trauma, hypoglycemia, electrolyte disorders, acidosis, infection, tumors, cerebral hematomas, and chemical ingestion (e.g., medications, illicit drugs, and alcohol) can all provoke isolated seizure activity. Additionally, seizures can occur and be unprovoked and recurrent; this disorder is referred to as *epilepsy*. The definition of epilepsy has evolved over several years. As of 2014, epilepsy is defined as 1) at least two unprovoked (or reflex) seizures occurring more than 24 hours apart; or 2) one unprovoked (or reflex) seizure and the probability of further seizures (probability is defined as a risk similar to the general recurrence risk (at least 60%) after two unprovoked seizures, occurring over the next 10 years); or 3) diagnosis of an epilepsy syndrome (e.g., benign rolandic epilepsy) (ILAE, 2014).

According to the CDC (2016b), epilepsy affects approximately 2.9 million Americans. New-onset epilepsy incidence increases with aging, particularly in those over 65 years of age. Disorders such as stroke and Alzheimer disease can cause seizures and increase the risk for developing epilepsy. Older adults commonly have an underlying disorder when evaluated for their first seizure. Complications of seizures may include brain damage, TBIs, aspiration, mood disorders, and status epilepticus (seizures that last longer than 20 minutes or subsequent seizures that occur before the individual has fully regained consciousness).

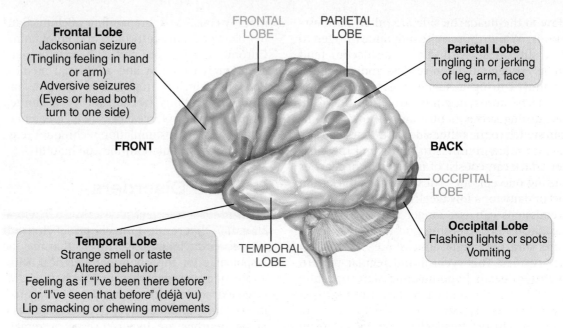

FRONTAL LOBE

PARIETAL LOBE

Frontal Lobe
Jacksonian seizure
(Tingling feeling in hand or arm)
Adversive seizures
(Eyes or head both turn to one side)

Parietal Lobe
Tingling in or jerking of leg, arm, face

FRONT

BACK

OCCIPITAL LOBE

Occipital Lobe
Flashing lights or spots
Vomiting

Temporal Lobe
Strange smell or taste
Altered behavior
Feeling as if "I've been there before" or "I've seen that before" (déjà vu)
Lip smacking or chewing movements

TEMPORAL LOBE

FIGURE 11-42 Manifestations of focal seizures depending on the region of the brain.

Benign Febrile Seizure

The most common type of seizure in children is febrile seizures that occur as a result of systemic viral or bacterial infection. These fevers are benign and self-limiting; however, CNS infection or inflammation and possible seizure triggers should be distinguished. These seizures usually occur between the ages of 6 months and 5 years. Most febrile seizures are generalized and simple (duration less than 15 minutes, do not recur in 24 hours). The seizure usually ends (usually within 2–3 minutes) by the time a caretaker seeks medical attention. The child usually has no residual effects of the seizure, and the child acts normally. Children with one febrile seizure are more likely to have recurrent febrile seizures. Antipyretics may help with reducing recurrence during the same illness, but they will not prevent recurrence in future febrile illness. Some febrile seizures are complex because they are prolonged (> 15 minutes) or have focal manifestations or postictal syndrome (paresis). Complex seizures can occur more than once in 24 hours. Children with complex febrile seizures may require longer observation and evaluation. Caregiver education is important in allaying concerns and should include how to handle any future seizures.

Clinical Manifestations

Seizures can be classified into two broad categories—focal and generalized. Focal seizures, also called *partial seizures*, occur in just one part of the brain. Approximately 60% of people with epilepsy have focal seizures. These seizures vary depending on the area of the brain affected, and they are frequently described by the area of the brain in which they

originate (**FIGURE 11-42**). In a simple focal seizure, the individual having the seizure remains conscious but experiences unusual feelings or sensations that can take many forms. The person may experience sudden and unexplainable feelings of joy, anger, sadness, or nausea. Additionally, he or she may hear, smell, taste, see, or feel things that are not real. In a complex focal seizure, the individual has changes in or loss of consciousness and memory, producing a dreamlike experience. People having a complex focal seizure may display strange, repetitious behaviors (e.g., blinking, twitching, moving one's mouth, walking in a circle) called *automatisms*. These seizures usually last just a few seconds. Some people with focal seizures, especially complex focal seizures, experience auras (unusual sensations just prior to an impending seizure). An aura is actually a simple focal seizure in which the person maintains consciousness. The symptoms an individual has and the progression of those symptoms tend to be similar with every seizure. Because the symptoms of focal seizures can easily be confused with other disorders (e.g., migraine headaches, narcolepsy, syncope, and psychiatric disorders), those disorders should be ruled out as part of the differential diagnosis. Focal seizures in older adults can be challenging to recognize because their symptoms are similar to those of delirium (e.g., confusion and sudden sleepiness), TIA, or syncope. Seizures in older adults can present as sudden falling with no recollection of the event or awakening from sleep confused or disoriented. Older adults also do not get an aura or have motor features (e.g., convulsions, lip smacking, or twitching).

Generalized seizures are a result of abnormal neuronal activity on both sides of the brain. They can include cortical and subcortical structures, but the whole cortex does not have to be involved. These seizures may cause loss of consciousness, falls, or massive muscle spasms. Many kinds of generalized seizures are possible. A person having an absence seizure (previously called a *petit mal seizure*) may appear to be staring into space and/or have jerking or twitching muscles (FIGURE 11-43). These seizures usually are brief, lasting less than 15 seconds. Tonic seizures cause stiffening of muscles of the body, generally those in the back and extremities. Clonic seizures cause repeated jerking movements of muscles on both sides of the body. Myoclonic seizures cause jerks or twitches of the upper body, arms, or legs (FIGURE 11-44). Atonic seizures ("drop attack") cause a loss of normal muscle tone, such that the affected person will fall down or may drop his or her head involuntarily. Tonic–clonic seizures (previously called *grand mal seizures*) cause a mixture of symptoms, including stiffening of the body and repeated jerks of the arms and/or legs and loss of consciousness (FIGURE 11-45). The individual having a generalized seizure may be confused, be fatigued, and fall into a deep sleep in the period following the seizure, referred to as the *postictal period*. Postictal paresis (i.e., Todd paralysis) includes focal neurologic deficits, such as hemiparesis, that can occur after a seizure.

Not all seizures can be easily defined as either focal or generalized. Some people have seizures that begin as focal seizures but then spread to the entire brain. Other people may have both types of seizures but with no clear pattern. Some seizures fall into an unknown type category.

Diagnosis and Treatment

A thorough history (including a description of the seizure activity if possible) and physical examination are critical in the diagnosis of seizure disorder even in comparison to diagnostic testing. The diagnostic tests often include an EEG, particularly for those individuals suspected of having epilepsy. Evaluation for an underlying cause can include a head CT, head MRI, and head PET. Metabolic disorders will be

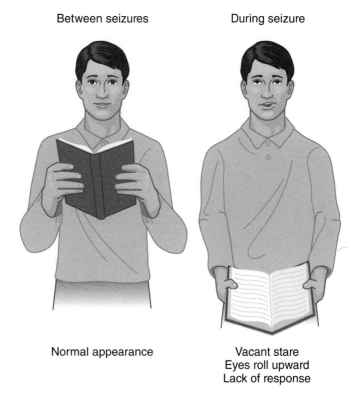

Between seizures   During seizure

Normal appearance

Vacant stare
Eyes roll upward
Lack of response

FIGURE 11-43 Absence seizures.

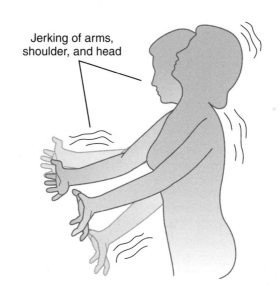

Jerking of arms, shoulder, and head

Episodes typically occur soon after awakening

FIGURE 11-44 Myoclonic seizures.

evaluated with serum analysis for electrolytes, blood urea nitrogen, creatinine, glucose, calcium, magnesium, and liver function tests.

Treatment focuses on preventing the occurrence and limiting the duration of the seizure activity. Seizure classification is important as it will guide the selection of antiseizure medications. There are over 20 classifications

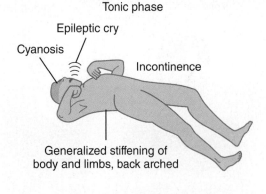

Tonic phase

Epileptic cry

Cyanosis

Incontinence

Generalized stiffening of body and limbs, back arched

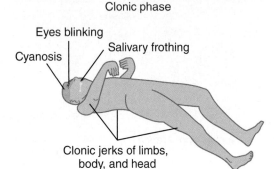

Clonic phase

Eyes blinking

Cyanosis

Salivary frothing

Clonic jerks of limbs, body, and head

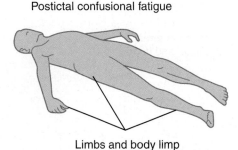

Postictal confusional fatigue

Limbs and body limp

FIGURE 11-45 Tonic–clonic seizures.

of seizures and epilepsy syndromes. Classification is usually determined by using the International League Against Epilepsy framework found at www.ilae.org. Treatment strategies can be grouped into two categories—those to manage acute seizures and those to prevent seizures. Most seizures resolve spontaneously within a few minutes, but employing safety precautions can prevent injury. During a seizure, positioning the individual on his or her side can prevent aspiration (vomiting is common). Additionally, the head should be protected. Items should not be forced in between the individual's teeth; doing so is more likely to cause harm than to help. Attempts should not be made to restrain the individual; this also is more likely to cause injury. Airway management and oxygen therapy may be necessary

to minimize hypoxia. If status epilepticus develops, medication (e.g., muscle relaxants or antiseizure agents) will often be administered intravenously to stop the seizure. Following a seizure, the individual should be allowed to sleep as desired.

For epilepsy, antiseizure agents will be administered daily to minimize the frequency and duration of seizure activity. These medications require close monitoring and accurate administration to ensure therapeutic dosing and limit side effects. Medication side effects are common reasons medications are discontinued. Seizure medications may have teratogenic effects, and folate use will reduce this risk. There are oral contraceptives that are inactivated by some seizure medications (e.g., enzyme-inducing antiseizure drugs). Women with epilepsy who are pregnant or want to become pregnant require close monitoring but generally have good outcomes. Psychiatric disorders, such as depression and anxiety, are more common in those with epilepsy than in the general population, and some antiseizure drugs are associated with increased suicide risks. Monitoring for mood changes is, therefore, important. If medications are not successful in controlling seizure activity, surgical resection or transection of the region in which the abnormal electrical activity originates might be necessary. Additionally, persons with seizure disorders should wear a medical alert bracelet and avoid precipitating factors (e.g., sleep deprivation, alcohol, illicit drugs, and excessive stimuli). Restricting driving may be necessary, which can greatly impact the quality of life for patients with epilepsy. Epilepsy is considered to be resolved for individuals who have remained seizure-free for the last 10 years, with no seizure medicines for the last 5 years.

Chronic Degenerative Disorders

Chronic degenerative disorders of the nervous system include those conditions in which neurologic function deteriorates over time. These conditions usually result in significant neurologic dysfunction that requires lifelong management. Such disorders are not usually preventable, and often treatment options are limited and not curative.

Multiple Sclerosis

Multiple sclerosis (MS) is a debilitating inflammatory, immune-mediated condition that involves a progressive and irreversible demyelination and axonal degeneration of the brain, spinal cord, and optic nerve. The prevalence rates are the highest among women, Whites, and persons living in temperate climates, and the incidence is higher if there is a family history of MS. MS is the most common disabling neurologic disease among young adults, often presenting in persons between 20 and 40 years of age. Some evidence suggests that smoking and obesity in childhood or adolescence increases risk, whereas increased sun exposure may decrease risk.

Genetic susceptibility to MS along with possible environmental factors (mostly unknown) are thought to lead to the development of MS. Variations of the major histocompatibility complex, particularly on the human leukocyte antigen (HLA) DRB1 locus, are associated with MS development. The HLA-DRB1 loci is involved in T cell activation and regulation. See chapter 2 for more on immunity.

A viral infection, possibly the Epstein-Barr virus, may be an environmental trigger, but many adults test positive for the virus and never develop MS. The cause of MS is mostly unknown and theoretic. MS leads to tissue injury through different mechanisms. A commonly accepted theory explaining demyelination is that MS begins as an inflammatory autoimmune disorder, and later injury occurs through mechanisms other than autoimmunity. Autoreactive lymphocytes mediate the destruction in MS with a predilection to affect the myelin sheath, but axonal and neuron destruction can also occur. The T cells are sensitized and reactive to proteins on myelin. The damage occurs in diffuse patches throughout the CNS and can affect the optic nerve and chiasm. The destruction can slow or stop nerve impulses. The damage affects mainly the white matter, and the lesions are called *plaques* because they are sharply delineated on imaging (**FIGURE 11-46**). Other immune involvement includes B cells, macrophages, immunoglobulins (IgG and IgM), and T helper cells; T regulatory cells are also present in MS lesions or in CSF. The immune system cells are thought to release various cytokines (e.g., tumor necrosis factor and interleukins). The blood–brain barrier is disrupted, oligodendrocytes and axons are destroyed, possibly through mechanisms other than inflammation. Oligodendrocytes that are not destroyed have few proliferative capacities and are ineffective in repairing the myelin. As the disease progresses, the brain's

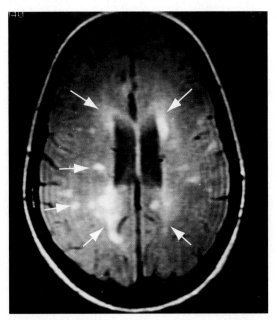

FIGURE 11-46 Multiple sclerosis demonstrated by MRI.
Courtesy of Leonard V. Crowley, MD, Century College.

cortex atrophies and scar tissue (plaques) develops throughout the white matter, resulting in chronic neurodegeneration. The pathophysiologic mechanisms and progression of this damage varies from person to person.

Clinical Manifestations

The course of MS is unpredictable. Some patients will have a mild course with little to no disability, whereas others will experience a steady deterioration with increasing disability. The disease, however, is typically characterized by remissions and exacerbations. Clinical manifestations of MS vary depending on the degree of damage and the specific nerves affected. Exacerbations may last for days to months. Fever, hot baths, sun exposure, and stress can trigger or worsen these episodes. Although remissions and exacerbations are common, the disease may continue to progress in some individuals without remissions. MS has a propensity to affect parts of the CNS, so certain clinical manifestations are often characteristic of MS. These characteristic manifestations and more common manifestations include:

- Sensory symptoms in limbs or face (e.g., numbness, tingling, tightness, coldness, and intense itching)
- Visual issues (e.g., vision loss, diplopia, nystagmus, abnormal gaze, abnormal eye movement including flutters and jerking)
- Motor spasticity (worse in the legs), weakness and coordination issues (e.g., gait

disturbance, difficulty with arm and hand coordination, intention tremors in limbs and the head, ataxia, balance problems, and vertigo)
- Bladder and bowel dysfunction (e.g., urgency, urinary and fecal incontinence, constipation, and stool leakage)
- Cognitive changes (e.g., decreased attention span, poor judgment, memory loss, difficulty reasoning and solving problems)
- Sleep issues as a result of symptoms (e.g., restless leg syndrome, nocturia, pain)
- Sexual dysfunction (e.g., decreased libido, erectile disorder, orgasmic dysfunction, and decreased genital sensation)
- Fatigue
- Brainstem symptoms (e.g., dysarthria, dysphagia, and respiratory issues such as poor cough)
- Pain (e.g., neuropathic extremity pain, back pain, and painful muscle spasms)

Some patients experience transverse myelitis, a condition caused by inflammation of the spinal cord that causes a loss of cord functioning that can last several hours to several weeks. Transverse myelitis usually begins as a sudden onset of lower back pain, muscle weakness, or paresthesia of the toes and feet and can rapidly progress to more severe symptoms, including paralysis. In most cases of transverse myelitis, people recover at least some function within the first 12 weeks after an attack begins. Transverse myelitis is also associated with neuromyelitis optica, a type of optic nerve inflammation. Some patients experience Lhermitte sign, which is a transient electric shocklike sensation that runs down the back and/or limbs upon flexion of the neck or head movement. Other complications of MS include epilepsy, paralysis (most often the legs), and depression.

Diagnosis and Treatment

There is no definitive test for MS, which can delay diagnosis of this condition. Diagnostic procedures for MS may consist of a history and physical examination (including a neurologic assessment), and MRIs of the brain with and without contrast are the best test to evaluate lesions. Additional testing may include a spine MRI, lumbar puncture with CSF analysis (this often shows high levels of protein, gamma globulin, and lymphocytes), nerve conduction studies, and autoimmune testing (e.g., erythrocyte sedimentation rate, antimyelin titers, and antinuclear antibody).

No cure for MS exists, but treatment can often slow its progression. Treatment strategies focus on minimizing symptoms and maximizing quality of life. These strategies include plasmapheresis (removal of abnormal antibodies from the blood) which is usually used for unresponsive exacerbations. Other strategies include medications such as corticosteroids (treat exacerbations), interferons (slow damage), disease-modifying agents, and immunomodulators (suppress immune response). Various components of the immune system are targeted with medications such as those that reduce the number of T cells in the periphery (e.g., siponimod), target B cells resulting in cytolysis (e.g., ocrelizumab), deplete B and T cells (e.g., cladribine), and prevent leukocyte mobilization to injured tissue (e.g., natalizumab). Other medications may be used to manage symptoms (e.g., antispasmodics, anticholinergics, laxatives, antiseizure, and antidepressants). Additionally, physical and occupational therapy, along with assistive devices (e.g., wheelchairs, walkers, and handrails), can maximize functioning. Coping strategies, support, proper nutrition, and adequate rest can promote and maintain overall health.

Parkinson Disease

Parkinson disease is a progressive condition involving loss of neurons in the substantia nigra and a depletion of the neurotransmitter dopamine in the brain. The lack of dopamine results in impairment in smooth, coordinated muscle movement. According to the NIH (2016d), approximately 50,000 Americans are diagnosed with Parkinson disease each year. Parkinson disease is the most common nervous system disorder of the elderly. The disorder occurs between the ages of 45 and 70 with a peak in the 60s. For unknown reasons, prevalence rates are twice as high in men as in women, and some evidence suggests that rates are higher in persons living in rural areas.

The basal ganglia, which is also known as the extrapyramidal system, is composed of a set of structures deep within the cerebrum that are involved in voluntary motor movement, posture, and cognitive and emotional functions. These structures include the substantia nigra, striatum, global pallidus, subthalamic nucleus, and thalamus. Various neurotransmitters mediate communication in this region. These include glutamate (excitatory), dopamine (generally excitatory, some inhibitory), GABA (inhibitory), and acetylcholine (excitatory or inhibitory). (See Table 11-1).

The cause of Parkinson disease is unknown, but in the presence of genetic vulnerability, sporadic alterations and activation by an environmental trigger (e.g., a virus) are probably associated with Parkinson disease development. These circumstances lead to a cascade of cellular level abnormalities such oxidative stress, mitochondrial dysfunction, excitotoxicity, and inflammation. The end result is neuronal depigmentation (due to loss of neuromelanin), neuronal loss, and glial cell abnormalities that can occur throughout various areas of the basal ganglia (e.g., globus pallidus and striatum), but the substantia nigra is the most commonly affected area. Norepinephrine-producing cells, which require dopamine as a precursor, may also be destroyed, explaining the issues with blood pressure regulation noted in Parkinson disease. Lewy bodies (unusual deposits of the alpha-synuclein protein) have been identified in the substantia nigra and other parts of the body (e.g., cerebral cortex and cardiac sympathetic plexus) in many cases, but their role in the disease is not yet understood. Lewy bodies are found in many other neurodegenerative disorders such as Alzheimer disease.

Clinical Manifestations

While Parkinson disease has been traditionally recognized as a motor system disorder, there is an increasing recognition of various neuropsychiatric and nonmotor manifestations. Clinical manifestations of Parkinson disease vary depending on the degree of dopamine deficit. When approximately 80% of the dopamine-producing cells are destroyed, movement issues develop. The key manifestations are tremor, rigidity, akinesia, and postural instability, which can remembered by the acronym TRAP (**FIGURE 11-47**). Tremor is the presenting symptom in almost 80% of patients with Parkinson disease and usually occurs in the limbs when they are at rest (i.e., resting tremor) and stops during purposeful movement. Finger–thumb rubbing (called *pill-rolling tremor*) may be present. Eventually, the tremor can be seen in the lips, tongue, and jaw, but rarely the head. The tremor may be worse when the affected individual is tired, excited, or stressed. Bradykinesia is a term that refers to a generalized slowness of movement and is often a cause of disability. Bradykinesia is described as difficulty with initiating or continuing movement (e.g., walking or getting out of a chair) and loss of dexterity (e.g., difficulty with buttoning clothes, tying shoelaces, and typing).

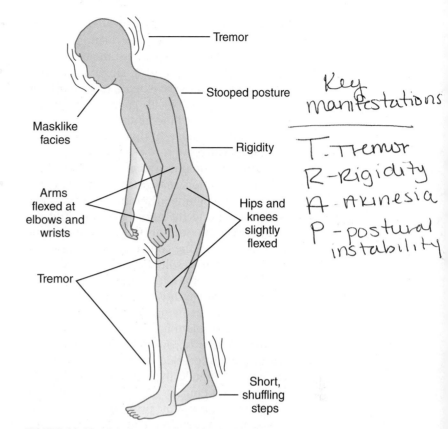

FIGURE 11-47 Clinical presentation of Parkinson disease.

Patients may have trouble standing from a sitting position. Eventually, the gait will freeze, and the affected individual will impulsively try to take quick and short steps (i.e. shuffling gait) in response. Resistance to passive movements characterizes the rigidity in Parkinson disease. Some patients will experience a specific type of rigidity termed *cogwheel rigidity* that occurs when an examiner moves a limb (e.g., an arm) through a range of motion, and there is a ratchet pattern of resistance and relaxation. A *ratchet pattern* is the term used as it is similar to a ratchet wrench, which hesitates before clicking forward into its next position. Rigidity results in stiffness and pain and contributes to the stooped posture and reduced arm swing when walking. Postural instability appears later in the disease course and is associated with an increased risk of falling and subsequent injury. If a person without Parkinson disease is pulled from behind at the shoulders, normal postural reflexes would maintain balance. With Parkinson disease, these reflexes are diminished and eventually are lost; the person who is pulled from behind will fall or take multiple steps backwards to try to maintain balance. Tremor, bradykinesia, and rigidity can at first be unilateral but later can become bilateral. Other manifestations of motor dysfunction include a masked facial expression, slowing, or stopping of automatic movements (e.g., blinking) and micrographia (small, cramped handwriting). Speech impediments include dysarthria, slowed, quieter speech (hypophonia), and a monotone voice.

Nonmotor manifestations are diverse and can include mood changes (e.g., anxiety and depression), cognitive dysfunction (e.g., decision making and memory retrieval), and dementia. The nonmotor manifestations tend to occur later in the course of the disease and can also be the result of medication side effects. Hallucinations (usually visual) can occur along with psychosis, often with delusions (e.g., of intruders living in the patient's house or a caregiver planning to hurt him or her). Hallucinations and psychoses can also be a result of medication side effects (e.g., dopamine agonists). Fatigue, hypersomnia during the day, and wakefulness at night are common complaints. Autonomic problems can result in orthostatic hypotension, constipation, dysphagia, excessive sweating, and sexual dysfunction (underactivity or hyperactivity, often due to Parkinson disease medication side effects). Pain is a common complaint and is described as burning, tingling, generalized, or localized (e.g., to the abdomen or joints). Vision changes, such as blurriness, can occur, and the skin can become oily (seborrhea).

Diagnosis and Treatment

Much like MS, Parkinson disease does not have a definitive test available for its diagnosis. Diagnostic procedures consist of a history, physical examination (including neurologic assessment), and other tests to rule out other conditions. There is no cure for Parkinson disease; instead, the goal of treatment is to control symptoms. Pharmacotherapeutic agents include levodopa, dopamine agonists (e.g., bromocriptine, pramipexole, and ropinirole), monoamine oxidase B (MAO-B) inhibitors (e.g., selegiline), and amantadine. The medications can increase the levels of dopamine via different mechanisms. The medications can be given as monotherapy or at times in combination. MAO-B inhibitors and amantadine are generally well tolerated and are often used for those patients with milder symptoms and when there is minimal impact of the disease on quality of life. Levodopa and

dopamine agonists can be used at any time during the disease, but they have an increased risk of side effects. Levodopa and dopamine are often given when symptoms are moderate to severe and affect quality of life. Levodopa is the most potent of anti-Parkinson medications. The therapeutic effects of levodopa use often diminish over time (termed *wearing off*), requiring increased doses to maintain effectiveness. Chronic levodopa use also results in motor fluctuations with patients improving for a period of time and then experiencing periods of worsening symptoms. Medications may eventually reach maximum dosing, and symptom control will be lost. Anticholinergics can control tremors, but risk of adverse events increases, especially in the elderly. Deep brain stimulation is a common surgical treatment for Parkinson disease. Additionally, physical and occupational therapy, along with assistive devices (e.g., wheelchairs, walkers, and handrails), can maximize functioning. Coping strategies, support, proper nutrition, and adequate rest can promote and maintain overall health. Caregiver burden is high in those caring for someone with Parkinson disease as with other chronic neurodegenerative disorders.

Amyotrophic Lateral Sclerosis

Amyotrophic lateral sclerosis (ALS)—also called *Lou Gehrig disease* after the famous baseball player who died from this condition—is a disease that involves damage to the motor neurons of the cerebral cortex and motor neurons of the brainstem and spinal cord. The exact number of cases in the United States is unknown, but in 2016, the NIH (2016a) estimated that 14,000-15,000 Americans had ALS. The only risk factors seem to be increasing age, as the condition usually begins around age 45, and a family history of the disorder. Smoking is being investigated as a possible risk factor. Men are affected at twice the rate of women. Although this condition is not necessarily common, it is a public concern because there is no way to prevent the continuous and rapid decline in motor function. In 2010, a national ALS registry was launched to collect, manage, and analyze data about people with ALS. This registry is intended to provide information that will illuminate the scope and epidemiology of the problem as well as guide practice and research.

ALS results in degeneration of cortical motor cells. Subsequently, loss of axons and abnormal glial cells (e.g., astrocytes and oligodendrocytes) affect the corticospinal tract and the abnormal glial cells (e.g., those with hypertrophic changes) replace the lost neurons. The spinal cord becomes atrophic, and large myelinated motor nerves degenerate. Neurotransmitter receptors (e.g., for acetylcholine) are consequently lost with the nerve degeneration. The innervated muscles atrophy. While most cases of ALS affect motor neurons, there are cases of ALS with dementia with neuronal loss in portions of the frontal and temporal lobe (i.e., frontotemporal dementia). Most cases of ALS are sporadic, while familial forms occur in about 10% of cases. Researchers are exploring several possible etiologies of ALS. The first possible cause is free radical damage. The inherited form of ALS often involves a mutation in a gene, superoxide dismutase 1, responsible for producing a strong antioxidant enzyme that protects cells from damage caused by free radicals. The second possible cause being explored is glutamate's influence. People who have ALS typically have higher than normal levels of glutamate, a neurotransmitter, in their CSF. Too much glutamate is toxic to some nerve cells. Finally, autoimmune responses are being studied as a possible trigger for ALS.

Clinical Manifestations

Clinical manifestations of ALS become progressively worse as more motor neurons are damaged. The manifestations may affect the limbs, the central or axial structures (head and trunk), and bulbar nerves located on medulla oblongata (cranial nerves IX, X, XI, XII). Sensory neurons and cranial nerve III are not affected. Cranial nerve III controls pupil constriction, lid elevation and eye muscle movements, which are also controlled by cranial nerves IV and VI (eye muscle movement only). Cognitive function may remain intact; however, frontotemporal dementia can be associated with ALS. The loss of upper motor neurons results in spastic paralysis and hyperreflexia (this reflects frontal lobe motor neuron damage), and the loss of lower motor neurons results in flaccid paralysis. Early manifestations of ALS include the following symptoms:

- Footdrop (difficulty lifting the front of the foot and toes; usually the first lower limb sign)
- Lower-extremity weakness

- Hand weakness or clumsiness (first sign in about 80% of cases)
- Muscle cramps and twitching in the upper extremities and the tongue
- Slurred speech (dysarthria) or dysphagia (both known as bulbar symptoms)

The disease frequently begins in the upper or lower extremities. The limb weakness is initially asymmetric but progressively spreads to other parts of the body. As it advances, muscles become progressively weaker until they are paralyzed. ALS eventually affects chewing, swallowing, speaking, and breathing. It causes death usually in 3 to 5 years of onset of symptoms.

Diagnosis and Treatment

As is true for the other degenerative neurologic disorders, there is no definitive test for ALS. Instead, diagnostic procedures are often used to rule out other conditions. Diagnosis is based on a history and physical examination (including a neurologic assessment). Diagnostic tests include electromyogram (in which an electrode is inserted into the muscles to measure electrical activity), nerve conduction studies, MRI studies (head and spinal cord), lumbar puncture with CSF analysis, and muscle biopsy.

ALS has no cure. Treatment strategies focus on slowing the progression and controlling symptoms, but options are limited. Riluzole (Rilutek), a benzothiazole, is a disease-modifying treatment used to slow ALS progression. This drug appears to slow the disease's progression in some people, perhaps by reducing levels of glutamate. Edaravone is a free radical scavenger and peroxynitrite (a strong oxidizing ion that causes tissue damage) scavenger that prevents oxidative damage, which also slows ALS progression. Additionally, stem cell therapy is being explored as a possible treatment. Antispasmodic agents may be given to treat muscle spasms. Physical, occupational, and speech therapy, along with assistive devices (e.g., wheelchairs and braces), can maximize muscle function. Because of risk for aspiration and dysphagia, nutritional support, including high-caloric foods, soft or pureed foods, thickened liquids, and parenteral feedings become critical to maintaining optimal health as the patient's muscles weaken. Respiratory management (e.g., oxygen therapy, pulmonary hygiene, respiratory treatments, noninvasive positive pressure ventilation, and mechanical ventilation) also becomes necessary as muscle weakness progresses. Palliative care can improve quality of life and should be discussed at diagnosis. Coping strategies and support for the patient and caregivers can be helpful as the condition worsens.

Myasthenia Gravis

Myasthenia gravis is an autoimmune condition in which acetylcholine receptors are impaired or destroyed by immunoglobulin G (IgG) autoantibodies. This acetylcholine receptor compromise leads to a disruption of normal communication between the nerve and the muscle at the neuromuscular junction. Myasthenia gravis is uncommon and affects all gender, ethnic, and age groups equally.

The exact trigger for the autoimmune response is unclear, but the thymus gland is thought to play a role. Persons with myasthenia gravis often have a thymus gland abnormality (e.g., hyperplasia and tumors). The autoantibodies against acetylcholine receptors (AChR) may come from the thymus gland as they are found in clusters in the thymus germinal center. AChRs, in most cases, are destroyed by IgG; however, a different type of IgG (IgG4) antibody destroys muscle-specific kinase (MuSK) receptors. The MuSK receptor is in the postsynaptic neuromuscular junction. Some affected individuals have autoantibodies directed at both receptors (AChR and MuSK receptors). A few people are seronegative for both autoantibodies but have the disorder with the same features. T cells are also involved in the immunologic attack and are thought to stimulate B cell antibody production.

Clinical Manifestations

Myasthenia gravis results in weakness of the voluntary skeletal muscles because of inadequate nerve stimulation. The weakness generally affects the ocular, limb, bulbar, and respiratory muscles. Muscle weakness and muscle fatigue fluctuates but typically worsens during periods of activity and improves after periods of rest. As the disease progresses, the muscle symptoms become continuous. Fatigue without muscle weakness is not consistent with myasthenia. The full extent of the disease is usually experienced within 3 years.

Certain muscle manifestations occur more commonly than others. Ocular dysfunction is seen in many patients. One type of myasthenia gravis (i.e., ocular myasthenia) affects only eyelid and extraocular eye muscles, resulting in ptosis, diplopia, difficulty maintaining gaze, and blurred vision, but the pupils are unaffected. Ocular symptoms can also occur with generalized myasthenia. Muscles that control chewing, talking, and swallowing (bulbar muscles) are often, but not always, involved in the disorder; if affected, the condition can result in dysarthria, dysphagia, chewing fatigue, and voice quality changes (e.g., hoarseness or hypophonia). Muscles that control facial expression can be affected and make the affected individual look expressionless (e.g., loss of smile, sneering expression). Muscles that control the neck may result in a drooping head. Limb weakness involves the arms more than the legs. Limb involvement is mostly proximal, but it can also affect the distal muscles. Respiratory muscle involvement may result in difficulty breathing and respiratory insufficiency.

Certain factors can worsen myasthenia gravis and cause a myasthenic crisis, including fatigue, illness, stress, extreme heat, alcohol consumption, and certain medications (e.g., beta blockers, calcium channel blockers, quinine, and some antibiotics). Myasthenic crisis is a potentially life-threatening complication that occurs when the muscles become too weak to maintain adequate ventilation.

Diagnosis and Treatment

Diagnosis of myasthenia gravis is primarily made based on the clinical presentation. Diagnostic procedures consist of a history and a physical examination (including a neurologic assessment). Serum testing for antibodies, particularly AChR antibodies and MuSK receptor antibodies, generally confirms the diagnosis. Several other antibodies can be evaluated (e.g., antistriated muscle antibodies). Nerve conduction studies and electromyograms are other diagnostic tests. A CT or MRI of the mediastinum is performed to evaluate the thymus. Screening is done for other autoimmune disorders of the thyroid and for rheumatoid disorders and systemic lupus erythematosus, which can coexist with myasthenia gravis.

There is no cure for myasthenia gravis, but treatment strategies can be employed to manage its symptoms. Medications used to treat this disorder include anticholinesterase agents (e.g., pyridostigmine), which improve neuromuscular transmission and increase muscle strength. Immunosuppressive drugs (e.g., glucocorticoids) may improve muscle strength by suppressing the production of abnormal antibodies. Other therapies include thymectomy, plasmapheresis, and high doses of immunoglobulins. Additional self-care strategies to maximize health and functioning include proper nutrition, adequate rest, assistive devices, coping strategies, and support. Since medications can precipitate life-threatening myasthenia crisis, education is necessary to avoid these drugs. Administration of anesthesia for any type of surgery or even the surgery alone poses a risk for myasthenic crisis. Patients with myasthenia gravis are resistant or sensitive to anesthetic drugs, particularly neuromuscular blocking agents (e.g., succinylcholine, vecuronium), so sedatives, hypnotics, and anesthetic medications should be very short acting. Close monitoring for potential myasthenic crisis is warranted.

Huntington Disease

Huntington disease (HD), or Huntington chorea, is a condition caused by a genetically programmed degeneration of neurons in the brain. According to the NIH (2016b), more than 15,000 Americans have HD. At least 150,000 others have a 50% risk of developing the disease, and thousands more of their family members live with the possibility of developing HD.

HD is an autosomal dominant disorder involving a defect on chromosome 4 in the *HTT* gene (i.e., *HD* gene). This defect causes a segment of DNA, called a *cytosine-adenine-guanine* repeat, to occur many more times than usual. Normally, this section of DNA is repeated 10–35 times within the DNA coding sequence, but it is repeated 36–120 times in persons with HD. This defect leads to progressive atrophy of the brain, particularly in the basal ganglia and the frontal cortex (**FIGURE 11-48**). The ventricles (brain) dilate, GABA levels diminish, and acetylcholine levels fall. As the gene is transmitted

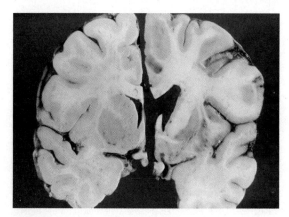

FIGURE 11-48 Neurologic changes of Huntington disease.
© Biophoto Associates/Science Source.

from one generation to the next, the number of repeats (called *cytosine-adenine-guanine repeat expansion*) tends to increase. With a larger number of repeats, the chance of developing symptoms at an earlier age increases. As the disease is transmitted in families, it becomes evident at younger and younger ages. The earlier HD symptoms appear, the faster the disease progresses. Most cases of HD appear in persons between 30 and 40 years of age, but HD may appear in childhood or adolescence in a small number of cases. In general, the duration of the illness ranges from 10 to 30 years. The most common causes of death for persons with HD are infection (most often pneumonia), injuries related to a fall, or other complications (e.g., suicide).

Clinical Manifestations

Clinical manifestations of HD consist of choreiform movements, psychiatric problems, and dementia. The manifestations are a reflection of the cerebral atrophy caused by neural degeneration. Initially, manifestations are insidious and vary from person to person. Family members may first notice that the individual experiences mood swings or becomes uncharacteristically irritable, apathetic, passive, depressed, or angry. Other behavioral symptoms may include antisocial behavior, hallucinations, paranoia, and psychosis. These symptoms may lessen as the disease progresses or, in some individuals, may persist and expand to include aggression or severe depression. HD may produce dementia as the individual's judgment, memory, and other cognitive functions become affected. Early signs often include having trouble driving, learning new things, remembering facts, answering questions, or making decisions. Some people may even display changes in handwriting. As the disease progresses, concentration on intellectual tasks becomes increasingly difficult.

In some people, the disease may initially manifest with uncontrolled, rapid, jerky movements (chorea, Greek for *dance*)—for example, tremors, grimaces, and twitching—in the fingers, feet, face, or trunk. These movements often intensify when the person is anxious. HD can also begin with mild clumsiness, unsteady gait, and rigidity. Some people develop chorea manifestations later, after the disease has progressed. Chorea often creates serious problems with ambulation, increasing the likelihood of falls. As the disease progresses, speech becomes slurred, and other functions (e.g., swallowing, eating, speaking, and walking) continue to decline. Many people with HD remain aware of their environment and are able to express emotions, but some cannot recognize their family members. Children with juvenile-onset HD often have minimal or no chorea, but they often have a rapid, progressive disease.

Diagnosis and Treatment

Because of its psychological manifestations, HD is often mistaken for various psychiatric disorders. Diagnostic procedures for this disease include a history, physical examination, psychiatric evaluation, genetic testing for the defective gene (either before or after the onset of symptoms), head CT, head MRI, and head PET.

There is no cure for HD, and no treatment to stop its progression. Treatment strategies focus on slowing the progression and managing symptoms to maximize functioning. Tetrabenazine (Xenazine) is the first medication specifically approved by the Food and Drug Administration for the treatment of HD signs and symptoms. This agent reduces the jerky, involuntary movements associated with HD by increasing the amount of dopamine available in the brain. Tranquilizers and antipsychotic agents can control movements, violent outbursts, and hallucinations. Antidepressant agents can control depression and the obsessive–compulsive rituals that some people with HD develop. Some evidence suggests that coenzyme Q10 may also slow the course of the disease. Physical, occupational, and speech therapy can maximize function. Coping strategies, support, adequate hydration, proper nutrition, and regular exercise for both the patient and caregivers can support optimal health. New therapies are currently under investigation, including stem cell therapy, new medications, and new combinations of existing medications.

Dementia

Dementia refers to a group of conditions in which cortical function is decreased, impairing cognitive skills (e.g., language, logical thinking, judgment, and learning) and motor coordination. Issues with memory are common with dementia and include short-term memory losses as well as confusion of historical events. Behavioral and personality changes may interfere with relationships, work, and activities of daily living. Vascular risk factors (e.g., atherosclerosis, diabetes, hypertension, hypercholesteremia, and obesity), infections, toxins (e.g., smoking), and genetic conditions may cause dementia.

Several types of dementia have been identified, each of which has only limited treatment options. Although great strides have been made in recent years, most types of dementia remain poorly understood.

Learning Points

Delirium

Delirium is an acute state of confusion that is characterized by a disturbance of consciousness and altered cognition. Manifestations often include hypervigilance, hyperactivity with agitation, tremulousness, and hallucinations. The state of confusion represents a change from an individual's usual baseline, develops over a short period of time (e.g., hours to days), and the onset can be gradual or sudden. The manifestations tend to fluctuate throughout the day. The most common causes are medical conditions such as electrolyte imbalance, dehydration, infections, or liver failure. Substance intoxication and withdrawal (e.g., alcohol, narcotics) and medication side effects—particularly psychoactive drugs—can cause delirium. The pathogenesis of delirium is poorly understood, and because there are so many conditions that can cause delirium there are probably many mechanisms involved in development. Delirium often occurs in hospital settings, particularly critical care units. The elderly have a higher risk for the development of delirium.

Alzheimer Disease

Alzheimer disease (AD) is the most common form of dementia among older adults. In AD, healthy brain tissue degenerates and atrophies (**FIGURE 11-49**). This atrophy causes a steady decline in memory and mental abilities. According to the CDC (2015a), as many as 5 million

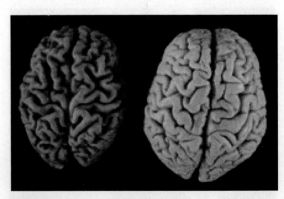

FIGURE 11-49 Alzheimer disease (left) compared to a normal brain (right).
Courtesy of Michael Hart.

Americans have AD; this prevalence is double the prevalence in 1980. AD has recently surpassed diabetes mellitus as the sixth leading cause of death among U.S. adults. Notably, mortality rates for AD are on the rise—unlike heart disease and cancer death rates, which continue to decline. Although AD is not a part of normal aging, risk for developing this disease does increase with age (onset usually occurs after 60 years of age). While uncommon, there are cases of early-onset AD (symptoms before the age of 65); some of these cases occur without family history, and less than 1% are inherited. The mode of transmission usually follows an autosomal dominant inheritance pattern. Prevalence rates are higher in women, in part because of their longer life expectancy relative to men. Some evidence suggests that AD rates are higher in those persons with less education, but the precise reason for this association remains unknown. Some researchers theorize that the more the brain is used, the more synapses are created, which provides a greater reserve with aging. Additional risk factors include family history, hypertension, hypercholesterolemia, diabetes mellitus, obesity, and history of TBI.

The exact etiology of AD is unknown, but a common feature is the overproduction and/or decreased clearance of *beta amyloid peptides*. Three pathologic characteristics are associated with AD. First, amyloid plaques, which contain fragments of a protein called beta-amyloid peptide, mix with a collection of additional proteins, neuron remnants, and other nerve cell pieces. Second, neurofibrillary tangles, found inside neurons, form as abnormal collections of a protein called *tau*. Normal tau is required for neuron microtubule (part of a bundle of neurofilaments) health; however, in AD, tau clumps together. As a result, neurons fail to function normally and eventually die. Third, connections among the neurons responsible for memory and learning are lost. Neurons cannot survive when their connections to other neurons are lost. Pathologic tau is shared between neurons, neurons die throughout the brain, and the affected regions begin to atrophy, or shrink. By the final stage of AD, damage is widespread and brain tissue has shrunk significantly. In inherited forms, early onset AD forms mutations that have been located on three genes—amyloid precursor protein (*APP*), presenilin 1 (*PSEN1*), and presenilin 2 (*PSEN2*). Genetic mutations for late-onset AD are varied and not well established, but an apolipoprotein E epsilon 4 (APOE4) mutation does confer a genetic risk factor.

Clinical Manifestations

The onset of AD tends to be insidious. Clinical manifestations commonly start with mild memory loss and confusion, but AD eventually leads to irreversible mental impairment that destroys a person's ability to remember, reason, learn, and imagine. This course may extend 10–20 years. To develop memories, an individual must record, retain, and retrieve information. Memory impairment in AD often follows a specific pattern. Memory can be divided into two broad categories—explicit and implicit. Each category includes various subtypes that are associated with various brain structures. The subtypes of memory include:

- Explicit memory (i.e., declarative memory) is for factual knowledge and involves awareness and consciousness. It is dependent on the hippocampus and parts of the temporal lobe and parts of the cortex for retention.
  1. Semantic memory refers to memories of facts (e.g., words, rules, and language)
  2. Episodic memory refers to memories of events (e.g., experiences and personal history that occur at a specific time and place)
- Implicit memory (i.e., nondeclarative memory) does not involve consciousness, and the hippocampus is not required for retention; however, it requires an intact amygdala, cerebellum, striatum, parts of the cortex, and reflex pathways.
  1. Procedural memory refers to memory of skills and habits that become unconscious and automatic once learned.
  2. Priming and perceptual learning involves the facilitation of recognition of a word or object as a result of activation of particular representations or associations (e.g., if the color blue is seen, one may think of sky, because blue and sky are related).
  3. Associative learning (relates to classical and operant conditioning) involves learning the relationship between one stimulus and another and having an emotive and motor response.
  4. Nonassociative learning refers to habituation and sensitization.

Memory, particularly explicit type, can be short term or long term. Working memory is sometimes categorized as a type of short-term memory and reflects attention and ability to concentrate; the information is usually kept for a short period of time while a reaction is planned. Memory can be long term (i.e., remote) where storage can last for years. Short-term memory can be easily disrupted (e.g., by drugs or trauma) in contrast to long-term memory, which is less easily disrupted.

All types of memory impairments eventually occur with AD. Initially, working and recent memory are often affected (e.g., inability to remember things a few minutes after they occur), which progresses to loss of other types of memory. Other individuals may report that the person affected with AD may repeat things, forget conversations or appointments, misplace things, and forget the names of family members and everyday objects. Procedural memory (e.g., how to brush teeth) is usually the last type of memory to be lost.

Problem solving, judgment, and executive functioning impairment can initially be subtle or very noticeable. These impairments will present as problems with abstract thinking (e.g., trouble balancing a checkbook, a problem that progresses to trouble recognizing and dealing with numbers); difficulty finding the right word to express thoughts or even follow conversations; difficulty reading and writing; disorientation, even in familiar surroundings; loss of judgment (e.g., not knowing what to do if food on the stove is burning); and difficulty performing familiar tasks (e.g., driving, cooking, bathing, eating, or dressing). Bowel and bladder incontinence can occur. Behavioral and personality changes can occur at any stage but are more common as AD progresses. These changes can include mood swings, paranoia, stubbornness, withdrawal, depression, anxiety, and aggression. Psychosis can occur, manifesting as hallucinations or delusions. Complications such as infections (primarily pneumonia and urinary tract infections), injuries related to falls, malnutrition, dehydration, and pressure injuries contribute to the mortality associated with AD.

Diagnosis and Treatment

Diagnosis of AD is often difficult and involves ruling out other conditions. Diagnostic procedures consist of a history and physical examination (including a neurologic assessment and mental status evaluation). Diagnostic clinical criteria have been developed by the National Institute on Aging and the Alzheimer's Association and can be found at www.nia.nih.gov/health/alzheimers-disease-diagnostic-guidelines. Neuroimaging can consist of a brain MRI and brain PET. While cortical changes can be seen with AD (e.g., cortical atrophy and white matter lesions), neuroimaging is usually performed to evaluate for other possible causes of dementia. Genetic testing is usually completed in individuals affected with early onset AD. Biomarkers to support the diagnosis of AD are under investigation.

There is no cure for AD, nor are there any therapies that will slow its progression. Medications can, however, manage symptoms and maximize functioning. Cholinesterase inhibitors (e.g., donepezil [Aricept], rivastigmine [Exelon], and galantamine [Razadyne]) can improve neurotransmitter levels in the brain in some cases. Memantine (Namenda) is specifically approved to treat AD. It blocks NMDA acid receptors, which are glutamate receptors. Memantine may be given in combination with a cholinesterase inhibitor. Other medications may be given to control aggression. Alternative therapies that may improve symptoms include vitamin B_6, vitamin B_{12}, vitamin E, ginkgo, and huperzine A, although the research evidence is mixed regarding their efficacy. Other strategies include memory aids (e.g., calendars), nutritional support, physical exercise, cognitive activities, safety precautions (e.g., supervision and removing clutter), maintaining a calm environment, and social interactions (e.g., adult day care). Coping strategies and support for both the patient and the caregiver can decrease stress and anxiety.

Vascular Dementia

Vascular dementia (i.e., vascular cognitive impairment) is the second leading cause of dementia after AD. Vascular dementia is a progressive syndrome that occurs as a result of any disorder that impairs cerebral blood flow. The incidence of vascular dementia is difficult to estimate because it often coexists with dementia due to other disorders such as AD. Vascular dementia without other causes of dementia (i.e., pure vascular dementia) accounts for 10% of all dementia cases. Disorders associated with development of vascular dementia include cerebrovascular diseases (e.g., stroke, intracranial hemorrhage) and cardiovascular disorders (e.g., embolization from the heart). A common cause and finding in vascular dementia is cerebral small-vessel disease (a cause of lacunar stroke) that occurs as a result of arteriolosclerosis or beta-amyloid deposition in small arteries. The major risk factors are the same as those for stroke, such as hypertension, diabetes, and smoking. Vascular dementia incidence has been decreasing due to improvements in prevention of risk factors and management of causative factors.

Because vascular dementia can occur after a stroke, the manifestations will be the same as the stroke. Cognition may have been relatively normal prior to a stroke, so onset of dementia after a stroke points to the vascular dementia etiology. Cognitive decline poststroke occurs in a stepwise manner, and memory may be less affected than in AD at times. A wide variation in clinical manifestations is seen as the stroke can affect any number of brain structures including those that regulate memory. Vascular dementia can occur without a stroke, and manifestations can be similar to AD. Diagnostic testing is similar to those tests used in stroke or AD (e.g., brain MRI). Treatment centers on treating the underlying vascular causes and risk factors (e.g., stroke or hypertension); however, these strategies will not improve dementia symptoms. AD can often coexist with vascular dementia, making it difficult to distinguish between the two, so medications used for AD are often used even though their effects on vascular dementia are inconclusive.

Dementia With Lewy Bodies

Dementia with Lewy bodies, which are made of the proteins ubiquitin and synuclein, is a common cause of dementia—the incidence is only superseded by AD and vascular dementia. The effects of the Lewy bodies are diffuse and affect the cortical neurons. Dementia with Lewy bodies (DLB) can affect up to 5% of the population. Risk factors, as with other dementias, include aging.

The pathogenesis of DLB is still unclear, but there seems to be structural changes and dysfunction of alpha-synuclein (a key component of Lewy bodies). This protein is found throughout all of brain tissue, and while its function is unclear, it is thought to be involved in neurotransmitter release. While not necessarily a key feature, neurofibrillary tangles and amyloid plaques (common to AD) can be present. The dysfunctional alpha-synuclein protein and Lewy bodies affect dopamine and cholinergic neurons resulting in similar manifestations to Parkinson disease. While mostly considered a sporadic disorder, various genetic mutations leading to sporadic or familial disease are being investigated. Some of these mutations are similar to those in AD such as amyloid precursor protein (*APP*), presenilin 1 (*PSEN1*), and presenilin 2 (*PSEN2*).

Clinical Manifestations

An essential manifestation in DLB is progressive dementia, which is often the presenting symptom. In contrast to AD, memory loss initially is not the most prominent feature, but rather attention and executive and visuospatial functioning are impaired early on. These characteristics can manifest as difficulty driving (e.g., getting lost, failing to see stop signs) and difficulty with job performance. In addition to dementia, other key features include cognitive fluctuations and changes in level of alertness which can manifest in varied ways, some subtle and others overt. A patient may develop an inability to perform an activity of daily living, may appear confused, or may behave in a bizarre manner. Somnolence or daytime napping for prolonged periods can occur. Visual hallucinations are another key feature, and when present aids in distinguishing DLB from AD as hallucinations do not usually occur in AD. The hallucination can include seeing people, animals, shapes, or colors. Sleep disorders involving rapid eye movement are a common feature and can manifest as dreaming and acting out the dream during sleep or as motor movements during sleep. For example, if the person is dreaming of danger, he or she may try to protect himself or herself, and motor movements could include punching or kicking. Parkinsonism features (e.g., bradykinesia, limb rigidity, gait disorder) are common in those with DLB. Other symptoms can include frequent falling, syncopal episodes, delusions, depression, and autonomic symptoms (e.g., orthostatic hypotension, urinary incontinence or retention, or constipation).

Diagnosis and Treatment

The diagnosis is made based on a history and physical examination. Clinical criteria that include key features (e.g., dementia, visual hallucinations, parkinsonism) have been developed and are used in diagnosing DLB. Diagnostic tests are similar to others used for dementia and are often done to exclude other possible explanations of the symptoms. Treatment strategies are focused on managing symptoms. Nonpharmacologic therapies are the same as for those with other types of dementia (e.g., memory aids, exercise, physical therapy, adult day care). Pharmacologic agents for DLB, which are also used in AD and Parkinson disease, can include such agents as cholinesterase inhibitors, memantine, and levodopa, although their efficacy in DLB is limited. Up to 50% of patients with DLB have an increased risk for severe sensitivity to first-generation antipsychotics (e.g., haloperidol), but sensitivity can also occur with second-generation antipsychotics. Therefore, use of antipsychotic agents (e.g., quetiapine) should be avoided. The severe neuroleptic sensitivity reaction will manifest as worsening of symptoms such as parkinsonism and confusion. Melatonin may be useful for sleep disorders.

Frontotemporal Dementia

Frontotemporal dementia (FTD) (formerly known as Pick disease) is a spectrum of disorders that leads to focal degeneration of the frontal and/or temporal lobes. FTD is a common cause of early-onset dementia (< 65 years of age), like early-onset AD. The pathogenesis is unknown. The disorder is inherited in many cases, but the pattern of inheritance is often unclear. Several disorders can lead to the development of FTD, but the most common ones are those associated with the tau protein or the TDP-43 protein. These two proteins, for unknown reasons, have an affinity for the frontal and temporal lobes. Neurons and myelin are lost and the lobes atrophy.

Clinical Manifestations

Clinical manifestations occur in three different forms and include behavioral-variant FTD (most common) and two forms of primary progressive aphasia (PPA), which includes nonfluent and semantic variant types. Key findings with behavioral variant FTD are progressive changes in personality and behavior. The affected individual may be disinhibited (e.g., subject to impulsivity and disregard for social norms), apathetic, unempathic, hyperoral (e.g., the patient might engage in lip smacking, excessive chewing, and food craving). In PPA with nonfluent type there are motor speech deficits (expressive language deficits), which can be manifested as hesitant speaking, ungrammatical speaking, difficulty articulating, and word searching. Patients with semantic variant PPA have difficulty understanding words or formulating a sentence (putting words together). Motor neuron disorder can occur before or after development of FTD. Motor neuron disorder is more likely to be associated with behavioral variant FTD and is not typically present in PPA. FTD with motor neuron disorder manifests as symptoms similar to ALS. The motor manifestations will be similar to those with ALS (e.g., muscle wasting). In addition to ALS, those with behavioral variant FTD can develop two other motor neuron disorders—

corticobasal syndrome and progressive supranuclear palsy. With corticobasal syndrome, limbs become stiff, and movements are uncoordinated, while progressive supranuclear palsy causes a stiff, erect posture, bradykinesia, rigidity, and difficulty with gaze.

Diagnosis and Treatment

Diagnostic testing will include neuropsychologic testing and neuroimaging studies similar to those for other forms of dementia (e.g., PET scan and brain MRI). Genetic testing may be performed to evaluate for familial FTD. As with many other forms of dementia, there is no cure, and treatment strategies are aimed at managing symptoms. Nonpharmacologic treatment can include regular exercise; supervised care; and speech, occupational, and physical therapy. Behavior modification techniques can include distraction and redirection. Caregiver support is important. Pharmacologic management is complex as many medications used in other forms of dementia are either ineffective or can cause adverse effects such as paradoxical worsening of behavior or motor symptoms. Affected individuals with FTD are more susceptible to adverse effects of medication.

Creutzfeldt-Jakob Disease

Creutzfeldt-Jakob disease (CJD) is a rare but rapidly progressive form of dementia caused by an infectious prion. A prion is an abnormal protein particle that causes proteins to fold abnormally, especially in nervous tissue. The prion renders the protein dysfunctional, creating plaques and vacuoles (empty spaces) (FIGURE 11-50).

CJD may be classified into two types (classic and variant) and three main categories (sporadic, hereditary, and acquired). Classic CJD accounts for 90% of the five recognized types. Although also caused by a prion, classic CJD is not related to bovine spongiform encephalopathy (commonly known as mad cow disease). However, the new variant is related to bovine spongiform encephalopathy. The most common form of classic CJD occurs sporadically, caused by the spontaneous transformation of normal prion proteins into abnormal prions. This sporadic disease occurs worldwide, including in the United States, at an annual rate of approximately 1 case per 1 million people (CDC, 2015b). Hereditary CJD is rare and occurs when the abnormal protein is inherited. Finally, acquired CJD is rare (accounting for fewer than 1% of cases worldwide) and occurs when the individual is exposed to infected

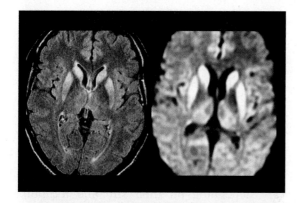

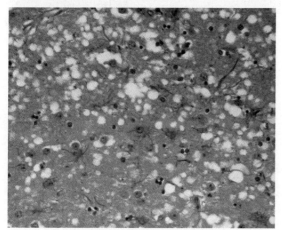

FIGURE 11-50 Creutzfeldt-Jakob disease.

A: © BSIP/Science Source; B: Courtesy of Dr. Al Jenny/CDC.

materials (e.g., via tissue transplants and ingestion). The prion is resistant to common methods of sterilization and disinfection.

Clinical Manifestations

CJD has a long incubation period (up to 40 years) after being introduced into the brain; however, it is rapidly progressing and always fatal (usually within 1 year of onset). The rapidly progressive course of CJD, along with myoclonus and gait issues, distinguish this disorder from other causes of dementia. Clinical manifestations develop rapidly and include the following symptoms: ataxia, lack of coordination, muscle twitching, myoclonic jerks or seizures, and spasticity. Visual changes (e.g., blurred vision) and speech impairment can occur. Neuropsychiatric manifestations can include personality changes, profound confusion or disorientation, anxiety, lethargy, and hallucinations.

Diagnosis and Treatment

Diagnostic procedures for CJD consist of a history, physical examination (including a neurologic assessment and mental status evaluation), EEG, head MRI, and other tests (e.g., lumbar puncture and serum tests) to rule out other forms of dementia. There is no known cure for CJD, although interleukins and other immunomodulator agents may slow the progression of the disease. Custodial care (nonmedical care that assists with activities of daily living) may be required early in the course of the disease. Medications may be needed to control aggressive behaviors, spasticity, pain, and seizure activity. Providing a safe environment, controlling aggressive or agitated behavior, and meeting physiologic needs may require monitoring and assistance in the home or in an institutionalized setting. Family counseling may help in coping with the changes required for home care.

AIDS Dementia Complex

Dementia is common in later stages of AIDS, a condition that is referred to as *AIDS dementia complex*, or HIV-associated encephalopathy. When HIV invades the brain tissue, its effects may be exacerbated by the other infections and tumors that are frequently associated with AIDS. Clinical manifestations include encephalitis, behavioral changes, and a gradual decline in cognitive function (e.g., trouble with concentration, memory, and attention). Persons with AIDS dementia complex also show progressive slowing of motor function with a loss of dexterity and coordination. In children with congenital HIV infection, the brain is often affected, causing mental retardation and delayed motor development. See chapter 2 for further discussion of immunity.

A staging system is used to describe the condition's progression. The staging system ranges from 0 (normal) to 4 (nearly vegetative).

Diagnostic procedures for AIDS dementia complex consist of a history, physical examination (including a neurologic assessment and mental status evaluation), head CT, head MRI, and biopsy. When left untreated, AIDS dementia complex can be fatal. Aggressive antiretroviral therapy is the cornerstone of treatment.

Cancers of the Nervous System

Nervous system malignancies can originate in the brain or spinal cord, or they may spread there from other sites. Regardless of the etiology, these cancers can result in significant neurologic dysfunction and death. Typical cancer diagnosis, staging, and treatments are usually utilized in such cases (see chapter 1 for more on cellular function).

Brain Tumors

Brain tumors, whether malignant or benign, can be life threatening because they often increase ICP and are difficult to access (**FIGURE 11-51**). Approximately one third of brain tumors are malignant. Brain tumors also account for only 2% of neoplasms, but they disproportionately contribute to a high rate of cancer morbidity and mortality (CBTRUS, 2018). Malignant brain tumors are the most common cancer in children and the most common cause of cancer death. In adolescents and young adults, malignant brain tumors are the third most common cancer. Brain tumors may be primary, but most are secondary tumors. Any cancer can spread to the brain, but the types that most commonly do so include breast cancer, lung cancer, and melanoma. Other cancers that less frequently cause brain metastasis include colon cancer, kidney cancer, and sarcoma. Primary tumors are thought to arise from genetic mutations. The risk for such mutations increases with age and exposure to ionizing radiation and occupational chemicals. In the United States, prevalence and mortality rates of brain tumors are highest among Whites and males (National Cancer Institute, 2016). Complications of brain tumors include neurologic deficits, seizures, personality changes, and death. The 5-year survival rate for brain tumors is nearly 34%.

The most common types of primary brain tumors in adults are glial tumors. These tumors are so named due to histologic features that are similar to glial cells (e.g., astrocytomas and glioblastomas) and meningiomas. Glial cells are tumors of the neuroepithelial tissue, and meningiomas are tumors of the meninges. Astrocytomas have varying degrees of malignancy. Grade I and II tumors tend to be benign or slow growing and are usually well differentiated,

while grade III and IV tumors (e.g., glioblastomas and grade IV astrocytomas) are malignant and poorly differentiated. Meningiomas are usually benign, but some are malignant. Pituitary tumors, lymphoma of the CNS, and craniopharyngiomas are less common types of primary brain tumors. In children, the most common types are astrocytomas, medulloblastomas (rapidly growing malignant tumors), and gliomas.

Clinical manifestations of brain tumors vary depending on their size and location. These manifestations reflect the local invasion of the tumor, compression of structures, decreased cerebral blood flow, and increased ICP associated with such tumors:

- Headaches—new onset or change in pattern of headaches or headaches that gradually become more frequent and more severe. Headaches that worsen with position changes or that are worse at night and awaken the affected individual
- Unexplained nausea or vomiting
- Seizures
- Changes in level of consciousness
- Neurocognitive dysfunction—mood, personality, or memory changes
- Weakness
- Cortical sensory loss—inability to recognize "writing" on the hand by touch only (i.e., graphesthesia) and inability to recognize an object by touch (i.e., stereognosis)
- Aphasia
- Vision problems (e.g., blurred vision, diplopia, or loss of peripheral vision)
- Ataxia and gait disturbances
- Developmental delays (in children)

Diagnostic procedures consist of a history, physical examination (including a neurologic assessment) and brain MRI with contrast. If a tumor was found on CT or other imaging studies, an MRI should still be done. Biopsy and other tests will be done to determine cancer histology. Treatment of brain tumors depends on the size and location of the originating cancer, if any. If possible, surgical removal of the tumor is recommended. Additional treatment options include radiation (external and radiosurgery), chemotherapy (e.g., temozolomide [Temodar]), and targeted drug therapy (e.g., bevacizumab [Avastin]). Regardless of the strategy, rehabilitation will be necessary to minimize residual neurologic dysfunction. Rehabilitation will likely require physical, occupational, and speech therapy.

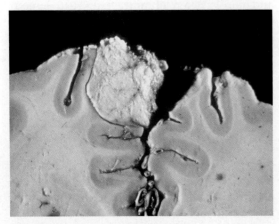

FIGURE 11-51 Brain tumor.

Mental Health Disorders

Mental health disorders encompass a wide range of problems that are generally characterized by abnormal thoughts, perceptions, emotions, behavior, and relationships with others. Symptoms vary greatly among the various disorders. The severity of mental health disorders can vary from mild and self-limiting issues to severe, chronic, and debilitating issues. Mental health disorders can negatively impact physical health, in addition to social well-being. Suicide can be one of the devastating consequences of a mental health disorder. The burden and incidence of mental health disorders is increasing in the United States and worldwide (NIMH, 2017; WHO, 2017). Nearly one in five adults (46.6 million in 2017–18.9% of all U.S. adults) live with mental illness, and less than half receive treatment (42.6%). Of those individuals, approximately 11.2 million (4.5% of all U.S. adults) have a serious mental illness. Approximately 49.5% of adolescents (age 13–18) have a lifetime prevalence of mental illness with 22.2% categorized as having severe impairment (NIMH, 2017). Those individuals with serious mental illness have impairment that significantly interferes or limits major life activities (e.g., working and relationships) and causes significant disabilities in comparison to those with milder or moderate illness severity. While mental illness affects all ages, the highest prevalence is in young adults (age 18–25), and then prevalence decreases. Women have a higher prevalence (22.3%) overall in comparison to men (15.1%). Prevalence is also higher in Whites and adults who report two or more races.

Many classifications of mental disorders have been defined by the American Psychological Association in the fifth edition of the *Diagnostic and Statistical Manual of Mental Disorders (DSM-5)* (APA, 2013). This manual is the common source used by clinicians to diagnose mental health disorders. The classification and diagnosis of mental disorders can be complex as definitions must be considered in relation to cultural, social, and familial norms and values. In other words, what is normal in one culture may be considered abnormal in other cultures. Understanding mental health in the context of culture is critical to avoid misdiagnosis. Cultural norms will also influence the level of social and societal acceptance and support a patient will receive.

Understanding of the development of mental health disorders is complex and multifactorial. While the existence of mental health disorders has been recognized as far back as 1844, understanding the pathogenesis has centered on theories that posit that mental disorders develop due to environmental and psychosocial problems. While this approach still holds true, it was only until the advent of advanced neuroimaging techniques (around the 1970s) that the biologic and physiologic basis of mental disorders was elucidated. Epidemiologic studies and breakthroughs in the association between genetics, epigenetics, and development of disease have also significantly contributed to understanding the pathophysiology of mental health disorders. Despite these advances, neurobiologic causal associations continue to remain challenging and complex to identify because many mental disorders often coexist (e.g., depression, anxiety, and substance abuse). Additionally, there continue to be challenges in determining whether neurobiologic and neurochemical alterations have caused the disorder, are a consequence of the disorder, are a combination of both, or neither. However, the scientific advances, particularly understanding of neurotransmitters, have led to identification and increasing use of effective and better tolerated pharmacotherapeutic agents for treating mental health disorders.

Over 100 mental health disorders are classified. This section of the chapter will discuss some of the more serious disorders (e.g., schizophrenia) and disorders that most clinicians will encounter (e.g., anxiety and depressive disorders). The neurobiologic basis of the disorders will be emphasized. Comprehending common neurochemical alterations (e.g., neurotransmitters) and abnormalities in brain structure and function in mental health disorders is also important in understanding disease development and symptomatology.

Depressive Disorders

Depressive disorders are categorized as mood disorders and have common features that include a sad, empty, or irritable mood. The concept of mood refers to a sustained feeling that is experienced internally and prevails for a time. The feelings in depressive disorders are accompanied by cognitive changes and somatic manifestations. An individual's mood can shift regularly, and this shift is considered normal. With depressive disorders, the sadness, emptiness, or irritability are persistent and affect the ability to function. Depression is one of the most common mental disorders in the United States and the world, and it is one of the main causes of disability worldwide (WHO, 2018). The incidence of a major depressive episode occurred in 7.1% of all U.S. adults while the rate was 13.3% for all U.S. adolescents (age 12–17) (NIMH, 2017). Many of these episodes, whether in adults or adolescents, resulted in severe impairment. The incidence of major depression declines with aging; however, depression is more common in older adults with a high burden of medical illness whether from acute or chronic medical conditions. Older adults living in assisted living or skilled nursing facilities or those who receive home care also have a higher incidence of depression. Women are more commonly affected in comparison to men. The incidence of major depressive episode is highest in adults age 18–25, in Whites, and adults who report one or more races. Other risks include a family history of depression.

The development of depression is complex and multifactorial. The recognition of a genetic basis in depression development is based on studies in monozygotic twins where concordance rates has varied between 38 and 62%. Concordance is used in twin studies and refers to the probability that both of the twins will both have a characteristic if one individual has the characteristic. The presence of depression in a first-degree relative increases the risk for its development by 2–4 times that of the general population. The heritability is higher for women than men and is more likely to be related to early age onset of depression (e.g., 18 years). Alterations in chromosomes 3 and 10 have been associated with five mental health disorders—major depressive disorder (MDD), bipolar disorder, schizophrenia, autism spectrum disorders, and attention-deficit/hyperactivity disorder. One of the polymorphisms is on the locus involved in calcium channel development (e.g., CACNB2). Calcium is important in neuronal signaling, growth, and development. Most genetic studies, however, have not produced strong associations or replicable findings that identify specific genetic mutations related to depression development. Epigenetic factors change gene expression (e.g., turning them on or off without alteration of the nucleotide base sequence) and are thought to contribute to depression development. The triggers that cause these epigenetic changes can be environmental, such as recurrent stress or traumatic life experiences. See chapter 1 for more on cellular function.

Alterations in the neuroendocrine system are associated with major depressive disorders. Hypothalamic-pituitary-adrenal axis hyperactivity is associated with depression. Stress triggers a response by the cortex and the amygdala, which then sends a signal to the hypothalamus. The hypothalamic response to this signal is the production of corticotropin-releasing hormone, which stimulates the release of adrenocorticotropin hormone (i.e., corticotropin hormone) from the anterior pituitary. The adrenal cortex is stimulated by corticotropin, resulting in the secretion of glucocorticoid (i.e., cortisol). Chronic stress will cause an overproduction of corticotropin-releasing hormone and results in hypercortisolemia. Prolonged hypercortisolemia can suppress neuron formation (i.e., neurogenesis) and glia cells and can result in atrophy of the hippocampus and amygdala. Stress may also lead to a deficit in the growth factor brain-derived neurotrophic factor, which is noted in depression. Brain-derived neurotrophic factor is involved in neuron growth, maturation, and survival, so deficits may lead to a reduction in neurons and hippocampal size. Stress can also result in activation of the immune system. Chronic inflammation may also contribute to depression development as C-reactive protein and cytokine (e.g., interleukin 6, tumor necrosis factor) levels can be higher in those with depression. The reason for this association is unclear.

Abnormal functioning of neurotransmitters is associated with depression. These associations were made when depressed individuals improved with the administration of antidepressants that modulated neurotransmitters (e.g., serotonin reuptake inhibitors). Reduction of neurotransmitter levels is also associated with depression. The monoamine hypothesis of depression postulates that decreased monoamine levels, particularly norepinephrine and serotonin (i.e., 5 hydroxytryptamine [5-HT]), cause depression (see **TABLE 11-4**). The raphe-serotonin system (the raphe nucleus is the location of serotonin synthesis) and the locus coeruleus–norepinephrine system (locus coeruleus is the location of norepinephrine cells) are both dysfunctional with depression (see FIGURE 11-52). Reduction in 5-HT serotonin receptors and serotonin transporter binding may be decreased in depressed individuals. Diminished tryptophan levels have been noted to cause depression relapses. Tryptophan, a serotonin precursor, is an essential amino acid and only comes from dietary sources (e.g., poultry

TABLE 11-4	Neurotransmitters and Neurocognitive Effects

Neurotransmitters/receptors	Synthesis	Neurocognitive effects
Monoamine neurotransmitters*		
Serotonin 7 serotonin receptors (5-HT$_1$–5-HT$_7$)	Synthesized from the essential amino acid tryptophan	Mood, memory processing, anxiety, sleep, cognition
Norepinephrine 2 receptors (alpha and beta)	Metabolized from dopamine	Sleep–wake cycle, mood, attention, vigilance, orientation to stimuli (e.g., aversive or novel)
Dopamine 5 receptors (D$_1$–D$_5$)	Synthesized from the amino acid tyrosine	Emotional response; capacity to feel pleasure and pain
Amino Acid Neurotransmitters		
GABA 2 receptors (A and B)	Synthesized from amino acid glutamate	Major inhibitor of neuron transmission; increasing GABA results in relaxation, antianxiety, anticonvulsant effects
Glutamate 3 receptors (NMDA, α-amino-3-hydroxy-5-methyl-4-isoxazolepropionic acid, and kainate)	Synthesized from the amino acid α ketoglutarate	Mainly excitatory Learning and memory
Acetylcholine Neurotransmitter		
Acetylcholine (muscarinic and nicotinic)	Synthesized from acetyl-Co-A and choline	Learning and memory

Text by Tusaie and Fitzpatrick, 2017. Table adapted from the American Psychiatric Association (APA). 2010. *Practice guidelines for the treatment of patients with major depressive disorder* (3rd ed). Washington, DC: Author.

* are derived from amino acids, but decarboxylase removes the acid component, leaving the structure as one amine (i.e., monoamine).

and eggs). Reduced dopamine transmission, another monoamine neurotransmitter, is also associated with depression. Low levels of the neurotransmitter GABA and decreases or increases in glutamate levels are also implicated in the development of depression. The NMDA receptor is activated by glutamate. NMDA receptors are altered by various psychoactive substances such as alcohol, dextromethorphan, and phencyclidine. Ketamine is an NMDA antagonist, and some studies have described its antidepressant effects. Studies on the long-term safety and efficacy of ketamine as a pharmacotherapeutic for depression are still necessary. Pharmacotherapeutic agents generally target neurotransmitters (see Table 11-6).

Other theories of depression pathogenesis include the neural network model. Communication between different regions of the brain (e.g., prefrontal cortex and amygdala) involved in autonomic, behavioral, and endocrine components of emotions is impaired in depressive episodes (see **FIGURE 11-53**). Brain functioning may be altered in different areas (e.g., overactivity or diminished activation) in various regions such as the cingulate cortex, thalamus, prefrontal cortex, or temporal lobe. Some studies have found that normal pruning (selective elimination of gray matter) during adolescence is accelerated, causing increased cortical gray matter volume loss in those with depression. The pruning also leads to decreased neural connections. Anatomic changes in addition to the smaller hippocampus noted in some patients with depression include smaller frontal lobes, particularly in the anterior cingulate and prefrontal cortex. Telomeres (nucleotide sequences at the ends of chromosomes) normally change with aging and become shorter. In some studies, abnormally short telomeres were noted in depressed patients, reflecting premature cellular aging.

Clinical Manifestations

Major depressive disorder (MDD) (i.e., unipolar depressive disorder or clinical depression) is the most common form of depression. The onset of MDD generally increases with puberty with a peak in the 20s. MDD can result in periods of remission where there are no symptoms. These periods of remission can even last for years with occasional episodes, but complete

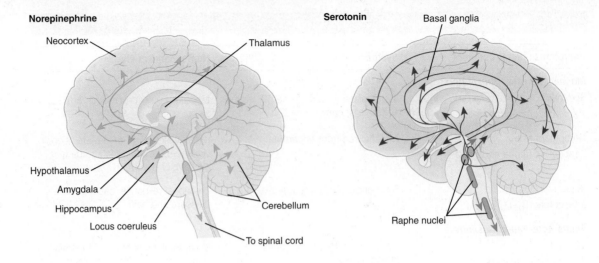

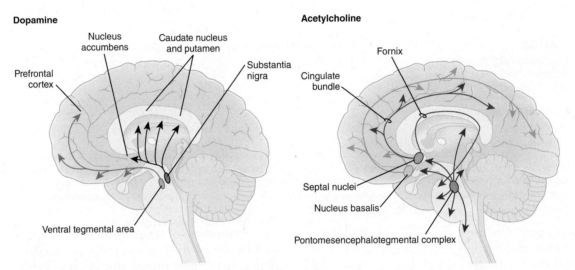

FIGURE 11-52 Systems of central neuromodulators.

Republished with permission of McGraw-Hill Education from Barrett et.al, Ganong's Review of Medical Physiology, 25e, 2015; permission conveyed through Copyright Clearance Center, Inc.

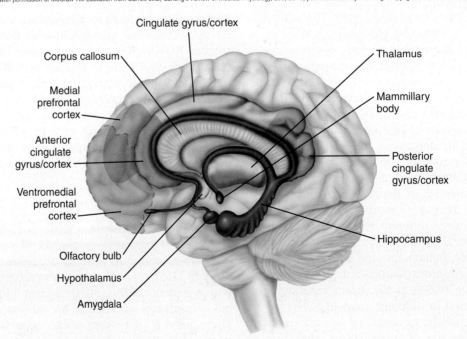

FIGURE 11-53 Major limbic structures.

TABLE 11-5	Age-Related Differences in Presentation of Depression			

Children	Adolescents	Adults	Older adults
Irritability	Behavior problems	Low self-esteem	Motor agitation
Temper tantrums	Poor hygiene	Work/interpersonal problems	Impaired cognition
Somatic (headache, stomachache)	Anhedonia	Insomnia	Delusions
Withdrawn	Hopelessness	Weight changes	Anxiety/panic
Insomnia	Suicidal ideation/actions	Suicidality	Pain
	Excessive sleep	Decreased libido	Chronic medical comorbidities
	Substance misuse	Substance misuse	

Adapted from the American Psychiatric Association (2010).

symptom resolution is not common. The clinical manifestations include:

- Depressed mood (feeling sad, empty, and/or hopeless)
- Loss of interest or pleasure in all or almost all activities (i.e., anhedonia)
- Significant weight loss (unintentional) or weight gain
- Insomnia or hypersomnia
- Psychomotor agitation (e.g., restlessness) or retardation (slowing down)
- Fatigue or loss of energy
- Feelings of worthlessness or excessive guilt
- Diminished ability to concentrate or indecisiveness
- Recent thoughts of death or suicide

Clinical manifestations of MDD can vary based on age (see **TABLE 11-5**).

For the diagnosis of MDD, five or more manifestations must be present within the same 2-week period. One of the five or more manifestations must be either a depressed mood or a loss of interest or pleasure. In other words, MDD is not the appropriate diagnosis if there is a suspicion of MDD and the patient has symptoms such as insomnia, fatigue, or feelings of worthlessness but denies having a depressed mood or a loss of interest. In MDD, the symptoms are present most of the day or nearly every day and cause impairment in functioning (e.g., work and relationships). Psychosis can occur with severe MDD, although the incidence is uncommon. The psychosis can include delusions and hallucinations.

In addition to MDD, other types of depressive disorders include **persistent depressive disorder** (i.e., dysthymia or chronic unipolar major depression). Persistent depressive disorder manifestations are similar to those of MDD, although they are not as numerous, and the

Learning Points

Grief Versus Depression

Individuals will lose a significant other at some point in their life and experience grief. Individuals who are grieving experience a sense of emptiness or loss. With time, the intensity of these feelings tend to decrease and are often experienced in cycles or waves. These waves of grief, often called *pangs of grief*, are usually triggered while reminiscing about the deceased. Those individuals who are grieving can have interspersed moments of positive feelings. The feelings and thoughts in grief tend to be centered around the deceased, and feelings such as guilt or worthlessness tend to be connected to the deceased (e.g., not expressing love enough or spending enough time with them). Thoughts of death while grieving are centered on wanting to reunite or join the deceased. These characteristics of grief are in contrast to depression during which the depressed mood and anhedonia are persistent, and positive emotions are not generally felt. A sense of pervasive unhappiness is also present with depression. The depressed mood is not associated with specific thoughts or worries. Self-esteem is usually normal with grief, while it is not with MDD. Those patients with MDD often self-loath and feel worthless about general things. Thoughts of death in MDD are related to the decreased self-esteem and inability to cope with MDD.

symptoms must be present most of the day or for most days for at least 2 years (for children or adolescents the time frame is 1 year). MDD episodes can precede or occur with persistent depressive disorder. **Premenstrual dysphoric disorder** is another type of depressive disorder, and symptoms must be present in the week before the onset of menses and have an impact on work and social functioning. Premenstrual dysphoric disorder symptoms also improve after menses and become minimal to absent. Manifestations of this disorder include significant mood lability, irritability, depressed mood, and anxiety. As with other forms of depression, physical and behavioral symptoms may be present. Depression may be due to secondary (i.e., underlying) factors such as in substance- or medication-induced depressive disorder. Many substances (e.g., cocaine, alcohol, and hallucinogens) and medications (e.g., amphetamines, antihypertensives, and systemic glucocorticoids) can cause depressive symptoms. The symptoms with substance use usually begin with the use of the substance and persist after the known physiologic effects of the drug have worn off. Depressive disorder due to another medical condition is another type of secondary depressive disorder. A wide range of medical conditions (e.g., systemic lupus erythematosus, obstructive sleep apnea, stroke, and multiple sclerosis) are associated with depression. The depressive symptom onset due to other medical conditions usually occurs shortly after the onset of the disease. Depressive disorders are not usually associated with manic and hypomanic symptoms.

In summary, many manifestations are similar in the different types of depressive disorders. The differences are mainly in timing issues (i.e., when episodes occur or duration) and underlying causes. Other mental health disorders can coexist with depressive disorders such as anxiety disorders, substance abuse disorders, or personality disorders (e.g., antisocial or borderline).

Diagnosis and Treatment

Diagnosis of depressive disorders is based on a history and physical examination (usually normal), using the *DSM-5* criteria. Despite advances in the understanding of neurobiologic changes in depressive disorders, diagnostic markers (e.g., imaging studies or laboratory tests) are not available. Diagnostic tests (e.g., thyroid function studies, a substance abuse toxicology screen, and a brain MRI) are done to evaluate for possible underlying disorders.

Treatment strategies include psychotherapy (e.g., cognitive behavioral therapy, interpersonal psychotherapy, and psychodynamic therapy). Various classes of pharmacotherapeutic agents are available (see **TABLE 11-6**). The most effective strategy for depression treatment includes a combination of psychotherapy and pharmacotherapy. Selective serotonin reuptake inhibitors are the most common initial drug therapy. Typically, tricyclic antidepressants and monoamine oxidase inhibitors have more adverse effects than other classes. While symptoms may improve after starting a medication (within 2 weeks), adequate relief is not usually achieved until about 6 weeks. Herbal supplements such as St. John's wort have been used in depression, but there are a variety of medication interactions such as those with serotonin reuptake inhibitor that can be potentially dangerous (e.g., serotonin levels can be become dangerously increased). Valerian has been used for a variety of mental health disorders, including depression, and while it is generally safe, its efficacy is uncertain. Other therapies include relaxation (e.g., imagery) and engagement in positive activities such as exercise, sleep hygiene, and following a healthy diet. Hospitalization may be necessary for safety and stabilization for those who are unable to care for themselves or are having suicidal ideation. Brain stimulation techniques are usually used in those patients with severe major depression. These techniques activate brain regions. Electroconvulsive therapy (ECT) involves the application of brief electrical brain stimulation with a goal of producing a generalized cerebral seizure that lasts about 15–70 seconds. General anesthesia is administered for the procedure. ECT is generally reserved for those with severe major depression. The procedure usually takes about 10 minutes, and the patient can resume activities after an hour. There is a stigma associated with use of ECT mainly due to misinformation and outdated perceptions of how the procedure is performed. Other brain-stimulating techniques include transcranial magnetic stimulation and vagus nerve stimulation. In the former, rapid alternating magnetic fields stimulate areas of the brain but do not induce a seizure; in the latter, an implantable device intermittently stimulates the vagus nerve.

Learning Points

Pharmacogenomics

Individual genetic testing can be performed to determine whether a medication will be effective, to provide guidance regarding dosing, and to identify potentially harmful medications. The study of how genetics impacts medications is known as pharmacogenomics. Genetic testing is increasingly being used in prescribing psychiatric medications, particularly for antidepressants. Other medication classes that can be tested include some benzodiazepines (e.g., clonazepam and alprazolam) and antipsychotics (e.g., quetiapine and risperidone).

Bipolar Disorders

Bipolar disorders (i.e., manic-depressive disorder), like depressive disorders, are categorized as mood disorders, and common features include episodes of mania, hypomania, and

TABLE 11-6 Antidepressant Classes and Mechanism of Action

Classification	Mechanism of action	Generic examples*
Selective serotonin reuptake inhibitors	Selectively inhibit neuronal uptake of serotonin (and norepinephrine and dopamine to a lesser degree), allowing more to remain in the synapse for use by neurons	Paroxetine, sertraline, fluoxetine, citalopram, and escitalopram
Serotonin and norepinephrine reuptake inhibitors	Inhibit neuronal uptake of serotonin and norepinephrine, allowing more to remain in the synapse for use by neurons	Duloxetine, desvenlafaxine, venlafaxine, and levomilnacipran
Norepinephrine and specific serotonergic modulators	Antagonistic action on noradrenergic receptors (presynaptic that prevent release), leading to enhanced norepinephrine and serotonin neurotransmission, and antagonistic action on specific serotonin receptors (those that cause side effects), making medication better tolerated	Mirtazapine
Norepinephrine-dopamine reuptake inhibitors	Inhibit neuronal uptake of norepinephrine and dopamine, allowing more to remain in the synapse for use by neurons	Bupropion
Serotonin reuptake inhibitors and 5-HT$_{1A}$ partial agonists	Selectively inhibit neuronal reuptake of serotonin (but not norepinephrine or dopamine), allowing more to remain in the synapse for use by neurons; and are a partial agonist of serotonergic 5-HT$_{1A}$ receptors, increasing transmission	Vilazodone**
Serotonin modulators	Inhibit neuronal reuptake of serotonin and various effects on agonistic and antagonistic receptors; some drugs in this class have effects on norepinephrine, dopamine, and acetylcholine	Vortioxetine**, nefazodone, and trazodone
Monoamine oxidase inhibitors	Nonselectively inhibit enzyme monoamine oxidase, preventing breakdown of serotonin, dopamine, and norepinephrine, thereby increasing concentration	Isocarboxazid, phenelzine, and selegiline
Tricyclics	Inhibit neuronal reuptake of serotonin and norepinephrine; some drugs in this class are variable in blocking serotonin versus norepinephrine; some drugs block anticholinergic, histamine, and adrenergic receptors	Amitriptyline and imipramine

* Partial list
** Mechanism of action not fully understood

major depression. A manic episode is a state of abnormal and persistently elevated, expansive, or irritable mood with persistently increased energy and activity. The mood can shift rapidly from excessive cheerfulness or euphoria to marked irritability. The mood disturbances affect the ability to function. The incidence of bipolar disorder in adults in the United States is approximately 2.8%, and it is 2.9% in adolescents (age 13–18) (NIMH, 2017). Many of these episodes in adults (82.9%) result in severe impairment. The incidence is slightly higher in women in comparison to men. Risk factors for bipolar disorder include a family history and advanced paternal age at conception.

The prevalence of bipolar disorder is higher in high-income countries.

Bipolar disorder pathogenesis is complex, multifactorial, and poorly understood. While bipolar disorder pathogenesis is related to depressive disorders, evidence of a close association with schizophrenia development in terms of family history and genetics is increasing. Bipolar disorder is thought to be on a spectrum between depressive disorders, schizophrenia, and other psychotic disorders. The genetic basis for the development of bipolar disorder is based on studies in monozygotic twins where the concordance rate has varied between 40 and 70%. The presence of a bipolar disorder in a first-degree relative increases the risk for development tenfold. Alterations in chromosomes (e.g., 3, 10, 18, 22) and calcium channel polymorphisms (e.g., CACNA1C) have been associated with bipolar disorder and schizophrenia. Many genes are likely involved in the development of bipolar disorder, each with small effects that render an individual susceptible. Epigenetic changes and environmental triggers (e.g., toxic substances, air pollution, and early life stressors) are implicated in bipolar development. As with depression, neural network connections are impaired with bipolar (e.g., as a result of accelerated pruning), particularly in the prefrontal cortex, limbic system, and amygdala. Chronic stress and hypercortisolemia may contribute to bipolar disorder development. Immune dysregulation may also contribute to the development as C-reactive protein and cytokine (e.g., interleukin 6, tumor necrosis factor) can be higher in those with bipolar disorder. In comparison to depression, monoamine concentrations are higher in mania.

Clinical Manifestations

Bipolar disorder symptom onset generally occurs before the age of 20, and the mood at onset is usually major depression (precedes mania). The severity of bipolar disorder varies. Some affected individuals have periods of mania with major depression, which can occur with or without periods of remission (i.e., euthymia—no mood disturbance). The clinical manifestations of mania are centered on mood lability (e.g., elevated, expansive, or irritable), increased activity, and increased energy. Mood in mania is often described as euphoric, excessive cheerfulness, or feeling on top of the world. These symptoms are persistent and affect functioning (e.g., work and social). The clinical manifestations of mania, according to the *DSM-5*, include:

- **Inflated self-esteem:** The individual has an exaggerated self-confidence and exhibits grandiosity (can become delusional) (e.g., he claims to know famous people, have a special relationship with God, embarks on complex tasks such as writing a novel, or senses that he possesses special talents).
- **Decreased need for sleep:** The patient feels energized, well rested, or wired despite having had little sleep (e.g., 3 hours). She is able to go days without sleep. This manifestation is distinguished from insomnia, which is an inability to sleep despite wanting to sleep or feeling tired.
- **Excessively talkative or feeling pressured to keep talking:** The patient has a loud and forceful speech quality, which is more important than the content conveyed; interruption is difficult; he talks continuously with disregard for others; his speech is intrusive; he makes increased dramatic gestures marked by singing and theatricality. He makes hostile comments, has angry outbursts, and he complains when he is irritable.
- **Flight of ideas or racing thoughts:** The patient abruptly changes topic from one to another, her speech can become incoherent and disorganized, and her thoughts race faster than she can express them.
- **Distractibility:** The individual easily diverts his focus of attention to unimportant or irrelevant external stimuli (e.g., background noises and the clothing he is wearing), making it difficult to follow instructions and have a conversation.
- **Increase in goal-directed activity or psychomotor agitation:** The individual plans excessively, participates in multiple activities at once, is restless, paces, and holds multiple conversations.
- **Excessive involvement in activities that have a high potential painful consequences:** The individual may embark on unaffordable spending sprees, reckless driving, and risky sexual behavior such as with strangers.

The depressive episodes in bipolar disorders manifest the same as in MDD, and the criteria are the same (e.g., depressed mood and anhedonia). Bipolar disorders are divided into two subtypes—**bipolar I** and **bipolar II**. A key distinction is the symptomatology and duration. For the diagnosis of bipolar I, manic symptoms of depression must last at least 1 week and be present most of the day, nearly every day. At least three symptoms must present (see manifestations list) or four if the mood is irritability. Bipolar II is characterized as hypomania. A **hypomanic** episode has the same symptoms and criteria for diagnosis as a manic episode, but the duration of the symptoms are four consecutive days (in comparison to the week for bipolar I). Additionally, those individuals with bipolar I almost always experience MDD (however, it is not required for diagnosis) in addition to manic and hypomanic episodes. In contrast, those individuals with bipolar II do not have manic episodes and have a least one episode of MDD and one episode of hypomania. Most (90%) with one episode of mania will have recurrent mood episodes (i.e., major depressive, manic, or hypomanic). Those individuals with four or more mood episodes, whether bipolar I or II, within 1 year are additionally described as having a rapid cycling pattern. Psychosis, particularly delusions, can occur during a manic or MDD episode of bipolar I. **Cyclothymic disorder** is characterized by features of distinct periods of hypomanic symptoms and depressive symptoms that are chronic and fluctuating over a period of 2 years for adults and 1 year for children and adolescents. In cyclothymic disorders, the hypomanic and depressive episodes never reach full criteria for diagnosis of MDD or bipolar disorder. As with depression, many of the same substances, medications, and medical conditions can cause secondary bipolar disorders (i.e., substance- or medication-induced bipolar disorder or bipolar disorder related to another medical condition). Most individuals with bipolar disorder have at least one other mental health disorder such as anxiety disorders, substance abuse disorders, or personality disorders (e.g., antisocial or borderline).

Diagnosis and Treatment

Diagnosis of bipolar disorders is based on a history and physical examination (usually normal), using the *DSM-5* criteria (bipolar disorder was discussed under *Clinical Manifestations*). Despite advances in the understanding of neurobiologic changes in bipolar disorders, diagnostic markers (e.g., imaging studies or laboratory tests) are not available. Diagnostics tests (e.g., thyroid function studies, a substance abuse toxicology screen, and a brain MRI) are performed to evaluate for possible underlying disorders.

Treatment strategies are centered on reducing or resolving symptoms and maintaining functioning. Pharmacotherapeutics are the mainstay of therapy with an intended effect of balancing depressive and manic episodes. Some medications can be used during the acute episodes, for maintenance, or both. The drug classes that can reduce mania and hypomania symptoms include lithium, antiepileptics, and second-generation antipsychotics (**TABLE 11-7**). Antidepressants, particularly tricyclic antidepressants or monoamine oxidase inhibitors, can induce hypomania or mania.

Other treatment strategies include psychotherapy (e.g., cognitive behavioral therapy, interpersonal psychotherapy, family therapy, and psychoeducation). Teaching coping strategies, symptom recurrence awareness, and adherence of medication therapy is important in bipolar disorders. Other therapies for MDD episodes (e.g., ECT) may be used if depression in bipolar disorder is refractory.

TABLE 11-7	Medications for Bipolar Disorder and Schizophrenia	
Classification	**Mechanism of action**	**Generic examples***
Lithium	The mechanism is largely unknown; it possibly affects multiple neurotransmitters (e.g., norepinephrine, serotonin, dopamine, and GABA, glutamate), inhibiting excitatory dopamine and glutamate. Lithium increases neurogenesis and confers neuroprotection (e.g., gray matter preservation).	Lithium
Second-generation atypical antipsychotics	This class provides an antagonistic/agonist action on neurotransmitter-specific dopamine and serotonin receptors, resulting in overall decreased dopamine transmission counterbalanced with reduction in side effects seen in typical antipsychotics that only block dopamine. Decreases in side effects make the medication better tolerated; some atypical antipsychotics additionally block norepinephrine, cholinergic, and histamine receptors. The type of receptor blocked and degree of blockage varies depending on the agent in this class.	Aripiprazole, lurasidone, olanzapine, quetiapine, and risperidone
Antiepileptics	The mechanism is not clearly understood; it may modulate neurotransmitters GABA, glutamate, or dopamine and alter signaling pathways.	Carbamazepine, lamotrigine, and valproate

*Partial list

Schizophrenia

Schizophrenia is categorized as a psychotic disorder that is chronic and recurrent. Characteristics include alterations in perception of reality (e.g., delusions, hallucinations), disorganized thinking, grossly disorganized or abnormal behavior, and disruptions in normal emotional states and expressions. Schizophrenia often impairs the ability to function. Schizophrenia is one of the most serious and disabling mental health disorders. The incidence of schizophrenia is estimated at less than 0.64% in the United States and less than 0.75% in the world (NIMH, 2018). Incidence is relatively similar between men and women, but the onset is usually earlier in men. Risk factors for schizophrenia include a family history, advanced paternal age at conception, living or having been brought up in an urban area, immigration, and prenatal and perinatal complications (e.g., maternal infections or neonatal hypoxia). Autoimmune disorders (e.g., celiac disease, thyrotoxicosis, and acquired hemolytic anemia) have been associated with a higher prevalence of schizophrenia.

The pathogenesis of schizophrenia is largely unknown, as it is with other mental health disorders. Schizophrenia, however, is likely the result of complex genetic, epigenetic, and environmental factors. The concordance rate in monozygotic twins is estimated at 40–50%. Schizophrenia is thought to be a polygenetic disorder (multiple genes) with small genetic additive effects. Alterations in chromosomes, particularly copy number variants (genes that are duplicated or deleted) at the long arm of chromosome 22 are found in higher rates in those individuals with schizophrenia. Gene polymorphisms at loci involved with dopamine and glutamine have been identified, and other gene locus alterations that modify pruning of brain synapses have been noted. Dopamine alterations (i.e., dopamine hypothesis) is one of the first theories in understanding neurotransmitter alterations and schizophrenia. Dopamine receptor (D2) activation in the limbic system results in increased dopamine and is associated with development of psychotic symptoms, and concomitant decrease in dopamine in the prefrontal cortex (D1 receptors) is associated with cognitive and emotional changes. Other receptor dysfunction includes hypofunctioning of the NMDA receptors, causing the inability to stimulate the receptor by glutamate (i.e., glutamate hypothesis of schizophrenia). The glutamate hypothesis was developed when it was noted that cognitive and psychotic manifestations occurred when NMDA antagonists (e.g., ketamine or phencyclidine) were taken. Serotonin antagonism noted through the use of recreational drugs (e.g., lysergic acid diethylamide [LSD] and ecstasy) that induced mind-altering effects led to a serotonin hypothesis in schizophrenia. GABA levels in schizophrenia are decreased. Anatomic brain changes in schizophrenia include abnormal neuronal connectivity as well as gray matter and cortical loss with reduction in volume in the hippocampus, amygdala, thalamus, and frontal lobe. The third and lateral ventricles (where CSF circulates) are enlarged, which results in reduction in volume of other structures (e.g., thalamus and parts of the cortex).

Clinical Manifestations

Schizophrenia is considered a syndrome composed of various diseases with similar characteristics. Symptom onset generally occurs in the late teens to young adulthood (e.g., before age 30). Clinical manifestations are categorized as positive, negative, and cognitive symptoms. The clinical manifestations, according to the *DSM-5*, include:

- **Positive symptoms:** An exaggeration of normal processes, including reality distortion and thought/behavior alterations
  - **Hallucinations:** A perception of sensory stimuli in the absence of an external source
    - Auditory (most common)—hearing voices, other sounds (e.g., music, machinery), visual (e.g., glowing shapes, flashes of color)
    - Somatic (e.g., feel body being touched)
    - Olfactory/gustatory (e.g., strange taste or smell)
  - **Delusions:** A false belief or fixed belief that is not amenable to change
    - **Persecutory (most common):** A belief that someone or some group will cause harm or harass
    - **Grandiose:** The patient's belief that he has exceptional abilities or talents
    - **Nihilistic:** The belief that a catastrophe will happen
    - **Somatic:** A preoccupation with body and health
    - **Bizarre:** Implausible beliefs, such as believing her body has been cloned by aliens
  - **Disorganized thoughts:** A thought disorder that is inferred from speech

such as switching from one topic to another, answering questions that are completely unrelated, getting off topic (tangentiality), or eventually answering questions but in a roundabout manner (circumstantiality)

- **Disorganized behavior:** Varies from agitation, aggression, and silliness
- **Catatonic behavior:** A marked decrease in reactivity to the environment (e.g., resistance to instructions, rigid or inappropriate posture, complete absence of verbal or motor response [i.e., mutism and stupor])
- **Negative symptoms:** An absence or diminution of normal processes, including disruption in normal emotional states and expression
  - **Affective flattening:** A reduced expression of emotion (e.g., in face, eye contact, and speech intonation) and reduced use of expressive motions (e.g., body language and gestures)
  - **Alogia:** Diminished speech output (e.g., decreased content and increased response time)
  - **Anhedonia:** Decreased ability to experience pleasure or recollect pleasure
  - **Asociality:** Lack of interest in social interactions, few relationships, or social activities
  - **Avolition:** Apathy (decrease in motivated self-initiated purposeful activities), impaired personal hygiene, and lack of persistence
- **Cognitive symptoms:** A lack of insight, difficulty with attentiveness, impaired visual and verbal learning and memory, impaired reasoning and judgment, and lack of social awareness

Criteria for diagnosis of schizophrenia include at least two of the following characteristics: 1) delusions, 2) hallucinations, 3) disorganized speech, 4) grossly disorganized or catatonic behavior, or 5) negative symptoms. At least one of the five characteristics must be delusion, hallucination, or disorganized speech. Other diagnostic criteria include marked impairment in functioning (e.g., work, interpersonal relations, and self-care), and the disturbances persist for at least 6 months. The progressive course in schizophrenia is variable, but a more favorable outcome occurs in only 20% of those affected. Others with schizophrenia have periods of exacerbations and

remissions that require lifelong support, while others deteriorate progressively. Positive symptoms can decline over time, reflecting the natural decline in dopamine that occurs with aging; negative symptoms tend to persist and cause significant morbidity. Cognitive deficits do not improve. Several other psychotic disorders are related to schizophrenia or have features similar to schizophrenia such as **schizoaffective disorder**, which is schizophrenia with manic episodes and a significant depressive component. **Schizotypal personality disorder** is characterized by odd or eccentric beliefs and/or perceptual disturbances that are not quite delusions or hallucinations or **delusional disorder** (the patient has delusions but the criteria for schizophrenia are not met). Substances, medications, and medical conditions can cause secondary psychotic disorders and episodes of psychosis. Most individuals with schizophrenia have at least one other mental health disorder such as anxiety disorders and often have a substance-related disorders, particularly tobacco abuse (> 50%).

Diagnosis and Treatment

Diagnosis of schizophrenia is based on a history and physical examination (usually normal), using the *DSM-5* criteria (discussed under *Clinical Manifestations*). Despite advances in the understanding of neurobiologic changes in schizophrenia, diagnostic markers (e.g., imaging studies or laboratory tests) are not available. Diagnostic tests (e.g., thyroid function studies, a substance abuse toxicology screen, and a brain MRI) are performed to evaluate for possible underlying disorders.

Treatment strategies are centered on reducing symptoms and maintaining functioning. Pharmacotherapeutics are the mainstay of therapy with an intended effect reducing symptoms and maintaining function. Some medications can be used during the acute episodes, for maintenance, or both. Antipsychotics are generally the first-line medication treatment, and they are effective for acute episodes and maintenance. Some patients develop treatment-resistant schizophrenia, so other medications (e.g., antiepileptics and NMDA receptor modulators) may be necessary. Brain stimulation (e.g., ECT) may also be used with resistant cases. In addition to antipsychotic medications, various psychosocial interventions are beneficial to address the deficits manifested with schizophrenia. The psychosocial interventions include family-based interventions with psychoeducation and problem solving. Many individuals with schizophrenia have difficulty with daily activities such as personal care, cooking, paying bills, transportation, and socializing. These deficits are often related to the negative symptoms, which do not respond as well to antipsychotic medications, so social skills training is important to address these various deficits. Psychotherapy (e.g., cognitive behavioral therapy), supported employment, and education and group therapy may improve quality of life.

Anxiety Disorders

Anxiety disorders include a group of mental health disorders characterized by fear, which is the emotional response to a real or perceived imminent threat, and anxiety, which is anticipation of future threat. Fear often triggers an autonomic response (i.e., fight or flight) and escape behaviors while anxiety is associated with muscle tension, vigilance, and avoidance behaviors. However, fear and anxiety responses and reactions overlap. Anxiety disorders can interfere with functioning (e.g., work, school, and social relationships). Anxiety disorders are the most prevalent of mental health disorders. The incidence of anxiety disorders for adults in the United States is 19%, and 31% of all adults will experience some type of anxiety disorder in their lifetime (NIMH, 2017). Of the adults with anxiety, most have mild impairment, approximately 22.8% have serious impairment, and 33.7% have moderate impairment. The incidence of anxiety disorders among adolescents (age 13–18) is estimated at 31.9% with 8.3% suffering severe impairment (NIMH, 2017). Anxiety disorders are more prevalent in women in comparison to men across all age groups. The risks for development of an anxiety disorder include a family history and an increased number of traumatic and undesirable events during childhood. Anxiety disorders more commonly occur in those who tend to be timid, shy, or have a negative affect.

Several types of anxiety disorders are possible, each with some commonalities and variations in pathogenesis, etiology, and manifestations. The anxiety disorders that will be discussed in this section include generalized anxiety disorder (GAD), panic disorder, and social anxiety disorder. Other types of anxiety disorders include separation anxiety disorder, selective mutism, agoraphobia, and specific phobias. Most of the biologic basis of anxiety disorders remains unknown. Genetic

links are evidenced by the increased incidence in families. Abnormal genotypes that increase susceptibility have been identified. These abnormalities include variations in the glutamic acid decarboxylase gene, which is responsible for enzyme coding that metabolizes L-glutamine acid into GABA. Further indications of a genetic link include evidence that hereditary traits are shared between GAD and depression. Other research, particularly in studies of panic disorder, postulates that individuals may inherit hyperexcitable brain areas that lead to susceptibility to panic with different stimuli. Some studies have revealed that those individuals with GAD and panic disorder have an increased sensitivity in detecting stimulation by panicogens (e.g., carbon dioxide, caffeine), which leads to panic symptoms. In GAD and social anxiety disorder, with visual cues (e.g., angry faces) there is an elevated activity in certain regions of the brain (e.g., the cingulate cortex and amygdala) leading to enhanced overall anticipatory response (e.g., anxiety and fear). This elevated activity also decreases after pharmacologic treatment. Neurotransmitter alterations—specifically serotonin, norepinephrine, GABA, and dopamine alterations—may be present in anxiety disorders. Additionally, glutamate and oxytocin (neuropeptide) alterations have been noted in social anxiety disorders. Oxytocin is a neuropeptide involved in social cognition (e.g., empathy, trust), and secretion may be reduced.

Clinical Manifestations

Anxiety disorders can develop in childhood but can also manifest in adolescence. Clinical manifestations vary depending on the type of anxiety disorder, which are caused and triggered by different stimuli. The description of each type of disorder and manifestations, as outlined in the *DSM-5*, include:

- **Panic disorder:** This disorder features recurrent or unexpected episodes of panic attacks, which are defined as an abrupt surge of intense fear/discomfort that peaks within minutes. Various autonomic responses can also be present such as palpitations, sweating, trembling, paresthesias, or nausea. The patient can experience shortness of breath, chest pain, dizziness, light-headedness, intense warmth, or chills. Feelings of being detached or unreality or of losing control or dying may be present. In addition to the presence of the symptoms, panic disorder leads to persistent worry about having more panic attacks and avoidance of situations or things that may cause the panic attacks.

- **GAD:** The patient experiences excessive worrying and anxiety about a number of life events (e.g., work, school, money, health). The worrying must be present more days than not for at least 6 months. The affected individual finds it difficult to control the worry. Accompanying symptoms include restlessness, fatigue, difficulty with concentration, irritability, muscle tension, or poor sleep (e.g., insomnia, unsatisfying sleep).
- **Social anxiety disorder:** The patient experiences fear or anxiety and avoidance of social situations (e.g., public speaking and meeting new people) that are persistent and usually last for at least 6 months. The affected individual feels she will be embarrassed or criticized. Significant distress is caused by the social situation and causes significant impairment.

As with other mental health disorders, substances, medications, and medical conditions can cause secondary anxiety disorders (i.e., substance- or medication-induced anxiety disorders or anxiety disorders related to another medical condition). Most individuals with anxiety disorder have other comorbid mental health disorders, such as depressive disorders or substance abuse disorders.

Diagnosis and Treatment

Diagnosis of anxiety disorders is based on a history and physical examination (usually normal), using the *DSM-5* criteria (discussed under *Clinical Manifestations*). Despite advances in the understanding of neurobiologic changes in anxiety disorders, diagnostic markers (e.g., imaging studies or laboratory tests) are not available. Diagnostics tests (e.g., thyroid function studies, a substance abuse toxicology screen, and a brain MRI) are performed to evaluate for possible underlying disorders.

Treatment strategies often include simultaneous pharmacotherapy along with psychotherapy, with cognitive behavioral therapy as one of the most efficacious types. Psychotherapy can be a monotherapy, but the reverse is generally not recommended (i.e., medication without psychotherapy). Usual therapeutic agents include antidepressants.

Benzodiazepines are effective but have a particularly high addictive potential. Antipsychotics can be used with resistant cases. Brain stimulation therapies (e.g., ECT) are used to treat depression, which can coexist with anxiety, but these therapies may also decrease anxiety symptomatology. Various behavioral techniques can be effective, such as relaxation techniques and breathing techniques. Other therapeutic approaches can include yoga, exercise, and massage.

Obsessive-Compulsive Disorders

Obsessive-compulsive disorders (OCD) are characterized by chronic, repetitive, intrusive thoughts or urges (i.e., obsessions) and repetitive mental or behavioral acts (i.e., compulsions). Attempts are made to ignore the obsessions, which can include performing a compulsive act for relief. Obsessions and compulsions cause distress and anxiety and are time consuming, taking up more than 1 hour per day. OCD causes impaired functioning. The incidence of OCD in adults in the United States is estimated at 1.2%, and almost half have serious impairment (NIMH, 2017). Those individuals with a family history of OCD are at higher risk for development. Those individuals with Tourette disorder or neurologic tics also have an increased incidence of OCD. The pathogenesis of OCD includes an interplay of genetics and environmental factors. Abnormal neural circuitry and abnormal neuronal activity in various regions in the brain (e.g., frontal cortex, anterior cingulate cortex, and striatum) have been noted in OCD.

Clinical Manifestations

The onset of OCD is usually in adolescence or young adulthood. Males have an earlier onset in comparison to females (e.g., some as early as 10 years old). The clinical manifestations are the obsessions and compulsions, and the types can vary but often have a theme. As an example, an affected individual may have obsessive thoughts about contamination with an accompanying cleaning compulsion. Other themes include symmetry obsession, where things need to be symmetrical with an accompanying compulsion to repeat, order, and count things. Other obsessions include a fear of losing things, worrying about harm coming to oneself or others, and thoughts about sex or religion. Compulsions can include hoarding unnecessary objects or constantly seeking reassurance. Individuals with

OCD can experience panic attacks. During compulsive acts, a sense of uneasiness is often present, which is not relieved until things are a specific way (e.g., certain things must feel, sound, or look just right). Avoidance of triggers is common (e.g., a person concerned with contamination may avoid using a public restroom). OCD often coexists with an anxiety or mood disorder, usually MDD. A higher incidence of OCD is present in those individuals with bipolar disorder, schizophrenia, and eating disorders.

Diagnosis and Treatment

Diagnosis of OCD is based on a history and physical examination (usually normal), using the *DSM-5* criteria, and obsessions, compulsions, or both may be present. There are no diagnostic markers, imaging studies or laboratory tests available to diagnose OCD.

Diagnostic tests such as thyroid function studies, a substance abuse toxicology screen, and a brain MRI are performed to evaluate for possible underlying disorders.

Therapeutic strategies can include psychotherapy, usually cognitive behavioral therapy with an emphasis on exposure and response prevention. Family therapy and psychoeducation are also important. Pharmacotherapeutic agents include antidepressants, usually selective serotonin reuptake inhibitors. Other antidepressants or other agents such as antipsychotic drugs may be used. Brain stimulation techniques such as ECT or transcranial magnetic stimulation may be used. Surgical techniques such as anterior cingulotomy and deep brain stimulation (implanting electrodes in the brain and a pulse generator that sends electrical impulses to different parts of the brain) may be used to relieve those with treatment-resistant OCD.

CHAPTER SUMMARY

The nervous system is a complex network that receives, organizes, and responds to internal and external stimuli—functions that are vital for achieving and maintaining homeostasis. The nervous system controls all sensory and motor functions. All thoughts, perceptions, emotions, and behaviors are regulated by the nervous system. Damage to this system—even when minor—can result in significant neurologic deficits. The nature and severity of those deficits can vary greatly. Such damage can result from trauma, infections, tumors, chemical imbalances,

genetic conditions, or environmental life stressors. Regardless of the neurologic disorder, an affected individual may face significant neurologic dysfunction and even death. Mental health disorders, in addition to negatively impacting physical health, often impact social functioning and social well-being. Supporting neurologic health involves strategies such as observing safety precautions (e.g., wearing safety equipment), avoiding illicit drug use, minimizing alcohol consumption, getting vaccinations, and maintaining adequate nutrition.

REFERENCES AND RESOURCES

AAOS. (2004). *Paramedic: Anatomy & physiology*. Sudbury, MA: Jones and Bartlett Publishers.

Alzheimer's Association. (2019). Vascular dementia. Retrieved from https://www.alz.org/alzheimers-dementia/what-is-dementia/types-of-dementia/vascular-dementia

American Heart Association (AHA). (2019). Heart disease and stroke statistics—2019—At-a-glance. Retrieved from http://www.professional.heart.org

American Psychological Association (APA). (2013). *Diagnostic and statistical manual of mental disorders* (5th ed.). Arlington, VA: American Psychiatric Association Publishing.

Learning, memory, language, & speech. In K. E. Barrett, S. M. Barman, H. L. Brooks, J. J. Yuan (Eds.), *Ganong's review of medical physiology* (26th ed.). New York, NY: McGraw-Hill. Retrieved from http://accessmedicine.mhmedical.com.ezproxy.fiu.edu/content.aspx?bookid=2525&sectionid=204291894

Centers for Disease Control and Prevention (CDC). (2015a). Alzheimer's disease. Retrieved from http://www.cdc.gov/aging/aginginfo/alzheimers.htm

Centers for Disease Control and Prevention (CDC). (2015b). Creutzfeldt-Jakob disease. Retrieved from http://www.cdc.gov/prions/cjd/index.html

Centers for Disease Control and Prevention (CDC). (2015c). Spina bifida. Retrieved from http://www.cdc.gov/ncbddd/spinabifida/data.html

Centers for Disease Control and Prevention (CDC). (2015d). Stroke. Retrieved from http://www.cdc.gov/stroke/facts.htm

Centers for Disease Control and Prevention (CDC). (2019b). Menigococcal vaccination. Retrieved from https://www.cdc.gov/meningococcal/vaccine-info.html

Centers for Disease Control and Prevention (CDC). (2016a). Data and statistics for cerebral palsy. Retrieved from http://www.cdc.gov/ncbddd/cp/data.html

Centers for Disease Control and Prevention (CDC). (2016b). Epilepsy fast facts. Retrieved from http://www.cdc.gov/epilepsy/basics/fast-facts.htm

Centers for Disease Control and Prevention (CDC). (2016c). Zika virus. Retrieved from http://www.cdc.gov/zika/geo/index.html

Centers for Disease Control and Prevention (CDC). (2019a). Traumatic brain injury. Retrieved from http://www.cdc.gov/TraumaticBrainInjury/get_the_facts.html

Central Brain Tumor Registry of the United States (CBTRUS). (2018). 2018 CBTRUS Fact sheet. Retrieved from http://www.cbtrus.org/aboutus/aboutus.html

Chiras, D. (2015). *Human biology* (8th ed.). Burlington, MA: Jones & Bartlett Learning.

Cochrane, T. I., & Williams, M. A. (2015). *Disorders of consciousness: Brain death, coma, and the vegetative and minimally conscious states.* Baltimore, MD: The Sandra and Malcolm Berman Brain and Spine Institute, LifeBridge Health.

Elling, B., Elling, K., & Rothenberg, M. (2004). *Anatomy and physiology.* Sudbury, MA: Jones and Bartlett Publishers.

Gould, B. (2015). *Pathophysiology for the health professions* (5th ed.). Philadelphia, PA: Elsevier.

Hart, M., & Loeffler, A. (2012). *Introduction to human disease: Pathophysiology for health professionals.* Burlington, MA: Jones & Bartlett Learning.

International Headache Society. (2018). Headache Classification Committee of the International Headache Society (HIS): The International Classification of Headache Disorders, 3rd edition. *Cephalalgia, 38*(1), 1–211. doi: 10.1177/0333102417738202

International League Against Epilepsy (ILAE). (2014). A practical definition of epilepsy. Retrieved from https://www.ilae.org/guidelines/definition-and-classification/definition-of-epilepsy-2014

International League Against Epilepsy (ILAE). (2017). *ILAE classification of the epilepsies (2017).* Position paper of the ILAE Commission for Classification and Terminology. Retrieved from https://www.ilae.org/guidelines/definition-and-classification

Krishnan, R. (2019) Unipolar depression in adults: Epidemiology, pathogenesis, and neurobiology. In D. Solomon (Ed.). *Uptodate.* Retrieved from https://www.uptodate.com/contents/unipolar-depression-in-adults-epidemiology-pathogenesis-and-neurobiology

Madara, B., & Pomarico-Denino, V. (2008). *Quick look nursing: Pathophysiology* (2nd ed.). Sudbury, MA: Jones and Bartlett Publishers.

McCance, K. L., & Huether, S. E. (2019). *Pathophysiology: The biologic basis for disease in adults and children* (8th ed.). St. Louis, MO: Elsevier.

Merikangas, K. R., He, J. P., Burstein, M., Swanson, S. A., Avenevoli, S., Cui, L., … Swendsen, J. (2010). Lifetime prevalence of mental disorders in U.S., adolescents: Results from the National Comorbidity Survey Replication—Adolescent Supplement (NCS-A). *Journal of the American Academy of Child and Adolescent Psychiatry, 49*(10), 980–989.

National Cancer Institute. (2016). Brain and other nervous system cancer. Retrieved from http://seer.cancer.gov/statfacts/html/brain.html#incidence-mortality

National Hydrocephalus Foundation. (2014). Facts about hydrocephalus. Retrieved from http://nhfonline.org/facts-about-hydrocephalus.htm

National Institutes of Health (NIH). (2011). Alzheimer's disease diagnostic guidelines. Retrieved from https://www.nia.nih.gov/health/alzheimers-disease-diagnostic-guidelines

National Institutes of Health (NIH). (2016a). Amyotrophic lateral sclerosis information page. Retrieved from https://www.ninds.nih.gov/Disorders/All-Disorders/Amyotrophic-Lateral-Sclerosis-ALS-Information-Page

National Institutes of Health (NIH). (2016b). Huntington's disease information page. Retrieved from https://www.ninds.nih.gov/Disorders/All-Disorders/Huntingtons-Disease-Information-Page

National Institutes of Health (NIH). (2016c). Multiple sclerosis information page. Retrieved from https://www.ninds.nih.gov/Disorders/All-Disorders/Multiple-Sclerosis-Information-Page

National Institutes of Health (NIH). (2016d). Parkinson's disease. Retrieved from https://www.ninds.nih.gov/Disorders/All-Disorders/Parkinsons-Disease-Information-Page

National Institute of Mental Health (NIMH). (2017). Mental health. Retrieved from www.nimh.nih.gov

National Institute of Mental Health (NIMH). (2018). Schizophrenia. Retrieved from https://www.nimh.nih.gov/health/statistics/schizophrenia.shtml

National Spinal Cord Injury Statistical Center (NSCISC). (2016). Spinal cord injury facts and figures at a glance. Retrieved from https://www.nscisc.uab.edu/Public/Facts%202016.pdf

Navalkele, B., Chandrasekar, P., & Levine, M. (2016). Zika virus. *Medscape.* Retrieved from http://emedicine.medscape.com/article/2500035-overview#a2

Professional guide to pathophysiology (3rd ed.). (2010). Philadelphia, PA: Lippincott Williams & Wilkins.

Rajajee, V. (2019). Management of acute severe traumatic brain injury. Wilterdink, J. L. (Ed.), *Uptodate.* Retrieved from https://www.uptodate.com/contents/management-of-acute-severe-traumatic-brain-injury

Ropper, A. H., Samuels, M. A., Klein J. P., & Prasad S. (Eds.). (2019). *Adams and Victor's principles of neurology* (11th ed.). New York, NY: McGraw-Hill.

Singer, R. J., & Ogilvy, C. S. (2019). Brain arteriovenous malformations. In J. F. Dashe (Ed.), *Uptodate.* Retrieved from https://www.uptodate.com/contents/brain-arteriovenous-malformations

Vos, B., Nieuwenhuijsen, K., & Sluiter, J. K. (2018). Consequences of traumatic brain injury in professional American football players: A systematic review of the literature. *Clinical Journal of Sport Medicine, 28*(2), 91–99. doi: 10.1097/JSM.0000000000000432

Waxman, S. G. (2017). *Clinical neuroanatomy* (28th ed.). New York, NY: McGraw-Hill.

World Health Organization (WHO). (2016). Zika virus. Retrieved from http://www.who.int/mediacentre/factsheets/zika/en/

World Health Organization (WHO). (2017). Mental disorders. Retrieved from www.who.int

World Health Organization (WHO). (2018). Depression. Retrieved from https://www.who.int/en/news-room/fact-sheets/detail/depression

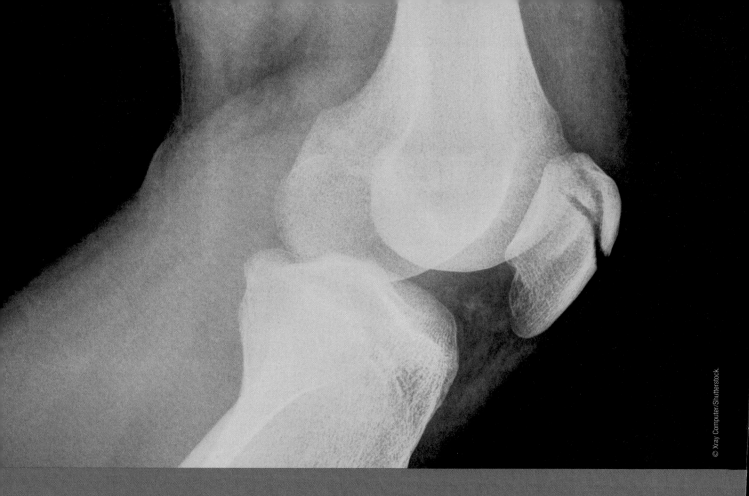

CHAPTER 12
Musculoskeletal Function

LEARNING OBJECTIVES

- Discuss normal musculoskeletal anatomy and physiology.
- Explain and summarize congenital musculoskeletal disorders.
- Explain and summarize traumatic musculoskeletal disorders.
- Summarize musculoskeletal injuries in child abuse.
- Differentiate disorders of the lower back.
- Differentiate metabolic bone disorders.
- Differentiate inflammatory joint disorders.

- Differentiate chronic muscle disorders.
- Differentiate bone and muscle neoplasms.
- Apply understanding of musculoskeletal system alterations in describing various common disorders such as traumatic injuries, metabolic bone disorders, inflammatory disorders, autoimmune disorders, chronic muscular disorders, and tumors.
- Develop diagnostic and treatment considerations for various musculoskeletal disorders.

The musculoskeletal system consists of bones, joints, muscles, ligaments, tendons, and other connective tissue that provide support for the body and protection of organs. The structures of the musculoskeletal system are essential for standing erect and collaborate with the nervous system to make movement possible. This system also gives the human body form and stability while protecting the body's vital organs. It plays a role in homeostasis by storing calcium and other minerals that can be mobilized when needed. Additionally, hematopoiesis occurs in the bones.

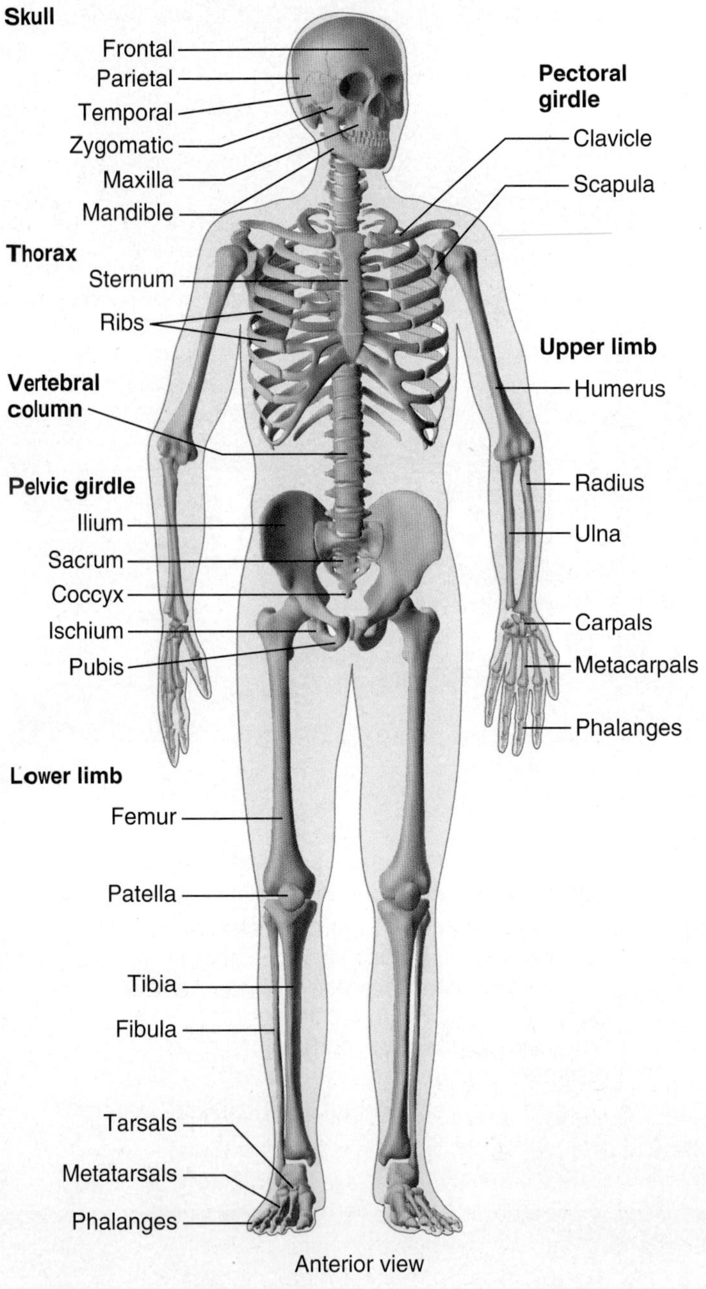

Connective tissues are the biologic material that supports and binds tissues and organs together. The chief components of connective tissue include elastic fibers and collagen (a protein substance). See chapter 3 for a discussion of hemtopoiesis.

Disorders of the musculoskeletal system may be either acute or chronic. Many of these conditions are easily treatable and leave no lasting effects (e.g., fractures). Other conditions, such as fibromyalgia, can leave the individual with chronic pain or significant disability. These disorders may have congenital, genetic, autoimmune, trauma, nutritional-deficit, and excessive-use causes.

Anatomy and Physiology

The musculoskeletal system is interconnected despite each component's unique structure and function. The skeletal system is a metabolically active organ system, which is composed of bones. Junctions between bones are known as joints. Bones are connected to bones with strong collagenous fibers known as ligaments, which keep the bones together and stable. Skeletal muscle tissues are attached to the bones with strong collagenous fibers known as tendons, which allow movement of the bones. Skeletal muscle tissue is the only type of muscle group that is consciously controlled. The other muscle groups are cardiac and smooth and are unconsciously controlled.

Bones

Bone is a specialized form of connective tissue. At first glance, the bone appears to be a dry, dead material. In fact, the word *skeleton* is derived from a Greek word that means "dried-up body." Looks can be deceiving, however, because nothing could be further from the truth. Bone is a living, metabolically active tissue. This tissue is the site of fat and mineral storage (especially calcium) as well as hematopoiesis. The human body contains 206 bones of varying shapes and sizes that make up the skeleton (**FIGURE 12-1**). The skeleton provides support and protection for vital organs such as the heart, lungs, and brain. It is organized into two divisions—axial and appendicular. The axial skeleton forms the long axis of the body and includes the skull, vertebral column, and rib cage. The appendicular skeleton consists of the bones that form the arms, shoulders, pelvis, and legs.

Skull
Frontal
Parietal
Temporal
Zygomatic
Maxilla
Mandible

Thorax
Sternum
Ribs

Vertebral column

Pelvic girdle
Ilium
Sacrum
Coccyx
Ischium
Pubis

Lower limb
Femur
Patella
Tibia
Fibula
Tarsals
Metatarsals
Phalanges

Pectoral girdle
Clavicle
Scapula

Upper limb
Humerus
Radius
Ulna
Carpals
Metacarpals
Phalanges

Anterior view

FIGURE 12-1 The human skeleton.

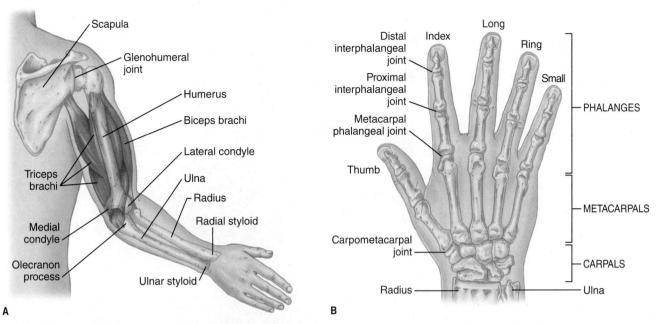

FIGURE 12-2 Classifications of bones. **(A)** The scapula is a flat bone, and the humerus, ulna, and radius are long bones. **(B)** The carpals, or wrist bones, are short bones.

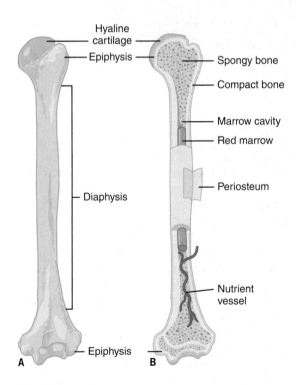

FIGURE 12-3 Long bones. **(A)** The humerus. Notice the long shaft and dilated ends. **(B)** Longitudinal section of the humerus showing compact bone, spongy bone, and marrow.

Five types of bone are found within the skeleton—long, short, flat, irregular, and sesamoid bones (**FIGURE 12-2**). Long bones (**FIGURE 12-3**) have bodies (diaphyses) that are

longer than they are wide, epiphyses at either end, and growth plates (i.e., epiphyseal plates) contained in a narrow area known as the metaphysis, which is between the diaphysis and epiphyses. There is a hard outer surface (compact bone) and inner regions (spongy bone) that are less dense than the outer regions and contain bone marrow. Spongy bone is further made of trabeculae (**FIGURE 12-4**) and a layer of cortical bone (i.e., thin outer layer of compact bone). The terms *compact* and *cortical* bone are often used interchangeably. Both epiphyseal ends of long bones are covered in hyaline cartilage to help protect the bone by reducing friction and absorbing shock. Long bones include not only the longest bones in the body (e.g., femur, humerus, and tibia) but also some of the smallest (e.g., metacarpals, metatarsals, and phalanges). Short bones are approximately as wide as they are long; their primary function is providing support and stability with little movement. Short bones consist of only a thin layer of compact bone along with spongy bone but contain relatively large amounts of bone marrow despite not having a shaft. The ends of short bones are not epiphyses, but rather, the ends are covered with a hyaline membrane. Examples of short bones include the carpals (wrists) and tarsals (ankles).

Flat bones are strong, level plates of bone that provide protection to the body's vital

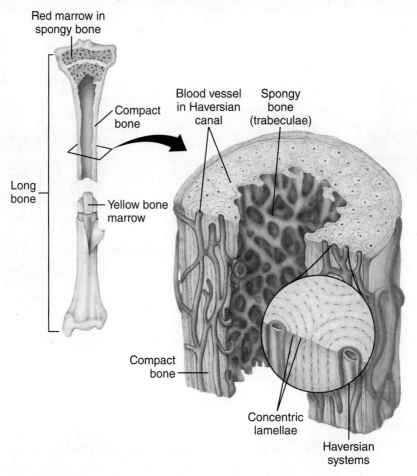

FIGURE 12-4 Shaft of the bone.

organs and serve as a base for muscular attachment. The anterior and posterior surfaces of flat bones are formed from compact bone to provide strength, and the center consists of spongy bone and varying amounts of bone marrow. In adults, most red blood cells are formed in flat bones. Examples of flat bones include the scapula, sternum, skull, pelvis, and ribs.

Irregular bones include bones that do not fall into any other category, due to their nonuniform shape. They primarily consist of spongy bone, with a thin outer layer of compact bone. Examples of irregular bones include the vertebrae, sacrum, and mandible.

Sesamoid bones are usually short or irregular bones embedded in a tendon. Sesamoid bones are often present in a tendon where it passes over a joint and serve to protect the tendon. Examples of sesamoid bones include the patella (a flat bone), pisiform (smallest of the carpals), and the two small bones at the base of the first metatarsal.

A layer of connective tissue called the *periosteum* covers compact bone surfaces. The periosteum serves as the site of muscle attachment (via tendons). The outer surface of the periosteum contains cells that aid in remodeling and repair (osteoblasts). The periosteum is richly supplied with blood vessels that enter the bone at numerous sites (Figure 12-4). These vessels travel through small tubes (Haversian canals or osteons) in the compact bone and flow through the spongy bone, providing nutrients and oxygen while removing waste products. The periosteum is supplied with nerve fibers.

Inside the shaft of long bones is a large cavity for bone marrow. The marrow cavities in most bones of a fetus or newborn contain red marrow. Red marrow, so named because of its color, serves as the site for hematopoiesis. As humans age, this red marrow is slowly replaced by fat, creating yellow marrow. Yellow marrow begins to form during adolescence and is present in most bones by adulthood. At this point, hematopoiesis continues in the vertebrae, pelvis, and a few other sites. The yellow marrow can be reactivated to produce blood

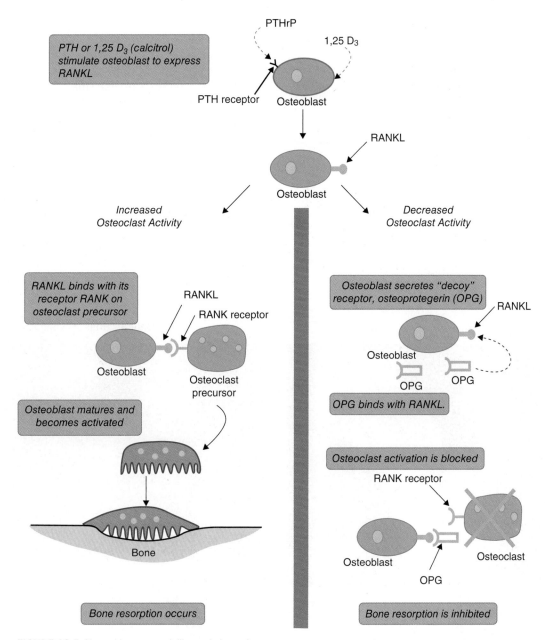

PTHrP

PTH or 1,25 D₃ (calcitrol) stimulate osteoblast to express RANKL

1,25 D₃

PTH receptor   Osteoblast

RANKL

Osteoblast

Increased Osteoclast Activity   Decreased Osteoclast Activity

RANKL binds with its receptor RANK on osteoclast precursor

RANKL

RANK receptor

Osteoblast

Osteoclast precursor

Osteoblast matures and becomes activated

Bone

Osteoblast secretes "decoy" receptor, osteoprotegerin (OPG)

RANKL

Osteoblast

OPG   OPG

OPG binds with RANKL.

Osteoclast activation is blocked

RANK receptor

Osteoblast

OPG

Osteoclast

Bone resorption occurs   Bone resorption is inhibited

FIGURE 12-5 Normal bone remodelling: a balanced process.

cells under certain circumstances (e.g., after an injury).

Bone Remodelling

Bone is a dynamic tissue that is constantly undergoing remodeling to repair aging bone, fractures, or to adjust for factors such as changes in activity. For example, spongy bone is remodeled to increase bone strength when a person's activity level increases after periods of inactivity. During remodeling, cells called *osteoclasts* (derived from monocytes/macrophages) break down (i.e., resorption) bone. Bone remodeling (**FIGURE 12-5**) begins with osteoclastic resorption, which involves cleaning up the bony

matrix organic material (proteins and collagen) and the inorganic materials (minerals). When the cleanup is finished, osteoblasts begin rebuilding bone to increase bone strength (**TABLE 12-1**). The osteoblasts begin their work by secreting the building blocks of the bone matrix, which consists of collagen and a gel called *ground substance* (made of proteoglycans and glycoproteins). These two substances (collagen and ground substance) make up the nonmineral bone matrix known as **osteoid**. Osteoblasts also secrete alkaline phosphatase, an enzyme that is involved in forming the inorganic mineral component of bone matrix hydroxyapatite crystals, which are composed of calcium, phosphate, and water. When these osteoblasts become surrounded by calcified extracellular material (i.e., calcifying osteoid), the complex is referred to as an *osteocyte* (i.e., a mature osteoblast). Bone tissue contains many of these osteocytes in small cavities (i.e., lacunae) that are connected by thin structures called *canaliculi*. The canaliculi are like small tunnels that allow information to travel between the osteocytes to control calcium and phosphate balance. The lacuna and canaliculi are organized into thin layers called *lamellae* (Figure 12-4; FIGURE 12-6). The osteocytes are essentially embedded in an extracellular material referred to as the *bone matrix*. The matrix consists of calcium phosphate crystals (hydroxyapatite) that make the bones hard and strong. It also contains collagen fibers that reinforce the bone, giving it flexible strength. Balance between the mineral components and collagen is necessary

TABLE 12-1	Structural Elements of Bone
Bone cells	**Function**
Osteoblasts	Build bone through collagen
Osteoclasts	Enable the matrix to be absorbed (i.e., resorption) and assist with the release of calcium and phosphate
Osteocytes	Mature osteoblasts that help maintain the bone matrix; also play a major role in the release of calcium into blood

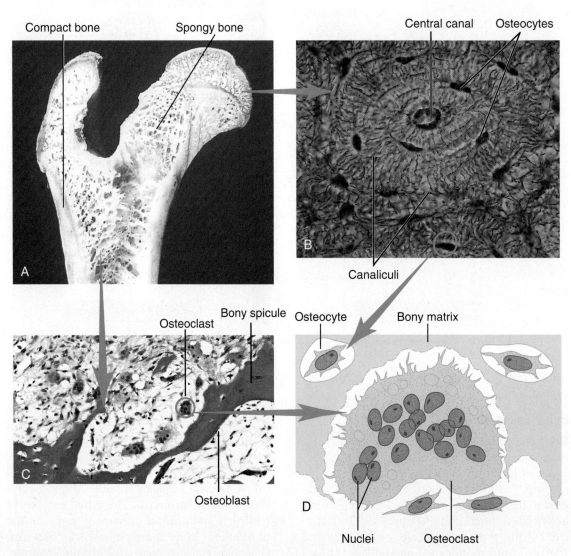

FIGURE 12-6 Bone. **(A)** Compact and spongy bone of the humerus. **(B)** Light micrograph of the lamellae (concentric circles) showing the osteocytes and canaliculi. **(C)** Photomicrograph of spongy bone showing osteoblasts and osteoclasts. **(D)** An osteoclast digesting the surface of a bony spicule (sharp body or spike).

for optimal bone function. Bone without adequate mineral quantities is extremely brittle; bone without adequate collagen is too flexible.

The process of bone remodeling is controlled by several cytokines (e.g., growth factors), hormones, and **osteoprotegerin** (OPG). OPG is a glycoprotein that is a key mediator of osteoblast and osteoclast activity (see Figure 12-5). OPG is produced by osteoblasts. OPG inhibits osteoclastic formation, and the effects of OPG are opposed by the cytokine **RANKL** (receptor activator of nuclear factor-kappa B ligand). When RANKL binds to an osteoclast, it causes resorption. When OPG blocks RANKL by acting as a RANKL receptor decoy, osteoclast resorption activity is blocked and, therefore, bone formation is promoted. Several disorders and conditions are caused by an imbalance in the OPG–RANKL system. As an example, estrogen blocks RANKL (i.e., it prevents resorption), and when estrogen levels drop in postmenopausal women, there is more bone resorption and a higher risk for osteoporosis. Glucocorticoids can increase RANKL and inhibit OPG, leading to increased bone resorption. Denosumab (i.e., Prolia) is a RANKL inhibitor that is used to treat osteoporosis.

Several hormones influence bone structure. Growth hormone produced by the anterior pituitary gland works with thyroid hormones to control normal bone growth. Growth hormone increases the rate of growth by causing cartilage and bone cells to reproduce and lay down their intercellular matrix as well as by stimulating mineralization within the matrix. Bones grow in two ways—appositional growth and endochondral growth. In appositional growth, new bone forms on the surface of a bone. In endochondral growth, bone eventually replaces new cartilage growth in the epiphyseal plate. Calcitonin (from the thyroid gland) and parathyroid hormone (PTH) regulate bone remodeling and mineralization of calcium. Calcitonin alters serum calcium levels by inhibiting osteoclast activity, which decreases calcium release from the bone, and by stimulating osteoblast activity, which increases calcium deposits in the bone. PTH is more important than calcitonin in calcium regulation, and PTH increases serum calcium levels by increasing osteoclast activity, which increases calcium release from the bone. Calcitonin and PTH also regulate calcium through effects on the kidneys and gastrointestinal tract. See chapter 10 for more details on endocrine function.

Vitamin D also plays a critical role in bone metabolism. This fat-soluble vitamin, in conjunction with PTH, controls the absorption of calcium from the intestine and increases calcium and phosphate reabsorption in the kidneys. Proper nutrition (including adequate intake of dietary calcium and vitamin D) and physical activity from childhood onward are essential for the development and maintenance of healthy bone.

Joints

Cartilage is a connective tissue that is tough and flexible. Three types of cartilage (fibrocartilage, elastic cartilage, and hyaline cartilage) can be found throughout the body in the ears, larynx, nose, and joints; hyaline cartilage is the most common type in the body. During fetal development, the skeleton forms from hyaline cartilage. The composition of cartilage is similar to bone with collagen fibers (e.g., type I and type II) and ground substance (made of proteoglycans). One distinction is the lack of calcification in cartilage in comparison to bone. Cartilage also does not have blood vessels or nerves; however, the gel substance of the matrix in cartilage allows for exchanges (e.g., nutrients and wastes), usually through diffusion between cartilage cells known as **chondrocytes**. Hyaline cartilage is the weakest of the three cartilages and is found on the weight-bearing joints such as those of long bones as well as the sternum and ribs. Elastic cartilage is made of elastin, which allows for flexibility, and is in places such as the auricle. Fibrous cartilage is the strongest of the three cartilages and consists of a significant amount of collagen intermixed with hyaline cartilage. Fibrous cartilage is tough, and movement is limited. Fibrocartilage is located in the symphysis pubis and intervertebral joints. Various changes in cartilage occur with aging, including a loss of water content and glycosaminoglycans. Glycosaminoglycans are components (e.g., chondroitin sulfate and hyaluronic acid) involved in joint lubrication, so the cartilage is rigid and fragile without it.

Joints are classified based on their degree of movement as moveable, slightly moveable, or immoveable. The most common type of joint is the freely moveable, or synovial joint (i.e., diarthrosis) (FIGURE 12-7). Synovial joints are complex and vary significantly, but they all share similar features. Synovial joints contain articular cartilage that is lubricated by a transparent viscous fluid (synovial fluid) secreted

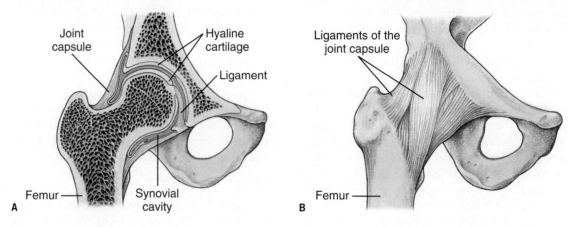

FIGURE 12-7 A synovial joint. **(A)** A cross-section through the hip joint (a ball-and-socket joint) showing the structures of the synovial joint. **(B)** Ligaments in the outer portion of the joint capsule help support the joint.

by the synovial membrane—a soft tissue that lines the noncartilaginous surfaces within joints. This lubricated cartilage has hyaluronic acid, which gives it an egg white consistency, and this consistency reduces friction by providing a slippery surface that enables bones to move freely. Hyaluronic acid can be used as a treatment by injecting it into joints to increase lubrication and decrease pain. In addition to lubrication, synovial fluid delivers nutrients to the cartilage during joint compression, which forces fluid out, and when pressure is relieved, fluid flows back in. Synovial fluid contains leukocytes (e.g., phagocytic cells) that fight infections in the joints. The second commonality among synovial joints is the presence of a joint capsule (i.e., the articular capsule), a structure that joins one bone to another. The outer layer of the synovial joint capsule consists of dense connective tissue that is attached to the periosteum of adjacent bones. An abundance of blood vessels, nerves, and lymphatic vessels surround the joint capsule. Many of these joints contain parallel bundles of dense connective tissue called *ligaments*. Ligaments connect bones to bones in a joint and provide support to the joint. The shoulder joint is an example of a ball-and-socket type synovial joint, and it is the most moveable joint in the whole body.

Slightly moveable joints, or amphiarthroses, can be seen in the vertebral column (**FIGURE 12-8**). An intervertebral disk unites the components of each vertebra. The inner portion of this disk (i.e., nucleus pulposus) serves as a gel-like cushion, absorbing the impact of walking and running. The outer, fibrous portion holds the disk in place and joins one vertebra to the next.

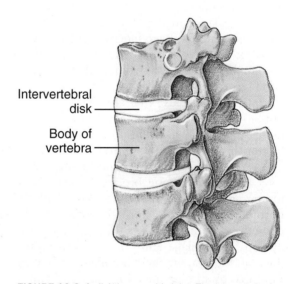

FIGURE 12-8 A slightly moveable joint. The intervertebral disks allow for some movement, giving the vertebral column flexibility.

The skull is an example of an immoveable joint, or synarthrosis (**FIGURE 12-9**). In the skull, the bones interlock to form immoveable joints called *sutures*. Sutures and fontanelles (the space where sutures interconnect) in the skull of an infant are not fused, allowing for movement during birth and expansion as the brain and child grows (**FIGURE 12-10**). The posterior fontanelle usually closes around 2 months of age, while the anterior fontanelle usually closes by the age of 2 years of age. Fibrous connective tissue extends the space between the interlocking bones, holding them together. Another immoveable joint is the pubic symphysis, where the two pubic bones come together and are held in position by fibrocartilage. The pelvic girdle is a site of profound changes due

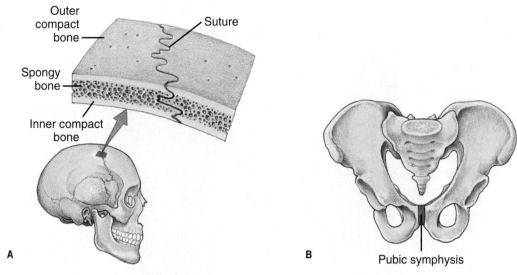

FIGURE 12-9 Immoveable joints. **(A)** Many of the bones of the skull are held in place by sutures. These bones are linked by fibrous tissue, and the joints are immoveable. **(B)** The pubic symphysis is another immoveable joint. During childbirth, it softens and expands to permit delivery.

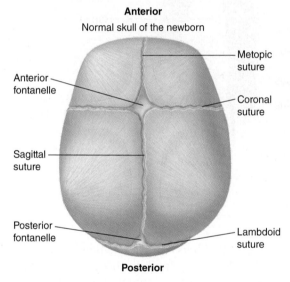

FIGURE 12-10 Normal skull of a newborn.

to pregnancy. Most of the changes are due to weight gain, uterine growth, progesterone effects such as softened cartilage in joints and estrogen and relaxin effects such as ligamentous laxity. The pelvic girdle changes include a widening of the symphysis pubis and sacroiliac joints. The pelvis also tilts forward. These anatomic changes can result in some normal discomforts of pregnancy, such as low back pain and carpal tunnel syndrome.

Muscles

Motion requires a skeleton with moveable joints and muscles acting on the bones. There are three types of muscles: skeletal, smooth, and cardiac. Skeletal muscles connect to bone. They are the most frequently occurring muscle type, making up approximately 40% of the body's weight. The more than 350 skeletal muscles are under the voluntary control of the brain (**FIGURE 12-11**). Smooth muscles line the walls of hollow organs and tubes; they are also found in the eyes, skin, and glands. Smooth muscles are involuntary, meaning they work without conscious control by the brain. Cardiac muscle makes up the heart and is under involuntary control.

Almost every muscle in the body attaches to bones through structures such as tendons. Tendons are specialized tough cords or bands of dense connective tissue that are continuous extensions of the periosteum.

In addition, most muscles cross one or more joints. Muscles contract to produce movement of the bones at the joints. They work in groups to produce smooth movements. When one muscle contracts to produce a movement, the antagonistic (opposing) muscles relax to allow the movement. Muscles contract in response to nerve stimulation. Because muscle fibers are elastic, the fibers return to their normal length after contracting. Not all skeletal muscles make bones move. Some muscles steady joints, allowing other muscles to act. These muscles assist with posture, permitting the body to sit or stand upright against gravitational pull. Like nerve cells, muscle fibers are excitable cells with high action potential, allowing them to respond to stimulation rapidly. See chapter 11 for more on neural function.

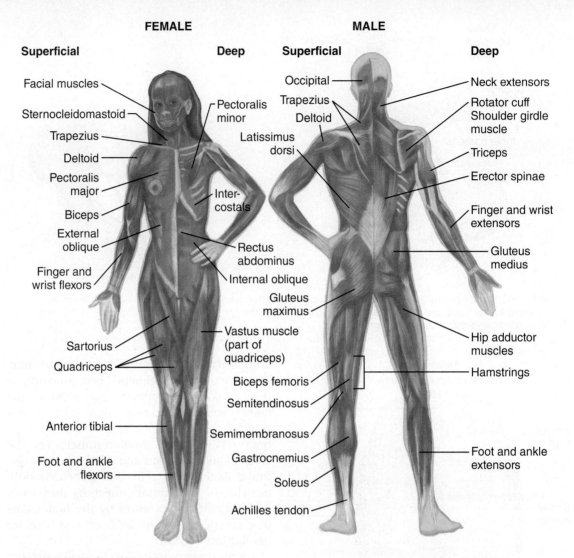

FIGURE 12-11 Skeletal muscles.

Skeletal muscles are composed of muscle fibers, connective tissue, blood vessels, and nerves (**FIGURE 12-12**). Each skeletal muscle fiber or cell (i.e., myocyte) is a cylinder with multiple nuclei. Within each fiber are myofibrils, thread-like structures extending for the entire length of the muscle fiber. Myofibrils contain two types of myofilaments (protein fibers)—actin and myosin. Actin myofilaments are involved in muscular contractions, cellular movement, and cell shape maintenance. Myosin myofilaments are darker and thicker than their actin counterparts. Myosin myofilaments are fibrous globulins (a type of protein) that work with actin to form actomyosin. The alignment of these two kinds of myofilaments gives the skeletal muscle its striated appearance (alternating light and dark bands) (**FIGURE 12-13**). Myofilaments are organized into repeated structural units called *sarcomeres* (Figure 12-12).

Muscle fibers contract when actin filaments slide over myosin filaments. In this process, the myosin filament pulls the actin filament. When calcium is released from inside the muscle fibers it then binds to troponin. The bound calcium and troponin cause movement of tropomyosin and expose an actin-binding site. The myosin attaches to the actin. Calcium is stored in the smooth endoplasmic reticulum, which forms an extensive network inside muscle fibers. Impulses from nerve cells at the neuromuscular junction result in release of neurotransmitters, such as acetylcholine, with subsequent depolarization and release of calcium. Once the calcium causes the head of the myosin to attach to the actin filament, adenosine triphosphate (ATP) in the muscle provides the energy needed to pull the actin filament inward. Relaxation occurs when there is no longer a signal or no ATP, calcium is pumped

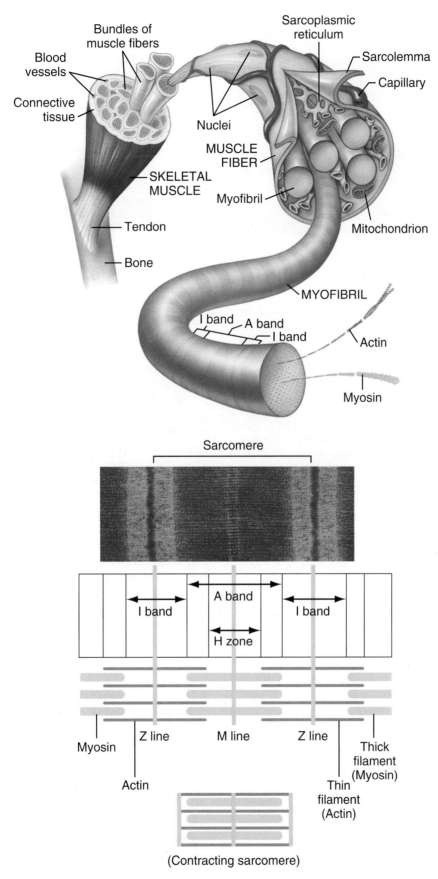

FIGURE 12-12 Structure of a skeletal muscle.

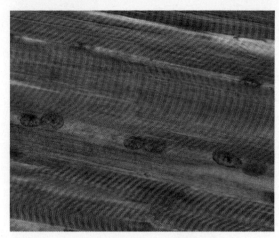

FIGURE 12-13 Striated pattern of skeletal muscle.
© Jose Luis Calvo/Shutterstock.

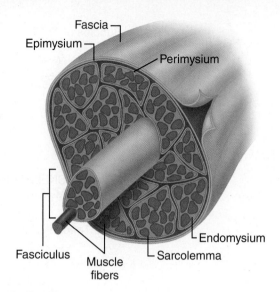

FIGURE 12-14 Muscle group.

back in, and tropomyosin covers the actin-binding sites. To meet the muscle cell's high-energy needs, ATP is recycled repeatedly in rapid succession. During vigorous activity, ATP stores become depleted, oxygen levels drop sharply, glucose production ceases, and lactic acid accumulates.

Each muscle fiber is enclosed by a cell membrane (sarcolemma) (**FIGURE 12-14**). Numerous muscle fibers are bundled together and surrounded by connective tissue called *endomysium*. Additional connective tissue called *perimysium* surrounds several of these bundles, grouping them together to form a muscle. Yet another layer of connective tissue called *epimysium* and fibrous connective tissue (fascia) surround these muscles. This fascia may also surround muscle groups. In the plantar portion of the foot, the fascia extends from the heel to the hallux (i.e., big toe). This fascia can become inflamed and cause plantar fasciitis, a common cause of foot and heel pain. Significant pressure or tension in the fascia of a limb (usually the legs) can compromise circulation and require an emergency fasciotomy (cutting of fascia) to restore circulation and save the limb.

Various normal physiologic changes can occur in the muscles with aging. The number of muscle fibers decreases with age, with less frequently used muscle declining quicker. The fibers also atrophy and are replaced with adipose tissue. Motor innervation is lost in a spotty manner. The consequence of all these changes is a decrease in muscle strength and efficiency over time. Muscle strength declines faster than mass. After the age of 50, muscle mass loss is approximately 10% and approaches 30% after the age of 80. Sarcopenia is the term to describe age-related muscle loss. The resulting effect is highly variable and dependent on physical activity and endurance prior to aging and on conditioning (i.e., exercising and training) with aging.

In addition to stimulating bone growth, growth hormone causes muscle growth. The number of muscle fibers or cells in a muscle remains relatively constant throughout the life span. Thus, increases in muscle sizes reflect increases in individual muscle fibers, rather than greater numbers of fibers. When muscles work harder, they respond by becoming larger and stronger. This increase in size and strength results from an increase in the amount of contractile protein inside the muscle fiber. Unfortunately, muscle protein is produced and destroyed quickly. In fact, approximately half of the muscle gained in a weight-lifting program is broken down 2 weeks after ceasing the activity. The only way to maintain the muscle gain is to continue the weight-lifting program.

Understanding Conditions That Affect the Musculoskeletal System

When considering alterations of the musculoskeletal system, organizing them based on their basic underlying pathophysiology and common anatomic location can increase understanding. In patients with musculoskeletal system disorders, multiple problems can occur that impair physical mobility, increasing the risk for injury and self-care deficits. Interventions are specifically selected to prevent complications of immobility (e.g., osteoporosis, renal calculi, thrombus, constipation, and pressure injuries). Musculoskeletal system disorders often cause acute or chronic pain and result in disability without prompt recognition and treatment.

Congenital and Developmental Musculoskeletal Disorders

Musculoskeletal disorders can be congenital in nature and can affect the bones (e.g., osteogenesis imperfecta), joints (e.g., developmental hip dysplasia), or muscle (e.g., muscular dystrophy). These congenital conditions may be apparent at birth or, alternatively, they may manifest as the child grows. During growth spurts in affected individuals, muscular development lags behind skeletal growth; this lag results in inadequate skeletal support. Some disorders are not congenital but rather occur during musculoskeletal development due to the vulnerabilities of the immature musculoskeletal structures (e.g., Osgood-Schlatter disease). Additionally, comorbidity of developmental abnormalities (e.g., Down syndrome and cerebral palsy) may become aggravated during growth periods. Musculoskeletal deformities require early treatment to prevent progression and complications.

Developmental Hip Dysplasia

Developmental dysplasia of the hip (DDH) occurs as a result of abnormal acetabular and proximal femur development. Previously, DDH was termed *congenital hip dislocation*; however, the disorder may manifest after birth (e.g., early infancy or childhood). Additionally, various instabilities can occur with the hip—not just dislocation (e.g., complete separation of two bones). Females are up to three times more likely to have DDH than males possibly due to females having an increased susceptibility to maternal hormone influences (e.g., relaxin). Risk factors for DDH include a breech position during the third trimester. Breech deliveries are more common with females, which may partially explain the higher incidence. A newborn may be born with stable hips; however, many newborns' hips are immature and may have laxity (looseness). In 90% of newborns who have physiologic laxity, resolution occurs spontaneously after a few weeks then development proceeds as normal. Tight infant swaddling with the hips fully adducted (toward midline) and extended (legs straight) has been associated with a higher incidence of DDH development. DDH can occur in the presence of other neuromuscular disorders, such as cerebral palsy or muscular dystrophy.

During normal intrauterine development, the hip joint (i.e., acetabulum, femur, and hip joint capsule) is formed by the 10th to 11th week of gestation. However, the femoral head grows fast and is still only partially covered by the acetabulum by the end of gestation. During the last month of gestation, the hip is subject to more forces that can continue to pull the femoral head away from the acetabulum. This pull worsens the lack of normal contact between these two structures that is necessary for normal hip development. In the presence of risk factors, DDH can develop. When the femoral head is not properly in the acetabulum, other structures such as the labrum (which is a soft tissue that covers the acetabulum) shift. The acetabulum can become shallow and ossified. Additional changes can ensue, including hypertrophy of joint structures, a thickening of the labrum, and contraction of hip muscles (e.g., iliopsoas).

Clinical Manifestations

DDH can include changes in the shape and position of the femoral head and acetabulum. The hip can be dislocated, or the femoral head can be partially outside the acetabulum. The femoral head is considered unstable if it is in the acetabulum at rest but can be moved out of the acetabulum with certain positions or during physical examination. The femoral head may be moved completely out (i.e., dislocatable) or partially out (i.e., subluxable). Dysplasia refers to an abnormality in shape. With DDH, the acetabulum is usually shallow and does not fully cover the femoral head. Most cases of DDH are unilateral and involve the left hip more than the right; however, DDH can be bilateral. The left hip is more frequently affected because a common position in utero is the left leg adducted against the mother's lumbosacral spine. The clinical manifestations of DDH can vary depending on the position, shape, and child's age and can include the following based on age:

Less Than 12 Months

- The hips are unstable—dislocated, subluxed—which occurs with different positions, or with inducement. With the Ortolani test, the unstable hip can be put back in place (i.e., reduced) when the hip is flexed and abducted. With the Barlow test, the hip that is in place but unstable can be dislocated or subluxed when the hips are flexed and adducted.

- Leg creases or folds (e.g., gluteal or thigh) are asymmetric.
- One femur appears shorter than the other when the knees are flexed and the heels are pushed toward the buttocks (i.e., Galeazzi sign) (FIGURE 12-15).
- The infant has limited hip abduction (usually < 45°). This sign is a better indicator in infants older than 3 months.

Older Than 12 Months (Walking)

- The child has an altered gait (i.e., manner of walking), such as Trendelenburg gait, in which the affected hip is higher (hiked up); the short leg is limp.
- The child has excessive lordosis.
- The adductors become more contracted, causing genu valgum (i.e., knock knees).
- The greater trochanter is prominent.

In some children, a dislocation may persist for a while without any symptoms. Dysplasia can occur even without dislocation, and the patient can be asymptomatic until adolescence or older in these circumstances. Under these circumstances, manifestations can include hip pain and symptoms of osteoarthritis.

Diagnosis and Treatment

DDH is diagnosed with a history and physical examination. Diagnostic imaging can include an ultrasound for young infants as the femoral head and acetabulum are still cartilaginous, so abnormalities may not be evident on

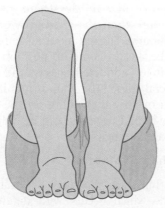

FIGURE 12-15 Galeazzi test.

X-ray. X-rays are used over ultrasound after 4–6 months of age when the structures have ossified.

Most cases of DDH will lead to no future problems if recognized and treated early. Hip examinations of newborn infants should occur after birth and routinely until the child is walking. Treatment strategies are aimed at reducing (resetting) the femoral head until the acetabulum can develop. This reduction can be accomplished with a splint (e.g., Pavlik harness), which is usually used for 2–3 months. DDH can be reduced manually (closed) or surgically (open), and a cast applied. Parents' teaching should include how to care for a child with a splint or cast and manifestations of potential treatment complications. The devices can cause skin breakdown, so the skin needs to be kept dry and clean.

Delivery via a cesarean section can reduce the amount of time an infant is in a breech position in utero and can reduce the incidence of DDH. After birth, parents can be taught proper swaddling techniques, such as making sure the infant can move, flex, and abduct the hips when swaddled. Any other devices, such as infant carriers, should allow hip flexion and abduction.

Osteogenesis Imperfecta

Osteogenesis imperfecta is a rare connective tissue disorder that results in fragile bones that fracture easily. This disorder is often referred to as *brittle bone disease.* The disorder is usually inherited in an autosomal dominant manner. Many subtypes (I–XI) can occur due to mutations in the collagen gene. The collagen affected is often type I collagen that is present in bones, tendons, ligaments, skin, and the sclerae. There are variable phenotypes. Some infants die in utero or shortly after birth (usually type II) as a result of multiple severe fractures and pulmonary failure.

Clinical manifestations include excessive (often > 100) and atypical (e.g., transverse) bone fractures. Bone deformities, such as in the skull, can result in nerve compression and neurologic symptoms. Bone deformities can range from mild to severe, and ligaments are lax. Bone deformities, such as short neck or cervical spine motion limitations, can cause airway problems. Cardiopulmonary abnormalities can include restrictive lung disease, heart valve and aortic abnormalities, and spine deviations such as kyphoscoliosis. Stature is often short, and some patients have short limbs (they have dwarfism). Hearing loss is common due to neural or conduction issues, such as fractures of the ossicles (bones in the ears) seen in some subtypes (e.g., type I). Osteoporosis development is premature. Teeth develop abnormally and wear away, a phenomenon termed *dentinogenesis imperfecta*. The sclera is blue (light to dark) in many subtypes. Type I is the mildest from of the disease with few fractures throughout life. Stature is usually normal; however, early and accelerated osteoporosis and hearing loss can occur. Bruising and bleeding disorders occur due to fragile capillaries and abnormal platelets.

Diagnosis is usually made based on a history and physical examination. In cases that are ambiguous, molecular genetic testing may be used to identify abnormalities of collagen type I, which are present in 90% of those patients with osteogenesis imperfecta. This type of genetic testing can be difficult to access as it is usually just conducted in research laboratories.

Therapies are directed at reducing chronic pain and maintaining functional capabilities by reducing fracture rate and preventing deformities. Care requires a multidisciplinary team, including clinicians specializing in osteogenesis imperfecta, surgeons, physical therapists, and occupational therapists. Bisphosphonate therapy is key in preventing bone resorption and bone turnover. Bone fractures are treated in the usual manner with fracture stabilization. Balancing safety and engagement in everyday activities can be challenging, and referral

for support services is important in improving quality of life for patients and their families. Life expectancy varies depending on the type.

Spinal Deviations

The spine consists of cervical, thoracic, lumbar, and sacral curves that exist to accommodate internal structures (e.g., abdominopelvic viscera) and allow the body to shift weight so that an upright position can be maintained. The vertebral bodies and intervertebral disks are the structures that form the spinal curves. Deviations in these normal curves can be a result of congenital or developmental disorders or degenerative spinal conditions, or from issues that originate outside the spine. The abnormal curvatures include scoliosis, lordosis, and kyphosis.

Kyphosis refers to an increase in the curvature of the thoracic spine outward (FIGURE 12-16). Often called *hunchback*, kyphosis is rarely present at birth. Instead, it can appear during the adolescent growth spurts as a disorder known as Scheuermann juvenile kyphosis. This kyphosis can appear as poor posture; although as opposed to poor posture, the curvature does not flatten when bending, extending, or lying supine. The disorder can affect the thoracic or thoracolumbar area. With Scheuermann juvenile kyphosis, pain is worse with activity and improves with rest. In adults, kyphosis usually develops secondary to osteoporosis, degenerative spine disease (e.g., arthritis or disk degeneration), or injury (e.g., vertebral fractures). Flexibility and ligamentous spinal support decreases

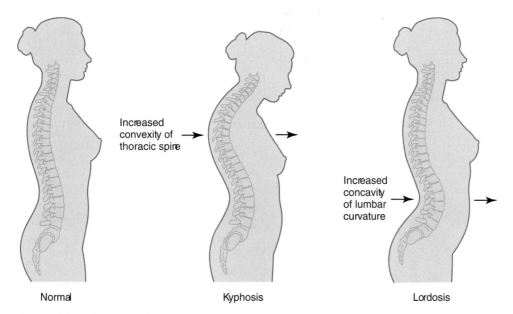

Normal   Kyphosis   Lordosis

FIGURE 12-16 Kyphosis and lordosis.

with aging, leading to an inability to correct and maintain posture and development of kyphosis. Severe kyphosis can impair lung expansion and ventilation. Additionally, patients with this disorder are at increased risk for injury because of alterations in their center of gravity. Other manifestations may include fatigue, back pain, and spine stiffness.

Lordosis refers to an exaggerated concave of the lumbar spine (Figure 12-16). Often called *swayback*, lordosis may develop during adolescent growth spurts or because of poor posture. Obesity and pregnancy can increase the tendency toward this posture because of an altered center of gravity and postural compensation. Lordosis is also commonly associated with dwarfism.

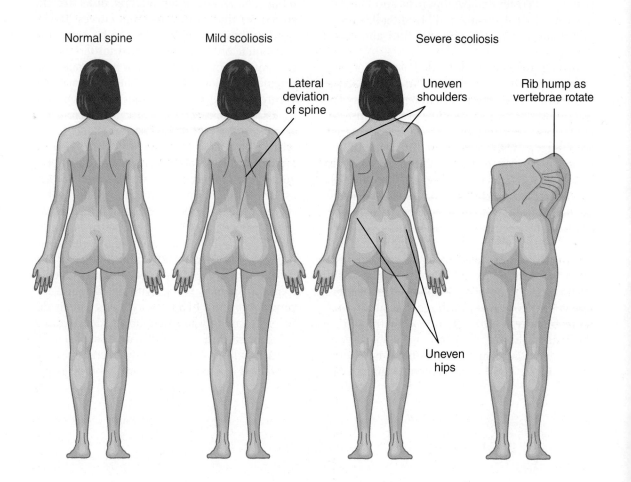

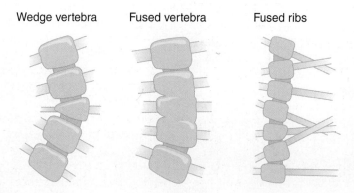

FIGURE 12-17 Scoliosis.

Scoliosis refers to a lateral deviation of the spine (FIGURE 12-17). This lateral curvature may affect the thoracic area, the lumbar area, or both. Scoliosis may also include a rotation of the vertebrae on their axis. Stress on the vertebrae causes an imbalance in osteoclast activity; therefore, the curvature increases during growth spurts. Scoliosis may also be associated with kyphosis and lordosis.

Scoliosis varies in severity and is more common in females. Most cases are idiopathic and occur during rapid growth periods in adolescence. Idiopathic cases prior to the age of 9 years are less frequent. While the cause is usually idiopathic, known causes may include genetic influences, embryonic developmental deformities, degenerative diseases, unequal leg lengths, spinal nerve compression, and asymmetric muscle support. The genetic influences are autosomal dominant; embryonic involvement usually includes the hemivertebrae; degenerative diseases include osteoporosis and osteoarthritis; and asymmetric muscle support includes partial paralysis, muscular dystrophy, cerebral palsy, poliomyelitis, trauma, and spinal tumors. Complications of scoliosis include pulmonary compromise, chronic pain, degenerative arthritis of the spine, intervertebral disk disease, and sciatica.

Clinical manifestations of spinal deviations will vary depending on the degree and location of the curvature. Spinal deviations are exaggerated in certain positions, such as when an affected person bends over (Adams forward bend test). The forward bend test is useful, particularly with scoliosis. Deviations may be best noted by viewing the patient from the side. The manifestations may include the following symptoms:

- Asymmetric hip and shoulder or scapulae alignment
- Asymmetric thoracic cage or waistline
- Asymmetric gait
- Abnormal curvature in certain positions when it should be flat (e.g., in juvenile kyphosis)
- Back pain or discomfort
- Fatigue
- Indications of respiratory compromise (e.g., dyspnea and reduced chest expansion)

Because of the prevalence of scoliosis in adolescent females, schools often conduct periodic scoliosis screening. Diagnostic procedures for spinal deviations consist of a history and physical examination, including the use of a scoliometer, which measures the angle of trunk rotation. Spinal X-rays are necessary to confirm a spinal deviation diagnosis. The Cobb angle is a quantitative measure determined with an X-ray for scoliosis and is reported as a degree. A Cobb angle of $> 10°$ is diagnostic of scoliosis. The Cobb angle measurement is also assessed with kyphosis, and while there are different reference ranges, $\geq 40°$ is usually a cutoff for older adults. The higher the Cobb angle, the higher the severity. Imaging tests may include a computed tomography (CT), magnetic resonance imaging (MRI), and other tests to evaluate for underlying causes (e.g., spinal tumor and spondylolisthesis).

Without treatment, the curvature associated with kyphosis, lordosis, and scoliosis often progresses in adulthood. Patient outcomes improve with early treatment. Treatment strategies may include exercises with a focus on flexibility, core strengthening, and posture. These exercises should be continued throughout life. Analgesics may be used to manage pain. Spinal bracing and surgical correction (with instrumentation or fusion) are additional options.

Traumatic Musculoskeletal Disorders

Traumatic musculoskeletal disorders are usually mild and easily treated; however, occasionally these conditions can result in life-threatening complications (e.g., fat embolism and osteomyelitis). Many of these conditions are caused by events like the ones that lead to traumatic neurologic disorders (e.g., falls, motor vehicle accidents, and sports-related injuries). Additionally, neurologic dysfunction may occur in conjunction with the musculoskeletal injury. These traumatic conditions are on the rise because of increasing numbers of children and adults participating in fitness, recreation, and sport activities. Factors contributing to these injuries include inappropriate or inadequate equipment, training, or warm-up techniques; more aggressive approaches to sports; and failure to allow minor injuries to heal. Traumatic injuries can be localized and involve only one area of the body or one anatomic structure such as a bone fracture, tendinitis, or bursitis. However, injury in one area often involves surrounding tissues such as the muscle or blood vessels.

Fractures

A fracture is a break in the rigid structure of the bone that occurs when any stress applied to the bone is greater than its strength (**FIGURE 12-18**). Fractures are the most common type of traumatic musculoskeletal disorders. They mainly occur as a primary condition because of falls, motor vehicle accidents, and sports-related injuries. Additionally, fractures can occur secondary to conditions that weaken the bone (e.g., osteoporosis, Paget disease, and bone cancer). While fractures can occur on any or many parts of the bone, certain regions are more prone to fracture. The physis is where long bones grow and are the areas prone to fractures in children; because of the increased vascularity, infections are more likely in this area. The metaphysis is composed mostly of softer (spongy and trabecular) bone tissue and is vulnerable to compressive-type forces and resultant compression fracture. Fractures are classified based on characteristics such as the direction of the fracture line, the number of fracture lines, or other characteristics (**FIGURE 12-19**). Fracture types include the following:

- **Simple fracture:** A fracture with a single break in the bone and in which bone ends maintain their alignment and position:
  - **Transverse fracture:** A fracture straight across the bone shaft
  - **Oblique fracture:** A fracture at an angle to the bone shaft
  - **Spiral fracture:** A fracture that twists around the bone shaft
- **Comminuted fracture:** A fracture characterized by multiple fracture lines and bone pieces
- **Greenstick fracture:** An incomplete fracture in which the bone is bent and only the outer curve of the bend is broken; commonly occurs in children because of minimal calcification and often heals quickly.
- **Compression fracture:** A fracture in which the bone is crushed or collapses into small pieces.

A variety of other terms may be used to describe a fracture. For example, fractures may be described based on the degree of break. Complete fractures occur when the bone is broken into two or more separate pieces; in contrast, in incomplete fractures, the bone is partially broken (e.g., greenstick fracture). Additionally, fractures may be described as open or closed.

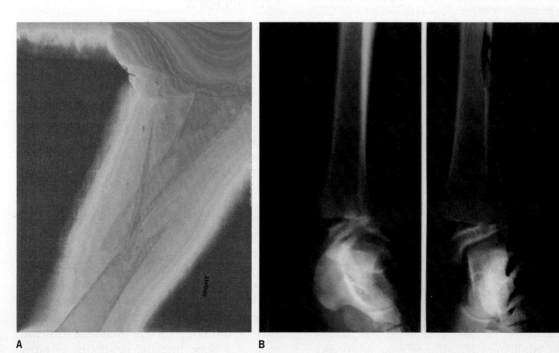

A   B

FIGURE 12-18 Fractures.
A: © Carolina K. Smith, MD/Shutterstock; **B:** © ESB Basic/Shutterstock.

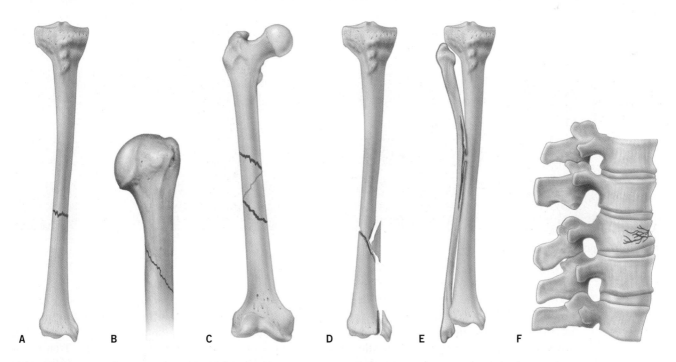

FIGURE 12-19 Classifications of fractures. **(A)** Transverse fracture of the tibia. **(B)** Oblique fracture of the humerus. **(C)** Spiral fracture of the femur. **(D)** Comminuted fracture of the tibia. **(E)** Greenstick fracture of the fibula. **(F)** Compression fracture of a vertebral body.

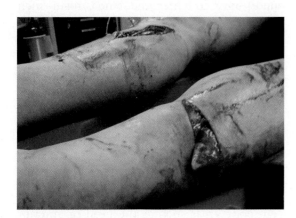

FIGURE 12-20 Open fracture.
Courtesy of Rhonda Hunt.

In open fractures, or compound fractures, the skin is broken (**FIGURE 12-20**). The bone fragments or edges may be angled and protrude out of the skin. Open fractures are characterized by more damage to soft tissue and are at risk for infection. In closed fractures, the skin is intact. Impacted fractures occur when one end of the bone is forced into the adjacent bone. Pathologic fractures result from a weakness in the bone structure secondary to conditions such as bone tumors or osteoporosis. Stress fractures, or fatigue fractures, occur from repeated excessive stress. These fractures are common in the tibia, femur, and metatarsals.

Intra-articular fractures are those that cross the articular cartilage and enter the joint. Finally, depressed fractures occur in the skull when the broken piece is forced inward on the brain.

When a bone breaks, blood from damaged vessels in the periosteum and bone marrow pours into the fracture and forms a hematoma, or blood clot (**FIGURE 12-21**). This first step in fracture healing is known as the inflammatory phase. Necrosis occurs to the broken ends of the bone because of the blood vessel damage. Over time, the necrotic tissue is reabsorbed and replaced by new bone. This reabsorbed necrotic bone makes fracture lines and is seen on an X-ray, usually within 10 days after an injury. The second step in healing is the reparative phase. Within a few days of the fracture, new blood vessels start to form outside the bone and fibroblasts (connective tissue from the periosteum) invade the clot. These fibroblasts secrete collagen fibers, which form a mass of cells and fibers called a *cartilaginous callus*. The callus bridges the broken bone ends together inside and outside. The callus takes 2–6 weeks to form. The third step in healing is the remodeling phase. At that point, osteoblasts from the periosteum invade the callus, which slowly convert the callus to bone. This ossification process can take from 3 weeks to several months (usually 4–6 weeks) to reach

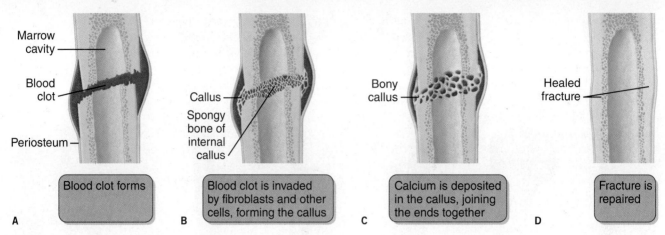

FIGURE 12-21 Stages of fracture repair.

completion. Healing time can vary depending on age (e.g., young children quickly remodel), nutritional status, blood supply, and fracture type and location. The callus is initially a large, often palpable structure, but osteoclasts gradually remodel the bone by removing the excess bone. This remodeling process leaves little to no evidence that the fracture occurred and may take as long as a year.

Multiple complications can result from fractures. The types of complications are dependent of the severity and location of the fractures (e.g., rib fractures can cause lung injury). Delayed union (nonhealing before 20 weeks), malunion, or nonunion, for example, may occur due to poor nutrition, inadequate blood supply, malalignment (e.g., inadequate reduction), infection, and premature weight-bearing. X-rays should reveal fracture healing progress. Nonunion refers to fractures that demonstrate no healing after treatment or on X-rays. Several factors, such as diabetes or smoking, can impair healing. Fractures can cause arterial damage, nerve injury, and deep vein thrombosis, particularly fractures of the lower extremity (e.g., hip, pelvis, femur, or tibia). Other fracture complications may include compartment syndrome, fat embolism, osteomyelitis, and osteonecrosis.

Compartment syndrome is a serious condition that results from increased pressure in a compartment, usually the muscle fascia in the case of fractures. This pressure impinges on the nerves and blood vessels present within the compartment, potentially compromising the distal extremity. Compartment syndrome requires prompt identification and treatment to prevent permanent tissue damage from anoxia. Clinical manifestations usually include

excruciating pain beyond what would be expected given the injury. Compartment syndrome can be diagnosed by measuring pressures inside the muscle fascia. Treatment usually includes removing the cast (if present) and performing an immediate fasciotomy to relieve the pressure.

A fat embolism occurs when fat has an opportunity to enter the bloodstream such as during surgery. Fatty marrow can enter the bloodstream after a fracture to one of the long bones or pelvic fractures. A fat embolism, while commonly caused by orthopedic injuries, can occur due to several conditions such as burns, liposuction, and soft tissue injuries. Although a fat embolism is a rare occurrence, the outcome can be fatal if the emboli travel to vital organs such as the lungs, brain, or heart. Fat emboli presents with a triad of hypoxemia, neurologic abnormalities (e.g., mental status changes), and a petechial rash on nondependent body areas such as the head or anterior thorax. Diagnosis is made with X-rays and CT of the chest. Other tests, such as imaging of the brain, may be indicated if neurologic symptoms are present. Treatment is supportive, and patients can spontaneously and fully recover. Fat embolism can be prevented with early immobilization of the fracture.

Osteomyelitis refers to an infection of the bone tissue. The infection causes a delay in healing. It is a serious complication of fractures because it often goes undetected, can take months to resolve, and can result in bone or tissue necrosis. In children, the vascular metaphysis is often the site where the infection spreads; in adults, the infection occurs through external contact with bone (e.g., open fracture or surgical fixation). In adults and children, a common organism is *Staphylococcus aureus* followed by group A beta hemolytic streptococci in children and *Pseudomonas aeruginosa* in adults. Osteomyelitis can also occur through mechanisms other than fractures such as bite wounds, pressure injuries, puncture wounds, or diabetic foot ulcers, and organisms may be different. The routes of spread can vary but are either through blood or direct inoculation with an organism. Acute osteomyelitis may cause pain, tenderness, erythema, increased warmth, and fever. Chronic osteomyelitis may have similar symptoms as acute osteomyelitis except for the absence of fever, and the pain may be intermittent. White blood cell count will be elevated in acute osteomyelitis. Inflammatory markers, such as the erythrocyte sedimentation rate and the C-reactive protein, will also increase with acute or chronic osteomyelitis. A CT scan or MRI is better than X-rays to make a diagnosis. Osteomyelitis is treated with potent antibiotic therapy (often delivered on a long-term basis) and surgery (e.g., debridement).

Osteonecrosis, or avascular necrosis, is death of bone tissue due to a loss of the blood supply to that tissue. It can result from displaced fractures or dislocations but can also occur due to atraumatic conditions such as corticosteroid use or alcoholism. Osteonecrosis may be asymptomatic or cause pain. While osteonecrosis can occur in various regions, locations with a higher incidence include the femoral head, knee, and scaphoid or lunate bone in the wrist. An X-ray or MRI is used to confirm diagnosis. Osteonecrosis often requires surgical replacement of the necrotic bone and/or joint.

The following clinical manifestations of a fracture reflect the tissue trauma caused by the bone fragments as well as the disruption of function:

- Deformity (e.g., angulation, shortening, and rotation)
- Swelling at the site (due to the inflammatory process triggered by the tissue trauma)
- Inability to move the affected limb
- Crepitus (grating sound or sensation, usually occurring with movement)
- Pain (results from tissue trauma and muscle spasms triggered by the bone fragments)
- Paresthesia
- Muscle flaccidity progressing to spasms

Diagnostic procedures for fractures consist of a history and physical examination with a focus on neurovascular assessment. X-rays are necessary and consist of anterior–posterior and lateral views. Additional X-ray views, such as an oblique angle, may be necessary depending on suspected fracture location. X-rays of the joint above and below the injury are usually performed. Treatment strategies include immediate immobilization with devices such as splints or traction (application of a force or weight pulling a limb). The fracture is reduced to restore the bone to its normal position. Reduction can be accomplished with closed manipulation by applying pressure or traction or with open manipulation via surgery. During surgery, devices such as pins, plates, rods, or screws may be placed to secure the bone fragments in position. These instruments may be either internal and permanent or externally fixated and gradually retracted. Any necrotic tissue or foreign material is also removed in a process called *debridement*. When a fracture is suspected, the individual with the injury should not consume anything by mouth in case surgery is deemed necessary. Surgical repair may be delayed up to a few days after the injury to allow the edema secondary to the inflammatory response to resolve. Immobilization of the fracture during this time and throughout the entire reparative phase is crucial to prevent complications and allow for development of new blood vessels. Long-term immobilization that permits bone healing to occur is accomplished with slings, casts, splints, or traction. Traction maintains bone alignment and prevents muscle spasms. As the fracture is healing, exercise is helpful to limit muscle atrophy, joint stiffness, and contracture formation as well as to maintain adequate circulation.

Dislocations

Dislocation refers to the separation of two bones where they meet at a joint (FIGURE 12-22). With this type of injury, the two bones are no longer in their normal position. The dislocation may involve a complete or partial loss of contact (i.e., subluxation). Such an injury causes deformity and immobility of the joints, and it may damage nearby ligaments and nerves. Dislocations usually result from a sudden impact to the joint, but they may also be congenital (e.g., developmental dysplasia of the hip) or pathologic (e.g., arthritis, ligament injuries, paralysis, or neuromuscular disease). Any joint can be affected, but dislocations are especially common in the inherently unstable shoulder joint. The shoulder commonly dislocates anteriorly

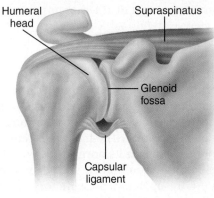

Humeral head · Supraspinatus · Glenoid fossa · Capsular ligament

Normal

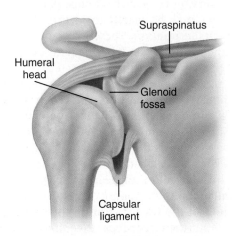

Supraspinatus · Humeral head · Glenoid fossa · Capsular ligament

Anterior dislocation

FIGURE 12-22 Anterior dislocation of the shoulder.

while posterior and inferior shoulder dislocations are not as common.

Clinical manifestations of a dislocated joint may include the following signs and symptoms:

- Visibly out-of-place, discolored, or deformed joint
- Limited movement
- Swelling or bruising
- Intense pain, especially with movement or weight-bearing
- Paresthesia near the injury (often distal to the injury)

Diagnostic procedures for dislocations consist of a history, physical examination, X-rays, and MRI. Treatment strategies focus on limiting tissue damage by initial immobilization and subsequent reduction of the joint. Treatment depends on the site and severity of the injury. Reduction may occur spontaneously, or gentle manipulation may be used to return the bones to their usual position (closed reduction). Surgical reduction may be necessary for extensive injury and when blood vessels or nerves are damaged. Depending on the amount of pain and swelling, a local anesthetic or **procedural sedation and anesthesia** (PSA) may be used.

The decision to administer PSA is dependent on the duration of the dislocation (e.g., medical personnel may be able to attempt

BOX 12-1 Application to Practice

Gina Dickerson is a 34-year-old woman who is being admitted to the orthopedic unit following a motor vehicle accident. She was driving her car through an intersection when someone ran a stop sign and hit her vehicle. Ms. Dickerson was diagnosed in the emergency department with a compound fracture of the left femur and a comminuted fracture of the left ankle.

When this patient arrived in the orthopedic unit at 1600, her left leg was immobilized with an air cast and ice bags were applied. She was medicated in the emergency department

with morphine sulfate, 2 mg intravenously at 1200. The unit admission assessment data revealed that Ms. Dickerson had no significant medical problems. Her vital signs on admission to the unit were as follows: temperature, 99.2° F; pulse, 90 beats per minute; respirations, 24 breaths per minute; oxygen saturation, 95% on room air; and blood pressure, 140/80 mmHg. She was scheduled for surgery in the morning to repair both fractures.

1. Explain the type of fractures this patient has incurred.

2. What are some complications that this patient is at high risk for developing and what are prevention strategies?
3. Develop a treatment plan that includes pharmacologic and nonpharmacologic strategies.
4. Explain how you would educate the patient pertaining to the healing process and possible time frame for recuperation.

reduction without sedation if it is recent), the location of the dislocation, the mechanism of injury, and associated injuries. PSA can be performed outside the operating room, but close patient monitoring is necessary as adverse cardiovascular and pulmonary effects can be life threatening. PSA is indicated for painful and anxiety-provoking procedures, for which deep relaxation would allow for the ability of the clinician to optimally perform the intervention. PSA is often used for closed reduction of fractures, joints, and several other nonorthopedic procedures such as laceration repair or drainage of an abscess. The various levels of sedation are defined by the American Society of Anesthesiologists (2014), and these levels range from minimal sedation to general anesthesia and dissociative sedation (e.g., use of ketamine) as a separate category. The deeper the sedation level, the higher the risk for cardiopulmonary compromise. General anesthesia has the highest risk and requires maintenance of mechanical ventilation. Close monitoring during PSA includes frequent evaluation of vital signs, oxygen saturation, end-tidal carbon dioxide level, and electrocardiogram monitoring.

After joint reduction, the joint will need to be immobilized with a splint or sling for several weeks. Analgesics and muscle relaxants may be required during this recovery period. After the splint or sling is removed, a gradual rehabilitation program (primarily physical therapy) designed to restore the joint's range of motion and strength is often needed. Strenuous activity involving the injured joint should be avoided until full movement, normal strength, and stability have been regained.

Some dislocations, such as those involving the hip, may need up to several months to heal.

Healing of dislocations is also slowed when ligament or soft-tissue damage is present. Preinjury function is usually restored, but some residual deficits may occur in more severe injuries.

Sprains

A sprain is an injury to a ligament that often involves stretching or tearing of the ligament. Sprains are caused when a joint is forced to move into an unnatural position (e.g., twisting one's ankle). Sprains are uncommon in children whose growth plates are still open and in adults with frail bones. Ligaments can be stronger than the area of the growth plate or a frail bone; hence, a fracture can occur before a ligament tear during an injury. Growth plate or physeal fractures are termed *Salter-Harris fractures*. Avulsion fractures, where the ligament or tendon pulls off a piece of bone, are more common in children. The severity of the sprain is described using a grading scale (**TABLE 12-2**; **FIGURE 12-23**). Of all sprains, ankle, knee, and wrist sprains occur most often. Such an injury triggers the inflammatory process, resulting in edema and pain at the site. Additionally, blood vessels may be damaged, resulting in bleeding and bruising, which appears soon after the injury or within 48 hours. Bleeding into the joint capsule can delay healing. If a tear occurs, granulation tissue develops along with the inflammation. Collagen fibers form to create a link between the torn ligament fragments, and eventually fibrous tissue binds them together. Sprained ligaments swell rapidly and are painful. Generally, the degree of pain reflects the severity of injury. Other clinical manifestations may include joint stiffness, limited function, disability, difficulty bearing weight, and discoloration (usually bruising).

TABLE 12-2	Sprain Grading System	

Grade	Degree of damage	Clinical findings and implications
Grade I	Partial tear, stable joint: Minimal damage or disruption	Tender without swelling No bruising Active and passive range of motion are painful Prognosis is good, with no expectation of instability or functional loss
Grade II	Partial tear with some ligamentous laxity: Moderate damage	Moderate swelling and bruising Very tender, with more diffuse tenderness than grade I Range of motion is very painful and restricted Joint may be unstable, and functional loss may result
Grade III	Complete tear with ligamentous laxity	Prognosis is variable (injury may require surgery) Requires a prolonged healing/rehabilitation period

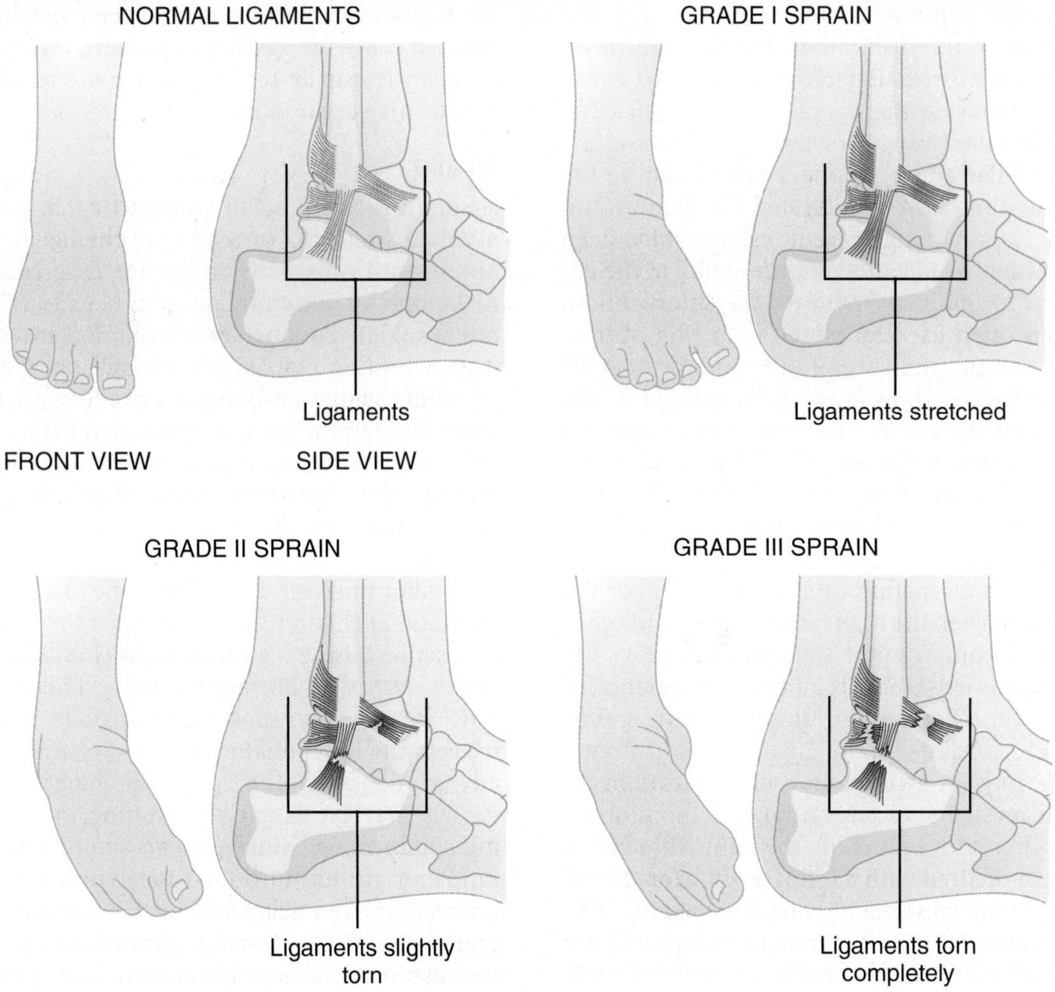

NORMAL LIGAMENTS

GRADE I SPRAIN

Ligaments

FRONT VIEW   SIDE VIEW

Ligaments stretched

GRADE II SPRAIN

GRADE III SPRAIN

Ligaments slightly
torn

Ligaments torn
completely

FIGURE 12-23 Sprain grading system.

Diagnostic procedures for sprains consist of a history and physical examination, including the contralateral, uninjured extremity. The stability of the joint is evaluated using manual stress maneuvers that are unique to each joint. As an example, the Lachman test is performed to evaluate the stability of the anterior cruciate ligament in the knee. In this exam, the injured knee is flexed to 30° while the patient is lying supine. With one hand, the examiner holds the femur in place just above the knee, and with the other hand, the tibia is gently pulled forward. If the tibia moves freely, then an anterior cruciate tear is likely as this ligament stabilizes anterior knee movement. An X-ray is indicated only if a fracture is suspected. MRI is a good diagnostic test to evaluate for soft tissue injuries and could be performed with severe injuries.

Although surgical repair might be necessary for ligament tears, most sprains can be managed at home. Treatment strategies include the following measures:

- Apply ice immediately to reduce pain and swelling. Wrap the ice in a cloth—do not place ice directly on the skin because it can worsen tissue damage.
- Immobilize the joint with a splint or an elastic wrap or bandage.
- Elevate the swollen joint above the level of the heart.
- Rest the affected joint for several days and gradually increase activity.
- Provide nonsteroidal anti-inflammatory drugs (NSAIDs; e.g., ibuprofen) to relieve pain and inflammation.

Treatment for Soft-Tissue Injuries

Treatment strategies for soft-tissue injuries such as sprains and strains can be remembered using the acronym PRICE.

P Protect the injured limb from further injury by not using the joint. The patient may need crutches or splints to accomplish this.

R Rest the injured limb, but do not avoid all activity; exercise other muscles to minimize deconditioning.

I Ice the affected area (e.g., with a cold pack, a slush bath, or a compression sleeve filled with cold water) as soon as possible after injury to limit swelling, and continue to ice the area for 10–15 minutes (any longer than that may cause tissue damage) four times a day for 48 hours.

C Compress the area with an elastic wrap or bandage; compressive wraps or sleeves made from elastic or neoprene are best.

E Elevate the injured limb above the level of the heart whenever possible to help prevent or limit swelling.

- Keep pressure off the injured area until pain subsides (usually 7–10 days for mild sprains and 3–5 weeks for severe sprains); however, duration is dependent on the affected joint. The injured person may require crutches when walking.
- Rehabilitate the injured area (usually including physical therapy) to regain joint motion and strength, beginning within 1 week.

Strains

A **strain** is an injury to a muscle, tendon, or the muscular tendon (myotendinous) junction that often involves stretching or tearing of the muscle or tendon. *Tendinitis* is usually the term used to describe acute tendon inflammation, and tendinopathy is used to describe persistent or chronic localized tendon pain with loss of function. Tendinitis and strains may occur suddenly or develop over time. A strain, often referred to as a *pulled muscle*, results from an awkward muscle movement or excess force that can be caused by an accident, improper use of a muscle or tendon, or overuse of a muscle or tendon. Tendinopathy is an overuse syndrome. Excessive physical activity, improper stretching prior to activity, and poor flexibility can contribute to this injury. Collagen changes in aging cause a decrease in elasticity, making older adults vulnerable to strains. The lower back is the most common site for strains. Strains also often occur at the muscle tendon connection in a muscle that is attached to two joints such as the hamstring or quadriceps. Some common locations for development of tendinopathy include the shoulder (rotator cuff), elbow (lateral epicondyle), thigh (hamstring, quadriceps), knee (patella), and ankle (Achilles tendon). In children or adolescents, strains tend to occur at growth plates. The severity of a muscle strain is described using a grading scale similar to that used for sprains (Table 12-2) except the range is from I to IV. A tear to a few muscle fibers (< 10%) is a grade I, and a complete tear of all fibers with fascia disruption is a grade IV strain (i.e., rupture).

Strains and tendinitis follow the same pathogenesis pathway as sprains (e.g., inflammation, granulation, and bleeding). Scar tissue may be present as the tissue heals. Tendinopathy is often referred to as *tendinitis*. Inflammation may be present during the development of tendinopathy, but inflammation is usually minimal or absent as the tendinopathy becomes persistent. In tendinopathy, there are few inflammatory cells, but the tendon structure changes and becomes thickened and scarred. With aging, the body is less able to self-repair the repetitive microtrauma that occurs with loading-type activities. Tendon injuries, like muscle injuries, are more likely with aging. Clinical manifestations of a strain include pain, stiffness, difficulty moving the affected muscle, skin discoloration (often bruising), and edema.

With tendinopathy, edema is usually absent and pain is over the affected tendon and occurs when palpated or when the tendon is loaded. If the tendon is superficially located (e.g., Achilles tendon), the tendon may appear and feel thick.

Diagnostic procedures for strains may consist of a history, physical examination, MRIs, and ultrasound. X-rays may be used with suspected bone involvement. Treatment in the acute phase of strains is similar to that for sprains. Tendon tears might require surgery, but most other treatment options can be managed by the patient and include the following:

- Applying ice immediately to reduce pain and swelling; wrapping the ice in cloth and not placing ice directly on the skin because it can worsen tissue damage.
- Using ice for the first 3 days; after that, either heat or ice may be helpful.
- Resting the affected muscle for at least a day.

- Keeping the affected muscle elevated above the level of the heart if possible.
- Avoiding use of the affected muscle until pain subsides; then, advancing activity slowly and in moderation.
- Using NSAIDs to relieve pain and inflammation.
- Using muscle relaxants to relieve muscle stiffness.
- Rehabilitating the injured area (usually including physical therapy) to regain muscle movement and strength as necessary.

Chronic tendinopathy can be difficult to treat and often requires many months of treatment. Rehabilitation (usually with a trained therapist) may result in decreased pain and improved function. Proper body mechanics should be emphasized. Investigational therapies for tendinopathy include topical nitroglycerin, prolotherapy (injection of substances such as dextrose or lidocaine in the tendon), sclerotherapy (injecting a substance in the tendon to reduce neovascularization), dry needling (inserting a needle to stimulate healing), injections of autologous blood/platelets, ultrasound therapy, shockwave therapy, and laser therapy.

Child Abuse

Child abuse and neglect are a significant health problem in the United States with one in four children having experienced abuse or neglect at some point in their life (CDC, 2017). In 2017, approximately 674,000 children were identified as victims of child abuse or neglect by child protective service agencies, and 1,720 abused or neglected children died. The risk for health consequences and chronic illnesses as a result of child abuse continue into adulthood. Physical abuse of children, one component of child abuse and neglect, results in musculoskeletal injuries, predominantly soft tissue injuries followed by fractures. The highest incidence of fractures is in children younger than 3 years old, and children under 12 months sustain the most fractures from physical abuse. Overall, abuse and neglect are three times higher in children under 12 months of age (Child Trends, 2018). In all 50 states, healthcare workers are required by law to report suspected child abuse to an appropriate agency, such as child protective services. Based on history or physical examination, physical abuse should be suspected in the following circumstances:

History
- Denial of trauma despite severe injury
- History that is inconsistent with the degree or type of injury
- Delay in seeking health care
- Injury attributed to attempts at resuscitating the child or blamed on other young children or pets, or explained as self-inflicted
- Conflicting or changing histories between caregivers or other observers

Physical Examination
- Bruising, particularly in premobile infants or in the pattern of an object (e.g., belt mark).
- Human bite marks.
- Bruising on the upper extremities, face, neck, or buttocks.
- Oral injuries, such as tongue lacerations or broken teeth.
- Burns, particularly those with sharply demarcating edges (no splash pattern) or those in the shape of an object or cigarette burns.
- Fractures, particularly of the ribs, upper torso (e.g., sternum), spinous process, or long bones.
- Multiple fractures in various healing stages.
- Epiphyseal separations.
- Abdominal and intracranial injuries (e.g., perforated bowel or subdural hematoma).

The injuries sustained from physical abuse are evaluated with the same diagnostic tests as for other traumatic injuries (e.g., X-rays, MRI, CT scans). Prior to treating injuries, photographs should be taken; however, parental permission may be necessary depending on state laws. Treatment strategies are the same as those used for other musculoskeletal trauma (e.g., fracture stabilization).

Bursitis

Bursitis is an inflammation of the fluid-filled, saclike structures that provide a cushion between bones, tendons, and muscles around a joint (FIGURE 11-24). The bursae have an inner lining of synovial cells, and a small amount of fluid is produced. This cushion reduces friction and facilitates the gliding motion of muscles over each other and over bony prominences. Over 150 bursae are located throughout the body. Trauma, prolonged pressure, strenuous physical exertion, and overuse of a joint can lead to bursitis. Bursitis can occur with inflammatory disorders such as gout or rheumatoid arthritis. Septic bursitis usually results from an infection from an injury that penetrates the skin or repetitive trauma and can less commonly be spread through blood. Septic bursitis is more common in individuals with alcoholism and diabetes and in those who are immunosuppressed. Superficial bursa, such as those over the olecranon or around the patella, are vulnerable to septic bursitis. Bursitis can occur with muscle and tendon disorders. Bursitis can occur in many different bursae, but the usual locations are the elbow (i.e., olecranon bursitis), the hip (i.e., trochanteric bursitis), and the knee (i.e., prepatellar or infrapatellar bursitis).

Inflammation occurs with acute types of bursitis, which usually results from trauma and disorders such as gout where crystals get deposited in the joint. Acute bursitis results in a sudden increase in pressure within the bursa with pain over the bursa that worsens with flexion of the joint (e.g., olecranon bursitis worsens with elbow flexion). Edema may be seen in bursae that are superficial; however, some bursae are deep, and edema may not be clinically evident. Chronic bursitis, as with tendinopathy, is usually the result of repetitive overuse or chronic joint inflammation (e.g., rheumatoid arthritis). With chronic bursitis, the pressure within the bursae is gradual, so the joint has time to adapt, resulting in less pain in comparison to acute bursitis. The bursa, however, are considerably swollen and thick. Septic bursitis manifestations include pain, erythema, swelling, and warmth.

Diagnosis is based on the history and physical examination findings. Imaging may not be necessary for superficial bursa. Imaging may be necessary for deeper bursa and to evaluate for underlying disorders. Bursitis may be evident on ultrasound and MRI but not on X-rays, which are usually performed to evaluate for underlying fracture. When an infection or crystals are suspected, aspiration and analysis of the bursal fluid can be completed. Treatment strategies include pain relief with NSAIDs. A local anesthetic and a glucocorticoid can be injected into the bursa. Ice or heating pads can also provide pain relief. Septic bursitis treatment includes antibiotics. Patients should be taught about avoiding activities or using protective equipment to promote healing and prevent recurrence. As an example, knee bursitis can occur in occupations that require excessive kneeling such as a janitor or carpet layer, and knee pads may be helpful.

Anatomic-Specific Injuries

Injuries to specific anatomic regions are common. Most injuries are a result of overuse. Playing sports or exercising and occupational demands are some of the many circumstances leading to an overuse injury. The injuries can occur to the tendon, ligament, bursa, or joint but often affect surrounding structures and tissues. These injuries can significantly affect quality of life and cause chronic or recurring pain and impair mobility. Healing and rehabilitation can take a long time. The following is an overview of some select anatomic-specific injuries with risk factors, etiologies, manifestations, and diagnostic techniques. Treatment strategies are often similar to other general musculoskeletal disorders and only the differences (if applicable) will be discussed.

Shoulder

Adhesive capsulitis (i.e., frozen shoulder) is caused by an idiopathic loss of active and passive range of motion. It is unclear whether the underlying pathophysiology is a result of an inflammatory or fibrosing condition. The disorder is often associated with other diseases, with a higher prevalence in those with diabetes mellitus, particularly type 1. The incidence is higher in women. Usually the disorder affects one shoulder and presents as severe, diffuse pain worse at night with stiffness and decreased range of motion (known as the freezing phase). This phase is then followed by slow improvement in range of motion and decreased pain. Recovery can take up to two years. Imaging studies are used to evaluate for other disorders.

Shoulder impingement syndrome (i.e., rotator cuff tendinitis or shoulder bursitis) is caused by compression of structures around the glenohumeral joint when the shoulder is elevated. Shoulder impingement syndrome is a common cause of shoulder pain. The main risk

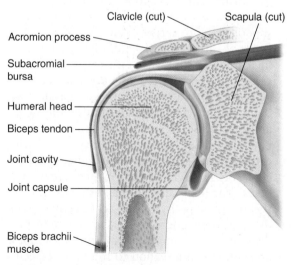

FIGURE 12-24 The bursa.

factors for development are repetitive work or sports activities at or above the shoulder level. The syndrome is not one specific injury by rather a result of edema, hemorrhage, fibrosis, and tendinitis that result in rotator cuff tear, tendon rupture, and bony changes. Clinical manifestations are shoulder pain that is worse with overhead activity and often occurs at night or when lying on the affected shoulder. Physical examination may reveal involvement of multiple structures (e.g., biceps tendon, subacromial bursa). Imaging studies are used to evaluate for other disorders.

Elbow

Epicondylitis is a tendinopathy of the tendon just distal and anterior to the epicondyle. The tendinopathy can occur laterally causing lateral epicondylitis (i.e., tennis elbow) or medially causing medial epicondylitis (i.e., golfer's elbow). Lateral epicondylitis is more common than medial. While initially there is a mild inflammatory process (clinically not visible) the underlying problem is a thickened and scarred tendon. Lateral epicondylitis will manifest as pain in the lateral elbow and forearm with activities involving gripping or wrist extension (e.g., backhand stroke in tennis) while medial epicondylitis manifests with pain in the medial elbow with activities involving wrist flexion and forearm pronation (e.g., golf swing). Inflammation and erythema are absent. Imaging studies are used to evaluate for other disorders.

Wrist

Carpal tunnel syndrome is a common disorder that results from compression of the median nerve as it travels into a space known as the carpal tunnel of the wrist. The carpal tunnel is made by a transverse carpal ligament superiorly and carpal bones inferiorly. The cause of carpal tunnel syndrome is a result of increased pressure within the carpal canal. The cause of the pressure, while unclear, seems to be related to anatomic compression and/or inflammation, which directly injures the nerve and compresses vessels leading to nerve ischemia. Multiple risk factors are associated with carpal tunnel syndrome development and include obesity, female gender, pregnancy, diabetes, rheumatoid arthritis, osteoarthritis of the hand, hypothyroidism, connective tissue diseases, occupational factors, and genetic predisposition. The median nerve provides motor and sensory innervation to the hand (specifically the first three fingers and radial half of

the fourth finger). The classic manifestations are pain or paresthesia, which is worse at night and wakens the patient at night. Sensory symptoms can radiate to the forearm and uncommonly to the shoulder (the neck is unaffected). Flexing or extending the wrist or raising the arm provokes the symptoms. Remissions and exacerbations are usually experienced. Motor symptoms, such as weakness or clumsiness, can occur with disease progression. The diagnosis is usually made clinically with a history and physical examination. Nerve conduction studies and electromyography can support the diagnosis. Treatment strategies include neutral wrist splinting, glucocorticoid injection, or oral glucocorticoids. Surgery to decompress the median nerve and occupational therapy may be necessary.

Stenosing tenosynovitis, also known as **de Quervain tendinopathy**, is a common cause of wrist pain in adults. The disorder involves wrist tendons on the radial side. The incidence is higher in women and is higher in pregnancy—probably as a result of hormonal influences. The injury is thought to occur because of overuse but generally the cause is unknown. Clinical manifestations are swelling and pain over the wrist on the distal radial side. Moving the wrist or thumb or attempts to make a fist (Finkelstein maneuver) causes pain. Crepitus may be felt. Imaging is generally not necessary. NSAIDs and a forearm-based thumb spica splint are initial treatment. Other strategies can include corticosteroid injections into the wrist or corrective surgery.

Hand

Dupuytren contracture (i.e., palmar fibromatosis) is the thickening and contracture of the palmar fascia as a result of fibroblast proliferation and abnormal collagen deposition. The ring finger is the most common area involved. The cause is unknown, but there is an association with other conditions (e.g., diabetes mellitus, smoking, and repetitive vibratory trauma). It is more common in men particularly of northern European ancestry, and genetic predisposition may be a factor. The clinical manifestations include the presence of a painless nodule and thickening over the affected area, which begins in the metacarpophalangeal joint. As the disease progresses the proximal interphalangeal joint is affected. Extension is limited but flexion is normal.

Trigger finger (i.e., stenosing flexor tenosynovitis) is a result of abnormal thickening of the flexor (palmar) tendon at the metacarpophalangeal joint. The fingers have a sophisticated pulley system that allows a back and forth gliding motion. The thickening of the flexor tendon causes the affected finger to snap or lock during flexion. Trigger finger can occur in any finger; however, it is most common in the ring and middle finger. The cause is idiopathic, but there is an association with other disorders (e.g., diabetes mellitus, rheumatoid arthritis). The clinical manifestations include pain (volar aspect) and a catching when the affected finger is flexed, and the patient may report that the finger is going out of its joint. A nodule may be palpated at the metacarpophalangeal joint. Patients can awaken with the finger in a flexed position, and swelling and stiffness may be present in the morning. As the day progresses, the finger gradually unlocks and straightens. Treatment can involve corticosteroid injection in the area, splinting, and possible surgery.

Hip

Slipped capital femoral epiphyses is a common cause of hip pain in adolescents (premenarche or shortly after puberty in males). The disorder occurs when the head of the femur (i.e., epiphysis) slips down and backwards off the neck of the bones. The reason for the slippage is not known; however, a higher incidence is seen in obese children. The clinical manifestations can occur after minor trauma, and the adolescent may complain of hip pain and an inability to walk. While the pain can be acute, it is often present for a few months and associated with a limp. The pain is usually dull and achy and worsens with physical activity. Range of motion—particularly internal rotation, abduction, and flexion—is decreased. The pain can be in the hip, thigh, or groin and even the knee. X-rays are usually performed to confirm diagnosis. The posterior displacement of the femoral epiphysis looks like ice cream slipping off a cone. The treatment is stabilization with non–weight-bearing until surgery, which involves the insertion of screws or pins.

Meralgia paresthetica (i.e., lateral femoral cutaneous nerve entrapment) is a result of compression of the nerve that supplies sensation to the upper, outer thigh. The compression usually occurs when the nerve is entrapped as it travels under the inguinal ligament. Obesity, diabetes mellitus, and age (mean age at diagnosis is 50) are risk factors. Other risk factors include large abdomens with overlying fat (the fat mechanically compresses the nerve), wearing tight belts or garments around the waist, and pregnancy. Clinical manifestations include burning pain, numbness, and tingling, usually over the upper, outer thigh. There are no motor symptoms as the lateral femoral nerve only has sensory fibers. Imaging tests are done to exclude other disorders. The disorder is benign and self-limiting, and treatment involves removal of the source of compression (e.g., weight loss and no belts). A nerve block and use of neuropathic pain medications such as gabapentin can be considered.

Knee

Osgood-Schlatter disease is an osteochondritis of the tibial tubercle that occurs in adolescents who have undergone a rapid growth spurt. In this disorder, there is a tendinitis of the patellar tendon and avascular necrosis (osteochondrosis) of the tibial tubercle. With the disorder (also known as tibial tubercle avulsion), the proximal anterior patellar tendon insertion eventually separates from the tibial tubercle. The separation is a result of an overuse injury caused by repetitive strain and chronic avulsion. The incidence is higher in males (ages 13–14 years) and those who play sports. Clinical manifestations include anterior knee ache that worsens over time to pain. A limp and activity impairment can occur. Pain is aggravated by direct trauma or any activities that stretch the patella tendon such as kneeling, running, jumping, and squatting. Rest alleviates the symptoms. The tibial tubercle may be prominent. Usually only one knee is affected, but the disorder can be symmetric. Diagnosis is made with a history and physical examination. Osgood-Schlatter disease is usually benign and resolves with conservative measures that include icing the knee after sports and analgesics (e.g., NSAIDs) for pain control. Sports can be continued to avoid deconditioning; however, pain after sports should resolve within 1 day. Quadriceps and hamstring stretching and strengthening are accomplished with physical therapy. Persistent pain may require surgery to remove ossicles that have developed as a result of the repetitive strain.

Low Back Pain

Almost 80% of adults will experience low back pain at some point in their lives. Most cases of back pain are due to strains (muscles and tendons). Strains usually cause acute pain that is self-limiting and resolves within a few weeks.

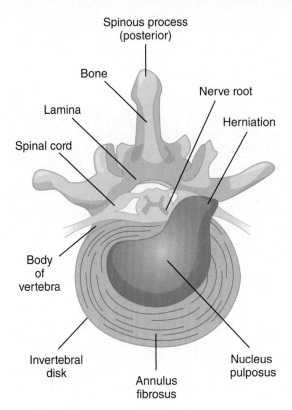

Spinous process
(posterior)

Bone

Nerve root

Lamina

Herniation

Spinal cord

Body
of
vertebra

Invertebral
disk

Annulus
fibrosus

Nucleus
pulposus

FIGURE 12-25 Herniated vertebral disk.

However, low back pain can become chronic (> 3 months) and is one of the leading causes of disabilities in the United States (NIH, 2018). Causes of low back pain can be categorized into mechanical and nonmechanical spinal disorders. Mechanical pain refers to pain that is caused by stress and strain on the spine, intervertebral disks, muscles, tendons, ligaments, and any other surrounding tissue. The causes of mechanical low back pain include the following:

- Muscle issues due to strain
- Intervertebral disks issues due to degeneration, rupture, herniation, or displacement (**FIGURE 12-25**)
- Facet joint issues due to degeneration or asymmetry
- Vertebral body issues due to fractures shifting
- Spine issues due to fractures, osteoporosis, or abnormal curvatures (e.g., lordosis)
- Vertebral canal issues due to canal narrowing (i.e., spinal stenosis)

Nonmechanical low back pain can be caused by neoplastic disorders, infections of the spine or chronic inflammatory disorders. Neoplastic disorders include multiple myeloma, metastatic cancer, and spinal cord tumors; infections include epidural abscess and

osteomyelitis; and chronic inflammatory disorders include psoriasis and ankylosing spondylitis. Women have a higher incidence of low back pain and other risk factors include smoking, obesity, advancing age, anxiety, and depressive disorders. Nonmechanical low back pain is discussed in various chapters (e.g., multiple myeloma in chapter 3).

Intervertebral disk issues often occur due to improper body mechanics, lifting heavy objects, repetitive use, or trauma (e.g., a fall or a blow to the back). Additional contributing factors include vertebral stress secondary to obesity, degenerative changes secondary to aging, and demineralization secondary to metabolic conditions (e.g., osteoporosis). The intervertebral disks begin to normally degenerate with aging due to wear and tear. When low back pain occurs, the disorder is termed *degenerative disk disease*, which is one of the most common causes of mechanical back pain. The matrix of the disks loses water, the disk height diminishes, and the bones get closer together. The degeneration can occur anywhere along the spine. The narrow disk space can be seen on imaging tests (e.g., X-rays and MRI), and this narrowing is termed **spondylosis**. Degenerated disks are susceptible to herniation. Each vertebra has two facet (i.e., zygapophyseal) joints located on each side of the spine. The facet joints are synovial joints that link the vertebrae together. Degeneration of the facet joints can also occur and is also termed *spondylosis*.

A **herniated intervertebral disk** describes a state in which the nucleus pulposus (the inner gelatinous component of the intervertebral disk) protrudes through the annulus fibrosus (the tough outer covering of the disk) and beyond it's boundary (Figure 12-25). This condition may also be called a *slipped disk, ruptured disk*, or a *herniated nucleus pulposus*. The tear in the annulus may occur suddenly or gradually. A disk can also bulge rather than herniate or rupture. Bulging disks do not extend beyond the boundaries of the annulus fibrosus. Protrusions into the extradural space can exert pressure on the spinal cord, interfering with nerve conduction (**FIGURE 12-26**). Sensory, motor, or autonomic function may be impaired depending on the location of injury. The most frequently involved vertebrae are in the lumbosacral region, but some injuries may involve the cervical disks. If pressure on nerve tissue or blood supply is prolonged or severe, permanent neurologic damage may result.

A thin portion of vertebrae known as the pars interarticularis connects the upper and lower facet joints. This pars interarticularis can be weak, particularly in the L5 vertebra, making this area vulnerable to stress fractures. A pars interarticularis fracture can be seen on imaging tests (e.g., X-rays and MRI), and this fracture is termed **spondylolysis** (see **FIGURE 12-27**). This type of stress fracture can occur at any age but is more common in young people who participate in sports that involve spinal hyperextension, such as gymnastics, or repetitive stress on the lower back, such as weightlifting. A genetic weakness may lead to an increased risk for spondylolysis. The fracture causes an instability and can cause the vertebral body to shift forward, which is seen on imaging tests and is termed **spondylolisthesis**. Other conditions causing instability and spondylolisthesis (anterior or posterior shift) include degenerative disorders of the disks or facet joints. Spondylolisthesis can occur anywhere in the spine but is more common in the L4–L5 region and the L5–S1 area. Spondylolisthesis can cause compression of the nerves exiting the spinal column.

Narrowing of the spinal canal results in a disorder known as **spinal stenosis**. Multiple factors can lead to spinal stenosis, with spondylosis and spondylolistheses with degeneration as the most frequent causes. The ligamentum flavum (a band of elastic tissue that serves as a covering in the spinal cord) thickens and contributes to spinal stenosis. Other disorders that can cause spinal stenosis include spinal neoplasms, fibrosis from trauma, or skeletal disorders such as Paget disease, ankylosing spondylitis, or rheumatoid arthritis. The disorder is more common in individuals over the age of 60 and is a common cause of disability due to aging. The clinical manifestations of

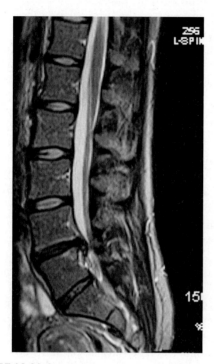

FIGURE 12-26 Spinal cord compression by a herniated disk.
Courtesy of Steven Goldstein, MD.

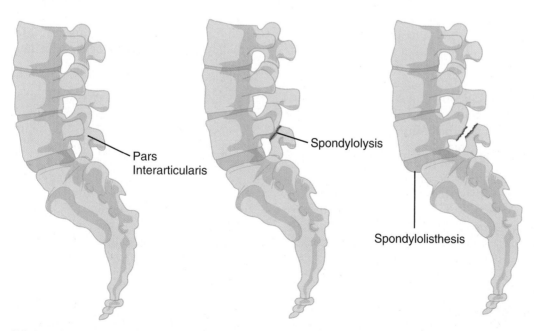

FIGURE 12-27 Spondylolysis and spondylolisthesis.
Spondylolysis and Spondylolisthesis, American Academy of Orthopaedic Surgeons, retrieved from https://orthoinfo.aaos.org/en/diseases--conditions/spondylolysis-and-spondylolisthesis/.

spinal stenosis are due to mechanical compression and ischemia of the nerve roots.

Clinical Manifestations

Low back pain manifestations are dependent on the underlying cause and the effects on surrounding tissues (e.g., nerves). Low back pain characteristics are similar to muscular, joint, or tendon issues in other anatomic locations, including pain with movement or palpation. Edema and erythema are not present. In addition to strains, vertebral compression fractures are a cause of low back pain, and patients may be asymptomatic or have pain that is localized over the fracture site. The fractures can occur without any preceding trauma and can be due to osteoporosis and factors that weaken the bone (e.g., chronic glucocorticoid use or advancing age). Other manifestations of back pain can include physical examination findings of **radiculopathy** (also referred to as a *pinched nerve*) and subjective complaints of **sciatica**. Radiculopathy is due to an impairment of a nerve root. Radiculopathy causes radiating pain, paresthesias (numbness or tingling), or muscle weakness that corresponds to the injured nerve root. Reflexes may be diminished or absent. Radiculopathy at L5 or S1 often causes sciatic nerve root issues. The sciatic nerve root distribution is down the buttocks to the posterior or lateral aspect of the leg down to the foot or ankle. Lumbosacral radicular pain can be elicited with maneuvers such as the straight leg raise. This test is conducted by laying the patient supine and passively elevating the leg with the foot dorsiflexed. This maneuver causes tension in the dura in the lumbosacral area. If positive the patient will complain of radicular signs when the hip is flexed between 30-70 degrees. Spinal stenosis can have manifestations that distinguish this disorder from other causes of low back pain. The hallmark manifestation of lumbar stenosis is pain localized to the calf and distal lower extremities that occurs with ambulation and resolves with sitting or leaning forward. This pain pattern is termed *pseudoclaudication* or *neurogenic claudication*. The symptoms of neurogenic claudication must be distinguished from vascular claudication. Vascular claudication is not relieved with flexing forward but is improved with standing upright. Rest immediately resolves pain from vascular claudication, while it may take longer with neurogenic claudication. Patients with lumbar stenosis can also have low back pain with sensory loss and motor weakness in the legs. See chapter 4 for more on cardiovascular function.

Serious underlying disorders or complications of common low back pain etiologies are uncommon (< 1% of low back pain cases); however, recognition of these manifestations is important. These conditions include cauda equina, spinal infections, and metastatic cancer. Cauda equina (Latin for *horse's tail*) refers to compression of the lumbar and sacral nerve roots. The most common cause of the compression is a ruptured or herniated intervertebral disk. Other less common causes include disorders such as tumors (malignant or benign), infections, or trauma. These nerve roots innervate the lower extremities, bowels, and bladder. Clinical manifestations include low back pain (usually bilateral along with pain radiating to one or both legs), motor weakness, and sensory loss or weakness. Bowel and bladder dysfunction can include loss of control (e.g., retention or incontinence). Rectal numbness, often referred to as *saddle anesthesia*, may be present. Metastatic cancer often spreads to the spine and should be suspected in individuals with a history of cancer, or the low back pain may be the initial presentation of metastasized cancer (e.g., multiple myeloma). Low back pain due to cancer may appear suddenly and can be severe, and a pathologic fracture may be present. Low back pain due to infections can be nonspecific, and general infection signs, such as fever and malaise, can occur. Spinal infections can be due to iatrogenic causes (e.g., spinal injection or epidural catheter), intravenous drug use, and other systemic infections near the spine.

Diagnosis and Treatment

Diagnostic procedures may consist of a history, physical examination, including neurologic assessment; spinal X-rays; spinal CT; spinal MRI; nerve conduction study; myelogram (injection of contrast medium into the spinal fluid, followed by X-rays); and electromyography. Treatment for low back pain due to muscular strain is similar to treatment for other muscle strains. In general, low back pain treatment includes analgesics such as NSAIDs; muscle relaxants; physical therapy, including back-strengthening exercises; heat and cold application; and traction. Most people will recover with such treatment and return to their normal functioning, but a small number of patients will need further treatment such as injections (e.g., corticosteroid and

BOX 12-2 Application to Practice

Review the following two musculoskeletal disorder cases.

Case 1: A 35-year-old, healthy White male is complaining of right-sided, low back pain for 1 day. The pain began suddenly after lifting a box weighting 35 pounds at work. The pain radiates down the back of his leg to his right ankle. He has tried ibuprofen and ice without relief. His pain is an 8 out of 10 (with 0 being no pain and 10 being the worst pain). He denies bowel or bladder dysfunction, paresthesia, motor weakness, or fever.

Past medical/surgical history: no major medical illnesses; no surgical history; no previous hospitalizations.

Social history: has smoked 1 pack of cigarettes a day for 15 years.

Medications: none.

Allergies: no known drug allergies.

Vital signs: temperature 98.7° F; pulse 90 beats per minute; respiration rate 18; blood pressure 126/78 mmHg; O_2 saturation 100%.

Physical examination revealed a well-nourished adult male without any acute distress. Significant right paraspinal tenderness at L4–L5 was present with no midline tenderness. Straight leg raise was positive at 30° to the right lower extremity. Straight leg raise was negative to the left lower extremity. The remainder of musculoskeletal examination was unremarkable (e.g., deep tendon reflexes,

strength, and sensation). Other systems examinations were unremarkable (e.g., heart, lungs, etc.).

1. What are your differential diagnoses? What are subjective and objective findings consistent with the various differentials for low back pain?
2. Would you consider imaging for this patient? If so, what imaging would be recommended and why?
3. What are the concerning manifestations of low back pain?
4. What are treatment strategies for this patient?
5. What education would be provided to the patient?
6. When should you refer this patient to a specialist?

Case 2: A 13-year-old male is complaining of mild recurrent bilateral anterior knee pain without fever, joint swelling, erythema, or limitation of ambulation for the past 3 months. He is accompanied by his mother.

Prenatal and birth history: unremarkable.

Developmental history: mother reports normal development.

Past medical/surgical history: no major medical illnesses; no surgical history; no previous hospitalizations.

Social history: actively involved on his school's soccer team for 2 years.

Family and environmental risks: none.

Immunization history: up to date.

Medications: none.

Allergies: no known drug allergies.

Vital signs: temperature 98.7° F; pulse 72 beats per minute; respiration rate 18; blood pressure 120/70 mmHg; O_2 saturation 100%.

Physical examination revealed a well-nourished adolescent male without any acute distress. Significant bilateral tenderness was noted when palpating the tibial tubercles, and extending his knees against resistance reproduced pain. The remainder of the musculoskeletal examination was unremarkable (e.g., deep tendon reflexes, strength, and sensation). Other systems examinations were unremarkable (e.g., heart, lungs, etc.).

1. What is the most likely diagnosis for this patient?
2. What is the pathogenesis of this disorder?
3. What additional information assists in making the diagnosis?
4. What are treatment strategies for this patient?
5. What education would the provided to the patient and mother?

Case 1 by Dana Sherman. Case 2 authored by or contributed by Deana Goldin, PhD, DNP, APRN, FNP-BC.

chemonucleolysis) into the site or surgical repair (e.g., diskectomy, laminectomy, and spinal fusion). Weight loss may be beneficial if the patient is overweight. Back pain due to serious underlying disorders such as spinal epidural abscess or vertebral osteomyelitis will require urgent management (e.g., emergency surgery and intravenous antibiotics).

Metabolic Bone Disorders

Metabolic bone disorders refer to a variety of bone conditions associated with mineral abnormalities. These abnormalities may be caused by genetic factors, medications, or dietary deficits. Metabolic bone disorders can be prevented and are usually treated easily once identified, but if left untreated, they can lead to significant complications (e.g., electrolyte disturbances and fractures).

Osteoporosis

Osteoporosis is a condition characterized by a progressive loss of bone strength due to a low bone mass (quantity of bone) and low bone quality, leading to an increased risk for fractures (FIGURE 12-28). Osteoporosis is one of the most common bone disorders, and approximately 53 million Americans have osteoporosis (9.9 million) and low bone mass (43.1 million), which increases risk for osteoporosis (National Osteoporosis Foundation, 2016). The rate of osteoporosis is higher in women; it is 1 in 2 for women and 1 in 5 for men. Whites and Asians have a higher incidence of osteoporosis. Blacks have a lower incidence of osteoporosis, but risk is equivalent to other ethnicities if a fracture develops. Osteoporosis can occur as a primary or secondary condition. Secondary osteoporosis, which is less common than primary, is caused by many conditions such as endocrine disorders (e.g., diabetes and thyroid disorders),

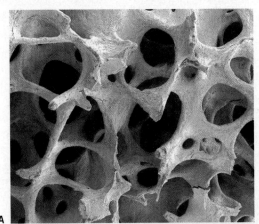

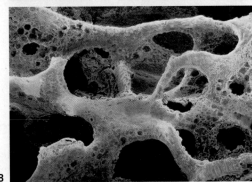

FIGURE 12-28 Osteoporosis. The loss of estrogen or prolonged immobilization weakens bone. In these situations, bone is dissolved and becomes brittle and easily breakable. **(A)** Normal bone. **(B)** Bone weakened by osteoporosis.

medications, and inflammatory bone disorders such as rheumatoid arthritis.

The loss of bone strength can occur due to multiple pathogenetic mechanisms that interact to either cause a decrease in osteoblast activity or an increase in osteoclast activity. This remodeling imbalance results in a net effect of greater bone removal than replacement. Bone density and bone quality are ultimately affected, leading to an increased fracture risk. The main factors contributing to this imbalance are aging and a deficiency of estrogen, usually a result of menopause. However, neither of these two factors alone is sufficient for development of osteoporosis as many older adults maintain relatively strong bones. Reactive oxygen species increase during aging contributing to the development of degenerative disorders, including osteoporosis. Reactive oxygen species are a normal byproduct of aerobic metabolism, and their accumulation leads to oxidative stress, which causes osteoblast apoptosis and results in decreased bone formation. Likewise, increased reactive oxygen species facilitates osteoclast generation, stimulation, and survival. Osteocytes are key regulators in the bone remodeling process and are located throughout the skeleton. With aging, osteocyte apoptosis increases initially, resulting in the central trabecular (i.e., cancellous or spongy) bone becoming more fragile (Figure 12-4). Since the osteocytes are dead, normal signals that osteocytes send to repair damaged bones are also lost. Mechanical stress on the bones is a necessary requisite for osteocyte viability and functionality. With aging, reduced strength and decreased activity further compound osteocyte loss. Other factors that occur with aging include a decrease in growth hormone and insulin growth factor, which causes increased RANKL binding (RANKL binds to osteoclasts and increases resorption) and decreased OPG (Figure 12-5). These hormonal changes alter osteoblast and osteoclast activities.

Low estrogen and androgen cause a loss of bone due to an increase in bone resorption. The estrogen deficiency that occurs after menopause causes an initial rapid decline in bone mass, particularly trabecular bone. Subsequently, a loss of cortical bone occurs but at a slower pace. Osteoporosis prevalence increases for women each decade after the age of 50. Low estrogen contributes to osteoporosis in men; however, men have a 30% higher baseline bone mass in comparison to women. The bone loss is more of a thinning in men as opposed to a complete loss, and this thinning occurs at a slow rate. Osteoporosis risk in men increases at a much later age (e.g., > 80). Men also have higher androgen levels, which also causes OPG production (OPG inhibits osteoclastic activity and blocks RANKL, promoting bone formation). Men with androgen disorders, such as idiopathic hypogonadotropic hypogonadism, are at higher risk for osteoporosis. Estrogen usually provides a protective effect by increasing OPG production and decreasing the effects of RANKL; therefore, deficiencies alter this balance. Higher RANKL levels seen with estrogen deficiency cause increased osteoclastic activity and reduced osteoclastic death. Estrogen and androgen deficiencies may also have a direct effect on T and B lymphocytes and cytokines that affect bone cells and alter resorption balance. However, the role of these hormone effects on the immune system and the development of osteoporosis is unclear.

Different types of bone density and structure (e.g., trabecular or cortical composition) are found throughout the various areas of the skeleton, and the density and structures change with aging. With osteoporosis, the bones become porous (FIGURE 12-29). Bone remodeling

occurs on the surface of bone. In adults, trabecular surface areas are greater initially, so trabecular bone loss is greater early in osteoporosis. This trabecular bone loss is accelerated with estrogen deficiency. With advancing age, cortical surface area is higher early in osteoporosis, so cortical bone loss occurs at a slower rate in comparison to trabecular bone loss. The vertebrae, hip (femoral neck), and wrist are likely to sustain a fracture due to osteoporosis. Vertebral fractures are more common in individuals younger than age 65 with osteoporosis as the vertebrae has more trabecular bone. After 65 years of age, incidence of hip fractures is higher because the hip has more cortical bone.

Other conditions, such as rheumatoid arthritis and metastatic cancer, alter the OPG–RANKL–RANK system that is critical in maintaining bone homeostasis. Cushing disease, thyroid dysfunction, hyperparathyroidism, bone tumors, malabsorption, and anorexia nervosa are also associated with osteoporosis. Glucocorticoid administration is a common secondary cause of osteoporosis because it increases RANKL and decreases OPG production. Additionally, glucocorticoids have direct effects on bone cells and suppress osteoblast production and activity, increase osteocyte apoptosis,

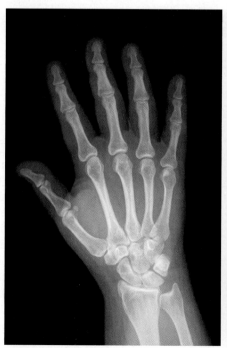 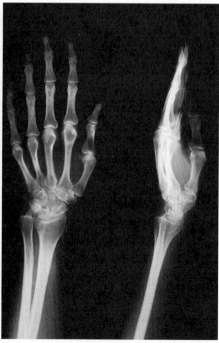

A   B

FIGURE 12-29 Bone changes of osteoporosis. (A) An X-ray of normal bones. (B) An X-ray of bones affected by osteoporosis.

A: © picbyst/Shutterstock; B: © Fmajor/E+/Getty Images.

and prolong osteoclast life span. After 3 months of glucocorticoid administration, bone changes and fractures can occur before bone mass is affected. Other medications can increase osteoporosis risk, including chemotherapy, thyroid replacements, heparin, and antacids. Dietary deficiencies or vitamin (C, D, E, K) and mineral malabsorption are associated with the development of osteoporosis. This development is especially true of calcium malabsorption, and its absorption decreases with aging. Deficient protein intake and excessive phosphorus also increase osteoporosis risk. Gastrointestinal procedures, such as a gastrectomy or gastrointestinal bypass, increase osteoporosis risk because of the nutritional deficits that often result from these surgeries. In addition, individuals with smaller bones and thin frames (genetically determined) are at increased risk. Other risk factors include smoking, excessive alcohol or caffeine consumption, being underweight, and family history.

Aging, estrogen deficiency, and various conditions can cause osteoporosis, but bone conditions (mass and quality) are also influenced during development. By age 30, the average adult has acquired most of his or her skeletal mass. A person with high bone mass as a young adult is more likely to have a higher bone mass later in life; therefore, achieving maximum bone mass in young adulthood is important for maintaining bone health throughout the life span. Adequate calcium consumption and physical activity (including weight-bearing exercises) early in life are particularly vital to achieve maximum bone mass and bone health in adulthood.

Clinical Manifestations

Osteoporosis is often asymptomatic in its early stages, and a fracture may be the first indication of its presence. Fractures can occur with little or no trauma. Vertebral fractures are more likely before the age of 65, and hip fractures are more likely after the age of 65. Other common fracture locations associated with osteoporosis include the wrist, humerus, ribs, and pelvis. As the disease progresses, clinical manifestations are a result of skeletal deformity, particularly vertebral collapse that causes a height reduction (as much as 6 inches) and kyphosis (**FIGURE 12-30**). Kyphosis can cause issues with activities that require bending and reaching. Pain and disability associated with osteoporosis are a result of fractures. Fractures significantly increase mortality in the elderly, especially in individuals who experience a hip fracture (20% of whom will die within a year of the fracture).

Myth Busters

Osteoporosis is a common condition associated with several myths that warrant discussion.

Myth 1: People with osteoporosis can feel their bones getting weaker.

Osteoporosis often has no apparent symptoms. In fact, breaking a bone may be the first clue that someone has osteoporosis. Some people may learn they have osteoporosis after they lose height from one or more vertebral fractures. These fractures can even occur without any noticeable pain. Thus, individuals at risk should be screened for this often-silent disease.

Myth 2: Children and teens do not need to worry about their bone health.

While it is true that osteoporosis typically appears in older populations, building strong bones and preventing osteoporosis begins in youth. Bone mass peaks around the third decade of life. Being physically active, getting enough calcium and vitamin D early, and maintaining these habits throughout life can build strong bones for later in life.

Myth 3: Osteoporosis is not serious.

This myth is important to dispel. The fractures that can result from osteoporosis can be painful and have serious complications. Older individuals are at particular risk for life-altering and life-threatening effects from these fractures. These individuals tend to be immobile for longer because of their extended healing time, which puts them at risk for problems associated with immobility (e.g., renal calculi, thrombus, constipation, decubiti, and incontinence).

Data from National Osteoporosis Foundation. (2016). What is osteoporosis and what causes it? Retrieved from https://www.nof.org/patients/what-is-osteoporosis/.

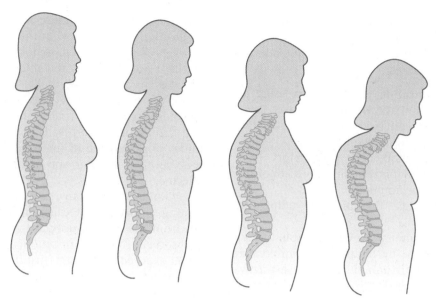

FIGURE 12-30 Kyphosis and height changes associated with osteoporosis.

Diagnosis and Treatment

Diagnostic procedures include a history with a focus on evaluation for falls. Early in the course of the disease, physical examination findings are normal. Bone mineral density is measured with a dual-energy X-ray absorptiometry (DEXA) scan. The DEXA scan results reflect bone density and do not reflect bone quality. With improvements in DEXA scans, information related to bone quality may be provided. Results of the DEXA scan that demonstrate osteoporosis risk and are diagnostic of osteoporosis are based on the World Health Organization criteria (1994). The results are reported as T-scores, which are the standard deviation (SD) differences between patients' bone mineral density (BMD) and that of a young adult reference population. The sites measured are usually the hip and spine. These criteria include:

- A BMD T-score that is 2.5 SDs or more below the young adult mean indicates osteoporosis.
- A BMD T-score that is 1–2.5 SDs or more below the young adult mean indicates **osteopenia** (i.e., low bone mass).
- A BMD T-score that is within 1 SD of the young adult mean is normal.

A DEXA scan report can also include Z-scores, which reflect the patient's BMD compared to an age-matched population. Low Z-scores (more than 2 SDs) may reflect coexisting problems that can contribute to osteoporosis. The FRAX fracture risk assessment tool can be used to identify patients between 40 and 90 years of age who are at risk for fractures. The FRAX tool estimates the 10-year probability of hip fracture and osteoporotic fracture for untreated patients. The tool uses various clinical data, such as previous fracture, age, alcohol use, and femoral neck BMD. The score can be obtained by entering data into an online calculator, which can be accessed at the FRAX website (www.sheffield.ac.uk/FRAX/). The FRAX score (expressed as a percentage) can be used with the BMD to identify those individuals at risk or can be used independently as a predictor of fracture.

Osteoporotic bone will appear radiolucent on X-rays but usually not until bone loss is significant (> 25%) (Figure 12-29). The initial presentation of osteoporosis is often a fracture, so X-rays are used in this context. An initial serum test will include a chemistry profile (e.g., glucose, potassium, etc.) with alkaline phosphatase, a complete blood count, calcium, phosphorus, and 25-hydroxyvitamin D. Other laboratory tests are performed (e.g., FSH, LH, and parathyroid hormone) based on suspicions for underlying disorders.

Screening for osteoporosis should be conducted periodically on those persons at risk because of the high prevalence rates of this disease and the silent nature of the disease. Women ages 65 and older should be routinely screened as part of their health prevention and maintenance (USPSTF, 2011). Screening is accomplished with a DEXA scan. The optimal screening frequency with a DEXA scan is not defined; however, the scan is usually not repeated before 2 years.

Treatment strategies focus on minimizing further bone loss and restoring bone density in some cases. These strategies may include the following measures:

* Proper nutrition, especially increasing dietary calcium and vitamin D intake
* Increasing physical activity, including weight-bearing activities
* Modifying modifiable risk factors (e.g., smoking cessation and limiting alcohol and caffeine consumption)
* Pharmacologic therapies, including the following:
  * Bisphosphonates, which inhibit bone resorption by binding to hydroxyapatite, in turn inhibiting osteoclast activity, suppressing osteoclast production, and increasing osteoclast apoptosis; and which improve osteoblast survival, usually with initial therapy
  * Parathyroid hormone/parathyroid hormone-related protein analog, which stimulates osteoblasts
  * Denosumab, a monoclonal antibody that inhibits RANKL
  * Selective estrogen receptor modulators, which mimic estrogen
  * Calcitonin, which increases calcium and phosphate deposits in the bone; however, it is not commonly used due to concerns regarding long-term safety and increased cancer rates.
* Safety measures (e.g., assistive devices, handrails, and removal of clutter).
* Surgical repair of fractures or weakened bones.

Rickets and Osteomalacia

Rickets is a softening and weakening of bones in children, usually because of an extreme and prolonged vitamin D, calcium, or phosphate deficiency. Rickets is the result of deficient mineralization that affects the growth plates. **Osteomalacia** is the result of deficient mineralization that affects the bone matrix. When the growth plates are open, rickets and osteomalacia usually occur. When the growth plates close, only osteomalacia occurs. Calcipenic rickets refers to the disorder developing as a result of calcium or vitamin D deficiencies. Phosphopenic rickets is a result of phosphate deficiencies, usually due to renal disease. If the blood levels of these minerals become too low, calcium and phosphate are released from the bones to maintain homeostasis. This shift of minerals out of the bone results in abnormal ossification of the bones. In the growth plate, cartilage developmental abnormalities cause cartilage accumulation and thickening. Chondrocytes function abnormally, further worsening the ossification process. Unmineralized osteoids accumulate under the periosteum, and this accumulation leads to skeletal deformities (e.g., bowing of the long bones in the legs). Both trabecular and compact bone are affected.

Vitamin D plays an essential role in promoting absorption of calcium and phosphorus from the gastrointestinal tract. Vitamin D is absorbed from food or produced by the skin when exposed to sunlight. Insufficient vitamin D production by the skin may occur in people who live in climates with little exposure to sunlight, who must stay indoors such as bedridden or institutionalized persons, who work indoors during the daylight hours, or who have dark skin. Dietary deficiency may occur with persons who are lactose intolerant, do not drink milk products, or follow a vegetarian diet. Infants who are only breastfed may also develop vitamin D deficiency because human milk does not supply the proper amount of vitamin D. Using strong sunscreen and limiting sun exposure to minimize skin cancer risk may also increase the risk for vitamin D deficiency. Conditions that reduce the digestion or absorption of fats (e.g., celiac disease, cystic fibrosis, and undergoing a gastrectomy) will make it more difficult for vitamin D to be absorbed into the body.

Insufficient dietary calcium and phosphorus intake can also lead to rickets, but this condition is rare in developed countries because calcium and phosphorus are found in both milk and green vegetables. Rickets may also occur because of genetic influences. Hereditary rickets occurs when the kidneys are unable to reabsorb phosphate. For this reason, rickets may occur in some individuals with renal disease. This metabolic bone disorder may occasionally occur in children who have liver disorders or who cannot convert vitamin D to its active form.

Clinical Manifestations

Clinical manifestations of rickets and osteomalacia develop slowly, as the bones weaken over time. Rickets may become apparent at the places of rapid bone growth (e.g., knee, forearm) that do not mineralize and cannot support the growing child. Manifestations in adults and children usually include the following signs and symptoms:

- Delayed fontanelle closure and craniotabes (softening and thinning of the skull)
- Skeletal deformities (e.g., bowed legs, asymmetric skull, scoliosis, kyphosis, pelvic deformities, and sternum projection) (FIGURE 12-31)
- Fractures
- Delayed growth in height or limbs; delayed motor development
- Dental problems (e.g., defects in tooth structure, dental caries, poor enamel, delayed teeth formation)
- Bone pain (usually a dull, aching pain or tenderness in the spine, pelvis, and legs)
- Muscle cramps, spasms, or weakness
- Difficulty with ambulation or waddling gait

Diagnosis and Treatment

Diagnostic procedures for rickets and osteomalacia include a history, physical examination, serum mineral levels (calcium, phosphate), 25-hydroxyvitamin D, serum parathyroid hormone levels, serum alkaline phosphatase, X-rays, and a bone density study. Serum minerals levels will be dependent on the underlying cause and the stage of the disease (initial versus advanced). In general, the 25-hyroxyvitamin D, calcium, and phosphate will be low and the parathyroid hormone and alkaline phosphatase will be high if the cause is nutritional deficiency. If the cause is a renal phosphate issue, then the serum phosphate is low (urine clearance high), and vitamin D, parathyroid, and calcium are relatively normal.

Treatment focuses on correcting or managing the underlying cause. Providing calcium, phosphorus, or vitamin D that is lacking will eliminate most symptoms. The body's vitamin D levels can be increased through dietary intake (e.g., fish, liver, and processed milk), exposure to moderate amounts of sunlight, or administration of vitamin D supplements. Severe vitamin D deficiency requires supplementation with high doses (e.g., 50,000 international units a week in adults) for approximately 2 months followed by a daily maintenance dose (e.g., 800 international units per day in adults). Calcium levels can be increased through dietary intake (e.g., dairy products; dark green, leafy vegetables; and nuts). Positioning or bracing may be used to reduce or prevent deformities associated with rickets and osteomalacia, although some skeletal deformities may require corrective surgery.

Paget Disease

Paget disease (i.e., osteitis deformans) is a progressive condition characterized by abnormal bone destruction and remodeling, which results in bone deformities (FIGURE 12-32). In

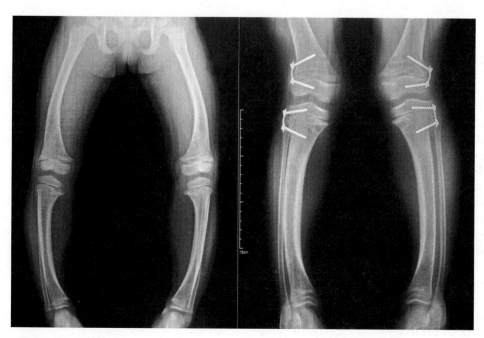

FIGURE 12-31 Rickets.
© Tee.wara/Shutterstock.

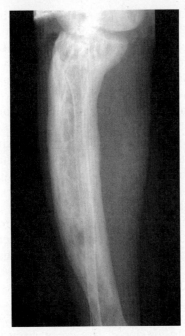

FIGURE 12-32 Bone deformities from Paget disease.
© Mediscan/Alamy Stock Photo.

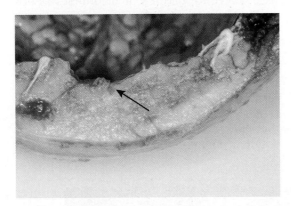

FIGURE 12-33 Paget disease.
© Dr. P. Marazzi/Science Source.

the usual bone metabolism process, old bone is recycled into new bone throughout the life span; however, the rate at which old bone is broken down and new bone forms is distorted with Paget disease. Notably, bone turnover proceeds at 20 times the normal rate. Excessive bone turnover occurs, resulting in the replacement of bone by fibrous tissue and abnormal bone. The new bone is bigger but weakened and filled with new blood vessels (**FIGURE 12-33**). Over time, Paget disease results in fragile, misshapen bones. This disease may be present in only one or two areas of the skeleton, or it may occur throughout the body. Paget disease often involves the pelvis, long bones (e.g., femur), tibia, skull, and vertebrae.

The exact cause of Paget disease is unknown, but several genetic loci that affect bone physiology and particularly RANK-RANKL activity have been identified. Another theory is that Paget is caused by environmental toxin such as a viral infection but data is limited. The pattern of inheritance is autosomal dominant. An estimated 1 to 3 million people are affected by Paget disease, but the actual numbers may be higher because this condition is often asymptomatic (Alikhan, Lohr, & Driver, 2015). Paget disease is more common in men, those of central European descent, and persons with a family history.

Paget disease proceeds through three phases (lytic, mixed lytic, and blastic), and multiple stages may be present in different regions of the body at any point. The disease begins with the lytic phase, in which normal bone is resorbed by osteoclasts that are more numerous, are larger, and have more nuclei. These abnormal osteoclasts increase bone turnover. The mixed lytic phase is characterized by rapid increases in bone formation from the numerous osteoblasts present. Although increased in number, these osteoblasts remain morphologically normal. In contrast, the new bone formed by them is abnormal, with collagen fibers being haphazardly deposited throughout the bone structure. In the final, blastic phase, the bones formed are weak and deformed. The bone marrow becomes infiltrated by excessive fibrous connective tissue and blood vessels, leading to a hypervascular bone state (Alikhan et al., 2015).

Clinical Manifestations

The clinical manifestations of Paget disease vary depending on the area affected. This condition is often insidious in onset and may be asymptomatic early in the course of the disease. Manifestations rarely occur before the age of 40 and are usually the result of skeletal issues. When present, some clinical manifestations include the following signs and symptoms:

- Bone pain (severity ranges from mild to severe and is persistent but worsens at night)
- Skeletal deformities (e.g., bowing of the legs, asymmetric skull, and enlarged head)
- Fractures with absent to minimal impact
- Headache
- Hearing and vision loss due to skull involvement
- Joint pain or stiffness as a result of deformity of articular bone or forces to an abnormal bone
- Neck pain
- Reduced height

- Warmth over the affected bone as a result of increased vascularity
- Paresthesia or radiating pain in the affected region (due to nerve compression)
- Hypercalcemia with generalized skeletal disease

Complications of Paget disease may include pathologic fractures, osteoarthritis, heart failure, osteosarcoma (bone cancer), and nerve compression. Heart failure is unusual but is related to hypercalcemia and increased cardiac workload as the body must pump more blood to the affected areas.

Diagnosis and Treatment

Diagnostic procedures for Paget disease consist of a history and physical examination. Imaging will include X-rays, which will reveal osteolytic lesions and sclerotic appearance of bone. Other X-ray findings depend on the disease stage and may include increased bone size, bowing, and transverse lucencies termed *fissure fractures*. A bone scan will determine the extent of the disease. Laboratory tests include serum alkaline phosphatase and serum calcium. Other imaging tests, such as a CT or MRI, can be performed. Mild cases may require just periodic monitoring and no treatment. Treatment strategies focus on reducing fractures and deformities. Pharmacologic therapies may include bisphosphonates, which increase bone density. Calcitonin may be considered but has considerable side effects including nausea and vomiting. NSAIDs can alleviate pain and inflammation, and analgesics can relieve pain. Calcium supplementation and vitamin D supplementation are often necessary. Surgery such as joint replacement and osteotomy may be required to correct severe bone deformities. Fractures may also require surgical management.

Inflammatory Joint Disorders

Inflammatory joint disorders encompass a group of arthritic conditions. These conditions involve inflammation that can be triggered by an autoimmune response, excessive use, increased physical stress, or injury. While osteoarthritis is discussed in this section, it is usually categorized as a noninflammatory joint disorder. The immune system is activated, and inflammatory mediators play a role in the destruction seen in osteoarthritis albeit at a different microscopic level and with a less pronounced response than other inflammatory joint disorders such as rheumatoid arthritis. Similar clinical manifestations can be seen across the various joint disorders, so distinguishing between them is best accomplished in a common section. Complications of these conditions often include chronic pain and disability. Treatment strategies focus on slowing the progression, managing pain, and promoting independence.

Osteoarthritis

Osteoarthritis (OA) (meaning inflammation of the joint), often used interchangeably with osteoarthrosis (meaning degeneration of the joint), is a localized joint disease characterized by deterioration of articulating cartilage and its underlying bone as well as bony overgrowth (**FIGURE 12-34**; **TABLE 12-3**). Osteoarthritis is also commonly termed *wear-and-tear arthritis* and *degenerative joint disease*; however, the pathogenesis is more complex than this simple terminology reflects. The Centers for Disease Control and Prevention (CDC, 2015b) estimates that nearly 27 million Americans have OA, with women having higher prevalence rates than men. OA is a significant contributor of disability, healthcare costs, and job loss in the United States.

Healthy cartilage allows the joint to move in a smooth, gliding motion, but most of the load placed on a joint is handled by other tissues such as the surrounding articular muscles and subchondral bone. In OA, all joint tissues are affected. The cartilage, however, is the key site of destruction and the site where early pathologic changes are seen. Loss of normal articular cartilage proteoglycan is a hallmark of OA. With OA, the surface of the cartilage becomes rough and worn, interfering with joint movement. The cartilage surface loosens and becomes disorganized. The normally quiet chondrocytes begin to proliferate in response to the breakdown. The tissue damage triggers the release of proinflammatory mediators (e.g., cytokines), causing a production of destructive proteolytic enzymes. The various proteases involved in OA joint destructions are categorized as matrix metalloproteinases (e.g., aggrecanases and collagenases), cysteine proteinases (e.g., cathepsin K), and serine proteinases (e.g., activated protein C). Therapies are being developed to inhibit some of these proteases and modify disease progression. The chondrocytes also produce proinflammatory mediators and proteases. Chondrocyte death increases, and the matrix is incapable of repair (usually cartilage

Normal synovial joint

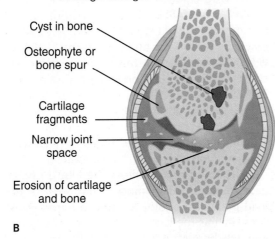

A

Pathologic changes in osteoarthritis

B

Pathologic changes in rheumatoid arthritis

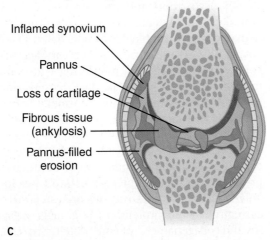

C

FIGURE 12-34 Pathologic changes associated with osteoarthritis and rheumatoid arthritis.

repair is limited in any circumstance). Eventually, the subchondral bone is exposed and damaged, and it thickens as abnormal (unmineralized) collagen is deposited. Cysts and

osteophytes (bone spurs) develop around joint margins as the bone attempts to remold itself. Pieces of the osteophytes and cartilage break off into the synovial cavity, causing the synovium to become inflamed (i.e., synovitis) and hypertrophy. The inflammation does not initiate OA but, rather, contributes to destruction through proinflammatory mediators and protease production. Additionally, nearby muscles and ligaments may become weakened and loose as their matrix and cells in those areas are activated to promote destruction or inhibit repair. These changes collectively cause narrowing of the joint space, joint instability, stiffness, and pain.

The joints most commonly affected by OA are the knees, hips, and joints in the hands and spine. Erosion of the cartilage also occurs secondary to excessive mechanical stress on the joint (e.g., aging, obesity, overuse, injury, and congenital musculoskeletal conditions) but as previously discussed, mechanical stress is not the only factor leading to cartilage destruction. Some disorders, such as obesity, may also contribute to OA development as a result of metabolic derangement and not simply mechanical stress. Non–weight-bearing joints such as the hands are commonly affected in obese individuals with OA. The proposed mechanism is not clear. Adipose tissue produces proinflammatory cytokines, which contributes to OA development. Adipose tissue also produces leptin, an adipokine, that may produce degradative enzymes (e.g., matrix metalloproteinases) and directly lead to joint destruction. Additionally, OA may occur as a primary condition in which the cause is idiopathic.

Clinical Manifestations

Disease onset is gradual and usually begins after the age of 40. Manifestations may be present in one or a few joints. The key manifestations are joint pain, stiffness, and decreased range of motion. OA often begins in the hands and then affects the knees, and other commonly affected joints include the hip and spine. Other joints affected less commonly are the shoulder, ankle, elbow, and wrist. The following clinical manifestations often develop slowly and worsen over time:

- Joint pain that is exacerbated during or after movement or weight-bearing and is relieved by rest. Pain and stiffness eventually become more constant (usually dull and achy) and unpredictable.

TABLE 12-3 | Comparison of Major Features of Common Types of Arthritis

	Rheumatoid arthritis	Osteoarthritis	Gout
Age and sex of usual patient	Young and middle-aged, female	Adults, older persons, both sexes but more common in females	Middle-aged, male
Major characteristic	Systemic disease with major effects in joints; causes chronic synovitis	Degeneration of articular cartilage	Disturbance of purine metabolism; acute episodes caused by crystals of uric acid in joints
Secondary effects of disease	Ingrowth of inflammatory tissue over cartilage destroys cartilage, leads to destruction of joint space; deformities common	Overgrowth of bone; thickening of periarticular soft tissues	Deposits of uric acid in joints with damage to joints (gouty arthritis); soft tissue tophi
Joints usually affected	Small joints of hands and feet	Central and peripheral joints—predilection for hand, knee, hip, spine	Small joints; joint at base of great toe often affected
Special features	Autoantibody against gamma globulin (rheumatoid factor)	No systemic symptoms or biochemical abnormalities	High blood level of uric acid

- Joint tenderness with light pressure. The joint tenderness is prominent at the joint line (the connection between two joints).
- Joint stiffness, especially upon rising in the morning, which dissipates within 30 minutes, or joint stiffness after a period of inactivity.
- Limited joint range of motion that occurs as osteophytes develop and the joint capsule thickens.
- Joint deformities that occur as the disease advances.
- Enlarged, hard joints due to bone thickening and hypertrophy of the joint capsule. The hard joints of the distal interphalangeal joint of the fingers are named *Heberden nodes* while hard joints of the proximal interphalangeal joints of the fingers are named Bouchard nodes.
- Minimal swelling that can be mistaken for enlarged joints.
- Crepitus (grating sound or sensation produced by gliding of bone and cartilage).

Diagnosis and Treatment

Diagnosis of OA is based on a history and physical examination. If there are typical manifestations, X-rays and MRI are not necessary for diagnosis. Young age, atypical joint location, weight loss, or other symptoms may be caused by another disorder and warrant further testing. Laboratory tests, such as erythrocyte sedimentation rate or other inflammatory markers, are normal in OA and are usually performed to exclude other diagnosis (e.g., rheumatoid arthritis).

There is currently no cure for OA. The goals of treatment are to increase joint strength, maintain joint mobility, reduce disability, and relieve pain. Treatment strategies may include a combination of physical therapy, weight loss/management, ambulatory aids (e.g., walkers and canes), orthopedic devices (e.g., braces and splints), pharmacologic agents, and surgery. Pharmacologic therapies may involve oral and topical analgesics, NSAIDs (including cyclooxygenase-2 inhibitors), and corticosteroids. As OA is a chronic disorder, long-term side effects of each pharmacotherapeutic agent need to be considered (e.g., NSAID use and peptic ulcer development). Analgesics should only be used in the presence of pain and not as a preventive measure. Acetaminophen is not considered an effective analgesic for OA. Additionally, synthetic synovial fluid and corticosteroids may be injected directly into the joint. Herbal therapies that may be helpful include glucosamine, chondroitin, and ginger, although research evidence is mixed regarding their efficacy. Pain management may focus on adequate rest, heat/cold application, topical agents that create a cool or hot sensation, water therapy (e.g., whirlpool and water aerobics), acupuncture, tai chi, and yoga. In some cases, surgery may be necessary to repair or replace damaged joints. These procedures may include arthroscopy to trim torn and damaged cartilage, osteotomy to change the alignment of a bone and relieve stress on the bone or joint, surgical fusion, and arthroplasty to completely or partially replace the damaged joint with an artificial joint.

Learning Points

Septic Arthritis

Septic arthritis refers to an infection in a joint. Recognition is important as complications such as amputation can occur. The organism (bacteria—*Staphylococcus aureus* and resistant forms) usually enters via the bloodstream (hematogenous spread) or through direct inoculation into the joint or as an extension of a bone infection. Septic arthritis is more likely to occur in patients with pre-existing arthritic disorders (e.g., gout or rheumatoid arthritis). The onset of symptoms is acute, and joints that are infected will be painful, swollen, and warm; and movement will be limited. Fever will be present. Diagnosis is usually made with synovial fluid analysis and culture (obtained prior to antibiotic administration). Treatment strategies include joint drainage and antibiotics.

Rheumatoid Arthritis

Rheumatoid arthritis (RA) is a systemic, autoimmune condition involving multiple joints. In RA, the inflammatory process primarily affects the synovial membrane, but it can also affect other organs (e.g., heart, skin, and eyes). RA rates in the United States have declined since 1990. According to the CDC (2016b), an estimated 1.5 million Americans have RA. Risk factors include family history, advancing age (although a juvenile form also exists), and smoking. RA is more common in women, and research is being conducted to explore the potential role that hormones might play in its etiology.

The exact cause of RA is unknown, but it is thought to be caused by a genetic vulnerability due to several genes that influence development and severity. The most commonly associated genes are the human leukocyte antigen (HLA) genes that participate in self-protein recognition. Epigenetic alterations, such as dysregulation in histones or expression of microRNAs, influence RA development. Other factors include environmental triggers, particularly smoking, possible infectious agents, other antigens, and the autoimmune process. See chapter 1 for details about cellular function.

RA begins with an initial acute inflammatory episode, after which the joint may appear to recover. The process is repeated, and the immune system is repeatedly activated. Systemic inflammation and autoantibody production are thought to occur years before the disease becomes clinically evident. The cell-mediated (particularly CD4 helper T cells) immune system activation leads to inflammatory cytokine (e.g., interleukin, tumor necrosis factor, and RANKL) release and eventual destruction of the joints and tissue. Each exacerbation includes synovitis, pannus formation (a mass of granulation tissue, fibroblasts, and synovial inflammatory cells), cartilage erosion (due to enzymes, mainly metalloproteinases, from the pannus), fibrosis, and **ankylosis** (joint fixation and deformity) (Figure 12-34; Table 12-3). Over time, the recurring inflammation has a cumulative effect—it thickens the synovium, which can eventually invade and destroy the cartilage and bone within the joint. In addition, the muscles, tendons, and ligaments that hold the joint together weaken and stretch. Synovial inflammation affects the vasculature, and vascular flow becomes impeded by surrounding debris (e.g., fibrin and platelets). Gradually, the joint loses its shape and alignment. The humoral immune system activation (B cells) causes production of autoantibodies that attack the host (self-antigens). Normal circulating antibodies, with continued antigen exposure, become autoantibodies and begin attacking the host, resulting in a type III hypersensitivity reaction. The autoantibodies are known as rheumatoid factors, and the most common classes are IgM and IgG antibodies and occasionally IgA. Autoimmune complexes form and can deposit in tissues. The immune complexes can vary, resulting in the characteristic remission and exacerbations seen in autoimmune disorders. The complement system is activated, further perpetuating inflammatory activity, increasing capillary permeability, and contributing to joint effusion. See chapter 2 for more on immunity.

Clinical Manifestations

Like other autoimmune disorders, RA is typically characterized by remissions and exacerbations. The disease onset is usually insidious, with vague articular and nonarticular manifestations that can mimic other conditions. Clinical manifestations are usually gradual, progressive, and involve multiple joints (i.e., they are polyarticular). The typical classic manifestations include pain, stiffness (particularly in the morning lasting more than 1 hour), and swelling of several joints in a symmetric pattern. The joints commonly affected are those of the hands, particularly the

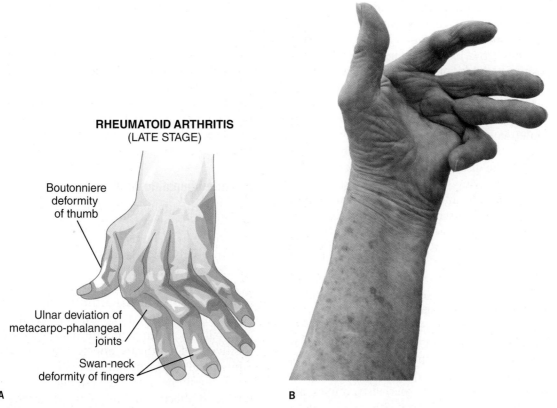

RHEUMATOID ARTHRITIS
(LATE STAGE)

Boutonniere
deformity
of thumb

Ulnar deviation of
metacarpo-phalangeal
joints

Swan-neck
deformity of fingers

A

B

FIGURE 12-35 Joint deformities associated with rheumatoid arthritis.

B: © Peterfactors/Dreamstime.com.

metacarpophalangeal (knuckles) and proximal interphalangeal joints of the fingers and the interphalangeal joints of the thumbs; the wrists; and the metatarsophalangeal joints of the toes. Other joints affected include the elbows, shoulders, ankles, and knees. Most patients with RA present initially with polyarthritis; however, some patients may have monoarthritis (affecting one joint such as a knee or shoulder) that then progresses to polyarthritis within months. The joint pain is characterized as aching and stiffness, which worsens when pressure is applied or with movement. The joint may also be swollen. Due to synovial thickening, the joint may feel boggy or mushy, and if an effusion is present, the joint may feel fluctuant. The joint is not red or warm. As the disease progresses, the joints can become deformed (e.g., they may have ulnar drift or swan neck deformities and boutonnière deformities of the fingers; FIGURE 12-35). The cervical spine can become involved in RA, but the other axial skeleton components are not usually affected (e.g., sacroiliac joint or thoracic/lumbar spine). Rheumatoid nodules may be seen and palpated in the subcutaneous tissue, usually on the elbows. Other nonarticular findings include anemia, fatigue, anorexia, weight loss,

and depression. RA can affect various organs such as the heart and lung (e.g., pleuropericarditis), the eyes (e.g., scleritis), vascular system (e.g., vasculitis), spleen (splenomegaly), and renal disease (e.g., amyloid deposits in kidneys). Sjögren syndrome (an immune system disorder characterized by dry eyes and dry mouth) can occur with RA.

Diagnosis and Treatment

Diagnostic procedures for RA may consist of a history and a physical examination. Serum rheumatoid factor and anticyclic citrullinated peptide antibodies tests will be positive; however, these antibodies can be negative upon initial presentation of patients with RA. Citrullination (i.e., deamination) is a process where amino acid arginine is converted to amino acid citrulline. Citrullinated proteins have a different structure and function than other proteins and are vulnerable to attack by the immune system. In RA, anticitrullinated protein antibodies develop against these citrullinated proteins and are measured in the serum as anticyclic citrullinated peptide antibodies. Another citrullinated peptide antibody can be measured against a specific mutated citrullinated vimentin (protein). Acute phase reactants, erythrocyte sedimentation rate, and serum C-reactive protein levels are usually high, reflecting the inflammatory state. Serum antinuclear antibody (ANA) is usually negative but can be positive in a third of patients with RA. Synovial fluid analysis will be positive for rheumatoid factor and other immune cells such as leukocytes, which are usually between 1,500 and 25,000/cubic mm (counts are usually low with osteoarthritis). Joint X-rays may be normal early in the disease, and with progression joint space narrowing, bone erosion, and eventual osteopenia become evident. MRI and ultrasounds may be used. Other blood tests will include a complete blood count with differential and platelet count as well as liver and kidney function evaluation.

There is no cure for RA, so treatment focuses on remission and slowing the progression of the disease to avoid irreversible damage and destruction of affected RA areas. Early, aggressive treatment for RA is important. Treatment strategies are complex and often require the support of an interprofessional team consisting of rheumatology specialists, nurses, and a wide range of therapists. Strategies may include the following measures:

- Adequate rest and pacing activities
- Physical and occupational therapy (including therapy directed at maintaining or increasing range of motion)
- Regular exercise
- Pharmacologic therapies, including the following:
  - Disease-modifying antirheumatic drugs early in the disease course to prevent, stop, and slow injury, including the following:
    - Immunosuppressant agents (e.g., methotrexate—usually the initial agent)
    - Antimalarial agents (e.g., hydroxychloroquine [Plaquenil])
    - Gold compounds
  - NSAIDs (to relieve pain and inflammation) in conjunction with disease-modifying antirheumatic drugs
  - Corticosteroids (either orally or as an intra-articular injection to decrease inflammation) in conjunction with disease-modifying antirheumatic drugs
  - Biologic response–modifying agents (e.g., infliximab [Remicade]) (which block tumor necrosis factor, an inflammatory cytokine associated with RA)
  - Herbal therapies, including thunder god vine, plant oils, and fish oil

- Nonpharmacologic pain management (e.g., relaxation techniques, tai chi)
- Application of heat and cold
- Splints and braces (to support joints, maintain proper alignment, and prevent deformities)
- Assistive devices (e.g., walkers and rails)
- Coping strategies and support
- Surgical repair (e.g., synovectomy and arthroplasty)

Juvenile Idiopathic Arthritis

Juvenile rheumatoid arthritis was reclassified as juvenile idiopathic arthritis (JIA) to reflect that there is a broad category of childhood arthritis with no relationship to seropositive rheumatoid arthritis. There are several types of JIA such as psoriatic arthritis, enthesitis, oligoarthritis, polyarticular arthritis, and systemic arthritis. Enthesitis affects multiple joints and is usually found in someone who is HLA-B27 positive. Oligoarthritis affects four or fewer joints, and polyarticular JIA affects five or more. Systemic JIA has systemic manifestations and affects multiple joints. Regardless of the type, a common feature is chronic arthritis (> 6 weeks) in a joint that occurs in the young (< 16 years old). The overall incidence is complicated as prior classifications were centered on juvenile rheumatoid arthritis, which encompassed three of the current types. The general mechanisms in the development of JIA include autoimmunity, genetic factors, immune dysfunction, and environmental factors.

The major clinical manifestation is joint swelling, which is a result of synovial thickening and fluid accumulation. Due to the thickening, structures surrounding the affected joints become deformed due to ligament and tendon stretching. Eventually inflammatory cells in the synovial fluid release degradative enzymes, and the articular cartilage (collagen and proteoglycan) breaks down. Inflammatory cytokines activate osteoclasts leading to bone demineralization and erosion. The articular damage, in addition to joint swelling, causes joint stiffness. The stiffness occurs after a period of inactivity such as after sleep and improves with activity. Other clinical manifestations will be dependent on the type as systemic arthritis is characterized by daily fever spikes, pink macular rash, and hepatosplenomegaly and lymphadenopathy. Patients with oligoarticular arthritis are at risk for the development of uveitis (middle eye [uvea] inflammation). Patients with polyarticular arthritis that is rheumatoid factor positive may develop rheumatoid nodules and many of the manifestations of adult rheumatoid arthritis. Psoriatic arthritis can present with integumentary findings such as onycholysis or nail pitting, although these findings can occur years after the arthritis.

Diagnostic tests will be similar to many of the other tests used for other forms of arthritis such as an ESR, CRP, rheumatoid factor, and ANA. Treatment strategies are also similar to those used for other arthritis such as NSAIDs, disease-modifying antirheumatic drugs, and biologics. Rehabilitation and family support may be necessary as some forms of JIA can significantly impact quality of life.

Gout

Gout is an inflammatory disease resulting from deposits of uric acid crystals (monosodium urate) in tissues and fluids within the body (**FIGURE 12-36**; Table 12-3). The body produces uric acid when it breaks down purines, a substance naturally found in the body as well as in certain foods (e.g., organ meats, shellfish, anchovies, herring, asparagus, and mushrooms). Normally, uric acid dissolves in the blood and is excreted by the kidneys. Gout results from an overproduction of uric acid (urate) or, more commonly underexcretion of uric acid by the kidneys or gastrointestinal system. Many people with hyperuricemia, however, never develop gout.

Gout affects approximately 8.3 million people in the United States and is considered the most common type of inflammatory arthritis. Gout is more frequent in males and certain ethnicities such as Pacific Islanders and Blacks (CDC, 2016a). It may occur as a primary inborn error of metabolism or secondary to some contributing factor. Factors contributing to its development include being overweight or obese, having certain diseases (e.g., hypertension, diabetes mellitus, renal disease, and sickle cell anemia), consuming alcohol (beer and spirits more than wine), using certain medications (e.g., thiazide or loop diuretics), and following a diet rich in meat and seafood. Dietary factors, however, may trigger rather than cause gout. Gout is more prevalent with advanced age with incidence increasing around the fourth decade. In women, the incidence increases after menopause as serum urate levels become comparable to those of men.

Gout typically follows four phases. Initially, the individual with gout is asymptomatic, though uric levels are climbing in the bloodstream and uric acid crystals are being deposited in the tissues (**FIGURE 12-37**). Over time, these crystals accumulate, damaging tissues. This damage or release of preformed crystal deposits triggers an acute inflammation that characterizes the second phase of gout, referred to as *acute flares* or *attacks*. Neutrophils (key mediators), monocytes/macrophages, and lymphocytes infiltrate the synovial fluid during the acute inflammatory gout flare. A flare is distinguished by pain, burning, redness, swelling, and warmth at the affected joint lasting days to weeks. Pain may be mild or excruciating. Most initial attacks occur in the lower extremities. The metatarsophalangeal joint of the big toe is the presenting joint for 50% of people with gout (i.e., podagra). The possible reasons for predisposition for the big toe metatarsophalangeal joint include coolness (reduces solubility of crystals), the repeated trauma of the joint that might alter the tissue, and reabsorption of joint fluids and urate by the toe when going from weight-bearing to lying down. Podagra often occurs at night possibly because during rest water is absorbed from the joint more rapidly than urate, thereby increasing amount of uric acid at night. After the acute attack subsides, the person may enter intercritical periods in which the disease remains clinically inactive until the next flare (the third phase). The person with gout continues to have hyperuricemia, which results in continued deposits of uric acid crystals in tissues, which, in turn, cause damage and bony erosions that can evolve to chronic gouty arthropathy. These intercritical periods

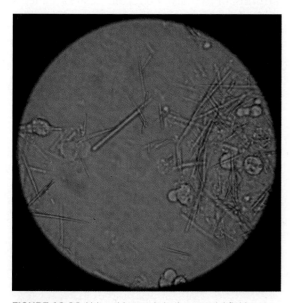

FIGURE 12-36 Uric acid crystals in the synovial fluid.

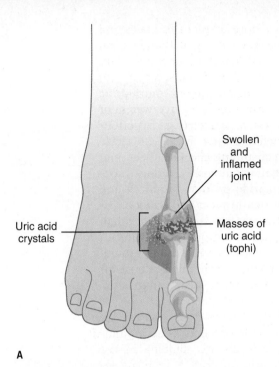

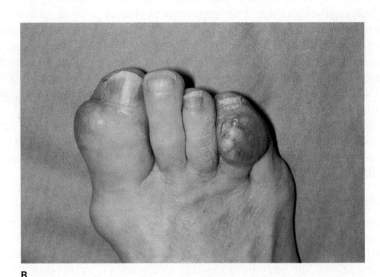

A

B

FIGURE 12-37 Gout.

B: © Dr. Ken Greer/Visuals Unlimited, Inc.

become shorter as the disease progresses. Reoccurring attacks are often precipitated by sudden increases in serum uric acid. In the final phase, chronic gout is characterized by chronic arthritis associated with soreness and aching of joints. People with gout may also develop **tophi** (large, hard nodules composed of uric acid crystals surrounded by granulomatous inflammation and deposited in soft tissue), usually in cooler areas of the body (e.g., toes, elbows, ears, and distal finger joints). The tophi cause chronic inflammation and are found in joints, bone, cartilage, tendons, and skin and, uncommonly, on organs. Because some renal calculi (kidney stones) are made of uric acid, renal calculi may also be associated with gout, and chronic urate nephropathy can also occur (see chapter 7 for details on urinary function).

Clinical Manifestations

Clinical manifestations of gout vary depending on the phase that the individual is experiencing. Usually gout is monoarticular (one joint), but multiple-joint (polyarticular) flares are likely with long-standing disease. Manifestations of acute gout attacks include the following symptoms:

- Intense pain at the affected joint (usually the big toe) that frequently starts during the night and is often described as throbbing, crushing, burning, or excruciating

- Joint warmth, redness, swelling, and tenderness (even to light touch)
- Fever

The severity of the flare usually peaks within 24 hours, and the resolution occurs within weeks even if the patient is not treated. After a first gout attack, patients may have no symptoms for varying lengths of time. Some people may go months or even years between gout attacks. Although some individuals develop chronic gouty arthritis, others have no further attacks. Patients with chronic arthritis develop joint deformities and limited joint mobility. With chronic gout, joint pain and other symptoms will be present most of the time. Tophi may form below the skin around joints or in other places with chronic gout. Tophi can cause a local inflammatory response, and draining them may reveal the presence of a chalky material.

Diagnosis and Treatment

Diagnostic procedures for gout include a history, physical examination, serum uric acid levels, urine uric acid levels (will be low in those with gout caused by underexcretion), synovial fluid analysis (presence of uric acid crystals), and joint X-rays (may demonstrate erosion). The level at which uric acid crystals precipitate is usually greater than 6.8 mg/dL. If joint fluid analysis cannot be conducted, then a clinical diagnosis can be made with a diagnostic scoring tool with weighted points assigned to each of the following seven clinical manifestations: male sex, previous arthritis flare, onset of joint flare within one day, joint redness, first metatarsal phalangeal joint involvement, hypertension or at least one cardiovascular disease, or serum urate level greater than 5.88 mg/dL. The greater the number of manifestations, the higher the score and the higher the probability of gout.

Treatment strategies focus on lowering uric acid levels, usually with medications and dietary changes. Medications often vary depending on the current phase of gout the patient is experiencing. Treatment strategies for gout may include avoiding triggers such as stress, high protein, and alcohol; as well as pharmacologic therapy for acute gout attacks and preventing the complications associated with frequent gout attacks.

Pharmacology for Acute Attacks

- NSAIDs to control inflammation and pain; higher doses to stop an acute attack
- Colchicine, an analgesic that is particularly effective in reducing gout pain
- Corticosteroids, usually oral, to relieve inflammation and pain; intraarticular injections can be considered

Pharmacology to Prevent Complications

- Xanthine oxidase inhibitors (e.g., allopurinol [Zyloprim]) to block uric acid production
- Uricosuric drugs (e.g., probenecid [Probalan]) to improve renal excretion of uric acid
- Uricase drugs (e.g., pegloticase) to lower uric acid level

When initiating urate-lowering medications, a gout flare can be precipitated, so an acute gout flare medication is often recommended (e.g., colchicine). The increased excretion caused by initiation of urate-lowering medications can also cause kidney stone formation, so increased hydration (e.g., 2 or more liters of fluids per day) is recommended at the beginning of therapy. Serum urate-lowering goals are in the vicinity of less than 6 mg/dL.

Ankylosing Spondylitis

Ankylosing spondylitis is a progressive inflammatory disorder affecting the sacroiliac joints, intervertebral spaces, and costovertebral joints. Ankylosing spondylitis is one of several groups of disorders categorized as spondyloarthritis. The inflammation associated with this condition starts in the vertebral joints where the ligaments, tendons, bones, and cartilage interface. As the inflammation persists, destruction of bone (an osteoclastic process) with new bone formation (an osteoblastic process) can occur in an attempt to remodel the damage. Fibrosis and calcification, or fusion, of the joints follows. The vertebral joints become fixed, or ankylosed, and lose mobility. Inflammation begins in the lower back at the sacroiliac joints and progresses up the spine. The vertebrae appear square, and the vertebral column becomes rigid (referred to as *bamboo spine*) and loses curvature (**FIGURE 12-38**).

The exact cause of ankylosing spondylitis is unknown, although genetic factors seem to be involved. In particular, people who have a gene called *HLA-B27* are at significantly increased risk of this condition. Ankylosing spondylitis is more common in males than in females and typically appears between 20 and 40 years of age. Ankylosing spondylitis is associated with psoriasis and inflammatory bowel disease. Complications include kyphosis, osteopenia, osteoporosis, vertebral fractures, respiratory compromise due to reduced lung expansion resulting from fusion of the rib cage, endocarditis (inflammation of the internal cardiac structures), and uveitis.

Clinical Manifestations

Clinical manifestations of ankylosing spondylitis reflect the decreased joint mobility. The individual may experience periods of remission and exacerbation. Inflammatory back pain characteristics are different than mechanical causes. The following five characteristics of inflammatory back pain include:

1. Onset before the age of 40
2. Insidious onset
3. Improves with exercise
4. No improvement with rest
5. Pain at night, which improves upon arising

Other characteristics and manifestations of ankylosing spondylitis include:

- Intermittent lower back pain (early)
- Lower back pain and buttocks pain that can be initially one-sided and that evolves to include the entire back
- Pain in other joints (especially the shoulders, hips, or lower extremities)
- Muscle spasms
- Fatigue
- Low-grade fever early in the course of the disease

Normal anatomy

Ankylosing spondylitis

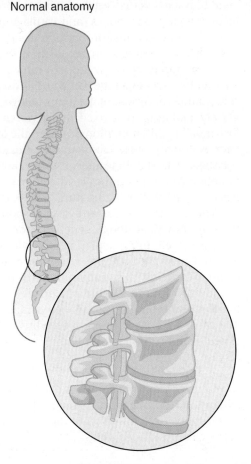

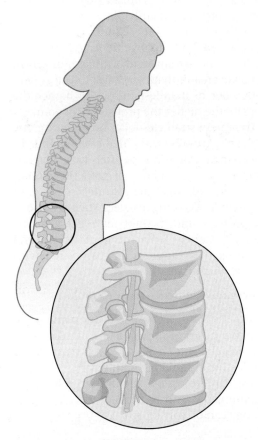

Normal S-curve of spine

Loss of normal curvature

FIGURE 12-38 Ankylosing spondylitis.

- Weight loss
- Kyphosis, loss of normal lumbar lordosis, and flexion deformity of the hips

Diagnosis and Treatment

Diagnostic procedures for ankylosing spondylitis may consist of a history and physical examination. Laboratory tests include evaluation for serum presence of the *HLA-B27* gene. Erythrocyte sedimentation rate, C-reactive protein, and alkaline phosphatase may be elevated. Spine X-rays, spine CT, and spine MRI may reveal findings such as bony erosions, ankylosis, changes in joint width, and sclerosis. An X-ray may reveal a bamboo-appearing spine, which is considered a late sign.

The goal of treatment is to relieve pain and stiffness as well as prevent or delay complications and spinal deformity. Treatment of ankylosing spondylitis is most successful when it is initiated before the disease causes irreversible damage (e.g., fusion), especially in positions

that limit function. Treatment strategies may include the following measures:

- NSAIDs (generally the initial therapy), tumor necrosis factor inhibitors to relieve inflammation, pain, and stiffness
- Muscle relaxants to treat muscle spasms
- Physical therapy, including range-of-motion exercises and positioning
- Surgical repair (e.g., hip arthroplasty)
- Health-promoting lifestyle behaviors (e.g., proper nutrition, adequate rest, stress management, and smoking cessation)
- Coping strategies and support

Chronic Muscle Disorders

Chronic muscle disorders include conditions that result from a wide range of causes (e.g., genetic predisposition, trauma, and infection). These conditions may lead to chronic pain, weakness, and paralysis. Chronic muscle disorders may be progressive, requiring lifelong treatment. Treatment is often aimed at managing symptoms because most of these conditions have no known cure.

Muscular Dystrophy

Muscular dystrophy (MD) refers to a group of inherited, noninflammatory disorders characterized by degeneration of skeletal muscle. Muscles become weaker as damage from these disorders worsens. Nine different forms of MD are distinguished (including Becker MD, Duchenne MD, myotonic MD, and limb-girdle MD), each with its own pattern of inheritance (e.g., X-linked recessive, autosomal dominant, and autosomal recessive) and pathogenesis (e.g., age of onset and progression). The commonality across all types is the presence of a muscle protein abnormality (dystrophin). The dystrophin protein is normally located on the plasma membrane of muscle fibers, and its function is to provide sarcolemma reinforcement and glycoprotein stabilizations so that the muscle

fibers do not degrade. Without dystrophin, the proteases digest the glycoprotein complex and cause muscle dysfunction, weakness, muscle fiber loss, and inflammation, and it may involve other tissues (e.g., cardiac and smooth muscle tissues). Over time, fat and fibrosis connective tissues replace skeletal muscle fibers in persons with MD.

Some types of MD are rare, while others are relatively common. Most types of MD are inherited, but some occur because of a genetic mutation (often spontaneous). Some types cause tremendous disability and rapid decline; whereas others are associated with minimal symptoms and hardly noticeable progression. Some types present in childhood, while others present in late adulthood. Duchenne MD is the most common and severe type, affecting only males (X-linked recessive). Complications of MD may include cardiomyopathy, recurrent respiratory infections, respiratory compromise, and death.

BOX 12-3 Application to Practice

A 48-year-old White male presents to the clinic for an evaluation of rapid onset of swelling of his left big toe and pain for the past 2 days. The pain is an 8 out 10 on a pain scale (0 indicates no pain and 10 indicates severe pain). The toe is red and warm. He denies injury or any decreased range of motion.

Past medical history: hypertension.
Surgical history: none.
Hospitalizations: none.
Immunization history: up to date.
Social history: No smoking or illicit drug use. Drinks one or two beers a day and one or two cocktails on the weekends.
Medications: hydrochlorothiazide 25 mg orally once a day.

Allergies: no known drug allergies.
Vital signs: Temperature 98.7° F; pulse 72 beats per minute; respiration rate 16 breaths per minute; blood pressure 120/80 mmHg; and O₂ saturation 99% on room air. His BMI is 31.

The review of symptoms is negative for fever, chills, nausea, vomiting, rash, headache, chest pain, palpitations, or shortness of breath.

Physical examination reveals a well-nourished adult male without any acute distress. Significant physical findings include a hot, erythematous, and tender left first metatarsophalangeal joint. Pedal pulses are palpable bilaterally. Gait is steady. Skin is fully intact.

Answer the following questions:

1. What is the most likely diagnosis of this patient? Explain the pathophysiology of this disorder.
2. What other information about this patient would be helpful in making the diagnosis?
3. What is the best test to confirm the diagnosis for this patient? Why?
4. What are the pharmacologic and nonpharmacologic treatment strategies that are suitable for this patient?
5. What recommendations should be made to prevent future musculoskeletal risks for this patient?

Deana Goldin, PhD, DNP, APRN, FNP-BC.

Clinical Manifestations

Clinical manifestations of MD vary depending on the type. All or a select group of the muscles may be affected. In general, manifestations may include the following signs and symptoms:

- Intellectual disability (in some types)
- Muscle weakness that slowly worsens to hypotonia
- Muscle spasms
- Delayed development of muscle motor skills
- Difficulty using one or more muscle groups
- Poor coordination
- Drooling
- Ptosis (eyelid drooping)
- Frequent falls
- Problems walking (e.g., delayed walking)
- Gowers maneuver (an affected child pushes to an erect position by using his or her hands to climb the legs)
- Progressive loss of joint mobility and contractures (e.g., clubfoot and foot drop)
- Unilateral calf hypertrophy
- Scoliosis or lordosis

Diagnosis and Treatment

Diagnostic procedures for MD may consist of a history, physical examination, muscle biopsy, electromyography, electrocardiogram, serum creatine kinase levels, test for serum presence of defective dystrophin, and genetic testing. Additionally, fetal chorionic villus testing can be performed prenatally at 12 weeks' gestation.

Learning Points

Statins and Effects on Muscles

Medications classified as statins are the primary pharmacotherapeutic agents used to lower serum cholesterol. Among the side effects of statins are various muscle syndromes that include myalgia (muscle pain), myopathy (muscle weakness not due to pain), myositis (muscle inflammation), and muscle injury (myonecrosis and/or rhabdomyolysis). Myalgia and myopathy incidence ranges from 2 to 11%, while muscle injury is rare ($< 0.5\%$). The muscle syndromes due to statins usually begin within weeks to a few months after initiation of therapy but can occur at any time. Discontinuation is the treatment, and it can take a few days to weeks for symptoms to dissipate completely. The myalgia and myopathy tend to be proximal, symmetric muscle weakness and/or soreness. The patient may complain of fatigue or tiredness.

There is no cure for MD; however, gene therapy may potentially be feasible. The goal of treatment is to maintain motor function and prevent deformities as long as possible. Treatment strategies may include physical therapy, proper nutrition, muscle relaxants, immunosuppressant agents (e.g., oral glucocorticoids), assistive devices (e.g., walker, braces, and splints), and surgical contracture release. Additionally, coping strategies and support for the patient and caregivers may be beneficial.

Fibromyalgia

Fibromyalgia is a syndrome predominantly characterized by widespread muscular pains and fatigue. This disorder affects joints, muscles, tendons, and surrounding tissues. No apparent inflammation or degeneration is associated with fibromyalgia. The cause remains uncertain, but fibromyalgia may be related to an altered pattern of central neurotransmission that results in sensitivity to substance P (a neurotransmitter responsible for pain sensation). Other pain-processing abnormalities that have been identified in patients with fibromyalgia include decreased levels of inhibitory neurotransmitters (e.g., serotonin and norepinephrine), enhanced temporal summation of pain (perceived intensity of pain increases with repetitive stimuli), altered endogenous opioid analgesic activity, and dopamine dysregulation. In fibromyalgia, the brain's pain receptors seem to develop a sort of pain memory and become more sensitive to pain signals (i.e., lowered pain threshold). Additional postulated causes include physical or emotional trauma, sleep disturbances, altered skeletal muscle metabolism, infections, and genetic predisposition. The CDC (2015a) estimates that approximately 5 million Americans have fibromyalgia, with the prevalence rates being highest among women.

Clinical Manifestations

Clinical manifestations may vary depending on the weather, stress, fatigue, physical activity, and time of day. In general, fibromyalgia is characterized by widespread pain, typically described as a constant, dull, muscle ache. Fatigue, sleep disturbances, depression, irritable bowel syndrome, headaches, and memory problems may also occur with this chronic disorder. Joint swelling or inflammation is absent.

Conditions often associated with fibromyalgia include RA, systemic lupus erythematosus, and ankylosing spondylitis.

Diagnosis and Treatment

Various classification criteria are available for fibromyalgia. The American College of Rheumatology (Ward et al., 2016) criteria centers on a widespread pain index (WPI) and symptom severity scale (FIGURE 12-39). The WPI reflects pain that can occur in 19 different body areas. The symptom severity scale score includes data pertaining to the degree of fatigue, waking unrefreshed, and cognitive symptoms (e.g., thinking or remembering), as well as the number of general somatic symptoms (e.g., depression, headache). Based on these criteria, a WPI rating of > 7 and symptom severity scale score of ≥ 5 or a WPI rating of 4 to 6 with a symptom severity scale score of ≥ 9 are consistent with fibromyalgia The pain must be in at least four different regions and present for at least 3 months. Diagnostic testing such as a complete blood count or erythrocyte sedimentation rate may be performed to evaluate for other diagnoses and are normal with fibromyalgia.

Treatment strategies focus on minimizing symptoms and improving overall health. These strategies may include stress reduction, regular exercise, adequate rest, proper nutrition, heat application, massage therapy, acupuncture, physical therapy, analgesics, antidepressant agents (e.g., tricyclic amitriptyline or selective serotonin reuptake inhibitors such as duloxetine), muscle relaxants, and antiseizure agents (specifically, pregabalin [Lyrica] or gabapentin). NSAIDs are not considered effective with fibromyalgia. Coping strategies, counseling, and support may be helpful as well.

Learning Points

Rhabdomyolysis is a syndrome that can occur due to multiple triggering events such as trauma to muscle, prolonged immobilization, extreme exertion in an unconditioned individual, hyperthermia, and infections. The syndrome is characterized by muscle cell death and release of cell content into the bloodstream. The usual triad of symptoms include muscle pain, weakness, and dark urine. The serum creatine kinase, particularly the skeletal muscle fraction, is markedly elevated (at least 5 times the normal). Myoglobinuria is released from damaged muscle and causes the dark urine. Several fluid and electrolyte imbalances can occur (e.g., hyperkalemia, hypocalcemia). Complications can include acute kidney injury, hypercalcemia, compartment syndrome, and rarely disseminated intravascular coagulation.

Widespread Pain Index

Please indicate if you have had pain or tenderness **during the past 7 days** in the areas shown below. Check the boxes in the diagram for each area in which you have had pain or tenderness.

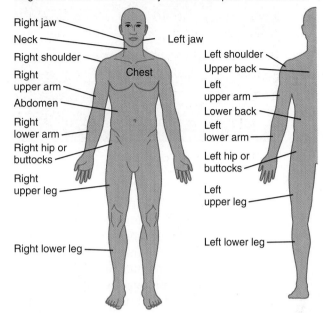

FIGURE 12-39 Widespread pain index: 19 points for fibromyalgia criteria.

Bone and Muscle Neoplasms

Tumors of the musculoskeletal system typically arise from the bone. Bone tumors can be malignant or benign. Bone tumors can be secondary, stemming from other cancers (e.g., breast, lung, and prostate). Bone tumors rarely occur as primary tumors. The exact cause of these primary tumors is unknown, but they are more common in men and Whites (National Cancer Institute, 2016). Paget disease increases the risk of developing primary bone cancer. The overall 5-year survival rate for bone cancer is approximately 67%.

Bone cancer usually occurs in areas of rapid bone growth and is described based on the type of cell in which the cancer originates. The mesodermal layer is where bone tumors originate and where fibroblast progenitors and reticulum cells are present. The fibroblasts are the progenitors of the osteoblasts and chondroblasts. Bone cancer types and clinical manifestations include osteogenic, chondrogenic, collagen, and myelogenic tumors.

Osteogenic tumors are a mix of osteoid and sarcoma tissue. An osteosarcoma is

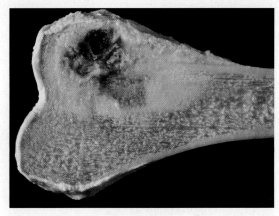

FIGURE 12-40 Osteosarcoma.
© CNRI/Science Source.

an aggressive tumor that begins in the bone cells, usually in the femur, tibia, or humerus (**FIGURE 12-40**). While uncommon, it is the most common primary bone malignancy. Osteosarcoma occurs most often in children and young adults but peaks again over the age of 65 (it is considered a secondary tumor in adults when occurring due to Paget disease or other disorder). The usual clinical manifestations are localized pain that initially is intermittent and progressively becomes longer in duration and more severe. Swelling may also be present. Systemic symptoms such as fever and weight loss are usually absent.

Chondrogenic tumors are cartilage-producing tumors. An osteochondroma is a tumor that develops adjacent to growth plates or joints. The most common benign bone tumor (it can, however, become malignant), it occurs most often in persons between 10 and 20 years of age. It usually presents as a painless mass near a joint or on the axial skeleton or as a painful mass with local trauma. Depending on location (usually the knee or humerus), range of motion may be decreased or pathologic fractures may be present.

A chondrosarcoma is a slow-growing tumor that begins in the cartilage cells commonly found on the ends of bones. It is the third most common primary malignant bone tumor and frequently affects older adults (the peak incidence is in the sixth decade of life). Initially, pain and swelling are local, dull, and intermittent. As the disease progresses, the pain increases in intensity and duration.

Collagen tumors are a mix of fibrous connective tissue. A fibrosarcoma is usually a solitary tumor that affects the metaphysis of the femur or tibia. It is rare and may be primary or secondary (e.g., due to Paget disease or radiation therapy). Fibrosarcoma is more common in adults between the ages of 30 and 50. Manifestations include local pain and swelling, a palpable mass, decreased range of motion, and pathologic fractures.

Myelogenic tumors originate in bone marrow cells. They include Giant cell tumors and multiple myeloma (see chapter 3 for more on hematopoietic function).

A giant cell tumor is usually benign and solitary. This type of tumor is more common in women than men (most other bone tumors are more common in men), and the most common ages affected are between 20 and 40 years of age. As with other tumors, local pain and swelling, pathologic fractures, and decreased range of motion are common manifestations.

Ewing sarcoma is an aggressive tumor (metastasis usually occurs within 1 year) whose origin is unknown. This type may begin in nerve tissue within the bone. Ewing sarcoma occurs most frequently in children and young adults, and it is 10 times more common in Whites than in other ethnic groups. The incidence is highest during rapid growth periods with a peak incidence between the ages of 10 and 20 years. Like osteosarcoma, pain is the most common manifestation. A mass may also be present. Systemic symptoms can include fever, anorexia, and malaise.

Diagnostic procedures for bone tumors may consist of a history, physical examination, X-rays, CT, MRI, positron emission tomography, bone scan, and biopsy. Treatment varies depending on the type and stage of the cancer. Surgical excision or amputation is often the treatment of choice. Radiation and chemotherapy may be used following surgery if the tumor is inoperable or in the presence of metastasis.

Muscle tumors are rare. **Rhabdomyosarcoma** is a malignant tumor of the striated muscle. These tumors are usually found in the head and neck, genitourinary tract, and extremities. The tumors are aggressive with rapid metastasis. They are more common in children and adolescents. The manifestations are dependent on the locations (e.g., orbital tumors can produce proptosis).

CHAPTER SUMMARY

The musculoskeletal system forms the framework for the body, provides support and protection, and allows for movement. Damage to this system is likely to cause issues with mobility. Musculoskeletal disorders vary from short lived and mild to long term and debilitating in nature. Although most of these disorders are not life threatening, many of them can result in life-altering effects. Musculoskeletal damage may be caused by trauma, genetic defects, metabolic imbalances, or daily and wear and tear. Supporting musculoskeletal health involves strategies such as weight management, proper nutrition, regular exercise, abstaining from smoking, and observing safety precautions (e.g., wearing safety equipment).

REFERENCES AND RESOURCES

AAOS. (2004). *Paramedic: Anatomy and physiology*. Sudbury, MA: Jones and Bartlett Publishers.

Alikhan, M., Lohr, K., & Driver, K. (2015). Paget disease. *Medscape*. Retrieved from http://emedicine.medscape.com/article/334607-overview#a3

American Society of Anesthesiologists. (2014). *Continuum of depth of sedation: Definition of general anesthesia and levels of sedation/analgesia*. Retrieved from https://www.asahq.org/standards-and-guidelines/continuum-of-depth-of-sedation-definition-of-general-anesthesia-and-levels-of-sedationan-algesia

Armstrong, A. D., & Hubbard, M. C. (2016). *Essentials of musculoskeletal care* (5th ed.). Burlington, MA: Jones & Bartlett Learning.

Centers for Disease Control and Prevention (CDC). (2015a). Fibromyalgia. Retrieved from http://www.cdc.gov/arthritis/basics/fibromyalgia.htm

Centers for Disease Control and Prevention (CDC). (2015b). Osteoarthritis. Retrieved from http://www.cdc.gov/arthritis/basics/osteoarthritis.htm

Centers for Disease Control and Prevention (CDC). (2016a). Gout. Retrieved from http://www.cdc.gov/arthritis/basics/gout.html

Centers for Disease Control and Prevention (CDC). (2016b). Rheumatoid arthritis (RA). Retrieved from http://www.cdc.gov/arthritis/basics/rheumatoid.htm

Centers for Disease Control and Prevention (CDC). (2017). Child abuse prevention. Retrieved from https://www.cdc.gov/features/healthychildren/index.html

Child Trends. (2018). Child maltreatment. Retrieved from https://www.childtrends.org/indicators/child-maltreatment

Chiras, D. (2015). *Human biology* (8th ed.). Burlington, MA: Jones & Bartlett Learning.

Cosman, F., de Beur, S. J., LeBoff, M. S., Lewiecki, E. M., Tanner, B., Randall, S., ... National Osteoporosis Foundation. (2014). Clinician's guide to prevention and treatment of osteoporosis. *Osteoporosis International: A Journal Established as Result of Cooperation Between the European Foundation for Osteoporosis and the National Osteoporosis Foundation of the USA, 25*(10), 2359–2381. doi:10.1007/s00198-014-2794-2

Crowley, L. V. (2017). *An introduction to human disease* (10th ed.). Burlington, MA: Jones & Bartlett Learning.

Elling, B., Elling, K., & Rothenberg, M. (2004). *Anatomy and physiology*. Sudbury, MA: Jones and Bartlett Publishers.

Gould, B. (2015). *Pathophysiology for the health professions* (5th ed.). Philadelphia, PA: Elsevier.

Madara, B., & Pomarico-Denino, V. (2008). *Quick look nursing: Pathophysiology* (2nd ed.). Sudbury, MA: Jones and Bartlett Publishers.

National Cancer Institute. (2016). Bone and joint cancer. Retrieved from http://seer.cancer.gov/statfacts/html/bones.html

National Institutes of Health (NIH). (2018). Low back pain fact sheet. Retrieved from https://www.ninds.nih.gov/Disorders/Patient-Caregiver-Education/Fact-Sheets/Low-Back-Pain-Fact-Sheet

National Osteoporosis Foundation. (2016). What is osteoporosis and what causes it? Retrieved from https://www.nof.org/patients/what-is-osteoporosis/

Osterhoff, G., Morgan, E. F., Shefelbine, S. J., Karim, L., McNamara, L. M., & Augat, P. (2016). Bone mechanical properties and changes with osteoporosis. *Injury, 47*(Suppl 2), S11–S20. doi:10.1016/S0020-1383(16)47003-8

Professional guide to pathophysiology (3rd ed.). (2010). Philadelphia, PA: Lippincott Williams & Wilkins.

Singer, F. R., Bone, H. G., Hosking, D. J., Lyles, K. W., Murad, M. H., Reid, I. R., & Siris, E. S. (2014). Paget's disease of bone: An Endocrine Society clinical practice guideline. *The Journal of Clinical Endocrinology & Metabolism, 99*(12), 4408–4422. https://doi.org/10.1210/jc.2014-2910

United States Preventive Services Task Force (USPSTF). (2011). Retrieved from https://www.uspreventiveservicestaskforce.org/Page/Document/RecommendationStatementFinal/osteoporosis-screening1

Ward, M. M., Deodhar, A., Akl, E. A., Lui, A., Ermann, J., Gensler, L. S., . . . Caplan, L. (2016). American College of Rheumatology/Spondylitis Association of America/Spondyloarthritis Research and Treatment Network 2015 recommendations for the treatment of ankylosing spondylitis and nonradiographic axial spondyloarthritis. *Arthritis & Rheumatology, 6*(2). doi: 10.1002/ART.39298

Wolfe, F., Clauw, D. J., FitzCharles, M., Goldenerberg, D., Häuser, W., Katz, R. S., . . . Walitt, B. (2016). 2016 Revisions to the 2010/2011 fibromyalgia diagnostic criteria [abstract]. *Arthritis Rheumatology, 68*(Suppl 10). Retrieved from https://acrabstracts.org/abstract/2016-revisions-to-the-20102011-fibromyalgia-diagnostic-criteria/

World Health Organization. (1994). *Assessment of fracture risk and its application to screening for postmenopausal osteoporosis: Report of a WHO study group [meeting held in Rome from 22 to 25 June 1992]*. Retrieved from http://www.who.int/iris/handle/10665/39142

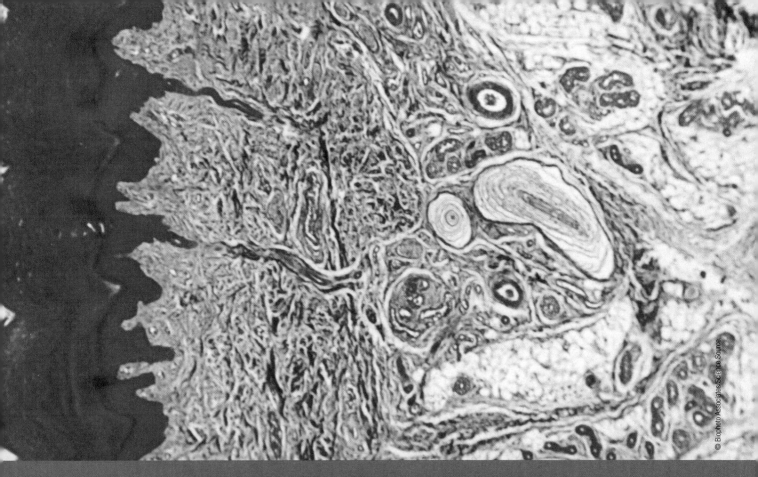
© Biophoto Associates/Science Source.

CHAPTER 13
Integumentary Function

The integumentary system protects the body from pathogen invasions, regulates temperature, senses environmental changes, and maintains water balance. This system comprises the skin, nails, hair, mucous membranes, and glands. Disorders of the integumentary structures can result in numerous issues because of the extensive functions of this system. Such disorders can stem from a wide range of causes, including congenital defects, advancing age, inflammation, infections, and cancers. The skin, just like a book cover, can provide an abundance of information pertaining to internal bodily functions. Many skin conditions, such as birthmarks, are mild and may not require treatment, whereas others, such as skin cancer, can be life threatening.

Anatomy and Physiology

The skin, along with the nails, hair, mucous membranes, and glands, constitutes the integumentary system. In addition to participating in sensory functions, the integumentary system plays a key role in immunity, temperature regulation, and water balance. Moreover, this system excretes a small amount of waste products. The integumentary system is the body's largest organ system, covering all external surfaces and accounting for approximately 15% of the body's weight.

The skin consists of three layers—the epidermis, the dermis, and the hypodermis (FIGURE 13-1). The epidermis, or outermost layer of the skin, comprises squamous epithelia, or flat sheets of cells. The dermis, the middle layer, is composed of dense, irregular connective tissue and very little fatty tissue. The dermis includes nerves, hair follicles, smooth muscle, glands, blood vessels, and lymphatic vessels. The hypodermis, or subcutaneous tissue, is the innermost layer of the skin, consisting of soft, fatty tissue as well as blood vessels, nerves, and immune cells (e.g., macrophages).

Epidermis

The epidermis consists of five distinct layers (FIGURE 13-2).

1. **Stratum corneum:** The outermost layer of body protection against environment. The **stratum corneum** is composed of waterproof keratin.
2. **Stratum lucidum:** The location of transitional cells that maintain function. Cells appear as stratum corneum cells.
3. **Stratum granulosum:** The location of cell loss or continued cell keratin production.
4. **Stratum spinosum:** The location of basal cell differentiation into cells such as keratinocytes. Keratin production commences in this layer. The cells continue migrating toward the stratum corneum.

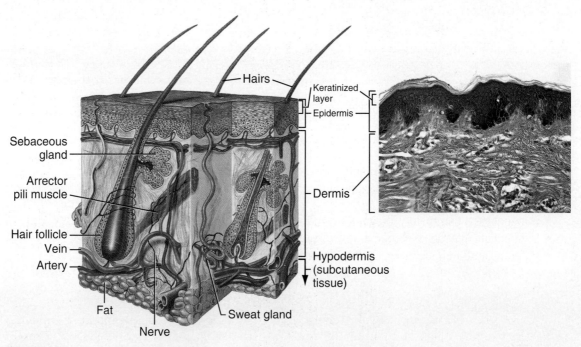

Hairs

Keratinized layer

Epidermis

Sebaceous gland

Arrector pili muscle

Dermis

Hair follicle

Vein

Artery

Hypodermis (subcutaneous tissue)

Fat

Sweat gland

Nerve

FIGURE 13-1 The layers of the skin.

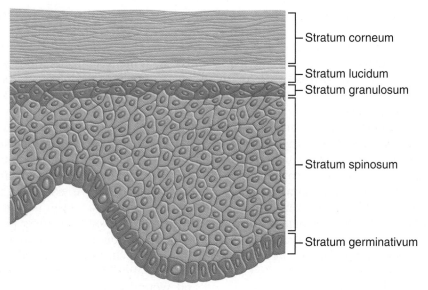

- Stratum corneum
- Stratum lucidum
- Stratum granulosum
- Stratum spinosum
- Stratum germinativum

FIGURE 13-2 The layers of the epidermis.

5. **Stratum germinativum:** The innermost layer attached to basal cells (the basement membrane) that separate the epidermis from dermis. Basal cells remain in the **stratum germinativum** and undergo mitosis to produce keratinocytes. Specialized cells, known as Merkel cells, are connected to afferent nerves with receptors responsible for the sensation of touch. Although located throughout the body, the Merkel cells are abundant in areas used often in detecting touch (fingers, toes, lips, mouth). The basement membrane is a selectively permeable membrane.

New cells proliferate from the innermost basal layer and push upward toward the stratum corneum. The outer layers often contain 25 sheets of dead cells that are continuously shed; however, the number of layers can vary around the body with the palms and soles having about 100 layers. Most of these cells (e.g., keratinocytes and melanocytes) produce keratin, a protein that strengthens skin, and melanin, a pigment that gives the skin, hair, and eyes color. The types of melanin are eumelanin and pheomelanin. Eumelanin (brown and black pigments) protects the skin from ultraviolet (UV) rays. Eumelanin causes tanning and freckles. Pheomelanin (yellow and red pigment) reacts to ultraviolet light, and this reaction possibly explains why fair-skinned people are more susceptible to skin cancer. Everyone has the same number of melanocytes. The difference in skin tones (light to dark) in individuals is explained by the amount of melanin produced, which is genetically determined.

Other important cells in the epidermis are Langerhans cells that are part of the skin's immunologic function. Langerhans cells are dendritic cells (antigen-presenting cells), formed in the bone marrow, that recognize foreign antigens and transport them to the lymphatic system. These cells also produce cytokines involved in the immune system (see chapter 2 for a discussion of immunity).

Dermis and Appendages

The dermis is the layer between the epidermis and subcutaneous layers. This layer has many structures and the protein collagen. The collagen is in a substance known as hyaluronic acid, which helps the skin to retain moisture. Many lotions and topical skin products contain hyaluronic acid to help with dry skin. Sebaceous glands produce sebum, which moisturizes and protects the skin. The sebaceous glands are located throughout the body except for the palms, soles, and sides of the feet. The glands' secretory activity is controlled by genetics and hormones such as testosterone, and the glands are inactive until adolescence. During adolescence, the glands increase in size and produce more sebum, leading to inflammation—one component of acne vulgaris. Two types of sweat glands—eccrine and apocrine glands—are located throughout the skin. Eccrine glands, which are also known as merocrine glands, secrete sweat (sodium chloride and water) through skin pores in response to the sympathetic nervous system. The eccrine gland function includes temperature regulation by secreting water. The eccrine glands are located throughout the body except on the lips and genitalia. Apocrine glands open into hair follicles in the axillae, scalp, face, and external genitalia. Skin bacteria convert apocrine secretions (oily) into chemicals that cause human body odor.

The dermis also consists of hair, which is keratinized and emanates from hair follicles. Hair phases—growth (anagen), atrophy (catagen), and rest (telogen)—are influenced by hormones. Hair follicles are often part of sebaceous glands, and together they form the pilosebaceous unit. Several disorders stem from the pilosebaceous unit, such as acne vulgaris. Other structures of the dermis include nerves, smooth muscle, blood vessels, and lymphatic vessels.

Subcutaneous Tissue

The subcutaneous layer—the hypodermis—connects the dermis to the muscle. The subcutaneous layer is made of fat cells (adipose tissue) and connective tissue that functions as a cushion for the body and provides insulation from cold temperatures. Blood vessels, nerves, and macrophages are also located in this layer.

Nails

Nails consist of hard, keratinized plates located on the fingers and toes. Nail growth is continuous and occurs in a structure known as the nail matrix. The end of growth is a crescent-shaped white area known as the lunula. The cuticle is at the lower part of the nail, and the paronychium is the tissue that surrounds the border. The nail bed is vascular, so it can be a window into oxygenation status (e.g., cyanosis, pallor, or clubbing). The nail can develop disorders such as onychomycosis, and nail bed abnormalities can be a sign of an underlying systemic disorder (e.g., leukonychia in liver or heart disease).

Understanding Conditions That Affect the Integumentary System

There are approximately 2,200 disorders of the skin, so when considering alterations of the integumentary system, organizing them based on their basic underlying pathophysiology can increase understanding. Skin disorders can be organized by how they occurred (e.g., infections, allergens, and trauma), and by the anatomic structure predominantly affected (e.g., sebaceous gland or the dermal layer). Disorders can be organized by those that are congenital or those that are due to aging. Skin disorders are easy to detect visually; however, determining the cause is usually based on a thorough history, as many skin alterations have a similar appearance. Skin disorders often occur in certain body distributions (e.g., trunk or extremities) while sparing body areas, so pattern and distribution are also important in diagnosing skin disorders. Impairments in skin integrity require interventions that are intended to either prevent such impairment, maintain skin integrity, or improve skin integrity. Because the skin provides a barrier to protect the body from invasion, skin disorders are a relevant risk for infection. Interventions to prevent and manage infections are directed at minimizing contamination, for example, by hand washing and wound care, and by supporting the immune system such as by proper nutrition. The skin can also be a window to the body's inside, and an understanding of skin alterations can provide relevant information in regards to potential or actual systemic disorders.

Congenital Integumentary Disorders

Congenital disorders of the integumentary system can vary widely in severity. Many conditions occur because of an error during embryonic development. These errors may occur randomly, due to environmental influences, or because of genetic abnormalities. Congenital disorders usually cause vascular tumors or malformations or melanocytes or melanin (i.e., pigmentary) abnormalities. They may cause either minor conditions with only aesthetic problems (e.g., birthmarks) or life-altering states (e.g., albinism). Occasionally, these seemingly benign conditions may be associated with other, more serious problems that warrant further investigation. Treatment is often unnecessary, but when needed, these options are usually limited.

Birthmarks

Birthmarks are skin anomalies that are present at birth or shortly after. Most are harmless and may even shrink or disappear with age. Birthmarks vary from barely noticeable to disfiguring. These abnormalities may be flat or raised, have regular or irregular borders, and have different shades of coloring including brown, tan, black, pale blue, pink, red, or purple. Birthmarks cannot be prevented and are not the result of anything done or not done during pregnancy. Two types of birthmarks are distinguished—vascular and pigmented.

Vascular Birthmarks

Vascular birthmarks can arise from blood vessels that have not formed correctly (i.e., vascular malformations), vessels that are proliferating (i.e., vascular tumors such as hemangiomas), or due to vessel dilation (e.g., nevus simplex). Due to the vascular alterations, these birthmarks are generally red. The various types of vascular birthmarks include nevus simplex, hemangiomas, and port-wine stains.

Macular stains, also called *nevus simplices, salmon patches, angel kisses,* and *stork bites*—are the most common type of vascular birthmark (**FIGURE 13-3**). Nevus simplex is due to vessel vasodilation. These faint red patches (flat, nonpalpable > 1 cm) are blanchable and often occur on the forehead, eyelids, posterior neck, nose, upper lip, or posterior head (**TABLE 13-1**). On a baby, these birthmarks may be more noticeable when crying. Most often, these marks fade on their own by 2 years of age, but they sometimes last into adulthood (e.g., back-of-neck patches).

Hemangiomas, also referred to as *strawberries* (although not all look like strawberries), are birthmarks that appear usually as a solitary bright red papule (raised, palpable, < 1 cm), a plaque (raised, palpable, > 1 cm), or a nodule due to the proliferation of the vascular endothelium in the skin (**FIGURE 13-4**). They are more common in girls than boys. They may be either superficial or deep. The deep hemangiomas may be bluish because they involve deeper blood vessels and may have a telangiectatic patch in the center. Hemangiomas grow (proliferate) during the first year of life and

then usually recede (regress) over time. Most involute by 5 years of age and the remainder by 9 years. Some hemangiomas, particularly larger ones, leave scars as they regress; these scars can be corrected by minor plastic surgery. Many hemangiomas are found on the head or neck, although they can appear anywhere on the body. Most are benign and not associated with other medical conditions, but they can ulcerate and cause complications if their location interferes with sight, feeding, breathing, or other bodily functions.

TABLE 13-1	Lesion Description	
Lesion	**Description**
Macule	Flat, nonpalpable, < 1 cm (circumscribed area)
Patch	Flat, nonpalpable, > 1 cm
Papule	Raised, palpable, < 1 cm (circumscribed area)
Nodule	Raised, palpable; deeper in dermis than papule, 1–2 cm (circumscribed area)
Plaque	Raised, palpable, > 1 cm (rough surface)
Vesicle	Serous, filled "blisters" < 1 cm
Bulla	Serous, filled "blisters" > 1 cm
Pustule	Like vesicle but fluid is pus
Cyst	Raised, palpable, filled with liquid (circumscribed area)

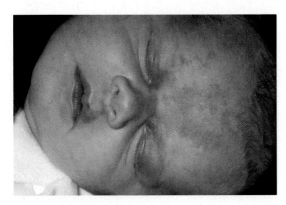

FIGURE 13-3 Macular stain.
© Dr. P. Marazzi/Science Source.

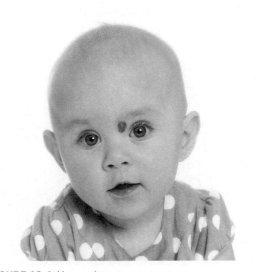

FIGURE 13-4 Hemangioma.
© Julie DeGuia/Shutterstock.

Port-wine stains, also called *nevus flammeus*, are discolorations that look like wine was spilled on an area of the body—hence their name (FIGURE 13-5). These birthmarks most often occur on the face, neck, arms, and legs. Port-wine stains are caused by malformations of the dermis capillaries and venules. Port-wine stains are patches that are blanchable and can be any size, but they grow only as the child grows. They tend to be unilateral and do not cross the midline (i.e., they stay on one side). They tend to darken over time and can thicken and have a cobblestone texture in mid-adulthood unless treated. Port-wine stains will not resolve spontaneously, and those occurring near the eye should be assessed for possible complications such as glaucoma, as well as other conditions (e.g., Sturge-Weber syndrome).

Pigmented Birthmarks

Pigmented birthmarks are made of a cluster of pigment cells, which cause color in skin. These birthmarks can be many different colors, from tan to brown, gray to black, or even blue. The most common pigmented birthmarks are café au lait spots, Mongolian spots, and moles.

Café au lait macules or spots are very common birthmarks that are the color of coffee with milk—hence their name (FIGURE 13-6). These birthmarks are macules (flat, nonpalpable, < 1 cm) or patches and can appear anywhere on the body. They sometimes increase in number as a child gets older. Café au lait macules are caused by increased melanin production. One café au lait macule alone is not usually a concern, but the child should be further evaluated if he or she has several patches larger than a quarter, which can be a sign of neurofibromatosis.

Mongolian spots, also called *congenital dermal melanocytosis*, are flat, bluish-gray macules or patches that are nonblanching and often found on the lower back or buttocks (FIGURE 13-7). Mongolian spots are caused because melanocytes that are not normally in the dermis (only in the basal layers) have not migrated up to the epidermis. These birthmarks are most common on individuals with darker complexions, such as children of Asian, American Indian, Black, Hispanic, and Southern European descent. Mongolian spots are usually benign, and they usually fade, often completely, by school age without treatment. However, some are associated with pediatric disorders (e.g., inborn errors of metabolism).

Mole (congenital nevi, hairy nevi) is a general term for melanocytic nevi or brown nevi (the singular is *nevus*). Most people get moles at some point in life. When present at birth or within a few months after birth, the mole is called a *congenital melanocytic nevus* and will last a lifetime. Large or giant congenital nevi are more likely to develop into skin cancer (melanoma) later in life; however, all moles should be monitored for cancerous changes.

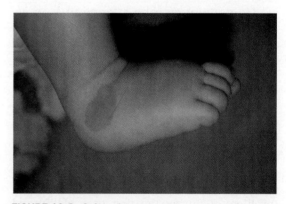

FIGURE 13-6 Café au lait spot.
Courtesy of Marnie Pasciuto-Wood.

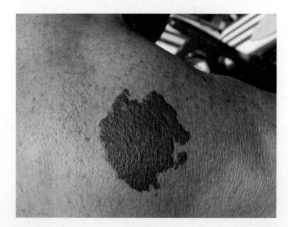

FIGURE 13-5 Port-wine stain.
© guentermanaus/Shutterstock.

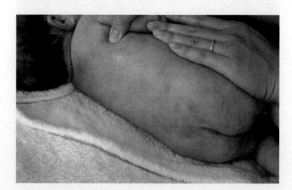

FIGURE 13-7 Mongolian spot.
Courtesy of Wassa Catlow.

Moles can be tan, brown, or black; can be flat or raised; and may have hair growth.

Diagnosis and Treatment

Diagnosis of birthmarks is often made during a physical examination. Treatment strategies vary depending on the type of birthmark, as some birthmarks cannot be treated. Macular stains and Mongolian spots usually fade away on their own. Hemangiomas are usually left untreated, as they typically shrink back into themselves by age 9. Laser therapy can be used for removal of some hemangiomas, such as small, superficial ones. Larger or more serious hemangiomas often are treated with steroids. Laser therapy is the treatment of choice for port-wine stains. Most port-wine stains lighten significantly after several laser treatments, although some return and need retreatment. Laser treatment is typically started in infancy when the stain and the blood vessels are smaller. Marks on the head and neck are the most responsive to laser treatment.

Pigmented birthmarks are usually left untreated, with the exception of moles and, occasionally, café au lait macules. Moles (particularly large or giant congenital nevi) are surgically removed. Café au lait macules can be removed with laser treatment but often return.

Some birthmarks can be disfiguring and embarrassing for children. Special opaque makeup can be used to conceal or minimize the appearance of some birthmarks. Additionally, support and coping strategies can be helpful.

Learning Points

Erythema Blanching

When there is erythema or skin discoloration, the lesion should be assessed for blanching. Pressure is applied for a few seconds over an area, which temporarily decreases blood flow and the area turns pale or white. When the pressure is released, the color should return and the erythema is described as *blanchable*. In nonblanchable erythema, pallor does not occur or the redness persists (this may appear differently in darker skin); in other words, the erythema does not fade when pressure is applied. Nonblanchable erythema is an indication of altered perfusion.

Disorders of Melanin

Melanin is a pigment that provides color and protection. Disorders involving melanin result in alterations in skin coloring and can leave the skin vulnerable to the harmful effects of UV light. Melanin disorders include albinism and vitiligo.

Albinism

Albinism is a condition that results in little or no melanin production (melanocyte numbers are adequate). Most cases are inherited in an autosomal recessive pattern. Melanin deficits cause a lack of pigment in the skin, hair, and the eyes (**FIGURE 13-8**). In addition to coloring and protection, melanin plays a role in the development of certain optical nerves. Therefore, all forms of albinism cause problems with eye development and function. Albinism is generally grouped into oculocutaneous albinism (OCA), which affects the skin, hair, and eyes; or ocular albinism (X-linked recessive), affects mainly the eyes, and hair and skin color are normal to near normal coloration. OCA is more common than ocular albinism.

Seven different types of OCA (OCA 1–7) are associated with mutations on different genes. The most common worldwide is OCA type 2, and in the United States, OCA type 1 and type 2 are the most prevalent forms. OCA type 1 is due to a defect in an enzyme, tyrosinase, which is necessary in melanin synthesis (i.e., melanogenesis). Tyrosinase defects can cause no melanin production to varying amounts of melanin production. OCA type 2 is due to a mutation in the *OCA2* gene (formerly called *P gene*). The *OCA2* gene regulates a pH-regulating protein that is necessary for tyrosinase enzyme function. Rare OCA mutations can occur in genes also associated with several syndromes such as Hermansky-Pudlak and Chédiak-Higashi syndromes. Hermansky-Pudlak syndrome is very rare (1 in 500,000–1,000,000 persons worldwide) and results in OCA, a bleeding disorder, and lung and bowel diseases. Chédiak-Higashi syndrome is also rare (200–500 cases worldwide) and results in OCA, recurrent bacterial

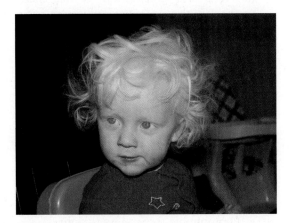

FIGURE 13-8 Albinism.
Courtesy of Cassandra Hartley.

infections, neurologic abnormalities, coagulation defects, and lymphoma-like abnormalities.

Clinical Manifestations

Clinical manifestations of albinism are usually—but not always—apparent in a person's skin, hair, and eye color. Regardless of the effect of albinism on appearance, all people with the disorder experience vision impairments. Manifestations may include the following conditions:

- **Skin changes:** Although the most recognizable form of albinism results in milky white skin (OCA 1), skin pigmentation can range from white to nearly the same as relatives without albinism (OCA 2). For some people with albinism, skin pigmentation never changes. For others, melanin production may begin or increase during childhood and adolescence, resulting in slight increases in pigmentation. Some people may synthesize melanin and develop freckles, moles (with or without pigment), or lentigines (large frecklelike spots) with exposure to the sun.
- **Hair changes:** Hair color can range from very white to brown. People who are Black or of Asian descent who have albinism may have hair color that is yellow, reddish, or brown. Hair color may also change by early adulthood.
- **Eye changes:** Eye color can range from very light blue to brown and may change with age. The lack of pigment in the irises makes them somewhat translucent, meaning they cannot completely block light from entering the eye. This translucence can cause very light-colored eyes to appear pink-red in some lighting because of light reflecting off the retina and passing back out through the iris again. The retina also has reduced pigmentation, which makes the back of the eye appear yellowish or orange; therefore, this pigmentary change gives a different color eye similar to when a flash photograph changes eye color.
- **Vision changes:** Multiple vision issues can result from the lack of melanin, including the following problems:
  - Nystagmus (rapid, involuntary back-and-forth eye movement)
  - Strabismus (inability of both eyes to stay directed at the same point or to move in unison, or crossed eyes)
  - Extreme nearsightedness or farsightedness
  - Photophobia (sensitivity to light)
  - Astigmatism (abnormally shaped cornea)
  - Functional blindness

Diagnosis and Treatment

Diagnostic procedures for albinism consist of a history, physical examination (including a thorough ophthalmologic exam), and genetic testing (most accurate). Although there is no cure for albinism, people with this disorder can take steps to improve vision and avoid damage from sun exposure:

- Using sunscreen with a high sun protection factor (SPF) against ultraviolet A and B (UVA and UVB, respectively) rays
- Wearing protective clothing (e.g., long-sleeved shirts, long pants, and hats)
- Limiting time outdoors, especially between 10:00 a.m. and 4:00 p.m., when the sun's UV rays are the most intense
- Wearing sunglasses (with UV protection), which may relieve light sensitivity
- Avoiding or caution in using medications that increase photosensitivity (e.g., antihistamines, statins)
- Performing routine skin self-examination and obtaining a routine skin examination by a healthcare provider (e.g., dermatologist)
- Wearing glasses to correct vision problems and eye position
- Having eye muscle surgery to correct abnormal eye movements (i.e., nystagmus)

Albinism does not impair intellectual development, although people with albinism often feel socially isolated and may experience discrimination. Coping strategies and support may be beneficial in addressing these issues. The visual issues may lead to educational challenges. Educational strategies may include sitting at the front of the classroom, using large-print books and notes, and printing materials with high-contrast colors (e.g., black and white).

Vitiligo

Vitiligo is a rare condition characterized by areas of hypopigmentation (**FIGURE 13-9**). This disorder occurs when melanocytes die or no longer form melanin, causing slowly enlarging hypopigmented macules and patches that are well demarcated. The lesions can vary in size from millimeters to a few centimeters. This condition affects people of all races but may be more noticeable and disfiguring in people with dark skin tones. Its exact cause is unknown, but potential causes of melanocyte destruction include genetic susceptibillity (multifactorial inheritance), autoimmunity, and oxidative stress.

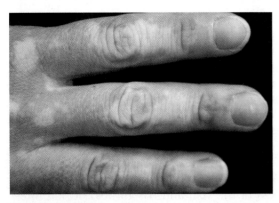

FIGURE 13-9 Vitiligo.
© Nadine Mitchell/Dreamstime.com.

Vitiligo is associated with autoimmune disorders such as pernicious anemia, autoimmune hypothyroidism, and Addison disease. Although any area of the body may be affected, depigmentation usually develops first on sun-exposed areas (e.g., hands, feet, arms, face, and lips). Vitiligo often first appears between 10 and 30 years of age, and in this age group, most report a family or personal history of autoimmune disorder. Onset at a younger age (e.g., < 12 years of age) is often associated with a family history of vitiligo or other depigmenting disorders. Vitiligo generally develops in one of three patterns. Nonsegmental vitiligo encompasses a focal pattern, meaning depigmentation is limited to one or a few areas of the body. The second pattern is generalized and depigmentation is widespread across many parts of the body, often symmetrically. The third pattern is considered segmental, and depigmentation occurs on one side of the body. Segmental pattern is not as common as the nonsegmental patterns and usually occurs with childhood-onset vitiligo.

The natural course of vitiligo is difficult to predict. Sometimes the patches stop forming without treatment. In most cases, pigment loss spreads and can eventually involve most of the skin's surface. In addition to patchy skin depigmentation, clinical manifestations may include depigmentation of the hair, mucous membranes, and retina.

Diagnosis and Treatment

Diagnosis of vitiligo is usually made clinically with a history and physical examination. Use of a Wood lamp will reveal depigmented areas that are bright blue–white. Due to the association with autoimmune thyroid disorder, diagnostic evaluation will include a thyroid function panel (e.g., thyroid stimulating

hormone, T3, T4) and antithyroperoxidase and antithyroglobulin antibodies. Evaluation for other autoimmune disorders may be necessary. Skin biopsy may be necessary if the diagnosis is questionable. There is no cure for vitiligo. The goal of treatment is to stop or slow the progression of pigment loss and attempt to return some pigment. Treatments to stabilize rapid progression of vitiligo may include the following measures:

- Intermittent or minipulse therapy (e.g., given two times a week for a few months)
- Low dose corticosteroids, oral or intramuscular
- Phototherapy

Treatment for repigmentation and coping strategies may include the following measures:

- Phototherapy (controlled exposure to intense UV light in a clinic or hospital)
- Pharmacotherapy, including the following medications:
  - Oral synthetic melanizing agents (e.g., trimethylpsoralen [Trisoralen])
  - Topical corticosteroid agents
  - Topical immunosuppressants, which are also known as calcineurin inhibitors (e.g., pimecrolimus [Elidel] and tacrolimus [Protopic])
  - Topical repigmenting agents (e.g., methoxsalen [Oxsoralen])
  - Oral or topical photochemotherapy (e.g., psoralen plus UVA radiation)
- Skin graft
- Autologous melanocyte transplant (still experimental)
- Permanent depigmentation of the remaining skin (a last resort reserved for extreme cases)
- Sun safeguards (e.g., sunscreen and protective clothing)
- Coping strategies and support:
  - Makeup or skin dyes
  - Tattooing (most effective around the lips)

Learning Points

Sunscreens

Ultraviolet (UV) radiation from the sun includes UVA and UVB rays. UVA are the most prevalent rays that reach the earth (95%) and is mainly responsible for photoaging and skin darkening but also causes burn but less than UVB. UVA rays have a possible role in skin cancer development. UVB rays are the remaining rays (5%) that reach the earth and are mainly responsible for sunburns, inflammation, and darkening. A way to remember the key effects are UV**A** causes **a**ging and UV**B** causes **b**urns. Sunscreens have ingredients (there are 17 different FDA-approved types) that act as filters to reflect or absorb UVA and UVB rays (i.e., they are broad spectrum). Sun protection factor (SPF) is a measure of the sunscreen's ability to absorb UVB rays. The minimum recommended by the FDA is SPF 15 (it absorbs 93% of UVB rays), and the American Academy of Dermatology recommends SPF 30 (absorbs 97% of UVB rays). There are no sunscreens that block 100%, but slightly higher numbers may block more. Regardless of SPF, sunscreen should be applied to all exposed skin (ears, feet, head etc.) and applied 15 minutes before sun exposure. Reapplication should occur every 2 hours, after swimming, or sweating. Some sunscreens may be water resistant and last longer with water exposure (up to 80 minutes).

Integumentary Changes Associated With Aging

The skin undergoes several changes with aging. Sensations of pain, vibration, cold, heat, pressure, and touch usually decrease over the course of the life span. These changes may be related to decreases in blood flow to touch receptors, decreased number of receptors (i.e., Meissner and pacinian corpuscles) or decreased blood flow to the brain that can occur with age. Decreases in these sensations can increase the risk of injury, including falls, pressure injuries, burns, hypothermia, and decreased pain perception. See chapter 14 for a discussion of sensory function.

In addition to sensory changes, the skin undergoes other aging-related changes. It loses elasticity, integrity, and moisture over time. Environmental factors, genetic makeup, and nutrition may all contribute to these changes. The greatest single contributing factor, however, is sun exposure (i.e., photoaging). Every month the epidermis sheds, but this shedding decreases with aging, prolonging the amount of time skin is exposed to carcinogens. There is also a decrease in protective macrophages. Natural pigments seem to provide some protection against sun-induced skin damage. Consequently, blue-eyed, fair-skinned people show more of these aging skin changes than people with darker, more heavily pigmented skin. The combined changes of decreased epidermal shedding and decreased macrophages along with carcinogen exposure increases the risk for integumentary cancers.

With aging, the epidermis thins, even though the number of cell layers remains unchanged. The number of melanocytes decreases, but the remaining melanocytes increase in size. Aging skin thus appears thin, pale, and translucent. Large pigmented spots called *age spots*, *liver spots*, or *lentigos* occur as a consequence of long-standing sun exposure causing increased melanin production. The lentigines may appear in sun-exposed areas (FIGURE 13-10). The basement membrane, which is normally undulated, flattens out, and the epidermal thinning makes the skin vulnerable to injuries (e.g., abrasions, blisters). Removing bandages in the elderly can easily cause tearing of the skin. The flattened basement membrane reduces the surface area for movement of necessary and protective skin nutrients. The decreased protective skin nutrients contribute to drying (i.e., xerosis) of the skin and risk for loss of skin integrity. **Seborrheic keratosis** is a benign tumor that is usually seen in older age. These tumors are due to immature keratinocyte proliferation in the epidermis. The cause is unknown, but there may be a genetic predisposition. The lesions are well demarcated and can be round or oval (FIGURE 13-11). The lesions appear stuck

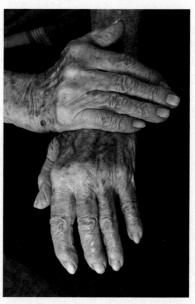

FIGURE 13-10 Lentigo.
Courtesy of Dean Ducas.

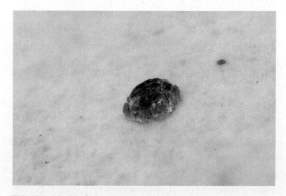

FIGURE 13-11 Seborrheic keratosis or senile wart.
© Lipowski Milan/Shuttestock.

on, and their surface looks like a wart. They are referred to as *senile warts* or *seborrheic verruca*, and they can have different colors (e.g., yellowish, dark brown). While they are usually asymptomatic because they are elevated, friction or trauma can cause pain and bleeding.

The dermal changes include decreases in collagen and elastin. In sun-exposed areas, these changes in the connective tissue reduce the skin's strength, elasticity, and resilience. These changes further contribute to thin skin and is the cause of wrinkling. Dermis blood vessels become fragile, which can lead to bruising (senile purpura), cherry angiomas (a benign collection of capillaries) (**FIGURE 13-12**), and other similar conditions.

Sebaceous glands also produce less sebum over time. Men experience a minimal decrease in sebum production, usually after the age of 80, whereas women gradually produce less sebum beginning after menopause. This decrease in sebum can make it difficult to maintain skin moisture, resulting in dryness and itching.

The subcutaneous fat layer, which provides insulation and padding, thins with age. This waning subcutaneous layer increases the risk of skin injury and reduces the ability to maintain body temperature (e.g., heat conservation). Additionally, this fat layer absorbs some medications, so loss of this layer changes the actions of these medications.

The number and functioning of sweat glands decreases, and dermal capillaries are decreased. These two factors reduce the ability to lose heat. These changes make older adults vulnerable to heat stroke.

Aging skin repairs itself more slowly than younger skin. Wound healing may take as much as four times longer to complete. This sluggish repair contributes to pressure injury formation and infections. The presence of chronic diseases (e.g., diabetes mellitus and arteriosclerosis) and other aging-related changes (e.g., impaired immunity and circulatory changes) may further delay healing.

The number of hair follicles and the rate of hair growth changes with aging. These changes cause thinning and hair loss. Melanocytes in the hair follicle decrease, so melanin concentration is diminished, causing white hair. Nail changes in older adults include nail plate thickening or thinning and loss of smoothness. These changes may be due to decreased nail bed circulation. The changes in the nail plate cause fissuring and splitting. The nail color can change and become yellow to grayish.

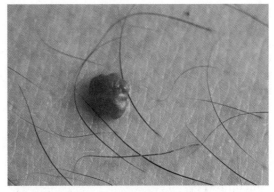

FIGURE 13-12 Pink senile angioma.
© FCG/Shutterstock.

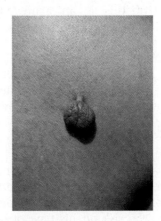

FIGURE 13-13 Skin tags.
© Somjit Chomram/Shutterstock.

Other skin abnormalities may also develop over time. Abnormalities such as skin tags and other blemishes are more common in older people. Skin tags are benign, soft brown or flesh-colored masses that usually occur on the neck (**FIGURE 13-13**). Most skin tags are painless, but they can become inflamed in the presence of constant friction (e.g., from clothing). Skin tags are more common in persons who are obese or have diabetes mellitus. Skin tags can be removed with surgery, cryotherapy, and cautery.

Inflammatory Integumentary Disorders

Dermatitis is a general term to describe a broad range of inflammatory skin diseases ranging in severity from mild itching to serious medical complications. *Eczema* is a term often used interchangeably with dermatitis as well as in reference to atopic dermatitis. Dermatitis can be acute with lesions that are characteristically pruritic, erythematous, inflamed, and papulovesicular. Chronic dermatitis lesions reflect long-term and recurrent skin lesions such as pruritus, xerosis, lichenification (i.e., thickened and roughened), hyperkeratosis (i.e., thickened), and fissuring (i.e., linear cracks). Physical manifestations can be similar, regardless of the cause, so a thorough history is important in identifying the diagnosis. Dermatitides are noncontagious conditions that may occur in isolation or in conjunction with other conditions. Most of these disorders can be resolved or managed easily with treatment; however, chronic disorders can recur frequently and be difficult to treat.

Contact Dermatitis

Contact dermatitis is an acute inflammatory reaction triggered by direct exposure to an irritant or allergen-producing substance (FIGURE 13-14). Contact dermatitis is not contagious or life threatening. It varies in severity depending on the substance, area affected, exposure extent, and individual sensitivity.

Irritant Contact Dermatitis

Irritant contact dermatitis is more common than allergic contact dermatitis. Chemicals, acids, rubber gloves, soaps, and many other environmental substances can cause irritant contact dermatitis. The risk of this type of dermatitis is high in occupations where there is frequent exposure to wetness (e.g., housekeepers, food handlers, healthcare workers). This type of contact dermatitis does not involve the immune system, but simply triggers the inflammatory response, which causes keratinocytic

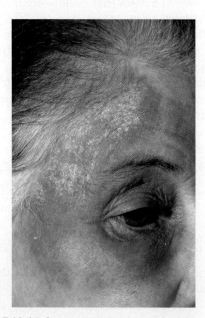

FIGURE 13-14 Contact dermatitis.
© Dr. Zara/BSIP/age fotostock.

production of inflammatory cytokines (e.g., tumor necrosis factor). Irritant contact dermatitis produces a reaction similar to a burn. The site of irritant contact dermatitis is often the hands but can be anywhere there has been irritant exposure. Manifestations tend to appear soon after exposure to the irritant (from minutes to about 24 hours). Manifestations typically include erythema and edema but may also include pain (e.g., burning, stinging), pruritus, and vesicles (i.e., serous, filled blisters < 0.5 cm). The lesions are localized to the area of exposure of the irritant and are well demarcated. Prolonged exposure or caustic substances can cause erosions, crusting, scaling, and necrosis. Irritant contact dermatitis can become chronic when there is repeated exposure to irritants (e.g., hairdressers using chemicals, dishwashers using soaps). The lesions with chronic irritant dermatitis can include fissures, xerosis, and crusting.

Allergic Contact Dermatitis

Allergic contact dermatitis results from contact with substances such as metals, chemicals, adhesives, cosmetics, and plants (e.g., poison ivy and poison sumac). Sensitization occurs on the first exposure to the substance, and subsequent exposures to the substance produce manifestations. With exposure, the haptens (allergens) penetrate the epidermis and bind to skin proteins resulting in a type IV hapten-specific T cell–mediated hypersensitivity reaction. The reaction is usually delayed, with manifestations appearing 48–72 hours after exposure. Typically, manifestations of allergic contact dermatitis include pruritus (a key symptom), erythema, and edema at the site, but vesicles may also be present. In severe cases, bullae (> 0.5 cm serous blister) may occur. As with irritant exposure, the lesions in allergen contact dermatitis are localized to the area that comes in contact with the allergen. However, allergic contact dermatitis may spread depending on the allergen or whether there is transfer of the allergen to another area. Lesions with chronicity are similar to other chronic skin dermatitis. See chapter 2 for a discussion of immunity.

Diagnosis and Treatment

Diagnosis is usually made clinically with a history, physical examination, and allergy testing (for allergic contact dermatitis). Treatment of contact dermatitis centers on identifying and removing the causative agent (e.g., rinsing the affected area). If the offending agent can be avoided, the rash usually resolves in 2–4 weeks. Self-care measures, such as wet compresses or drying agents (e.g., oatmeal compresses), and anti-inflammatory creams (e.g., corticosteroid agents) can help soothe skin and reduce inflammation. Topical calcineurin inhibitors may be used in acute cases that are not responsive to topical steroids or with chronic cases. Calcineurin is an enzyme that activates T cells. Systemic anti-inflammatory agents may be used in severe cases. Protective strategies may include use of gloves; however, rubber gloves can irritate the dermatitis. Regular use of creams and emollients may offer some protection against irritants. Workplace modifications, such as using milder detergents and cleansers, may be necessary.

Atopic Dermatitis

Atopic dermatitis, often referred to as *eczema*, is a chronic inflammatory condition (**FIGURE 13-15**). It has an inherited tendency with 70% of patients reporting a positive family history of atopy (i.e., with eczema, asthma, or allergic rhinitis). Atopic dermatitis commonly begins in infants but usually resolves by early adulthood. It tends to be characterized by remissions and exacerbations and may be accompanied by asthma and allergic rhinitis. The exact cause is unknown, but atopic dermatitis may result from an immune system malfunction, similar to hypersensitivity (an elevation of immunoglobulin E is usually present). There is a genetic impairment of the epidermal skin barrier and an increase in water loss that are

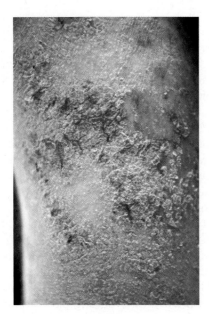

FIGURE 13-15 Atopic dermatitis.
Courtesy of Paul Matthews.

thought to be caused by several mechanisms: 1) deficiencies in filaggrin (a protein involved in the maintenance of hydration and water retention), 2) protease imbalances (e.g., kallikrein), 3) disruption of the junctions that keep intercellular spaces sealed, 4) microbial colonization, and 5) an increased immune-mediated response. Atopic dermatitis is thought to be the first of a series of allergic diseases that affect the epithelial surfaces (referred to as the *atopic march theory*)—including food allergies, asthma, and allergic rhinitis (Spergel, 2010).

Complications may include secondary bacterial, viral, or fungal skin infections, neurodermatitis (permanent scarring and discoloration from chronic scratching), and eye problems (e.g., conjunctivitis). Atopic dermatitis may affect any area, but the pattern exhibited tends to be age specific. The skin lesions primarily affect the face, scalp, and extensor surfaces (knees, elbows) in young children (e.g., < 2 years of age). The flexural surfaces of knees (popliteal fossa) and elbows (antecubital space) are the most commonly affected sites in older children and adults. Clinical manifestations may be made worse by exposure to allergens (especially to pollen, mold, dust, or animals), cold and dry air, upper respiratory infections, contact with irritants, dry skin, emotional stress, and extreme temperatures. The key manifestations of atopic dermatitis are xerosis and pruritus, which may be severe especially at night. Acute atopic dermatitis lesions include papules and vesicles that can ooze serous fluid and crusting. Chronic atopic dermatitis lesions include dry, scaly, excoriated erythematous papules, lichenification, and fissuring.

Diagnosis and Treatment

Diagnosis of atopic dermatitis is made clinically based on the history and physical examination. Allergy testing to identify triggers and skin biopsy (to rule out other causes) may be done. Serum IgE and eosinophil count, while not necessary for diagnosis, may be elevated. In children, the condition usually improves with age (starting around age 5–6 years), but flare-ups may occur. Treatment focuses on decreasing the inflammatory process. These strategies may include the following measures:

- Avoiding factors that can worsen manifestations, including:
  - Long, hot baths or showers
  - Dry skin
  - Stress

BOX 13-1 Application to Practice

Irritant, allergic, and atopic dermatitis have similar clinical manifestations. Recognizing similarities and differences may aid in determining diagnosis. In this activity, determine whether the manifestations listed are present in irritant, allergic, or atopic dermatitis and identify the key manifestations for each dermatitis. The manifestations may be present in more than one type of dermatitis.

General manifestations: Pain; pruritus; xerosis; erythema; edema; appearance of manifestations immediately after exposure to a trigger; delay of manifestations after exposure to a trigger.

Lesion appearance: Vesicles; papules; crusting; lichenification; fissuring; well-demarcated lesions.

Lesion distribution: Lesions confined to one area; lesions affecting multiple areas.

- Sweating
- Rapid changes in temperature
- Low humidity
- Solvents, cleaners, soaps, or detergents
- Wool or synthetic fabrics or clothing
- Dust or sand
- Cigarette smoke
- Certain foods (e.g., eggs, milk, fish, soy, and wheat)—it is controversial whether elimination or reduction of certain foods is beneficial
- Avoiding scratching
- Moisturizing the skin by applying ointments (e.g., petroleum jelly) 2–3 times per day
- Using a humidifier
- Employing the following strategies when washing or bathing:
  - Keeping water contact brief and using gentle soap
  - Not excessively scrubbing or drying the skin
  - After bathing, applying lubricating creams, lotions, or ointment on the skin while it is damp to trap moisture in the skin
- Using the following pharmacologic agents:
  - Antihistamine agents (may be topical or oral)
  - Corticosteroid agents (may be topical or oral)
  - Immunomodulators (topical calcineurin inhibitors or oral agents)
  - Phosphodiesterase 4 inhibitor (topical)
  - Antibiotics (may be topical or oral if infection is present)
  - Allergen-desensitizing injections
- Receiving phototherapy

Learning Points

Topical Skin Agents

Topical skin products and medications are made of different types of bases (i.e., the vehicles). The base choice is important in healing response and duration of healing. In general, most drying agents are used for moist, weeping lesions and oil-based bases are used for dry, lichenified lesions. Bases in order of moisturizing (oil) effects to drying effects include ointments, creams, lotions, solutions, and gels. Ointments are semiocclusive and increase medication absorption but are greasy and messy, decreasing patient acceptance. Ointments are not useful for lesions in the hair. Drying agents such as lotions and solutions are soothing due to the cooling effects. Gels are thin and greaseless bases and are good for use in hair.

Urticaria

Urticaria, or hives, consist of raised, erythematous skin lesions (welts) (FIGURE 13-16). These lesions are a result of a type I hypersensitivity reaction with mast cell mediation (can be IgE or non–IgE mediated). Urticaria occurs when histamine release is initiated by various substances. This reaction is often triggered by food (e.g., shellfish and nuts) or medicine (e.g., antibiotics) ingestion. Urticaria may also be a result of emotional stress, excessive perspiration, diseases, and infections (e.g., mononucleosis). Other urticarial mechanisms are type II hypersensitivity with tissue-specific cytotoxic cells (e.g., urticarial vasculitis). Type III hypersensitivity urticarial processes involve immune complexes (e.g., autoimmune diseases). In many cases, no specific trigger can be identified. The resulting skin lesions are usually short-lived and harmless, but breathing can be impaired when the swelling occurs

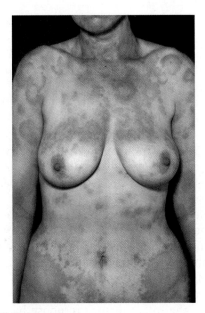

FIGURE 13-16 Urticaria.

© LeventKonuk/iStockphoto.com.

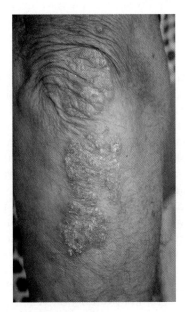

FIGURE 13-17 Psoriasis.

Courtesy of Yale Residents' Slide Collection, Dermatology Department, Yale University School of Medicine.

around the face (angioedema). Additionally, a type I hypersensitivity reaction can progress to an anaphylactic reaction and shock. The diffuse erythematous plaques (welts) may grow large, spread, and are circumscribed but can fuse together. These plaques are often pale in the center and are blanchable. The plaques are often intensely pruritic. Individual lesions usually resolve within 24 hours, but new ones develop. Urticaria can be acute, lasting less than 6 weeks, or chronic, lasting for 6 weeks or longer. See chapter 2 for a discussion of immunity.

Diagnosis and Treatment

Diagnosis of urticaria is made clinically with a a history and physical examination. Diagnostic procedures can include allergy testing and skin biopsy. If there are suspicions of the presence of systemic disorders associated with urticaria, additional procedures may be necessary. Usually urticarial lesions from systemic disorders are painful, prolonged (e.g., individual lesions last for > 24 hours), and recurrent. Treatment focuses on ceasing the inflammatory reaction and maintaining respiratory status (if appropriate). Mild urticaria may disappear without any treatment. Treatment strategies to reduce itching and swelling include the following measures:

- Avoiding hot baths or showers
- Avoiding irritating the area (e.g., with tight-fitting clothing or rubbing)

- Taking H_1 antihistamines, usually second generation (e.g., cetirizine, loratadine), however first-generation agents (e.g., diphenhydramine or hydroxyzine) are available for parenteral administration for a rapid relief
- Taking H_2 antihistamines (e.g., ranitidine) for acute urticaria, but reports are conflicting as to the efficacy
- Administering glucocorticoids to inhibit inflammatory response (not mast cell degranulation) for short periods (e.g., < 1 week)

Severe reactions, especially if angioedema is present, may require epinephrine (adrenaline) or corticosteroid injections. Additionally, airway maintenance may be necessary, including an artificial airway, oxygen therapy, and mechanical ventilation. Epinephrine (adrenaline) and other bronchodilator agents can also be administered directly into the respiratory tract to improve ventilation.

Psoriasis

Psoriasis is a common, chronic inflammatory condition that affects the life cycle of the skin cells (**FIGURE 13-17**). Psoriasis is an immune-mediated disease that occurs in genetically susceptible individuals. There are alterations and dysregulation of the innate immune system (e.g., dendritic cells) and adaptive immune system (e.g., T cells) with altered keratinocyte function and vascular dysfunction.

Key innate and adaptive immunologic processes that are thought to occur in psoriasis include:

- Immune cells (e.g., dendritic, macrophages, and neutrophils in the skin) are activated.
- Immune cells, particularly plasmacytoid dendritic cells, produce proinflammatory cytokines such as interferon alfa, which activates other immune cells (e.g., myeloid dendritic cells).
- Immune cells that were activated, particularly myeloid dendritic cells, produce cytokines such as tumor necrosis factor alpha and various interleukins (IL) such as IL 12 and 23. IL 23 plays a major role in creating a T-cell response. Myeloid dendritic cells alter keratinocyte function (via IL 20) and induces vasodilation through nitric oxide production.
- T cells, particularly CD4+ T cells and T helper type 17, also produce cytokines such as interleukin 17A. Cytokines collaborate and cause keratinocytes to proliferate and further produce proinflammatory cytokines and antimicrobial peptides.
- A vicious loop of cytokine production by immune cells and keratinocytes maintain the inflammatory process.

Key keratinocyte alterations and processes that are thought to occur in psoriasis include:

- IL, particularly 20 and 22, produced by immune cells, contributes to keratinocyte hyperplasia with resulting epidermal thickening and keratinocyte developmental defects. Cellular proliferation is significantly increased in this disorder, such that cells build up too rapidly on the skin's surface (FIGURE 13-18).
- The process of skin cells growing in the innermost layers of the skin (i.e., basal cell layer) and then rising to the surface (i.e., stratum corneum) normally takes weeks, but with psoriasis, this process occurs over 3–4 days. The dead cells cannot be shed fast enough, causing thickening.
- The ILs also increase cellular response of antimicrobial polypeptides (e.g., cathelicidins) produced by keratinocytes that contribute to the integumentary inflammatory response.
- Keratinocytes produce substances that sustain the inflammatory response by affecting the immune system.

Key vascular change that is thought to occur in psoriasis includes:

- Tortuous and leaky blood vessels in the integument as a result of increased endothelial cellular expression of nitric oxide (vasodilator), prostaglandin (vasodilator), and vascular endothelial growth factor (which stimulates angiogenesis).

Psoriasis occurs in families, so there is a hereditary predilection. Several human leukocyte alleles are associated with the development of psoriasis. The mode of transmission is multifactorial. Environmental factors such as stress, cold, trauma, infections, obesity, excessive

NORMAL SKIN

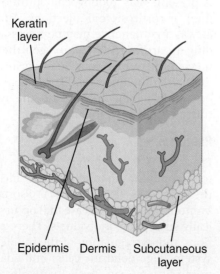

Keratin layer

Epidermis   Dermis   Subcutaneous layer

PSORIASIS

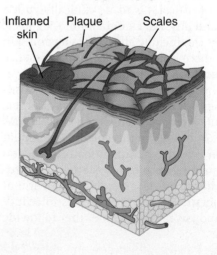

Inflamed skin   Plaque   Scales

FIGURE 13-18 Cellular changes associated with psoriasis.

alcohol consumption, and certain medications are known to trigger psoriasis; however, the mechanism by which this occurs is unclear. Psoriasis can affect people of any age, but onset peaks between 30–39 and then again between 50–69 years of age. The onset may be sudden or gradual, and many patients will experience remissions and exacerbations. See chapter 2 for a discussion of immunity.

The following factors may trigger a psoriasis exacerbation or make the condition more difficult to treat:

- Bacterial or viral infections in any location
- Dry air or dry skin
- Skin injuries (e.g., cuts, burns, and insect bites)
- Use of certain medicines (e.g., antimalaria agents, beta blockers, and lithium)
- Stress
- Too little or too much sunlight
- Excessive alcohol consumption

The severity of psoriasis varies widely, from being a mere nuisance to being disabling; as many as 30% of persons with psoriasis also have arthritis, a combination referred to as *psoriatic arthritis*. In general, psoriasis may be severe in persons who have a weakened immune system (e.g., those with AIDS, those with autoimmune conditions, or those who are receiving chemotherapy).

Clinical Manifestations

There are different forms of psoriasis with chronic plaque psoriasis as the most common type. The major different clinical types include:

- **Plaque (chronic):** Thick, red plaques covered by flaky, silver-white scales (the most common type); lifting the scale causes bleeding (i.e., Auspitz sign). The bleeding occurs because of the abnormal blood vessels' proximity to the scales. The lesions are usually symmetrically distributed and sharply defined. The usual location of the lesions is the scalp, extensor surface of elbow, knees, and the gluteal cleft (i.e., "butt crack"). In darker skin tones, lesions may appear purplish or darker.
- **Erythrodermic (acute or chronic):** Intense erythema and scaling that covers a large area usually from head to toe. The lesions are usually pruritic and painful. There is high risk for infections and fluid and electrolyte abnormalities due to the large skin surface area affected.

- **Guttate:** Small, pink-red papules and plaques that usually appear abruptly and acutely with no necessary prior history of psoriasis; may occur postinfection (e.g., streptococcal pharyngitis). Guttate means droplike and refers to the small size of the lesions (< 1 cm). The usual location of the lesions is the trunk and proximal extremities. Guttate psoriasis may remit, recur, or progress to plaque psoriasis.
- **Inverse:** Erythema and irritation usually with no scaling that occur in the intertriginous areas such as armpits, groin, and skin folds; referred to as *inverse* as the location of the lesions are opposite of the usual extensor surface areas that are affected.
- **Pustular:** Papules or plaques with pustules surrounded by erythema. This type can be acute in onset, and severe forms can be associated with infectious signs such as malaise and fever. Systemic complications can include sepsis and respiratory, renal, or hepatic abnormalities. This type may present without a prior history of psoriasis. Pustular psoriasis may remit for years and also recur after a few years.

Other manifestations may include joint pain or aching (psoriatic arthritis). Nail changes such as thickening, yellow-brown spots, dents (pits) on the nail surface and separation of the nail from the base (onycholysis) may occur, and the nail changes can occur prior to skin manifestations. At times only the nails are involved in psoriasis. There is an increased recognition of risk or association with comorbid diseases such as cardiovascular disease, hypertension, inflammatory bowel disease, and other autoimmune disorders. Therefore, manifestations of these disorders may be present with the skin lesions.

Diagnosis and Treatment

Diagnosis is made clinically with a history and physical examination. Skin biopsy may be done to rule out other causes. Other tests may be conducted to rule out conditions that mimic psoriasis (e.g., seborrheic dermatitis and tinea corporis).

No cure exists for psoriasis, but treatment can improve symptoms significantly in most cases. The goal of psoriasis treatment is to interrupt the process that leads to cell buildup and improve manifestations. Treatment is usually multipronged and includes three main approaches—topical treatments, phototherapy, and systemic medications:

- Topical treatments:
  - **Corticosteroid agents:** To slow cell turnover, decrease inflammation by suppressing the immune system
  - **Vitamin D analogues:** To slow down the skin cell growth and immune modulations (inhibit T cells and inflammatory mediators)
  - **Anthralin (Dritho-Scalp):** To normalize DNA activity in skin cells, remove scales, and smooth skin
  - **Retinoids:** To normalize DNA activity in skin cells and possibly decrease inflammation
  - **Calcineurin inhibitors:** To disrupt the activation of T lymphocytes, thereby reducing inflammation and plaque buildup
  - **Salicylic acid:** To promote shedding of dead skin cells and reduce scaling
  - **Coal tar:** To reduce scaling, itching, and inflammation, although the mechanism of action remains unknown
  - **Moisturizers:** To reduce dryness, itching, and scaling (ointment-based moisturizers are the most effective, especially when applied while skin is moist after washing)
  - **Dandruff shampoo:** To reduce cellular turnover
- Phototherapy:
  - **Sunlight:** UV light, whether natural or artificial, to cause activated T lymphocytes in the skin to die, slowing cell turnover, reducing scaling, and decreasing inflammation
  - **Broadband ultraviolet B (UVB) phototherapy:** To slow cellular growth
  - **Narrowband UVB phototherapy:** A newer and more effective treatment than broadband UVB treatment
  - **Photochemotherapy, or psoralen plus ultraviolet A:** Psoralen (a light-sensitizing medication) administration before exposure to UVA light to increase the response to the light
  - **Excimer laser:** A controlled beam of UVB light of a specific wavelength that is directed to only the involved skin
- Systemic therapy: Oral or injected pharmacotherapy (primarily reserved for severe or resistant cases and used for brief periods because of the potential serious side effects)
  - **Retinoids:** Related to vitamin A; used in an attempt to reduce the production of skin cells
  - **Methotrexate:** Decreases the production of skin cells (alters DNA synthesis) and suppresses inflammation (suppresses T-cell activity)
  - **Cyclosporine:** Systemic calcineurin inhibitor; suppresses the immune system (T-cell suppression) similarly to methotrexate
  - **Hydroxyurea:** Suppresses the immune system but not as effectively as methotrexate and cyclosporine
  - **Phosphodiesterase 4 inhibitor:** Reduces cytokines
  - **Immunomodulator drugs:** Biologics; block interactions between certain immune system cells such as tumor necrosis factor alpha inhibitors (e.g., etanercept), anti-IL-17 (e.g., ixekizumab); anti-IL-12 and IL-23 (e.g., ustekinumab)
  - **Janus kinase inhibitors:** Protein kinase C inhibitors, selective tyrosine kinase 2 inhibitors; interrupt cellular signaling thereby reducing the inflammatory response; in clinical trials

In addition to these main strategies, stress management (e.g., coping strategies and support) and avoiding psoriasis triggers may be beneficial. Due to the chronicity and the potentially disfiguring nature of psoriasis, it is important to recognize and address psychosocial distress that may arise. Psoriasis can be difficult to manage and referrals to counseling and support groups such as the National Psoriasis Foundation may be helpful.

Infectious Integumentary Disorders

Skin infections are common and may be caused by a number of pathogens (e.g., bacteria, viruses, and parasites). These organisms usually gain access through a breach in the skin or mucous membranes. They often trigger the inflammatory response as well. Such infections can occur in any of the skin layers or structures (e.g., hair follicles, nails); they may be acute or chronic, and they vary widely in severity. In most cases, infectious integumentary disorders resolve easily with treatment.

Bacterial Infections

Any number of bacteria present in the body as part of the normal flora or encountered externally may cause bacterial skin infections. These infections can vary in severity from mild to life threatening. Bacteria in the *Staphylococcus* and *Streptococcus* genera are common culprits in integumentary infections. These infections can result in numerous conditions.

Folliculitis

Folliculitis refers to infections involving the hair follicles. Folliculitis is characterized by tender pustules and erythematous papules that form around hair follicles, often on the scalp, neck, buttocks, and face (any area with hair). *Pseudomonas aeruginosa* (gram negative) causes hot tub folliculitis, which is due to inadequate chemical treatment of swimming pools, whirlpools, or hot bubs. Pruritus often accompanies folliculitis.

Furuncles

Furuncles, or boils, are infections that begin in the hair follicles and then spread into the surrounding dermis. Furuncles most commonly occur on the face, neck, axillae, groin, buttocks, and back. A furuncle lesion starts as a firm, red, painful nodule that develops into a large, painful mass, which frequently drains large amounts of purulent exudate. **Carbuncles** are clusters of furuncles.

Impetigo

Impetigo (nonbullous and bullous) is a common and highly contagious skin infection, which is most often seen in children. Impetigo is commonly caused by staphylococci and less commonly streptococci. Although it can occur without an apparent breach, this infection typically arises from a break in the skin (especially from animal bites, human bites, insect bites, and trauma). Impetigo spreads easily to others by direct contact with skin or contaminated objects (e.g., eating utensils, towels, clothing, and toys). Lesions (nonbullous impetigo) usually begin as small vesicles with surrounding erythema that become pustules, enlarge, and rupture, forming the characteristic honey-colored crust (**FIGURE 13-19**). In bullous impetigo, the vesicles develop into bullae (blisters that are > 0.5 cm) with clear yellow fluid that becomes cloudy and darker. The bullae rupture causes a thin brown crust to form. With bullous impetigo, there are fewer lesions than in the nonbullous type, and the trunk is often affected. Bullous impetigo is also caused by staphylococci strains that cause the release of an exfoliating toxin against the desmoglein protein (maintains tissue integrity). In contrast,

nonbullous impetigo is a result of the normal response to an infection rather than a toxin. Impetigo lesions can spread throughout the body through self-transfer of the exudate. Pruritus is common, and lymphadenopathy can occur near the lesions.

Ecthyma is an ulcerative type of impetigo. The ulceration can extend deep into the dermis. Causes are similar to impetigo and can be the result of untreated or poorly treated impetigo.

Cellulitis

Cellulitis refers to an infection deep in the dermis and subcutaneous tissue. It usually results from a direct invasion of the pathogens through a break in the skin, especially those breaches where contamination is likely (e.g., intravenous drug use and bites) or spreads from an existing skin infection. Cellulitis appears as a swollen, warm, tender area of erythema (**FIGURE 13-20**). Cellulitis is also unilateral, smooth, and has indistinct borders. Linear streaks of erythema (lymphangitic

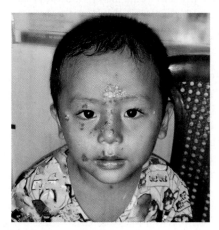

FIGURE 13-19 Impetigo.
© Zay Nyi Nyi/Shutterstock.

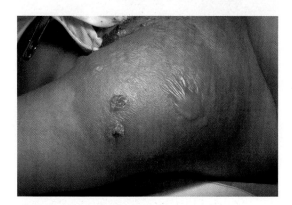

FIGURE 13-20 Cellulitis.
Courtesy of CDC/Allen W. Mathies, MD/California Emergency Preparedness Office (Calif/EPO), Immunization Branch.

BOX 13-2 Application to Practice

Stasis dermatitis is often mistakenly diagnosed as cellulitis. This misdiagnosis leads to unnecessary treatment of stasis dermatitis with antibiotics. The clinical manifestations can be similar, and patients with stasis dermatitis are at risk for developing cellulitis. Both types of dermatitis are erythematous and are commonly present in the lower extremities. Both can present with vesicles and weeping (acute stasis dermatitis).

Some tips to help in distinguishing between cellulitis and stasis dermatitis are as follows:

- **Cellulitis** tends to be unilateral. Systemic symptoms such as fever may be present. Cellulitis tends to be smooth, is generally tender, and progresses rapidly. Inciting factors for cellulitis include immunocompromise, medications, and outdoor activities.
- **Stasis dermatitis** tends to be bilateral. Pitting edema is present. The skin is hyperpigmented, scaly, and edematous. Stasis dermatitis is generally nontender and chronic. Inciting factors for stasis dermatitis include venous insufficiency.

---

streaks) may be seen near the cellulitis along the lymphatic vessels. These streaks occur as a result of lymphatic inflammation. Additionally, systemic manifestations of infection are usually present (e.g., fever, leukocytosis, malaise, and arthralgia). If left untreated, cellulitis can lead to necrotizing fasciitis, septicemia, and septic shock.

Necrotizing Fasciitis

Necrotizing fasciitis is a serious infection that is generally rare. One out of four people who develop this infection will die because of it. Also known as flesh-eating bacteria, necrotizing fasciitis can aggressively destroy skin, fat, muscle, and other tissue (**FIGURE 13-21**). This infection typically involves a highly virulent strain of gram-positive, group A, beta-hemolytic *Streptococcus* that invades through a minor cut or scrape. The bacteria begin to grow and release harmful toxins that directly destroy the tissue, disrupt blood flow, and break down material in the tissue. The first sign of infection may be a small, reddish, painful area on the skin. This area quickly evolves into a painful bronze- or purple-colored patch that grows rapidly. The center of the lesion may become black and necrotic. Exudate is often present. The wound may quickly grow, in less than an hour. Systemic manifestations may include fever, tachycardia, hypotension, and confusion. Complications of necrotizing fasciitis include gangrene, multisystem organ failure, and shock.

Diagnosis and Treatment

Diagnostic procedures for all bacterial skin infections center on the identification of the causative organism, usually through cultures. Antibiotics (systemic or oral) are started empirically to avoid systemic complications. Care should be taken when draining any wounds, as this procedure can spread the infection. Other strategies may include maintaining adequate hydration, wound care, surgical debridement, drainage, hyperbaric oxygen therapy, antipyretic agents, and analgesic agents. Hospitalization may be necessary for patients at risk for complications (e.g., elderly or immunocompromised patients), those with evidence of severe infections (e.g., systemic symptoms, hypotension, or tachycardia), or those with an inability to tolerate oral antibiotics. With cellulitis, elevation of the extremity is important to facilitate drainage.

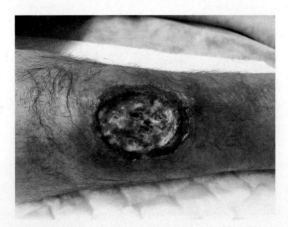

FIGURE 13-21 Necrotizing fasciitis.
© TisforThan/Shutterstock.

Viral Infections

A number of viruses can cause a multitude of skin issues, each with its own manifestations and treatments. These infections can result in numerous conditions, including herpes simplex 1, herpes zoster, verrucae, molluscum contagiosum, and pityriasis rosea.

Herpes Simplex 1

Herpes simplex 1 (HSV-1), or a cold sore, is a viral infection typically affecting the lips, mouth, and face. This common infection usually begins in childhood. HSV-1 can also involve the eyes, leading to conjunctivitis. Herpes keratitis (corneal infection) is a common cause of blindness that is caused by HSV-1. Additionally, infection with this pathogen can result in meningoencephalitis. The virus is transmitted by contact with infected saliva. The primary infection may be asymptomatic or present with multiple painful vesicles with surrounding inflammation and erythema. The oral lesions can be on the lips, mouth, or throat. With primary infection, fever and malaise may occur. The incubation period (i.e., from exposure to symptoms) is between 1 and 26 days. After the primary infection, the virus remains dormant in the affected sensory nerve ganglion (e.g., trigeminal nerve). Reactivation may be a result of an infection, stress, or sun exposure. When reactivated, HSV-1 causes painful blisters or ulcerations, which are preceded by a burning or tingling sensation or pruritus that can occur about 2 days before the vesicles. Reactivation usually causes lesions around the lips that are not as numerous, and symptoms are not as severe in comparison to the primary infection. The lesions resolve spontaneously within 3 weeks, but healing can be accelerated by administration of oral or topical antiviral agents.

Herpes Zoster

Herpes zoster, or shingles, is caused by the varicella-zoster virus. This condition appears in adulthood after a primary infection of varicella (chickenpox) has occurred in childhood. The virus lies dormant on a cranial nerve or a spinal nerve dermatome until it becomes activated years later. Because the virus affects only a specific nerve, the condition typically presents with unilateral manifestations—for example, pain, paresthesia, and a vesicular rash that develops in a line over the area innervated by the affected nerve (FIGURE 13-22). The rash may appear red or silvery, and it occurs on one side

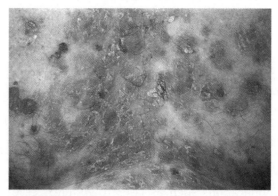

FIGURE 13-22 Herpes zoster.
Courtesy of Dr. Dancewiez/CDC.

of the head or torso depending on the nerve affected. The skin often becomes extremely sensitive, and pruritus may be present. The rash may persist for weeks to months. In some cases, especially in older persons, postherpetic neuralgia or pain may continue long after the rash disappears. Blindness may result if the eye is affected. Antiviral agents can limit the condition's duration and severity, and antidepressant and anticonvulsant agents have been beneficial in relieving the neuralgia associated with shingles. The CDC (2018) estimates that up to 30% of individuals may develop herpes zoster, so vaccination with one dose of zoster vaccine live (Zostavax) or two doses of recombinant zoster vaccine (Shingrix) is recommended. A person can receive the herpes zoster vaccine even if he or she already had the disease. Vaccines are also available to prevent varicella, and they are usually administered during childhood. Individuals vaccinated with the varicella vaccine (licensed in the United States in 1995) have a lower chance of developing herpes zoster.

Verrucae

Verrucae, or warts, are caused by a number of human papillomaviruses. These skin lesions can develop at any age and often resolve spontaneously. They can be transmitted through direct skin contact between people or within the same person. The incubation period is approximately 2–6 months. The human papillomavirus replicates in the skin cells, causing irregular thickening. Lesions that vary in color, shape, and texture depending on their type can appear. There are three categories of warts: 1) verruca vulgaris (common wart); 2) verruca plana (flat warts because they appear as flat-topped papules) and; 3) verruca plantaris (plantar warts because they appear on the plantar surface of the foot) (FIGURE 13-23). Plantar surface warts are a common cause of forefoot pain. When warts are pared with a file such as an emery board, small capillaries that are thrombosed may become visible. The presence of the thrombosed capillaries further confirms the diagnosis of a wart, as calluses and corns may look like warts but will not have these vessels. Treatment includes a wide range of local applications such as laser treatments, cryotherapy with liquid nitrogen, electrocautery, and topical medications (e.g., keratolytic, cytotoxic, and antiviral agents), but the verrucae may return after treatment.

Molluscum Contagiosum

Molluscum contagiosum is caused by a poxvirus. Molluscum contagiosum is common in children and is spread by direct skin contact between people and within the same person. The infection can also spread through fomites (inanimate object that when contaminated with organism can transfer the organism to a host). Examples of fomite transmission would be towels, sponge, or razors. In adolescents and adults, the virus is usually sexually transmitted (lesions are most likely in genital areas) or through contact sports. The incubation period is 1 week to 6 months. Molluscum

lesions are dome-shaped white papules that are shiny, firm, and have a craterlike center (FIGURE 13-24). Lesions can become inflamed. The lesions often resolve without treatment, and it can take up to 1 year for complete resolution. A wide range of treatment is available that includes cryotherapy with liquid nitrogen, curettage (physical removal with a curette), and topical medications (e.g., keratolytic agents, cantharidin, and antimitotic agents); however, evidence is lacking to determine effectiveness of these treatments.

Pityriasis Rosea

Pityriasis rosea is disorder that is thought to be caused by a virus as the lesions often occur after a viral infection. There is also an absence or association with bacterial and fungal organisms. The human herpes virus and H1N1 influenza virus have been implicated; however, there is inadequate evidence to firmly conclude these organisms as causative. The lesions are benign and noncommunicable. The disorder begins with a lesion termed the *herald patch* that is solitary, salmon-colored, fine, scaly, and clearly demarcated (FIGURE 13-25).

The herald patch usually appears on the chest, neck, or back. After this initial patch, several other similar-appearing patches, scaly papules, and plaques of varying sizes usually start to appear after a few days to 2 weeks. The lesions are on the trunk and proximal areas of the extremities. The distribution of the lesions on the back are said to appear like a Christmas tree. Usually erythema and pruritus is present, but some cases are asymptomatic. In children, the distribution of lesions is often atypical and appears inversely to adults; lesions appear

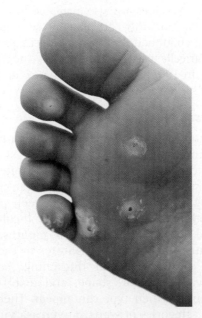

FIGURE 13-23 Plantar warts.
© Sdominick/iStock/Getty Images.

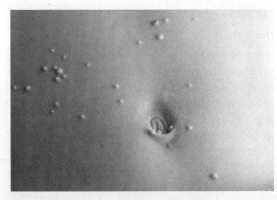

FIGURE 13-24 Molluscum contagiosum lesions around a person's navel.
© Jarrod Erbe/Shutterstock.

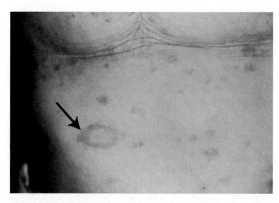

FIGURE 13-25 Pityriasis rosea.
Courtesy of CDC.

on the face and distal extremities with sparing of the trunk. In children, the lesions may also be vesicular, pustular, urticarial, or purpuric. The lesions can take up to 2 months to resolve; however, darker pigmented individuals may have postinflammatory hyperpigmented lesions that last for several months. The diagnosis is made by the characteristics of the lesion but a potassium hydroxide (KOH) microscopic examination may distinguish the disorder from tinea corporis (i.e., ringworm). The lesions of pityriasis rosea are similar to those caused by secondary syphilis, so serologic testing for syphilis may be indicated in those at risk (e.g., those who are sexually active). Treatment is not necessary but the rash can appear dramatic, so education and reassurance of the benign nature are necessary. If pruritus is present, topical corticosteroids and antipruritics may be used.

Parasitic Infections

A number of parasitic infections can occur on the skin, including those caused by fungi. Fungi can include yeasts, of which *Candida albicans* is a common infection-causing pathogen. Fungi can also include pathogens that cause tinea infections. The tinea pathogens are generally part of three genera: *Microsporum*, *Epidermophyton*, or *Trichophyton*. These conditions are usually diagnosed through microscopic examination of skin scrapings processed with KOH. The presence of hyphae confirms the diagnosis. See chapter 8 for a discussion of candida infections.

Many of the causative organisms feed off the dead skin cells of the host and may use the host as a breeding ground. Some of the numerous parasitic skin infections are profiled in the following sections.

Tinea

Tinea (i.e., dermatophytosis) causes several types of superficial fungal infections. The organisms live and disrupt the keratinized cells of the epidermis. Tineas are described based on the area of the body affected. These fungi typically grow in warm, moist places (e.g., showers and locker rooms). Tinea corporis is an infection of the body. Tinea corporis typically manifests as a circular, erythematous, scaling patch or plaque. The center of the plaque clears, and there is a circular raised border, giving the common name of ringworm (**FIGURE 13-26**). Tinea capitis is an infection of the scalp commonly encountered in school-aged children. Along with the typical rash associated with tinea, hair loss at the site is common. Tinea pedis, also called *athlete's foot*, is the most common dermatophytosis. Tinea pedis involves the feet, especially between the toes. The manifestations of tinea pedis are usually hyperkeratotic and erythematous lesions of the foot. The lesions create the appearance that a person is

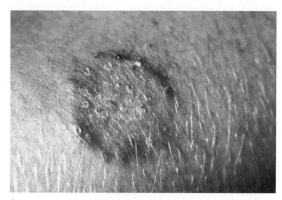

A

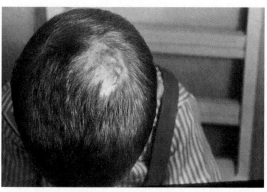

B

FIGURE 13-26 Tinea. **(A)** Ringworm on the arm.
(B) Ringworm on the scalp.
A: Courtesy of Dr. Lucille K. Georg/CDC; **B:** Courtesy of CDC.

wearing a moccasin. Tinea pedis between the toes generally causes erythematous erosions and fissures or scales. Tinea in the midfoot area usually causes vesicles or bullae with erythema. Tinea cruris is an infection of the inner thigh that usually causes tiny vesicles with an erythematous, sharply demarcated border. Tinea cruris can spread around the genital area but usually does not spread to the scrotum. Candidal infections of the groin are differentiated as they cause papules and pustules and can affect the scrotum. Most of the tineas described, regardless of location, can cause pruritus and pain. Tinea unguium (i.e., onychomycosis) is an infection of the nails, typically the toenails (in fingernails the fungi is usually *Candida albicans*). This infection begins at the tip of one or two nails and then usually spreads to other nails. The nail initially turns white and then brown, causing it to thicken and crack. Clippings of the nails can be sent for culture. Several topical and systemic antifungal agents are available to treat tinea infections, but several weeks of treatment may be necessary to resolve the infection.

Tinea versicolor (i.e., pityriasis versicolor) is a superficial, benign, noncommunicable fungal infection. In contrast to other tinea infections, tinea versicolor is not a dermatophytosis as it is caused by yeasts from the *Malassezia* genus (normal skin flora). The disorder has a higher incidence in tropical countries due to the heat and humidity. Excessive sweating also contributes to the development. Tinea versicolor is more prevalent in adolescents and young adults. The lesions appear as macules and patches and thin plaques that are hyper- or hypopigmented (hence the name *versicolor*). The distribution is usually on the trunk and distal extremities (similar to pityriasis rosea) as the yeast depends on lipids and there is greater sebum production in the upper body. However, the face is commonly involved in children. The lipid dependency also explains the age distribution as less sebum is produced with aging. Diagnosis is made clinically and confirmed through microscopy with KOH preparation. In some cases, a Wood lamp may reveal yellow-greenish fluorescence. Treatment includes topical antifungals (e.g., selenium sulfide or azoles). Lesions can take months to clear even with successful treatment, and recurrence is common.

Scabies

Scabies is a result of a mite (*Sarcoptes scabiei*) infestation. The male mites fertilize the females and then die. The female mites burrow into the epidermis, laying eggs over a period of several weeks in a series of tracts. After laying the eggs, the female mites die. When the larvae subsequently hatch from the eggs, they migrate to the skin's surface. They burrow into the skin in search of nutrients and mature to repeat the cycle. This burrowing appears as small, light brown streaks on the skin (**FIGURE 13-27**). The burrowing and fecal matter left behind by the mites triggers the inflammatory process, leading to erythema and intense pruritus, which is worse at night. The lesions are many small erythematous papules. The distribution usually involves the sides and webs of the fingers. Many other body areas such as the wrists, axillae, around the areola, and genitalia (it can include the scrotum) can become affected. Other locations are the wrists, axillae, around the areola, and genitalia (it can include the scrotum). If there are a lot of mites (millions as opposed to the usual 15) then thick scales, crusting, and fissuring may be present. The mites can survive for only short periods without a host, so transmission usually results from close contact (between household members or through sexual contact). Several topical treatments for scabies are available, but multiple applications are usually needed to successfully eradicate the infestation. Clothing, linens, and other fabrics will likely require treatment as well although transmission is more likely due to close contact.

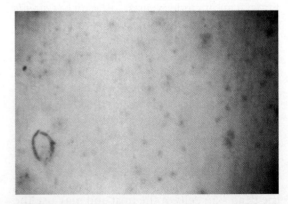

FIGURE 13-27 Scabies.
Courtesy of CDC.

Pediculosis

Pediculosis refers to lice infestation, which can take three forms—*Pediculus humanus corporis* (body louse), *Phthirus pubis* (pubic louse), and *Pediculus humanus capitis* (head louse). Lice are small, brown, parasitic insects that feed off human blood and cannot survive for long without the human host (**FIGURE 13-28**). The female lice lay eggs (nits) on the hair shaft close to the scalp (**FIGURE 13-29**). The nits appear as small white, iridescent shells on the hair. After hatching, the lice bite and suck the host's blood; in turn, the site of the bite develops a highly pruritic macule or papule. Hyperpigmentation can occur and is due to inflammation. The lesions of pediculosis can also occur around seams of clothing as the lice lay eggs in seams and live on clothing. Pediculosis is easily transmitted through close contact. Several topical treatments are available, but multiple applications are usually needed to successfully eradicate the infestation. Clothing, linens, and other fabrics will likely require treatment as well.

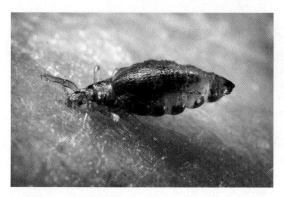

FIGURE 13-28 Louse.

Courtesy of CDC/James Gathany/Frank Collins, PhD.

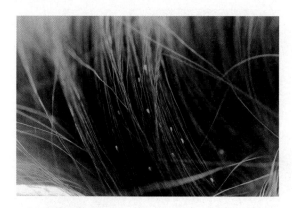

FIGURE 13-29 Nits.

Callista Images/Cultura/Getty Images; © hirun/iStock/Getty Images.

Traumatic Integumentary Disorders

Traumatic integumentary disorders can result from a wide range of injuries. Skin trauma can produce multiple skin conditions, depending on the nature of the injury (**FIGURE 13-30**). Such injuries may range from mild to life threatening in severity, depending on the location and extent of the injury. Regardless of the nature or extent of the injury, all traumatic skin conditions increase the risk for infection because they create a breach in the body's protective barrier. Although numerous traumatic skin conditions are possible (e.g., lacerations and abrasions), this section will focus on burns.

Burns

A burn is a skin injury that results from exposure to either a thermal (heat) or a nonthermal source. Such sources may include dry heat (e.g., fire), wet heat (e.g., steam or hot liquids), radiation, friction, heated objects, natural or artificial UV light, electricity, and chemicals (e.g., acids, alkaline substances, and paint thinner). The burn injury triggers the inflammatory reaction and results in tissue destruction. The severity of the condition varies depending on the location, extent, and nature of the injury. Severity is described, in part, in terms of the levels of the skin that are damaged (**FIGURE 13-31**):

- Superficial (first-degree) burns affect only the epidermis. These burns cause pain, erythema, and edema.
- Partial-thickness—superficial or deep (second-degree)—burns affect the epidermis and dermis. Partial thickness burns cause pain, erythema that blanches, edema, and blistering (usually within a day). Hypopigmentation may remain but scarring does not occur. Deeper partial-thickness burns will also damage hair follicles and glands and are painful with pressure only. The burn causes blistering and can have a cheesy whitish to red appearance with no blanching. Hypertrophic scarring is common, and resolution can take up to 9 weeks.
- Full-thickness (third-degree) burns extend into deeper tissues (full dermis and subcutaneous). These burns cause white or

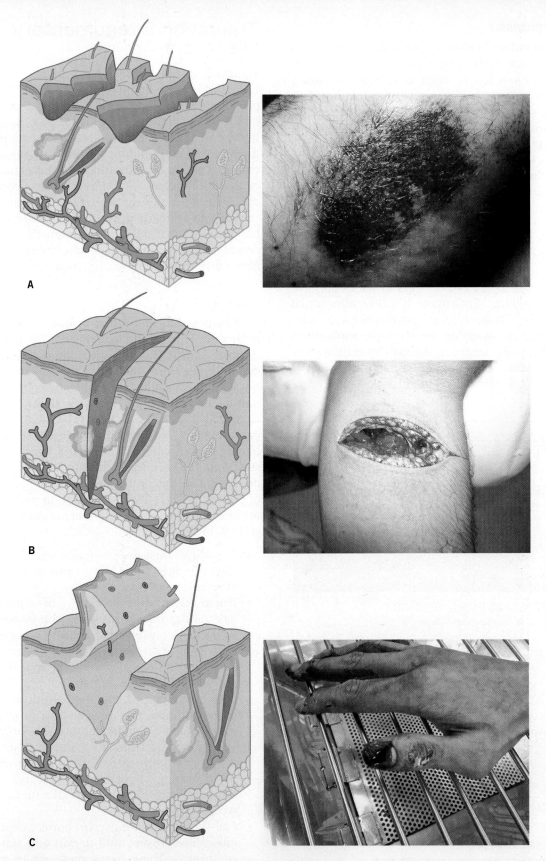

FIGURE 13-30 Types of wounds. **A.** Abrasion. **B.** Laceration. **C.** Avulsion.

A: © Kondor83/Shutterstock; **B:** © E.M. Singletary, M.D. Used with permission.; **C:** © NeeooN/Shutterstock.

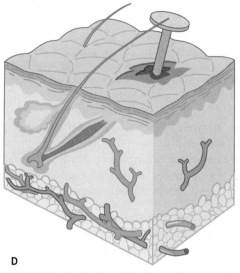
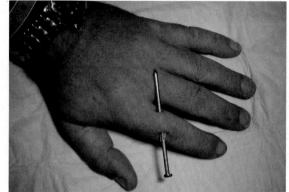

D

FIGURE 13-30 (*Continued*) **D.** Penetrating wound.

D: © E.M. Singletary, MD. Used with permission.

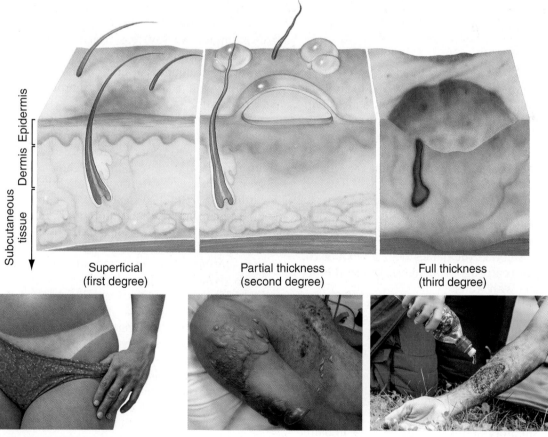

FIGURE 13-31 Burn classification.

Bottom 1: © Amy Walters/Shutterstock; **Bottom 2:** Courtesy of Rhonda Hunt; **Bottom 3:** © microgen/iStock/Getty Images.

blackened, charred dead skin (i.e., eschar) that may be numb. Eschar is inelastic, dry (no vesicles), and does not blanch. Scarring is severe and often includes contractures.

- Deep-tissue-extension (fourth-degree) burns can extend to underlying muscle and bone.

Clinical Manifestations

Complication development is usually related to burn severity. Burns may result in any of the following complications:

- Local infection (particularly *Staphylococcus* infection)
- Sepsis
- Hypovolemia (burns can damage blood vessels and plasma proteins, causing fluid shifts; see chapter 6)
- Shock (may result from sepsis or hypovolemia)
- Hypothermia (heat is lost through large injuries)
- Respiratory problems (inhaling hot air or smoke can burn the tissues making up the airway, causing inflammation)
- Scarring
- Contractures

Diagnosis and Treatment

Burns are diagnosed based on a history and physical examination that includes identifying the type of burn and the body surface area of the burn. Treatment varies and is dependent on the location and severity of the burn.

Treatment of a severe burn at the scene of the injury includes:

- Removing the source of the burn. If someone is on fire, have the person stop, drop, and roll. Wrap the person in thick material to smother the flames (e.g., a wool or cotton coat, rug, or blanket). Douse the person with water.
- Leaving burned clothing that is stuck to the skin. The clothing may be soaked with sterile water or saline and then removed, and surgical removal may be necessary in severe cases.
- Ensuring the person is breathing. Initiate cardiopulmonary resuscitation if necessary. Continue to monitor the patient's respiratory status—it can become impaired as edema worsens.

At the emergency department, a thorough evaluation of severe burns starts with a primary and secondary survey. The primary assessment proceeds in an ABCDE format.

ABCDE—Burn Assessment

A **a**irway management
B **b**reathing and ventilation
C **c**irculation and **c**ardiac status
D **d**isability, neurologic **d**eficit, and gross **d**eformity
E **e**xposure (completely disrobe the patient, examine for associated injuries, and maintain a warm environment)

Airway, respiratory, and ventilation compromise should be suspected with inhalation injury. Airway edema can develop rapidly and be life threatening, so maintaining a patent airway is a priority. Suspicions of airway compromise should arise when there is a history indicating smoke, soot, or toxic fume exposure. Physical signs may include facial burns, singed hair, oral area evidence of soot, and sputum that appears like soot. Other clinical signs are similar to airway compromise in other conditions (e.g., hoarseness, stridor). Airway management can be accomplished with oral airway devices, endotracheal intubation, or creation of a surgical airway (e.g., tracheotomy). Circumferential burns to the neck or trunk may cause a tourniquet-type effect and impair chest wall movement, so a bedside escharotomy may be necessary.

Circulation and cardiac status evaluation includes focusing on oxygenation (e.g., use of pulse oximeter) and perfusion. Due to the burn injury and subsequent catecholamine response, the heart rate may be slightly tachycardic (e.g., 100–120 heartbeats per minute). Vital signs should be monitored frequently to assess for signs of shock (e.g., tachycardia, usually beyond 120 heartbeats per minute) and hypotension. Administration of intravenous fluids (which may include colloids or crystalloids) is based on specific formulas. Adults with burns greater than 20% of total body surface area (TBSA) and children with burns greater than 10% TBSA will be administered fluids based on body weight and percentage of burn. Fluid bolus administration should be avoided as it may exacerbate edema. Exposure in the primary survey involves awareness of the altered thermoregulatory abilities. While the patient is evaluated, all clothing, jewelry, and contact lenses need to be removed. Remove any items that can act as a tourniquet as edema will occur. The environment should be warm, and blankets can be used to prevent hypothermia. If cooling of the burn is necessary, only cool—not cold—water should be used.

The secondary assessment involves evaluating nonburn injuries that could be life threatening and require attention prior to beginning evaluation of the burn injury. At this stage, laboratory evaluation such as complete blood count and blood chemistry can be conducted, and other imaging, such as a chest X-ray) can be done as necessary.

After the primary and secondary assessment, attention can be placed on evaluating the burn injury, including depth and body surface area affected. The goal of burn wound care is to promote healing and prevent infection. The general treatment of severe burns includes:

- Wound care, which is dependent on the depth of the burn. There are several types of dressings and techniques (e.g., open, closed) available.
- Cleansing the wound with tap water or sterile solutions (there is no evidence for benefit or harm between types). Tap water, if used, should be running (not stored) and meet the standards of the World Health Organization.
- Rupturing blisters only under circumstances where it may be beneficial such as when a deeper burn may be underneath.
- Protecting the burn area from pressure and friction.
- Limiting the risk for infection and promoting healing by meticulous wound care.
- Providing a clean and dust-free hospital environment, as infections in the hospital usually occur through surface contact, air, and water.

Full-thickness burns will not heal on their own, so excision and grafting are necessary. Excision can be tangential, meaning only the overdevitalized tissue is removed, and it is done at an angle. Fascial excision involves removal of all layers of the eschar and tissue all the way to the fascia. Fascial excision is usually necessary for deep burns and high-voltage electrical conduction burns. Deep partial-thickness burns (less than full thickness) may also recover quicker with excision and grafts. Skin grafts promote tissue regeneration, prevent scarring, and aid the healing process.

Other treatments will include pain management with oral and intravenous analgesics and sedation. Physical therapy will be necessary to reduce the effects of scar tissue and reduce contractures. Surgery may be necessary for the contractures. Provide an increased dietary intake of protein and carbohydrates to promote healing and meet the increased caloric needs. Prophylactic antibiotic administration should not be used as resistance may develop.

Minor and/or smaller surface area burns can be evaluated in the same manner that other nonthermal wounds are assessed. A minor burn is defined by the American Burn Association (2018) as a partial thickness of < 10% TBSA for patients 10–50 years of age, < 5% TBSA in patients under 10 years of age or over 50 years of age, or a full thickness < 2% TBSA without other injuries. Attention should be paid to the depth, as third-degree and deeper burns will not heal on their own and require surgical management. Circumferential burns, even if in a small area, such as the finger, can act like a tourniquet, cutting off blood supply and, therefore, may require further evaluation and possible surgical management. The burn should be treated in a specialized burn center if a second-degree burn is located on the hands, feet, face, groin, buttocks, or a major joint.

Minor burns can be managed on an outpatient basis. Superficial burns usually heal in less than 2 weeks. Treatment for minor burns includes:

- Removing the source of the burn.
- Running cool water over the area or soaking it in a cool water bath (not ice water) if the skin is unbroken. Keep the damaged area submerged for at least 5 minutes. Applying a clean, cold, wet bandage or towel will also help reduce pain.
- Evaluation to determine whether debridement is necessary prior to dressing.
- Debridement can be accomplished with gentle mechanical techniques (e.g., brushing, scraping, or cutting). Enzymatic topical products (e.g., collagenase) can also be used for debridement.
- Coverage with a dry, sterile bandage or clean dressing.
- Protection from pressure and friction.
- Administration of analgesics and nonsteroidal anti-inflammatory drugs to relieve pain and swelling.
- Daily cleansing with mild soap and tap water.
- Application of moisturizing lotion (on intact skin) once the skin has cooled.

- Application of topical antibiotics. However, if a burn is superficial, topical antibiotics are usually not necessary.
- Tetanus vaccination.

A patient with a minor burn injury will need to be taught how to change their dressing and be taught how to watch for signs of infection. The patient should be evaluated soon after the injury and followed closely (e.g., daily). At follow-up, the burn should be reevaluated. Pruritus is common as a burn is healing and can be managed with oral antihistamines. If the minor burn does not heal within 3 weeks, a referral may be necessary to a surgeon as additional measures become necessary. Hypertrophic scarring is more likely the longer it takes for a wound to heal. Hypertrophic scarring can be avoided or minimized with pressure garments, massage, and moisturization.

Pressure Injuries

Pressure injuries are defined as injuries to the skin and soft tissue that have occurred as a result of unrelieved pressure. The result is damage to the underlying tissue. *Pressure injury* has replaced the common term, *pressure ulcers*, to reflect that deep-tissue injury can occur without ulceration. Pressure injuries occur when an external force is applied to the skin. When the pressure applied is greater than arteriolar pressure of the skin (32 mmHg), then tissue hypoxia can occur. Pressure injuries in vulnerable patients can occur in as short as 1 hour if the pressure applied is high enough and sustained. As an example of applied pressures, there is 300 mmHg of pressure over the ischial tuberosities when a person sits. The muscle tissue is the most vulnerable to injury caused by pressure followed by the subcutaneous fat and dermis. Therefore, pressure injuries can start deep internally and not be evident on the surface. These deep injuries can then progress to the surface. The hypoxia that can occur from pressure is not the only factor contributing to injury. Compression of small vessels and injury from reperfusion also contribute to hypoxia and damage to the skin. Shearing forces (such as when a patient is inclined with the head of the bed up) contribute to the injury as muscle and fat are stretched downward. Moisture and friction can contribute to alteration in skin integrity and have been associated with contributing to ulcer formation. Moisture alone, such as from urine or perspiration, can lead to skin

softening and breakdown (i.e., maceration), and then an ulcer can form. Friction, such as that caused by sliding a patient across a surface, leads to abrasions (Figure 13-30) and, therefore, leads to a breach in skin integrity and potential ulcer formation. These macerations and abrasions as described are not pressure injuries.

Pressure injuries are usually located over bony prominences such as the sacrum, coccyx, heels, elbows, and trochanters. Pressure injuries can also occur from pressure caused by medical devices. Risk factors for the development of pressure injuries includes immobility (the most significant factor), malnutrition, inadequate tissue perfusion (e.g., hypotension, vasoconstriction), and sensory loss (e.g., neuropathy). The sensory loss is a risk as a patient loses the ability to sense the discomfort or pain from prolonged pressure. Various tools (e.g., Braden scale) can be used to predict risk for pressure injury development.

Clinical Manifestations

Pressure injuries are described based on their stage (e.g., from 1 to 4) (**FIGURE 13-32**) The staging is a reflection of the extent of an injury, the depth, and other injury features. The National Pressure Ulcer Advisory Panel (2016) developed the staging system, and the descriptions are as follows:

- **Stage 1:** Intact skin with nonblanchable erythema. The area is localized and does not include purple or maroon discoloration,

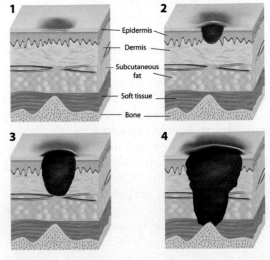

FIGURE 13-32 The stages of pressure injuries.
© Alila Medical Media/Shutterstock.

which may indicate a deep-tissue pressure injury. Prior to visual changes, there may be blanchable erythema, changes in sensation, temperature, or firmness.

- **Stage 2:** Partial thickness loss of skin with exposed dermis. The wound is viable, pink or red, and moist. The wound may present as an intact or ruptured serum-filled blister. Deeper structures such as adipose (fat) and deeper tissues are not visible. There is no granulation tissue (granulation tissue is an intermediary to healing and when healthy is shiny red and granular), slough (adherent or non-adherent non-viable tissue that is usually yellowish), and eschar (necrotic granulation tissue that is leathery, dry, hard).
- **Stage 3:** Full-thickness skin loss. Adipose is visible in the ulcer and granulation tissue and an epibole (rolled wound edges) are often present. The depth of tissue damage varies by anatomic location; areas of significant adiposity can develop deep wounds. Undermining and tunneling may occur. Fascia, muscle, tendon, ligament, cartilage and/or bone are not exposed. If slough or eschar obscures the extent of tissue loss, it is an unstageable pressure injury.
- **Stage 4:** Full-thickness skin and tissue loss with exposed or directly palpable fascia, muscle, tendon, ligament, cartilage, or bone in the ulcer. Slough and/or eschar may be visible. Epibole (rolled edges), undermining (tissue destruction that occurs at the wound perimeter), and/or tunneling (wound extension in one direction that is deep) often occur. Depth varies by anatomic location. If slough or eschar obscures the extent of tissue loss, it is an unstageable pressure injury.
- **Unstageable pressure injury:** Obscured full-thickness skin and tissue loss. The extent of the tissue damage within the ulcer cannot be confirmed because it is obscured by slough or eschar. If slough or eschar is removed, a stage 3 or stage 4 pressure injury will be revealed. Stable eschar (i.e. dry, adherent, intact without erythema or fluctuance) on the heel or ischemic limb should not be softened or removed.

Deep tissue injuries can occur with intact skin. These injuries at inception do not quite fit into any stages. These injuries may appear as a persistent, nonblanchable deep red, maroon, or purple discoloration (nonintact or intact skin) or epidermal separation revealing a dark wound bed or blood-filled blister. Pain and temperature changes may preceed this type of injury. The wound may evolve rapidly, and the extent will be visible and then can be staged, or resolution may occur without tissue loss.

Learning Points

Pressure Injuries in Dark Skin Tones

Usual skin tone changes reflective of pressure injuries such as blanching and erythema may not be evident in darker skin tones. When evaluating a blanch response in a darker skinned person, apply pressure and look for a darkened area or a shiny, taut induration. Underlying vasodilatory changes that cause erythema in lighter skin may present as hyperpigmentation or hypopigmentation, and redness may not be visible. Feeling for temperature and texture changes (e.g., increased warmth or soft bogginess) are necessary for pressure injuries. Moisturizing the skin may intensify skin color changes.

Diagnosis and Treatment

Diagnosis is based on a history and physical examination using the staging criteria. Impaired skin integrity (e.g., ulcers, abrasions) due to other causes such as diabetes, arterial or venous insufficiency, or chemical irritation (e.g., urine) should be distinguished as treatment will vary. See chapter 4 for a discussion of vascular ulcers.

Treatment for pressure injuries is focused on reduction or elimination of pressure through redistribution with proper position and use of supportive surfaces. Pressure injury prevention points are as follows:

- Frequently turn and reposition patients in bed or in a chair.
- Turn the patient to a side-lying position, and with a hand, check that the sacrum is off the bed. The head of bed should be no higher than 30° to prevent shearing. If the head of the bed is higher than 30°, then a polyurethane foam dressing should be on the sacrum.
- If pressure injuries are present, do not position the person on the affected areas.
- Ensure that heels are not on the bed.
- Use pressure-redistributing cushions for sitting on chairs or wheelchairs.
- Use breathable dressings or thin foam under medical devices.
- Bed surfaces may be enhanced with non-powered support devices such as foam mattresses or overlays.
- Specialized beds may be necessary (e.g., air-fluidized beds).
- Meticulous skin assessment is important in early identification.

- Daily cleansing with pH-balanced solutions will minimize injury.
- Use skin moisturizers daily.
- Ensure adequate nutrition and hydration.

Wound management is dependent on the pressure injury stage. Dressings are used to prevent infection and promote healing. Wounds that are especially moist and exudative will cause further skin breakdown and slow epithelial cell proliferation, while exceptionally dry wounds will slow epithelial cell migration and slow wound healing. The longer the wound is open, the greater the chance of infection and scarring. Absorptive dressings such as foams are best for moist injuries, and hydrogels or other dressings that maintain moisture are best for dry wounds. Stage 1 injuries are covered with a transparent film as a protective barrier. Stage 2 injuries require maintenance of a moist environment. Various dressings can be used to maintain the moist environment. These include hydrocolloids or hydrogels, which are both occlusive, and transparent films, which are semiocclusive. Stage 3 and 4 injuries generally require debridement (chemical enzymatic or mechanical) for the wound to heal. After debridement, an appropriate moist dressing is applied. Wounds, as in burns, may require skin grafting or mucocutaneous flaps for rapid healing. Adjunctive therapies for wound healing may be useful, but data is limited on their effectiveness. These therapies can include electrical stimulation, negative-pressure wound therapy, therapeutic ultrasound, hyperbaric oxygen or direct oxygen application and use of topical growth factors.

Chronic Integumentary Disorders

Numerous chronic conditions can affect the integumentary system. Several have been discussed and categorized based on their underlying pathophysiology (e.g., psoriasis and inflammatory disorders). These conditions vary in severity. Although most are not life threatening, many can have a significant impact on an individual's appearance.

Acne Vulgaris

Acne vulgaris is an inflammatory skin disorder of the pilosebaceous unit (i.e., hair follicles and sebaceous glands). Acne vulgaris commonly affects adolescents and young adults, but it can occur at any age. The four key factors in the pathogenesis of acne vulgaris are 1) follicular hyperkeratinization, 2) increased sebum production, 3) bacteria in the follicle, and 4) inflammation (FIGURE 13-33). The pathogenesis of acne vulgaris occurs when sebum production from the sebaceous gland increases under the influence of androgens. This period occurs during prepuberty and sebum accumulates, hyperkeratinization occurs, and the hair follicle becomes blocked. Microcomedones, which are a mixture of sebum and keratin and are not visible on the surface, develop. The microcomedones are lipid rich and provide an environment for the growth of *Cutibacterium acnes* (formerly known as *Propionibacterium acnes*), an anaerobic bacterial organism that is part of the normal skin flora. The bacteria stimulate the immune response with resulting inflammation. The microcomedones become closed comedones (whiteheads). The follicles start to widen and open to the skin, and open comedones (blackheads) develop. Blackheads are a mixture of keratinocytes, lipids, and melanin (which gives it a dark color). The follicles eventually rupture with further inflammation ensuing and resulting in inflammatory lesions of papules, pustules, cysts, and nodules (FIGURE 13-34). Acne vulgaris commonly appears on areas with increased hormone-responsive sebaceous glands such as the face, neck, and shoulders (upper arms), but it may also occur on the trunk, arms, legs, and buttocks. It varies widely in severity, with severe cases sometimes resulting in significant scarring. Postinflammatory hyperpigmentation is more likely to occur in darker skin tones and is the result of increased melanin production due to inflammation. Risk factors for acne vulgaris include the following:

- Family history
- Hormonal changes (e.g., changes that occur with menstrual periods, pregnancy, birth control pill use, and stress)
- Use of oily cosmetic and hair products, which block pilosebaceous follicles and cause comedo formation
- Use of certain medications (e.g., corticosteroids, testosterone, estrogen, and phenytoin)
- High levels of humidity and sweating
- Helmets, bra straps, and shoulder pads, which can cause occlusion of pilosebaceous follicles and comedo formation

NORMAL HAIR FOLLICLE

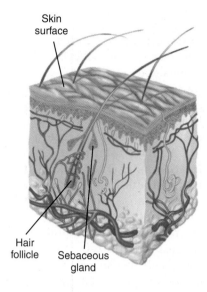

Skin surface

Hair follicle

Sebaceous gland

Duct clogged by dead cells, sebum starts to accumulate

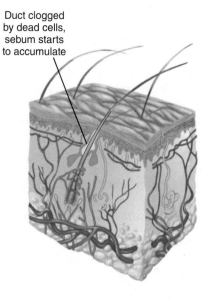

Bacterial infection, inflammation triggered

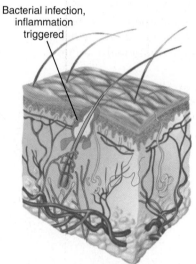

PIMPLE

Follicle ruptures, pustule with fluid formed

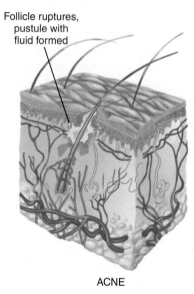

ACNE

FIGURE 13-33 Pathogenesis of acne vulgaris.

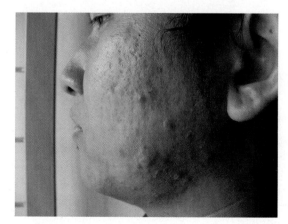

FIGURE 13-34 Acne vulgaris.

Diagnosis and Treatment

Diagnosis for acne vulgaris is made clinically with a history and physical examination. Diagnostic testing may be necessary if there are underlying disorders causing or contributing to the acne (e.g., polycystic ovarian syndrome). Treatment varies depending on the severity. Treatment includes behavioral and medical (e.g., medications and techniques such as laser) strategies. Behavioral strategies include the following:

* Cleaning skin gently with a mild, nondrying soap to remove all dirt or makeup once or twice a day, including after exercising;

while avoiding excessive or repeated skin washing

- Shampooing hair daily, especially if it is oily
- Combing or pulling hair back to keep it away from the face, but avoiding tight headbands
- Avoiding squeezing, scratching, picking, or rubbing acne because it can lead to skin infections and scarring
- Avoiding touching affected areas
- Avoiding oily cosmetics or creams; using water-based or noncomedogenic formulas instead
- Limiting sun exposure

Pharmacotherapeutic strategies target mechanisms that lead to the pathogenesis (**TABLE 13-2**). While monotherapy with one agent may be sufficient, there are circumstances where multiple agents—such as a topical retinoid with topical antimicrobial—are used. Hormonal therapies are reserved for women and include oral contraceptives with antiandrogenic ingredients such as drospirenone (spironolactone analogue). Oral isotretinoin (Accutane) is generally used for severe, difficult-to-manage nodular acne. There is a high risk for teratogenicity with oral isotretinoin, so contraception so contraception is important during use. The various medications are available over the counter or may require prescriptions.

Pharmacotherapeutic strategies, in addition to those in table 13-2, include the following:

- Alternative therapies, including tea tree oil, zinc, guggul, and brewer's yeast
- Photodynamic therapy (laser/light procedure) and photopneumatic therapy (pressure and light)
- Chemical skin peels
- Microdermabrasion or dermabrasion
- Intralesional glucocorticoids for nodular acne

- Soft-tissue fillers (e.g., collagen and fat)

Rosacea

Rosacea is a chronic inflammatory skin condition that typically affects the face. It is poorly understood, but rosacea is prevalent in persons who are fair skinned, persons who bruise easily, and women. Proposed pathogenesis includes an innate immune dysfunction. The dysfunction causes an abnormal skin response to microorganisms in or on the skin, such as *Demodex* mites. The immune dysfunction leads to the production of chemicals (e.g., cathelicidin) that cause vasoactive and other inflammatory manifestations. There are four subtypes of rosacea—erythematotelangiectatic, papulopustular (classic presentation), phymatous, and ocular. Rosacea may present as erythema, prominent spiderlike blood vessels (telangiectasia), or swelling (**FIGURE 13-35**). Acnelike (papules and pustules) eruptions can occur, but unlike acne, there are no comedones. Additional manifestations may include a

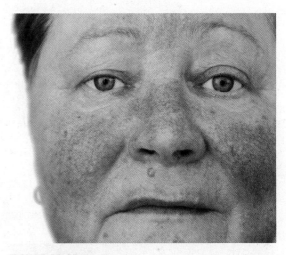

FIGURE 13-35 Rosacea.
© Lipowski/iStock/Getty Images.

TABLE 13-2	Pharmacotherapeutic Strategies				
Pathogenesis	**Retinoids**	**Acids/benzoyl peroxide**	**Antibiotics**	**Hormonal therapies**	
Hyperkeratinization and desquamation (peeling)	+ (topical or oral)	+ Azelaic acid or salicyclic acids		+	
Increased sebum production	+ (oral)			+	
P. acnes proliferation		+ Azelaic acid Benzoyl peroxide	+ (topical or oral)		
Inflammation	+ (topical or oral)	+ Azelaic acid	+ (oral)		

+ indicates effective.

Myth Busters

There are a couple of myths in regard to acne that warrant clearing up (no pun intended).

Myth 1: Eating greasy foods and chocolate worsens acne.

Contrary to popular belief, greasy foods and chocolate have little effect on acne. Studies are ongoing to determine whether other dietary factors—including high-starch foods (such as bread, bagels, and chips), which increase blood sugar—may play a role in acne.

Myth 2: Acne is a result of the skin being dirty.

Acne is not caused by dirt. In fact, scrubbing the skin too hard or cleansing with harsh soaps or chemicals irritates the skin and can make acne worse. The frequent cleansing also does not reduce sebum production. Simple cleansing of the skin to remove excess oil and dead skin cells is all that is required.

Modified from Story, L. (2017). *Pathophysiology: A Practical Approach* (3rd ed.). Burlington, MA: Jones & Bartlett Learning.

---

burning or stinging sensation and red, watery eyes. Further eye examination may reveal infiltrates in the cornea and sclera. A thickening of the skin on the nose (rhinophyma) is more common in men, and the phymatous changes can also occur on the chin, forehead, or cheeks. If left untreated, rosacea is progressive, but most people with this condition experience remissions and exacerbations. Exacerbation triggers are specific to the individual but may include sun or wind exposure, sweating, stress, spicy food, alcohol, hot beverages, hot baths, and cold weather.

Diagnosis and Treatment

Diagnosis of rosacea is made clinically with a history and physical examination. Skin biopsy is indicated if there are suspicions of another disorder. There is no known cure for rosacea. Instead, treatment strategies center on identifying and avoiding possible triggers, so that affected individuals can reduce exacerbations. These strategies may include the following measures:

- Avoiding excessive scrubbing when cleaning the skin
- Avoiding sun exposure (e.g., wearing protective hats and clothing, limiting exposure time especially between 10:00 a.m. and 4:00 p.m.) and using sunscreen that protects against both UVA and UVB rays every day
- Avoiding prolonged physical exertion in hot weather
- Managing stress (e.g., through deep breathing and yoga)
- Limiting spicy foods, alcohol, and hot beverages
- Avoiding any other triggers

- Applying topical or oral antibiotics, such as topical metronidazole (antifungal) or ivermectin (antiparasitic) to control skin eruptions (pustules and papules)
- Applying retinoic acid cream or gel (e.g., Retin-A) or oral isotretinoin (Accutane) for pustules and papules
- Administering topical vasoconstrictors (e.g., brimonidine tartrate or oxymetazoline)
- Performing laser/light therapies to help reduce the redness
- Performing surgical reduction of enlarged nose tissue
- Applying green- or yellow-tinted prefoundation creams and powders to reduce the appearance of redness.

Integumentary Cancers

Skin cancer is an abnormal growth of skin cells. According to the Centers for Disease Control and Prevention (CDC, 2016), skin cancer is the most frequently occurring cancer in the United States, and the number of cases continues to rise. Prevalence rates are highest in males, Whites, persons with fair complexion, and those with a family history. The overall 5-year survival rate is approximately 92%. UV exposure, either natural or artificial, is by far the most significant risk factor for this type of cancer. For this reason, most skin cancers occur on areas that have the most sun exposure (e.g., the arms and neck).

Three major types of skin cancer are distinguished and include basal cell carcinoma, squamous cell carcinoma, and melanoma. A discussion of each follows.

- **Basal cell carcinoma** (BCC), the most common type, develops from abnormal growth of the cells in the lowest layer of the epidermis. BCC has a low metastatic potential, but BCC can cause significant local tissue destruction, and ulceration is common. BCC cell has different clinical manifestations (e.g., nodular, superficial). Nodular is one of the more common types and presents as a flesh-colored papule that appears pearly or translucent (**FIGURE 13-36**). The lesion often has rolled borders (i.e., the borders are higher than the middle).

- **Squamous cell carcinoma** (SCC) involves changes in the squamous cells, which are found in the middle layer of the epidermis. The lesions have a varied presentation in comparison to BCC. Lesions can be papules, plaques, nodular, smooth, hyperkeratotic, or ulcerative. There is a higher potential for metastasis in comparison to BCC, but the incidence is low. **Actinic keratosis** (i.e., solar keratosis) is a skin lesion that is benign and is a result of proliferation of epidermal keratinocytes. These lesions are considered part of a continuum of SCC. Actinic keratosis lesions have the potential to progress to SCC. Actinic keratosis lesions can be similar to SCC.

- **Melanoma** develops in the melanocytes. It is the least common type but the most serious due to metastasis to other areas. There are several subtypes of melanomas, and the lesions have a varied presentation (**FIGURE 13-37**). The ABCDE rules were initially developed for early identification of melanoma and are often used in mole evaluation.

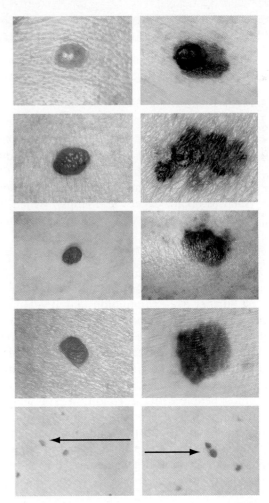

FIGURE 13-37 Skin cancers.

Courtesy of The Skin Cancer Foundation (www.skincancer.org).

Manifestations

Skin cancers can vary widely in appearance; they can be small, shiny, waxy, scaly, rough, firm, red, crusty, bleeding, and so on (Figure 13-37). Given the many possible presentations, any suspicious skin lesion should be biopsied. The following features may be considered suspicious:

- Asymmetry—part of the lesion is different from the other parts
- Borders that are irregular
- Color that varies from one area to another with shades of tan, brown, or black (sometimes white, red, or blue)
- Diameter that is usually (but not always) larger than 6 mm in size
- Sensory changes
- Any skin growth that bleeds or is crusting or will not heal
- Any skin growth that changes in appearance over time (e.g., shape, color)

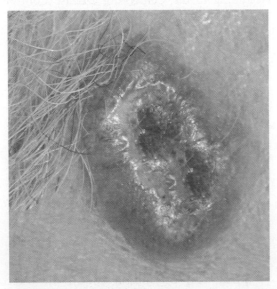

FIGURE 13-36 Basal cell carcinoma.

[Handwritten note in left margin:] Check labs & CXR for melanoma, not BCC/SCC.

Most skin cancers can be prevented by limiting or avoiding exposure to UV light (e.g., by using sunscreen and wearing protective clothing). Early detection is crucial to positive outcomes; with early detection, even the most aggressive forms can be successfully treated. Diagnostic procedures for skin cancer typically include a history, physical examination, and biopsy. Removal of the cancerous growths offers the best prognosis. Treatment strategies may include the following measures:

- Cryosurgery
- Excisional surgery
- Laser therapy
- Mohs surgery (the skin growth is removed layer by layer, examining each layer under the microscope, until no abnormal cells remain)
- Curettage and electrodessication (layers of cancer cells are scraped away using a circular blade [curette], and then an electric needle is used to destroy any remaining cancer cells)
- Radiation therapy
- Chemotherapy

Learning Points

Identifying Skin Cancers

All skin lesions, such as moles, should be monitored for any suspicious changes. These changes can be readily identified—their diagnosis is as easy as A, B, C, D, and E.

A	**a**symmetry—part of the lesion is different from the other
B	**b**orders—irregular
C	**c**olor—varies from one area to another with shades of tan, brown, or black (sometimes white, red, or blue)
D	**d**iameter—usually (but not always) larger than 6 mm in size (the diameter of a pencil eraser)
E	**e**volution—a lesion that is changing in size, shape, or color, or a new lesion

Hair Disorders

Alopecia is defined as hair loss and is associated with several disorders. Hair loss can occur as a result of growth issues, inflammatory damage to hair follicles, or abnormalities in the hair shaft. There are scarring and nonscarring types of alopecia. The scarring types are termed *cicatricial alopecia* and are due to inflammation of the scalp with resulting permanent hair loss. Nonscarring alopecia has mild or absent inflammation. The nonscarring alopecia can be further divided by the hair loss distribution with focal hair loss, diffuse hair loss, and patterned hair loss. Focal patches of complete hair loss can be caused by **alopecia areata**, which is an autoimmune T cell mediated disorder of the hair follicle in genetically susceptible individuals. Alopecia areata in some patients can cause total loss of hair (scalp and body). Diffuse hair loss distribution is commonly caused by **telogen effluvium**. The cause of telogen effluvium is a premature shift of hair entering the telogen (resting) cycle of growth from the anagen growth phase. Most hair (about 90%) is in the anagen growing phase and only a small amount (10%) is in the telogen phase. The hair loss can be acute or chronic and there is a significant amount of shedding. The scalp is usually visible, but the whole head is not usually affected. The third distribution of nonscarring alopecia is patterned. Male pattern hair loss (androgenetic alopecia), female pattern hair loss, and trichotillomania are examples of patterned distribution of hair loss. Male pattern loss usually proceeds in the frontotemporal area where there are andogen sensitive hair follicles (sides and back of head have androgen insensitive follicles). Female pattern hair loss usually involves thinning on the frontal and crown areas while the occiput is spared. Both male and female pattern hair loss are more likely to occur in genetically susceptible individuals. Trichotillomania is a mental health disorder characterized by repeatedly pulling hair out. As hair is pulled from different areas the distribution is usually irregular and has different shapes.

Nail Disorders

Nail disorders can cause an alteration in nail growth. Nail disorders can occur with systemic diseases (e.g., splinter hemorrhages with psoriasis), trauma, infection, cancer, or inherited skin/nail disorders. Fungal infections are termed *onychomycosis* and leads to nail thickening, discoloration, and abnormal shaping. Bacterial infections are a common type of infection caused by *S. aureus*. The nail fold (i.e., around the base or sides of the nail) is often the site of infection and is termed *paronychia*. Viral infections can cause warts due to human papilloma virus around the nail but also in the nail bed. Herpetic whitlow is due to herpes simplex virus that can affect the hand and periungal (around toes/fingers) area. Herpes whitlow often occurs in children who suck their finger and have oral herpes or in healthcare workers through direct contact. Squamous cell carcinoma and melanoma can occur in the nails. Similar to the ABCDE for skin cancer evaluation, there is an ABCDEF mnemonic for nail changes that should raise suspicion for melanoma.

ABCDEF—Nail Changes

A **a**ge of patient (peak 50–70 years of age)

B **b**and of dark (brown or black) pigmentation on nail bed; **b**readth greater than 3 mm; border irregular or blurred

C **c**hange in the band (e.g., size, rapid growth)

D **d**igit involved (multiple digits are more common)

E **e**xtension of the pigmented band (e.g., nail fold)

F **f**amily history of melanoma

Nail disorders are diagnosed with a history and physical, and, if necessary (e.g., if melanoma is suspected), a biopsy. Nail infections can additionally be diagnosed with a KOH preparation and sending nail clippings for pathologic evaluation or culture. Nail disorders are treated based on their underlying disorder.

CHAPTER SUMMARY

The integumentary system plays a vital role in homeostasis and well-being by protecting the body from invasion by pathogens, maintaining water balance, sensing changes in the environment, and regulating body temperature. Conditions affecting this system can cause issues with any or all of these functions. Some of these conditions can be prevented through measures such as limiting UV light exposure through using sunscreen that protects against UVA and UVB rays, wearing protective clothing, and limiting time outdoors, especially between 10:00 a.m. and 4:00 p.m., when the sun's rays are the most intense. Early diagnosis and treatment of other conditions can improve prognosis.

REFERENCES AND RESOURCES

AAOS. (2004). *Paramedic: Anatomy and physiology*. Sudbury, MA: Jones and Bartlett Publishers.

American Burn Association. (2018). *Advanced burn life support provider manual*. Chicago.

Berlowitz, D. (2018). Epidemiology, pathogenesis, and risk assessment of pressure-induced skin and soft tissue injury. In K. A. Collins (Ed.), *Uptodate*. Retrieved from https://www.uptodate.com/contents/epidemiology-pathogenesis-and-risk-assessment-of-pressure-induced-skin-and-soft-tissue-injury

Centers for Disease Control and Prevention (CDC). (2016). Skin cancer. Retrieved from http://www.cdc.gov/cancer/skin/

Centers for Disease Control and Prevention (CDC). (2018). Shingles (herpes zoster). Retrieved from https://www.cdc.gov/shingles/surveillance.html

Chiras, D. (2015). *Human biology* (8th ed.). Burlington, MA: Jones & Bartlett Learning.

Elling, B., Elling, K., & Rothenberg, M. (2004). *Anatomy and physiology*. Sudbury, MA: Jones and Bartlett Publishers.

Feldman, S. R. (2018). Epidemiology, clinical manifestations, and diagnosis of psoriasis. In A. O. Ofori (Ed.), *Uptodate*. Retrieved from https://www.uptodate.com/contents/epidemiology-clinical-manifestations-and-diagnosis-of-psoriasis

Gould, B. (2015). *Pathophysiology for the health professions* (5th ed.). Philadelphia, PA: Elsevier.

International Society for Burn Care (ISBI). (2016). ISBI practice guidelines for burn care. *Burns, 42,* 953–1021.

Keller, E. C., Tomecki, K. J., & Alraies, M. C. (2012). Distinguishing cellulitis from its mimics. *Cleveland Clinic Journal of Medicine, 79*(8), 547–552.

Lyons, F., & Ousley, L. (2015). *Dermatology for the advanced practice nurse*. New York, NY: Springer.

National Institutes of Health (NIH). (2019a). Chediak-Higashi syndrome. Retrieved from https://ghr.nlm.nih.gov/condition/chediak-higashi-syndrome

National Institutes of Health (NIH). (2019b). Hermansky-Pudlak syndrome. Retrieved from https://ghr.nlm.nih.gov/condition/hermansky-pudlak-syndrome

National Pressure Ulcer Advisory Panel. (2016). NPUAP pressure injury stages. Retrieved from https://www.npuap.org/resources/educational-and-clinical-resources/npuap-pressure-injury-stages/

Professional guide to pathophysiology (3rd ed.). (2010). Philadelphia, PA: Lippincott Williams & Wilkins.

Robinett, R. H., & Chop, W. C. (2015). *Gerontology for the health care professional* (3rd ed.). Burlington, MA: Jones & Bartlett Learning.

Sommers, M. S. (2011). Color awareness: A must for patient assessment. *American Nurse Today, 6*(1). Retrieved from https://www.americannursetoday.com/color-awareness-a-must-for-patient-assessment/

Spergel, J. (2010). From atopic dermatitis to asthma: The atopic march. *Annuals of Allergy, Asthma, and Immunology, 105*(2), 107–109.

Weston, W. L., & Howe, W. (2019). Atopic dermatitis (eczema): Pathogenesis, clinical manifestations, and diagnosis. In R. Corona (Ed.), *Uptodate*. Retrieved from https://www.uptodate.com/contents/atopic-dermatitis-eczema-pathogenesis-clinical-manifestations-and-diagnosis

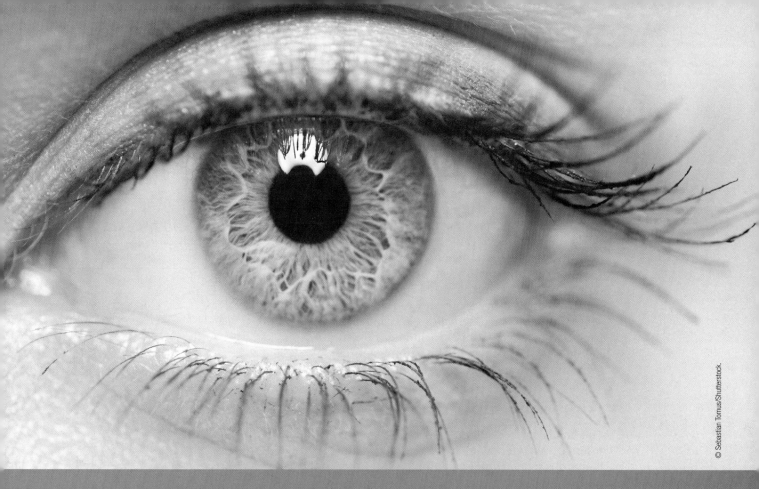

CHAPTER 14
Sensory Function

LEARNING OBJECTIVES

- Discuss normal sensory anatomy and physiology.
- Explain mechanisms of acute and chronic pain.
- Differentiate eye and ear sensory disorders that are age related or due to infections and inflammation.
- Differentiate acute and chronic sensory emergencies.
- Summarize how various sensory disorders lead to sensory deficit.

- Explain the clinical consequences of sensory deficit disorders.
- Apply understanding of sensory disorder alterations in describing various common disorders such as infections, trauma, glaucoma, macular degeneration, otosclerosis, and Meniere disease.
- Develop diagnostic and treatment considerations for various sensory disorders.

The human body has a complex surveillance system that senses changes in the internal and external environments. This vigilant system utilizes numerous receptors throughout the body to detect even subtle alterations; these receptors are located in the skin, internal organs, and other tissue. The stimuli perceived by these receptors give rise to sensations, including those related to the general and special senses (**TABLE 14-1**). The general senses include pain, light touch, pressure, temperature, and proprioception (position), while the special senses include taste, smell, sight, hearing, and balance. Disorders of the sensory structures can result in sensory dysfunction. These disorders can result from a wide range of causes including congenital defects, advancing age, infections, neurologic disorders, and cancers.

Anatomy and Physiology

The ability to sense changes in ever-changing internal and external environments allows the body to respond to those stimuli and to function. Sensations are detected by receptors, which then convert the stimuli into nerve impulses. These impulses travel to the brain by cranial or spinal nerves to be processed and appreciated (**FIGURE 14-1**). The human body contains five types of receptors for the general and special senses: 1) mechanoreceptors (activated by mechanical stimuli such as touch or pressure), 2) chemoreceptors (activated by chemicals in the blood, food, or air), 3) thermoreceptors (activated by heat or cold), 4) photoreceptors (activated by light), and 5) nociceptors (activated by painful stimuli). General sense receptors can occur as exposed or encapsulated nerve endings (**FIGURE 14-2**).

The exposed nerve endings detect pain, temperature, and light touch and are located in the skin, bones, and internal organs. One or more layers of cells surround encapsulated nerve endings. A variety of encapsulated nerve

TABLE 14-1	Summary of the General and Special Senses	
Sense	**Stimulus**	**Receptor**
General senses	Pain	Naked nerve endings
	Light touch	Merkel disks; naked nerve endings around hair follicles; Meissner corpuscles; Ruffini corpuscles; end bulbs
	Pressure	Pacinian corpuscles
	Temperature	Naked nerve endings
	Proprioception	Golgi tendon organs; muscle spindles; receptors similar to Meissner corpuscles in the joints
Special senses	Taste	Taste buds
	Smell	Olfactory epithelium
	Sight	Retina
	Hearing	Organ of Corti
	Balance	Crista ampullaris in the semicircular canals; maculae in utricle and saccule

Reproduced from Story, L. (2017). *Pathophysiology: A Practical Approach* (3rd ed.). Burlington, MA: Jones & Bartlett Learning.

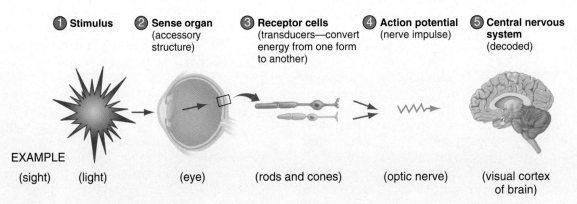

① Stimulus   **②** Sense organ (accessory structure)   **③** Receptor cells (transducers—convert energy from one form to another)   **④** Action potential (nerve impulse)   **⑤** Central nervous system (decoded)

EXAMPLE

(sight)   (light)   (eye)   (rods and cones)   (optic nerve)   (visual cortex of brain)

FIGURE 14-1 The general sensory pathway.

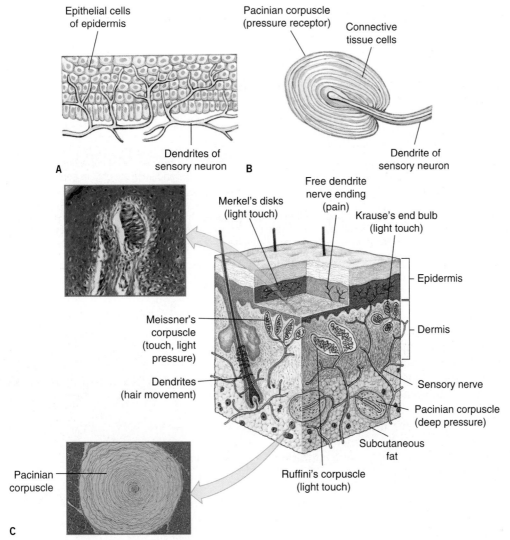

FIGURE 14-2 General sense receptors are either **(A)** exposed nerve endings or **(B)** encapsulated nerve endings. **(C)** The skin houses many of the receptors for the general senses. The pacinian corpuscle, often located in the dermis of the skin, detects pressure. The Meissner corpuscle, found just beneath the epidermis, detects light touch.

© Astrid & Hans-Friender Michler/Science Source; © Carolina Biological Supply Co/Visuals Unlimited, Inc.

endings, including pacinian corpuscles, Meissner corpuscles, Krause end-bulbs, and Ruffini corpuscles, are located throughout the body for a variety of senses. Many of these sensory receptors (especially those for pain, temperature, and pressure) will stop generating impulses after an extended exposure to stimuli through adaptation.

Pain Mechanisms

Pain is associated with many conditions and, therefore, warrants further discussion. Pain is a protective mechanism, warning the body when something is wrong. In addition, acute pain is the most common reason people seek medical attention and can be used to aid diagnosis. Likewise, patients with chronic pain frequently access the healthcare system to obtain relief from the debilitating effects of chronic pain. Pain is a subjective feeling, and the perception of pain and the level at which it is sensed (**pain threshold**) can be influenced by affective (emotional, feelings), behavioral, cognitive (thinking, reasoning, beliefs, and attitudes), sensory (perceptual), and physiologic factors. Unrelieved pain can delay healing, stimulate the stress response, and result in **pain tolerance**.

The transmission of a pain stimulus (nociceptive signal) to the periphery, spinal cord, and brain (ascending pathway) and then back to the periphery (descending pathway) is complex. Various theories have been proposed over the last 200 years (e.g., specificity theory was developed around 1895) to describe the mechanisms of pain (**TABLE 14-2**).

TABLE 14-2	Summary of Proposed Theories of Pain
Theory	**Mechanism**
Specificity theory	The somatosensory system is divided. Each sensation has a specific receptor (e.g., tactile, hot, cold, and pain) that is sensitive to one stimulus and is associated with one sensory pathway that projects to specific cortical structures.
Intensity	The number of impulses in neurons determines stimulus intensity. This theory disputed distinct pathways.
Pattern theory	Sensory impulses have specific and particular patterns and the peripheral nerve firing is dependent on spatial and temporal profile that modulates the stimulus and intensity of pain perception. This theory explains concepts of central sensitization, allodynia, and hyperalgesia.
Gate control theory	Sensory impulses are transmitted to the dorsal horn of the spinal cord. The substantia gelatinosa through large and small fibers modulate transmission to specialized cells (transmission cells) and small fibers ("open the gate") and allow impulse transmission and large fibers ("close the gate") and inhibit transmission.

These theories served as the basis for subsequent pain research; however, each of these theories is incomplete in explaining the complex phenomenon of pain. The early theories' primary focus was acute and somatic pain. Pain is now understood as multidimensional with several components interacting and modulating the experience and expression of pain. The dimensions of pain include the sensory discriminative dimension, which describes intensity, location, quality, and duration. Affective–motivational dimensions include unpleasantness and subsequent response. The cognitive–evaluative dimension consists of appraisal, cultural values, context, and cognition.

Pain Transmission

An understanding of pain transmission from stimulus to brain and back to the periphery is important as the target of analgesics is usually one of these areas or mechanisms. The pain pathway involves first-, second-, and third-order neurons (FIGURE 14-3).

The first-order neuron receptors detect painful stimuli prior to any injury or alteration in tissue integrity. The pain signal will then travel to the dorsal horn of the spinal cord. The primary neuron afferent (i.e., ascending) fibers will make a synaptic connection in the spinal cord with second-order neurons that process the painful stimuli. The dorsal horn in the spinal cord is like a meeting place for the synaptic connections. Several afferent impulses from cutaneous, muscle, and visceral stimuli converge in the dorsal horn. The dorsal horn has many intricate connections (e.g., first and second-order neurons, interneurons) and neurotransmitters, making it a crucial stopping

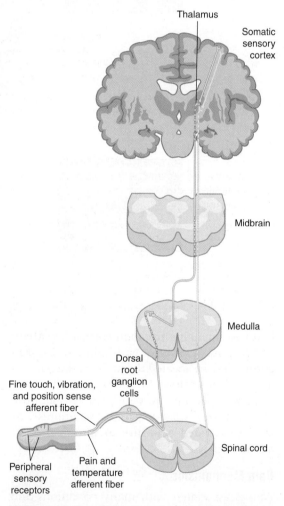

FIGURE 14-3 Simplified pathway from peripheral receptor up to somatosensory cortex.

point before transmission to the brain. The second-order neurons then send pain signals up two different tracts—the spinothalamic and the spinoreticular. The spinothalamic tracts send afferent impulses to the ventrobasal complex of the thalamus, and the impulses then go to the somatosensory cortex. In the somatosensory cortex, the sensory–discriminative component of pain is modulated. The second-order neurons in the spinoreticular tracts send afferent impulses to the centromedian complex of the thalamus and then impulses go to the limbic system and frontal lobe. The motivational–affective component of pain is modulated in these regions. These brain centers are the location of the third-order neurons where pain information is integrated and processed.

Along the pathway at all levels, there are various excitatory and inhibitory influences. The sensory (afferent) fibers from the periphery to the spinal cord are made of nociceptive and nonnociceptive fibers. The nociceptive fibers consist of large, myelinated $A\delta$ fibers and thin, unmyelinated C fibers. The $A\delta$ fibers transmit impulses quickly and are associated with sharp pain, and C fibers transmit impulses slowly and are associated with later, dull or diffuse pain. The nonnociceptive fibers ($A\beta$) consist of large, myelinated fibers that transmit impulses quickly; however, they are inhibitory and reduce and block nociceptive input. Stimulation of nonnociceptive fibers leads to an analgesic effect and is the principle behind transcutaneous electrical nerve stimulation modalities and massage for pain reduction.

In addition to the nociceptive and nonnociceptive fibers, interneurons influence the passage of the stimuli from the periphery to the spinal cord. Inflammatory markers are released in the periphery. These markers include chemical mediators such as potassium, prostaglandins, bradykinin, histamine, substance P, and serotonin. These substances recruit nociceptors, causing a lower pain threshold (sensitization) or allodynia (when an innocuous stimulus causes pain). Sensitization, which is also known as hyperalgesia, can be peripheral or central. Sensitization can occur in the spinal cord (i.e., central sensitization). With central sensitization in the spinal cord, neurons known as wide-dynamic-range neurons are excitable and spontaneously discharge. Sensitization can also be the result of a decrease in inhibitory mechanisms. The wide-dynamic-range neurons are dependent on N-methyl-D-aspartate receptors. Several medications and drugs used recreationally act as N-methyl-D-aspartate antagonists. These include ketamine, dextromethorphan (cough suppressant), and methadone (used in opioid addiction). Sensitization is a phenomenon that occurs in chronic pain syndromes where repeated stimulation of C fibers causes a sensitizing effect in the dorsal horn. With chronic pain, subsequently less provocation is needed to cause pain, or perceived pain increases even with a constant stimuli at the same level. Peripheral sensitization is usually short lived and responsive to anti-inflammatories, while central sensitization requires different types of treatments such as anticonvulsants (e.g., gabapentin, lamotrigine, or topiramate). To make the matter of pain mechanisms more complex, at times neurons act in the opposite intended manner to a neurotransmitter during certain physiologic conditions. Opioids, which are normally used to manage pain, can in some circumstances cause hyperalgesia.

Various endogenous inhibitory mechanisms reduce pain. The activation of nonnociceptive afferent fibers causes activation of inhibitory interneurons resulting in analgesia. Areas that have inhibitory effects include the periaqueductal gray region in the midbrain and magnus raphe nucleus in the medulla. These areas have serotonergic and noradrenergic inhibitory mechanisms. An example of this inhibitory effect is the use of tricyclic antidepressants that block serotonin uptake and can be used in chronic pain syndromes (e.g., migraines). Brain imaging techniques have revealed that various changes in cortical regions respond to cognitive manipulation. Cognitive manipulation includes techniques such as distraction, hypnosis, and information, which are used to modulate pain expectation and relief. Brain plasticity (ability of brain to change) is a phenomenon that is evident when understanding the various responses to pain.

Types of Pain

Pain can be categorized in various ways, including by perception (somatic, visceral), duration (acute, chronic), or characteristics (e.g., neuropathic). The body perceives two types of pain, each with its own cause, location, and characteristics. Somatic pain results from noxious stimuli to the skin, joints, muscles, and tendons. These stimuli may include cutting, crushing, pinching, extreme temperature, and irritating chemicals. Somatic pain can be superficial or deep. Somatic pain is generally easy to pinpoint and is often described as aching, throbbing, or cramping. In contrast, visceral pain results from noxious stimuli to internal organs. Visceral pain mechanisms are different than the previously discussed somatic afferent mechanisms. On visceral organs (e.g., thoracic, pelvic, abdominal), the nociceptors are sparsely distributed. The afferent fibers from visceral organs travel to the central nervous system through the autonomic nervous system (e.g., vagus and spinal nerves). The stimuli causing visceral pain are different than those causing somatic pain and may include expansion and hypoxia. Visceral pain is usually vague and diffuse. The pain is often described as squeezing, deep, or colicky. It may even be sensed on body surfaces at distant locations from the originating organ, a phenomenon called *referred pain* (FIGURE 14-4). The exact mechanism by which referred pain arises is unknown, but it is thought to result from the brain's misinterpretation of the visceral impulses as somatic impulses because both types of impulses enter the spinal cord at the same location (e.g., dorsal ganglion). Referred pain qualities are similar to somatic qualities. Due to autonomic nervous system involvement, visceral pain is often accompanied by symptoms such as nausea, vomiting, and sweating. The term *phantom pain* describes pain that exists after the removal of a body part. The affected person may feel the discomfort of the removed part. The severing of neurons may result in spontaneous firing of spinal cord neurons because normal sensory input has been lost. This type of pain can be extremely distressing but usually resolves with time. Intractable pain describes chronically progressing pain that is unrelenting and severely debilitating. This type of pain does not usually respond well to typical pharmacologic pain treatments (e.g., analgesics and narcotics). Intractable pain is common with severe injuries, especially those crushing in nature. Neuropathic pain describes pain that results from damage to peripheral nerves by disease (e.g., diabetes mellitus) or injury; it tends to be both chronic and intractable. Patients with neuropathic pain also experience losses of the senses of touch and pressure. This condition causes an unusual sensation of paresthesia (numbness) and pain at the same time. The resulting pain is often described as a prickly, stabbing, or burning sensation.

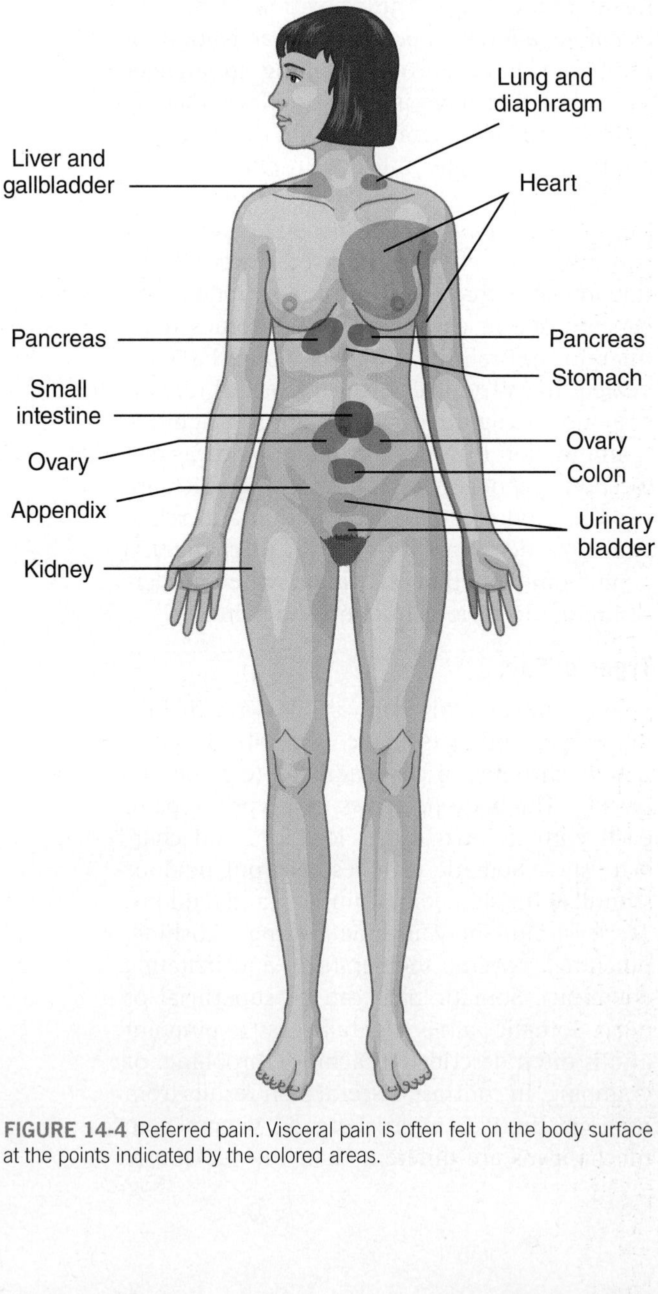

FIGURE 14-4 Referred pain. Visceral pain is often felt on the body surface at the points indicated by the colored areas.

Learning Points

Brain–Gut Axis, Pain, and the Microbiome

Irritable bowel syndrome (IBS) is a functional gastrointestinal disorder associated with abdominal contractions and pain, yet there is no identifiable injury or dysregulation to explain the pain. So how or why does the visceral abdominal pain occur? The central nervous system and enteric nervous system have a bidirectional communication. Essentially, the brain influences the autonomic, motor, sensory, and secretory functions of the intestines, and the intestines, through these same connections, communicate (modulate) with the brain. However, this activity still does not necessarily explain the pain. While mechanisms are poorly understood, intestinal microbiome alterations (e.g., lack of stability and diversity) may play an important role in IBS development. The altered intestinal microbiome affects the gastrointestinal nervous system and immune system. These two affected systems (nervous and immune) send visceral and sensory pain signals to the brain (particularly the limbic and frontal regions). This initiates an autonomic response and alters cognitive and affective response. This theory is one of several pertaining to the development of IBS.

Pain can be categorized as acute or chronic. Acute pain is usually defined as less than 6 months in duration, and chronic is pain that lasts for 6 months or longer. While acute pain is a warning sign that something is wrong, chronic pain has no functional purpose. Acute pain is commonly associated with autonomic nervous system responses (e.g., increased heart rate, increased blood pressure), while there is a lack of an autonomic response with chronic pain. Chronic pain is often challenging to manage due to the complex mechanisms (e.g., physiologic, psychological, and social) sustaining the pain.

Eyes

The human eye is a remarkable organ that allows us to perceive the environment in which we live. Human eyes are globe-shaped organs located in orbits in the anterior skull. Each eye consists of three distinct layers (**FIGURE 14-5**; **TABLE 14-3**).

The outermost layer of the eye is composed of a durable, fibrous material called the *sclera* (white area) and a clear lens on the anterior side called the *cornea*. Tendons and muscles attach to the sclera to control eye movement. The cornea allows light to enter the eye.

The middle layer of the eye consists of the choroid, which contains melanin that absorbs any stray light. The anterior portion of the choroid forms the ciliary body, whose smooth muscle fibers control the shape of the lens,

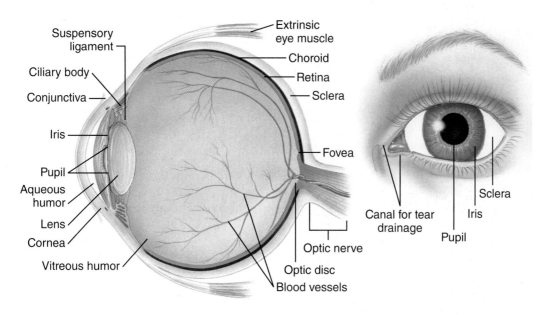

FIGURE 14-5 Anatomy of the eye.

TABLE 14-3	Structures and Functions of the Eye	

Structure	Substructure	Function
Wall		
Outer layer	Sclera	Provides insertion for extrinsic eye muscles
	Cornea	Allows light to enter; bends incoming light
Middle layer	Choroid	Absorbs stray light; provides nutrients to eye structures
	Ciliary body	Regulates the lens, allowing it to focus images
	Iris	Regulates the amount of light entering the eye
Inner layer	Retina	Responds to light, converting light to nerve impulses
Accessory structures and components	Lens	Focuses images on the retina
	Vitreous humor	Holds the retina and lens in place
	Aqueous humor	Supplies nutrients to structures in contact with the anterior cavity of the eye
	Optic nerve	Transmits impulses from the retina to the brain

Reproduced from Story, L. (2017). *Pathophysiology: A Practical Approach* (3rd ed.). Burlington, MA: Jones & Bartlett Learning.

allowing it to focus on incoming light. The iris is the colored portion of the eye, and the pupil is the dark opening in the center of the iris. The choroid layer and the pigmented section of the retina give the pupil its black appearance. The iris contains smooth muscle fibers that control the diameter of the pupil to regulate light entering the eye. The pupil opens and closes reflexively in response to light intensity.

The innermost layer of the eye is the retina. It contains an outer, pigmented layer and an inner layer consisting of photoreceptors and nerve cells (FIGURE 14-6). The retina is weakly attached to the choroid, making it vulnerable to damage. It contains two types of photoreceptors—rods and cones. The nearly 150 million rods in each eye are sensitive to low light and function at night. By comparison, each eye contains approximately 6 million cones, which can operate only in bright light and are responsible for visual acuity and color vision.

The axons of the ganglion cells come together at the back of the eye to form the optic nerve (cranial nerve II). The optic nerve exits the eye through an area with no photoreceptors and is known as the optic disc (blind spot).

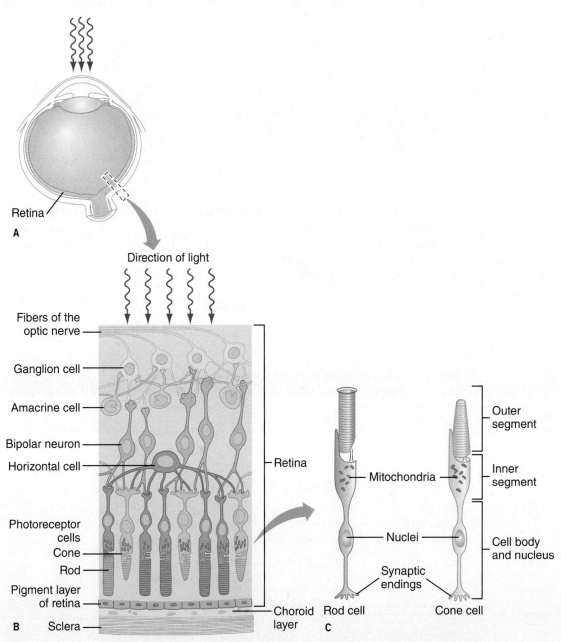

FIGURE 14-6   The retina. (A) Cross-section through the wall of the eye, showing (B) the arrangement of the cellular components of the retina, and (C) the structure of the rods and cones.

Retinal arteries and veins also pass through the optic disc. Lateral to the optic disc is the macula, and the center contains an area known as the fovea centralis, which contains only cones and is the site of visual acuity. The optic nerve extends from the optic disc to the optic chiasm and then branches into the left and right optic tract. These tracts are composed of nasal and temporal fibers. The nasal fibers cross to opposite sides while the temporal fibers remain on the same side. Each of these can become injured and lead to visual field defects. Visual images are cast upside down onto the retina, and impulses are transmitted via the optic tracts to the visual cortex located in the occipital lobe of the brain. The retina processes some of the image, and then the brain processes the rest.

The lens is a transparent, flexible structure that lies behind the iris in the eye. Smooth muscles at the anterior portion of the choroid attached to the lens alter its shape, thereby allowing it to focus on various objects. The lens separates the eye's interior into two cavities—the anterior and posterior chambers. The anterior chamber is in front of the lens, while the posterior chamber is behind the lens. The anterior chamber contains a watery liquid called *aqueous humor* that provides nutrients to the cornea and lens and carries away cellular waste products. A clear, gelatinous material called *vitreous humor* fills the posterior chamber. The pressures exerted by these liquids give the eye its shape.

The inner surface of the eyelid and the exposed surface of the eye are covered by a fragile membrane called the *conjunctiva* and kept moist by the lacrimal glands located in the upper lateral portion of eye. Blinking cleans the eye by sweeping the fluid across the eye. Tears drain on the inner side of the eye through two lacrimal ducts. Lining the lashes are meibomian glands that act as an exocrine gland that produces an oily substance (meibum) that keeps tears and water from evaporating. Eyelid opening and closure controls the amount of light entering the eye.

Ears

The human ear serves to detect and process sound as well as detect body position and maintain balance. The human ear has three separate divisions—outer, middle, and inner ear (**FIGURE 14-7**; **TABLE 14-4**). The outer ear consists of the auricle (or pinna), ear lobe, and external ear canal. The middle ear includes the tympanic membrane and the ossicles. The inner ear comprises the cochlea, semicircular canals, saccule, and utricle.

Sound enters the ear through the auricle (**FIGURE 14-8**). The auricle, an irregularly shaped

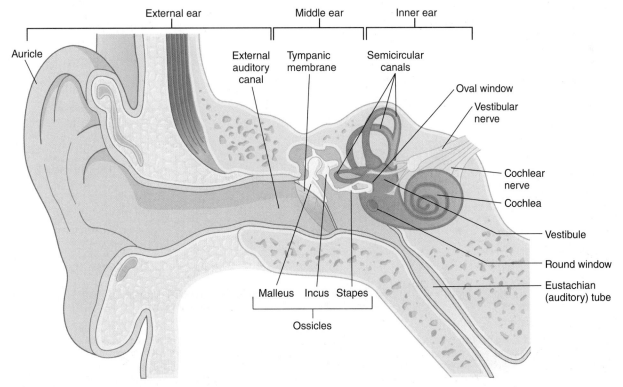

FIGURE 14-7 The structures of the ear.

TABLE 14-4 | **Structures and Functions of the Ear**

Part	Structure	Function
Outer ear	Auricle	Funnels sound waves into the external auditory canal
	Ear lobe	No role
	External auditory canal	Directs sound waves to the eardrum
Middle ear	Tympanic membrane, or eardrum	Vibrates when struck by sound waves
	Ossicles	Transmit sound to the cochlea in the inner ear
Inner ear	Cochlea	Converts fluid waves to nerve impulses
	Semicircular canals	Detect head movement
	Saccule and utricle	Detect head movement and linear acceleration

Reproduced from Story, L. (2017). *Pathophysiology: A Practical Approach* (3rd ed.). Burlington, MA: Jones & Bartlett Learning.

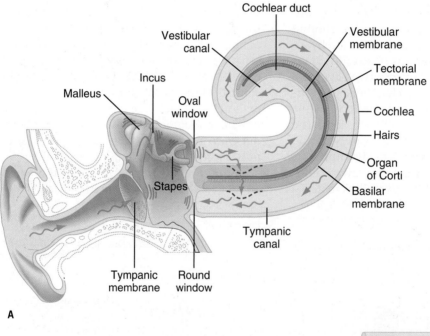

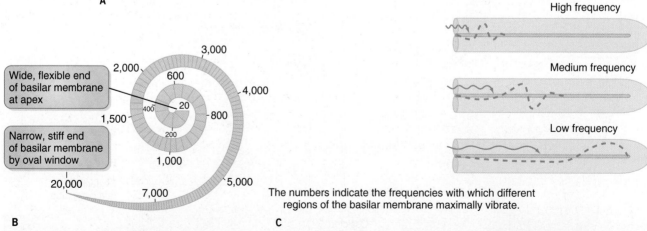

The numbers indicate the frequencies with which different regions of the basilar membrane maximally vibrate.

FIGURE 14-8 Transmission of sound through the ear. The cochlea is shown unwound here to simplify matters. **A.** Vibrations are transmitted from the stirrup (stapes) to the oval window. Fluid pressure waves are established in the vestibular canal and pass to the tympanic canal, causing the basilar membrane to vibrate. **B.** A representation of the basilar membrane, showing the points along its length where the various wavelengths of sound are perceived. Notice that the basilar membrane is narrowest at the base of the cochlea at the oval window end and widest at the apex. **C.** High-frequency sounds set the basilar membrane near the base of the cochlea into motion. Hair cells send impulses to the brain, which interprets the signals as a high-pitch sound. Low-frequency sounds stimulate the basilar membrane where it is widest and most flexible.

cartilage, channels sound into the ear. Sound travels through the external ear canal until it reaches the tympanic membrane. The process of sound waves going from the outer ear to the tympanic membrane comprises conductive hearing. The tympanic membrane, or eardrum, separates the outer and middle ear. Sound hits the tympanic membrane, creating vibrations that are then transmitted to the ossicles. The ossicles consist of three bones—the malleus (hammer), the incus (anvil), and the stapes (stirrup). The malleus lies near the tympanic membrane; vibrations from the membranes cause it to rock back and forth. This rocking causes the incus to vibrate, which in turn causes the stapes to move in and out against the oval window. The oval window is the opening to the inner ear, covered with a membrane. The vibrations created by the tympanic membrane are amplified as they are transmitted through the structures to the inner ear. Movement of the oval window causes fluid within the cochlea to vibrate, creating waves. The cochlea is a spiral-shaped structure that houses the organ of Corti (FIGURE 14-9). The organ of Corti contains hearing receptors in the form of hair cells. Vibrations at the organ of Corti stimulate hair movement. Dendrites wrap the bases of these hair cells. Hair movement causes the dendrites to form nerve impulses that travel to the temporal lobe of the brain via the vestibulocochlear nerve, which is also known as cranial nerve VIII. The process of sound traveling from the middle ear to inner ear and then to the brain comprises sensorineural hearing. See chapter 11 for details on neural function.

The inner ear also holds the vestibular apparatus (FIGURE 14-10), which consists of two parts—the semicircular canals and the vestibule. The semicircular canals are three ringlike, fluid-filled structures that house receptors for body position and movement. The fluid in the semicircular canals works much like a carpenter's level. Movement of the head causes the fluid in the semicircular canal to move; this movement then stimulates dendrites to send impulses to the brain to report the movement. The vestibule is a bony chamber positioned between the cochlea and the semicircular canals; it houses receptors that respond to body position and movement. The vestibule contains the utricle and the saccule, both of which have receptor organs. Nerve impulses generated in the vestibular apparatus travel to a cluster of nerve cell bodies in the brainstem and travel to the cerebellum. At the brainstem, these impulses are combined with input from the eyes,

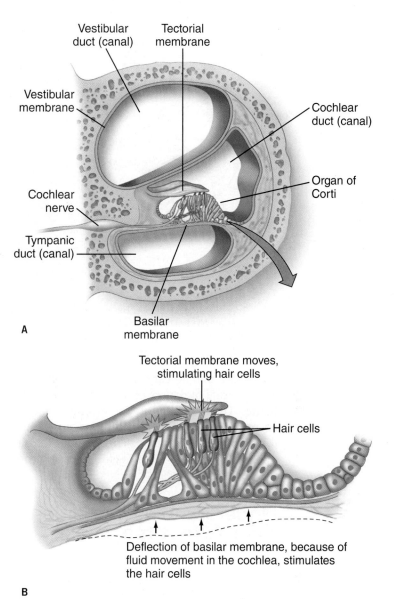

FIGURE 14-9 Cross-section of the cochlea. **A.** Notice the three fluid-filled canals and the central position of the organ of Corti. **B.** Hair cells of the organ of Corti are embedded in the overlying tectorial membrane. When the basilar membrane vibrates, the hair cells are stimulated.

skin, joints, and muscles. This center then directs the information to many areas of the brain. The majority of the information travels on a pathway to the cerebral cortex, increasing awareness of position and movement. Another pathway leads to the muscles of the limbs and torso; information sent via this pathway enables them to maintain balance and correct body position if necessary. See chapter 11 for details on neural function.

The middle ear also opens into the pharynx via the eustachian tube. The eustachian tube acts as a pressure valve. Normally, it remains closed, but the tube may open up with activities such as yawning and swallowing. Opening the eustachian tube allows air to flow in and

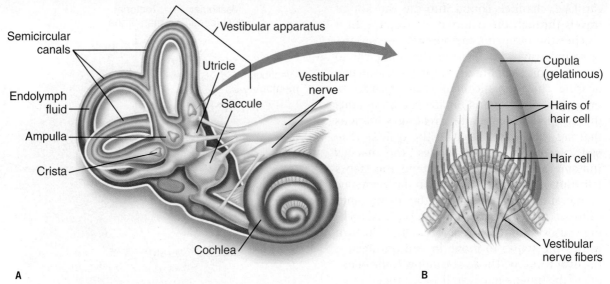

FIGURE 14-10 Vestibular apparatus. **A.** This illustration shows the location of the cristae in the ampullae of the semicircular canals. The semicircular canals are filled with endolymph. **B.** When the head spins, the endolymph is set into motion. This action deflects the gelatinous cupula of the crista, thereby stimulating the receptor cells.

out of the middle ear, equalizing the internal and external pressures on the tympanic membrane. The function of the eustachian tube becomes apparent when the ears pop while taking off in an airplane. This popping sensation is a result of pressure being released from the eustachian tubes.

Understanding Conditions That Affect the Senses

When considering sensory conditions, organizing them based on their basic underlying pathophysiology can increase understanding. Eye and ear underlying pathophysiology can be infectious/inflammatory, traumatic, chronic, congenital, or age-related. Eye and ear disorders will cause alterations in perception, and prompt recognition and treatment are critical to avoiding permanent deficits.

Congenital Sensory Disorders

Congenital sensory disorders vary widely in severity. Many different conditions may arise when an error occurs during embryonic development. These, be due to environmental influences, occur because of genetic abnormalities which can occur randomly, or be hereditary. They may result in minor conditions with only aesthetic problems (e.g., microtia) or life-altering states (e.g., congenital cataracts). Treatment is often unnecessary, but when needed, treatment options are usually limited.

Eyes

Congenital eye conditions are rare. These conditions vary widely in severity, but vision impairment is present to some degree in most cases. These conditions seldom happen in isolation and are often associated with other disorders.

Congenital Cataracts

Congenital cataracts involve a clouding of the lens that is present at birth or develops over time. This clouding of the usually clear lens results in hazy vision. In most cases, no specific cause can be identified. However, congenital cataracts have been associated with several genetic and chromosomal conditions (e.g., Down syndrome, Turner syndrome, and galactosemia) as well as intrauterine infection exposure (e.g., congenital rubella, syphilis, toxoplasmosis, and herpes simplex). Cataracts can also be hereditary and usually follow an autosomal dominant inheritance pattern (see chapter 1 for details on cellular function).

In addition to clouding of the lens, clinical manifestations usually include a failure of an affected infant to demonstrate visual awareness and the presence of nystagmus (rapid, involuntary back-and-forth eye movement) and strabismus (crossed eyes). Asymmetry of the red reflex or a white pupillary reflex (i.e., leukocoria) may be present. Diagnostic procedures for congenital cataracts consist of a history and physical examination (including a thorough ophthalmologic exam). Additional tests may be necessary to determine other associated conditions.

In some cases, congenital cataracts are mild and do not affect vision; these cases require no treatment. Moderate to severe cataracts that affect vision will require cataract extraction surgery, followed by placement of an artificial intraocular lens. Patching to force the child to use the weaker eye may be required to prevent amblyopia (lazy eye). Treatment for any underlying disorder may also be needed.

Ears

Congenital conditions affecting the ears usually result from an absence or malformation of the external ear. These conditions may or may not affect hearing. Anotia refers to the absence of the auricle, while microtia refers to an underdeveloped, small auricle (FIGURE 14-11). Persons with anotia and microtia may also lack an external ear canal (atresia). These conditions are more common in males than in females and are often associated with other congenital conditions affecting the head (e.g., hemifacial microsomia, Goldenhar syndrome, and

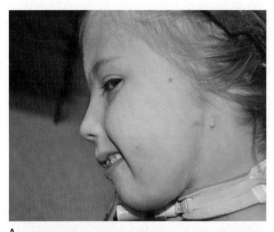

A

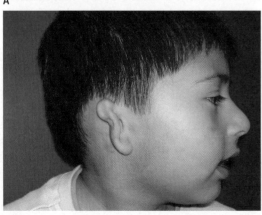

B

FIGURE 14-11 **A.** Anotia. **B.** Microtia.

Courtesy of Dr. Arturo Bonilla, Microtia—Congenital Ear Deformity Institute (http://microtia.org).

Treacher Collins syndrome). There are also several middle and inner ear malformations such as fixation of the ossicles (e.g., malleus and incus), and an absence of the labyrinth. Cochlear malformations may also be present. Such congenital ear conditions may be unilateral or bilateral. In addition to these structural abnormalities, congenital hearing loss can occur because of damage associated with maternal rubella and syphilis infection during pregnancy.

Sensory Conditions Associated With Aging

The way in which the body senses and responds to sensory input changes with age. In general, the senses become less acute and less able to distinguish details. These sensory changes vary in severity but can have a tremendous impact on lifestyle and quality of life. Aging increases the threshold needed to perceive sensory input, so the amount of sensory input needed to be aware of the sensation becomes greater. Physical changes in the body part related to the sensation account for most of the other sensation changes. Hearing and vision changes can be the most dramatic, but all senses can be affected by aging. Equipment such as glasses and hearing aids or changes in lifestyle can compensate for many of the sensory aging changes.

Eyes

Age-related eye changes may begin as early as 30 years of age. Such changes include less tear production as well as structural deteriorations. All of the eye structures change to some degree with aging. The cornea becomes thicker and the curvature decreases, causing astigmatism and blurry vision. The cornea becomes less sensitive, so injuries may go unnoticed. By age 60, pupils decrease to about one-third of the size they were at age 20. The pupil may also react more slowly in response to darkness or bright light than it did in one's youth. The lens becomes yellowed, less flexible, and slightly cloudy, and there is loss of accommodating ability. These lens changes lead to problems with focus, difficulty adapting to darkness, and decreased color vision. The amount of light needed to see things clearly increases as rods are lost in the retina. The vitreous humor liquefies and decreases in volume, increasing the risk for retinal detachment. The fat pads supporting the eye decrease and the eye sinks back into the skull. The eye muscles weaken, decreasing the ability to rotate the eye fully and limiting the visual field. Visual acuity also may gradually decline.

Glasses or contact lenses may help correct these age-related vision changes. Nearly all persons 55 years of age or older need glasses at least part of the time. However, the severity of changes varies. Only 15–20% of elderly persons have vision deficits severe enough to impair driving ability, and only 5% become unable to read.

The most common eye problem associated with aging is difficulty focusing the eyes due to a loss of the lens' normal ability to accommodate, a condition called *presbyopia*. The condition usually begins around the age of 40. Presbyopia results in difficulty focusing on objects that are at reading distance. Other lens changes (i.e., thickening and opacity) cause intolerance to glare, and difficulty adapting to darkness and brightness may be experienced, making driving at night difficult. Inability to distinguish colors can also become more pronounced with age. Keeping a red light on in darkened rooms (such as the hallway or bathroom) may make it easier to see than using a regular night light because it produces less glare than a white light bulb.

Ears

All the ear structures thicken and change with aging, affecting balance and hearing. Hearing may decline slightly, especially regarding high-frequency sounds. Such age-related hearing loss is called *presbycusis*. Some hearing loss is almost inevitable, but an estimated 30% of all people older than age 65 have significant hearing impairment. Hearing acuity (sharpness) may decline slightly beginning at about 50 years of age, possibly caused by changes in the auditory nerve. In addition, the brain may have a slight decreased ability to process or translate sounds into meaningful information. Impacted cerumen is another cause of impaired hearing and is more common with increasing age.

Sensorineural hearing loss involves damage to the inner ear, auditory nerve, or the brain. Presbycusis is a type of sensorineural hearing loss caused by a disorder of the cochlea. While the inciting event is often unclear, the main structures affected are the inner ear sensory structures (e.g., hair cells). Presbycusis is accelerated in people who were exposed to excessive noise or smoking when they were younger. Manifestations of presbycusis include progressive and symmetric high-frequency hearing loss. Tinnitus, vertigo, and balance issues can also be present. This type of hearing loss may or may not respond to treatment, but hearing aids can improve function. Conductive hearing loss occurs when an individual has problems transmitting sound through the outer and middle ear to the inner ear and can occur due to such disorders as cerumen impaction, psoriasis, and otosclerosis. Surgery or a hearing aid may be helpful for this type of hearing loss, depending on the specific cause.

Infectious and Inflammatory Sensory Disorders

Infectious sensory disorders can result from a wide range of causative agents, often triggering the inflammatory response. These conditions may be acute or chronic and vary widely in severity. In most cases, infectious sensory disorders resolve with treatment and no sequelae. However, some eye infections can cause a loss of vision and need prompt identification and treatment.

Eyes

Eye infections can result from a variety of pathogenic organisms, usually bacteria and viruses. Many of these infections are self-limited, and most respond well to treatment. However, severe or untreated infections can lead to visual impairment. These conditions can also be caused by other events that can trigger the inflammatory process (e.g., trauma, allergens, and irritants).

Conjunctivitis

Conjunctivitis, or pinkeye, refers to an infection or inflammation of the conjunctiva, the lining of the inside of the eyelids and the sclera up to the cornea (FIGURE 14-12). Conjunctivitis may be caused by viruses, bacteria, allergens,

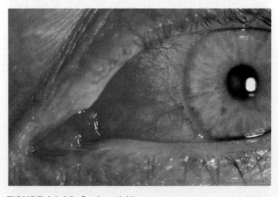

FIGURE 14-12 Conjunctivitis.
Courtesy of John T. Halgren, MD, University of Nebraska Medical Center.

chemical irritants, and trauma. Each cause produces slightly different manifestations. Regardless of its cause, conjunctivitis can generate edema, eye discharge, and eye redness, The eye redness with conjunctivitis is diffuse involving the conjunctiva under the lid and over the globe. Eye redness mainly located around the limbus, which is where the cornea transitions into the sclera may indicate another more serious diagnosis such as angle closure glaucoma or keratitis. Blurry vision may occur due to the secretions, but once the secretions are removed acuity should be normal and if not, another diagnosis should be considered (e.g., keratitis). The pupil and fundoscopic exam are also normal in conjunctivitis. Photophobia (i.e., sensitivity to light) may also be indicative of more serious eye infections such as keratitis. **Viral conjunctivitis** is the most common cause and is usually due to adenovirus). Viral infections normally produce a watery or mucuslike discharge that is usually scant and stringy or ropelike. The eye also feels gritty, like there is sand in it. Viral conjunctivitis usually starts in one eye and then goes to the other eye. Viral conjunctivitis can be accompanied by other viral syndromes such as an upper respiratory tract infection. **Bacterial conjunctivitis** is usually due to *Streptococcus pneumoniae*, *Haemophilus*, *Moraxella catarrhalis* in children, and *Staphylococcus aureus* in adults. Bacterial infections usually produce a mucopurulent yellow-green exudate (puslike) in one eye or both eyes. Bacterial conjunctivitis can be accompanied by other disorders such as otitis media. **Gonococcal conjunctivitis** is a sexually transmitted form of conjunctivitis that can cause blindness. The cause is the bacteria *Neisseria gonorrhoeae*. Transmission is usually from the genitalia to the hands and then the eyes. The discharge usually begins within 12 hours after infection and is profuse and purulent. Irritation and redness appear rapidly. The eye is markedly edematous with lid swelling, and the conjunctiva looks like a bulging blister (i.e., chemosis). Gonorrhea can be transmitted to a newborn's eye during birth, so the Centers for Disease Control and Prevention (CDC) recommends that all newborns be treated with erythromycin ointment regardless of whether the mother has a gonorrheal infection. **Trachoma conjunctivitis** is caused by the bacteria, *Chlamydia trachomatis* (serotypes A–C). The infection is highly contagious, and transmission occurs through contact with infected eyes, noses, and throats. Trachoma is a leading cause of infectious blindness worldwide (WHO, 2019) and is endemic in remote areas and areas with lack of resources such as clean water and sanitation. The infection can lead to conjunctival and eyelid scarring, causing the eyelids to turn inward (entropion) and the lashes to rub the eye. Entropion can further lead to ulceration and scarring. *Chlamydia trachomatis* (serotypes D–K) is another type of bacterial conjunctivitis. However, rather than being caused by poor hygiene, the D–K serotypes are sexually transmitted. This type of chlamydial conjunctivitis is usually unilateral, and the manifestations are usually chronic. The manifestations are a mucus discharge, irritation, and redness. Screening for chlamydia in pregnant women has decreased the incidence of vaginally transmitted newborn chlamydial conjunctivitis. Use of ocular antibiotics, as in gonorrhea, is not effective for chlamydia conjunctivitis. **Allergic conjunctivitis** is due to allergens (e.g., dust and pollen) that stimulate an IgE response. The discharge is usually watery (excessive tearing) that is bilateral and accompanied by redness and grittiness (symptoms similar to the viral type). Itching is a symptom that is manifested in allergic conjunctivitis as opposed to other causes. Allergic conjunctivitis can be accompanied by rhinitis and occurs more often in patients with a history of atopy. See chapter 2 for a discussion of immunity.

Diagnostic procedures for conjunctivitis focus on identifying the causative agent and include a history and physical examination. Cultures are usually only done with cases of conjunctivitis suspected to have been caused by *Neisseria gonorrhoeae*. A rapid (10-minute) viral test for adenovirus can be used to aid in differentiating viral from bacterial causes. Many cases of conjunctivitis will resolve without treatment. Treatment may vary depending on the underlying cause. Symptomatic relief for all conjunctivitis can include warm, moist compresses to soothe the discomfort associated with conjunctivitis. Cool compresses can improve edema if present. Artificial tears can be used for relief. Viral conjunctivitis treatment is symptomatic and includes topical antihistamines or decongestants. Allergic conjunctivitis treatment is also symptomatic with avoidance of allergens. Pharmacologic agents for allergic conjunctivitis can include antihistamines with vasoconstrictors or with mast-cell–stabilizing properties. Topical glucocorticoids can be used but have serious side effects (e.g., scarring and

BOX 14-1 Application to Practice

Review the various conjunctivitis cases and determine the most likely cause, including pathogen and mode of transmission. Discuss data that supports your decision and treatment strategies.

Case 1: A 5-year-old girl has had a cough and runny nose (yellowish discharge) for the past 3 days. Her mother brought her for an evaluation as her left eye became pink and the right eye is also starting to get pink. Her daughter keeps rubbing them. The mother says there was a little discharge that was like mucus, but she wiped it away before coming to get checked. The physical examination reveals an active, alert girl. Her ears and lungs are within normal limits (WNL). Yellowish discharge is noted from the nose, and her oropharynx is mildly erythematous; however, there is no tonsillar enlargement or exudate. Her eyes have conjunctival erythema and mild edema—the left eye greater than the right eye. Mild crusting at the lid but no discharge is noted.

Case 2: A 40-year-old woman is complaining of itching, redness, and watery discharge in both her eyes. She feels like she has sand in her eyes. She also starting sneezing and has a clear nasal discharge. She thinks the symptoms started after petting a cat 2 days before at a friend's house. She stated this reaction never happened before around animals, but she does get hay fever a few times a year. She has a past medical history of eczema. The physical examination reveals alert woman in no acute distress. Her ears, nose, throat, and lungs are WNL. There is evidence of bilateral stringy "ropelike" discharge and conjunctival erythema.

Case 3: An 18-month-old boy has a runny nose (yellowish discharge) and has been rubbing his left ear for 3 days. His parents kept him home from day care and brought him in for an evaluation as both his eyes became pink and were full of crust and yellowish discharge this morning. He has been fussy, not eating well, and had a temperature of 100°F. The physical examination reveals a fussy, alert boy. His throat and lungs are WNL. There is evidence of yellowish discharge from the nose, and his left ear canal is clear, but the tympanic membrane is bulging and red, and fluid is noted behind the tympanic membrane. His eyes have a yellowish discharge and conjunctival erythema bilaterally.

---

perforation) that can affect vision and should be used cautiously. Bacterial conjunctivitis is treated with antibiotics (e.g., topical ointment or eye drops). Chlamydia conjunctivitis (sexually transmitted) is treated with oral antibiotics (e.g., doxycycline). Trachoma conjunctivitis eradication efforts were initiated by WHO in 1993 and include the SAFE strategy, which stands for surgery (for eyelid inversion), antibiotics, facial cleanliness, and environmental improvement. Gonococcal conjunctivitis requires immediate referral, hospitalization, and treatment with systemic and topical antibiotics. Viral and bacterial conjunctivitis are highly contagious through direct contact, and steps are necessary to prevent transmission of the infection (e.g., hand washing, limiting contact, proper eye hygiene, and discarding contaminated ophthalmic products).

Keratitis

Keratitis refers to an inflammation of the cornea that can be triggered by an infection or trauma (**FIGURE 14-13**). Common traumatic causes of keratitis include artificial ultraviolet exposure, welding, contact lens overuse, and abrasions; and common viral infections that cause it include herpes simplex, varicella zoster, Epstein-Barr virus, and cytomegalovirus. Herpes simplex 1 virus can be self-transmitted from the mouth and cause an ulcerated form of keratitis. Bacterial infections are caused by *S. aureus* and *Pseudomonas aeruginosa*. Clinical manifestations reflect the inflammatory

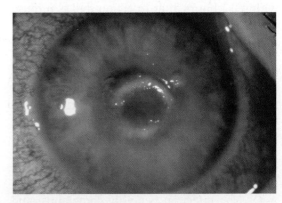

FIGURE 14-13 Keratitis.

Courtesy of Christopher J. Rapuano, MD, Cornea Service, Wills Eye, Professor, Jefferson Medical College of Thomas Jefferson University, Philadelphia, PA.

process and include severe eye pain, erythema, drainage (clear or mucopurulent), excessive tearing, photophobia, sensation of a foreign body, and visual disturbances. The cornea may also have an opacity.

Diagnostic procedures for keratitis focus on identifying the causative agent and include a history and physical examination. A fluorescein staining may reveal an ulceration. Corneal infections can cause ulceration, scarring, and vision loss, so prompt referral to an ophthalmologist is necessary. As an example, bacterial keratitis most often occurs in those who wear contact lenses and a corneal ulceration can form within 24 hours. Treatment varies depending on the underlying etiology, but strategies often include ophthalmic or oral antibiotics and corticosteroid agents.

Diagnostic Link

Fluorescein Staining

A quick procedure to evaluate the integrity of the eye surface is the use of fluorescein staining. Fluorescein is an orange dye that comes in a solution or strips (like pH paper). The fluorescein stains the basement membrane (epithelial cells), and the injury (e.g., abrasions, ulceration) will be evident with the staining. The technique involves, pulling the lower lid and moistening the fluorescein strip with saline or the moist conjunctiva or placing a drop of fluorescein solution on the lower lid. If a strip is used, the provider gently touches the inner lower lid with the strip, and the dye goes around the surface of the globe when the patient blinks. A cobalt blue light on most ophthalmoscopes or a Wood lamp is used to look at the eye. The injury will appear yellow or green reflecting increased uptake of the dye. Fluorescein solutions can grow *Pseudomonas*, so the solution should be properly stored and maintained.

Blepharitis

Blepharitis is an inflammation of the eyelid margin caused by infection (e.g., *S. aureus*). Blepharitis can also be caused by alterations in the Meibomian glands due to chronic inflammatory skin conditions such as rosacea, seborrheic dermatitis (dandruff), and psoriasis. Irritants such as smoking, contact lenses, and cosmetics, as well as medications such as retinoids can also cause or be associated with blepharitis. In blepharitis, the inflammation can be anterior—at the base of the eyelashes—or posterior—at the inner portion of the eyelid along the level of the Meibomian glands. Blepharitis can be acute or chronic. In chronic blepharitis, the duct epithelial lining becomes keratinized, and the gland secretions change

and become toxic to the eye. These glandular changes can promote infections. Incidence of blepharitis is higher in adults in comparison to children, and the incidence increases with age.

Clinical Manifestations

Clinical manifestations of blepharitis include erythematous, edematous, and pruritic eyelids with flaking or scaling of the eyelid skin. The eyelashes may also be crusted in the morning. The conjunctivae may be pink (more on the palpebral surface), and there may be a gritty or burning sensation. Blurred vision is transient and improves with blinking. Because the Meibomian gland is important in eye lubrication, a common complication is dry eye; however, a person may complain of excessive tearing as a manifestation. Paradoxically, excessive tearing is a common presentation in dry eye syndromes as the tears are a reflex, but the tears produced may be imbalanced (e.g., decreased water composition). With blepharitis, the eyelashes can be altered (e.g., they can be misdirected, there can be loss, or there can be abnormal growth). The eyelids can turn toward the inside of the eye (i.e., **entropion**) or turn toward the outside of the eye (i.e., **ectropion**).

Diagnosis and Treatment

Diagnosis is usually made clinically with a history and physical examination. Treatment includes good hygiene. Warm compresses followed by lid massaging may promote Meibomian gland emptying and increase secretions. After compresses and massage, the lid should be washed gently with diluted baby shampoo and rinsed. Artificial tears can be used for dry eyes. Patients who do not respond to conservative treatment or have severe symptoms may need topical ophthalmic antibiotics (e.g., bacitracin or erythromycin). Oral antibiotics, topical glucocorticoids, and topical cyclosporine are alternatives for refractory cases.

Hordeolum and Chalazion

A **hordeolum**, which is commonly called a *stye*, is an acute infection of the eyelid that presents as an abscess and nodule. The infection is usually caused by *S. aureus*. The infection can be in two small eyelid glands called the *gland of Zeis* (sebaceous gland) and the Moll gland (the apocrine sweat gland) in the eyelash follicle or the lid margin. Infections of the eyelash follicle or lid margin are termed *external hordeola*. The infection and inflammation can also be in the Meibomian gland (internal hordeola). Some hordeola are not infectious but rather are a result of chronic inflammatory skin conditions such as seborrheic dermatitis and rosacea. Clinical manifestations of a hordeolum are a painful, erythematous, edematous nodule along the lid margin or under the conjunctival side of the eyelid. Treatment usually includes warm compresses several times a day to help with drainage along with gentle massage. Hordeola often resolve spontaneously within a few days. Contact lens use and makeup should be avoided while the hordeolum is present. The effectiveness of topical antibiotics and topical glucocorticoids are questionable.

Chalazion is a localized eyelid swelling caused by glandular obstruction (e.g., in the Meibomian gland or the gland of Zeis) that results in a painless, mildly erythematous lid nodule. Chalazion can be noninfectious, but a hordeolum can become a chalazion. The nodule occurs as a result of an inflammatory granulomatous reaction to lipids in the gland secretions. Chalazion resolution is usually longer than resolution of a hordeolum and can take days to weeks. Treatment for chalazion is similar to hordeolum treatment and includes warm compresses. Some chalazions will require incision and drainage.

Dacryocystitis

A blockage of the nasolacrimal duct can lead to an infection in the lacrimal sac known as dacryocystitis. The nasolacrimal duct disorder can be congenital or acquired (e.g., facial trauma). Dacryocystitis most commonly occurs in infants and adults over 40 years of age. The infection can be acute or chronic. Clinical manifestations include purulent discharge, tearing, edema, erythema, and pain in the lacrimal sac area. Acute dacryocystitis is treated with systemic antibiotics, applying warm compresses, and gentle massage. Chronic dacryocystitis generally requires surgery known as dacryocystorhinostomy, which involves forming a new drainage (fistula) into the nasal cavity.

Ears

Ear infections can result from a variety of pathogens, usually bacterial or viral. These conditions are classified based on the area of the ear infected and typically resolve with treatment.

Otitis Media

Acute otitis media (AOM) describes an infection or inflammation of the middle ear. AOM is a common condition in young children and is a frequent reason for an acute care visit. The prevalence is highest between the age of 6 months and 2 years old, but most children have experienced an episode by the age of 5. The introduction of the 13-valent pneumococcal vaccine for infants in 2010 has reduced the incidence of AOM. Most common causative organisms in descending order of prevalence include *Haemophilus influenzae*, *Streptococcus pneumoniae*, *Moraxella catarrhalis*, and group A streptococci. Other organisms that are not as common include *Staphylococcus aureus* and *Escherichia coli*. Viral causes include influenza viruses, respiratory syncytial virus, and human metapneumoviruses. The infection can also be polymicrobial with more than one bacteria or a combination of bacterial and viral organisms. Children are at higher risk for AOM as the eustachian tubes of young children are narrower, straighter, and shorter than those of adults and older children. This developmental variation in anatomy decreases the ability of fluid to drain from the young child's middle ear adequately. In addition to these structural differences, a young child's immune system is less equipped to manage infections than that of an adult or older child. Another cause of fluid accumulation in the middle ear is adenoid enlargement, usually due to inflammation. Because of their close proximity to the eustachian tubes, enlargement of the adenoids can compress the tubes. See chapter 2 for a discussion of immunity.

Typically, AOM begins as a viral upper respiratory infection, so it is more common in the winter months than in the rest of the year. The viral infection migrates to the middle ear, causing accumulation of fluid behind the tympanic membrane. This fluid buildup provides a prime medium for secondary bacterial growth. Additional risk factors include child care in group settings, feeding infants in the supine position, environmental smoke exposure, pacifier use, a history of allergic rhinitis, and presence of orofacial deformities (e.g., cleft lip or palate).

A complication of AOM is **otitis media with effusion** (OME) (i.e., serous otitis media). OME refers to the presence of fluid in the middle ear without an acute infection. The effusion can last for weeks to months even after other acute otitis media manifestations have resolved. OME can also be caused by eustachian tube dysfunction and possibly allergies. Other complications of AOM include rupture of the tympanic membrane, scar tissue formation, and conductive hearing loss (fluid in the middle ear does not allow tympanic membrane vibration). Additionally, the infection can spread to nearby structures and cause mastoiditis, cholesteatoma (a benign epithelial cell tumor in the middle ear and mastoid), meningitis, and osteomyelitis.

Clinical Manifestations

Clinical manifestations can vary depending on age; in some cases, the infection may be asymptomatic. Clinical manifestations of AOM frequently include ear pain caused by pressure in the middle ear, mild hearing deficits, or rubbing and pulling at the ear. The child may be crying and irritable and may have sleep disturbances. Other nonspecific symptoms include nausea, vomiting, diarrhea, and headache. Indications of infection will include fever, malaise, and chills. Physical examination findings reflect inflammation as the tympanic membrane is red and bulging. Due to the middle ear effusion, the tympanic membrane may be opaque and air–fluid levels may be visible behind the membrane. Tympanic membrane mobility will be absent or decreased. Manifestations of OME include hearing loss that is generally mild and intermittent, sensation of ear fullness, tinnitus, or problems with balance (e.g., falling, stumbling). Physical examination findings in OME will include an impaired tympanic membrane mobility and air–fluid levels with amber or translucent fluid behind the tympanic membrane. The tympanic membrane may also appear opaque and retracted.

The diagnosis of AOM and OME is made clinically based on the history and physical. The otologic examination usually includes visualization of the tympanic membrane, and tympanometry (which measures tympanic membrane movement), and acoustic reflectometry (reflection of sound). Tympanometry and acoustic reflectometry will simply provide information regarding the presence or absence of an effusion and not if the fluid is infected or uninfected. The aspiration of middle ear fluid (tympanocentesis) for culture can confirm a diagnosis, but this culture is not usually necessary unless there is serious illness (e.g., immune deficits). Culture of the drainage, if present, may be done.

Treatment for AOM focuses on eradicating any infection present, decreasing the amount of fluid in the middle ear, and managing pain. Strategies may include oral or otologic antibiotics and analgesics. Otologic therapy is usually

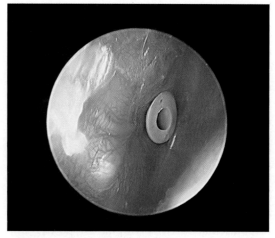

FIGURE 14-14 Tympanostomy tubes.
Courtesy of Andrew Heaford and Richard Smith, University of Iowa.

not effective unless the tympanic membrane has ruptured. Oral decongestant and antihistamine agents are controversial as they may cause prolongation of the middle ear effusion. Antipyretics may be necessary to control fever. OME can cause hearing loss, and this loss can place children at risk for issues with speech and learning. While OME can resolve without treatment, routine hearing evaluation and treatment may be necessary in those with chronic OME (> 3 months). Drainage tubes (tympanostomy tubes) can be inserted to facilitate fluid drainage for children with recurrent AOM or OME (**FIGURE 14-14**). Removal of the adenoids may also be performed with the placement of tympanostomy tubes.

Otitis Externa

Otitis externa, or swimmer's ear, refers to an infection or inflammation of the external ear canal or auricle. Otitis externa is usually bacterial in origin (often *P. aeruginosa*) but may also be fungal (usual polymicrobial). With otitis externa, inflammation alters the skin's natural cerumen protective function. Otitis externa generally arises from moisture in the ear that creates an environment for bacterial or fungal growth or introduction of the organisms from external sources. Risk factors include swimming in contaminated water, scratching the outside or inside of the ear, and insertion of foreign objects (e.g., cotton swabs, earphones, and ear plugs) into the ears. Allergies and dermatologic diseases (e.g., psoriasis) may also cause external otitis. Most cases are mild and respond well to treatment, but occasionally this condition can lead to malignant otitis externa, which causes hearing loss, cellulitis, necrosis, osteomyelitis, and meningitis.

Clinical Manifestations

Clinical manifestations of otitis externa include ear pain that worsens with auricle movement, purulent exudate, pruritus, a sensation of fullness in the ear, and hearing deficits. The ear canal is usually edematous and erythematous upon examination. The exudate may be various colors such as yellow or white. Fungal infections may cause a different color exudate such as a dark coating with *Aspergillus*. Severe cases can also cause erythema outside the ear (preauricular area), lymphadenopathy, and fever.

Diagnosis and Treatment

Diagnosis is made clinically based on history and physical examination. Most episodes of otitis externa respond well to empiric antibiotic treatment, so exudate analysis (e.g., culture and sensitivity) is not necessary. However, a culture should be considered if the otitis is recurrent, chronic, or severe or if the patient is immunocompromised (e.g., with HIV). Because of the easy access to the external ear canal, treatment strategies are typically applied locally (i.e., topically). These strategies may include otologic antibiotic, antifungal, corticosteroid, and analgesic agents. Additionally, the external ear canal may be cleaned (e.g., via lavage of warm saline) and a cotton wick may be inserted to increase medication penetration and absorb drainage. Prevention strategies include drying the ears after swimming or applying ear drops after swimming, avoiding insertion of foreign objects into the ear, wearing ear plugs, and treating pools properly.

Traumatic Sensory Disorders

Traumatic sensory disorders can result from a wide range of injuries and can vary widely in severity. Often the patient's prognosis depends on prompt treatment.

Eyes

Eye trauma can result from numerous types of injuries. Any of the eye structures can be involved, including the eyelid, cornea, or the entire eye globe. These conditions may vary in severity from mild (e.g., black eye) to sight threatening (e.g., orbital compartment syndrome and acute closed-angle glaucoma). The eye is highly vulnerable to injury, and vision deficits can result from such damage. Corneal abrasions and corneal foreign bodies are common causes of eye injury and will be discussed separately. Other eye injuries may result from direct physical trauma or chemical burns and include chemical burns, hyphemas, and subconjunctival hemorrhage.

Chemical burns can be due to acidic substances (e.g., acetic acid present in hair wave neutralizer, hydrochloric acid in pool cleaner, and grout cleaner) and alkalotic substances (e.g., ammonia hydroxide in fertilizers, hair dyes, and sodium hypochlorite in bleach). The degree of burn is dependent on the duration of the exposure and the type of chemical. Alkaline substances are usually more caustic than acidic substances. Treatment involves continuous irrigation (it can take as long as 60 minutes) until the pH of the eye fluid neutralizes. Irrigation can be accomplished with saline or water either manually with an intravenous tubing or with a scleral lens device (e.g., a Morgan lens).

A **hyphema** is a pooling of blood in the anterior chamber (**FIGURE 14-15**). A hyphema is sight-threatening and can be easily confused with a subconjunctival hemorrhage (**FIGURE 14-16**), which is a benign tear of a blood vessel. A hyphema is usually caused by blunt trauma and often accompanies other injuries such as head trauma and orbital fractures. Spontaneous hyphemas are rare but can occur in the absence of trauma in diabetes mellitus or coagulation disorders.

A **subconjunctival hemorrhage** is a tearing of the fragile vessels under the conjunctiva. This bleeding is usually a benign condition caused by coughing, sneezing, and straining. There are no symptoms other than the visible blood in the subconjunctiva and resolution occurs without treatment within 2 weeks. However, a subconjunctival hemorrhage associated

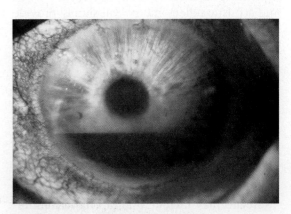

FIGURE 14-15 Hyphema.

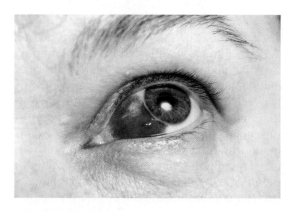

FIGURE 14-16 Subconjunctival hemorrhage.
© Haoka/Shutterstock.

with trauma, pain, vision change (e.g., loss or double) or in a person with a bleeding disorder warrants emergency evaluation.

Clinical Manifestations

Clinical manifestations vary depending on the nature of the injury and prompt recognition of sight-threatening injuries must be done quickly. Traumas—whether blunt or penetrating—are always suspect for severe injury to the eye and possible other nearby structures, such as the cervical spine and airway. Manifestations that are likely to reflect a serious eye injury include eye pain, visual changes (e.g., decreased acuity, blurry vision, and diplopia), floaters, black spots, or appearance of cobwebs). Physical examination findings may include pupillary changes (e.g., pupil dilation, pupils that are unresponsive to light, anisocoria—unequal pupils); iridodialysis (tearing away of the iris from its insertion); obscuring of the optic disc, retina, and vessels; and absence of red reflex. Some manifestations of orbital compartment syndrome, which occurs with a rapidly elevated intraorbital pressure, are proptosis (bulging eye), inability to open eyelids, and the outer eye globe feeling tight when touched.

Diagnosis and Treatment

Early diagnosis and treatment can prevent or limit the severity of visual deficits. Diagnostic procedures consist of a history and physical examination (including an ophthalmic examination, often by an ophthalmologist). Treatment strategies may include the following measures:

- Flushing the irritant out of the eye with sterile saline
- Avoiding rubbing the eye (can worsen the damage)
- Leaving an embedded object in the eye
- Covering the eye with a sterile dressing or cloth
- Applying eye patches to protect the eye during the healing process
- Repairing any damage surgically

Corneal Abrasion and Corneal Foreign Body

Corneal abrasion and corneal foreign body are the most common type of eye injuries and occur across all ages. Incidence is estimated that 2% of primary care visits are eye complaints, and a majority are due to abrasions and foreign bodies. An abrasion is defined as a disruption of the surface epithelial layer of the cornea. The disruption is usually caused by trauma (i.e., chemical or physical). The many mechanisms of injury can include blowing debris such as sand or dust; foreign bodies such as glass, metal, or wood; direct trauma with fingernails (especially with contact lenses insertion and removal), airbag deployment; and inadequate eye protection while in a tanning bed, welding, or in bright sunlight, including snow blindness.

Clinical Manifestations

Regardless of the injury mechanism, patients with corneal abrasions will complain of severe eye pain, photophobia, and foreign body sensation. The eye pain occurs as a result of the corneal epithelium innervation by the trigeminal nerve (cranial nerve V). The manifestations of corneal abrasion may appear immediately after a direct trauma (e.g., piece of wood in the eye), may be delayed if the object was small (e.g., sand blowing), or even be intermittent (symptoms occur, abate, and then recur).

Physical examination findings may include a decreased visual acuity depending on the location of the abrasion (an injury close to the pupil is more likely to cause acuity changes than one farther away from it). The eye is first examined with a penlight. With an abrasion, the pupil should be reactive. Other findings with a penlight may include mild redness around the cornea (i.e., a ciliary flush), tears, and a visible foreign body. The fundoscopic examination with a corneal abrasion should be normal. After examining externally with a penlight, the exam can then proceed with fluorescein staining. The foreign body does not stain, but the disrupted cornea will appear yellow or green. The upper eyelid should be everted and inspected. Retained foreign body under the eyelid will cause parallel vertical lines at the top of the cornea. Abrasions that have been present for a prolonged period (e.g., > 12 hours) may cause corneal edema. Edema may also be present due to the patient rubbing or pressing their eye. The presence of other manifestations such as pupillary changes, impaired visual acuity, discharge other than tears, corneal opacity or white spots on the cornea, hyphemas, purulence in the anterior chamber (hypopyon), or a foreign body that is penetrating (e.g., piece of metal even if small) are signs of another or underlying serious eye injury, and emergent referral to an ophthalmologist or emergency eye care center is critical.

Diagnosis and Treatment

The diagnosis of a corneal abrasion is made based on the history and physical examination. If recognized and treated early, most abrasions will heal. Lack of treatment can result in corneal ulceration and visual impairment. Treatment includes the administration of topical antibiotics and daily evaluation until the eye heals. Follow-up is usually within 24 hours. If a corneal foreign body is detected, an attempt to remove it can be made with irrigation or a swab after instillation of a topical analgesic. However, some foreign objects need to be removed with other instruments. Metals with iron often leave a rust ring, and metal causes an infiltrate. The eye may need to be debrided if the abrasion does not heal within a few days. Pain control may include topical ophthalmic nonsteroidal anti-inflammatory drugs or short-term (e.g., 1 day) oral opioids for slower healing abrasions or larger abrasions. Eye patching is not recommended for small, uncomplicated abrasions as the patch itself may be irritating and may cause visual field problems leading to falls. Driving while wearing a patch is also dangerous. Patching increases risk of infection in contact lens wearers with an abrasion. Patching may decrease pain in large abrasions (> 50% of cornea). Large abrasions may require the use of topical cycloplegics. Complications of corneal abrasions can include recurrent erosion, ulceration, and infections that could then lead to vision impairment.

Ears

Ear trauma can result from a variety of injuries to any of the internal or external ear structures. These injuries may stem from direct physical trauma such as from motor vehicle accidents, foreign objects, and insects; barotrauma due to exposure to excessively loud noises such as explosions and gunshots; or pressure changes such as those that occur when scuba diving. Such events can result in permanent hearing deficits. Clinical manifestations of ear trauma may include otorrhea (e.g., bloody or clear exudate), tinnitus, dizziness, balance disturbance, ear pain, hearing deficits, nausea, vomiting, edema, a sensation that an object is in the ear, and pressure in the ear. Physical examination findings may include a ruptured tympanic membrane, hemotympanum, or fluid in the middle ear. Nystagmus and ataxia may occur. Hematomas behind the auricle (i.e., Battle sign) indicate a basilar skull fracture and can appear up to 2 days after an injury.

Treatment strategies vary depending on the nature of the injury. Perforated tympanic membranes with minimal hearing loss (e.g., cannot hear a whisper) and those that affect < 25% of the eardrum usually resolve within 4 weeks. Larger surface–area tympanic rupture and those patients with significant hearing loss may require surgical repair (i.e., tympanoplasty). While the tympanic membrane is healing, water should be kept out of the ears and topical ear antibiotics applied.

Other strategies for ear trauma may include the following measures:

- Removing the object if it is visible and easily removed
- Flushing the ear with sterile water or saline to remove small objects (alcohol or mineral oil may be used to kill insects, limiting the trauma during their removal)
- Performing surgery to remove objects or repair the damage
- Limiting exposure to loud sounds as structures heal

Chronic Sensory Disorders

Numerous chronic conditions can affect the sensory organs. These conditions may cause significant sensory deficits. Some disorders can be prevented or their progression delayed by wearing sunglasses; however, several conditions are congenital or hereditary.

Eyes

Many chronic conditions affecting the eyes are progressive and can result in visual deficits. Most of these conditions can be prevented. Early treatment may delay progression and even correct the disorder. These conditions may cause significant visual deficits, and while for some, such as cataracts, there are effective treatments; for other disorders, such as

BOX 14-2 Application to Practice

One night, Tammy, a 24-year-old female, was cleaning her ears with a cotton swab as she does every night as a part of her hygiene routine. She was in a hurry to go out on a date. Her hand slipped as she was cleaning her ears with the cotton swab, and the swab went deep into her right ear. Her ear immediately began to bleed. She continued to get dressed for her date, assuming the bleeding would stop, but it did not. She decided to cancel the date and have her ear checked by a healthcare provider at the after-hours clinic.

At the clinic, the healthcare provider told Tammy that she had probably perforated her tympanic membrane, and it would likely heal in a few weeks. The bleeding continued for the next 24 hours, so Tammy called the clinic again. The healthcare provider at the clinic referred her to an ear, nose, and throat specialist the next day. During her visit with the specialist, Tammy explained the incident with the cotton swab, and the specialist reminded her—as she had heard many times before—"Never put anything smaller than your elbow in your ear." Upon examination, the specialist determined that Tammy had a severe perforation of her tympanic membrane that required surgical repair with skin grafting to prevent permanent severe hearing loss.

Postsurgical repair, Tammy continues to have significant hearing loss in her right ear. The risk for graft rejection remains. Steps to protect her hearing are vital and include limiting exposure to excessive noise and avoiding ototoxic medications.

Modified from Story, L. (2017). *Pathophysiology: A Practical Approach* (3rd ed.). Burlington, MA: Jones & Bartlett Learning.

---

macular degeneration, treatments delay progression but are not curative.

Glaucoma

Glaucoma refers to a group of eye conditions that lead to damage to the optic nerve. The cause of glaucoma is unclear. The damage is often caused by increased intraocular pressure, but it can also result from decreased blood flow to the optic nerve (FIGURE 14-17). However, optic nerve damage can even occur with normal intraocular pressure. Pressures inside the eye can climb when the outflow of aqueous humor becomes blocked or when production of aqueous humor increases to an abnormal level. Pressures can also rise due to disorders in the outflow structures (e.g., trabecular meshwork). These increased pressures cause ischemia and degeneration of the optic nerve.

Glaucoma is the second leading cause of blindness (after diabetic retinopathy) in the United States. There are four types of glaucoma:

1. **Open-angle glaucoma:** Open-angle glaucoma is the most common type and is a chronic eye disorder. For reasons that are unclear, intraocular pressure increases gradually over an extended period. This type of glaucoma tends to run in families, and rates are six to eight times higher among Black individuals than among people of other races. A mutation in the myocilin gene is associated with open-angle glaucoma in adults and the juvenile form. The gene produces a protein called *myocilin* that is involved in regulating intraocular pressure. Patients with open-angle glaucoma often do not have symptoms and the disorder is usually found during a routine eye examination. Clinical manifestations, if present, typically include painless, insidious, bilateral changes in peripheral vision (i.e., abnormal visual field). The visual field should be evaluated with specialized equipment (e.g., automated perimetry) as confrontation testing by a clinician is inadequate. Ophthalmoscopic examination findings include the presence of cupping of the optic disc (i.e., hollowed out appearance). Because the vision changes (e.g., tunnel vision, blurred vision, halos around lights, and decreased color discrimination) are gradual and there are typically no other manifestations, open-angle glaucoma can often be overlooked or misdiagnosed as presbyopia. The progression from vision changes to blindness can take about 25 years.

2. **Closed-angle glaucoma:** Closed-angle glaucoma is a chronic eye disorder that is a result of blockage of aqueous humor outflow. The blockage is a result of narrowing (i.e., narrow-angle glaucoma or closed-angle glaucoma) or complete closure (acute-angle glaucoma). Closed-angle

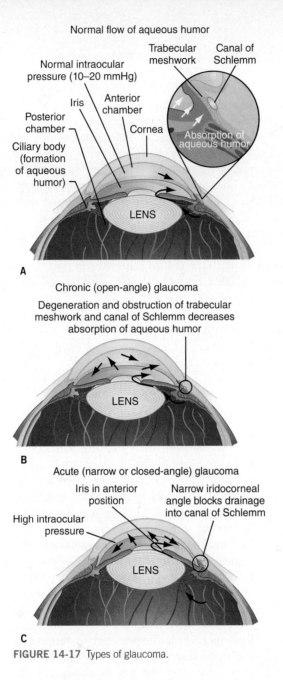

Normal flow of aqueous humor

Trabecular meshwork

Canal of Schlemm

Normal intraocular pressure (10–20 mmHg)

Iris

Anterior chamber

Posterior chamber

Cornea

Ciliary body (formation of aqueous humor)

Absorption of aqueous humor

LENS

A

Chronic (open-angle) glaucoma

Degeneration and obstruction of trabecular meshwork and canal of Schlemm decreases absorption of aqueous humor

LENS

B

Acute (narrow or closed-angle) glaucoma

Iris in anterior position

Narrow iridocorneal angle blocks drainage into canal of Schlemm

High intraocular pressure

LENS

C

FIGURE 14-17 Types of glaucoma.

glaucoma can be caused by an anatomically forward lens that rests against the iris and causes the pupil to block the aqueous humor. Some patients are born with narrow anterior chambers or have shallow anterior chambers. In certain Asian populations and Inuit Eskimos, their anatomic eye structure is associated with a narrow angle with less trabecular meshwork, which predisposes them to closed-angle glaucoma. Over time, pressure builds up, further causing the iris to bow forward. Scarring develops, and the trabecular meshwork becomes damaged and covers

part or all of the flow. The optic nerve becomes damaged over time. When the flow is partially blocked, the patient may be asymptomatic. When flow is blocked suddenly, it is **acute closed-angle glaucoma**, which is a medical emergency. The patient with acute closed-angle glaucoma will be symptomatic and have severe eye pain, decreased vision, headache, and nausea and vomiting, and halos can appear around lights. The pupil will be nonreactive, the conjunctiva may be erythematous, and the cornea becomes edematous and cloudy. Patients with closed-angle glaucoma are at risk for developing acute-angle glaucoma attacks. The acute blockage can be caused by trauma, sudden pupil dilation (e.g., exposure to bright light after prolonged exposure to darkness), prolonged pupil dilation (e.g., medications for eye examinations), and emotional stress. Closed-angle glaucoma is typically unilateral, but it may affect both eyes.

3. **Congenital glaucoma:** This type of glaucoma is present at birth. It results from abnormal development of outflow channels (trabecular meshwork) of the eye. Congenital glaucoma follows an X-linked, recessive hereditary pattern. It may go unnoticed for a few months after birth. Clinical manifestations may include excessive lacrimation, photophobia, corneal edema, gray-white appearance to the cornea, enlarged eye globe, and vision deficits.

4. **Secondary glaucoma:** Secondary glaucoma may result from the use of certain medications (e.g., corticosteroids and anticholinergic agents), eye diseases (e.g., uveitis and nearsightedness), systemic diseases (e.g., arteriosclerosis and diabetes mellitus), and trauma.

Diagnostic procedures for glaucoma consist of a history and physical examination (including an ophthalmic examination). The ophthalmic examination typically involves a gonioscopy (use of a special lens to see the outflow channels of the angle), tonometry (which measures intraocular pressure), optic nerve imaging, pupillary reflex response, retinal examination, slit lamp examination (using a microscope and light to examine the anterior eye structures), visual acuity testing, and visual field measurement.

Treatment focuses on decreasing intraocular pressure. Early detection and treatment are crucial to preserve vision, so those persons at risk for glaucoma should be routinely screened for this condition (usually once a year). Treatment strategies vary depending on the type.

Strategies for open-angle glaucoma may include the following measures:

- Topical ophthalmic medications (usually a combination of two or three types), including the following:
  - Beta blockers (to reduce aqueous humor production)
  - Alpha agonists (to reduce production and increase drainage of aqueous humor)
  - Carbonic anhydrase inhibitors (to reduce aqueous humor production)
  - Prostaglandin-like compounds (to increase aqueous humor outflow)
  - Miotic or cholinergic agents (to increase aqueous humor outflow)
  - Epinephrine compounds (to increase aqueous humor outflow)
  - Alpha-2 adrenergic agonists (to protect the optic nerve)
  - Oral medications (not generally effective when used alone), including carbonic anhydrase inhibitors
  - N-methyl-D-aspartate receptor antagonists (may protect the optic nerve)
- Laser surgery to open aqueous humor outflow
- Filtering surgery (to remove a small section of the trabecular meshwork)
- Drainage implants

The main strategy for treating closed-angle glaucoma is iridotomy (a surgical laser procedure to open a new channel in the iris).

The main strategy for treating congenital glaucoma is surgery to open the aqueous humor outflow channels (e.g., laser, filtering, and drainage implants).

Strategies to treat secondary glaucoma include the following measures:

- Chronic disease management
- Treatment or elimination of the underlying causes
- Previously discussed glaucoma pharmacologic and surgical treatments

Cataracts

A cataract is opacity or clouding of the lens (FIGURE 14-18). Cataracts can occur as a congenital condition (previously discussed) or develop later in life. Over time, proteins in the lens break down, making the lens cloudy. The lens

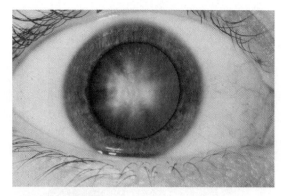

FIGURE 14-18 Cataracts.
Courtesy of National Eye Institute/NIH.

Learning Points

Red Flags for Red Eye

Many disorders cause a red eye. Several, which have been discussed, are sight-threatening and require immediate referral to an ophthalmologist. A summary of the red eye emergencies discussed include gonococcal conjunctivitis, infectious keratitis, hyphemas, hypopyon, and acute closed-angle glaucoma. With the exception of gonococcal conjunctivitis, each of these red eye disorders is accompanied by eye pain (some severe) and vision changes. Other manifestations accompanying a red eye that are warning signs of serious eye disorders are ciliary flush, photophobia, corneal opacity (e.g., infectious keratitis), fixed pupil, or presence of headache with nausea (e.g., angle closure glaucoma)

does not shed dead cells like other epithelial tissue, and therefore the normal degenerative aging changes create a vulnerability to cataract development. Risk factors for adult-onset cataracts include family history, advancing age, smoking, ultraviolet light exposure (natural or artificial), metabolic conditions (e.g., diabetes mellitus), certain medications (e.g., corticosteroids), and eye injury (e.g., trauma and infection). Cataracts may affect one or both eyes and do not necessarily affect eyes symmetrically. In addition to the cloudy appearance of the lens, clinical manifestations may include the following signs and symptoms:

- Cloudy, fuzzy, foggy, or filmy vision (FIGURE 14-19)
- Color intensity loss
- Diplopia
- Impaired night vision, gradually progressing to impaired day vision
- Halos around lights
- Photosensitivity
- Frequent changes in eyeglass or contact prescription

Diagnostic procedures for cataracts consist of a history and physical examination

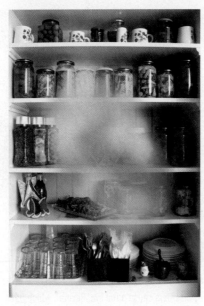

FIGURE 14-19 Visual changes associated with cataracts.
© Fenias/Dreamstime.com.

(including an ophthalmic examination). The ophthalmic examination typically involves visual acuity testing, retinal examination, and slit lamp examination.

Surgery is the only effective treatment for cataracts. Surgical procedures may include removal of the cataract (e.g., phacoemulsification) or a lens transplant. Surgery is typically performed one eye at a time, as an outpatient procedure with a local anesthetic. Recovery time is usually short, and the prognosis is good. Additional strategies may include managing or eliminating contributing factors.

Macular Degeneration

Macular degeneration refers to a deterioration of the macular area of the retina, causing a loss in central vision. Macular degeneration is caused by impaired blood supply to the macula that results in cellular waste accumulation and ischemia. The most significant risk factor for this condition is advancing age. Macular degeneration runs in families and is most prevalent in females and Whites. Additional risk factors include smoking, high-fat diet, heavy alcohol use, and chronic diseases such as cardiovascular disorders (e.g., stroke, ischemic disease) and myeloproliferative disorders (e.g., polycythemia vera).

Two types of macular generation—dry (atrophic) and wet (neovascular or exudative)—are distinguished. Dry macular degeneration—the most common form—occurs when the blood vessels under the macula become thin and brittle. Small yellow deposits (drusen) form under the macula. These deposits increase in size and number, blurring vision and creating a dim spot in the central vision. Wet macular degeneration occurs in only approximately 10% of people with macular degeneration. In this type, brittle vessels break down, and new, abnormal, fragile blood vessels grow under the macula (choroidal neovascularization). These vessels leak blood and fluid, leading to macula damage. Although it is not as common as dry macular degeneration, this form causes more vision loss. Dry macular degeneration progresses gradually (over years) in contrast to the wet form, which results in a sudden, rapid vision loss (over weeks or months).

Macular degeneration is often asymptomatic initially. The most common manifestation of the dry form is blurry vision or gradual loss of central vision. The most frequent manifestations of the wet form are distortion of straight lines, dark spots in central vision (i.e., scotoma), and sudden loss of central vision.

Diagnosis and Treatment

Diagnostic procedures for macular degeneration consist of a history and physical examination (including an ophthalmic examination). The ophthalmic examination usually involves visual acuity using the Amsler grid, retinal examination, fluorescein angiogram (uses dye and a camera to evaluate retinal blood flow), and optical coherence tomography (noninvasive retinal imaging).

No treatment exists for dry macular degeneration. However, a combination of vitamins, antioxidants, and zinc—often called the *Age-Related Eye Disease Study 2* (AREDS2) formula (Chew et al., 2013)—may slow the progression of both the wet and dry forms of the disease. Smokers should not use this treatment, but smoking cessation decreases progression of wet and dry macular degeneration. The AREDS2 contains the following nutrients:

- 500 milligrams (mg) of vitamin C
- 400 international units of vitamin E
- 80 mg of zinc
- 2 mg of copper
- 10 mg of lutein
- 2 mg of zeaxanthin

Although there is no cure for wet macular degeneration, the following treatment strategies may be used:

- Laser surgery—specifically, laser photo-coagulation (lasers destroy the abnormal blood vessels)
- Photodynamic therapy (light activates an injected drug to destroy leaking blood vessels)
- Antiangiogenesis or antivascular endothelial growth factor therapy (medications injected into the eye slow the formation of new blood vessels in the eye)

Low-vision aids (e.g., magnifying glasses and large print) and occupational therapy can also improve independence and quality of life.

Ears

Many chronic conditions affecting the ears are progressive and can result in hearing deficits. Some of these conditions are preventable. With early treatment, most cases can be managed.

Otosclerosis

Otosclerosis refers to an abnormal bone growth in the middle ear, usually involving an imbalance in bone formation (osteoblastic) and resorption (osteoclastic) along with increased vascular proliferation. The cause of otosclerosis is unknown. The disorder can be inherited with an autosomal dominant inheritance pattern with incomplete penetrance and varying degrees of expressivity. In this condition, an abnormal, dense, spongelike bone grows in the middle ear, preventing the ear structures from vibrating in response to sound waves. As the abnormal bone grows, low-frequency hearing loss progressively worsens. While any part of the bony labyrinth can be affected, the oval window area where the stapes is located is commonly affected. While rare, nerve loss due to extension of the otosclerotic process beyond the stapes (e.g., cochlea otosclerosis) can occur and cause a sensorineural hearing loss. Otosclerosis is most common in young adults, with typical age of presentation between 20 and 40 years. Women are often evaluated earlier as pregnancy may trigger otosclerosis and lead to a faster progression, but the incidence rate in men may be equal to women. Otosclerosis is more prevalent in Whites. Typically, otosclerosis affects both ears and is asymmetric. Tinnitus may be a sign of sensorineural involvement, and vertigo may be present as well if there is involvement of other parts of the otic capsule.

Diagnosis and Treatment

Diagnostic procedures consist of a history, physical examination, and temporal-bone computed tomography (CT). Audiometric testing is important in the diagnosis of otosclerosis. Treatment for otosclerosis focuses on minimizing hearing loss or improving hearing. These strategies may include the following measures:

- Medications such as oral fluoride, calcium, or vitamin D, which may help to control the hearing loss, although their efficacy remains in question
- Bisphosphonates typically used in osteoporosis to inhibit osteoclastic activity (i.e., decrease bone resorption) and possibly to help control the bony abnormalities
- Hearing aids to treat hearing loss
- Surgery to remove the stapes (stapedectomy) and replace it with a prosthesis to cure the condition
- Laser surgery to create an opening in the stapes (stapedotomy) with or without the placement of the prosthetic device

Cholesteatoma

Cholesteatoma is a benign tumor in the middle ear. Most cases are acquired, and rarely is the tumor congenital. The tumor forms because of the presence of desquamated squamous epithelial cells that have abnormally migrated to the middle ear or through the deposition of the cells as a complication of middle ear surgery such as tympanostomy tubes. The tumor usually forms because the tympanic membrane is retracted and forms a pocket. The cause of cholesteatoma is unclear. However, factors that contribute to tympanic membrane retraction and tumor formation include eustachian tube dysfunction and chronic middle ear inflammation (e.g., chronic otitis media). Normally, squamous epithelial cells migrate from the tympanic membrane out toward the external auditory canal. The tympanic membrane retraction causes a reverse migration with the squamous epithelial cells causing a keratinization and debris, forming a cholesteatoma, which is a saclike growth in the middle ear. The cholesteatoma causes inflammation and increased osteoclastic activity with bone resorption, and these changes further impair eustachian tube function and disrupt middle ear drainage pathways. The poor drainage causes an environment that fosters bacterial infections. The infections lead to more inflammation and a vicious cycle of destruction that can extend to the whole middle ear and mastoid process. Complications can include mastoiditis, meningitis, and brain abscess.

BOX 14-3 Application to Practice

Review the various hearing disorder cases and determine whether the disorder causes a conductive, sensorineural, or combination of both types of hearing loss. Once you identify the type of hearing loss, explain the part of the ear that is affected and describe the disorder.

Case 1: A 45-year-old woman noticed that she feels like her left ear is full and she cannot hear as well from her left ear as from her right. She states these symptoms started after she was cleaning the inside of her ears with a cotton-tip applicator. Physical exam reveals a right ear that is WNL. Her left ear canal has dark cerumen occluding her ear canal.

Case 2: A 15-year-old is complaining of right ear pain and a feeling of fluid in his right ear for the past 3 days. He feels likes it is getting worse. He says his hearing is slightly decreased in the right ear in comparison to the left. He stated these symptoms started after he came back from a camping trip where he went swimming in a lake several times. Physical exam reveals a left ear that is WNL. His right ear is painful when the auricle is tugged. The ear canal is edematous and erythematous. Whitish exudate is present in the right ear, and due to the amount of exudate, the tympanic membrane was only partially visible. The portion seen was intact and nonerythematous.

Case 3: An 80-year-old man states that he has been gradually having a harder time understanding what people are saying when he is with several people (e.g., like a party). He also states that he has a harder time understanding his grandchildren, and some words he hears well and other he does not. He states his hearing loss is equal in both ears. Physical exam is noncontributory and WNL.

Clinical Manifestations

Clinical manifestations include recurrent or persistent otorrhea, conductive hearing loss, and tinnitus. Vertigo may be present in more extensive disease, but this form is rare. Facial nerve injury such as facial twitching or palsy may occur due to nerve compression. Physical examination findings depend on the cause of the cholesteatoma and can include retracted tympanic membrane, ossicle erosion, debris with a whitish, cystic appearance in the middle ear, a polyp, purulent otorrhea, and a perforated tympanic membrane.

Diagnosis and Treatment

Diagnostic procedures consist of a history and physical examination with audiometric testing. Imaging studies can include a CT scan of the temporal bone. Treatment initially focuses on managing infections with removal of ear debris, keeping the ear canal dry, and topical otic antibiotics. Topical steroids may be considered to reduce inflammation, but the steroids may delay resolution of the infection. The infections caused by cholesteatoma can be difficult to treat, and the treatments often fail even with the addition of systemic antibiotics. Surgery is the only cure, and the goal is to reverse the causes of infection and inflammation. Various surgical techniques, such as tympanoplasty with mastoidectomy, are available. Unfortunately, recurrence rates can be as high as 40% despite corrective surgery, so routine examinations are critical to identify and treat recurrences quickly.

Meniere Disease

Meniere disease is a disorder of the inner ear that results from endolymph swelling. *Meniere syndrome* is the term used when the disorder is secondary to other inner ear disorders. The endolymph swelling stretches the membranes and interferes with the hair receptors in the cochlea and vestibule. The exact cause is unknown, but Meniere disease or syndrome may be associated with metabolic disturbances, hormonal imbalances, autoimmune diseases (e.g., systemic lupus erythematosus and rheumatoid arthritis), head injuries, otitis media, and syphilis. Additional risk factors include allergic rhinitis, alcohol abuse, stress, fatigue, certain medications (e.g., aspirin), and respiratory infections. Clinical manifestations of Meniere disease typically occur in waves of acute episodes that last several months, followed by periods of relief. The attacks may be triggered by changes in barometric pressure or any of the risk factors. These manifestations include intermittent episodes of vertigo, tinnitus, unilateral hearing loss (initially low frequency), and a sensation of ear fullness. Other manifestations include nausea, vomiting, diarrhea, headache, and uncontrollable eye movement. Repeated episodes can lead to permanent hearing loss. The hearing loss is sensorineural.

Diagnosis and Treatment

Diagnostic procedures for Meniere disease or syndrome consist of a history, physical examination (including a neurologic assessment), hearing test, balance test, electrocochleography (which measures fluid accumulation in the ear), electronystagmography, caloric stimulation, head CT, and head magnetic resonance imaging. In electronystagmography, balance sensors are placed in the inner ear to assess balance in relation to eye movement, and in caloric stimulation, a warm or cold solution is instilled into the inner ear to test eye reflexes. The vestibular evoked myogenic potential, which involves neurophysiologic tests to evaluate the otolithic organs (utricle and saccule), is an emerging technology for diagnosing Meniere disease. There is no cure for Meniere disease. Instead, treatment focuses on relieving inner ear pressure and relieving symptoms. Strategies may include the following measures:

- Antihistamine agents (to decrease fluid accumulation)
- Benzodiazepines (to improve vertigo)
- Anticholinergic agents (to decrease fluid accumulation)
- Diuretics (to decrease fluid accumulation)
- Antiemetic agents (to improve nausea and vomiting)
- Limiting dietary sodium intake (to decrease fluid retention)
- Avoiding triggers (e.g., alcohol and stress)
- Middle ear injections of gentamicin (an ototoxic antibiotic that can reduce balance structures) or corticosteroids (to reduce swelling)
- Partial or complete surgical removal of the endolymph or inner ear
- Vestibular nerve resection
- Hearing aids
- Meniett device (for difficult-to-treat vertigo; it improves fluid exchange by applying pulses of pressure to the ear canal through a ventilation tube)
- Physical therapy to improve balance

Sensory Organ Cancers

Any of the sensory organs can develop cancer, but such disease is rare. The severity varies depending on the type of cancer, and treatment often follows the typical cancer management regimens (e.g., chemotherapy, radiation, and surgery). Ear cancer is extremely rare and typically involves skin cancer of the auricle. For this reason, ear cancer will not be included in this discussion. See chapter 3 for a discussion of hematopoietic function. See chapter 13 for a discussion of integumentary function.

Eyes

An uncommon condition, eye cancer can affect any part of the eye, from the eyelid to the intraocular structures. The most common intraocular cancers in adults are melanoma and lymphoma. The most frequent eye cancer in children is retinoblastoma. Cancer can also metastasize to the eye from other parts of the body. According to the American Cancer Society (2019), eye cancer is most common in Whites and has an overall 5-year survival rate of nearly 80%. Clinical manifestations of eye cancer typically include some sort of visual disturbance (e.g., losing part of the visual field, blurry vision, or seeing flashing lights).

Diagnosis and Treatment

Most cases of eye cancer are found during a routine ophthalmic examination (e.g., finding dark spots on the iris). Additional diagnostic procedures may include a history, ultrasound, fluorescein angiography (imaging of blood vessels in the eye using contrast dye), biopsy, and other tests to detect and evaluate metastasis (e.g., CT and magnetic resonance imaging).

Treatment varies depending on the cancer type, location, and size. Surgery is the foundation of most eye cancer treatment. It may entail removal of all (enucleation) or part of the eye (e.g., iridectomy and choroidectomy). Additionally, radiation may be used (e.g., teletherapy and brachytherapy). A prosthetic eye may be used if the entire eye is removed.

Miscellaneous Sensory Organ Conditions

Several sensory organ conditions that do not fall under the previously discussed categories warrant discussion.

Eyes

A few eye conditions that do not fit previously discussed categories can occur. These conditions may be manifestations of other problems or happen alone. Some of these conditions are minor, causing minimal deficits. Other conditions can cause severe visual deficits.

Vision Screening in Children

Early identification of vision disorders in children can lead to an improved outcome for vision development. Several national organizations (e.g., the American Academy of Pediatrics and the U.S. Preventive Services Task Force) recommend vision screening at all child healthcare maintenance visits. The type of screening will vary based on age. As an example, children below 1 year of age will be screened by evaluating eye movement response, an external eye examination, pupillary response, and red reflex evaluation. As children get older (i.e., > 1 year) and depending on the cooperative abilities of the child, instrument-based screening (i.e., photo screening), ophthalmoscopic examination, and use of eye charts (e.g., HOTV chart) can be used. Healthcare visits may decrease as a child gets older because vaccinations are not as frequent, so the American Academy of Pediatrics recommends visual acuity measurement at the ages of 5, 6, 8, 10, 12, and 15 years.

Strabismus

Strabismus, or crossed eyes, is a gaze deviation of the eye (FIGURE 14-20). With strabismus, the eyes do not coordinate or align properly to focus on the same object together in the retina, resulting in diplopia. Strabismus can be due to problems with the eye muscles, abnormalities in innervation of the eye muscles, or in the brain where eye muscle coordination is controlled. This condition most often appears at birth or shortly after (usually by 3 years old). In children, the brain will begin to ignore the input from one of the eyes. If the brain continues to ignore one eye, the eye will never function properly, and permanent visual deficits may result (e.g., amblyopia). A weak or hypertonic eye muscle, a short muscle, or a neurologic deficit can cause strabismus. These defects can be associated with farsightedness, chromosomal defects such as Down syndrome, intrauterine infection exposure (e.g., congenital rubella), eye cancers such as retinoblastoma, and traumatic brain injuries. Adults may develop strabismus from various diseases such as autoimmune hyperthyroidism (i.e., Graves disease), a stroke, or myasthenia gravis. The eye affected, which can be one or both (they can alternate), can deviate in, out, up, or down.

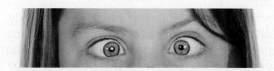

FIGURE 14-20 Strabismus.
© JPRFPhotos/Shutterstock.

Diagnostic procedures for strabismus consist of a history and physical examination, including an ophthalmic examination and a neurologic examination. Treatment focuses on strengthening the weak eye and realigning the eyes. It often involves resting the normally aligned eye to strengthen the misaligned eye. Strategies usually include prism glasses, eye muscle exercises, eye patching, and surgery.

Amblyopia

Amblyopia, or lazy eye, is the loss of one eye's ability to see details (i.e., fine depth perception). It is the most common cause of vision problems in children. Amblyopia occurs when the brain and the eyes do not work together properly; that is, the brain favors one eye. The preferred eye has normal vision, but because the brain ignores the other eye, vision does not develop normally. Usually, visual acuity in children reaches adult levels by age 5. The normal eye attempts to compensate for the affected eye, creating a vicious cycle in which the normal eye becomes stronger and the affected eye becomes weaker. The brain stops growing between 5 and 10 years of age, at which time the condition becomes permanent. Amblyopia can be classified by the underlying cause. Strabismus is the most frequent cause of amblyopia and is therefore called *strabismic amblyopia*. Other causes include a family history, bilateral astigmatism, congenital cataracts (i.e., deprivation amblyopia), farsightedness, and nearsightedness (i.e., refractive amblyopia).

Diagnostic procedures for amblyopia consist of a history and physical examination (including an ophthalmic examination). Much like with strabismus, treatment focuses on strengthening the weak eye and realigning the eyes. It often involves resting the normal eye to strengthen the weaker eye. Strategies usually include wearing prism glasses, eye muscle exercises, eye patching, ophthalmic medication (atropine may be used to dilate the pupil of the normal eye to "chemically patch" it), and surgery.

Retinal Detachment

Retinal detachment is an acute condition that occurs when the retina separates from its supporting structures (i.e., the underlying retinal pigment epithelium and highly vascular choroidal layer). This separation can happen spontaneously or because of severe nearsightedness (myopia), trauma, diabetes mellitus, inflammation, degenerative aging changes, and scar tissue. Retinal detachment occurs when vitreous humor leaks through a retinal tear and accumulates underneath the retina. Leakage can also occur through tiny holes where the retina has thinned due to aging or other retinal disorders. Less commonly, fluid can leak directly underneath the retina without a tear or break (e.g., vitreous traction pulls on the retina). A tear is the most common cause of retinal detachment. As vitreous humor collects underneath the retina, it peels away from the underlying choroid. These detached areas may expand over time, like wallpaper that, once torn, slowly peels off a wall. In turn, the retina becomes ischemic, and photoreceptor degeneration is rapid and progressive, causing vision loss.

Clinical Manifestations

Retinal detachment is typically painless. Clinical manifestations often include flashes of light (i.e., photopsia) in the peripheral visual field, blurred vision, floaters (e.g., looks like a cobweb), and darkening vision (like a curtain drawing across a visual field).

Diagnosis and Treatment

Diagnostic procedures consist of a history and physical examination (including an ophthalmic examination, often performed by an ophthalmologist). The ophthalmic examination may involve an electroretinogram (a record of the electrical currents in the retina produced by visual stimuli), fluorescein angiography, intraocular pressure measurements, ophthalmoscopy, a refraction test, retinal photography, color discrimination, visual acuity testing, slit lamp examination, and eye ultrasound.

Retinal detachment is a medical emergency requiring immediate treatment. Surgery is often the best treatment option. Several surgical options are available. In cryopexy, intense cold is applied to the area with an ice probe to form scar tissue, which holds the retina to the underlying layer. Laser surgery seals the tears or holes in the retina. Pneumatic retinopexy involves placing a gas bubble in the eye to help the retina float back into place. A scleral buckle indents the eye wall, and vitrectomy removes gel or scar tissue pulling on the retina. These procedures may be performed alone or in combination with each other.

Ears

A few ear conditions that do not fit previously discussed categories can occur. These conditions may be manifestations of other problems (e.g., neurologic disorders) or happen alone. Most of these conditions, while mild and causing only minor issues, can be bothersome to patients. Thorough evaluation is necessary to identify disorders that may be caused by life-threatening disorders (e.g., brainstem infarction).

Tinnitus

Tinnitus describes hearing abnormal noises in the ear in the absence of an outside sound source. Multiple theories explain the mechanism of tinnitus. Each of these theories point to a disruption of normal neural firing pathways that can happen anywhere from the cochlea to the auditory cortex. These noises may be described as a ringing, buzzing, humming, whistling, roaring, or blowing. The sound can be heard in one or both ears and can be heard in the head, around the head, or even from a distance. Tinnitus can be intermittent or continuous. Tinnitus is often accompanied by sensorineural hearing loss. Tinnitus is a common problem, affecting approximately 50 million Americans (American Tinnitus Association, 2018). It is not a condition itself, but rather a symptom of an underlying issue. Although tinnitus can be bothersome, it does not usually warrant significant concern. Tinnitus is more common in adults and smokers. There is a higher incidence in men in comparison to women. Tinnitus is associated with over 200 disorders that include presbycusis, exposure to excessive noise, cerumen impaction, otosclerosis, Meniere disease, stress, head injury, acoustic neuroma (a benign tumor on the acoustic nerve), atherosclerosis, hypertension, carotid stenosis, arteriovenous malformation, caffeine, and ototoxic medications (e.g., many antibiotics, aspirin, chemotherapies, and diuretics).

Diagnosis and Treatment

Diagnostic procedures for tinnitus focus on identification of the underlying cause. These procedures may consist of a history, physical examination (including a complete hearing test and otoscopic examination), and additional tests as necessary to identify the cause. Treating the underlying disorder (e.g., removing cerumen and controlling blood pressure) will resolve tinnitus in most cases. If there is no resolution, the goal for most patients will be to lessen perception of tinnitus and improving quality of life. Additional strategies may include the following measures although some, including medications, have variable effectiveness:

- Tricyclic antidepressants to reduce tinnitus symptoms
- Alprazolam (Niravam, Xanax), a benzodiazepine, to reduce tinnitus symptoms
- Acamprosate (Campral), a drug used to treat alcoholism, to relieve tinnitus
- Masking tinnitus symptoms with white noise machines and hearing aids
- Behavioral therapies, including:
  - Tinnitus retraining therapy
  - Biofeedback
  - Stress reduction
  - Cognitive behavioral therapy
- Avoiding factors that can worsen tinnitus (e.g., caffeine, smoking, and ototoxic medications)

Vertigo

Vertigo refers to an illusion of motion. Vertigo is not the same as feeling lightheaded, or as though one might faint (presyncopal episode). In contrast, people experiencing vertigo have a sensation that they or the room are spinning or moving. Two types of vertigo—peripheral and central—are distinguished. Peripheral vertigo occurs when there is a problem with the vestibular labyrinth, semicircular canals, or vestibular nerve. Central vertigo occurs when there is a problem in the brain, particularly in the brainstem or cerebellum. Peripheral vertigo is more common than vertigo from a central nervous system disorder. The three most common causes of peripheral vertigo are **benign paroxysmal positional vertigo** (BPPV), Meniere disease (i.e., endolymph swelling), and vestibular neuritis (i.e., vestibular nerve inflammation usually due to virus). Some other causes can include herpes zoster oticus (i.e., Ramsay Hunt syndrome), medications (e.g., aminoglycosides), acoustic neuroma, and otitis media.

BPPV occurs when the calcium carbonate crystals (otoconia) that are normally in the utricle gel (Figure 14-10) dislodge and travel to the semicircular canals (most common is the posterior canal). The accumulation of this calcium debris (i.e., canalithiasis) causes abnormal movement of the fluid (e.g., the fluid moves when the person does not), and this movement causes a false signal to the brain. The end result is the sensation of vertigo. The vertigo is usually triggered when the patient gets out of bed, bends forward, or bends backwards. Nausea can occur but patients do not usually vomit with BPPV. The sensation of vertigo with BPPV is short lived, usually lasting seconds; however, episodes are recurrent and can last for months.

Diagnosis of BPPV is based on the clinical examination, including a history and physical. The Dix-Hallpike maneuver (**FIGURE 14-21**) confirms the diagnosis. The maneuver encompasses having the patient sit upright and turning the head to one side. The patient is then brought down into a supine position quickly with the head still turned and hanging over the edge of the exam table. The same procedure is done turning the head in the opposite direction. With BPPV, this maneuver may provoke vertigo and nystagmus if there is posterior canal dysfunction. Patients with BPPV do not have ear pain, tinnitus, hearing loss, or any other neurologic symptoms (e.g., headache, abnormal gait, pupillary changes). Presence of these symptoms is suggestive of central vertigo, which requires urgent evaluation.

Vestibular neuritis (i.e., neuronitis) occurs usually due to a viral infection in the inner ear, which affects the vestibular portion of cranial nerve VIII. Vestibular neuritis generally occurs after a viral infection, but bacterial infections can also be a cause. Manifestations

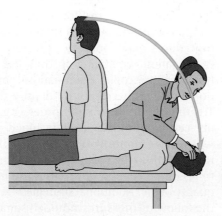
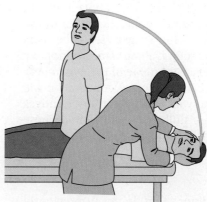
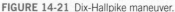

FIGURE 14-21 Dix-Hallpike maneuver.

appear rapidly, are severe, and include vertigo that is persistent. Nausea and vomiting may be present, and while the patient can walk, their gait may be unstable. The symptoms can last a few days. If there is unilateral hearing loss, the patient may have labyrinthitis, which affects both branches of cranial nerve VIII (i.e., vestibulocochlear nerve). Vestibular neuritis and labyrinthitis can occur together. Nystagmus is usually spontaneous. The diagnosis is made based on clinical examination, including a history and physical. Due to the presence of central nervous system features (e.g., gait imbalance) that may be present in cerebellar causes of vertigo, brain imaging should also be obtained.

Central vertigo is not as common as peripheral vertigo and includes central nervous system manifestations (e.g., diplopia, ataxia, and dysarthria) that are not usually present with peripheral vertigo. Some causes of central vertigo include migraines, multiple sclerosis, seizures, brainstem ischemia, and cerebellar infarction and hemorrhage. Some of these disorders are discussed in more detail chapter 11.

Peripheral vertigo treatment is based on the underlying cause. For BPPV and vestibular neuritis, pharmacology is the mainstay of treatment. The medications used for this purpose include anticholinergic agents, antihistamines (especially meclizine [Antivert]), benzodiazepines, and antiemetics.

Corticosteroids may also be given for vestibular neuritis. Particle repositioning maneuvers, which are similar to the Dix-Hallpike maneuver, can be a treatment for BPPV. The maneuvers are done in an attempt to move the debris so that it will move from the canals. These maneuvers can be taught to patients, so they can do them at home. Safety precautions should also be taken to prevent injury from falls (e.g., changing positions slowly and mobility assistance).

Learning Points

Peripheral and Central Nystagmus

Nystagmus is a repetitive, rhythmic, involuntary back-and-forth movement of the eyes. Central vertigo is associated with nystagmus that involves the eyes moving equally in both directions (like a pendulum). Nystagmus from central disorders tends to be relatively constant, and the movement can occur in all types of directions (horizontal, vertical, or rotational) and can change direction. The nystagmus continues even when the eyes fixate on an object. Body movement does not trigger the nystagmus, and the nystagmus occurs independently from the vertigo. Peripheral vertigo is associated with episodic nystagmus that at first is slow in one direction, and then the eyes try to correct with a quick jerking movement back to the other direction. Peripheral nystagmus, however, is usually unidirectional. The movement also tends to be horizontal or rotational. The nystagmus stops when the eyes fixate on an object, and the nystagmus will usually accompany the vertigo if it is due to peripheral vertigo.

CHAPTER SUMMARY

The sensory organs work together to sense changes in the body's internal and external environment. This information is then relayed to the nervous system for interpretation and response. Disorders of these organs can significantly affect the body's sensory function and can even be life altering. Some of these conditions can be prevented by restricting noise exposure (e.g., wearing protective ear coverings and minimizing music volume) and shielding the eyes (e.g., by wearing protective eye goggles and ultraviolet-protective sunglasses). Early diagnosis and treatment of other conditions can improve prognosis.

REFERENCES AND RESOURCES

AAOS. (2004). *Paramedic: Anatomy and physiology.* Sudbury, MA: Jones and Bartlett Publishers.

American Cancer Society. (2019). Eye cancer. Retrieved from http://www.cancer.org/cancer/eyecancer/

American Tinnitus Association. (2018). Demographics. Retrieved from https://www.ata.org/understanding-facts/demographics

Chang, C. (2012). Cholesteatoma. In A. K. Lalwani (Ed.), *CURRENT Diagnosis & treatment in otolaryngology—Head & neck surgery* (3rd ed.). New York, NY: McGraw-Hill. Retrieved from http://accessmedicine.mhmedical.com.ezproxy.fiu.edu/content.aspx?bookid=386&sectionid=39944092

Chew, E., Clemons, T., Agron, E., Sperduto, R., Sangiovanni, J., Kurinij, N., & Davis, M. (2013). Long-term effects of vitamins C and E, beta-carotene, and zinc on age-related macular degeneration: AREDS report no. 35. *Ophthalmology, 120,* 1604–1611.

Chiras, D. (2015). *Human biology* (8th ed.). Burlington, MA: Jones & Bartlett Publishers.

Domingo, E., & Zabbo, C. P. (2018). Corneal abrasion [updated October 27, 2018]. In *StatPearls* [Internet]. Treasure Island, FL: StatPearls Publishing. Retrieved from https://www.ncbi.nlm.nih.gov/books/NBK532960/

Driscoll, C. W., & Carlson, M. L. (2012). Otosclerosis. In A. K. Lalwani (Ed.), *CURRENT diagnosis & treatment in otolaryngology—Head & neck surgery* (3rd ed.). New York, NY: McGraw-Hill. Retrieved from http://accessmedicine.mhmedical.com.ezproxy.fiu.edu/content.aspx?bookid=386&sectionid=39944093

Elling, B., Elling, K., & Rothenberg, M. (2004). *Anatomy and physiology*. Sudbury, MA: Jones and Bartlett Publishers.

Furman, J. M., & Barton, J. J. S. (2015). Evaluation of the patient with vertigo. In J. L. Wilterdink (Ed.), *Uptodate*. Retrieved from https://www.uptodate.com/contents/evaluation-of-the-patient-with-vertigo

Gould, B. (2015). *Pathophysiology for the health professions* (5th ed.). Philadelphia, PA: Elsevier.

Jacobs, D. S. (2017). Corneal abrasions and corneal foreign bodies: Management. In J. F. Wiley (Ed.), *Uptodate*. Retrieved from https://www.uptodate.com/contents/corneal-abrasions-and-corneal-foreign-bodies-management?source=history_widget

Jacobs, D. S. (2018). Corneal abrasions and corneal foreign bodies: Clinical manifestations and diagnosis. In J. F. Wiley (Ed.), *Uptodate*. Retrieved from https://www.uptodate.com/contents/corneal-abrasions-and-corneal-foreign-bodies-clinical-manifestations-and-diagnosis?source=history_widget

Marchand, S. (2019). Basic anatomy and physiology of pain mechanisms. In R. Mitra (Ed.), *Principles of rehabilitation medicine*. New York, NY: McGraw-Hill. Retrieved from http://accessmedicine.mhmedical.com.ezproxy.fiu.edu/content.aspx?bookid=2550&sectionid=206762272

Marom, T., Tan, A., Wilkinson, G. S., Pierson, K. S., Freeman, J. L., & Chonmaitree, T. (2014). Trends in otitis media-related health care use in the United States, 2001–2011. *JAMA Pediatrics, 168*(1), 68–75. doi: 10.1001/jamapediatrics.2013.3924

Moayedi, M., & Davis, D. (2013). Theories of pain: From specificity to gate control. *Journal of Neurophysiology, 109*(1), 55–12.

Pflipsen, M., Massaquoi, M., & Wolf, S. (2016). Evaluation of the painful eye. *American Family Physician, 93*(12), 991–998.

Professional guide to pathophysiology (3rd ed.). (2010). Philadelphia, PA: Lippincott Williams & Wilkins.

Riordan-Eva, P. (2019). Disorders of the eyes & lids. In M. A. Papadakis, S. J. McPhee, & M. W. Rabow (Eds.), *Current medical diagnosis & treatment 2019*. New York, NY: McGraw-Hill. Retrieved from http://accessmedicine.mhmedical.com.ezproxy.fiu.edu/content.aspx?bookid=2449&sectionid=194433247

World Health Organization (WHO). (2019). Trachoma. Retrieved from https://www.who.int/blindness/causes/trachoma/en/

Glossary

α_2 **CS$_2$** A common form of sickle cell disease, with hemoglobin SC.

α_2 β**S$_2$** A common and severe form of sickle cell disease, with hemoglobin SS.

abdominal and pelvis The test of choice for nephrolithiasis (noncontrast low dose).

acquired type von Willebrand disease Type of von Willebrand disease that occurs in persons with Wilms tumor, congenital heart disease, systemic lupus erythematosus, and hypothyroidism.

acromegaly Increase in bone size caused by excessive growth hormone levels in adulthood.

actinic keratosis A skin lesion that is benign and is a result of proliferation of epidermal keratinocytes. Also called solar keratosis.

active transport The movement of a substance from an area of lower concentration to an area of higher concentration, against a concentration gradient.

acute cholangitis Stasis and infection in the biliary tract resulting from gallstones.

acute cholecystitis Gallbladder inflammation as a result of cystic duct obstruction.

acute closed-angle glaucoma A medical emergency caused by rapid increase in intraocular pressure.

acute gastritis Type of gastritis that usually develops suddenly and is likely to be accompanied by nausea and epigastric pain. It can be a mild, transient irritation, or it can be a severe ulceration with hemorrhage.

acute postinfectious glomerulonephritis Type of glomerulonephritis that usually occurs after an infection with group A beta-hemolytic streptococci.

acute retroviral syndrome Stage of HIV infection with the following clinical manifestations: high viral load (e.g., > 1 million copies), decreased CD4+, and a high transmission potential.

acute tubular injury See acute tubular necrosis.

acute tubular necrosis A common cause of intrarenal acute kidney injury. It is most common caused by ischemia due to decreased renal perfusion.

adenosine diphosphate One of the substances the body uses to activate platelets; it leads to aggregation (clustering).

adhesive capsulitis Shoulder disorder caused by an idiopathic loss of active and passive range of motion. Also called frozen shoulder.

AIDS A deadly, sexually transmitted disease caused by the human immunodeficiency virus (HIV), a retrovirus.

albinism A recessive condition that results in little or no melanin production.

allergic conjunctivitis Eye irritation caused by allergies involving excessive tearing and accompanied by redness, itching, and grittiness.

alopecia areata An autoimmune T cell mediated disorder of the hair follicle in genetically susceptible individuals. In some patients it can cause total loss of hair (scalp and body).

ammonia A metabolic waste managed by the kidneys. This highly toxic product results from the breakdown of amino acids in the liver.

amygdala Portion of the limbic system often referred to as the aggression center as stimulation can lead to anger, violence, fear, and anxiety.

anaphylactic shock Type of distributive shock that is a consequence of an allergic reaction. The allergic reaction leads to a cascade of events similar to that of septic shock, except the mediators differ. Additionally, bronchospasms and laryngeal edema that can impair the patient's respiratory status occur.

aneuploidy An abnormal separation during cell division leading to too many or too few chromosomes.

angiogenesis New blood vessels to meet the needs of a growing tumor.

ankylosing spondylitis A progressive inflammatory disorder affecting the sacroiliac joints, intervertebral spaces, and costovertebral joints.

ankylosis Joint fixation and deformity.

anti–glomerular basement membrane (anti-GBM) glomerulonephritis A type of immune response (type II hypersensitivity) that often results in rapid and progressive renal failure.

anxiety disorders Mental health disorders characterized by fear, which is the emotional response to a real or perceived imminent threat, and anxiety, which is anticipation of future threat. Fear often triggers an autonomic response (i.e., fight or flight) and escape behaviors, while anxiety is associated with muscle tension, vigilance, and avoidance behaviors.

aspiration pneumonia Type of pneumonia that frequently occurs when the gag reflex is impaired because of a brain injury or anesthesia. It can also occur because of impaired lower esophageal sphincter closure secondary to nasogastric tube placement or disease (e.g., gastroesophageal reflux disease).

asymptomatic bacteriuria Condition when urine contains bacteria (i.e., $\geq 10^5$ colony-forming units/mL), with or without pyuria and without symptoms of a UTI.

atypical pneumonia Type of pneumonia caused by organisms such as *Mycoplasma pneumoniae*, *Chlamydia pneumoniae*, and *Legionella* species. pneumonia from these pathogens may not respond to usual antibiotics, and symptoms and X-ray findings may be slightly different than pneumonia from typical pathogens.

autonomic dysreflexia Loss of coordinated heart rate and vascular response to various stimuli secondary to a previous spinal cord injury.

bacterial conjunctivitis Eye infection caused by bacteria.

basal cell carcinoma The most common type of skin cancer, it develops from abnormal growth of the cells in the lowest layer of the epidermis. It has a low metastatic potential, but it can cause significant local tissue destruction and ulceration.

base pair Nitrogen bases (steps) of the nucleotide are either purine (adenine and guanine) or pyrimidine (thymine and cytosine).

benign paroxysmal positional vertigo Condition that occurs when the calcium carbonate crystals (otoconia) that are normally in the utricle gel dislodge and travel to the semicircular canals. This causes abnormal movement of the fluid, and this movement sends a false signal to the brain, resulting in the sensation of vertigo.

bipolar I Subtype of bipolar disorder in which manic symptoms last at least 1 week and are present most of the day, nearly every day.

bipolar II Subtype of bipolar disorder characterized by hypomania.

blepharitis An inflammation of the eyelid margin caused by infection.

BUN Blood urea nitrogen; an indication of liver and kidney function.

café au lait macules Common type of birthmark that is the color of coffee with milk.

calcium The most abundant mineral in the body. It is necessary for bone and teeth formation, muscle contractility, coagulation, and other body processes.

carbuncles Clusters of boils.

cardiogenic shock Type of shock in which the left ventricle cannot maintain adequate cardiac output. Compensatory mechanisms of heart failure are triggered; however, these mechanisms increase cardiac workload and oxygen consumption, resulting in decreased contractility. Consequently, tissue and organ perfusion decrease, leading to multisystem organ failure.

cardiomyopathy Disease related to the heart muscle that reduces cardiac function.

carpal tunnel syndrome A common disorder that results from compression of the median nerve as it travels into a space known as the carpal tunnel of the wrist.

CD4+ helper T cells Cells of the immune system that are targeted by the HIV virus.

cellulitis An infection deep in the dermis and subcutaneous tissue. It usually results from a direct invasion through a breach in the skin, especially those breaches where contamination is likely.

chalazion A localized eyelid swelling caused by glandular obstruction.

chemical burns Burns that can be due to acidic substances (e.g., acetic acid present in hair wave neutralizer, hydrochloric acid in pool cleaner, and grout cleaner) and alkalotic substances (e.g., ammonia hydroxide in fertilizers, hair dyes, and sodium hypochlorite in bleach). The degree of burn is dependent on the duration of the exposure and the type of chemical.

chemokine receptor (CCR5) A coreceptor that allows the HIV virus to attack macrophages.

choledocholithiasis Gallstones present in the common bile duct.

chondrocytes Cartilage cells.

chondrogenic tumors Cartilage-producing tumors.

chromatid Each of the separate identical copies created when the chromosome replicates; they attach to each other through a centromere.

chromatin DNA that is combined and wrapped around the histone proteins.

chromosomal mosaicism When aneuploidy only occurs in some of the body cells of the offspring, but others are normal. It can occur in many disorders such as Turner, Klinefelter, and Down syndromes.

chromosome A nucleotide in DNA.

chronic gastritis Type of gastritis that develops gradually and is likely to be accompanied by a dull epigastric pain and a sensation of fullness after minimal intake. It can be asymptomatic.

chronic glomerulonephritis Condition that is a result of progressive types of glomerulonephritis that usually lead to chronic kidney disease.

chronic venous insufficiency A venous disorder caused by venous pressure that is prolonged and persistent. The increased venous pressure causes the capillary pressure to increase, causing fluid and pigment to leak out, leading to edema and skin discoloration.

chylothorax An accumulation of a milky white fluid composed of fat droplets and lymph.

clinical latency or chronic HIV infection stage The stage if HIV infection that occurs after the brief early infection episode, in which the individual may remain asymptomatic for months to years and the virus continues replicating, but not as fast as during the acute phase.

collagen tumors Tumors that are a mix of fibrous connective tissue.

community-acquired pneumonia Pneumonia that is acquired outside the hospital or healthcare setting.

compensatory Stage of shock in which bodily responses become activated when arterial pressure and tissue perfusion decrease. It represents an effort to maintain cardiac and cerebral function.

coxsackievirus Type of enterovirus implicated in two conditions known as herpangina and hand-foot-and-mouth disease.

creatinine Blood levels of this substance are an indication of renal function because it is entirely excreted by the kidneys.

CXCR4 The virus GP120 must attach to this receptor in order to attach to the T cells.

cyclothymic disorder A disorder with distinct periods of hypomanic symptoms and depressive symptoms that are chronic and fluctuating over a period of 2 years for adults and 1 year for children and adolescents.

cytotoxic edema Brain tissue membrane alterations that cause water accumulation.

de Quervain tendinopathy A common cause of wrist pain involving wrist tendons on the radial side. The injury is thought to occur because of overuse.

delusional disorder A disorder in which the patient has delusions but the criteria for schizophrenia are not met.

diabetes insipidus Excessive fluid excretion in the kidneys caused by deficient antidiuretic hormone levels.

diabetic ketoacidosis A pH imbalance characterized by increased ketones in the urine caused by insufficient insulin; if cells are starved for energy, the body may begin to break down fat-producing toxic acids (ketones).

diffuse Lesions that involve all or most ($> 50\%$) of the glomeruli.

diffusion The movement of solutes (particles dissolved in a solvent) from an area of higher concentration to lower concentration.

dilated cardiomyopathy Type of cardiomyopathy that affects systolic function. It is the most common type of cardiomyopathy.

distal convoluted tubule The tubule of the kidney responsible for reabsorption of sodium, water, and bicarbonate, and secretion of hydrogen, potassium, urea, ammonia, and certain drugs.

distributive shock Type of shock in which vasodilation causes hypovolemia.

DNA Deoxyribonucleic acid.

DNA methylation Addition of a methyl group to DNA cytosine, which causes a gene to become inactive or silent, leading to inhibition of transcription.

Doppler ultrasound Type of ultrasound that can be used to provide hemodynamic data of the velocity and direction of blood flow through the valves, pulmonary artery, and veins.

duodenal ulcers Type of ulcer that is commonly associated with excessive acid or *H. pylori* infections.

Dupuytren contracture A thickening and contracture of the palmar fascia as a result of fibroblast proliferation and abnormal collagen deposition.

dwarfism Short stature caused by deficient levels of growth hormone, somatotropin, or somatotropin-releasing hormone.

echocardiograms A noninvasive test frequently used to evaluate the structure and function of the heart. It produces images and recordings through ultrasound (high-frequency sound waves).

eclampsia An acute and life-threatening complication of pregnancy, characterized by tonic–clonic seizures, usually occurring in a patient who had developed preeclampsia.

ecthyma An ulcerative type of impetigo, in which the ulceration can extend deep into the dermis.

ectropion In blepharitis, when the eyelids turn toward the outside of the eye.

embolic strokes Type of stroke that is a result of arterial occlusion, but the source of the thrombus is from particles of debris that have originated outside the brain. The obstruction can be due to clots but also other debris (e.g., fat, air, or foreign body).

empyema Grossly purulent effusions in the plural space.

endocytosis The act of bringing a substance into a cell.

endothelin Under the influence of this substance, the blood vessel quickly vasoconstricts reflexively when a vessel is injured.

entropion In blepharitis, when the eyelids turn toward the inside of the eye.

epicondylitis A tendinopathy of the tendon just distal and anterior to the epicondyle. The tendinopathy can occur laterally, causing lateral epicondylitis (i.e., tennis elbow) or medially, causing medial epicondylitis (i.e., golfer's elbow).

epigenetic Determinant of gene expression (how the genes are read). These changes can determine whether a gene is on or off.

Epstein-Barr virus This virus is the most common cause of infectious mononucleosis. Also known as human herpesvirus 4.

erythropoietin Hormone produced by the kidney that promotes the formation of red blood cells in the bone marrow.

exhale To breathe out.

exocytosis The release of materials from a cell, usually with the assistance of a vesicle.

exudative effusions Fluid accumulations that occur when there is a localized lung or pleural alteration such as inflammation or decreased lymphatic drainage.

facilitated diffusion The movement of substances from an area of lower concentration to an area of higher concentration with the assistance of a carrier molecule.

fibrin An insoluble protein that strengthens the platelet plug. It is derived from fibrinogen.

fibrinogen Released by platelets along with calcium, this substance is necessary for secondary hemostasis.

fibromyalgia A syndrome predominately characterized by widespread muscular pain and fatigue. Fibromyalgia affects muscles, tendons, and surrounding tissue, but not the joints.

focal Lesions that involve some ($< 50\%$) of the glomeruli.

focal segmental glomerulosclerosis A histological description for sclerotic lesions that occur in parts of the glomeruli (segmental) and some of the glomeruli (focal).

folic acid While the red blood cell is developing, this substance and vitamin B_{12} are necessary in addition to EPO. They are necessary for cellular DNA synthesis.

folliculitis Infections involving the hair follicles. Folliculitis is characterized by tender, swollen areas that form around hair follicles, often on the neck, breasts, buttocks, and face.

forebrain The structural region that comprises the cerebrum, which controls the higher thought processes, and diencephalon.

functional Type of incontinence that occurs in many older adults, especially people in nursing homes, in which a physical or mental impairment prevents them from making it to the toilet in time.

furuncles Infections that begin in the hair follicles and then spread into the surrounding dermis. The lesions start as firm, red, painful nodules that develop into large, painful masses, which frequently drain large amounts of purulent exudate. Also called boils.

fusion The second part of the life cycle: the joining of the virus protein (glycoprotein 41) and the CD4+ membrane, which then allows entry.

gastric atrophy The final phase of chronic gastritis, during which glandular structures are lost.

gastroenteritis Inflammation of the stomach and intestines, usually because of an infection or allergic reaction.

genes Segments of deoxyribonucleic acid (DNA) that serve as a template of protein synthesis.

genetic Traits passed to offspring via chromosomes, or genes.

genome The complete set of DNA and genes (i.e., genetic instructions).

genotype Transmitted genetic information that forms the blueprint of a person.

gestational hypertension Onset of hypertension at 20 weeks or more of gestation with resolution 12 weeks after birth.

gigantism Tall stature caused by excessive growth hormone levels prior to puberty.

global When a whole glomerulus is affected.

glomerular filtration rate (GFR) The best measure of renal functioning; it measures the speed at which blood moves through the glomerulus. It can be calculated using a formula that incorporates serum creatinine levels, age, gender, and ethnicity. Usually it is approximately 125 mL/min.

glycoprotein 120 (GP-120) Substance on the outer surface of the HIV virus that binds to the CD4+ on dendritic cells (an antigen-presenting cell located on skin and mucosal tissue).

Goodpasture disease See anti–glomerular basement membrane (anti-GBM) glomerulonephritis.

Goodpasture syndrome See anti–glomerular basement membrane (anti-GBM) glomerulonephritis.

gout An inflammatory disease resulting from deposits of uric acid crystals in tissues and fluids within the body.

gross total incontinence A continuous leaking of urine, day and night, or the periodic uncontrollable leaking of large volumes of urine. In these cases, the bladder has no storage capacity.

heart failure A condition in which the heart is unable to pump an adequate amount of blood to meet metabolic needs. This pump inadequacy leads to decreased cardiac output, increased preload, and increased afterload. These three events result in decreased contractility and stroke volume. Often referred to as congestive heart failure.

hemangiomas Vascular birthmarks that appears as a bright red patch or a nodule of extra blood vessels in the skin. Also called a strawberry.

hemothorax Blood in the pleural space (usually due to trauma).

hepatic encephalopathy A buildup of ammonia caused by liver dysfunction that produces neurologic impairment.

hepatopulmonary syndrome Condition caused by liver damage that alters the pulmonary vasculature, resulting in hypoxemia.

hepatorenal syndrome Condition involving kidney function decline as a result of splanchnic artery vasodilation and other poorly understood changes in renal arterial circulation.

herniated intervertebral disk A state in which the nucleus pulposus protrudes through the annulus fibrosus. Also called slipped disk and ruptured disk.

herpes simplex 1 (HSV-1) A viral infection typically affecting the lips, mouth, and face. This common infection usually begins in childhood. Also called cold sore.

herpes zoster A viral infection caused by the varicella-zoster virus. The condition appears in adulthood years after a primary infection of varicella (chickenpox) in childhood. The virus lies dormant on a cranial nerve or a spinal nerve dermatome until it becomes activated years later; it affects this nerve only. Also called shingles.

hindbrain The structural region that comprises the cerebellum and pons.

hippocampus Portion of the brain that helps in the formation of new memories and is involved in short-term memories becoming long-term memory. Damage to this structure can lead to difficulties forming new memories.

histones Proteins that basically are the spools that DNA wraps itself around.

hordeolum An acute infection of the eyelid that presents as an abscess and nodule. Also called a stye.

hospital-acquired pneumonia Pneumonia that is acquired in a healthcare setting.

hypercalcemia Condition in which ionizing calcium levels climb above 5 mEq/L. It results from excessive intake of ionizing calcium or release of ionizing calcium from the bone as well as inadequate excretion.

hyperchloremia An excess amount of chloride in the blood (more than 108 mEq/L). It is usually a result of an underlying condition and without its own clinical manifestations.

hyperglycemia An excess amount of glucose in the blood (more than 180 mg/dL). It can be a result of an underlying condition (e.g., diabetes mellitus) or use of medications (e.g., corticosteroid agents).

hyperkalemia Serum potassium level greater than 5 mEq/L. It is unusual in the healthy individual and may be a medical emergency.

hypermagnesemia Condition in which magnesium levels increase to more than 2.5 mEq/L. This rare electrolyte imbalance usually results from renal failure or excessive laxative or antacid use.

hypernatremia Condition that results from high serum sodium levels (more than 145 mEq/L). The excessive sodium levels generally lead to high serum osmolality (more than 295 mOsm/kg) because of the imbalance between sodium and water.

hyperosmolar hyperglycemic nonketotic state Dangerous complication of type 2 diabetes caused by extremely high blood glucose levels.

hyperphosphatemia Condition in which phosphorus levels climb above 4.5 mg/dL.

hypertensive emergency Blood pressure systolic $\geq$ 180 and/or diastolic >120 mmHg but the patient is symptomatic and/or with evidence of acute/ongoing target organ damage.

hypertensive urgency Blood pressure systolic $\geq$ 180 and/or diastolic >120 mmHg in a patient who is relatively asymptomatic (e.g., mild headache) and there is no evidence of acute target end-organ damage (e.g., ischemia).

hypertonic solutions Intravascular solutions that have a higher concentration of solutes than those in the intravascular compartment. They cause fluid to shift from the intracellular space to the intravascular space.

hypertrophic cardiomyopathy Type of cardiomyopathy that mainly affects diastolic function.

hyphema A pooling of blood in the anterior chamber of the eye.

hypocalcemia Condition in which ionized calcium levels fall below 4 mEq/L. It occurs from increased losses or decreased intake of ionized calcium.

hypochloremia Condition in which chloride levels fall below 98 mEq/L. It rarely occurs in the absence of other electrolyte abnormalities and, therefore, does not have its own set of clinical manifestations.

hypoglycemia A low serum glucose level.

hypokalemia Condition in which potassium levels drop below 3.5 mEq/L. Usually, it results from excessive loss, inadequate intake, or increased potassium cellular uptake.

hypomagnesemia Condition in which magnesium levels drop below 1.8 mEq/L.

hypomanic A manic episode with a duration of symptoms of 4 consecutive days.

hyponatremia Condition that results from low serum sodium levels (less than 135 mEq/L). Serum osmolality levels also fall below 275 mOsm.

hypophosphatemia Condition in which phosphorus levels drop below 2.5 mg/dL.

hypotonic solutions An intravascular solution that has a lower concentration of solutes than that found in the intravascular compartment. Administration of these solutions causes fluid to shift from the intravascular space to the intracellular space.

IgA nephropathy A common cause of primary glomerulonephritis in adolescents and young adults. IgA immune complexes are deposited in the mesangium.

IgA vasculitis A systemic immune condition that affects mainly small vessels throughout the body. The vessels affected are usually in the skin and cause palpable purpura (i.e., Henoch-Schönlein purpura).

impetigo (nonbullous and bullous) A common and highly contagious skin infection. Although it can occur without an apparent break, it typically arises from a breach in the skin. It spreads easily to others by direct contact with skin or contaminated objects. Lesions usually begin as a small vesicle that enlarges and ruptures, forming the characteristic honey-colored crust.

inactivated Vaccines that are made from whole or fractions of viruses or bacterial antigens or the toxin produced by the bacteria.

incomplete penetrance Term that describes autosomal dominant disorders and, less commonly, autosomal recessive disorders that have a genotype, but the features (phenotype) of the disorder may never develop.

inhale To breathe in.

initiation Exposure of a normal cell to an environmental substance or event (e.g., chemicals, viruses, or radiation) that causes DNA damage or mutation.

integrase A viral enzyme that allows the viral DNA to become integrated into the CD4+ cell's own DNA.

intervertebral disk issues Conditions that often occur due to improper body mechanics, lifting heavy objects, repetitive use, or trauma (e.g., a fall or a blow to the back). Additional contributing factors include vertebral stress secondary to obesity, degenerative changes secondary to aging, and demineralization secondary to metabolic conditions (e.g., osteoporosis).

intravenous pyelogram Type of urinary imaging that is infrequently used due to the need to administer intravenous contrast and high-radiation exposure.

irreversible The final stage of shock that features end-organ damage, leading to respiratory and cardiac failure.

ischemic heart disease Problems caused by narrowed heart arteries, which result in decreased blood flow to the heart muscle.

isotonic solutions Intravascular solutions that have concentrations of solutes equal to those in the intravascular compartment. Because of these solute concentrations, these solutions allow fluid to move equally between compartments.

karyotype A representation of a person's individual set of chromosomes.

key vascular change

kyphosis An increase in the curvature of the thoracic spine outward. Also called hunchback.

lacunar strokes Small-vessel strokes. They are a cause of 25% of ischemic strokes.

Legionnaires' disease A specific type of pneumonia that is caused by *Legionella pneumophila*. The bacteria thrive in warm, moist environments, particularly air-conditioning systems and spas. It is not contagious. Most people acquire this type of pneumonia from inhaling the bacteria as they are spread by an air-conditioning system or spa.

lipoedema A type of edema caused by excess deposition of fat cells in an irregular and disproportional manner. It occurs mostly in women, and is usually in the legs, thighs, and buttocks. Eventually, it can cause venous and lymphatic problems.

live, attenuated Vaccines created from weakened wild viruses or bacteria that can replicate without causing diseases. They create an almost identical immune response as active infection.

loop of Henle Looped tubule responsible for secreting urea from the blood into the filtrate and reabsorbing water and sodium from the filtrate back into the blood.

lordosis An exaggerated concave of the lumbar spine. Also called swayback.

lymphedema Swelling, usually in the arms and legs, because of lymph obstruction. It can occur on its own or as a result of another disease or condition.

macular stains The most common type of vascular birthmarks. These faint red marks often occur on the forehead, eyelids, posterior neck, nose, upper lip, or posterior head. Also called salmon patch, angel kiss, and stork bite.

Meckel diverticulum A common congenital malformation of the GI tract that results in herniation of all layers of the small bowel wall, not just the mucosa as in diverticular disease.

melanoma Type of skin cancer that develops in the melanocytes. It is the least common but most serious type due to metastasis. There are several subtypes, and the lesions have a varied presentation.

membranous nephropathy A cause of primary nephrotic syndrome that reflects histologic changes that occur in the basement membrane, which becomes thickened.

meralgia paresthetica Lateral femoral cutaneous nerve entrapment that is a result of compression of the nerve that supplies sensation to the upper, outer thigh.

metastasis The spreading of cancer within the body.

microRNA Noncoding proteins whose function is decreasing mRNA translation or stability, essentially functioning as regulators. There are many types; some have an oncogenic effect, leading to cancer.

microvascular angina Type of angina caused by dysfunction in the coronary microvasculature (i.e., prearterioles and arterioles). Patients are usually younger and more often women in comparison to patients with angina from coronary artery disease.

midbrain The smallest region of the brain, which acts as a sort of relay station for auditory and visual information. It controls the visual and auditory systems as well as eye movement.

Middle East respiratory syndrome An emerging illness caused by a coronavirus family. It is currently isolated to four countries in the Arabian Peninsula.

minimal change disease Type of primary nephrotic syndrome in children, with podocyte loss and minor changes on renal biopsy. Renal function may be normal or impaired due to intravascular volume depletion, and complement levels are normal.

mixed Type of incontinence in which symptoms of more than one type of urinary incontinence are experienced.

MOGE(S) One example of a cardiomyopathy classification incorporating genetic information. It includes morphofunctional phenotype, organ involvement, genetic or family inheritance pattern, etiologic description, and functional status.

mole A brown nevus. They can be tan, brown, or black; can be flat or raised; and may have hair growth.

molluscum contagiosum Dome-shaped white papule that is shiny, firm, and has a craterlike center. It is caused by a poxvirus. It is common in children and is spread by direct skin contact.

Mongolian spots Birthmarks that are a flat, bluish-gray area often found on the lower back or buttocks. These birthmarks are most common on individuals with darker complexions.

multipotent Type of stem cell that can only make cells from their same germ layer.

muscular dystrophy A group of inherited disorders characterized by degeneration of skeletal muscle. Muscles become weaker as damage worsens. There are nine different forms.

myelogenic tumors Tumors that originate in bone marrow cells. They include giant cell tumors and multiple myeloma.

myxedema Advanced hypothyroidism. This condition is rare, but when it occurs, it can be life threatening.

Clinical manifestations include marked hypotension, respiratory depression, hypothermia, lethargy, and coma.

necrotizing Refers to cellular death.

necrotizing fasciitis A rare, serious infection that can aggressively destroy skin, fat, muscle, and other tissue. One out of four people with this infection will die because of it. Also called flesh-eating bacteria.

neurogenic shock Type of distributive shock in which a loss of sympathetic tone in vascular smooth muscle and autonomic function lead to massive vasodilation. Blood pools in the venous system, leading to decreased venous return, cardiac output, and hypotension.

neurogenic shock Type of distributive shock in which a loss of sympathetic tone in vascular smooth muscle and autonomic function lead to massive vasodilation. Blood pools in the venous system, leading to decreased venous return, cardiac output, and hypotension.

nitric oxide Under normal circumstances, this substance and prostacyclin block platelets from adhering to the cell membrane; it is also secreted by the endothelial cells.

nucleotide A double helix strand (it looks like a twisted rope ladder) made of a sugar molecule and phosphate (forms the ladder sides) attached to a nitrogen containing base (forms the ladder steps).

Osgood-Schlatter disease An osteochondritis of the tibial tubercle that occurs in adolescents who have undergone a rapid growth spurt. In this disorder, there is a tendinitis of the patellar tendon and avascular necrosis (osteochondrosis) of the tibial tubercle.

osmosis The movement of water or another solvent across the cellular membrane from an area of low solute concentration to an area of high solute concentration.

osteoarthritis A localized joint disease characterized by deterioration of articulating cartilage and its underlying bone as well as bony overgrowth. The surface of the cartilage becomes rough and worn, interfering with joint movement. Also called wear-and-tear arthritis and degenerative joint disease.

osteogenic tumors Tumors that are a mix of osteoid and sarcoma tissue. An osteosarcoma is an aggressive tumor that begins in the bone cells, usually in the femur, tibia, or humerus.

osteoid The nonmineral bone matrix made up of collagen and ground substance.

osteomalacia A softening and weakening of bones in adults, usually because of an extreme and prolonged vitamin D, calcium, or phosphate deficiency.

osteopenia Bone mass that is less than expected for age, ethnicity, or gender.

osteoporosis A condition characterized by a progressive loss of bone calcium that leaves the bones brittle.

osteoprotegerin A glycoprotein that is a key mediator of osteoblast and osteoclast activity. It is produced by osteoclasts and osteoblasts, and it inhibits osteoclastic formation.

otitis media with effusion An infection or inflammation of the middle ear. It is a common condition in young children.

overflow Incontinence as a result of an inability to empty the bladder.

Paget disease A progressive condition characterized by abnormal bone destruction and remodelling, which results in bone deformities.

pain threshold The perception of pain.

pain tolerance The amount of pain that an individual can physically and emotionally withstand.

pediculosis A lice infestation that can take three forms—*Pediculus humanus corpus* (body louse), *Pediculus pubic* (pubic louse), and *Pediculus humanus capitis* (head louse). Lice are small, brown, parasitic insects that feed off human blood and cannot survive for long without the human host.

penumbra The tissue that surrounds the infarcted core tissue following an ischemic stroke. This tissue can possibly be saved.

persistent depressive disorder This disorder's manifestations are similar to those of major depressive disorder, although they are not as numerous; symptoms must be present most of the day or for most days for at least 2 years. Also called dysthymia or chronic unipolar major depression.

Peyer patches Areas of immune cells such as lymphocytes, plasma cells, and macrophages that are located beneath the villus in lymph nodules.

phenotype The outward, physical expression of genes, such as eye color.

pityriasis rosea A disorder that begins with a lesion termed the *herald patch* that is solitary, salmon-colored, fine, scaly, and clearly demarcated. It is though to be caused by a virus.

pluripotent Type of stem cell that can develop into any kind of cell and ultimately will develop into the over 200 specialized cells (e.g., cardiac cells, nerve cells) of the adult human.

polyploidy When there is more than the normal (euploid) number of pairs of chromosomes in a cell.

port-wine stains Vascular birthmarks that look like wine was spilled on an area of the body. These birthmarks most often occur on the face, neck, arms, and legs.

portopulmonary hypertension Increase in vessel pressures in the hepatic artery and the portal vein. This increased pressure is often associated with liver disease.

preeclampsia Condition in which proteinuria is present with gestational hypertension.

premenstrual dysphoric disorder A severe form of premenstrual syndrome that is characterized by severe depression, tension, and irritability.

primary amenorrhea Lack of menstruation caused by genetic or anatomic abnormalities; the mechanism involves the hypothalamus, pituitary gland, ovaries, or other parts of the genital tract.

Prinzmetal angina A type of angina that occurs due to vasospasm in the coronary arteries without atherosclerosis. The incidence is rare, and patients are likely to be younger (i.e., < 50 years).

procedural sedation and anesthesia Technique in which sedation is administered in conjunction with analgesics, allowing the patient to undergo a painful procedure.

progressive State of shock that begins when the compensatory mechanisms fail to maintain cardiac output.

Tissues become hypoxic, cells switch to anaerobic metabolism, lactic acid builds up, and metabolic acidosis develops.

proliferative An increase in glomerular cells (e.g., mesangial, endothelial, basement membrane).

promotion Phase of carcinogenesis in which the mutated cells are exposed to factors that promote their growth. It may occur just after initiation or years later, and it can be reversible if the promoting factors are removed.

prostacyclin Under normal circumstances, this substance and nitric oxide block platelets from adhering to the cell membrane; it is also secreted by the endothelial cells.

protease Once out of the cell, this enzyme breaks up the protein into smaller chains, which then form mature, infectious HIV.

proximal convoluted tubule The tubule of the kidney that enlarges into a double-membrane chamber called the Bowman capsule (i.e., glomerular capsule).

radiculopathy A pinched nerve.

RANKL Receptor activator of nuclear factor-kappa B ligand. When it binds to an osteoclast, it causes resorption.

rapidly progressive glomerulonephritis A rare clinical syndrome with serious consequences if not diagnosed early. It is a manifestation of severe glomerular injury.

renal ultrasound Type of urinary imaging that is useful in evaluation of urinary tract obstruction and hydronephrosis.

reverse transcriptase The enzyme that converts the viral RNA to DNA.

rhabdomyosarcoma A malignant tumor of the striated muscle usually found in the head and neck, genitourinary tract, and extremities. The tumors are aggressive with rapid metastasis.

rheumatoid arthritis A systemic, autoimmune condition involving multiple joints. The inflammatory process primarily affects the synovial membrane, but it can also affect other organs.

rickets A softening and weakening of bones in children, usually because of an extreme and prolonged vitamin D, calcium, or phosphate deficiency.

scabies A result of a mite infestation. The female mites burrow into the epidermis, laying eggs over a period of several weeks. The larvae hatch from the eggs and then migrate to the skin's surface. The larvae burrow in search of nutrients and mature to repeat the cycle. The burrowing and fecal matter left by the mites triggers the inflammatory process, leading to erythema and pruritus.

schizoaffective disorder Schizophrenia with manic episodes and a significant depressive component.

schizotypal personality disorder Disorder characterized by odd or eccentric beliefs and/or perceptual disturbances that are not quite delusions or hallucinations.

sciatica A radiating, aching pain, sometimes with tingling and numbness, that starts in the buttock and extends down the back or side of one leg.

sclerosing Glomerular scar formation.

scoliosis A lateral deviation of the spine. This lateral curvature may affect the thoracic or lumbar area, or both. Scoliosis may also include a rotation of the vertebrae on their axis.

seborrheic keratosis A benign tumor that is usually seen in older age. These tumors are due to immature keratinocyte proliferation in the epidermis.

secondary amenorrhea Absence of menses for more than 3 months in a female who had regular menstrual cycles or absence of menses for 6 months in a female who had irregular menses.

segmental When only a portion ($<$ 50%) of the glomerulus is affected.

septic shock Type of distributive shock in which a bacterium's endotoxins activate an immune reaction. Inflammatory mediators are triggered, increasing capillary permeability and fluid shifts from the vascular compartment to the tissue. Falling cardiac output leads to multisystem organ failure.

serotonin A neurotransmitter, released by platelets in the clotting process, that acts as a vasoconstrictor.

severe acute respiratory syndrome A rapidly spreading respiratory illness that presents similarly to atypical pneumonia. Prevalence rates are higher in Asian countries. It is caused by a coronavirus, SARS-CoV. Transmission occurs through inhalation of respiratory droplets, close contact, or oral–fecal contact. It has high mortality and morbidity rates.

shoulder impingement syndrome A common cause of shoulder pain caused by compression of structures around the glenohumeral joint when the shoulder is elevated. Also called rotator cuff tendinitis or shoulder bursitis.

slipped capital femoral epiphyses A common cause of hip pain in adolescents. The disorder occurs when the head of the femur (i.e., epiphysis) moves down and backwards off the neck of the bones.

spinal stenosis Narrowing of the spinal canal.

spondylolisthesis A vertebral stress fracture that causes an instability and can cause the vertebral body to shift forward.

spondylolysis A pars interarticularis fracture.

spondylosis Narrowing of the intervertebral disk space.

spontaneous (nontraumatic) pneumothorax Type of pneumothorax that develops when air enters the pleural cavity from an opening in the internal airways.

squamous cell carcinoma Type of carcinoma that involves changes in the squamous cells. The lesions have a varied presentation ans can be papules, plaques, nodular, smooth, hyperkeratotic, or ulcerative.

stable angina Type of cardiac chest pain that is a result of ischemia that is initiated by increased demand (activity) and relieved with the reduction of that demand (rest).

stasis dermatitis Condition in which the skin is hyperpigmented, scaly, and edematous. It tends to be bilateral, with pitting edema present. It is generally nontender and chronic. Inciting factors include venous insufficiency.

strain An injury to a muscle or tendon that often involves stretching or tearing of the muscle or tendon.

stratum corneum The outermost layer of the epidermis composed of waterproof keratin.

stratum germinativum The innermost layer of the epidermis, which is attached to basal cells (the basement membrane) that separate the epidermis from dermis.

Streptococcus pyogenes A group A beta-hemolytic (GABHS) bacteria that is responsible for up to 30% of pharyngitis cases in children and up to 15% in adults

stress Loss of urine from pressure exerted on the bladder by coughing, sneezing, laughing, exercising, or lifting something heavy. This occurs when the sphincter muscle of the bladder weakens.

stress ulcers Peptic ulcer disease that develops because of a major physiologic stressor on the body (e.g., large burns, trauma, sepsis, surgery, or head injury).

subconjunctival hemorrhage A tearing of the fragile vessels under the conjunctiva, usually a benign condition caused by coughing, sneezing, and straining. There are no symptoms other than the visible blood in the subconjunctiva, and resolution occurs without treatment within 2 weeks.

syndrome of inappropriate antidiuretic hormone secretion A condition in which water is retained, and total body water increases as a result of the increased levels of antidiuretic hormone. Dilutional hyponatremia and hypoosmolality occurs as a result of excess total body water.

telogen effluvium Cause of diffuse hair loss distribution due to a premature shift of hair entering the telogen (resting) cycle of growth from the anagen growth phase.

tension pneumothorax The most serious type of pneumothorax; it occurs when the pressure in the pleural space is greater than the atmospheric pressure. This increased pressure is due to trapped air in the pleural space or entering air from a positive-pressure mechanical ventilator.

thrombin This enzyme mediates conversion of fibrinogen to fibrin through activation of the coagulation cascade. This process represents secondary hemostasis.

thrombotic strokes Strokes that are a result of localized arterial occlusion. The process can occur gradually (e.g., over several years as occurs in atherosclerosis) or acutely (e.g., platelets form a thrombus on plaque).

thromboxane A^2 A potent vasoconstrictor that acts in opposition to prostacyclin. It promotes further platelet activation and aggregation.

tinea versicolor A superficial, benign, noncommunicable fungal infection of the skin.

tophi Large, hard nodules consisting of uric acid crystals deposited in soft tissues, usually in cooler areas of the body.

trachoma conjunctivitis Eye infection caused by the bacteria, *Chlamydia trachomatis* (serotypes A–C). It is highly contagious, and transmission occurs through contact with infected eyes, noses, and throats.

transient incontinence Urinary incontinence resulting from a temporary condition.

transient ischemic attacks A temporary episodes of cerebral ischemia that result in symptoms of neurologic deficit. They are often called ministrokes because these neurologic deficits mimic a cerebral vascular accident or stroke except that these deficits resolve within 24 hours (1–2 hours in most cases).

transudative effusions Type of effusion that is caused by systemic processes, such as heart failure, cirrhosis, or kidney disease. They result because of changes in hydrostatic and osmotic pressure that shift fluid into the pleural space.

traumatic pneumothorax Type of pneumothorax that is caused by any blunt or penetrating injury to the chest. These injuries can inadvertently occur during certain medical procedures.

trigger finger A result of abnormal thickening of the flexor (palmar) tendon at the metacarpophalangeal joint that causes the affected finger to snap or lock during flexion. Also called stenosing flexor tenosynovitis.

tropical sprue A small intestine disease characterized by malabsorption of nutrients, and a differential diagnosis is celiac disease; however, this disorder is probably infectious in origin (bacterial, viral, parasitic, or amoebic) and occurs in tropical regions.

type 1 von Willebrand disease The most common (70–80%) and mildest form von Willebrand disease. It follows an autosomal dominant inheritance pattern. The level of von Willebrand factor in the blood is reduced. It is often very mild, and most cases go undiagnosed.

type 2 von Willebrand disease The form von Willebrand disease that occurs in 15–20% of cases. It can be either autosomal dominant or recessive, and four subtypes exist. The building blocks (multimers) that make up the von Willebrand factor are smaller than usual or break down easily. Bleeding with this type is usually moderate to severe.

type 3 von Willebrand disease This form of von Willebrand disease follows an autosomal recessive inheritance pattern. Severe bleeding problems are seen with this type due to the lack of measurable von Willebrand factor and factor VIII. It is the rarest form.

type III hypersensitivity Immune complex–mediated type of hypersensitivity, in which circulating antigen–antibody complexes accumulate and are deposited in the tissue. This accumulation triggers the complement system, causing local inflammation and increased vascular permeability, so more complexes accumulate.

type IV hypersensitivity Cell-mediated type of hypersensitivity, which involves a delayed processing of the antigen by the macrophages. Once processed, the antigen is presented to the T cells, resulting in the release of lymphokines that cause inflammation and antigen destruction.

unipotent Type of stem cell that can only make a single cell type such as precursors to egg or sperm cells.

unstable angina A change in cardiac chest pain; the pain becomes unpredictable, occurs at rest, or increases in frequency or intensity. It is considered a preinfarction state.

urea One of the three most significant metabolic wastes managed by the kidneys.

urge A sudden, intense urge to urinate, followed by an involuntary loss of urine.

uric acid A metabolism by-product managed by the kidneys that is a result of the breakdown of nucleotides, the building blocks of DNA.

uterine sarcoma A malignant uterine tumor that arises from the myometrium or connective tissue. These tumors are rare, accounting for only 3% of uterine cancers, and the incidence increases with aging.

variable expressivity A genetic disorder in which the clinical manifestations vary widely among affected individuals.

varicose veins Dilated, tortuous, engorged veins that develop because of improper venous valve function. The most common location in which varicose veins occur is the legs, but they can be found in the esophagus (esophageal varices) and the rectum (hemorrhoids). Also called varicosity.

vasogenic edema Type of cerebral edema caused by blood–brain barrier vascular alterations that allow large molecules (e.g., proteins) to go into the extracellular volume.

venous stasis ulcers Ulcers resulting from malfunctioning venous valves that increase pressure in the veins.

ventilator-associated pneumonia Pneumonia that develops 48 hours after intubation.

verrucae A viral infection caused by any of a number of the human papillomaviruses. They can develop at any age and often resolve spontaneously. They can be transmitted through direct skin contact between people or within the same person.

vestibular neuritis Vestibular nerve inflammation, usually due to virus.

viral conjunctivitis Eye infection caused by a virus.

viral pneumonias Forms of pneumonia that are usually mild and heal without intervention, but that can lead to a virulent bacterial pneumonia.

vitamin B$_{12}$ While the red blood cell is developing, this substance and folic acid are necessary in addition to EPO. They are necessary for cellular DNA synthesis.

vitiligo A rare condition characterized by small patchy areas of hypopigmentation. It occurs when the cells that produce melanin die or no longer form melanin, leading to slowly enlarging white patches of irregular shapes on the skin.

von Willebrand factor (vWF) A factor secreted by the endothelial lining, which, in response to injury, binds to the basement membrane.

Zollinger-Ellison syndrome Condition caused by duodenal or pancreatic neuroendocrine tumors, referred to as gastrinomas, that secrete gastrin. The tumors are sometimes cancerous.

Index